9 TH EDITION

NURSING CARE PLANS
DIAGNOSES, INTERVENTIONS, & OUTCOMES

MEG GULANICK, PhD, APRN, FAAN
Professor Emeritus
Marcella Niehoff School of Nursing
Loyola University Chicago
Chicago, Illinois

JUDITH L. MYERS, MSN, RN
Formerly, Assistant Professor of Nursing
Grand View University
Des Moines, Iowa

ELSEVIER

ELSEVIER

1600 John F. Kennedy Blvd.
St. Louis, Missouri 63043

Notices

Knowledge and best practice in this field are constantly changing. As new research and experience broaden our understanding, changes in research methods, professional practices, or medical treatment may become necessary.

    Practitioners and researchers must always rely on their own experience and knowledge in evaluating and using any information, methods, compounds, or experiments described herein. In using such information or methods they should be mindful of their own safety and the safety of others, including parties for whom they have a professional responsibility.

    With respect to any drug or pharmaceutical products identified, readers are advised to check the most current information provided (i) on procedures featured or (ii) by the manufacturer of each product to be administered, to verify the recommended dose or formula, the method and duration of administration, and contraindications. It is the responsibility of practitioners, relying on their own experience and knowledge of their patients, to make diagnoses, to determine dosages and the best treatment for each individual patient, and to take all appropriate safety precautions.

    To the fullest extent of the law, neither the Publisher nor the authors, contributors, or editors, assume any liability for any injury and/or damage to persons or property as a matter of products liability, negligence or otherwise, or from any use or operation of any methods, products, instructions, or ideas contained in the material herein.

Previous editions copyrighted 2014, 2011, 2007, 2003, 1998, 1994, 1990, and 1986.

Library of Congress Cataloging-in-Publication Data
Names: Gulanick, Meg, editor. | Myers, Judith L., editor.
Title: Nursing care plans : diagnoses interventions, & outcomes / [edited by] Meg Gulanick, Judith L. Myers.
Description: 9th edition. | St. Louis, Missouri : Mosby, an imprint of Elsevier Inc., [2017] |
    Includes bibliographical references and index.
Identifiers: LCCN 2016038099 | ISBN 9780323428187 (pbk. : alk. paper)
Subjects: | MESH: Patient Care Planning | Nursing Diagnosis | Nursing Care | Outcome Assessment
    (Health Care) | Handbooks
Classification: LCC RT49 | NLM WY 49 | DDC 610.73–dc23 LC record available at
    https://lccn.loc.gov/2016038099

Executive Content Strategist: Lee Henderson
Content Development Manager: Lisa Newton
Senior Content Development Specialist: Danielle M. Frasier
Publishing Services Manager: Jeff Patterson
Book Production Specialist: Carol O'Connell
Design Direction: Ashley Miner

Printed in the United States of America

Last digit is the print number: 9   8   7   6   5   4   3

Working together
to grow libraries in
developing countries

www.elsevier.com • www.bookaid.org

CONTRIBUTORS

We wish to express our ongoing gratitude to those who contributed to previous editions of this book, especially the following:

Virginia B. Bowman
Judy Lau Carino
Debra L. Cason
Pamela Cianci
Marianne T. Cosentino
Sandra Coslet
Paula Cox-North
Jennifer L. Crosby
Gail DeLuca
Lisa C. Dobogai
Amy Dolce

Linda Flemm
Patricia J. Friend
Katrina Gallagher
Nadia Goraczkowski-Jones
Rebecca Hagensee
Mary Ellen Hand
Margo S. Henderson
Connie Huberty
Judi Jennrich
Linda Kamenjarin
Tamara M. Kear

Catherine A. Kefer
Vicki A. Keough
Lucina Kimpel
Katherine T. Leslie
MariJo Letizia
Mary Jo Mikottis
Shelby J. Neel
Linda Denise Oakley
Linda Ohler
Kelly Oney
Judy K. Orth

Sue Penckofer
Joanne Pfeiffer
Dottie Roberts
Kathy G. Supple
Terry D. Takemoto
Geraldine Tansey
Stacy VandenBranden
Carol White
Jeffrey Zurlinden

We also want to acknowledge the prior editors of this classic book: Deidra Gradishar, Susan Galanes, Audrey Klopp, and Michele Knoll Puzas, who provided the foundation for *Nursing Care Plans: Diagnoses, Interventions, & Outcomes* as it is known today.

REVIEWERS

Sophia Beydoun, RN, MSN
Diane Daddario, MSN,
    ANP-C, ACNS-BC, RN-BC,
    CMSRN
Jennifer Duhon, RN, MS

Nancy W. Ebersole, RN,
    PhD
Arline El-Ashkar, MSN, RN,
    CAN
Linda P. Grimsley, DSN, RN

LaWanda Herron, PhD,
    MSN, FNP-BC
Jamie Lynn Jones, MSN,
    RN, CNE

Mary Lou Roark, MSN, RN
Denise Sevigny, MSN, RN,
    CNE

Nursing Care Plans: Diagnoses, Interventions, & Outcomes is a well-established and premier resource book used by nurses to plan care for an increasingly diverse population of patients. This book continues to be the most comprehensive care planning book on the market, with a total of 220 care plans between the printed book and the Evolve website. These care plans cover the most common nursing diagnoses and clinical problems nurses encounter in patients requiring medical-surgical nursing care. The care plans focus on patients with both acute and chronic health problems in the acute care, ambulatory, and home care settings.

One of our primary goals for this 9th edition has been to incorporate QSEN (Quality and Safety Education for Nurses) language throughout the text. The QSEN competencies relating to nursing diagnoses and interventions include Patient-Centered Care; Teamwork and Collaboration; Evidence-based Practice; and Safety. These competencies can be found highlighted in the rationales throughout the chapters. Because of the profession's emphasis on teamwork and collaboration, the term collaborative intervention previously used in our book has been updated to interprofessional collaboration. This change is consistent with the move in health care from multidisciplinary teams to interprofessional education and collaboration.

Nursing Care Plans: Diagnoses, Interventions & Outcomes continues to offer "several books in one." The book and its accompanying Evolve website contain 70 of the most commonly used nursing diagnoses (Chapter 2), in tandem with an introductory chapter on how to use care plans to provide safe, individualized, and quality care (Chapter 1). Chapter 3 provides 8 of the most common health promotion and risk factor management care plans needed to help a patient adopt new health behaviors. This chapter uses multifaceted, evidence-based strategies known to facilitate successful behavior change. Realizing that many patient conditions require attention to specialized yet commonly used interventions, Chapter 4 provides 10 of these overarching plans, including preoperative and postoperative care, central venous access, enteral nutrition, and parenteral nutrition. Other care plans that can relate to a variety of patients include hearing loss, visual impairment, death and dying, and substance abuse disorder. This book also includes 132 of the most commonly used medical-surgical adult health care plans. New to this part of the book (Chapters 4–14) is an expanded table of contents that lists every nursing diagnosis presented within each medical diagnosis. Listing every nursing diagnosis can assist students in making comparisons between how some NANDA diagnoses can be developed and used for various related factors and etiologies. This book provides detailed introductions to each care plan to serve as a foundation for understanding care for a specific nursing diagnosis or medical disorder. These introductions are a strength of this book. Content on patient safety and preventable complications using nursing bundles addresses national initiatives and discusses the nursing responsibility in preventing complications such as falls, pressure ulcers, infection, and the like. For example, key measures from the OSHA (Occupational Safety and Health Administration's) Safe Patient Handling initiatives are now incorporated into relevant care plans.

In Chapter 2, new care plans have been added for the NANDA International (NANDA-I) diagnoses of frail elderly syndrome and readiness for enhanced decision making. Frail elderly syndrome is a progressive condition that has both biological and psychosocial contributing factors. When the deficits associated with frail elderly syndrome are combined with the normal physiological processes of aging, the older adult has an increased risk for disability and mortality. Nurses have a key role in helping patients reverse this condition. Decisions related to our health warrant careful consideration and thoughtful reflection. Readiness for enhanced decision making assists health care professionals when working with patients deciding whether to reduce their risk factors such as smoking or overweight. However, this care plan can also be used to address more complex decision-making issues, such as determination of cancer therapy, genetic testing, refusal of blood products or surgical procedures, writing of advanced directives, organ donation, and end-of-life issues.

The previous chapters on men's health and women's health have now been combined into one chapter (Chapter 12). Included in this chapter is a new and timely care plan on gender dysphoria, a condition where a person experiences clinically significant discomfort or distress due to the discrepancy that exists between a person's gender identity and that person's sex assigned at birth. This is not a lifestyle, personal choice, or political decision, but a very real biological phenomenon. This care plan aims to educate nurses on how to work with patients seeking to cope with their gender incongruity distress, as well as to assist the person to find a gender role that is comfortable for them.

The essential format for the book and for the individual care plans has not changed from the 8th edition. These care plans include assessments and therapeutic interventions across the continuum of care. Chapter 2 also contains a section on patient education and continuity of care for each nursing diagnosis. Ongoing Assessments throughout this book contain the latest information on methods of assessment and for laboratory and diagnostic tests. Revised and expanded outcomes include new measurable and specific terms for each nursing diagnosis. Therapeutic Interventions include up-to-date information on independent and collaborative clinical management and on drug therapy related to nursing diagnoses and medical disorders. The rationales for the Ongoing Assessments and Therapeutic Interventions include current care and patient safety standards and clinical practice guidelines in nursing and other health care disciplines. Related care plans are referenced where applicable, making it easy to cross-reference content throughout the book. We continue to include the latest editions of Nursing Interventions Classification (NIC) and Nursing Outcomes Classification (NOC) labels at the beginning of each care plan. The index includes entries for all nursing diagnoses, all medical diagnoses, and all synonyms for the medical diagnoses, providing an easy-to-use, practical tool for accessing the book's content.

We continue to use the Evolve website as an adjunct to the printed book. The expanded website now includes 54 additional care plans on a wide range of disorders (see the inside back cover of this book for a full list).

We are grateful to the many contributors to previous editions of this book. Their work continues to be the foundation for the nurses who have contributed to the revisions for this edition.

Meg Gulanick, PhD, APRN, FAAN
Judith L. Myers, MSN, RN

CONTENTS

Using Nursing Care Plans to Individualize and Improve Care

Introduction

According to the American Nurses Association (ANA), nursing is the diagnosis and treatment of human responses to actual and potential problems. A broad foundation of scientific knowledge, including the biological and behavioral sciences, combined with the ability to assist patients, families, and other caregivers in managing their own health needs, defines the scope of nursing practice. Nursing care in this context transcends settings, crosses the age continuum, and supports a wellness philosophy focused on self-care. In many ways, the roles of nurses are enhanced by opportunities to provide nursing care in the more natural, less institutional paradigms that are demanded by restructured health care financing. Studies continue to document that society places its highest trust in nurses. To deserve this trust, nurses will need to continuously strive to improve health care quality. The current challenges in seizing these opportunities include the following: (1) recognition of the growing chasm between what currently "exists" in health care and what "should be" to achieve the safe, high-quality, effective, and patient-centered care that every patient deserves; (2) the importance of working effectively in interprofessional teams to deliver patient-centered care; (3) the need for more effective professional communication; (4) the need to help patients better navigate through difficult acute and chronic care issues; (5) the ability of the nursing educational system to increasingly prepare nurses for settings outside the hospital environment as well as within the complex hospital setting; (6) the ability of nurses themselves to be comfortable with the responsibility of their roles; (7) the need to increase the recruitment and retention of nurses from diverse backgrounds to meet the needs of an increasingly diverse population; and (8) the availability of tools to assist nurses in assessing, planning, and providing care. *Nursing Care Plans: Diagnoses, Interventions, and Outcomes* is such a tool.

Components of These Nursing Care Plans

Each care plan in this book begins with an expanded definition of the title problem or diagnosis (Fig. 1-1). These definitions include enough information to guide the user in understanding what the problem or diagnosis is, information regarding the incidence or prevalence of the problem or diagnosis, a brief overview of the typical management and/or the focus of nursing care, and a description of the setting in which care for the particular problem or diagnosis can be expected to occur.

Each problem or diagnosis is accompanied by one or more cross-references, some of which may be synonyms (see Fig. 1-1). These cross-references assist the user in locating other information that may be helpful in deciding whether this particular care plan is indeed the one the user needs.

For each care plan, appropriate nursing diagnoses are developed, which include the following components:
- Common related factors (those etiologies associated with a diagnosis for an actual problem) (Fig. 1-2)
- Defining characteristics (assessment data that support the nursing diagnosis) (see Fig. 1-2)
- Common risk factors (those situations or conditions that contribute to the patient's potential to develop a problem or diagnosis) (Fig. 1-3)
- Common expected outcomes (see Fig. 1-3)
- Ongoing assessment (see Fig. 1-3)
- Therapeutic interventions (both independent and interprofessional) (Fig. 1-4)

Each nursing diagnosis developed is based on the NANDA International (NANDA-I) label unless otherwise stated. Wherever possible, expanded rationales assist the user in understanding the information presented; this allows for use of *Nursing Care Plans: Diagnoses, Interventions, and Outcomes* as a singular reference tool. The interventions and supporting rationales for each care plan represent current research-based knowledge and evidence-based clinical practice guidelines for nursing and other health care professionals. Many care plans also refer the user to additional diagnoses that may be pertinent and would assist the user in further developing a care plan. Each diagnosis developed in these care plans also identifies the Nursing Interventions Classification (NIC) interventions and the Nursing Outcomes Classification (NOC) outcomes.

QSEN (Quality and Safety Education for Nurses) core competencies are highlighted throughout the book.

Thrombosis, Deep Vein
Venous Thromboembolic Disease; Phlebitis; Phlebothrombosis

Thrombophlebitis is the inflammation of the wall of a vein, usually resulting in the formation of a blood clot (thrombosis) that may partially or completely block the flow of blood through the vessel. Venous thrombophlebitis usually occurs in the lower extremities. It may occur in superficial veins, which, although painful, is not life threatening and does not require hospitalization, or it may occur in a deep vein, which can be life threatening because clots may break free (embolize) and cause a pulmonary embolism. Three factors contribute to the development of deep vein thrombosis (DVT): venous stasis, hypercoagulability, and endothelial damage to the vein. Prolonged immobility is the primary cause of venous stasis. Hypercoagulability is seen in patients with deficient fluid volume, oral contraceptive use, smoking, and certain malignancies. Venous wall damage may occur secondary to IV infusions, certain medications, fractures, and contrast x-ray studies. DVT most commonly occurs in lower extremities, where it is often asymptomatic and resolves in a few days. In the inpatient setting, all patients are required to be assessed for venous thromboembolism (VTE). The Joint Commission has a VTE bundle to guide prophylaxis and treatment for this high-risk condition. More proximal DVTs are associated with more severe symptoms and carry a higher risk for dislodgement and migration. Treatment is supportive, usually with anticoagulant therapy. Goals are to reduce risk for complications and prevent recurrence.

Figure 1-1 Expanded definition and cross-references of a care plan.

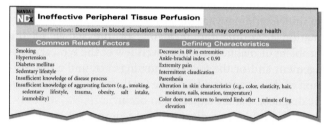

Figure 1-2 Common related factors and defining characteristics of the nursing diagnosis.

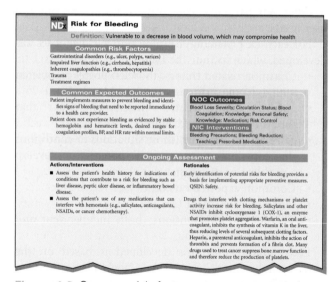

Figure 1-3 Common risk factors, common expected outcomes, and ongoing assessment of the nursing diagnosis.

Therapeutic Interventions

Actions/Interventions	Rationales
▲ Administer anticoagulant therapy as prescribed (continuous IV heparin/subcutaneous low-molecular-weight heparin; oral anticoagulants).	Anticoagulants are given to prevent further clot formation. The type of medication varies per protocol and severity of the clot. These medications are based on recommendations from national organizations. QSEN: Safety; Evidence-based practice.
▲ If bleeding occurs while on IV heparin: • Stop the infusion. • Recheck the PTT level stat. • Reevaluate the dose of heparin on the basis of the PTT result.	Laboratory data guide further treatment. The guide for the PTT level is 1.5 to 2 times normal. QSEN: Safety.
▲ Convert from IV anticoagulation to oral anticoagulation after the appropriate length of therapy. Monitor INR, PT, and PTT levels.	PT or INR levels should be in an adequate range for anticoagulation before discontinuing heparin.

Figure 1-4 Therapeutic interventions of the nursing diagnosis.

Nursing Diagnoses Taxonomy, and Interventions and Outcomes Classifications

As *Nursing Care Plans: Diagnoses, Interventions, and Outcomes* continues to mature and reflect the changing times and needs of its readers, as well as the needs of those for whom care is provided, nursing diagnoses continue to evolve. The body of research to support diagnoses, their definitions, related and risk factors, and defining characteristics is ever increasing and gaining momentum. Nurses continue to study both independent and interprofessional interventions for effectiveness and desirable outcomes.

The taxonomy of nursing diagnoses as a whole continues to be refined; its use as an international tool for practice, education, and research is testament to its importance as an organizing framework for the body of knowledge that is uniquely nursing. As a taxonomy, nursing diagnosis and all its components are standardized. This standardized language for nursing diagnoses, outcomes, and interventions is being incorporated into many computer programs for nursing documentation in an electronic medical record. Nurses must remember that care plans developed for each diagnosis or cluster of diagnoses for particular patients must be individualized. The patient-centered tailoring of the care plan is the hallmark of nursing practice.

NIC presents an additional opportunity for clarifying and organizing what nurses do. With NIC, nursing interventions have been systematically organized to help nurses identify and select interventions. In this ninth edition, NIC information continues to be presented along with each nursing diagnosis within each care plan, giving the user added ability to use NIC taxonomy in planning for individualized patient care. According to the developers of NIC, nursing interventions are "any treatment, based upon clinical judgment and knowledge, that a nurse performs to enhance patient/client outcomes" (Bulechek et al., 2013). These interventions may include direct or indirect care and may be initiated by a nurse, a physician, or another care provider. Student nurses, practicing nurses, advanced practice nurses, and nurse executives can use nursing diagnoses and NIC as tools for learning, organizing, and delivering care; managing care within the framework of redesigned health care and within financial constraints through the development of critical paths; identifying research questions; and monitoring the outcomes of nursing care both at an individual level and at the level of service provision to large populations of patients.

Nurse investigators at the University of Iowa developed NOC, a taxonomy of patient outcomes that are sensitive to nursing interventions. The authors of this outcomes taxonomy state, "For the nursing profession to become a full participant in clinical evaluation research, policy development, and interdisciplinary work, it is essential that patient outcomes influenced by nursing care be identified and measured" (Moorhead et al., 2013). In this context, an outcome is defined as the status of the patient or family that follows and is directly influenced by nursing interventions.

The following portion of this chapter guides the user of this text through the steps of individualized care plan development. It also contains recommendations about how this book can be used to ensure safe and quality care, as a tool for quality improvement work and creating seamless nursing care delivery regardless of where in the continuum of health care the patient happens to be, for the development of patient education materials, and as the basis of critical path development.

Using *Nursing Care Plans: Diagnoses, Interventions, and Outcomes*

Developing an Individualized Care Plan

The nursing care plan is best thought of as a written reflection of the nursing process: What does the assessment reveal? What should be done? How, when, and where should these planned interventions be implemented? What is the desired outcome? That is, will the delivery of planned interventions result in the desired goal? The nurse's ability to carry out this process in a systematic fashion, using all available information and resources, is the fundamental basis for nursing practice. This process includes correctly identifying existing needs, as well as recognizing potential needs and/or risks. Planning and delivering care in an individualized fashion to address these actual or potential needs, as well as evaluating the effectiveness of that care, is the basis for excellence in nursing practice. Forming a partnership with the patient and/or caregiver in this process and humanizing the experience of being a care recipient is the essence of nursing.

The Assessment

All the information that the nurse collects regarding a particular patient makes up the assessment. This assessment allows a nursing diagnosis, or clinical judgment, to be made. This, in turn, drives the identification of expected outcomes (i.e., what is desired by and for this particular patient in relation to this identified need) and the care plan. Without a comprehensive assessment, all else is a "shot in the dark."

Nurses have always carried out the task of assessment. As science and technology progress, information is more abundant than at any other time in history; however, length of contact with each patient becomes shorter, so astute assessment skills are essential to a nurse's ability to plan and deliver effective nursing care.

Assessment data are abundant in any clinical setting. What the nurse observes; what a history (written or verbal) reveals; what the patient and/or caregiver reports (or fails to report) about a situation, problem, or concern; and what laboratory and other diagnostic information is available are all valid and important data.

Methods useful in gathering these diverse data include interview, direct and indirect observation, physical assessment, medical records review, and analysis and synthesis of available laboratory and other diagnostic studies. The sum of all information obtained through any or all of these means allows the nurse to make a nursing diagnosis.

Gordon's (1976) definition of a nursing diagnosis includes only those problems that nurses are capable of treating, whereas others have expanded the definition to include any health-related issue with which a nurse may interface. In *Nursing Care Plans: Diagnoses, Interventions, and Outcomes* the nursing diagnosis terminology conforms to the NANDA-I *Nursing Diagnoses: Definitions and Classification,* 2015-2017 unless otherwise stated.

Performing the Assessment

A nurse has knowledge in the physical and behavioral sciences, is a trusted member of the health care team, and is the interprofessional team member who has the most contact with a patient. Because of these qualities, a nurse is in a key position to collect data from the patient and/or caregiver at any point at which the patient enters the health care continuum, whether in the home, in a hospital, in an outpatient clinic, or in a long-term care facility.

Interviewing is an important method of gathering information about a patient. The interview has the added dimensions of providing the nurse with the patient's subjective input on not only the problem but also what the patient may feel about the causes of the problem, how the problem has affected the patient as an individual, and what outcomes the patient wants in relation to the particular problem, as well as insight into how the patient and/or caregiver may or may not be capable of participating in management of the problem.

Good interviewing skills are founded on rapport with the patient, the skill of active listening, and preparation in a systematic, thorough format, with comprehensive attention given to specific health-related problems. The nurse as the interviewer must be knowledgeable of the patient's overall condition and the environment in which the interview will take place. A comprehensive interview that includes exploration of all the functional health patterns is ideal and will provide the best overall picture of the patient. When time is a limiting factor, the nurse may review existing medical records or other documents before the interview so that the interview can be focused. Care must be taken, however, not to "miss the forest for the trees" by conducting an interview in a fashion that precludes the discovery of important information the patient may have to share.

During an interview the patient may report the following types of information:
- Bothersome or unusual signs and symptoms (e.g., "I have been having cramps and bloody diarrhea for the past month.")

- Changes noticed (e.g., "It's a lot worse when I drink milk.")
- The impact of these problems on his or her ability to carry out desired or necessary activities (e.g., "I know every washroom at the mall. It's tough having lunch with friends.")
- Issues associated with the primary problem (e.g., "It's so embarrassing when my stomach starts to rumble loudly.")
- The impact of these problems on significant others (e.g., "My daughter cannot understand why a trip to the zoo feels like a challenge.")
- What specifically caused the patient to seek attention (e.g., "The amount of blood in the past couple of days really has me worried, and the pain is getting worse.")

In addition, the patient may share the following:

- Previous experiences or history (e.g., "My brother has had Crohn's disease for several years; this is how he started out.")
- Health beliefs and feelings about the problem (e.g., "I have always figured it would catch up with me sooner or later, with all the problems like this in our family.")
- Thoughts about what would help solve the problem (e.g., "Maybe I should watch my diet better.")
- What has been successful in the past in solving similar problems (e.g., "They kept my brother out of surgery for years with just a diet and medicine.")

From this scenario, it is clear that the interviewing nurse would want to explore issues of elimination, pain, nutrition, knowledge, and coping.

Information necessary to begin forming diagnoses has been provided, along with enough additional information to guide further exploration. In this example, the nurse may choose *diarrhea* as the diagnosis. Using NANDA-I–approved related factors for diarrhea, the nurse will want to explore stress and anxiety, dietary specifics, medications the patient is taking, and the patient's personal and family history of bowel disease.

The defining characteristics for *diarrhea* (typical signs and symptoms) have been provided by the patient to be cramping; abdominal pain; bowel urgency; loose, liquid stools; hyperactive bowel sounds; and changes in the appearance of the stool. These defining characteristics support the nursing diagnosis *diarrhea*.

To explore related concerns such as pain, nutrition, knowledge, and coping, the nurse should refer to defining characteristics for *imbalanced nutrition: less than body requirements; deficient knowledge; acute pain; and ineffective coping*. The nurse should then interview the patient further to determine the presence or absence of defining characteristics for these additional diagnoses.

To continue this example, the nurse might ask the patient the following questions: Have you lost weight? Of what does your typical breakfast/lunch/dinner consist? How is your appetite? Describe your abdominal cramping.

How frequent is the discomfort? Does it awaken you at night? Does it interfere with your daily routine? On a scale of 1 to 10, with 10 being the worst pain you have ever had, how bad is the cramping? Can you tell me about your brother's Crohn's disease? Have you ever been told by a doctor that you have Crohn's or a similar disease? How are you handling these problems? Have you been able to carry out your usual activities? What do you do to feel better? In asking these questions, the nurse can decide whether the four additional diagnoses (*imbalanced nutrition: less than body requirements; deficient knowledge; acute pain; and ineffective coping*) are supported as actual problems or are problems for which the patient may be at risk.

Family, caregivers, and significant others also can be interviewed. When the patient's condition makes him or her incapable of being interviewed, these may be the nurse's only sources of interview information.

Physical assessment provides the nurse with objective data regarding the patient and includes a general survey followed by a systematic assessment of the physical and mental conditions of the patient. Findings of the physical examination may support subjective data already given by the patient or may provide new information that requires additional interviewing. In reality, the interview continues as the physical assessment proceeds and as the patient focuses on particulars. The patient is then able to enhance earlier information, remember new information, become more comfortable with the nurse, and share additional information.

Patient comfort and cooperation are important considerations in performing the physical examination, as are privacy and an undisturbed environment. Explaining the need for assessment and what steps are involved is helpful in putting the patient at ease and gaining cooperation.

Methods used in physical assessment include inspection (performing systematic visual examination), auscultation (using a stethoscope to listen to the heart, lungs, major vessels, and abdomen), percussion (tapping body areas to elicit information about underlying tissues), and palpation (using light or heavy touch to feel for temperature, normal and abnormal structures, and any elicited subjective responses). The usual order of these assessment techniques is inspection, palpation, percussion, and auscultation, except during the abdominal portion of the physical examination. Percussion and palpation may alter a finding by moving gas and bowel fluid and changing bowel sounds. Therefore percussion and palpation should follow inspection and auscultation when the abdomen is being examined.

To continue the example, the nurse may note, through inspection, that the patient is a thin, pale, well-groomed young woman who is shifting her weight often and has a strained facial expression. When asked how she feels at the present, the patient gives additional support to the diagnoses *ineffective coping* and *deficient knowledge* ("I don't understand what is wrong with me; I feel tired and stressed out all the time lately"). Physical examination reveals a

10-pound weight loss, hyperactive bowel sounds, and abdominal pain, which is expressed when the nurse palpates the right and left lower quadrants of the patient's abdomen. These findings further support the nursing diagnoses *diarrhea, imbalanced nutrition: less than body requirements;* and *acute pain.*

Using General Versus Specific Care Plan Guides

General

At this point, the nurse has identified five nursing diagnoses: *diarrhea, imbalanced nutrition: less than body requirements, acute pain, deficient knowledge,* and *ineffective coping. Nursing Care Plans: Diagnoses, Interventions, and Outcomes* is organized to allow the nurse to build a care plan by using the primary nursing diagnoses care plans in Chapter 2. A nurse can also select, by medical diagnosis, a set of nursing diagnoses that have been clustered to address a specific medical diagnosis and then further individualize it for a particular patient.

Using the first method from Chapter 2, the nurse had every possible related factor and defining characteristic from which to choose to tailor the care plan to the individual patient. It is important to individualize these comprehensive care plans by highlighting those related factors, defining characteristics, assessment suggestions, and interventions that actually pertain to specific patients. Nurses should add any that may not be listed, customize frequencies for assessments and interventions, and specify realistic time frames for outcome achievement. (The blanket application of these standard care plans negates the basic premise of tailoring care to meet individual needs.) To complete the example used to demonstrate individualizing a care plan using this text, the nurse should select the nursing interventions based on the assessment findings, proceed with care delivery, and evaluate whether selected patient outcomes have been achieved.

Specific

Using the clustered diagnoses usually labeled by a medical diagnosis found in Chapters 5 to 14 (e.g., inflammatory bowel disease), the nurse has the added benefit of a brief definition of the medical diagnosis; an overview of typical management, including the setting (home, hospital, outpatient); synonyms that are useful in locating additional information through cross-referencing; and associated nursing diagnoses with related factors and defining characteristics. Again, it is important that aspects of these care plans be selected and applied (i.e., individualized) based on specific assessment data for a particular patient.

As a tool that guides nursing care delivery, the care plan must be updated and revised periodically to remain useful in care provision. Revisions are based on goal attainment, changes in the patient's condition, and response to inter-

ventions. In today's fast-paced, outpatient-oriented health care system, revision will be required often.

As the patient moves through the continuum of care, a well-developed care plan can enhance the continuity of care and contribute to seamless delivery of nursing care, regardless of the setting in which the care is provided. This will serve to replace replication with continuity and ultimately increase the patient's satisfaction with care delivery.

A Focus on Optimizing Health

Chapter 3 provides an additional type of care plan with its focus on *Health Promotion and Risk Factor Management.* Typical nursing care plans throughout this book focus on sick care and helping patients manage their medical illnesses. This chapter is unique in that it showcases patients who are actively engaged in health-seeking behaviors. To reflect this positive approach, the nursing diagnoses reflect a more positive, active title—beginning with *Readiness for.* The nurse realizes that making changes to one's lifestyle is very complex. Thus the nurse needs to use multifaceted evidence-based strategies known to reflect successful behavior changes. It is these strategies that serve as the assessment and therapeutic intervention foci for these health promotion care plans. These strategies include a combination of methods to enhance awareness of risk factors, increase motivation for change, set realistic goals, focus on tailoring the regimen, incorporate self-monitoring, enhance self-efficacy, provide skills in problem solving, include social support and rewards, and address relapse prevention. These care plans demonstrate the important partnership nurses have with patients in assisting them to develop the knowledge and skills needed for making healthy lifestyle decisions and enacting health behaviors.

Other Common Themes

Many patient conditions warrant attention to specialized yet commonly used interventions such as central venous access devices, blood component therapy, and parenteral and enteral nutrition. These care plans have a dedicated space in Chapter 4, where they can be easily accessed and incorporated into specialty care plans for a wide variety of medical problems. Other common themes that do not reflect on only one chapter are hearing loss, visual impairment, common mood disorders, substance use, and death and dying (end-of-life issues). The nurse who encounters these problems can simply refer to the care plans in this chapter to guide interventions. Finally, the broad-based care plan *Surgical Experience: Preoperative and Postoperative Care* is found in this chapter.

Ensuring Quality and Safety

Ever since the 1999 Institute of Medicine (IOM) published its landmark report, *To Err Is Human: Building a Safer*

Health System, there has been a major focus on transforming the health care environment. The 2001 IOM report *Crossing the Quality Chasm* identified issues with quality and safety and recommended six aims for U.S. health care. With nurses as the largest provider of health care in this country, quality and safety must be "their job." Follow-up reports by the IOM (2003) delineated areas needed by practitioners to gain further expertise in quality and safety issues.

The Robert Wood Johnson Foundation funded work called Quality and Safety Education for Nurses (QSEN) to provide the knowledge and tools needed to deliver high-quality, safe, effective, and patient-centered care. This QSEN initiative was developed to integrate quality and safety competencies into nursing education. These competencies include patient-centered care, quality, teamwork and collaboration, safety, evidence-based practice, and informatics. Although the initial work focused on the knowledge, attitude, and skill competencies needed for entry level roles, the project has expanded to graduate nurses, who will be the future leaders in practice, administration, education, and research. This expansion is in keeping with the IOM's report on the *Future of Nursing* (2011). While nurses are committed to providing vigilant care to individual patients and families, it is imperative that attention also be directed to continuously improve the quality and safety of the health care systems in which nurses work.

The QSEN core competencies are beginning to be incorporated into nursing textbooks. They are also carefully integrated into many of the plans of care in *Nursing Care Plans: Diagnoses, Interventions, and Outcomes.* Because this book's focus is on individual care, not system issues, the predominant QSEN competencies identified are patient-centered care, safety, teamwork and collaboration, and evidence-based practice. In most care plans a few specific nursing assessments and therapeutic interventions are highlighted as an example of a QSEN competency. In other more acute care plans, one or more of the QSEN competencies are assumed to be of concern in each assessment and intervention and thus are not highlighted throughout; such competencies include safety in *acute respiratory distress syndrome,* various types of *shock, impaired swallowing, risk for falls,* and *seizures;* patient-centered care in *self-care deficit* and *impaired verbal communication;* and evidence-based practice in *central venous access device.*

Nurses are well positioned to positively influence patient outcomes. These efforts are in concert with those of physicians and hospital administrators in pursuit of high-quality, safe care. Accreditation and regulatory bodies, professional nursing and medical societies, and quality improvement organizations alike are partnering to provide a culture of safety for patients and families. For example, in 2002 The Joint Commission (TJC) established its National Patient Safety Goals (NPSGs) program to help accredited organizations address specific areas of concern in regard to patient safety. Some of the general performance measures identified as a means of reducing errors included "do not use" abbreviations, hand-off communication, standardized drug concentrations, infusion-pump free-flow protection, Centers for Disease Control and Prevention (CDC) hand hygiene guidelines, surgical site marking, "time-out" before surgery, and medication reconciliation. Although an extremely important part of medical and nursing practices, these procedures would not be described in a typical nursing care plan. Similarly, general guidelines for implementing evidence-based practices to prevent health care–associated infections caused by multiple-drug–resistant organisms, to prevent central line–associated bloodstream infections, and to prevent surgical site infections, although critical to patient safety, are also not routinely found in a typical care plan.

In contrast, the Patient Safety Indicators recommended by the Agency for Healthcare Research and Quality (AHRQ) provide information about potentially preventable complications and adverse events for a variety of diagnoses or procedures, and these are incorporated into relevant care plans in *Nursing Care Plans: Diagnoses, Interventions, and Outcomes.* Some examples include attention to fall assessment and prevention, pressure ulcer assessment and prevention, pain management, prevention of pulmonary embolism or deep vein thrombosis, prevention of postoperative sepsis, prevention of hospital-acquired pneumonia, and avoidance of selected infections as a result of medical care. Moreover, TJC provides National Quality Improvement Goals and Guidelines that when followed by health care providers have resulted in faster patient recoveries with fewer complications. Some of these areas of care include pneumonia care, acute myocardial infarction care, heart failure care, blood clot prevention, and surgical infection prevention care. These measures are highlighted in the respective care plans.

Finally, when evidence-based practice and clinical practice guidelines are used to guide health care decisions and deliver care, the best patient outcomes are achieved. Such guidelines, when available, are well integrated into the plans of care in *Nursing Care Plans: Diagnoses, Interventions, and Outcomes.* Nurses are reminded that a key element in evidence-based clinical decision-making is the responsibility to personalize the evidence to apply to a specific patient's values and circumstances. Even the best research evidence cannot be followed blindly.

Tools for Performance Improvement

This book can also be used to identify outcome criteria in quality improvement projects and in the development of monitoring tools. For example, a nursing department, home health agency, or interprofessional pain management team may be interested in monitoring and improving its pain management outcomes. Using the Chapter 2 care plan for *acute pain,* the process of pain management can be monitored simply by using each assessment and intervention as a measurable indicator. The outcome of pain management assessment and intervention can also be studied through direct observation, records review, and patient satisfaction measures. There has been increasing focus on the interrelatedness of services and systems. The care plans in this text include independent and collaborative assessment suggestions and interventions, which facilitate use of the care plans as tools for quality improvement activities. Nurses, other health care professionals, clinical managers, and risk management and quality improvement staff will find that the care plans in this text provide specific, measurable detail and language. This aids in the development of monitoring tools for a broad scope of clinical issues.

Finally, when benchmarks are surpassed and there is desire to improve an aspect of care, the plans of care in *Nursing Care Plans: Diagnoses, Interventions and Outcomes* contain state-of-the-art information that will be helpful in planning corrections or improvements. These outcomes can be measured after implementation. The similarities between the nursing process (assess, plan, intervene, and evaluate) and accepted methods for quality improvement (measure, plan improvements, implement, and remeasure) make these care plan guides natural tools for use in performance improvement activities.

Development of Patient Education Materials

Education of patients and their families and/or significant others has always been a priority role for nurses. *Nursing Care Plans: Diagnoses, Interventions, and Outcomes* is an excellent source book for key procedural and self-care information to share with patients for more than 200 medical problems. It also provides guidance for teaching both the population of ill patients and healthier clients seeking health promotion and disease prevention strategies. Educational content is provided using two formats. For the Chapter 2 general nursing diagnoses, a separate section on Education/Continuity of Care is found near the end of each plan of care. This chapter also provides a more general overview of key educational assessments and interventions pertaining to all learners, as found in the *deficient knowledge* care plans. The subsequent chapters using the clustered medical diagnoses have the patient education material integrated throughout the care plan, rather than in a separate section at the end. These interventions, along with associated rationales, follow the *Ask Me 3* directive on health literacy, which recommends that patient education sessions provide answers to the following questions: What is my main problem? What do I need to do? Why is it important for me to do this? For some medical problems that require a larger focus on education and self-management, a separate nursing diagnosis of *deficient knowledge* may be found within the care plan.

A Basis for Clinical Paths

Clinical paths (also called critical paths, critical pathways, or care maps) are interprofessional care plans to which time frames have been added. The clinical path is designed to track the care of a patient based on average and expected lengths of stay in an acute care setting. Clinical paths can also be developed for the home care and long-term care settings. The path provides guidelines about the sequence of care provided by the various members of the health care team responsible for the care of the patient. Interventions in a specific clinical path may include patient education, diet therapy progression, medications, consultations and referrals to other members of the health care team, activity progression, and discharge planning. The nurse is usually responsible for implementing and monitoring the patient's progress and noting deviations from the suggested time frame.

Clinical paths are useful in organizing care delivered to a specific population of patients for whom a measurable sequence of outcomes is readily identifiable. For example, most patients having total hip replacement sit on the edge of the bed by the end of the operative day and are up in a chair by noon on the first postoperative day. They also resume a regular diet intake and stand by the end of the first postoperative day. They progress to oral analgesics by the third postoperative day and are ready for discharge on the fifth postoperative day. Every patient with total hip replacement may not progress according to this path because of individual factors such as other medical diagnoses, development of complications, or simple individual variation. However, most will, and therefore a clinical path can be a powerful tool not only in guiding care but also in monitoring use of precious resources and making comparative judgments about outcomes of one physician group, hospital unit, or facility against external benchmarks. This may facilitate consumer decision making and enable those who finance health care to base judgments about referrals on outcome measures of specific physicians, hospitals, surgical centers, and other places.

The care plan forms the basis of a clinical path. *Nursing Care Plans: Diagnoses, Interventions, and Outcomes* can be used as the clinical basis from which to begin the development of the clinical path. Because nursing care plans in this text are organized by nursing diagnoses, adaptation of these care plans into clinical paths may require organizing the information differently.

References

Bulechek G, Butcher H, Dochterman J, Wagner C, editors: *Nursing Interventions Classification (NIC)*, ed 6, St. Louis, 2013, Mosby.

Gordon M: Nursing diagnosis and the diagnostic process. *American Journal of Nursing* 76:1298, 1976.

Moorhead S, Johnson M, Maas M, Swanson E, editors: *Nursing Outcomes Classification (NOC)*, ed 5, St. Louis, 2013, Mosby.

Nursing Diagnosis Care Plans

NANDA-I NDx Activity Intolerance

Definition: Insufficient physiological or psychological energy to endure or complete required or desired daily activities

Most activity intolerance is related to generalized weakness and debilitation secondary to acute or chronic illness and disease. This is especially apparent in older patients with a history of orthopedic, cardiopulmonary, diabetic, or pulmonary-related problems. The aging process itself causes reduction in muscle strength and function, which can impair the ability to maintain activity. Activity intolerance may also be related to factors such as obesity, malnourishment, anemia, side effects of medications (e.g., beta-blockers), or emotional states (e.g., depression or lack of confidence to exert oneself). Nursing goals are to reduce the effects of inactivity, promote optimal physical activity, and assist the patient with maintaining a satisfactory quality of life.

Common Related Factors

Generalized weakness
Sedentary lifestyle
Insufficient sleep or rest periods
Immobility
Bed rest
Imbalance between oxygen supply and demand

Defining Characteristics

Fatigue
Generalized weakness
Abnormal heart rate (HR) or blood pressure (BP) response to activity
Exertional discomfort
Exertional dyspnea

Common Expected Outcomes

Patient reports ability to perform required activities of daily living (ADLs).
Patient verbalizes and uses energy-conservation techniques.
Patient exhibits tolerance during physical activity as evidenced by rating of perceived exertion of 3 or less (on a scale of 0 to 10), HR less than or equal to 120 beats/min (or within 20 beats/min of resting HR), systolic BP within 20 mm Hg increase over resting systolic BP, respiratory rate less than 20 breaths/min, absence of chest pain or dyspnea.

NOC Outcomes

Activity Tolerance; Energy Conservation; Fatigue Level; Fatigue: Disruptive Effects; Knowledge: Treatment Regimen; Self-Care: Activities of Daily Living (ADLs)

NIC Interventions

Energy Management; Teaching: Prescribed Exercise

Ongoing Assessment

Actions/Interventions

■ Assess the patient's level of physical activity and mobility.

Rationales

This information will serve as a basis for formulating realistic short-term and long-term goals. The nurse incorporates this information in the planning and evaluation of care and communicates the information to the interprofessional team. QSEN: Patient-centered care.

Actions/Interventions

- Determine the patient's perception of causes of activity intolerance.

- Assess nutritional status.
- Monitor the patient's sleep pattern and amount of sleep achieved over the past few days.
- Evaluate the patient's routine and over-the-counter medications.

- Assess the need for ambulation aids: bracing, cane, walker, equipment modification for ADLs.

- Assess the patient's baseline cardiopulmonary status before initiating activity using the following measures:
  - HR
  - Orthostatic BP changes

- Assess the patient's perception of effort required to perform desired activity.

- Observe and document response to activity. Signs of abnormal responses to be reported include the following:
  - Increased HR of 20 to 30 beats/min over resting rate, or 120 beats/min
  - Palpitations/noticeable change in heart rhythm
  - Greater than 20 mm Hg increase in systolic BP
  - Greater than 10 mm Hg decrease in systolic BP
  - Dyspnea, labored breathing, wheezing
  - Excessive weakness, fatigue
  - Lightheadedness, dizziness, pallor, diaphoresis
  - Chest discomfort
- Assess emotional response to limitations in physical abilities.
- Use portable pulse oximetry to assess for oxygen desaturation during activity.

Rationales

Etiological factors may be temporary or permanent as well as physical or psychological. Determining the cause can help direct intervention. QSEN: Patient-centered care.

Adequate energy reserves are required for activity.

Difficulties with sleeping need to be addressed before successful activity progression can be achieved.

Fatigue may be a medication side effect or an indication of a drug interaction. The nurse should pay particular attention to the patient's use of beta-blockers, calcium channel blockers, tranquilizers, alcohol, muscle relaxants, and sedatives. QSEN: Patient-centered care.

Assistive devices can increase mobility by helping the patient overcome limitations. Some aids may require more energy expenditure for patients who have reduced upper arm strength (e.g., walking with crutches). Adequate assessment of energy requirements is indicated. QSEN: Safety.

Close monitoring serves as a guide for optimal progression of activity. HR should not increase more than 20 to 30 beats/min above resting with routine activities. This number will change depending on the intensity of activity the patient is attempting (e.g., climbing one flight of stairs versus walking on a flat surface). Older patients are more susceptible to orthostatic drops in BP with position changes (20 mm Hg drop in systolic BP or 10 mm Hg drop in diastolic BP). QSEN: Safety.

The Borg Scale uses ratings from 6 to 20 to determine rating of perceived exertion. A rating of 9 (very light) to 13 (somewhat hard) is an acceptable level for most people performing ADLs. Higher ratings are used for high-intensity physical exercise.

Close monitoring serves as a guide for optimal progression of activity. Effective monitoring reduces the risk of harm to the patient. QSEN: Safety.

Depression over inability to perform desired/required activities can be a source of stress and aggravation.

Supplemental oxygen may help compensate for the increased oxygen demands during physical activity.

■ = Independent ▲ = Interprofessional Collaboration

Nursing Diagnosis Care Plans

Therapeutic Interventions

Actions/Interventions	Rationales
■ Establish guidelines and goals of activity with the patient and caregiver.	Motivation is enhanced if the patient participates in goal setting. Depending on the etiological factors of the activity intolerance, some patients may be able to live independently and work outside the home. Other patients with chronic debilitating disease may remain homebound. QSEN: Patient-centered care.
■ Evaluate need for additional help at home (e.g., housekeeper, neighbor to shop, family assistance).	Coordinated efforts are more meaningful and effective in assisting patient in conserving energy.
■ Encourage adequate rest periods, especially before meals, other ADLs, exercise sessions, and ambulation.	Rest between activities provides time for energy conservation and recovery. HR recovery following activity is greatest at the beginning of a rest period.
■ Assist with ADLs as indicated; however, avoid patient dependency as much as possible.	Assisting the patient with ADLs allows for conservation of energy. Caregivers need to balance providing assistance with facilitating progressive endurance that will ultimately enhance the patient's activity tolerance and self-esteem.
■ Provide bedside commode as indicated.	Use of the commode requires less energy expenditure than using a bedpan or ambulating to the bathroom.
■ Encourage physical activity consistent with the patient's energy resources.	This approach promotes a sense of autonomy while being realistic about capabilities.
■ Assist patients with planning activities for times when they have the most energy.	Activities should be planned to coincide with the patient's peak energy level. Not all self-care and hygiene activities need to be completed in the morning. Likewise, not all housecleaning needs to be completed in 1 day. QSEN: Patient-centered care.
■ Progress activity gradually, as with the following: • Active range-of-motion (ROM) exercises in bed, progressing to sitting and standing • Sitting up in chair 30 minutes three times daily • Walking in room 1 to 2 minutes three times daily • Walking in the hall 25 feet or walking through the house, then slowly progressing to walking outside the house, saving energy for return trip	The hazards of bed rest, especially in the elderly, are serious. Deconditioning of the cardiovascular system can occur in days. Appropriate progression prevents overexerting the heart while promoting attainment of short-range goals. Duration and frequency should be increased before intensity. QSEN: Safety.
■ Encourage active ROM exercises. Encourage the patient to choose activities that gradually build endurance. If further reconditioning is needed, confer with rehabilitation personnel.	Exercise maintains muscle strength, joint ROM, and exercise tolerance. Physically inactive patients need to improve functional capacity through repetitive exercises over a longer period of time. Strength training is valuable in enhancing endurance for many ADLs. QSEN: Teamwork and collaboration.
■ Provide emotional support while increasing activity. Promote a positive attitude regarding abilities.	Patients may be fearful of overexertion and potential damage to the heart. Appropriate supervision during early efforts can enhance confidence.
■ Provide the patient with the adaptive equipment needed for completing ADLs.	Appropriate aids will enable the patient to achieve optimal independence for self-care and reduce energy consumption during activity.

Education/Continuity of Care

Actions/Interventions	Rationales
■ Teach the patient and caregivers to recognize signs of physical overactivity.	Knowledge promotes awareness of when to reduce activity. QSEN: Safety.

ⓔvolve **For additional care plans, go to http://evolve.elsevier.com/Gulanick/.**

Actions/Interventions

▲ When the patient is hospitalized, arrange for a physical therapist to assess the need for family or significant others to bring in an ambulation aid (e.g., walker, cane) from home.

■ Assist in assigning priority to activities to accommodate energy levels.

■ Teach energy-conservation techniques, such as the following:
  • Sitting to do tasks
  • Pushing rather than pulling
  • Sliding rather than lifting
  • Working at an even pace
  • Placing frequently used items within easy reach
  • Using wheeled carts for laundry, shopping, and cleaning needs
  • Organizing a work-rest-work schedule

■ Teach appropriate use of environmental aids (e.g., bed rails, elevating head of bed while patient gets out of bed, chair in bathroom, hall rails).

■ Teach ROM and strengthening exercises.

■ Encourage the patient to verbalize concerns about discharge and home environment.

■ Refer to community resources as indicated.

Rationales

Integrating the contributions of members of the interprofessional team helps the patient and family achieve health goals. QSEN: Teamwork and collaboration.

With a reduced functional capacity, pacing of priority tasks first may better meet the patient's needs.

Energy-conservation techniques reduce oxygen consumption, allowing more prolonged activity. For example, standing requires more work than sitting and evenly paced work allows enough time so that not all work is completed in a short period.

These aids conserve energy and reduce the risk for falls. QSEN: Safety.

Exercise promotes increased venous return, prevents contractures, and maintains/increases muscle strength and endurance.

Verbalization can reduce feelings of anxiety and fear as well as open doors for ongoing communication.

Continuity of care is facilitated through the use of community resources. Supervised programs in a structured environment may be beneficial.

Related Care Plans

Sedentary lifestyle, Chapter 2
Impaired physical mobility, Chapter 2

NANDA-I
NDx Ineffective Airway Clearance

Definition: Inability to clear secretions or obstructions from the respiratory tract to maintain a clear airway

Maintaining a patent airway is vital to life. Coughing is the main mechanism for clearing the airway. However, the cough may be ineffective in both normal and disease states secondary to factors such as pain from surgical incisions or trauma, respiratory muscle fatigue, or neuromuscular weakness. Other mechanisms that exist in the lower bronchioles and alveoli to maintain the airway include the mucociliary system, macrophages, and the lymphatics. Factors such as anesthesia and dehydration can affect function of the mucociliary system. Likewise, conditions that cause increased production of secretions (e.g., pneumonia, bronchitis, chemical irritants) can overtax these mechanisms. Ineffective airway clearance can be an acute (e.g., postoperative recovery) or chronic (e.g., from cerebrovascular accident [CVA] or spinal cord injury) problem. Older patients, who have an increased incidence of emphysema and a higher prevalence of chronic cough or sputum production, are at high risk.

■ = Independent   ▲ = Interprofessional Collaboration

Common Related Factors

Decreased energy and fatigue
Infection
Foreign body in airway
Excessive mucus
Exudate in the alveoli
Retained secretions
Airway spasm
Presence of artificial airway
Allergic airway
Asthma
Chronic obstructive pulmonary disease
Neuromuscular impairment

Defining Characteristics

Adventitious breath sounds
Diminished breath sounds
Alteration in respiratory pattern and rate
Cyanosis
Dyspnea
Ineffective cough
Excessive sputum
Orthopnea
Restlessness

Common Expected Outcome

Patient will maintain clear, open airways as evidenced by normal breath sounds, normal rate and depth of respirations, and ability to effectively cough up secretions after treatments and deep breaths.

NOC Outcome
Respiratory Status: Airway Patency
NIC Interventions
Cough Enhancement; Airway Management; Airway Suctioning

Ongoing Assessment

Actions/Interventions	Rationales
■ Assess airway for patency.	Maintaining the airway is always the first priority. QSEN: Safety.
■ Auscultate lungs after coughing for presence of adventitious breath sounds, as in the following:	As fluid and mucus accumulate, abnormal breath sounds can be heard that may indicate an obstructed airway.
• Decreased or absent breath sounds	Decreased sounds may indicate presence of a mucous plug or other major airway obstruction.
• Wheezing	Wheezing may indicate partial airway obstruction or resistance.
• Coarse crackles	Crackles may indicate presence of secretions along larger airways.
■ Assess respirations; note quality, rate, rhythm, depth, flaring of nostrils, dyspnea on exertion, evidence of splinting, use of accessory muscles, and position for breathing.	Abnormality indicates respiratory compromise. An increase in respiratory rate and rhythm may be a compensatory response to airway obstruction.
■ Assess changes in level of consciousness.	Increasing confusion, restlessness, and/or irritability can be early signs of cerebral hypoxia. Lethargy and somnolence are late signs. QSEN: Safety.
■ Assess changes in HR, BP, and temperature.	Tachycardia and hypertension may be related to increased work of breathing or hypoxia. Fever may develop in response to retained secretions or atelectasis or may be a manifestation of an infectious or inflammatory process.
■ Assess cough for effectiveness and productivity.	Coughing is the most helpful way to remove secretions. An ineffective cough compromises airway clearance and prevents mucus from being expelled. Possible causes of ineffective cough may be respiratory muscle fatigue, severe bronchospasm, or thick and tenacious secretions.

Actions/Interventions

- Assess secretions, noting color, viscosity, odor, and amount.

- ▲ Send a sputum specimen for culture and sensitivity testing, as appropriate.
- ▲ Use pulse oximetry to monitor oxygen saturation; assess arterial blood gases (ABGs).

- Assess hydration status: skin turgor, mucous membranes, tongue.
- Assess for abdominal or thoracic pain.
- ▲ If the patient is on mechanical ventilator, monitor for peak airway pressures and airway resistance.

- Assess use of herbal remedies (e.g., echinacea for upper respiratory infections, goldenseal for pneumonia, ma huang for bronchospasm).

- Assess the patient's knowledge of disease process.

Rationales

Abnormalities may be a result of infection, bronchitis, chronic smoking, or other condition. A sign of infection is discolored sputum (no longer clear or white); an odor may be present. Thick, tenacious secretions increase airway resistance and work of breathing and may be indicative of dehydration.

Respiratory infections increase the work of breathing; antibiotic treatment is indicated.

Pulse oximetry is a useful tool to detect changes in oxygenation. Oxygen saturation should be maintained at 90% or greater. Increased partial pressure of carbon dioxide in arterial blood ($Paco_2$) and decreased partial arterial oxygen tension (Pao_2) and pulse oximetry readings can result from increased pulmonary secretions and respiratory fatigue. QSEN: Safety.

Airway clearance is impaired with inadequate hydration and subsequent secretion thickening.

Pain can result in shallow breathing and an ineffective cough.

Increases in these parameters signal accumulation of secretions or fluid and potential for ineffective ventilation. QSEN: Safety.

Drug interactions with prescribed medications and contraindications need to be evaluated (e.g., ma huang contains ephedrine, which should not be used by patients with hypertension, heart disease, prostatic hyperplasia, or diabetes).

Patient education will vary depending on the acute or chronic disease state as well as the patient's cognitive level.

Therapeutic Interventions

Actions/Interventions

- Assist the patient in performing coughing and breathing maneuvers (e.g., take a deep breath, hold for 2 seconds, and cough two or three times in succession).

- Instruct the patient in the following:
  - Optimal positioning (sitting position)
  - Use of pillow or hand splints when coughing
  - Use of abdominal muscles for more forceful cough
  - Use of quad and huff techniques
  - Use of incentive spirometry
  - Importance of ambulation and frequent position changes
- Use upright position (if tolerated, head of bed at 45 degrees; sitting in chair). If patient is bedridden, routinely check the patient's position so the patient does not slide down in bed.
- ▲ If cough is ineffective, use nasotracheal suctioning as needed based on presence of adventitious lung sounds and/or increased ventilatory pressure.
  - Explain procedure to patient.

Rationales

Coughing is the most helpful way to remove most secretions. Deep breathing promotes oxygenation before controlled coughing. The patient may be unable to perform independently and may require assistance.

Controlled coughing techniques help mobilize secretions from smaller airways to larger airways because the coughing is done at varying times. The sitting position and splinting the abdomen promote more effective coughing by increasing abdominal pressure and upward diaphragmatic movement. Ambulation helps maintain adequate lung expansion, mobilizes secretions, and reduces atelectasis. QSEN: Safety.

Upright position prevents abdominal contents from pushing upward and inhibiting lung expansion. This position promotes better lung expansion and improved air exchange. QSEN: Safety.

Suctioning is indicated when patients are unable to remove secretions from the airways by coughing because of weakness, thick mucous plugs, or excessive or tenacious mucus production. It can also stimulate a cough. Frequency of suctioning should be based on patient's clinical status, not on preset routine, such as every 2 hours. Oversuctioning can cause hypoxia and injury to bronchial and lung tissue. QSEN: Safety.

■ = Independent   ▲ = Interprofessional Collaboration

Actions/Interventions

- Use well-lubricated soft catheters.

- Use curved-tip catheters and head positioning (if not contraindicated).
- Instruct the patient to take several deep breaths before and after each nasotracheal suctioning procedure and use supplemental oxygen, as appropriate.
- Stop suctioning and provide supplemental oxygen (assisted breaths by resuscitation bag as needed) if the patient experiences bradycardia, an increase in ventricular ectopy, and/or significant desaturation.
- Use universal precautions: gloves, goggles, and mask, as appropriate.

■ Maintain humidified oxygen as prescribed.

■ Encourage increased fluid intake within the limits of cardiac reserve and renal function.

▲ Administer medications (e.g., antibiotics, inhaled steroids, mucolytic agents, bronchodilators, expectorants) as ordered, noting effectiveness and side effects.
▲ Consult a respiratory therapist for chest physiotherapy and nebulizer treatments as indicated (hospital and home care or rehabilitation environments).

▲ Coordinate optimal time for postural drainage and percussion (i.e., at least 1 hour after eating).
■ For patients with reduced energy, pace activities. Maintain planned rest periods. Promote energy-conservation techniques.
▲ For acute problems, anticipate bronchoscopy.

▲ If secretions cannot be cleared, anticipate the need for an artificial airway (intubation). After intubation, suction the airway as determined by the presence of adventitious sounds, increased peak airway pressures, and visible secretions in the tubing.
■ For patients with complete airway obstruction, institute appropriate basic life support measures.

Rationales

Suctioning with a well-lubricated catheter minimizes irritation and prevents trauma to mucous membranes.
These facilitate secretion removal from a specific side (right versus left lung).
Hyperoxygenation before, during, and after suctioning decreases hypoxia related to suctioning procedure.

Oxygen therapy is indicated to increase oxygen saturation and reduce potential complications.

These precautions prevent transmission of pathogenic microorganisms.
Increasing humidity of inspired air will decrease viscosity of secretions and facilitate their removal.
Maintaining hydration increases ciliary action to remove secretions and reduces viscosity of secretions. It is easier for the patient to mobilize thinner secretions with coughing.
A variety of medications are available to treat specific problems. Most promote clearance of airway secretions and may reduce airway resistance.
Chest physiotherapy includes the techniques of postural drainage and chest percussion to loosen and mobilize secretions from smaller airways that cannot be removed by coughing or suctioning. A nebulizer may be used to humidify the airway to thin secretions to facilitate their removal; it may also be used to deliver bronchodilators and mucolytic agents. QSEN: Teamwork and collaboration.
This measure reduces aspiration. QSEN: Safety.

Fatigue is a contributing factor to ineffective coughing. Effective coughing is hard work and may exhaust an already compromised patient.
Bronchoscopy obtains lavage samples for culture and sensitivity testing and removes mucous plugs.
Being prepared for an emergency helps prevent further complications. Intubation may be needed to facilitate removal of tenacious or copious amounts of secretions and provide source for augmenting oxygenation. QSEN: safety.

These measures are used to relieve airway obstructions and to sustain life until definitive treatment can be provided.

Education/Continuity of Care

Actions/Interventions

■ Teach coughing, breathing, and splinting techniques.

■ Instruct the patient in how to use prescribed medications and inhalers, as appropriate.

Rationales

These techniques facilitate clearance of secretions and prevent atelectasis. Dyspnea may be reduced with the use of pursed-lip or diaphragmatic breathing.
Instruction promotes safe and effective medication administration. QSEN: safety.

Actions/Interventions	Rationales
■ In the home setting, instruct caregivers regarding the need for humidification and adequate hydration.	Adequate fluid intake enhances liquefaction of pulmonary secretions and facilitates expectoration of mucus. Thin secretions are easier to clear from the airway.
■ Instruct caregivers in suctioning techniques. Provide opportunity for return demonstration. Adapt techniques for the home setting.	Instruction promotes safe and effective removal of secretions from the airway.
■ For patients with debilitating disease (e.g., CVA, neuromuscular impairment) being cared for at home, instruct caregivers in chest physiotherapy, as appropriate.	Chest physiotherapy loosens and mobilizes secretions.
■ Teach the patient about environmental factors that can precipitate respiratory problems.	Chemical irritants and allergens can increase mucus production and bronchospasm.
■ Explain effects of smoking, including secondhand smoke. Refer the patient and/or significant others to a smoking-cessation group, as appropriate.	Chemical irritants and allergens can increase mucus production and bronchospasm. Smoking cessation programs and groups can provide specialized information and ongoing support.
▲ Refer to the pulmonary clinical nurse specialist, home health nurse, or respiratory therapist as indicated.	Use of consultants may be required to ensure that patient needs are met and outcomes achieved. QSEN: Teamwork and collaboration.
■ Refer to the American Lung Association Call Center and support groups (e.g., Better Breathers Club).	Support groups provide emotional support and information that may assist patients in coping with chronic illness.

Related Care Plans

Pneumonia, Chapter 6
Tracheostomy, ⊖volve
Pulmonary tuberculosis, ⊖volve

Anxiety

Definition: Vague, uneasy feeling of discomfort or dread accompanied by an autonomic response (the source often nonspecific or unknown to the individual); a feeling of apprehension caused by anticipation of danger. It is an alerting signal that warns of impending danger and enables the individual to take measures to deal with the threat.

Anxiety represents an emotional response to environmental stressors and is therefore part of the person's stress response. Each individual's experience with anxiety is different. Some people are able to use the emotional edge that anxiety provokes to stimulate creativity or problem-solving abilities; others can become immobilized to a pathological degree. These pathological anxiety disorders include panic attacks, social phobias, specific phobias, obsessive-compulsive disorder, and post-traumatic stress disorder. Anxiety is generally categorized into four levels: mild, moderate, severe, and panic. Mild anxiety can enhance a person's perception of the environment and readiness to respond. Moderate anxiety is associated with a narrowing of the person's perception of the situation. The person with moderate anxiety may be more creative and more effective in solving problems. Severe anxiety is associated with increasing emotional and physical feelings of discomfort. Perceptions are further narrowed. The person with severe anxiety begins to manifest excessive autonomic nervous system signs of the fight-or-flight stress response. The person in a panic stage of anxiety has distorted perceptions of the situation. His or her thinking skills become limited and irrational. The person may be unable to make decisions. In the severe and panic stages of anxiety, the nurse needs to intervene to promote patient safety. The nurse can encounter the anxious patient anywhere in the hospital or community. The presence of the nurse may lend support to the anxious patient and provide strategies for effectively coping with anxious moments or panic attacks.

Common Related Factors

Major change (e.g., economic status, environment, health status, role function, role status)
Maturational or situational crises
Stressors
Substance abuse
Conflict about life goals or values
Unmet needs
Heredity

Defining Characteristics

Behavioral:
- Decrease in productivity
- Worried about change in life event
- Insomnia
- Restlessness

Affective:
- Apprehensiveness
- Feeling of inadequacy
- Irritability

Cognitive:
- Confusion
- Alteration in concentration
- Diminished ability to learn or problem-solve

Physiological:
- Facial tension
- Hand tremors
- Increase in perspiration
- Voice quivering

Sympathetic:
- Anorexia
- Diarrhea
- Dry mouth
- Facial flushing
- Increased blood pressure, heart rate, respiratory rate

Parasympathetic:
- Abdominal pain
- Fatigue
- Nausea
- Urinary frequency, urgency

Common Expected Outcomes

Patient uses effective coping mechanisms.
Patient describes a reduction in the level of anxiety experienced.
Patient maintains a desired level of role function and problem-solving.

NOC Outcomes
Anxiety Level; Anxiety Self-Control; Coping
NIC Interventions
Anxiety Reduction; Coping Enhancement; Relaxation Therapy; Presence; Emotional Support

Ongoing Assessment

Actions/Interventions	Rationales
■ Assess the patient's level of anxiety.	The patient with mild anxiety will have minimal or no physiological symptoms of anxiety. Vital signs will be within normal ranges. The patient will appear calm but may report feelings of nervousness such as "butterflies in the stomach." The patient with moderate anxiety may appear energized, with more animated facial expressions and tone of voice. Vital signs may be normal or slightly elevated. The patient may report feeling tense. With severe anxiety, the patient will have symptoms of increased autonomic nervous system activity, such as elevated vital signs, diaphoresis, urinary urgency and frequency, dry mouth, and muscle tension. At this stage the patient may experience palpitations and chest pain. The patient may be agitated and irritable and report feeling overloaded or overwhelmed by new stimuli. In the panic level of anxiety, the autonomic nervous system increases to the level of sympathetic neurotransmitter release. The patient becomes pale and hypotensive and experiences poor muscle coordination. The patient reports feeling completely out of control and may display extremes of behavior from combativeness to withdrawal.
■ Use the State-Trait Anxiety Inventory to differentiate between the patient's anxiety level as a temporary response state and a long-standing personality trait.	The State-Trait Anxiety Inventory, developed by Spielberger, is considered a definitive tool for measuring anxiety in adults. The tool is written at the sixth-grade reading level and is available in more than 40 languages. QSEN: Evidence-based practice.
■ Determine how the patient uses coping strategies and defense mechanisms to cope with anxiety.	Coping strategies may include reading, journaling, or physical activity such as taking a walk. People use defense mechanisms to preserve the ego and manage anxiety. Some defense mechanisms are highly adaptive in managing anxiety, such as humor, sublimation, or suppression. Other defense mechanisms may lead to less-adaptive behavior, especially with long-term use. These defense mechanisms include displacement, repression, denial, projection, and self-image splitting. QSEN: Patient-centered care.

Therapeutic Interventions

Actions/Interventions	Rationales
■ Acknowledge awareness of the patient's anxiety.	Because a cause for anxiety cannot always be identified, the patient may feel as though the feelings being experienced are counterfeit. Acknowledgment of the patient's feelings validates the feelings and communicates acceptance of those feelings.
■ Maintain a calm manner while interacting with the patient.	The health care provider can transmit his or her own anxiety to the hypersensitive patient. The patient's feeling of stability increases in a calm and nonthreatening atmosphere.

■ = Independent ▲ = Interprofessional Collaboration

Nursing Diagnosis Care Plans

Actions/Interventions	Rationales
■ Orient the patient to the environment and new experiences or people as needed.	Orientation to and awareness of the surroundings promote comfort and may decrease anxiety experienced by the patient. Anxiety may escalate to a panic level if the patient feels threatened and unable to control environmental stimuli.
■ Use simple language and brief statements when instructing the patient about self-care measures or about diagnostic and surgical procedures.	When experiencing moderate to severe anxiety, patients may be unable to comprehend anything more than simple, clear, and brief instructions.
■ Reduce sensory stimuli by maintaining a quiet environment; keep "threatening" equipment out of sight.	Anxiety may escalate to a panic state with excessive conversation, noise, and equipment around the patient. Increasing anxiety may become frightening to the patient and others.
■ Encourage the patient to talk about anxious feelings and examine anxiety-provoking situations if they are identifiable.	Talking about anxiety-producing situations and anxious feelings can help the patient perceive the situation realistically and recognize factors leading to the anxious feelings.
■ Suggest that the patient keep a log of episodes of anxiety. Instruct the patient to describe what is experienced and the events leading up to and surrounding the event. The patient should note how the anxiety dissipates.	Recognition and exploration of factors leading to or reducing anxious feelings are important steps in developing alternative responses. The patient may be unaware of the relationship between emotional concerns and anxiety. If the patient is comfortable with the idea, the log may be shared with the health care provider, who may help the patient develop more effective coping strategies. Symptoms often provide the health care provider with information regarding the degree of anxiety being experienced.
■ Support the patient's use of coping strategies that the patient has found effective in the past.	Using anxiety-reduction strategies enhances the patient's sense of personal mastery and confidence. QSEN: Patient-centered care.
■ Assist the patient in developing new anxiety-reducing skills (e.g., relaxation, deep breathing, positive visualization, and reassuring self-statements).	Learning new coping methods provides the patient with a variety of ways to manage anxiety.
■ Assist the patient in developing problem-solving abilities. Emphasize the logical strategies that the patient can use when experiencing anxious feelings.	Learning to identify a problem and to evaluate the alternatives to resolve that problem helps the patient cope more effectively and decrease anxiety.
■ Instruct the patient in the appropriate use of antianxiety medications.	Short-term use of antianxiety medications can enhance patient coping and reduce physiological manifestations of anxiety. QSEN: Evidence-based practice.
• Benzodiazepines	Drugs in this group work through enhancing the action of the inhibitory neurotransmitter gamma-aminobutyric acid (GABA). These drugs are recommended for short-term use, not to exceed 3 to 4 months. Physical dependence and tolerance are problems associated with prolonged use of these drugs.
• Buspirone HCL (BuSpar)	This drug has fewer side effects and less risk for dependence than the benzodiazepines. The drug has a slower onset of action and may take 1 to 2 weeks to produce a noticeable therapeutic effect.
• Selective serotonin reuptake inhibitors (SSRIs)	The Food and Drug Administration (FDA) has approved several drugs in this group for use in the management of panic disorder. Their use in treatment of other types of anxiety is being investigated.

Actions/Interventions

- Nonselective beta-blockers and alpha-2–receptor agonists

- Teach the patient to limit use of central nervous system stimulants.

Rationales

Beta-blockers are effective in managing the physical symptoms of anxiety that occur with the social phobias (e.g., stage fright). The alpha-2 agonists are used to manage anxiety associated with withdrawal from nicotine and opioids.

Stimulants (e.g., caffeine and nicotine) can increase physical symptoms of anxiety.

Education/Continuity of Care

Actions/Interventions

- Assist the patient in recognizing symptoms of increasing anxiety; explore alternatives to use to prevent the anxiety from immobilizing him or her.

- Remind the patient that anxiety at a mild level can encourage growth and development and is important in mobilizing changes.
- ▲ Refer the patient to members of the interprofessional team for management of anxiety that becomes disabling for an extended period.

Rationales

The ability to recognize anxiety symptoms at lower intensity levels enables the patient to intervene more quickly to manage his or her anxiety. The patient will be able to use problem-solving abilities more effectively when the level of anxiety is low. Knowledge of anxiety and effective coping strategies can help the patient's feelings of control over anxiety-producing situations.

Cognitive appraisal of mild anxiety can help the patient perceive the anxiety as an opportunity to develop new strengths that enhance coping.

Additional, long-term professional care may be needed when anxiety becomes severe and interferes with daily functioning. The types of disorders requiring this level of care include panic disorders, obsessive-compulsive disorder, and post-traumatic stress disorder. QSEN: Teamwork and collaboration.

Risk for Aspiration

Definition: Vulnerable to entry of gastrointestinal secretions, oropharyngeal secretions, solids, or fluids to the tracheobronchial passages, which may compromise health

Aspiration is the entry of secretions or materials such as foods or liquids into the trachea and lungs and occurs when protective reflexes are decreased or compromised. Aspiration from the oropharynx into the lungs can result in aspiration pneumonia. Depending on the acidity of the aspirate, even small amounts of gastric acid contents can damage lung tissue, resulting in chemical pneumonitis. Both acute and chronic conditions can place patients at risk for aspiration. Acute conditions, such as postanesthesia effects from surgery or diagnostic tests, occur predominantly in the acute care setting. Chronic conditions, including altered consciousness from head injury, spinal cord injury, neuromuscular weakness, hemiplegia and dysphagia from stroke, use of tube feedings for nutrition, and artificial airway devices such as tracheostomies, may be encountered in the home, rehabilitative, or hospital setting. Older and cognitively impaired patients are at high risk. Aspiration is a common cause of death in comatose patients. Patients should be evaluated for aspiration risk upon admission and periodically during the patient's stay.

■ = Independent   ▲ = Interprofessional Collaboration

Common Risk Factors

Decrease in level of consciousness
Depressed gag reflex
Ineffective cough
Impaired ability to swallow
Presence of oral/nasal tube (e.g., tracheal, feeding)
Enteral feedings
Increase in gastric residual
Treatment regimen
Decrease in gastrointestinal motility
Delayed gastric emptying
Facial, oral, or neck surgery or trauma
Barrier to elevating upper body

Common Expected Outcome

Patient maintains a patent airway as evidenced by normal breath sounds, absence of coughing, no shortness of breath, and no aspiration.

NOC Outcomes
Aspiration Prevention; Respiratory Status: Ventilation
NIC Interventions
Aspiration Precautions; Respiratory Monitoring

Ongoing Assessment

Actions/Interventions	Rationales
■ Monitor level of consciousness	A decreased level of consciousness is a prime risk factor for aspiration. QSEN: Safety.
■ Assess presence or absence of cough and gag reflexes.	The lungs are normally protected against aspiration by reflexes such as cough and gag. When these reflexes are absent or reduced, the patient is at increased risk. QSEN: Safety.
■ Evaluate swallowing ability by assessing for the following: • Coughing, choking, throat clearing, gurgling, or "wet" voice during or after swallowing • Residual food in mouth after eating • Regurgitation of food or fluid through the nares	Impaired swallowing increases the risk for aspiration. There remains a need for valid and easy-to-use methods to screen for aspiration risk. QSEN: Safety.
▲ Assess results of swallowing studies as ordered.	For high-risk patients, performance of a videofluoroscopic swallowing study may be indicated to determine the nature and extent of any swallowing abnormality.
■ In patients with tracheostomies, observe for food particles in tracheal secretions.	Food is not normal in the tracheobronchial passages. It signifies aspirated material.
■ Auscultate bowel sounds to evaluate bowel motility, and assess for abdominal distention and firmness.	Decreased gastrointestinal motility increases the risk for aspiration because food or fluids accumulate in the stomach. Older patients have a decrease in esophageal motility, which delays esophageal emptying. When combined with the weaker gag reflex of older patients, aspiration is a higher risk.
■ Assess for presence of nausea or vomiting.	Nausea or vomiting places patients at great risk for aspiration, especially if the level of consciousness is compromised. Antiemetics may be required to prevent aspiration of regurgitated gastric contents.

Actions/Interventions

▲ Assess pulmonary status for clinical evidence of aspiration. Auscultate breath sounds for development of crackles and/or wheezes. Monitor chest x-ray films as ordered.

▲ In patients with nasogastric (NG) or gastrostomy tubes:

- Check placement before feeding, using tube markings, x-ray study (most accurate), pH of gastric fluid, and color of aspirate as guides.

- Check residuals before feeding, or every 4 hours if feeding is continuous. Hold feedings if amount of residuals is large, and notify the physician.

- Test sputum with glucose oxidase reagent strips.

■ In patients with endotracheal or tracheostomy tubes, monitor the effectiveness of the cuff. Collaborate with the respiratory therapist, as needed, to determine cuff pressure.

Rationales

Aspiration of small amounts ("silent aspiration") can occur without coughing or sudden onset of respiratory distress, especially in patients with a decreased level of consciousness. Pulmonary infiltrates on chest x-ray films indicate some level of aspiration has already occurred.

Effective use of these strategies reduces the risk of harm to the patient. QSEN: Safety.

A displaced tube may erroneously deliver tube feeding into the airway. Chest x-ray verification of accurate tube placement is most reliable. Gastric aspirate is usually green, brown, clear, or colorless, with a pH between 1 and 5.

Large amounts of residuals indicate delayed gastric emptying and can cause distention of the stomach, leading to reflux emesis. The amount of residuals may vary depending on the volume and rate of infusion; however, the evaluation can be unreliable. Feedings are often held if residual volume is greater than 50% of the amount to be delivered in 1 hour.

Significant amounts of glucose in sputum may be indicative of aspiration.

An ineffective or overinflated cuff can increase the risk for aspiration. Properly inflated cuffs are the best protection. QSEN: Teamwork and collaboration.

Therapeutic Interventions

Actions/Interventions

■ Keep suction setup available (in both hospital and home settings) and use as needed.

■ Notify the physician or other health care provider immediately of noted decrease in cough/gag reflexes or difficulty in swallowing.

■ Position patients with a decreased level of consciousness supine on their side.

■ Supervise or assist the patient with oral intake. Never give oral fluids to a comatose patient.

■ Offer foods with consistency that the patient can swallow. Use thickening agents if recommended by a speech pathologist or dietitian.

■ Encourage the patient to chew thoroughly and eat slowly during meals.

Rationales

Tracheal suction may be necessary to maintain a patent airway. Secretions can rapidly accumulate in the posterior pharynx and upper trachea, increasing risk for aspiration. QSEN: Safety.

Early intervention protects the patient's airway and prevents aspiration. Anyone identified as being at high risk for aspiration should be kept NPO (nothing by mouth) until further evaluation is completed. QSEN: Safety.

This positioning (rescue positioning) decreases the risk for aspiration by promoting the drainage of secretions out of the mouth instead of down the pharynx, where they could be aspirated. QSEN: Safety.

Supervision helps detect abnormalities early and enables implementation of strategies for safe swallowing. Withholding fluids and foods as needed prevents aspiration.

Thickened semisolid foods such as pudding and hot cereal are most easily swallowed and less likely to be aspirated. Liquids and thin foods (e.g., creamed soups) are most difficult for patients with dysphagia. Integrating the contributions of members of the interprofessional team helps the patient and family achieve health goals. QSEN: Safety.

Well-masticated food is easier to swallow; food cut into small pieces may also be easier to swallow.

■ = Independent ▲ = Interprofessional Collaboration

Actions/Interventions	Rationales
■ For patients with reduced cognitive abilities, remove distracting stimuli during mealtimes. Instruct the patient not to talk while eating.	Concentration must be focused on chewing and swallowing. When talking and eating or drinking at the same time, there is higher risk for the airway being opened while food is in the pharynx.
■ Place whole or crushed pills in soft foods (e.g., custard). Verify with a pharmacist which pills should not be crushed. Substitute medication in elixir form as indicated.	Mixing pills with food helps reduce risk for aspiration. QSEN: Safety; Teamwork and collaboration.
■ Place medication and food on the strong side of the mouth when unilateral weakness or paresis is present.	Careful food placement facilitates chewing and successful swallowing.
■ Offer liquids *after* food is eaten.	Ingesting food and fluids together increases swallowing difficulties.
■ Position the patient at a 90-degree angle, whether in bed or in a chair or wheelchair. Use cushions or pillows to maintain position. Maintain the patient in an upright position for 30 to 45 minutes after feeding.	The upright position facilitates the gravitational flow of food or fluid through the alimentary tract. If the head of the bed cannot be elevated because of the patient's condition, use a right side-lying position after feedings to facilitate passage of stomach contents into the duodenum. QSEN: Safety.
■ Provide oral care before and after meals.	Oral care before meals reduces bacterial counts in the oral cavity. Oral care after eating removes residual food that could be aspirated at a later time. QSEN: Safety.
▲ In patients with artificial airways:	
• Perform oral suctioning as needed.	Suctioning reduces the volume of oropharyngeal secretions and reduces aspiration risk.
• Brush teeth twice a day, and swab mouth with sponge applicators every 2 to 4 hours between brushing.	Oral care reduces the risk for ventilator-associated pneumonia by decreasing the number of microorganisms in aspirated oropharyngeal secretions. QSEN: Safety.
▲ In patients with NG or gastrostomy tubes:	
• Place dye (e.g., methylene blue) in NG feedings only with a physician's order.	Detection of the color in pulmonary secretions would indicate aspiration. However, regular amounts of some dyes may discolor skin, body fluids, and tissues as well as increase morbidity and mortality risks, especially in patients with increased intestinal permeability or metabolic disorders such as sepsis.
• Elevate the head of the bed to 30 to 45 degrees while feeding the patient and for 30 to 45 minutes afterward if feeding is intermittent. Turn off the feeding before lowering the head of the bed. Patients with continuous feedings should be in an upright position.	Upright positioning reduces aspiration by decreasing reflux of gastric contents.
▲ Consult a speech pathologist, as appropriate.	A speech pathologist can be consulted to perform a dysphagia assessment that helps determine the need for videofluoroscopy or modified barium swallow and to establish specific techniques to prevent aspiration in patients with impaired swallowing. QSEN: Teamwork and collaboration.

Education/Continuity of Care

Actions/Interventions	Rationales
■ Explain to the patient and caregiver the need for proper positioning.	Upright positioning decreases the risk for aspiration.
■ Instruct in proper feeding techniques.	Both the patient and caregiver need to be active participants in implementing the treatment plan to optimize safe nutritional intake. QSEN: Patient-centered care; Safety.

Actions/Interventions

- Instruct in upper airway suctioning techniques to prevent accumulation of secretions in the oral cavity.

- Instruct in signs and symptoms of aspiration.

- Demonstrate to the patient, caregiver, or family what should be done if the patient aspirates (e.g., chokes, coughs, becomes short of breath). For example, use suction if available, and the abdominal thrust maneuver if the patient is unable to speak or breathe. If liquid aspiration, turn the patient three-fourths prone with the head slightly lower than the chest. If the patient has difficulty breathing, call the emergency medical system (9-1-1).

▲ Refer the patient to a home health nurse, rehabilitation specialist, or occupational therapist as indicated.

Rationales

Patient safety is a priority. Suctioning reduces the volume of oropharyngeal secretions and reduces aspiration risk. QSEN: Safety.

Information aids in appropriate assessment of high-risk situations and determination of when to call for further evaluation. QSEN: Safety.

Respiratory aspiration requires immediate action by the caregiver to maintain the airway and promote effective breathing and gas exchange. Being prepared for an emergency helps prevent further complications. QSEN: Safety.

Use of consultants may be required to ensure that outcomes are achieved. QSEN: Teamwork and collaboration.

Risk for Bleeding

Definition: Vulnerable to a decrease in blood volume, which may compromise health

A patient may experience bleeding when disease or the effects of disease treatments disrupt the normal mechanisms that support hemostasis. Some diseases such as hemophilia interfere with genetic expression of normal clotting factors. Risk for bleeding occurs with disorders that decrease the quantity or quality of circulating platelets (thrombocytopenia). Cancers of the blood and blood-forming organs are associated with a decrease in production of platelets from the bone marrow. Immune thrombocytopenic purpura (ITP) is associated with increased destruction of platelets. Impaired liver function leads to a decrease in the synthesis of clotting factors. Any condition that disrupts the "closed circuit" integrity of the circulatory system increases the risk for bleeding. Examples of these conditions include major organ surgery, traumatic injury, and the many inflammatory or ulcerative disorders of the gastrointestinal system (e.g., peptic ulcer disease, inflammatory bowel disease). Drugs that suppress bone marrow function or interfere with the action of normal clotting factors increase the patient's risk for bleeding as a side effect. These drugs include anticoagulants, nonsteroidal anti-inflammatory drugs (NSAIDs), and cancer chemotherapy agents. Herbal preparations may contribute to the risk for bleeding through direct effect on clotting factors or interactions with anticoagulants.

Common Risk Factors

Gastrointestinal disorders (e.g., ulcer, polyps, varices)
Impaired liver function (e.g., cirrhosis, hepatitis)
Inherent coagulopathies (e.g., thrombocytopenia)
Trauma
Treatment regimen

■ = Independent ▲ = Interprofessional Collaboration

Common Expected Outcomes

Patient implements measures to prevent bleeding and identifies signs of bleeding that need to be reported immediately to a health care provider.

Patient does not experience bleeding as evidenced by stable hemoglobin and hematocrit levels, desired ranges for coagulation profiles, BP, and HR rate within normal limits.

NOC Outcomes
Blood Loss Severity; Circulation Status; Blood Coagulation; Knowledge: Personal Safety; Knowledge: Medication; Risk Control

NIC Interventions
Bleeding Precautions; Bleeding Reduction; Teaching: Prescribed Medication

Ongoing Assessment

Actions/Interventions

■ Assess the patient's health history for indications of conditions that contribute to a risk for bleeding such as liver disease, peptic ulcer disease, or inflammatory bowel disease.

■ Assess the patient's use of any medications that can interfere with hemostasis (e.g., salicylates, anticoagulants, NSAIDs, or cancer chemotherapy).

■ Monitor BP and HR. Observe for signs of orthostatic hypotension.

■ Assess skin and mucous membranes for evidence of petechiae, bruising, hematoma formation, or oozing of blood.

▲ Monitor laboratory values for coagulation status as appropriate: platelet count, prothrombin time/international normalized ratio (PT/INR), activated partial thromboplastin time (aPTT), fibrinogen, bleeding time, fibrin degradation products, vitamin K, activated coagulation time (ACT).

▲ Monitor hematocrit (Hct) and hemoglobin (Hgb).

▲ Monitor stool (guaiac) and urine (Hemastix) for occult blood.

Rationales

Early identification of potential risks for bleeding provides a basis for implementing appropriate preventive measures. QSEN: Safety.

Drugs that interfere with clotting mechanisms or platelet activity increase risk for bleeding. Salicylates and other NSAIDs inhibit cyclooxygenase 1 (COX-1), an enzyme that promotes platelet aggregation. Warfarin, an oral anticoagulant, inhibits the synthesis of vitamin K in the liver, thus reducing levels of several subsequent clotting factors. Heparin, a parenteral anticoagulant, inhibits the action of thrombin and prevents formation of a fibrin clot. Many drugs used to treat cancer suppress bone marrow function and therefore reduce the production of platelets.

Tachycardia and hypotension are initial compensatory mechanisms commonly noted with bleeding. Orthostasis (a drop of 20 mm Hg in systolic BP or 10 mm Hg in diastolic BP [DBP] when changing from supine to sitting position) indicates reduced circulating fluids. The patient with orthostasis may experience lightheadedness when changing position. QSEN: Safety.

Patients with reduced platelet counts or impaired clotting factor activity may experience bleeding into tissues that is out of proportion to the injury. Prolonged oozing of blood from surgical incisions or areas of skin trauma is associated with coagulation abnormalities.

The blood-clotting cascade is an integrated system requiring intrinsic and extrinsic factors. Derangement in any of these factors can affect clotting ability. These laboratory tests provide important information about the patient's coagulation status and bleeding potential. The specific laboratory values to be monitored will depend on the patient's specific clinical condition. For patients receiving anticoagulants, increased levels of PT/INR and aPTT above therapeutic values are associated with increased risk for bleeding. Reduced platelet counts may develop in patients receiving heparin therapy. QSEN: Evidence-based practice.

When bleeding is not visible, decreased Hgb and Hct levels may be an early indicator of bleeding.

These tests are used to detect bleeding from the gastrointestinal or urinary tracts that may not be visible.

ⓔvolve **For additional care plans, go to http://evolve.elsevier.com/Gulanick/.**

Therapeutic Interventions

Actions/Interventions	Rationales
■ Instruct the at-risk patient about precautionary measures to prevent tissue trauma or disruption of the normal clotting mechanisms.	Effective use of precautionary measures reduces the risk of bleeding. QSEN: Safety.
• Use a soft toothbrush and nonabrasive toothpaste. Avoid the use of toothpicks and dental floss.	This method of providing oral hygiene reduces trauma to oral mucous membranes and the risk for bleeding from the gums.
• Avoid rectal suppositories, thermometers, enemas, vaginal douches, and tampons.	Use of these invasive devices or medications may cause trauma to the mucous membranes that line the rectum or vagina.
• Avoid straining with bowel movements, forceful nose blowing, coughing, or sneezing.	These activities may cause trauma to the mucosal linings in the rectum, nasal passages, or upper airways.
• Be cautious with the use of sharp objects such as scissors and knives. Use an electric razor for shaving (not razor blades).	The patient needs to avoid situations that may cause tissue trauma and increase the risk for bleeding.
■ Instruct the patient and family about signs of bleeding that need to be reported to a health care provider.	Early evaluation and treatment of bleeding by a health care provider reduce the risk for complications from blood loss.
▲ Administer appropriate antidotes as prescribed for bleeding associated with excessive anticoagulant use.	Protamine sulfate reverses the effect of heparin. Vitamin K will counteract the action of warfarin.
▲ If coagulation laboratory values are abnormal, administer blood products as prescribed: red blood cells (RBCs), fresh frozen plasma (FFP), cryoprecipitate, and platelets.	Blood product transfusions replace blood clotting factors; RBCs increase oxygen-carrying capacity; FFP replaces clotting factors and inhibitors; platelets and cryoprecipitate provide proteins for coagulation.

Education/Continuity of Care

Actions/Interventions	Rationales
■ Encourage the patient to use normal saline nasal sprays and emollient lip balms.	These applications reduce drying and cracking of mucous membranes and therefore reduce the risk for bleeding.
■ Educate the sexually active patient to use water-soluble lubricants during intercourse.	Lubricants are used to reduce friction and tissue trauma that increase the risk for bleeding.
■ Teach the patient about measures to reduce constipation such as increased fluid intake and dietary fiber.	The passage of hard, dry feces that occurs with constipation may cause trauma to the mucous membranes of the colon and rectum. Increasing fluid intake and dietary fiber soften the fecal mass for easier defecation. Pharmacological stool softeners may be needed.
■ Teach the patient to monitor the color and consistency of stools.	Bright red blood in the stools is an indicator of lower gastrointestinal bleeding. Stool that has a dark greenish black color and a tarry consistency is associated with upper gastrointestinal bleeding.
■ Instruct women to report to their health care provider an increase in menstrual bleeding as indicated by an increase in the number of sanitary pads used.	Changes in coagulation may lead to increased blood loss with regular menstruation.
■ Teach the patient to inspect skin and mucous membranes for oozing of blood.	Oozing of blood is often an early sign of coagulation abnormalities that increase the risk for bleeding.
■ Encourage the patient to read over-the-counter medication labels and avoid products that contain aspirin or NSAIDs such as ibuprofen and naproxen.	These drugs not only decrease normal platelet aggregation but also decrease the integrity of gastric mucosa through inhibition of cyclooxygenase 1 (COX-1) inhibitor and therefore increase the risk for gastrointestinal bleeding. QSEN: Safety.
■ Instruct the patient and family about limiting use of herbal preparations that are associated with an increased risk for bleeding. Examples of such herbal preparations are dong quai, feverfew, ginger, ginkgo biloba, and chamomile.	Many herbal preparations interfere with platelet aggregation through inhibition of serotonin release from the platelet. Other herbal preparations increase the effect of antiplatelet and anticoagulant medications, thus increasing the risk for bleeding.

■ = Independent   ▲ = Interprofessional Collaboration

Nursing Diagnosis Care Plans

Actions/Interventions

■ Teach the patient and family about using appropriate precautions and safety equipment with daily activities, sports, etc.

■ Teach the patient and family about measures to control bleeding from superficial skin trauma that bleeds.

Rationales

These measures reduce the risk for trauma and injury that contribute to the risk for bleeding. QSEN: Safety.

The patient and family need to know how to treat bleeding from skin trauma. Application of direct pressure to the site of injury will reduce bleeding. Use of ice packs may reduce hematoma formation and excessive bruising. QSEN: Safety.

NANDA-I
NDx Risk for Unstable Blood Glucose Level

Definition: Vulnerable to variation of blood glucose/sugar levels from the normal range, which may compromise health

Serum glucose is regulated by a complex interaction of insulin and glucagon. Insulin is secreted by the beta cells of the islets of Langerhans in the pancreas in response to elevated levels of blood glucose. This pancreatic hormone facilitates the movement of glucose across the cell membranes to be used for metabolic activity. The alpha cells of the islets of Langerhans secrete glucagon when blood glucose levels are low. Glucagon facilitates the conversion of stored glycogen to glucose. When cells are unable to use blood glucose as a metabolic fuel, glucagon stimulates the breakdown of fatty acids and protein. Elevated blood glucose levels (hyperglycemia) may occur in a variety of clinical situations. Diabetes mellitus is the most common disorder associated with elevated blood glucose levels. Prolonged physiological stress contributes to hyperglycemia through increased levels of cortisol as part of the neuro-endocrine stress response. Intravenous infusions containing dextrose may cause elevated blood glucose. Many drugs have hyperglycemia as a side effect.

Hypoglycemia occurs most often as the result of excess insulin administration in the person with diabetes mellitus. In the person without diabetes, hypoglycemia may occur with excess alcohol consumption, prolonged fasting and starvation states, adrenal insufficiency, and eating disorders such as anorexia nervosa. Hypoglycemia after meals may be related to gastric bypass surgery or excess consumption of refined carbohydrates and is the result of increased insulin secretion. This care plan focuses on general nursing care for the person who experiences fluctuations in blood glucose.

Common Risk Factors

Average daily physical activity is less than recommended for gender and age
Excessive stress
Excessive weight loss
Ineffective medication management
Insufficient diabetes management
Insufficient dietary intake

Common Expected Outcome

Patient maintains blood glucose levels within defined target ranges.

NOC Outcomes

Blood Glucose Level; Hyperglycemia Severity; Hypoglycemia Severity; Knowledge: Medication; Knowledge: Prescribed Diet; Knowledge: Prescribed Activity

NIC Interventions

Hyperglycemia Management; Hypoglycemia Management; Teaching: Prescribed Exercise; Teaching: Prescribed Diet; Teaching: Prescribed Medication

 evolve **For additional care plans, go to http://evolve.elsevier.com/Gulanick/.**

Ongoing Assessment

Actions/Interventions	Rationales
■ Assess for signs of hyperglycemia.	Hyperglycemia results when inadequate insulin is present to facilitate glucose transport across the cell membrane. Excess glucose in the bloodstream creates an osmotic effect that results in increased thirst (polydipsia), increased hunger (polyphagia), and increased urination (polyuria). The patient may also report nonspecific symptoms of fatigue and blurred vision.
■ Assess for signs of hypoglycemia.	Manifestations of hypoglycemia may vary among individuals but are consistent in the same individual. The signs are the result of both increased adrenergic activity and decreased glucose delivery to the brain. The patient may experience tachycardia, diaphoresis, tremors, dizziness, headache, fatigue, hunger, and visual changes.
■ Assess medications taken regularly.	Many medications cause fluctuations in blood glucose as a side effect. For example, hyperglycemia is a side effect of beta-blockers, corticosteroids, thiazide diuretics, estrogen, isoniazid, lithium, and phenytoin. Hypoglycemia is a side effect associated with regular use of salicylates, disopyramide, insulin, sulfonylurea agents, and pentamidine.
▲ Monitor blood glucose levels as fasting and postprandial levels.	Normal fasting blood glucose for an adult is 70 to 105 mg/dL. Critical values for hypoglycemia are less than 40 to 50 mg/dL. Critical values for hyperglycemia are greater than 400 mg/dL. Patients receiving total parenteral nutrition (TPN) may have a higher than normal blood glucose value because the solution contains up to 50% dextrose. Patients with reactive hypoglycemia will have a blood glucose level less than normal after eating a meal.
▲ Monitor serum insulin levels.	Hyperinsulinemia occurs early in the development of type 2 diabetes mellitus. Obesity and insulin receptor dysfunction in peripheral tissues stimulates insulin secretion from the pancreas. Insulinomas and some extra-pancreatic tumors cause increased insulin levels and contribute to hypoglycemia.
■ Assess eating patterns and knowledge of the prescribed diet.	Nonadherence to dietary guidelines for a specific clinical condition can result in fluctuations in blood glucose. For example, the patient with diabetes may experience either hyperglycemia or hypoglycemia when medication, exercise, and food intake are not balanced. The patient who has had gastric surgery may experience hypoglycemia following intake of large amounts of carbohydrates. QSEN: Patient-centered care.
■ Assess the pattern of physical activity.	Physical activity has an insulin-like effect and may lower blood glucose levels. Energy stores are depleted during prolonged periods of intense, physical exercise and contribute to hypoglycemia.
■ Assess alcohol intake.	Excessive alcohol consumption, without food intake, blocks release of glycogen from the liver, causing hypoglycemia.

■ = Independent   ▲ = Interprofessional Collaboration

Therapeutic Interventions

Actions/Interventions	Rationales
■ Assist the patient in identifying eating patterns that need changing.	This information provides the basis for individualized dietary instruction related to the clinical condition that contributes to fluctuations in blood glucose levels. QSEN: Patient-centered care.
▲ Refer the patient and family to a registered dietitian for individualized diet instruction.	An individualized meal plan is based on the patient's body weight, blood glucose values, activity patterns, and specific clinical condition. Modifications in the patient's food intake will contribute to stabilization of blood glucose levels. For example, the patient with diabetes needs a meal plan that balances intake of protein, carbohydrates, and fat. The patient who experiences postprandial hypoglycemia may need a meal plan that limits the intake of highly refined carbohydrates. QSEN: Teamwork and collaboration.
▲ Administer insulin medications as directed.	Insulin is required to lower blood glucose levels in type 1 diabetes mellitus, and for many patients with type 2 diabetes mellitus. Patients receiving TPN may require insulin to maintain stable blood glucose in response to high dextrose concentration in the solution.
▲ Administer food or other sources of glucose as directed for hypoglycemia.	A rapidly absorbed form of glucose is indicated to manage hypoglycemia. These forms of glucose may include oral intake of hard candy or fruit juice. For the patient who cannot take something orally, intravenous injection of glucose may be indicated.

Education/Continuity of Care

Actions/Interventions	Rationales
■ Review the progress toward goals during each patient visit.	Patient involvement in the treatment plan enhances adherence to treatment regimens. Interest in learning new health behaviors increases when the patient helps set the agenda for change and feels like an active participant. QSEN: Patient-centered care.
■ Teach the patient about following a prescribed meal plan.	A prescribed meal plan will help the patient maintain stable blood glucose levels. The patient with hyperglycemia will need to follow a balanced meal plan. A patient with hypoglycemia usually benefits from a meal plan that includes six small meals a day rather than three larger meals.
■ Teach the patient about taking prescribed medications to lower blood glucose.	The patient with diabetes mellitus needs to learn about taking insulin or oral hypoglycemic drugs to lower blood glucose.
■ Instruct the patient experiencing hypoglycemia about appropriate actions to raise blood glucose.	In most cases of hypoglycemia, food intake is the appropriate action to raise blood glucose levels. For the patient with diabetes, eating a rapidly absorbed source of glucose is appropriate. For the patient without diabetes, a meal plan that includes six small meals a day is preferred. QSEN: Safety.
■ Teach the patient to balance exercise with food intake.	Exercise balances glucose levels by facilitating uptake of glucose into cells. The patient needs to understand the relationship of exercise, food intake, and blood glucose levels.

Ⓔvolve **For additional care plans, go to http://evolve.elsevier.com/Gulanick/.**

Actions/Interventions

▲ Refer the patient and family to an exercise physiologist, physical therapist, or cardiac rehabilitation nurse for specific exercise instructions.

■ Teach the patient about measuring capillary blood glucose.

■ Instruct the patient to carry medical alert information.

Rationales

Specific exercises can be prescribed for the patient based on any physical limitations the patient may have. QSEN: Teamwork and collaboration.

Capillary blood glucose monitoring provides the patient with immediate information about blood glucose levels. This information allows the patient to initiate appropriate actions to return blood glucose levels to a normal range.

Medical personnel need to be able to identify the patient as having a clinical condition associated with unstable blood glucose. QSEN: Safety.

Disturbed Body Image

Definition: Confusion in mental picture of one's physical self

Body image is the attitude a person has about the actual or perceived structure or function of all or parts of his or her body. This attitude is dynamic and is altered through interaction with other people and situations, and it is influenced by age and developmental level. As an important part of one's self-concept, body image disturbance can have a profound impact on how individuals view their overall selves.

Throughout the life span, changes in a person's body related to normal growth and development can result in changes in the person's body image. For example, a woman may experience disturbed body image during pregnancy. Physical changes associated with aging may result in body image disturbance for the older adult.

Societal and cultural norms for ideal body shape, size, and appearance have a significant influence on a person's body image. Variations from the norm can result in body image disturbance. The value that an individual places on a body part or function may be more important in determining the degree of disturbance than the actual alteration in the structure or function. Therefore, the loss of a limb may result in a greater body image disturbance for an athlete than for a computer programmer. The loss of a breast to a fashion model or a hysterectomy in a nulliparous woman may cause serious body image disturbances even though the overall health of the individual has been improved. Removal of skin lesions, altered elimination resulting from bowel or bladder surgery, or head and neck resections are other examples of changes that can lead to body image disturbance. Chronic illness can contribute to changes in the person's body image related to decline in body function.

The nurse's assessment of the perceived alteration and importance placed by the patient on the altered structure or function will be very important in planning care to address body image disturbance.

Common Related Factors

Alteration in body function (due to anomaly, disease, medication, pregnancy, radiation, surgery, trauma, etc.)
Alteration in self-perception
Cultural incongruence
Developmental transition

Defining Characteristics

Preoccupation with change or loss
Depersonalization of body part or loss by use of impersonal pronouns
Hiding of body part
Avoids looking at or touching one's body
Focusing behavior on changed body part/function
Alteration in body structure or body function
Refusal to acknowledge change
Change in social involvement

■ = Independent   ▲ = Interprofessional Collaboration

Common Expected Outcome

Patient demonstrates enhanced body image and self-esteem as evidenced by ability to look at, touch, talk about, and care for actual or perceived altered body part or function.

NOC Outcomes
Body Image; Self-Esteem; Adaptation to Physical Disability

NIC Interventions
Body Image Enhancement; Self-Esteem Enhancement; Grief Work Facilitation; Coping Enhancement

Ongoing Assessment

Actions/Interventions	Rationales
■ Assess the patient's perception of change in the structure or function of the body part (also proposed change).	The extent of the patient's response is more related to the value or importance the patient places on the part or function than the actual value or importance. Even when an alteration improves the overall health of the patient (e.g., an ileostomy for an individual with precancerous colon polyps), the alteration may result in a body image disturbance. QSEN: Patient-centered care.
■ Assess the perceived impact of change on ADLs, social behavior, personal relationships, and occupational activities.	Changes in body image can have an impact on the patient's ability to carry out daily roles and responsibilities.
■ Assess the impact of body image disturbance in relation to the patient's developmental stage.	Adolescents and young adults may be particularly affected by changes in the structure or function of their bodies at a time when developmental changes are normally rapid and at a time when developing social and intimate relationships is particularly important.
■ Assess the patient's behavior regarding the actual or perceived changed body part or function.	There is a broad range of behaviors associated with body image disturbance, ranging from totally ignoring the altered structure or function to preoccupation with it.
■ Assess the patient's verbal remarks about the actual or perceived change in body part or function.	Negative statements about the affected body part may indicate limited ability to integrate the change into the patient's self-concept.

Therapeutic Interventions

Actions/Interventions	Rationales
■ Acknowledge the normalcy of the patient's emotional response to the actual or perceived change in body structure or function.	Experiencing stages of grief over loss of a body part or function is normal and typically involves a period of denial, the length of which varies among individuals.
■ Help the patient identify actual changes.	Patients may perceive changes that are not present or real, or they place an unrealistic value on a body structure or function. QSEN: Patient-centered care.
■ Encourage verbalization of positive or negative feelings about the actual or perceived change.	It is worthwhile to encourage the patient to separate feelings about changes in body structure or function from feelings about self-worth. Expression of feelings can enhance the patient's coping strategies.

Actions/Interventions

■ Assist the patient in incorporating actual changes into ADLs, social life, interpersonal relationships, and occupational activities.

■ Demonstrate positive caring in routine activities.

Rationales

The more visible the change in body structure or function, the more concern the patient may have about the response of others to the change. Opportunities for positive feedback and success in social situations may hasten adaptation to changes in body image.

Professional caregivers represent a microcosm of society; therefore, the patient will scrutinize their actions and behaviors. Positive comments by the nurse may help the patient develop more positive responses to the changes in his or her body.

Education/Continuity of Care

Actions/Interventions

■ Teach the patient about the normalcy of body image disturbance and the grief process.

■ Teach the patient adaptive behavior (e.g., use of adaptive equipment, wigs, cosmetics, clothing that conceals the altered body part or enhances remaining part or function, use of deodorants).

■ Help the patient identify ways of coping that have been useful in the past.

■ Refer the patient and family to support groups and social media composed of individuals with similar alterations.

Rationales

The patient experiencing a body image change needs new information to support cognitive appraisal of the change.

Adaptive behaviors help the patient compensate for the actual changed body structure and function.

Asking patients to remember other body image issues (e.g., getting glasses, wearing orthodontics, being pregnant, having a leg cast) and how they were managed may help the patient adjust to the current issue. QSEN: Patient-centered care.

Lay people in similar situations offer a different type of support, which is perceived as helpful (e.g., United Ostomy Association, Y Me?, I Can Cope, Mended Hearts).

NANDA-I NDx

Bowel Incontinence

Definition: Change in normal bowel habits characterized by involuntary passage of stool

Bowel incontinence, also called fecal incontinence, may occur as a result of injury to nerves and other structures involved in normal defecation or as the result of diseases that alter the normal function of defecation. Treatment of bowel incontinence depends on the cause. Injury to rectal, anal, or nerve tissue from trauma, childbirth, radiation, or surgery can result in bowel incontinence. Infection with resultant diarrhea or neurological disease such as stroke, multiple sclerosis, and diabetes mellitus can also result in bowel incontinence. In older patients, dementia can contribute to bowel incontinence when the individual cannot respond to normal physiological cues for defecation. Normal aging causes changes in the intestinal musculature

that may contribute to bowel incontinence. Fecal impaction, as a result of chronic constipation or denial of the defecation urge, can result in involuntary leakage of stool past the impaction. Loss of mobility can result in functional bowel incontinence when the person is unable to reach the toilet in a timely manner. Loss of bowel continence is an embarrassing problem that leads to social isolation, and it is one of the most common reasons that older patients are admitted to long-term care facilities. Goals of management include reestablishing a continent bowel elimination pattern, preventing loss of skin integrity, and/or planning management of fecal incontinence in a manner that preserves the individual's self-esteem.

■ = Independent   ▲ = Interprofessional Collaboration

Common Related Factors

Abnormal increase in abdominal pressure or intestinal pressure
Chronic diarrhea
Colorectal lesion
Deficient dietary habits
Difficulty with toileting self-care
Dysfunctional rectal sphincter
Environmental factor (e.g., inaccessible bathroom)
Generalized decline in muscle tone
Immobility
Impaction
Incomplete emptying of bowel
Laxative abuse
Upper motor or lower motor nerve damage
Pharmaceutical agent
Stressors

Defining Characteristics

Inability to recognize rectal fullness
Inability to expel formed stool despite recognition of rectal fullness
Bowel urgency
Constant passage of soft stool
Fecal staining of bedding or clothing
Inability to delay defecation
Does not recognize urge to defecate

Common Expected Outcome

Patient is continent of stool or reports decreased episodes of bowel incontinence.

NOC Outcomes
Bowel Continence; Bowel Elimination; Self-Care: Toileting
NIC Interventions
Bowel Incontinence Care; Bowel Management; Bowel Training; Self-Care Assistance: Toileting

Ongoing Assessment

Actions/Interventions	Rationales
■ Assess the patient's normal bowel elimination pattern.	Ascertaining what is "normal" for each patient allows the patient to be a full partner in providing care. There is a wide range of "normal" for bowel elimination; some patients have two bowel movements per day, whereas others may have a bowel movement as infrequently as every third or fourth day. Most people feel the urge to defecate shortly after the first oral intake (e.g., coffee or breakfast) of the day; this is a result of the gastrocolic reflex. QSEN: Patient-centered care.
■ Determine the cause of incontinence (i.e., review related factors).	Knowledge of etiological factors provides direction for subsequent interventions. For some patients, there may be multiple contributing factors. QSEN: Evidence-based practice.
■ Perform manual check for fecal impaction.	When the patient has a fecal impaction (hard, dry stool that cannot be expelled normally), liquid stool may leak past the impaction.
■ Assess current medications or treatments that may contribute to bowel incontinence.	Hyperosmolar tube feedings, bowel preparation agents, pelvic and/or abdominal irradiation, some chemotherapeutic agents, and certain antibiotic agents may cause explosive diarrhea that the patient cannot control.
■ Assist in preparing the patient for diagnostic measures.	These procedures are done to determine the causes of bowel incontinence. Tests include flexible sigmoidoscopy, barium enema, colonoscopy, and anal manometry (study to determine function of rectal sphincters).
■ Assess the degree to which the patient's daily activities are altered by bowel incontinence.	Patients may restrict their own activity or become isolated from work, family, and friends because they fear uncontrolled bowel elimination, soiling of clothing, odor, and embarrassment.

Actions/Interventions

■ Assess the use of diapers, sanitary napkins, incontinence briefs, fecal collection devices, and underpads.

■ Assess perineal skin integrity.

■ Assess the patient's ability to go to the bathroom independently.

■ Assess the patient's environment for availability of an accessible toilet facility.

■ Assess fluid and fiber intake.

Rationales

Patients or caregivers may use familiar products (e.g., sanitary napkins) to collect fecal material and protect clothing from staining.

Stool can cause chemical irritation to the skin, which may be exacerbated by the use of diapers, incontinence briefs, and underpads.

Soiling accidents may occur as a result of the patient's inability to get to the bathroom. This knowledge will provide direction for rearranging the environment, planning for trips to the bathroom, or providing a bedside commode.

Inadequate access to toileting facilities in the home (e.g., bathroom on upper level), in the work environment, at the shopping mall, and the like can aggravate the incontinence experience.

Fiber and fluid intake can result in changes in normal bowel evacuation.

Therapeutic Interventions

Actions/Interventions

■ Ensure fluid intake of at least 3000 mL/day, unless contraindicated.

▲ Provide high-fiber diet under the direction of a dietitian, unless contraindicated.

■ Encourage intake of natural bulking agents to thicken stools, for example, foods such as banana, rice, and yogurt.

■ Manually remove the fecal impaction, if present.

■ Encourage mobility or exercise, if tolerated.

■ Provide a bedside commode and assistive devices (e.g., cane, walker) or assistance in reaching the commode or toilet.

▲ Institute a bowel program.

  • Encourage bowel elimination at the same time every day.
  • After breakfast (or a warm drink), administer a suppository and perform digital stimulation every 10 to 15 minutes until evacuation occurs.
  • Place the patient in an upright position for defecation.

■ Wash the perineal area after each evacuation with soap and water. Dry thoroughly. Apply a moisture barrier ointment.

Rationales

Moist stool moves through the bowel more easily than hard, dry stool and prevents impaction. If the patient has a significant amount of diarrhea, fluids provide important volume replacement. QSEN: Safety.

Fiber aids in bowel elimination because it is insoluble and absorbs fluid as the stool passes through the bowel; this creates bulk. Bulky stool stimulates peristalsis and expulsion of stool from the bowel. QSEN: Teamwork and collaboration.

If bowel incontinence is related to diarrhea, these foods help provide bulk to the stool by absorbing fluids from the stool.

Presence of fecal impaction can interfere with establishment of a regular bowel routine.

Increasing mobility stimulates peristalsis and aids in bowel evacuation.

Immediate access to appropriate toileting facilities reduces unnecessary "accidents."

Facilitating regular time for bowel evacuation prevents the bowel from emptying sporadically (i.e., decreases incontinence). QSEN: Patient-centered care.

Shortly after breakfast is a good time because the gastrocolic reflex is stimulated by food or fluid intake.

For some causes, direct stimulation of the rectal sphincter and lower colon may be required to initiate peristalsis.

Flexion of the thighs (e.g., sitting upright with feet flat on floor) facilitates muscular movement that aids in defecation.

Any fecal material left on the skin can cause skin excoriation and pain. Perineal or perianal pain from irritation may result in fear of defecating and cause the patient to deny the urge to defecate. Repeated denial of the urge to defecate results in impaction and eventually in bowel incontinence. QSEN: Patient-centered care.

■ = Independent   ▲ = Interprofessional Collaboration

Actions/Interventions

■ Discourage the use of pads, diapers, or collection devices for long-term management of bowel incontinence.

■ Use fecal collection systems selectively over pads or diapers.

Rationales

Fecal containment devices can be useful in the short term to prevent soiling. Effective treatment of underlying contributing factors and a bowel training program will provide long-term management of the problem.

These devices (fecal collectors—pouches that adhere to the skin around the rectum—or rectal tube collection systems—rectal tubes that stay in the rectum via inflated balloons and drain liquid stool into a collection bag) allow for collection and disposal of stool without exposing the perianal skin to stool; odor and embarrassment are controlled because the stool is contained. These devices work best for patients who are in bed the majority of time.

Education/Continuity of Care

Actions/Interventions

■ Teach the patient or caregiver the importance of fluid and fiber in maintaining soft, bulky stool.

■ Teach the patient the importance of establishing a regular time for bowel evacuation.

■ Teach the caregiver the use of a fecal incontinence device, if appropriate.

■ Teach the patient to manage perianal irritation prophylactically by washing with soap and water, drying thoroughly after each bowel movement, and applying a moisture barrier ointment containing zinc oxide or dimethicone.

Rationales

Teaching the patient or caregiver methods to manage bowel incontinence improves personal efficacy and can enhance compliance with the therapeutic regimen.

Information helps the patient and family understand the rationale for therapy and aids the patient in assuming responsibility for self-care later. QSEN: Patient-centered care.

Use of specific devices may be challenging. The caregiver needs the opportunity to learn to manage the device with appropriate guidance and feedback.

Patients and caregivers need to prevent skin irritation and pain that can result from fecal incontinence.

Related Care Plans

Constipation, Chapter 2
Diarrhea, Chapter 2
Inflammatory bowel disease, Chapter 8

NANDA-I NDx Ineffective Breathing Pattern

Definition: Inspiration and/or expiration that does not provide adequate ventilation

Ineffective breathing patterns are considered a state in which the rate, depth, timing, rhythm, or chest/abdominal wall excursion during inspiration, expiration, or both do not maintain optimum ventilation for the individual. Most acute pulmonary deterioration is preceded by a change in breathing pattern. Respiratory failure may be associated with changes in respiratory rate, abdominal and thoracic patterns for inspiration and expiration, and depth of ventilation. Breathing pattern changes may occur in a multitude of conditions: heart failure, airway obstruction, respiratory infection, neuromuscular impairment, trauma or surgery resulting in musculoskeletal impairment/pain, diaphragmatic paralysis, cognitive impairment and anxiety, metabolic abnormalities (e.g., diabetic ketoacidosis, uremia, or thyroid dysfunction), peritonitis, drug overdose, pleural inflammation, and chronic respiratory disorders such as asthma or chronic obstructive pulmonary disease (COPD).

 For additional care plans, go to http://evolve.elsevier.com/Gulanick/.

Common Related Factors

Neuromuscular impairment
Spinal cord injury
Neurological impairment
Musculoskeletal impairment
Respiratory muscle fatigue
Body position that inhibits lung expansion
Fatigue
Pain
Anxiety

Defining Characteristics

Dyspnea/orthopnea
Tachypnea/bradypnea
Use of three-point position to breathe (bending forward while supporting self by placing one hand on each knee)
Nasal flaring
Abnormal breathing pattern (e.g., rate, rhythm, depth)
Altered chest excursion
Use of accessory muscles to breath
Pursed-lip breathing or prolonged expiratory phase
Increase in anteroposterior chest diameter

Common Expected Outcome

The patient maintains an effective breathing pattern, as evidenced by relaxed breathing at normal rate and depth and absence of dyspnea.

NOC Outcomes
Respiratory Status: Ventilation; Vital Signs
NIC Interventions
Airway Management; Respiratory Monitoring

Ongoing Assessment

Actions/Interventions	Rationales
■ Assess respiratory rate, rhythm, and depth.	Respiratory rate and rhythm changes are early warning signs of impending respiratory difficulties. QSEN: Safety.
■ Assess for use of accessory muscles (scalene and sternocleidomastoid).	Work of breathing increases greatly as lung compliance decreases. As moving air in and out of the lungs becomes increasingly more difficult, the breathing pattern alters to include use of accessory muscles to increase chest excursion to facilitate effective breathing. In COPD, the patient relies more on accessory muscles than on the diaphragm for breathing. QSEN: Safety.
■ Monitor for diaphragmatic muscle fatigue or weakness (paradoxical motion).	Paradoxical movement of the abdomen (an inward versus outward movement during inspiration) is indicative of respiratory muscle fatigue and weakness.
■ Note retractions or flaring of nostrils.	These signs signify an increase in respiratory effort.
■ Assess the position that the patient assumes for breathing.	A three-point position (bending forward while supporting self by placing one hand on each knee) or orthopnea is associated with breathing difficulty.
■ Inquire about precipitating and alleviating factors.	Knowledge of these factors is useful in planning interventions to prevent or manage future episodes of breathing difficulties.
■ Assess the ability to clear secretions.	An obstructed airway may cause a change in breathing pattern.
■ Assess sputum for quantity, color, consistency, and odor.	These may be indicative of a cause for the alteration in breathing pattern.
▲ If sputum is discolored (no longer clear or white), send the specimen for culture and sensitivity testing, as appropriate.	An infection may be present if sputum is found to be yellow, green, or dirty gray in color. Respiratory infections increase the work of breathing, resulting in fatigue and changes in breathing pattern. Antibiotic treatment may be indicated.
■ Assess the level of anxiety.	Hypoxia and the sensation of "not being able to breathe" are frightening and may cause worsening hypoxia.

■ = Independent   ▲ = Interprofessional Collaboration

Actions/Interventions	Rationales
■ Monitor for changes in the level of consciousness.	Restlessness, confusion, and/or irritability can be early indicators of insufficient oxygen to the brain. Lethargy and somnolence are late signs of hypoxia. QSEN: Safety.
■ Assess skin color and temperature.	Pale or cyanotic color indicates increased concentration of deoxygenated blood and indicates that the breathing pattern is no longer effective to maintain adequate oxygenation of tissues. Cool, pale skin may be secondary to a compensatory/vasoconstrictive response to hypoxemia.
■ Monitor pulse oximetry and ABGs as appropriate. Note changes.	Pulse oximetry is a useful tool to monitor oxygen saturation and detect early changes in oxygenation. Increasing $Paco_2$ and decreasing Pao_2 are signs of respiratory failure. As the patient's condition begins to fail, the respiratory rate decreases and $Paco_2$ begins to increase. QSEN: Safety.
■ Assess for thoracic or upper abdominal pain.	Pain can result in shallow breathing.
▲ Assess nutritional status (e.g., weight, albumin level, electrolyte level).	Malnutrition may result in premature development of respiratory failure because it reduces respiratory mass and strength. It blunts ventilatory responses to hypoxia and impairs pulmonary and systemic immunity. Overfeeding increases production of carbon dioxide, which increases respiratory drive and respiratory muscle fatigue.

Therapeutic Interventions

Actions/Interventions	Rationales
■ Position the patient for optimal breathing pattern, ideally in a semi-Fowler's or high-Fowler's position, unless contraindicated.	A sitting position allows adequate diaphragmatic and lung excursion as well as chest expansion.
■ Encourage sustained deep breaths by: • Using demonstration (emphasizing slow inhalation, holding end inspiration for a few seconds, passive exhalation, and pursed-lip breathing) • Using an incentive spirometer (place close for convenient patient use) • Asking the patient to yawn	These techniques promote deep inspiration, which increases oxygenation and prevents atelectasis. Controlled breathing techniques may also help slow respirations in patients who are tachypneic. Prolonged expiration prevents air trapping.
■ Encourage diaphragmatic breathing for the patient with chronic disease.	This breathing technique relaxes muscles and increases the patient's oxygen level.
■ Evaluate the appropriateness of inspiratory muscle training.	This training improves conscious control of respiratory muscles and inspiratory muscle strength.
■ Encourage the patient to clear his or her own secretions with effective coughing. If secretions cannot be cleared, suction as needed.	Productive coughing is the most effective way to remove most secretions. If patient is unable to perform independently, suctioning may be needed to promote airway patency and reduce work of breathing.
■ Plan activity and rest to maximize the patient's energy.	Fatigue is common with the increased work of breathing. Activity increases metabolic rate and oxygen requirements. Rest helps mobilize energy for more effective breathing and coughing efforts.
■ Avoid high concentration of oxygen in patients with COPD unless ordered. Maintain oxygen saturation at or above 90%.	Hypoxia stimulates the drive to breathe in the patient who is a chronic retainer of carbon dioxide. When applying oxygen, close monitoring is imperative to prevent unsafe increases in the patient's Pao_2, which could result in apnea. An oxygen saturation of less than 90% leads to tissue hypoxia, acidosis, dysrhythmias, and decreased level of consciousness.

Actions/Interventions

- Provide reassurance and allay anxiety by staying with the patient during acute episodes of respiratory distress.

- ▲ Splint the chest/abdomen with a pillow when coughing and use pain management as appropriate.
- ▲ Administer respiratory medications as ordered.

- Anticipate the need for intubation and mechanical ventilation if the patient is unable to maintain adequate gas exchange with the present breathing pattern.

Rationales

The presence of a trusted person may help the patient feel less threatened and can reduce anxiety, thereby reducing oxygen requirements. Anxiety increases dyspnea, respiratory rate, and work of breathing.

Splinting optimizes deep breathing and coughing efforts. Pain relief enhances the ability to deep breath and cough.

Beta-adrenergic agonist medications relax airway smooth muscles and cause bronchodilation to open air passages. Corticosteroids are effective anti-inflammatory drugs for treatment of reversible airflow obstruction.

Early intubation and mechanical ventilation are recommended to prevent full decompensation of the patient and a potentially life-threatening situation. Mechanical ventilation provides supportive care to maintain adequate oxygenation and ventilation. QSEN: Safety.

Education/Continuity of Care

Actions/Interventions

- Teach the patient or caregivers appropriate breathing, coughing, and splinting techniques.

- Teach patients to pace activities and to avoid unnecessary tasks when dyspneic.
- Instruct about medications: indications, dosage, frequency, and potential side effects. Include review of metered-dose inhaler and nebulizer treatments, as appropriate.
- Explain the use of oxygen therapy, including the type and use of equipment and why its maintenance is important.
- Assist the patient or caregiver in learning signs of respiratory compromise. Refer significant others or caregivers to participate in basic life support class for cardiopulmonary resuscitation, as appropriate. Provide emergency phone numbers.

Rationales

These techniques facilitate adequate clearance of secretions and prevent atelectasis. Dyspnea also may be reduced by techniques such as pursed-lip or diaphragmatic breathing.

Energy-conserving methods reduce fatigue, dyspnea, and oxygen consumption.

Knowledge promotes safe and effective medication administration.

Issues related to home oxygen use, storage, and precautions need to be addressed for safe and effective treatment.

This instruction prevents delays in seeking help and facilitates appropriate management in life-threatening situations. Patient and family members may not remember phone numbers in an emergency situation. QSEN: Safety.

Related Care Plans

Ineffective airway clearance, Chapter 2
Pneumonia, Chapter 2
Pulmonary tuberculosis, ⊜volve

NANDA-I
NDx **Decreased Cardiac Output**

Definition: Inadequate blood pumped by the heart to meet the metabolic demands of the body

Common causes of reduced cardiac output include myocardial infarction, hypertension, valvular heart disease, congenital heart disease, cardiomyopathy, pulmonary disease, arrhythmias, drug effects, fluid overload, decreased fluid volume, and electrolyte imbalance. Older patients are especially at risk because the aging process causes reduced compliance of the ventricles, which further reduces contractility and cardiac output. Patients may have acute, temporary problems or experience chronic, debilitating effects of decreased cardiac output. Patients may be managed in an acute care, ambulatory care, or home care setting.

■ = Independent ▲ = Interprofessional Collaboration

Common Related Factors

Altered preload
Altered afterload
Altered contractility
Alteration in HR, rhythm, and conduction
Altered stroke volume

Defining Characteristics

Altered HR and rhythm:
- Tachycardia/bradycardia
- Heart palpitations

Altered preload:
- Increase or decrease in central venous pressure (CVP)
- Increase or decrease in pulmonary capillary wedge pressure (PCWP)
- Jugular vein distention
- Edema weight gain
- Fatigue

Altered afterload:
- Alteration in BP
- Clammy skin
- Decreased peripheral pulses
- Prolonged capillary refill
- Oliguria
- Dyspnea

Altered contractility:
- Adventitious breath sounds
- Coughing
- Decrease in ejection fraction
- Paroxysmal nocturnal dyspnea (PND)
- Presence of S_3/S_4 heart sounds

Behavioral/emotional:
- Anxiety
- Restlessness

Common Expected Outcome

Patient has adequate cardiac output as evidenced by systolic BP within 20 mm Hg of baseline; HR 60 to 100 beats/min with regular rhythm; urine output 30 mL/hr or greater; strong peripheral pulses; warm, dry skin; eupnea with absence of pulmonary crackles; and orientation to person, time, and place.

NOC Outcomes

Cardiac Pump Effectiveness; Cardiopulmonary Status; Circulation Status; Knowledge: Disease Process; Knowledge: Treatment Regimen

NIC Interventions

Cardiac Care; Hemodynamic Regulation; Teaching: Disease Process

Ongoing Assessment

Actions/Interventions

- Assess for any changes in level of consciousness.

- Assess HR and BP.

Rationales

Hypoxia and reduced cerebral perfusion are reflected in restlessness, irritability, and difficulty concentrating. Older patients are especially susceptible to reduced perfusion.

Most patients have compensatory tachycardia and significantly reduced BP in response to reduced cardiac output. Older patients have reduced response to catecholamines; thus their response to reduced cardiac output may be blunted, with less increase in HR.

Actions/Interventions	**Rationales**
■ Assess skin color, temperature, and moisture.	Cold, pale, clammy skin is secondary to compensatory increase in sympathetic nervous system stimulation and low cardiac output and oxygen desaturation.
■ Assess peripheral pulses, including capillary refill.	Pulses are weak with reduced stroke volume and cardiac output. Capillary refill is slow, sometimes absent.
■ Assess for fluid balance and weight gain. Weigh the patient daily before breakfast. Inspect for pedal and sacral edema.	Compromised regulatory mechanisms may result in fluid and sodium retention. Body weight is a more sensitive indicator of fluid or sodium retention than intake and output.
■ Assess urine output. Determine how often the patient urinates.	The renal system compensates for low BP by retaining water. Oliguria is a classic sign of decreased renal perfusion. Diuresis is expected with diuretic therapy.
■ Assess for presence of S_3 or S_4 heart sounds.	S_3 denotes reduced left ventricular ejection and is a classic sign of left ventricular failure. S_4 occurs with reduced compliance of the left ventricle, which impairs diastolic filling.
■ Assess respiratory rate and rhythm and breath sounds. Determine any occurrence of PND or orthopnea.	Rapid, shallow respirations are characteristic of reduced cardiac output. Crackles reflect accumulation of fluid secondary to impaired left ventricular emptying. They are more evident in the dependent areas of the lung. Orthopnea is difficulty breathing when supine; PND is difficulty breathing at night.
▲ Assess B-type natriuretic peptide (BNP).	BNP is a substance secreted from the lower chambers of the heart in response to increased filling pressure and volume that occur when heart failure develops or worsens. This test aids in differentiating cardiac from noncardiac causes of dsypnea.
▲ If hemodynamic monitoring is in place, assess CVP, pulmonary artery diastolic pressure (PADP), and pulmonary capillary wedge pressure (PCWP), as well as cardiac output and cardiac index.	CVP provides information on filling pressures of the right side of the heart; PADP and PCWP reflect left-sided fluid volumes. Cardiac output provides an objective number to guide therapy. These direct measurements serve as optimal guides for therapy. QSEN: Safety.
▲ Assess oxygen saturation with pulse oximetry both at rest and during and after ambulation.	Change in oxygen saturation is one of the earliest indicators of reduced cardiac output. Hypoxemia is common, especially with activity.
■ Monitor electrocardiogram (ECG) for rate, rhythm, and ectopy.	Cardiac dysrhythmias may occur from low perfusion, acidosis, or hypoxia. Tachycardia, bradycardia, and ectopic beats can further compromise cardiac output. Older patients are especially sensitive to the loss of atrial kick in atrial fibrillation.
■ Assess for reports of fatigue and reduced activity tolerance.	Fatigue and exertional dyspnea are common problems with low cardiac output states. Close monitoring of the patient's response serves as a guide for optimal progression of activity.
■ Assess for chest pain.	Low cardiac output can further reduce myocardial perfusion, resulting in chest pain.
■ Assess contributing factors so an appropriate care plan can be initiated.	Specific causes guide treatment.

■ = Independent   ▲ = Interprofessional Collaboration

Nursing Diagnosis Care Plans

Therapeutic Interventions

Actions/Interventions

▲ Maintain optimal fluid balance. For patients with decreased preload, administer fluid challenge as prescribed, closely monitoring effects.

▲ For patients with increased preload, restrict fluids and sodium as ordered.

▲ Administer medication as prescribed, noting response and watching for side effects and toxicity. Clarify with the physician parameters for withholding medications.

▲ Maintain hemodynamic parameters at prescribed levels.

▲ Maintain adequate ventilation and perfusion, as in the following:
- Place the patient in a semi-Fowler's to high-Fowler's position.
- Place the patient in a supine position.

- Administer oxygen therapy as prescribed.

■ Maintain physical and emotional rest, as in the following:
- Restrict activity.
- Provide quiet, relaxed environment.
- Organize nursing and medical care.
- Monitor progressive activity within limits of cardiac function.

▲ Administer stool softeners as needed.

▲ Monitor sleep patterns; administer a sedative as needed.

▲ If dysrhythmia occurs, determine the patient's response, document, and report if significant or symptomatic.
- Have antidysrhythmic drugs readily available.
- Treat dysrhythmias according to medical orders or protocol, and evaluate response.

▲ If invasive adjunct therapies are indicated (e.g., intra-aortic balloon pump, pacemaker), maintain within the prescribed protocol.

Rationales

Volume therapy may be required to maintain adequate filling pressures and optimize cardiac output.

Fluid restriction decreases extracellular fluid volume and reduces demands on the heart.

Depending on etiological factors, common medications include digitalis therapy, diuretics, vasodilator therapy, antidysrhythmics, angiotensin-converting enzyme inhibitors, and inotropic agents.

For patients in the acute setting, close monitoring of these parameters guides titration of fluids and medications. QSEN: Safety.

When fluid overload is the cause, upright positioning reduces preload and ventricular filling.

For hypovolemia, supine positioning increases venous return and promotes diuresis.

The failing heart may not be able to respond to increased oxygen demands. Oxygen saturation needs to be greater than 90%.

Activity restriction and a quiet environment reduce oxygen demands. Attention to priority care delivery optimizes use of the patient's limited energy resources. Careful activity progression prevents overexertion and stress on the cardiopulmonary system.

Straining for a bowel movement further impairs cardiac output.

Rest is important for conserving energy.

Both tachydysrhythmias and bradydysrhythmias can reduce cardiac output and myocardial tissue perfusion.

Electrical/mechanical assist devices may be indicated to support cardiac output when more basic therapies fail. Nurse needs to follow protocols for managing each device. Effective attention to prescribed protocol reduces the risk for harm to the patient. QSEN: Safety.

Education/Continuity of Care

Actions/Interventions

■ Explain symptoms and interventions for decreased cardiac output related to etiological factors.

■ Explain the drug regimen, purpose, dose, and side effects.

Rationales

Thorough understanding of specific causes for each patient's disease is necessary for appropriate follow-through of treatment plan. QSEN: Patient-centered care.

Information provides rationale for therapy and aids the patient in assuming responsibility for self-care later. QSEN: Patient-centered care.

Actions/Interventions

- Explain diet restrictions, for example, with respect to fluid and sodium intake.
- Explain the progressive activity schedule and signs of overexertion.

Rationales

Diet changes and restrictions can be especially challenging to patients and may require ongoing monitoring.

Close monitoring of one's response to progressive activity reduces the risk for overexertion. QSEN: Safety.

Related Care Plans

Deficient fluid volume, Chapter 2
Acute coronary syndromes/myocardial infarction, Chapter 5
Heart failure, chronic, Chapter 5
Shock, cardiogenic, Chapter 5
Chest trauma, Chapter 6
Dysrhythmias, ⊝volve

NANDA-I NDx **Caregiver Role Strain**

Definition: Difficulty in performing family/significant other caregiver role

The focus of this care plan is on the supportive care rendered by family members, significant others, or caregivers responsible for meeting the physical/emotional needs of the patient. Rapid hospital discharges for even the most complex health problems result in both acute and chronic illnesses being essentially managed in the home environment. Today's health care environment places high expectations on the designated caregiver, whether a family member or someone for hire. For many older patients, the only caregiver is a fragile spouse overwhelmed by his or her own health problems. The degree of potential burden related to caregiving is influenced by many factors including frequency, severity, and distress of patient symptoms, and complexity of medications and treatments. Even in cultures in which care of the ill is the anticipated responsibility of family members, the complexities of today's medical regimens, the chronicity of some disease processes, and the burdens of the caregiver's own family or environmental milieu provide an overwhelming challenge.

Caregivers have special needs for knowledge and skills in managing the required activities, access to affordable community resources, and recognition that the care they are providing is important and appreciated. Moreover, caregivers can be considered "secondary patients" who are at high risk for injury and adverse events. Nurses can assist caregivers by providing the requisite education and skill training and offering support through home visits; special clinic sessions; telephone access for questions and comfort; innovative strategies, such as telephone or social media, "chat groups," or blogs; opportunities for respite care; and guidance in engaging in activities that promote their own health (nutrition, exercise, sleep, stress management).

■ = Independent ▲ = Interprofessional Collaboration

Common Related Factors

Care recipient:
  Illness severity
  Unpredictable illness course
  Unrealistic expectations
Caregiver:
  Complexity of care activities
  Knowledge deficit regarding management of care
  Change in nature of care activities
  Caregiver has health problems
  Caregiver has no respite from caregiving demands
  Caregiver has competing role commitments
  Economic hardship
Insufficient resources
Insufficient social support
Pattern of ineffective relationship between caregiver and care recipient

Defining Characteristics

Difficulty performing/completing required tasks
Apprehensiveness about future ability to provide care
Apprehensiveness about well-being of care recipient if unable to provide care
Preoccupation with care routine
Insufficient time to meet personal needs
Insufficient coping strategies
Difficulty watching care receiver with illness
Caregiver expresses negative feeling about patient or relationship
Caregiver neglects patient care
Caregiver expresses change in own health status (e.g., fatigue, gastrointestinal upset, headache, weight changes, disturbed sleep, frustration, stress)

Common Expected Outcomes

Caregiver expresses satisfaction with caregiver role.
Caregiver demonstrates competence and confidence in performing the caregiver role by meeting care recipient's physical and psychosocial needs.
Caregiver reports that formal and informal support systems are adequate and helpful.
Caregiver demonstrates flexibility in dealing with problem behavior of care recipient.

NOC Outcomes
Caregiver Well-Being; Caregiver Role Endurance; Caregiver–Patient Relationship
NIC Intervention
Caregiver Support

Ongoing Assessment

Actions/Interventions	Rationales
■ Assess the caregiver–care recipient relationship.	A healthy family or caregiver relationship based on familiarity and compassion provides a strong foundation for the evolving dynamics of caregiving. Mutually rewarding relationships foster a therapeutic caregiving experience. Dysfunctional relationships can result in ineffective, fragmented care or even lead to neglect or abuse. QSEN: Patient-centered care.
■ Assess the family communication pattern.	Open communication in the family creates a positive environment, whereas families with communication issues or who conceal feelings create problems for caregiver and care recipient.
■ Assess the family resources and support systems.	Family and social support are related positively to coping effectiveness. Some cultures are more accepting of this responsibility. However, factors such as blended family units, aging parents, geographical distances between family members, and limited financial resources may hamper coping effectiveness.
■ Determine the caregiver's knowledge and ability to provide patient care, including bathing, skin care, safety, nutrition, medications, and ambulation.	Information provides a starting point for educational sessions. Basic instruction may reduce caregiver's anxiety and improve the relationship.

Actions/Interventions

- Assess the caregiver's appraisal of the caregiving situation, level of understanding, and willingness to assume caregiver role.

- Assess for neglect and abuse of the care recipient.

- Assess the caregiver's physical and mental health status that can affect caregiving.

Rationales

Caregivers need to have a realistic perspective of the situation and the scope of responsibility. The demands may be temporary, as in recovering from surgery or physical injury, or the situation may be long-term, in which both the caregiver and recipient need to accept a new normal in their lives. Individual responses to caregiving situations are mediated by an appraisal of the personal meaning of the situation. For some, caregiving is viewed as "a duty"; for others, it may be an act of love. QSEN: Patient-centered care.

Safe and appropriate care are priority nursing concerns. The nurse must remain a patient advocate to prevent injury to the care recipient and strain on the caregiver. QSEN: Safety.

Even though strongly motivated to perform the role of caregiver, the person may have physical impairments (e.g., vision problems, musculoskeletal weakness, limited upper body strength) or cognitive impairments that affect the quality of the caregiving activities. QSEN: Patient-centered care.

Therapeutic Interventions

Actions/Interventions

- Encourage the caregiver to identify available family and friends who can assist with caregiving.

- Encourage caregiver to make list of all personal needs in order to fulfill them and not feel deprived.

- Suggest that the caregiver use available community resources such as respite, home health care, adult day care, geriatric care, housekeeping services, home health aides, Meals On Wheels, companion services, and others, as appropriate.

- Encourage the caregiver to set aside time for self. Assist the caregiver in identifying pleasant activities and positive experiences.

- Teach the caregiver coping and stress management techniques.

Rationales

Caring for a family member can be a mutually rewarding and satisfying family experience. Successful caregiving should not be the sole responsibility of one person. It often "takes a village" or network of people. Their contributions can be special skills, time, money, or knowledge of additional resources. In some situations, there may be no readily available resources; however, often family members hesitate to notify other family members or significant others because of unresolved conflicts in the past.

Identifying regular life obligations can be an important step in finding a balance between caregiving duties and one's personal responsibilities. QSEN: Patient-centered care.

Resources provide opportunity for multiple competent providers and services on a temporary basis or for a more extended period. Respite care helps family members cope with the burden of care

Finding time for oneself is difficult for the primary caregiver. Just as airlines advise parents to place oxygen masks on themselves before helping their children, caregivers need to be reminded to put themselves first if they are to be able to provide the best care possible. Having own "respite" time helps conserve physical and emotional energy.

Supportive interventions can be offered by peers or professionals. They should provide opportunities to discuss issues as well as successes and feelings regarding caregiving.

■ = Independent ▲ = Interprofessional Collaboration

Actions/Interventions

■ Encourage caregiver participation in support groups.

■ Encourage the care recipient to thank the caregiver for care given.
■ Make positive statements about caregiver's efforts.

■ Provide time for the caregiver to discuss problems, concerns, and feelings. Ask the caregiver how he or she is managing.

■ Inquire about the caregiver's health. Provide suggestions for ways to adjust the daily routines to meet the physical limitations of the caregiver.

Rationales

Groups that come together for mutual support can be quite beneficial in providing education and anticipatory guidance. Groups can meet in the home, in a social setting, by telephone, or through social media.
Feeling appreciated decreases feelings of strain.

Caregivers have identified how important it is to feel appreciated for their efforts. The patient may not be able to express this himself or herself.
As a caregiver, the nurse is in an excellent position to provide emotional support and provide guidance throughout this challenging period. Attention should be directed to assisting caregiver in problem-solving activities that focus on tangible issues such as time management, role overload, and emotional control.
The caregiver may have his or her own health challenges that can become aggravated during the caregiving process.

Education/Continuity of Care

Actions/Interventions

■ Provide educational information on the disease process and management strategies.

■ Provide information and training for caregiver to respond to care recipient's nursing diagnoses (e.g., incontinence, risk for falls). Demonstrate caregiving skills, and allow sufficient time before return demonstration.

■ Provide information on appropriate web-based interventions, social media sites, and peer networks.

■ Teach caregiver strategies to access and maximize health care, caregiver resources, and community resources/financial aid if needed.

Rationales

Caregivers may have an unrealistic picture of the extent of care required at the present time. Home care therapies are becoming increasingly complex (e.g., home dialysis, ventilator care, terminal care, Alzheimer's care) and require careful attention to the educational process.

Increased knowledge and skills increase the caregiver's confidence and decrease strain. Psychoeducational interventions are more effective when provided in multiple sessions over time, and focus on problem-solving skills. QSEN: Patient-centered care.

These sites can be beneficial in offering support and information by people facing the same circumstances, and may positively influence the caregiving outcomes.
Caregiver resources such as AARP, the Caregiver Action Network, and the National Alliance for Caregiving can be beneficial for meeting a variety of needs.

NANDA-I NDx **Impaired Verbal Communication**

Definition: Decreased, delayed, or absent ability to receive, process, transmit, and/or use a system of symbols

Human communication takes many forms. People communicate verbally through the vocalization of a system of sounds that has been formalized into a language. They communicate using body movements to supplement, emphasize, or even alter what is being verbally communicated. In some cases, such as American Sign Language (the formal language of the deaf community) or Signed English, communication is conducted entirely through hand gestures that may or may not be accompanied by body movements and pantomime. Language can be read by watching an individual's lips to observe words as they are shaped. Humans communicate through touch, intuition, written means, art, and sometimes a combination of all of the mechanisms. Communication implies the sending of information as well as the receiving of information. When communication is received, it ceases to be the sole product of the sender as the entire experiential history of the receiver takes over and interprets the information sent. At its best, effective communication is a dialogue that not only involves the transmission of information but also clarification of points made, expansion of ideas and concepts, and exploration of factors that fall out of the original thoughts transmitted. Communication is a multifaceted, kinetic, reciprocal process. Communication may be impaired for any number of reasons, but rarely are all avenues for communication compromised at one time. The task for the nurse, whether encountering the patient in the hospital or in the community, becomes recognizing when communication has become ineffective and then using strategies to improve transmission of information.

Common Related Factors

Physiological condition (e.g., brain tumor, decreased circulation to brain, weakened musculoskeletal system)
Oropharyngeal defect
Cultural incongruence
Physical barrier (e.g., tracheostomy, intubation)
Insufficient stimuli

Defining Characteristics

Difficulty expressing thoughts verbally (e.g., aphasia, dysphasia, apraxia, dyslexia)
Difficulty comprehending communication
Difficulty forming words (e.g., aphonia, dyslalia, dysarthria)
Difficulty in selective attending
Difficulty in use of body expressions or facial expressions
Difficulty in maintaining communication
Dyspnea
Inability to speak language of caregiver

Common Expected Outcome

Patient uses a form of communication to get needs met and to relate effectively with people and his or her environment.

NOC Outcomes

Communication: Expressive; Communication: Receptive; Information Processing

NIC Interventions

Active Listening; Communication Enhancement: Hearing Deficit; Communication Enhancement: Speech Deficit

Ongoing Assessment

Actions/Interventions	**Rationales**
■ Assess the following:	Assessing the patient's preferences for communication allows the patient to be a full partner in providing care. QSEN: Patient-centered care.
• The patient's primary and preferred means of communication (e.g., verbal, written, gestures)	Patients may have skill with many forms of communication, yet they will prefer one method for important communication.

Nursing Diagnosis Care Plans

Actions/Interventions	Rationales
• Ability to understand the spoken word	It is important for health care workers to understand that the construct of gestured language has an entirely different structure from verbal and written English. Signed English is not the true language of the deaf community but an instructional mechanism developed to teach the structure of English so that individuals with hearing impairments may read and write it. Some members of the deaf community learn to do so effectively. American Sign Language is the true language of the deaf community. U.S. federal law requires the use of an official interpreter to communicate with people who choose to receive informed consent and other important medical information in their own language.
• The patient's preferred language for verbal and written communication	Patients may speak a language quite well without being able to read it effectively. Discharge self-care and follow-up information must be communicated and reinforced with written information that the patient can use. In recognition of the vast array of cultures and physical challenges that patients face, it is the nurse's responsibility to communicate with the patient effectively. The nurse incorporates this information in the planning and evaluation of care and communicates the information to the interprofessional team.
• Ability to understand written words, pictures, and gestures	In some cases, the only way to be certain that communication has been effective is to arrange for a certified interpreter to validate information from both sides of the dialogue.
■ Assess conditions or situations that may hinder the patient's ability to use or understand language, such as the following:	A variety of clinical conditions may alter the patient's ability to communicate effectively. QSEN: Patient-centered care.
• Alternative airway (e.g., tracheostomy, oral or nasal intubation)	When air does not pass over vocal cords, sounds are not produced.
• Orofacial/maxillary problems (e.g., wired jaws)	The patient forms words by coordinated movement of the mouth and tongue. When this movement is impaired, communication may be ineffective.
■ Assess for the presence of expressive dysphasia (inability to convey information verbally) and receptive dysphasia (word meaning may be scrambled during the processing of information by the patient's brain).	The patient with expressive dysphagia has nonfluent speech; however, his or her verbal comprehension is often intact. The ability to read and write may be impaired with this type of dysphagia. The patient with receptive dysphagia has fluent speech, but the content of his or her communication is often meaningless. The primary disturbance is an inability to understand all forms of language.
■ Assess for the presence and history of dyspnea.	Patients who are experiencing breathing problems may reduce or cease verbal communication that may complicate their respiratory efforts.
■ Assess the patient's energy level.	Fatigue/shortness of breath can make communication difficult or impossible.

Therapeutic Interventions

Actions/Interventions	Rationales
■ Anticipate patient needs, and pay attention to nonverbal cues.	The nurse should set aside enough time to attend to all of the details of patient care. Care measures may take longer to complete when there is a communication deficit.
■ Provide an alternative means of communication for times when interpreters are not available (e.g., a phone contact who can interpret the patient's needs).	An alternative means of communication (e.g., flash cards, symbol boards, electronic messaging) can help the patient express ideas and communicate needs.
■ Encourage the patient's attempts to communicate; praise attempts and achievements. Clarify your understanding of the patient's communication with the patient or an interpreter.	Patients need feedback about the success of their communication attempts. Feedback promotes effective communication by allowing the sender of the message to verify that the message sent was the message received. Positive feedback enhances the patient's efforts to overcome communication barriers.
■ Avoid talking with others in front of the patient as though he or she comprehends nothing.	Excluding the patient from an interaction increases the patient's sense of frustration and feelings of helplessness.
■ Keep distractions such as television and radio at a minimum when talking to the patient.	Removing environmental distractions keeps the patient focused, decreases stimuli going to the brain for interpretation, and enhances the patient's ability to communicate effectively.
■ Do not speak loudly unless the patient is hearing impaired.	Loud talking does not improve the patient's ability to understand if the barriers are primarily language, dysphasia, or a sensory deficit.
■ Maintain eye contact with the patient when speaking. Stand close, within the patient's line of vision (generally midline).	Patients may have a defect in their field of vision or may need to see the nurse's face or lips to enhance understanding of what is being communicated.
■ Give the patient ample time to respond. Avoid finishing sentences for the patient. Allow the patient to complete his or her sentence and thought, but if the patient appears to be having difficulty, ask the patient for permission to help. Say the word or phrase slowly and distinctly if help is requested. Be calm and accepting during attempts; do not say you understand if you do not.	This communication approach may reduce frustration and enhance trust. It may be difficult for patients to respond under pressure; they may need extra time to organize responses, find the correct word, or make necessary language translations. QSEN: Patient-centered care.
■ If the patient's ability to speak is limited to "yes" and "no" answers, try to phrase questions so that the patient can use these responses.	Patients can become easily frustrated when they cannot communicate in a simple manner.
■ Use short sentences, and ask only one question at a time.	This technique allows the patient to stay focused on one thought. Sudden shifts from one subject to another do not allow time for the brain to keep pace with the messages.
■ Speak slowly and distinctly, repeating key words to prevent confusion. Supplement verbal communication with meaningful gestures.	This approach provides the patient with more channels through which information can be communicated.
■ Give concrete directions that the patient is physically capable of doing (e.g., "point to the pain," "open your mouth," "turn your head").	Simple, one-action directions enhance comprehension for the patient with language impairment.
■ When the patient has difficulty with verbal expressions, support the work the patient is doing in speech therapy by providing practice sessions often throughout the day. Begin with simple words (e.g., "yes," "no," "this is a cup"), then progress.	Practice with language skills in a supportive environment will increase the patient's communication. Reinforcement by repetition and practice enhances learning.
■ When the patient cannot identify objects by name, give practice in receiving word images (e.g., point to an object, and clearly enunciate its name: "cup" or "pen").	Visual cueing reinforces language comprehension.
■ Correct errors.	Not correcting errors reinforces undesirable performance and makes correction more difficult later.

■ = Independent ▲ = Interprofessional Collaboration

Actions/Interventions

- Create a list of words that the patient can say; add new words to it as needed. Share this list with family members, significant others, and members of the interprofessional health care team.
- Provide the patient with word-and-phrase cards, writing pad and pencil, or picture board. Use eye blinks or finger movements for "yes" or "no" responses.
- Carry on a one-way conversation with a totally dysphasic patient.

▲ Consider the use of an electronic speech generator in post-laryngectomy patients.

Rationales

Sharing information with others broadens the group of people with whom the patient can communicate. QSEN: Teamwork and collaboration.

Supplemental communication devices are especially helpful for intubated patients or those whose jaws are wired.

It may not be possible to determine what information the patient understands. The nurse should not assume that the patient understands nothing about his or her environment.

Adaptive devices can facilitate communication with patients who cannot produce vocal speech.

Education/Continuity of Care

Actions/Interventions

- Inform the patient, significant others, or caregiver of the type of dysphasia the patient has and how it affects speech, language skills, and understanding.

- Offer significant others the opportunity to ask questions about the patient's communication problem.

- Encourage family members and caregivers to talk to the patient even though the patient may not respond. Suggest that the family engage the patient often throughout the day for short periods. Encourage the family to look for cues that the patient is overstimulated or fatigued.
▲ Consult with a speech therapist for discharge planning.

- Assist the patient in seeking an evaluation of his or her home and work settings.

- Encourage the patient and family members to seek information about improving communication from the American Speech-Language-Hearing Association, http://www.asha.org/.
- Refer deaf patients and their families to their local hearing society for community support, education, and sign language training.

Rationales

Many family members assume that a patient's ability to think and process information has been affected by a brain injury or tumor; this may or may not be true, and, if true, some of the effects may be amenable to remediation. Changes in cognitive function often accompany language dysfunction in the patient with a brain injury. A decreased attention span may limit the patient's ability to concentrate during a long conversation. QSEN: Patient-centered care.

It is important for the family to know that there are many ways to send information to someone and that time may be needed to understand the special needs of the patient.

Meaningful interactions with others decrease the patient's sense of isolation and may assist in recovery from dysphasia. Overstimulation and fatigue hinder effective communication.

Outpatient speech therapy can support the patient's efforts to recover language skills. Integrating the contributions of members of the interprofessional team helps the patient and family achieve health goals and allows for shared decision-making to achieve quality patient care. QSEN: Teamwork and collaboration.

This evaluation will help the patient make decisions about the need for assistive devices such as talking computers, telephone typing devices, and interpreters.

Community resources and social media can offer additional information and support to patients and families coping with impaired language and communication skills.

Specialized services may be required to meet the communication needs of patients and families in the deaf community.

NANDA-I NDx **Chronic Confusion**

Definition: An irreversible, long-standing, and/or progressive deterioration of intellect and personality characterized by decreased ability to interpret environmental stimuli and decreased capacity for intellectual thought processes, and manifested by disturbances of memory, orientation, and behavior

Chronic confusion is not limited to any one age-group, gender, or clinical problem. Chronic confusion can occur in a variety of settings, including the home, hospital, and long-term care facilities. Although often associated with older adults with dementia, younger adults with chronic illnesses also may be affected. Depression, multiple sclerosis, brain infections and tumors, repeated head trauma (as seen in athletes sustaining concussions), abnormalities resulting from hypertension, diabetes mellitus, anemia, endocrine disorders, malnutrition, and vascular disorders are examples of illnesses that may be associated with chronic confusion. The person with chronic confusion experiences a gradual but progressive decline in cognitive function. Over months or years, the person has increasing problems with memory, comprehension, judgment, abstract thinking, and reasoning. The loss of cognitive ability may result in problems for the person with communication, ADLs, and emotional stability. Chronic confusion can have a profound impact on family members and family processes as the patient requires more direct supervision and care. This care plan discusses the management of chronic confusion in any setting. It also identifies the importance of addressing the needs of the caregivers.

Common Related Factors

Alzheimer's disease
Multi-infarct dementia
Cerebrovascular accident
Brain injury (e.g., cerebrovascular impairment, neurological illness, trauma, tumor)
Korsakoff's psychosis

Defining Characteristics

Alteration in interpretation
Alteration in response to stimuli
Chronic cognitive impairment
Normal level of consciousness
Alteration in short-term or long-term memory
Alteration in personality
Organic brain disorder
Impaired social functioning

Common Expected Outcomes

Patient will remain safe and free from harm.
Family or significant others will verbalize understanding of disease process and prognosis and the patient's needs, identify and participate in interventions to deal effectively with the situation, and provide for maximal independence while meeting safety needs of the patient.

NOC Outcomes

Cognitive Orientation; Decision Making; Distorted Thought Self-Control; Knowledge: Dementia Management

NIC Interventions

Delusion Management; Dementia Management; Environmental Management: Safety; Family Involvement Promotion; Validation Therapy

Ongoing Assessment

Actions/Interventions

■ Assess the degree of impairment:

Rationales

The degree of confusion will determine the amount of reorientation and intervention the patient will need to evaluate reality accurately. The patient may be awake and aware of his or her surroundings. QSEN: Patient-centered care.

■ = Independent   ▲ = Interprofessional Collaboration

Actions/Interventions

- Evaluate responses on diagnostic examinations (e.g., memory impairments, reality orientation, attention span, calculations).

- Test the ability to receive and send effective communications.
- Note deterioration and changes in personal hygiene or behavior.

- Talk with significant others regarding baseline behaviors, length of time since onset or progression of the problem, their perception of the prognosis, and other pertinent information and concerns for the patient.

- Determine the patient's anxiety level in relation to the situation. Note behavior that may be indicative of a potential for violence.

- Assess for sundown syndrome.

Rationales

Decreased attention span and memory loss can contribute to the patient's inability to accurately respond to environmental stimuli. A common screening tool is the Mini-Mental State Examination (MMSE). The Confusion Assessment Method (CAM) is a valid and reliable instrument that can help monitor changes in the patient's cognitive function. This tool is effective when assessing older adults. QSEN: Evidence-based practice.

Ability/willingness to respond to verbal direction/limits may vary with degree of reality orientation.

This information assists in developing a specific plan for grooming and hygiene activities. QSEN: Patient-centered care.

Assessment can identify areas of physical care in which the patient needs assistance. These areas include nutrition, elimination, sleep, rest, exercise, bathing, grooming, and dressing. It is important to distinguish ability and motivation in the initiation, performance, and maintenance of self-care activities. Patients may either have the ability and minimal motivation, or motivation and minimal ability.

Confusion, disorientation, impaired judgment, suspiciousness, and loss of social inhibitions may result in socially inappropriate/harmful behaviors to self or others. The patient may have poor impulse behavior control. QSEN: Safety.

This phenomenon associated with confusion occurs in the late afternoon. The patient exhibits increasing restlessness, agitation, and confusion. Sundowning may be a sign of sleep disorders, hunger, thirst, or unmet toileting needs.

Therapeutic Interventions

Actions/Interventions

- Prevent further deterioration and maximize level of function:
  - Provide a calm environment; eliminate extraneous noise and stimuli.

  - Communicate using simple, concrete nouns in positive terms.

  - Maintain consistency in the patient's environment and daily schedule.

  - Refrain from correcting or contradicting the patient's perceptions and experiences.

Rationales

The confused patient may misinterpret increased levels of visual and auditory stimulation. The confused patient may perceive pictures on walls or even shadows as threatening. High noise levels can disrupt sleep and add to levels of anxiety and stress.

This communication technique can reduce anxiety experienced in unfamiliar surroundings. For example, asking the confused patient to "Stay sitting in the chair" is more positive than saying "Don't get up."

Consistency in placement of furnishings promotes orientation and memory. Following the same schedule each day reduces stress and anxiety caused by change.

Challenges to the patient's thinking can be perceived as threatening and result in a defensive reaction. The confused patient will become more anxious and even combative. QSEN: Safety.

Actions/Interventions

- Encourage the family and significant others to provide ongoing orientation and input about current news and family happenings.

- Maintain reality-oriented relationships and environment (e.g., display clocks, calendars, personal items, seasonal decorations).

- Encourage participation in resocialization groups.

- Allow the patient to reminisce, existing in his or her own reality, if not detrimental to the patient's well-being.
- Provide safety measures (e.g., close supervision, identification bracelet, medication lockup, lower temperature on hot water tank).

■ Provide repetitive hand activities.

Rationales

Increased orientation ensures a greater degree of safety for the patient. The confused patient may not completely understand what is happening. The caregiver's facial expression and tone of voice may enhance the patient's level of comfort.

Orientation to one's environment increases one's ability to trust others. Encourage the patient to check the calendar and clock often to orient himself or herself. Familiar personal possessions increase the patient's comfort level and decrease the sense of alienation that the patient may feel in a strange environment.

Encouraging the patient to assume responsibility for his or her own behavior will increase his or her sense of independence. It is important for the patient to learn socially appropriate behavior through group interactions. This approach provides an opportunity for the patient to observe the impact his or her behavior has on those around him or her. It also facilitates the development of acceptable social skills.

Depending on the cause, long-term memory is usually retained longer than short-term; reminiscing can be enjoyable to the patient.

Effective use of these strategies reduces the risk of harm to the patient. The confused patient may lack appropriate insight and judgment about environmental risks. QSEN: Safety.

Engaging in safe, repetitive activities occupies the patient's mind and hands. The activities may reduce agitation and provide a release of energy. The confused patient may find it calming to fold and refold towels and washcloths. A box filled with pieces of cloth, balls of yarn, and stuffed animals can promote contentment as the patient removes items from the box and replaces them.

Education/Continuity of Care

Actions/Interventions

■ Assist the family and significant others in developing coping strategies.
- Determine family members' availability and willingness to participate in meeting the patient's needs. Refer family members to the interprofessional health team.

- Identify appropriate community resources (e.g., Alzheimer's or brain injury support groups, Meals On Wheels, adult day care, home care agency, respite care).
- Evaluate family members' attention to own needs, including the grieving process.

Rationales

The family needs to let the patient do all that he or she is able to do. This approach to the patient will maximize the patient's level of functioning and quality of life for both the patient and the family members. The family may need legal and financial guidance to ensure that the patient's needs are met appropriately. QSEN: Teamwork and collaboration.

Community resources provide support, assist with problem-solving, and reduce the demands associated with caregiving.

Caregiver strain can lead to increasing frustration with the confused patient. The frustration can precipitate anger and abuse.

■ = Independent   ▲ = Interprofessional Collaboration

Nursing Diagnosis Care Plans

Actions/Interventions

- Provide written information for significant others on living with chronic confusion.

Rationales

This information assists significant others with understanding the disorder and its impact on their lives.

Related Care Plans

Caregiver role strain, Chapter 2
Impaired memory, Chapter 2
Alzheimer's disease/dementia, Chapter 7

NANDA-I NDx Constipation

Definition: Decrease in normal frequency of defecation accompanied by difficult or incomplete passage of stool and/or passage of excessively hard, dry stool

Constipation is a common, yet complex problem; it is especially prevalent among older patients. Diet, exercise, and daily routine are important factors in maintaining normal bowel patterns. Too little fluid, too little fiber, inactivity or immobility, and disruption in daily routines can result in constipation. Use of medications, particularly opioid analgesics or overuse of laxatives or enemas, can cause constipation. Patients who ignore the need to defecate for long periods are at risk for developing constipation. Psychological disorders such as stress and depression can cause constipation. Because privacy with defecation is an issue for most people, being away from home, hospitalized, or otherwise being deprived of adequate privacy can result in constipation. Because "normal" patterns of bowel elimination vary so widely from individual to individual, some people believe they are constipated if a day passes without a bowel movement; for others, every third or fourth day is normal. Chronic constipation can result in the development of hemorrhoids; diverticulosis (particularly in older patients who have a high incidence of diverticulitis); straining at stool; and although rare, perforation of the colon. Constipation is usually episodic, although it can become a lifelong, chronic problem. Because tumors of the colon and rectum can result in obstipation (complete lack of passage of stool), it is important to rule out these possibilities. Nonpharmacological management (fluids, activity, and fiber) remains the most effective treatment for constipation.

Common Related Factors

Functional
  Abdominal muscle weakness
  Average daily physical activity is less than recommended for gender and age
  Habitually ignores urge to defecate
  Irregular defecation habits
  Recent environmental change
Mechanical
  Obesity
  Postsurgical bowel obstruction
Pharmacological
  Laxative abuse
  Pharmaceutical agent
Physiological
  Insufficient fluid intake
  Insufficient fiber intake
Psychological
  Confusion
  Depression

Defining Characteristics

Decrease in stool frequency or volume
Hard, formed stool
Straining with defecation
Liquid stool
Anorexia
Abdominal pain
Distended abdomen
Headache
Pain with defecation
Rectal pressure

 For additional care plans, go to http://evolve.elsevier.com/Gulanick/.

Common Expected Outcomes

Patient passes soft, formed stool at a frequency perceived as "normal" by the patient.

Patient or caregiver verbalizes measures that will prevent recurrence of constipation.

NOC Outcomes

Bowel Elimination; Medication Response; Self-Care: Toileting

NIC Interventions

Bowel Management; Constipation/Impaction Management; Bowel Training

Ongoing Assessment

Actions/Interventions	Rationales
■ Assess the usual pattern of elimination, including frequency and consistency of stool.	"Normal" frequency of defecation varies from twice daily to once every third or fourth day. Hard formed feces is characteristic of constipation. QSEN: Patient-centered care.
■ Evaluate laxative and enema use, type, and frequency.	Chronic use of laxatives and enemas causes the muscles and nerves of the colon to function inadequately in producing an urge to defecate. Over time, the colon becomes atonic and distended, and does not respond normally to the presence of stool. The patient becomes dependent on laxatives and enemas for defecation.
■ Evaluate the patient's usual dietary habits, eating habits, eating schedule, and liquid intake.	Change in mealtime, type of food, and disruption of the patient's usual schedule can lead to constipation.
■ Assess the patient's activity level.	Prolonged bed rest, lack of exercise, and inactivity contribute to constipation.
■ Evaluate current medication usage that may contribute to constipation.	Drugs that can cause constipation include opioids, antacids with calcium or aluminum base, antidepressants, anticholinergics, antihypertensives, general anesthetics, hypnotics, and iron and calcium supplements. Many of these drugs slow peristalsis.
■ Assess the need for privacy for elimination.	Many patients report that being away from home limits their ability to have a bowel movement. Those who travel or require hospitalization may have difficulty having a bowel movement away from the sense of privacy in their own home.
■ Evaluate for fear of pain with defecation.	Hemorrhoids, anal fissures, or other anorectal disorders that are painful can cause the patient to ignore the urge to defecate, which over time results in a dilated rectum that no longer responds to the presence of stool.
■ Assess the degree to which the patient responds to the urge to defecate.	Ignoring the defecation urge eventually leads to chronic constipation because the rectum no longer senses or responds to the presence of stool. The longer the stool remains in the rectum, the drier and harder (and more difficult to pass) it becomes.
■ Assess for a history of neurogenic diseases, such as multiple sclerosis or Parkinson's disease.	Neurogenic disorders may decrease peristaltic activity.

Therapeutic Interventions

Actions/Interventions	Rationales
■ Encourage a daily fluid intake of 2000 to 3000 mL/day, if not contraindicated medically.	Adequate fluid is necessary to keep the fecal mass soft. However, patients, especially older patients, may have cardiovascular limitations that require that less fluid be taken.

■ = Independent   ▲ = Interprofessional Collaboration

Actions/Interventions

- Encourage a minimum of 20 g of dietary fiber (e.g., raw fruits, fresh vegetables, whole grains) per day.

- Encourage physical activity and regular exercise. Encourage isometric abdominal and gluteal exercises.
- Encourage a regular time for elimination.

- Digitally remove the fecal impaction.

- Suggest the following measures to minimize rectal discomfort:
  - Warm sitz bath

  - Hemorrhoidal preparations

- For hospitalized patients, the following should be employed:
  - Orient the patient to the location of the bathroom, and encourage its use, unless contraindicated.

  - For bedridden patients; assist the patient in assuming a high-Fowler's position with knees flexed.
  - Close the bathroom door or pull curtains around the bed.
- For patients with neurogenic bowel problems:
  - Abdominal massage—Using the heel of the hand or a tennis ball, apply and release pressure firmly but gently around the abdomen in a clockwise direction.
  - Digital anorectal stimulation—A gloved lubricated finger is gently inserted into the rectum and slowly rotated in a circular motion. This is done for about 15 to 20 seconds until flatus/stool is passed.

Rationales

Fiber passes through the intestine essentially unchanged. When it reaches the colon, it absorbs water and forms a gel, which adds bulk to the stool and makes defecation easier.

Ambulation promotes peristalsis. Abdominal exercises strengthen abdominal muscles that facilitate defecation.

Many people defecate following the first daily meal or coffee, as a result of the gastrocolic reflex.

Stool that remains in the rectum for long periods becomes dry and hard; debilitated patients, especially older patients, may not be able to pass these stools without manual assistance.

The warmth of the water relaxes muscles before defecation attempts.

These over-the-counter preparations shrink swollen hemorrhoidal tissue to promote comfort with bowel movements.

A sitting position with knees flexed straightens the rectum, enhances use of abdominal muscles, and facilitates defecation.

This position best uses gravity and allows for effective Valsalva maneuver.

Providing privacy helps the patient relax for defecation.

Abdominal massage has been reported to be useful in neurogenic bowel disorder but not for constipation in older adults.

Digital stimulation increases muscular activity in rectum by raising rectal pressure to aid in expelling fecal matter.

Education/Continuity of Care

Actions/Interventions

- ▲ Consult with a dietitian regarding dietary sources of fiber.

- Explain to the patient and caregiver the importance of the following:

  - A balanced diet that contains adequate fiber, fresh fruits, vegetables, and grains
  - Adequate fluid intake (eight glasses per day or 2000 to 3000 mL/day).

Rationales

The dietitian can recommend sources of fiber consistent with the patient's usual eating habits. A patient unaccustomed to a high-fiber diet may experience abdominal discomfort and flatulence; a gradual increase in fiber intake is recommended. QSEN: Teamwork and collaboration.

These steps lead to reestablishing regular bowel habits.

Twenty grams of fiber per day is recommended.

Increased hydration promotes a softer fecal mass.

Actions/Interventions

- A regular time for evacuation and an adequate time for defecation

- Regular exercise and activity

- Privacy for defecation

▲ Teach the use of pharmacological agents as ordered:

- Bulk fiber (Metamucil and similar fiber products)

- Stool softeners (e.g., Colace)
- Chemical irritants (e.g., castor oil, cascara, Milk of Magnesia)
- Suppositories

- Oil retention enema

Rationales

Successful bowel training relies on routine. Facilitating a regular time for bowel elimination prevents the bowel from emptying sporadically.

Exercises strengthen abdominal muscles and stimulate peristalsis.

Privacy allows the patient to relax, which can help promote defecation.

The use of laxatives or enemas is indicated for short-term management of constipation. QSEN: Evidence-based practice.

These laxatives increase fluid, gaseous, and solid bulk of intestinal contents.

These laxatives soften stool and lubricate intestinal mucosa.

These laxatives irritate the bowel mucosa and cause rapid propulsion of contents of small intestine.

These laxatives aid in softening stools and stimulate rectal mucosa; best results occur when given 30 minutes before usual defecation time or after breakfast.

This intervention softens stool.

Ineffective Coping

Definition: Inability to form a valid appraisal of the stressors, inadequate choices of practiced responses, and/or inability to use available resources

For most people, everyday life includes its share of stressors and demands, ranging from family, work, and professional role responsibilities to major life events such as divorce, illness, and the death of loved ones. How one responds to such stressors depends in part on the person's coping resources. Such resources can include optimistic beliefs, social support networks, personal health and energy, problem-solving skills, and material resources. Sociocultural and religious factors may influence how people view and handle their problems. Some cultures may prefer privacy and avoid sharing their fears in public,

even to health care providers. As resources become limited and problems become more acute, this strategy may prove ineffective. Vulnerable populations such as older patients, those in adverse socioeconomic situations, those with complex medical problems such as substance abuse, or those who find themselves suddenly physically challenged may not have the resources or skills to cope with their acute or chronic stressors. Such problems can occur in any setting (e.g., during hospitalization for an acute event, in the home or rehabilitation environment as a result of chronic illness, or in response to another threat or loss).

Common Related Factors

High degree of threat
Inaccurate threat appraisal
Ineffective pattern of tension release strategies
Insufficient social support
Inadequate resources
Inadequate opportunity to prepare for stressor
Inadequate confidence in ability to deal with a situation
Situational crises
Maturational crises

Defining Characteristics

Ineffective coping strategies
Inability to make decisions
Inability to ask for help
Insufficient goal-directed behavior
Insufficient problem-solving
Inability to meet role expectations
Substance abuse
Alteration in concentration
Fatigue
Destructive behavior toward self or others
Frequent illness
Alteration in sleep pattern

■ = Independent ▲ = Interprofessional Collaboration

Nursing Diagnosis Care Plans

Common Expected Outcomes

Patient uses available resources and support systems.
Patient describes and initiates effective coping strategies.
Patient describes positive results from new behaviors.

NOC Outcomes
Coping; Stress Level; Decision Making;
  Information Processing
NIC Interventions
Coping Enhancement; Decision-Making Support

Ongoing Assessment

Actions/Interventions	Rationales
■ Assess for the presence of defining characteristics.	Behavioral and physiological responses to stress can be varied and provide clues to the level of coping difficulty.
■ Assess for specific stressors.	Accurate appraisal can facilitate development of appropriate coping strategies. Because a patient has an altered health status does not mean the coping difficulties he or she exhibits are only (if at all) related to that. Persistent stressors may exhaust the patient's ability to maintain effective coping.
■ Determine the patient's perception of the stressful situation.	Patients may feel that the threat is greater than their resources to handle it and feel a loss of control over solving the threat or problem. The patient's cultural heritage and previous experiences may affect the patient's understanding of and response to the current situation. This information provides a foundation for planning care and selecting appropriate interventions. QSEN: Patient-centered care.
■ Assess for past use of coping mechanisms including decision-making and problem-solving.	Successful adjustment is influenced by previous coping success. Patients with a history of maladaptive coping may need additional resources. Likewise, previously successful coping skills may be inadequate in the present situation.
■ Evaluate resources and support systems available to the patient.	Patients may have support in one setting, such as during hospitalization, yet lack sufficient support for effective coping in the home setting. Coping resources may include significant others, health care providers such as home health nurses, community resources, and spiritual counseling.
■ Assess the level of understanding and readiness to learn new coping methods.	Appropriate problem-solving requires accurate information and understanding of options. Often patients who are ineffectively coping are unable to hear or assimilate needed information.

Therapeutic Interventions

Actions/Interventions	Rationales
■ Establish a working relationship with the patient through continuity of care.	An ongoing relationship establishes trust, reduces the feeling of isolation, and may facilitate coping.
■ Provide opportunities to express concerns, fears, feelings, and expectations.	Verbalization of actual or perceived threats can help reduce anxiety and open doors for ongoing communication.

Actions/Interventions

- Convey feelings of acceptance and understanding. Avoid false reassurances.

- Encourage the patient to identify his or her own strengths and abilities.

- Assist patients with accurately evaluating the situation and their own accomplishments.

- Provide information the patient wants and needs. Do not provide more than the patient can handle.

- Encourage the patient to set realistic goals.

- Assist the patient with problem-solving in a constructive manner.
- Reduce stimuli in an environment that could be misinterpreted as threatening.

- Provide outlets that foster feelings of personal achievement and self-esteem.
- Point out signs of positive progress or change.

Rationales

An honest relationship facilitates problem-solving and successful coping. False reassurances are never helpful to the patient and only may serve to relieve the discomfort of the care provider.

During crises, patients may not be able to recognize their strengths. Fostering awareness can expedite use of these strengths.

It can be helpful for the patient to recognize that he or she has the skills and reserves of strength to effectively manage the situation. The patient may need help coming to a realistic perspective of the situation. QSEN: Patient-centered care.

Patients who are coping ineffectively have reduced ability to assimilate information and may need more guidance initially.

Setting realistic goals helps the patient gain control over the situation. Guiding the patient to view the situation in smaller parts may make the problem seem more manageable. QSEN: Patieint-centered care.

Constructive problem-solving can promote independence and a sense of autonomy for the patient.

In the acute hospital setting, patients are often exposed to new equipment and environments. The presence of and noise associated with medical equipment can increase anxiety and make coping more challenging.

Opportunities to role-play or rehearse appropriate actions can increase confidence for behavior in actual situations.

Patients who are coping ineffectively may not be able to assess their progress toward effective coping.

Education/Continuity of Care

Actions/Interventions

- Instruct the patient and family about the need for adequate rest and balanced diet.
- Teach the use of relaxation, exercise, and diversional activities as methods to cope with stress.
- ▲ Consult with social worker, psychiatric liaison, and pastoral care for additional and ongoing support resources.

- Assist in the development of an alternative support system. Encourage participation in self-help groups, if available.

Rationales

Inadequate diet and fatigue can themselves be stressors and limit effective coping.

A variety of brief interventions can be used toward assisting patients with reducing their level of stress.

Specialized services may be required to meet specific needs of the patient, promote effective coping and allow for shared decision-making to achieve quality patient care. QSEN: Teamwork and collaboration.

Relationships with people who have common interests and goals can be beneficial. Participation in a self-help group may provide the patient with new strategies for effective coping.

■ = Independent   ▲ = Interprofessional Collaboration

Nursing Diagnosis Care Plans

Readiness for Enhanced Decision-Making

Definition: A pattern of choosing a course of action for meeting short- and long-term health-related goals, which can be strengthened.

Throughout life people make a variety of decisions, some being more important than others. Decisions related to our health warrant careful consideration and thoughtful reflection. Some people put off decision-making, either by endlessly searching for information, by simply conforming to peer or expert pressure, or by resorting to the flip of a coin. This approach for making health care decisions can have serious consequences. Many different techniques for decision-making have been developed that usually include first clarifying the purpose for the decision, gathering necessary data from reliable sources, identifying possible options, reviewing one's values and what is important, evaluating each choice in terms of its benefits and consequences, and finally making the thoughtful decision. This care plan focuses on the patient who is ready to make an important decision. It can be used to assist health care professionals when working with patients deciding whether to reduce their risk factors, such as quitting smoking, managing their weight, or engaging in a serious physical activity regimen. However, this care plan can also be used to address more complex decision-making issues, such as determination of cancer therapy, genetic testing, refusal of blood products or surgical procedures, writing of advance directives, organ donation, end-of-life issues, withholding of treatments, and the like. In these more complex situations, shared decision-making in the medical encounter may be an ideal model in which both patient and health care professionals share information, take steps to build consensus about preferred treatment or action, and reach an agreement.

Defining Characteristics

Expresses desire to enhance decision-making
Expresses desire to enhance risk-benefit analysis of decisions
Expresses desire to enhance understanding of and meaning of their choices for decision-making
Expresses desire to enhance use of reliable evidence for decisions
Expresses desire to enhance congruency of decisions with goal
Expresses desire to enhance congruency of decisions with values

Expected Outcomes

Patient demonstrates needed knowledge for making decision.
Patient verbalizes the possible alternatives and potential consequences of each alternative for given decision-making situation.
Patient verbalizes satisfaction with the decision made for given situation.

NOC Outcomes
Decision-Making; Participation in Health Care Decisions
NIC Interventions
Decision-Making Support; Self-Efficacy Enhancement; Health System Guidance

Ongoing Assessment

Actions/Interventions	Rationales
■ Assess the patient's understanding of the situation needing a decision.	A key first step in making a decision is to clearly define the nature of the decision to be made. The nurse can assist the patient by using questions or statements to encourage expression of thoughts, feeling, and concerns.
■ Evaluate the patient's decision-making ability.	Decision-making requires the cognitive skills needed to make a correct decision for individuals based on their personal values and ultimate goal. Biases often enter into the decision-making process and the patient should be assisted to recognize them when evident. For example, some people may prematurely terminate their search for evidence and simply accept the first alternative that seems right. Others might place more value on recent information, ignoring more important distant information. Others may tend to conform to group pressure. And some may selectively search only for evidence that supports certain conclusions, disregarding other facts that support different conclusions. QSEN: Patient-centered care.
■ Explore the identification of specific life values and goals.	Everyone has a unique set of values and goals that the person believes to be important. Depending on which values are considered important, different opinions may seem more or less attractive. Health beliefs or values are also influenced by diverse cultural norms. Patients may delay a treatment for various reasons, including an acceptance of the disease as an inevitable fate or "God's will," a mistrust of Western medicine, fear, etc. QSEN: Patient-centered care.
■ Assess the accuracy of the patient's knowledge and what further information may be needed.	Gathering relevant information is key to decision-making. Consumers can easily be misled by media information. Without guidance from a health care professional, patients may make important decisions about treatment or prevention based on inaccurate, incomplete, or misunderstood information about their health situation.
■ Determine if there are differences between the patient's view of the condition and the view of the health care providers.	Accurate appraisal may give some perspective as to the challenges involved in the decision-making process. QSEN: Patient-centered care.

Therapeutic Interventions

Actions/Interventions	Rationales
■ Use appropriate questions to assist the patient in identifying the decision to be made.	The nurse can be helpful by posing reflective clarifying questions that assist the patient to identify the nature of the decision.
■ Assist the patient to clarify values and expectations that may assist in making critical life choices.	Using questions or statements can help encourage expression of thoughts, feeling, and expectations that can serve as the basis for further decision-making. QSEN: Patient-centered care.

■ = Independent   ▲ = Interprofessional Collaboration

Actions/Interventions

- Encourage consultation with the interprofessional team, as needed. Suggest getting a second opinion for more complex decisions.

- Work with the patient to identify options/alternative views to consider in a clear and supportive manner.
- Assist the patient to list and evaluate the advantages and disadvantages of each alternative.

- Assist patients to make the best decision for them.

- Help the patient evaluate how decisions are in agreement or in conflict with those of family members/significant others.

- Inform the patient/family how to challenge a decision made by a health care provider, as needed.

- Help patients explain their decisions to others as needed.

- Introduce the patient to persons/groups who have successfully undergone the same experience.

Rationales

Decision-making is hard. Getting a well-informed opinion from respected health care professionals can improve decision-making. Although some decision points (smoking vs not smoking) are ongoing, certain diseases such as cancer have decision points that occur only once (e.g., whether to have irradiation with lumpectomy vs. mastectomy for breast cancer, and following surgery, whether to have adjuvant chemotherapy and/or radiation). Here several different treatment options exist with different possible outcomes. Second opinions can provide clarification of treatment outcomes. Today these can even be obtained electronically from major medical centers across the country. QSEN: Teamwork and collaboration.

Decision-making is the act of choosing between a number of viable alternatives or paths of action.

This step requires patients to draw upon their information and emotions to imagine what it would be like if each of the proposed alternatives were carried out. In this cost-benefit analysis, the outcome of each possible option (both positive and negative) is examined. The patient also needs to decide how much risk will be taken in making the decision. This will depend on the benefits of making a right decision versus the seriousness of making a wrong decision. This step involves thinking not only about how bad the worst outcome may be but also how likely that outcome is to happen. QSEN: Patient-centered care.

It can be helpful for the patient to recognize that he or she has the knowledge and skills to effectively make a decision. The decision is in the hands of the patient, depending on his or her personal values. The nurse is in an ideal position to offer positive reinforcement and emotional support during the decision-making process.

Sometimes family members have conflicting interests based on finances, property, inheritance rights, and other concerns that influence their decision-making abilities. The right to refuse treatment can be more difficult if contrary to the wishes of family/significant others, especially if the treatment appears to have some effectiveness, or has been in place for some time.

The traditional concept of the doctor-patient relationship placed the patient in a passive compliant role. Today's medical environment demands more patient autonomy and supports a patient-centered approach with the patient as a collaborator. Most patients do not want the responsibility for making decisions totally on their own. However, as competent adults, they have the right to disagree with the treatment plan, and to consent to or refuse medical treatment. QSEN: Patient-centered care.

The nurse can serve as an important liaison between patient, family, and the interprofessional team. With the complexity of the health care system and care decisions patients need to make, the nurse serves as an important advocate.

Guidance will add available resources for decision-making efforts.

NANDA-I NDx **Diarrhea**

Definition: Passage of loose, unformed stools

Diarrhea may result from a variety of factors, including intestinal malabsorption disorders, increased secretion of fluid by the intestinal mucosa, and hypermotility of the intestine. Diarrhea may be a clinical sign of infection (i.e., viral, bacterial, or parasitic); inflammatory bowel diseases (e.g., Crohn's disease); side effects of drugs (e.g., antibiotics); increased intestinal osmotic loads (e.g., tube feedings); radiation; or increased intestinal motility such as with irritable bowel disease. Diarrhea may be an acute, short-lived episode of increased bowel elimination or it may be a long-term, chronic problem for the patient.

Problems associated with diarrhea include fluid and electrolyte imbalances, impaired nutrition, and altered skin integrity. In older patients, or those with chronic disease, diarrhea can be life threatening. Treatment is based on addressing the cause of the diarrhea, replacing fluids and electrolytes, providing nutrition, and maintaining skin integrity. Health care workers and other caregivers must take precautions (e.g., diligent hand washing) to avoid transmission of infection associated with some causes of diarrhea.

Common Related Factors

Psychological
    Stress
    Anxiety
Situational
    Laxative abuse
    Enteral feedings
    Exposure to toxin/contaminant
    Travel
    Treatment regimen
Physiological
    Gastrointestinal inflammation
    Gastrointestinal irritation
    Malabsorption
    Infection
    Parasite

Defining Characteristics

Abdominal pain
Cramping
Loose liquid stools, > 3 in 24 hours
Bowel urgency
Hyperactive bowel sounds

Common Expected Outcomes

Patient passes soft, formed stool no more than three times per day.
Patient has negative stool cultures.

NOC Outcomes
Bowel Continence; Bowel Elimination; Fluid Balance; Medication Response
NIC Interventions
Diarrhea Management; Enteral Tube Feeding; Medication Management

Ongoing Assessment

Actions/Interventions	**Rationales**
■ Assess for abdominal pain, cramping, frequency, urgency, loose or liquid stools, and hyperactive bowel sensations.	These assessment findings are commonly associated with diarrhea.
▲ Culture stool.	Testing will identify possible etiological organisms for the diarrhea. QSEN: Evidence-based practice.

■ = Independent   ▲ = Interprofessional Collaboration

Nursing Diagnosis Care Plans

Actions/Interventions	Rationales
■ Inquire about the following:	These assessments help to identify specific situations that may be the cause of the diarrhea. QSEN: Patient-centered care; Evidence-based practice.
• Tolerance to milk and other dairy products	Diarrhea is a common manifestation of lactose intolerance. Patients with lactose intolerance have insufficient lactase, the enzyme that digests lactose. The presence of lactose in the intestines increases osmotic pressure and draws water into the intestinal lumen.
• Medications the patient is or has been taking	Laxatives and antibiotics may cause diarrhea. *Clostridium difficile* can colonize the intestine after antibiotic use and lead to pseudomembranous enterocolitis. *Clostridium difficile* is a common cause of nosocomial diarrhea in health care facilities. Magnesium and calcium supplements can also cause diarrhea.
• Food intolerances	Foods may stimulate intestinal nerve fibers and cause increased peristalsis. Some foods will increase intestinal osmotic pressure and draw fluid into the intestinal lumen. Spicy, fatty, or high-carbohydrate foods; caffeine; sugar-free foods with sorbitol; or alcohol may cause diarrhea.
• Methods of food preparation	Inadequately cooked food, food contaminated with bacteria during preparation, foods that are not maintained at appropriate temperatures, or contaminated tube feedings may cause diarrhea.
• Osmolality of tube feedings	Hyperosmolar food or fluid draws excess fluid into the gut, stimulates peristalsis, and causes diarrhea.
• Change in eating schedule	Changes in eating pattern can result in changes in intestinal function and lead to diarrhea.
• Current stressors	Some individuals respond to stress with hyperactivity of the gastrointestinal tract.
■ Check for a history of the following:	These assessments help to identify specific situations that may be the cause of the diarrhea.
• Previous gastrointestinal surgery	After bowel resection, a period (1 to 3 weeks) of diarrhea is normal. Patients who have gastric partitioning surgery for weight loss may experience diarrhea as they begin refeeding. Diarrhea is a manifestation of dumping syndrome in which an increased osmotic bolus entering the small intestine draws fluid into the intestinal lumen.
• Gastrointestinal diseases	Diseases such as Crohn's disease and gastroenteritis can result in malabsorption and lead to chronic diarrhea.
• Abdominal radiation	Radiation causes sloughing of the intestinal mucosa, decreases usual absorption capacity, and may result in diarrhea.
• Foreign travel, ingestion of unpasteurized dairy products, or drinking untreated water	Patients may acquire intestinal infections from eating contaminated foods or drinking contaminated water.
■ Assess for fecal impaction.	Liquid stool (apparent diarrhea) may seep past a fecal impaction.
■ Assess the relationship of therapeutic or diagnostic regimens to diarrhea.	Preparation for radiography or surgery and radiation or chemotherapy predispose to diarrhea by altering the mucosal surface and transit time through the bowel.
■ Assess hydration status, including:	Diarrhea may cause significant changes in fluid balance that increases the patient's risk for deficient fluid volume. QSEN: Safety.
• Input and output	Diarrhea can lead to profound dehydration.

Actions/Interventions	Rationales
• Skin turgor	Decreased skin turgor and tenting of the skin occur in dehydration.
• Moisture of mucous membranes	Dehydration causes dry mucous membranes.
■ Assess the condition of perianal skin.	Diarrheal stools may be highly corrosive as a result of increased enzyme content. The perianal skin may become irritated and prone to break down. QSEN: Safety.
■ Explore the emotional impact of diarrhea and/or soiling accidents.	Control of bowel elimination is a developmental task of early childhood. Loss of control of bowel elimination that occurs with diarrhea can lead to feelings of embarrassment and decreased self-esteem. QSEN: Patient-centered care.

Therapeutic Interventions

Actions/Interventions	Rationales
▲ Give antidiarrheal drugs as ordered.	Most antidiarrheal drugs suppress gastrointestinal motility, thus allowing for more fluid absorption. Supplements of beneficial bacteria ("probiotics") or yogurt may reduce symptoms by reestablishing normal bacterial flora in the intestine.
■ Provide the following dietary alterations:	Changes in food intake can be beneficial in reducing diarrhea.
• Bulk fiber (e.g., cereal, grains, Metamucil) • "Natural" bulking agents (e.g., rice, apples, matzos, cheese)	Bulking agents and dietary fibers absorb fluid from the stool and help thicken the stool.
• Avoidance of stimulants (e.g., caffeine, carbonated beverages)	Stimulants may increase gastrointestinal motility and worsen diarrhea.
■ Encourage fluids to 1.5 to 2 L/24 hr plus 200 mL for each loose stool in adults unless contraindicated; consider nutritional support.	Increased fluid intake replaces fluid lost in the liquid stool.
■ Evaluate the appropriateness of protocols for bowel preparation on basis of age, weight, condition, disease, and other therapies.	Older, frail patients or those patients already fluid depleted may require less bowel preparation or additional intravenous fluid therapy during bowel preparation for surgery or diagnostic procedures.
■ Provide perianal care after each bowel movement.	Gentle cleansing of the perianal skin after each bowel movement will prevent excoriation. Barrier creams can be used to protect the skin.
■ For patients with enteral tube feeding, employ the following:	These nursing actions reduce the risk of diarrhea with enteral tube feedings. QSEN: Safety.
• Change feeding tube equipment according to institutional policy, but no less than every 24 hours.	Contaminated equipment can cause diarrhea.
• Administer tube feeding at room temperature.	Extremes of temperature can stimulate peristalsis.
• Initiate tube feeding slowly.	Starting a tube feeding at a slow infusion rate allows the gastrointestinal system to accommodate intake and adjust to the osmotic load of the formula.
• Decrease the rate or dilute feeding if diarrhea persists or worsens.	Decreasing the rate of infusion or osmolarity of the feeding prevents hyperosmolar diarrhea.
▲ For patients with diarrhea from intestinal infection, anticipate the need for contact precautions.	Contact precautions are necessary to minimize the risk of transmission of microorganisms to others. QSEN: Safety.

■ = Independent   ▲ = Interprofessional Collaboration

Education/Continuity of Care

Actions/Interventions	Rationales
■ Teach the patient or caregiver the following dietary measures to control diarrhea: • Avoid spicy, fatty foods, alcohol, and caffeine. • Broil, bake, or boil foods; avoid frying. • Avoid foods that are disagreeable.	These dietary changes can slow the passage of stool through the colon and reduce or eliminate diarrhea.
■ Encourage reporting of diarrhea that occurs with prescription drugs.	There are usually several antibiotics with which the patient can be treated; if the one prescribed causes diarrhea, this should be reported promptly.
■ Teach the patient or caregiver to use antidiarrheal medications as ordered.	Appropriate use of antidiarrheal medications can promote effective bowel elimination.
■ Teach the patient or caregiver the importance of fluid replacement during diarrheal episodes.	Fluid intake is necessary to prevent dehydration. QSEN: Safety.
■ Teach the patient or caregiver the importance of good perianal hygiene after each bowel movement including: • Wet wiping or cleansing is most effective. • Do not use wipes that contain alcohol or perfumes. • Dry perianal area thoroughly by patting and not rubbing area. • Use barrier creams to prevent excoriation.	Hygiene reduces the risk of perianal skin excoriation and promotes comfort.
■ Teach the patient and caregiver the importance of hand washing after toileting or perianal hygiene.	Most acute diarrhea is caused by enteric infection. Good hand washing will prevent the spread of the infectious agents. QSEN: Safety.
■ Explain the need to avoid unnecessary use of antibiotics.	Many antibiotics reduce the normal bacterial flora in the intestinal tract, causing more harmful bacteria to multiply. Supplements of beneficial bacteria (e.g., yogurt) can reduce antibiotic-associated diarrhea and symptoms.

Related Care Plans

Bowel incontinence, Chapter 2
Risk for electrolyte imbalance, Chapter 2
Deficient fluid volume, Chapter 2
Enteral nutrition, Chapter 4
Bariatric surgery, Chapter 8
Inflammatory bowel disease, Chapter 8

NANDA-I
NDx **Risk for Electrolyte Imbalance**

Definition: Vulnerable to changes in serum electrolyte levels, which may compromise health

Many clinical disorders and their treatments place the patient at risk for imbalances in serum electrolyte concentrations. Imbalanced dietary intake may contribute to electrolyte imbalances. Electrolyte losses may occur from draining wounds and fistulas, especially gastrointestinal fistulas. Imbalances in sodium and chloride concentrations occur most often in situations related to fluid imbalances, especially gastrointestinal fluid losses such as vomiting, diarrhea, or suctioning. Alterations in secretion of antidiuretic hormone and aldosterone put the patient at risk for sodium imbalances. The risk for potassium imbalances increases in patients receiving diuretics. Diarrhea, renal failure, and altered aldosterone secretion also contribute to the patient's risk for potassium imbalance. Alterations in thyroid and parathyroid function put the patient at risk for calcium imbalances. Magnesium imbalances often occur in the same situations as calcium and potassium imbalances. Changes in aldosterone secretion influence magnesium balance. Electrolyte imbalances affect a variety of functions in the body. The patient with an electrolyte imbalance may experience problems with fluid balance, muscle tone and strength, bone density, electrical conduction in the heart, wound healing, and renal stones. This care plan focuses on imbalances of sodium, potassium, calcium, and magnesium.

Common Risk Factors

Diarrhea
Compromised regulatory mechanisms
Endocrine regulatory dysfunction
Excessive fluid volume
Deficient fluid volume
Renal dysfunction
Treatment regimen
Vomiting

Common Expected Outcomes

Patient will maintain normal serum electrolyte balance as evidenced by sodium level of 136 to 145 mEq/L; potassium level of 3.5 to 5.1 mEq/L; chloride level of 98 to 107 mEq/L; total calcium level of 9 to 10.5 mg/dL; ionized calcium level of 4.6 to 5.1 mg/dL; and magnesium level of 1.8 to 3 mg/dL.

NOC Outcomes
Electrolyte Balance; Risk Control
NIC Interventions
Electrolyte Management; Electrolyte Monitoring

Ongoing Assessment

Actions/Interventions

■ Assess for clinical conditions or situations associated with risk for electrolyte imbalances.

  • Drug therapy

Rationales

Prevention of electrolyte imbalances begins with the identification of situations that put the patient at risk for imbalance. QSEN: Patient-centered care; Safety.

Side effects of diuretic therapy include potassium, calcium, and magnesium imbalances. Thiazide and loop diuretics may cause hypokalemia. Hypercalcemia is a side effect of thiazide diuretics. Potassium-sparing diuretics, angiotensin-converting enzyme (ACE) inhibitors, and angiotensin receptor blockers (ARBs) may cause hyperkalemia. Prolonged use of corticosteroids is associated with hypokalemia.

■ = Independent   ▲ = Interprofessional Collaboration

Actions/Interventions	Rationales
• Dietary intake	The patient's fluid and food intake has a direct influence on the risk for electrolyte imbalances. Sodium imbalances can occur with excesses or deficiencies in fluid intake.
• Gastrointestinal fluid losses	Vomiting, diarrhea, and gastrointestinal suctioning contribute to hyponatremia, hypokalemia, and hypomagnesemia.
• Wound drainage and extensive tissue injury	Patients with draining wounds, especially gastrointestinal fistulas, are at risk for loss of sodium and magnesium. Extensive tissue injury as may occur with trauma or burns may cause hyperkalemia, initially. Later, the patient may be at risk for hypokalemia and hyponatremia.
• Endocrine dysfunction	Changes in secretion of antidiuretic hormone from the posterior pituitary gland place the patient at risk for sodium imbalances. Alterations in thyroid gland and parathyroid gland increase the patient's risk for calcium imbalances. Disorders associated with changes in cortisol and aldosterone secretion from the adrenal cortex put the patient at risk for imbalances in potassium and sodium.
• Renal disease	Disorders associated with impaired renal function place the patient at risk for imbalances in sodium, potassium, and calcium. For example, hyperkalemia and hypocalcemia are common electrolyte imbalances in the patient with chronic kidney disease.
• Cancer	Patients with cancer are at risk for electrolyte imbalance related to tumor activity, metastasis, and complications of treatments. For example, hypercalcemia occurs with tumor metastasis to bones. Acute tumor lysis syndrome, as a complication of cancer drug therapy, puts the patient at risk for hyperkalemia and hypocalcemia.
■ Monitor serum electrolyte levels: • Sodium 136 to 145 mEq/L • Potassium 3.5 to 5.1 mEq/L • Chloride 98 to 107 mEq/L • Total calcium 9 to 10.5 mg/dL • Ionized calcium 4.6 to 5.1 mg/dL • Magnesium 1.8 to 3 mg/dL	Early detection of changes in serum electrolyte levels allows for prompt initiation of measures to prevent further imbalances. Normal values for electrolytes may vary based on the testing procedures used in the clinical laboratory. Patient values need to be compared to the normal values used by the clinical laboratory conducting the test. QSEN: Evidence-based practice.

Therapeutic Interventions

Actions/Interventions	Rationales
▲ Administer balanced electrolyte intravenous (IV) solutions as prescribed.	Lactated Ringer's solution has an electrolyte concentration equivalent to that of extracellular fluid. Isotonic saline (0.9% sodium chloride) may contribute to hypernatremia if used for an extended time. Excessive use of sodium-free IV solutions (e.g., D_5W [5% dextrose in water]) puts the patient at risk for hyponatremia.
■ Anticipate measures to reduce electrolyte excesses.	Drug therapy such as Kayexalate and hemodialysis may be indicated to treat patients at risk for excesses of electrolytes such as potassium.
▲ Irrigate nasogastric tubes with isotonic saline, as prescribed.	Irrigation of nasogastric tubes with plain water increases electrolyte losses. Plain water draws electrolytes from mucosal tissue into the stomach, where they are removed with suctioning.

Actions/Interventions

- Anticipate the administration of electrolyte replacements.

Rationales

Oral or IV administration of electrolytes may be prescribed to maintain electrolyte balance for patients at risk for imbalances. QSEN: Safety.

Education/Continuity of Care

Actions/Interventions

- Teach the patient about dietary sources of electrolytes.

- Teach patients using potassium-wasting diuretics about potassium replacements.

- Teach the patient to limit use of over-the-counter antacids and laxatives.

- Teach the patient about dietary sources of sodium and the use of salt substitutes.

Rationales

A balanced diet provides the patient with sources of electrolytes to prevent imbalances. Whole grains, nuts, fruits, and vegetables are good sources for magnesium and potassium. Dairy products; dark green, leafy vegetables; and legumes are good sources of calcium. Vitamin D is necessary for absorption of calcium from the intestines.

The patient needs to understand the importance of preventing hypokalemia as a side effect of these drugs. Potassium replacement may include dietary sources or prescribed oral replacements such as potassium chloride (KCl).

Excessive use of calcium- or magnesium-based antacids or laxatives may increase the patient's risk for imbalances in these electrolytes.

Sodium is present in a variety of foods. Patients need to learn to read labels to identify all sources of sodium in foods. Most salt substitutes replace sodium with potassium. Excessive use of this substance may increase the risk for hyperkalemia.

Related Care Plans

Parenteral nutrition, Chapter 4
Chronic kidney disease, Chapter 11
Syndrome of inappropriate antidiuretic hormone (SIADH), ⊜volve
Diabetes insipidus, ⊜volve
Thyroidectomy, ⊜volve

NANDA-I
NDx Risk for Falls

Definition: Vulnerable to increased susceptibility to falling, which may cause physical harm and compromise health

Falls are a major safety risk for adults, especially older adults. According to the Centers for Disease Control and Prevention (CDC), approximately one in three community-dwelling adults older than age 65 fall each year, and women fall more frequently than men in this age-group. This number increases to approximately 75% of nursing home residents because of their older age, frailty, chronic medical conditions, and cognitive impairments. Fall-related injuries are the most common cause of accidental death in individuals older than 65 years. Injuries sustained as a result of a fall include soft tissue injury, fractures (hip, spine, and wrist), and traumatic brain injury. Fall-related injuries are associated with prolonged hospitalization for older adults. For those surviving a fall, the quality of life is significantly changed after a fall-related injury.

The morbidity, mortality, and economic burdens resulting from patient falls pose serious risk management issues facing the health care industry. Patient falls are caused by multiple factors. Prevention of falls is an important dimension of the nursing care of patients in hospitals and

■ = Independent   ▲ = Interprofessional Collaboration

long-term care settings. The Joint Commission's National Patient Safety Goals require that all inpatient health care settings have admission and daily fall risk assessment tools, as well as a fall prevention program for those patients found to be at high risk for falls. Implementation of successful fall prevention programs is an essential part of nursing care in any health care setting and requires a multifaceted approach. The Agency for Healthcare Research and Quality (AHRQ) provides a comprehensive tool kit that reviews risk assessment instruments for various settings, selected prevention strategies, and recommendations from evidence-based practice and research implications. Nurses also have a major role in educating patients, families, and caregivers about the prevention of falls across the care continuum.

Common Risk Factors

History of falls
Age > 65 years
Living alone
Use of assistive devices (e.g., walker, cane, wheelchair)
Lower limb prosthesis
Acute illness
Orthostatic hypotension
Impaired hearing/visual impairments
Urinary or bowel incontinence
Impaired mobility
Alteration in cognitive functioning
Alcohol consumption
Pharmaceutical agent
Cluttered environment
Insufficient lighting
Unfamiliar setting
Exposure to unsafe environmental conditions (wet floors, ice)
Use of restraints
Use of throw rugs
Difficulty with gait
Impaired balance
Neuropathy
Decreased lower extremity strength
Sleeplessness

Common Expected Outcomes

Patient will not sustain a fall.
Patient and caregiver will implement strategies to increase safety and prevent falls in the home.

NOC Outcomes

Fall Prevention Behavior; Knowledge: Fall Prevention; Risk Control; Risk Detection

NIC Interventions

Fall Prevention; Environmental Management: Safety; Teaching: Prescribed Exercise; Medication Management

Ongoing Assessment

Actions/Interventions	Rationales
■ Assess for factors known to increase the level of fall risk on admission, after any change in the patient's physical or cognitive status, whenever a fall occurs, periodically during a hospital stay, or at defined times in long-term care settings:	The level of risk and subsequent fall precautions can be determined using standard risk assessment tools that incorporate these intrinsic and extrinsic factors. Examples of commonly used tools include Morse Fall Scale, and the Hendrich II Fall Risk Model. QSEN: Evidence-based practice; Safety.
• History of falls	Evidence indicates that a person who has sustained one or more falls in the past 6 months is more likely to fall again.
• Mental status changes	Confusion and impaired judgment increase the patient's risk for falls.
• Age-related physical changes	Normal changes associated with aging increase the patient's risk for falling. These changes include decreased visual capacity, impaired color perception, change in center of gravity, unsteady gait, decreased muscle strength, decreased endurance, altered depth perception, and delayed response and reaction times.
• Sensory deficits	Impaired vision and hearing limit the patient's ability to recognize hazards in the environment.
• Use of mobility assistive devices	Improper use and maintenance of mobility aids such as canes, walkers, and wheelchairs increases the patient's risk for falls.
• Disease-related symptoms	Increased incidence of falls has been demonstrated in people with symptoms such as orthostatic hypotension, urinary incontinence, dizziness, weakness, and confusion.
• Medications	Side effects of drugs and the drug interactions that occur with polypharmacy increase the patient's risk for falls. Drugs that affect BP and level of consciousness are associated with the highest fall risk.
• Unsafe clothing	Poor-fitting shoes, long robes, or long pants legs can limit a person's ambulation and increase fall risk.
■ Assess the patient's environment for factors known to increase fall risk such as unfamiliar setting, inadequate lighting, wet surfaces, waxed floors, clutter, and objects on floor.	Patients who are not familiar with the placement of furniture and equipment in their room are more likely to experience a fall. Anything that blocks or limits a clear, straight path for ambulation can contribute to a person's fall risk.

Therapeutic Interventions

Actions/Interventions	Rationales
■ For the patient in the hospital or long-term care setting:	The nurse develops an individual plan of care that integrates the best clinical evidence with clinical expertise. QSEN: Evidence-based practice; Safety.
• Post signs or use wristband identification to identify the patients at risk for falls and to remind health care providers to implement fall precaution behaviors.	All health care providers need to recognize the patient who is at risk for falls. All care providers are responsible for implementing actions to promote patient safety and prevent falls.
• Move the patient to a room close to the nurses' station.	Nearby location provides for more frequent observation and faster response to call needs.
• Place items used by the patient within easy reach, such as the call light, urinal, water, and telephone.	Stretching to get items from bedside tables that are out of reach can disrupt the patient's balance and contribute to falls.
• Answer call lights immediately. Help the incontinent patient to toilet every 1 to 2 hours.	Patients who experience delay in having their call lights answered are more likely to get out of bed without assistance and will increase their risk for falls.

■ = Independent ▲ = Interprofessional Collaboration

Actions/Interventions

- Place mechanical beds in the lowest possible position. If needed, place the patient's sleeping surface as close to the floor as possible.
- Use side rails on beds only as needed. For beds with split side rails, leave at least one of the rails at the foot of the bed down.

- Avoid the use of restraints to reduce falls.

- Ensure appropriate room lighting, especially at night.

- Encourage the patient to wear shoes or slippers with nonskid soles when ambulating.
- Orient the patient to the layout of the room. Limit rearranging the furniture in the room.
- Provide heavy furniture that will not tip over if used for support by the patient when ambulating. Keep the primary ambulation path clear and as straight as possible. Avoid clutter on the floor surface.
- Use bed and chair alarms to alert staff when the patient gets up without assistance.
- Provide the patient with a chair that has a firm seat and arms on both sides. Consider locked wheels as appropriate.
- ▲ Collaborate with the interprofessional health team to evaluate the patient's medications that contribute to falling. Consider peak effects for prescribed medications that affect level of consciousness.

- ■ For patients or residents with impaired ability to follow direction who are at risk for falls, consider the use of a sitter to provide continuous one-on-one observation.
- ■ Encourage the patient to participate in a program of regular exercise and gait training.

- ■ Encourage the patient to wear eyeglasses and hearing aids and to have these checked routinely.

- ▲ Collaborate with the interprofessional team (physical therapy; occupational therapy) to assist with gait techniques and provide the patient with assistive devices for transfer and ambulation. Initiate home safety evaluation as needed.

Rationales

Keeping beds in the lowest position reduces the risk for falls and serious injury. In some health care settings, placing the mattress on the floor significantly reduces fall risk.

There are both benefits and risks associated with bed rails. Potential benefits include aid in turning and repositioning within the bed, providing a handhold for getting out of bed, and providing an easy access to bed controls. Patients who are disoriented or confused have been known to climb over side rails and fall. Research demonstrates that when one of four rails is left down, the patient is less likely to fall. QSEN: Evidence-based practice.

Studies support that routine use of restraints does not reduce incidence of falls.

Older adults with reduced visual capacity will benefit from adequate lighting, especially in an unfamiliar environment. Using a night-light helps increase visibility if the patient must get up at night.

Nonskid footwear provides sure footing for the patient with diminished foot and toe lift when walking.

The more familiar the patient is with the layout of the room, the less likely the patient is to trip over furniture.

Patients with balance and gait problems are not as skilled at ambulating around objects that obstruct a straight path.

Audible alarms can remind the patient not to get up alone.

This chair style is easier to get out of, especially when the patient experiences weakness and impaired balance when transferring from bed to chair.

A review of the patient's medications by the prescribing health care provider and the pharmacist can identify side effects and drug interactions that increase the patient's fall risk. Polypharmacy in the older adult is a significant risk factor for falls. QSEN: Teamwork and collaboration.

Sitters are responsible for ensuring a safe environment. QSEN: Safety.

Evidence suggests that people who engage in regular exercise and activity will strengthen muscles, improve balance, and increase bone density. Increased physical conditioning reduces the risk for falls and limits injury that is sustained when a fall occurs.

Fall risk can be reduced if the patient uses appropriate aids to promote visual and auditory orientation to the environment. Poor vision can greatly increase fall risk.

The use of gait belts by all health care providers can promote safety when assisting patients with transfers from bed to chair. Canes, walkers, and wheelchairs can provide the patient with improved stability and balance when ambulating. Raised toilet seats can facilitate safe transfer on and off the toilet. QSEN: Teamwork and collaboration; Safety.

Actions/Interventions	Rationales
■ Provide high-risk patients with a hip pad.	These pads when properly worn may reduce a hip fracture should a fall occur.
■ Participate in national reporting initiatives, such as the American Nurses Association National Database of Nursing Quality Indicators.	These databases provide hospitals with the ability to view their fall and injury rates in relation to similar hospitals. QSEN: Evidence-based practice.

Education/Continuity of Care

Actions/Interventions	Rationales
■ Educate the patient and family caregivers about risk factors for falls in the home. Suggest home adaptations to increase safety.	Approximately 40% of older adults living in the community sustain at least one fall per year. Falls are the leading cause of accidental death in the home setting. Falls are frequently caused by hazards that are easy to fix. QSEN: Safety.
• Place bright, nonskid strips on the edges of stair treads. Install handrails on both sides of the stairs from top to bottom.	Older adults have problems differentiating shades of the same color and have diminished depth perception. These physiological changes make it difficult to see the edge of a stair tread that is a uniform color.
• Ensure that all rugs are securely fastened to the floor or removed.	Loose throw rugs increase the risk for slipping and falling.
• Install nonslip surfaces in tubs and showers. Place grab bars near the tub or shower and toilet. Consider use of a shower chair. Use soap on a rope to prevent dropping it.	Wet surfaces in bathrooms increase the risk for falls. Grab bars provide support when moving.
• Rearrange furniture to have a clear pathway between rooms, especially to the bathroom. Keep traffic patterns free of clutter and electrical cords.	People with diminished strength or who use mobility devices are less able to negotiate around obstacles in their path.
• Increase lighting at the top and bottom of stairs. Use night-lights in bathrooms, bedrooms, and hallways.	Older adults have poor vision at night and in dimly lit areas. Improved lighting reduces fall risk.
• Secure all handrails.	Handrails should be on both sides of the stairs and the length of the stairs.
• Rearrange items in kitchen so frequently used ones are in easy reach (waist level).	Easy access reduces temptation to stand on stools or chairs to secure needed items.
• Instruct to wear shoes both inside and outside the house.	Wearing slippers or going barefoot increases fall risk.
▲ Refer the family to community resources for assistance in making home safety modifications.	Many community service organizations provide financial assistance to help older adults make safety improvements in their homes.
■ Educate the patient and family caregivers about the correct use and maintenance of mobility assistive devices.	Incorrect use or improper maintenance of canes, walkers, and wheelchairs can increase the risk for falls. The devices need to be properly fitted to the patient. Falls can occur if brakes on wheelchairs are not used correctly. QSEN: Safety
■ Suggest the patient wear an alarm device in case of a fall.	A variety of devices are available to alert providers to come to the scene to assist a patient who falls and cannot get up. QSEN: Safety.

■ = Independent   ▲ = Interprofessional Collaboration

Actions/Interventions

- Instruct the patient and families in what to do after a fall.
  - If the patient has an obvious injury, notify medical assistance immediately.
  - If the patient has a significant blow to head or any loss of consciousness, initiate immediate medical assistance.
  - If the patient is on anticoagulant therapy but shows no signs of active bleeding, notify the health care provider.
  - If the patient is on anticoagulant therapy and there is active bleeding after fall, call 9-1-1.

Rationales

Prompt evaluation of the consequences of a fall will facilitate early treatment and minimize the risk of harm to the patient. QSEN: Safety.

NANDA-I
NDx **Interrupted Family Processes**

Definition: Change in family relationships and/or functioning

Interrupted family processes occur as a result of the inability of one or more members of the family to adjust or perform. The result of this inability to adjust is family dysfunction and an interruption in the development of the family. Family development is closely related to the developmental changes experienced by adult members. Over time, families must adjust to change within the family structure brought on by both expected and unexpected events, including illness or death of a member/changes in social or economic strengths precipitated by divorce, retirement, and loss of employment. The addition of new family members through birth or adoption may require adaptation to new roles and status for existing family members. Health care providers must also be aware of the changing constellation of families: gay couples raising children, single parents with children, older grandparents responsible for grandchildren or foster children, and other situations.

Common Related Factors

Developmental transitions
Developmental crisis
Situational transitions
Situational crisis
Alteration in family finances
Change in family social status
Power shift among family members
Shift in health status of a family member
Shift in family roles

Defining Characteristics

Change in communication patterns
Change in participation for decision-making
Decrease in available emotional support
Ineffective task completion
Change in expressions of conflict within family
Changes in expressions of conflict with or isolation from community resources
Alteration in family satisfaction
Decrease in mutual support

Common Expected Outcomes

Family develops improved methods of communication.
Family uses resources available for problem-solving.
Family expresses understanding of mutual problems.

NOC Outcomes
Family Coping; Family Functioning; Family Normalization
NIC Interventions
Coping Enhancement; Family Process Maintenance; Family Support

Ongoing Assessment

Actions/Interventions	Rationales
■ Assess for precipitating events (e.g., divorce, illness, life transition, crisis).	The Family Inventory of Life Events (FILE) is an assessment tool to identify recent family events. The data from this assessment may suggest the level of family stress. Depending on the stressor, a variety of strategies may be required to facilitate coping. QSEN: Evidence-based practice.
■ Assess family members' perceptions of the problem.	Resolution of family problems is possible if each person's perceptions are understood. Understanding another's perceptions can lead to clarification and problem-solving. A variety of standardized assessment tools are available to gather data about the perceptions of family members. QSEN: Patient-centered care.
■ Evaluate strengths, coping skills, and current support systems.	Genograms and ecomaps can be used as tools to help the family identify family structure, the strength of family relationships, sources of support, and use of community resources.
■ Assess the developmental level of family members.	The developmental stage of family members will influence family functioning. Developmental transitions may be a source of stress within the family.

Therapeutic Interventions

Actions/Interventions	Rationales
■ Provide opportunities for family members to express concerns, fears, expectations, or questions.	Providing such opportunities promotes communication among family members and may facilitate more effective coping. The feelings of one family member, such as loneliness, anger, or worry, may influence others in the family system.
■ Help family members perceive problems as "family" problems.	This approach promotes a sense of connectedness and reduces the tendency to blame individual family members. QSEN: Patient-centered care.
■ Encourage members to empathize with other family members.	Empathy can increase understanding of others' feelings and fosters mutual respect and support.
■ Assist the family in setting realistic goals and delineating responsibilities.	Setting realistic goals helps the family gain control over the situation. Clarification of family responsibilities can promote independence and a sense of autonomy.
■ Assist the family in breaking down problems into manageable parts.	Guiding them to view the problems in smaller parts may make the situation more tolerable.
■ Encourage family members to seek information and resources that increase coping skills.	Practical information and positive role models can be effective in helping family members develop new ways to adjust to changes and preserve family integrity.
▲ Consult with a social worker or family therapist.	Integrating the contributions of members of the interprofessional team helps the family develop and sustain new patterns of family interactions and problem-solving. QSEN: Teamwork and collaboration.

■ = Independent   ▲ = Interprofessional Collaboration

Education/Continuity of Care

Actions/Interventions

- Provide information regarding stressful situations, as appropriate (e.g., pattern of illness, time frames for recovery, expectations).
- Provide the family with information about community resources that may be helpful in the long term.

Rationales

Information helps the family understand what they are experiencing and gives them a window to future expectations.

Groups that come together for mutual support or information exchange (e.g., telephone hotlines, self-help groups, educational opportunities, social services agencies, counseling centers) can be beneficial helping the family dealing with particular situations.

Fatigue

Definition: An overwhelming sustained sense of exhaustion and decreased capacity for physical and mental work at the usual level

Fatigue is a subjective complaint with both acute and chronic illnesses. In an acute illness, fatigue may have a protective function that keeps the person from sustaining injury from overwork in a weakened condition. As a common symptom, fatigue is associated with a variety of physical and psychological conditions. Fatigue is a prominent finding in many viral infections such as hepatitis. Patients with rheumatoid arthritis, fibromyalgia, systemic lupus erythematosus, myasthenia gravis, and depression report fatigue as a profound symptom that reduces their ability to participate in their own care and fulfill role responsibilities. Fatigue has become the most common and distressing complaint for patients with cancer, especially during treatment. The patient with a chronic illness experiencing fatigue may be unable to work full-time and maintain acceptable performance on the job. The economic impact on the individual and the family can be significant. The social effects of fatigue occur as the person decreases his or her participation in social activities. Recently, attention has focused on sleep-disordered breathing as a cause for daytime somnolence, fatigue, and decreased alertness. Common screening methods are available.

Chronic fatigue syndrome is a poorly understood condition that is characterized by prolonged, debilitating fatigue, neurological problems, general pain, gastrointestinal problems, and flulike symptoms. Although the exact cause of chronic fatigue syndrome is not known, one theory suggests that the disorder may represent an abnormal response of the immune system to highly stressful physiological or psychological events. This illness is also known as "systemic exercise intolerance disease."

Common Related Factors

Sleep deprivation
Physical condition (e.g., disease states, anemia, pregnancy)
Physical deconditioning
Increase in physical exertion
Malnutrition
Chemotherapy/radiation therapy
Nonstimulating lifestyle
Stressors
Anxiety
Depression
Environmental barrier
Negative life event
Occupational demands

Defining Characteristics

Nonrestorative sleep patterns
Impaired ability to maintain usual level of physical activity
Impaired ability to maintain usual routines
Tiredness/lethargy
Drowsiness
Listlessness
Increase in rest requirements
Increase in physical complaints
Insufficient energy
Alteration in concentration
Guilt about difficulty maintaining responsibilities
Disinterest in surroundings

Common Expected Outcomes

Patient verbalizes reduction of fatigue as evidenced by reports of increased energy and ability to perform desired activities.

Patient demonstrates use of energy-conservation principles.

NOC Outcomes

Fatigue Level; Fatigue: Disruptive Effects; Activity Tolerance; Endurance; Energy Conservation; Self-Care: Activities of Daily Living (ADL)

NIC Interventions

Energy Management; Exercise Promotion; Nutrition Management; Sleep Enhancement

Ongoing Assessment

Actions/Interventions	Rationales
■ Assess the patient's description of fatigue: timing (afternoon versus all day), severity, relationship to activities and aggravating/alleviating factors.	Specific information about the patient's experience of fatigue can help the nurse develop an individualized approach. A quantitative rating scale (e.g., 0 to 10) can help the patient describe the amount of fatigue experienced. This method allows the nurse to compare changes in the patient's fatigue level over time. It is important to determine whether the patient's level of fatigue is constant or varies over time. QSEN: Patient-centered care.
■ Assess for possible causes of fatigue, such as: • Recent physical illness • Pain, especially chronic • Emotional stress/depression • Medication side effects • Anemia • Sleep disorders • Imbalanced nutritional intake • Increased responsibilities and demands at home or work	Etiological factors may be temporary or permanent, physical or psychological. Identifying the related factors with fatigue can aid in determining possible causes and establishing a collaborative care plan.
■ Assess the patient's ability to perform ADLs, instrumental activities of daily living (IADLs), and demands of daily living (DDLs).	Fatigue can limit the patient's ability to participate in self-care and perform his or her role responsibilities in the family and society, such as working outside the home. QSEN: Patient-centered care.
■ Assess the patient's emotional response to fatigue.	Fatigue is a very distressing symptom that significantly affects quality of life. Depending on the acute or chronic nature of the fatigue, anxiety and depression are common emotional responses associated with fatigue. These emotional states can add to the patient's fatigue level and create a vicious cycle. QSEN: Patient-centered care.
■ Evaluate the patient's routine prescription and over-the-counter medications.	Fatigue may be a medication side effect or an indication of a drug interaction. The nurse should give particular attention to the patient's use of beta-blockers, calcium channel blockers, tranquilizers, alcohol, muscle relaxants, and sedatives.
■ Assess the patient's nutritional intake of calories, protein, minerals, and vitamins.	Fatigue may be a symptom of protein-calorie malnutrition, vitamin deficiencies, or iron deficiencies.
■ Evaluate the patient's sleep patterns for quality, quantity, time taken to fall asleep, and feeling on awakening. Also assess for sleep apnea.	Changes in the patient's sleep pattern may be a contributing factor in the development of fatigue. The cycle of interrupted sleep results in reduced rapid eye movement (REM) sleep, which the body requires for rest and to replenish itself. Screening for sleep-disordered breathing may be indicated.

■ = Independent ▲ = Interprofessional Collaboration

Actions/Interventions

- Assess the patient's usual level of exercise and physical activity.
- Evaluate laboratory and diagnostic test results:
  - Blood glucose
  - Hemoglobin and hematocrit
  - Blood urea nitrogen
  - Oxygen saturation, resting and with activity
  - Thyroid-stimulating hormone
- Assess the patient's expectations for fatigue relief, willingness to participate in strategies to reduce fatigue, and level of family and social support.

Rationales

Both increased physical exertion and limited levels of exercise can contribute to fatigue.

Changes in these physiological measures can be compared with other assessment data to understand possible causes of the patient's fatigue.

Eliciting the patient's values, preferences, and expressed needs allows the patient to be a full partner in providing care. Social support will be necessary to help the patient implement changes to reduce fatigue. QSEN: Patient-centered care.

Therapeutic Interventions

Actions/Interventions

- Encourage the patient to keep a 24-hour fatigue and activity log for at least 1 week.

- Assist the patient with developing a schedule for daily activity and rest. Stress the importance of frequent rest periods.

- Minimize environmental stimuli, especially during planned times for rest and sleep.

- ▲ Teach energy-conservation techniques. Refer to an occupational therapist as needed.

- Implement the use of assistive and adaptive devices for ADLs and IADLs:
  - Long-handled sponge for bathing
  - Long shoehorn
  - Sock-puller
  - Long-handled grabber
- Assist the patient with setting priorities for desired activities and role responsibilities and refraining from performing nonessential activities.

- Promote adequate nutritional intake.

Rationales

Recognizing relationships between specific activities and levels of fatigue can help the patient identify excessive energy expenditure. The log may indicate times of day when the patient feels the least fatigued. This information can help the patient make decisions about arranging his or her activities to take advantage of periods of higher energy levels. QSEN: Patient-centered care.

A plan that balances periods of activity with periods of rest can help the patient complete desired activities without adding to levels of fatigue. Not all self-care activities need to be completed at one time, such as the morning. Likewise, not all housework needs to be completed in a day.

Bright lighting, noise, visitors, frequent distractions, and clutter in the patient's physical environment can inhibit relaxation, interrupt rest/sleep, and contribute to fatigue.

Patients and caregivers may need to learn skills for delegating tasks to others, setting priorities, and clustering care to use available energy to complete desired activities. Organization and time management can help the patient conserve energy and reduce fatigue. The occupational therapist can reinforce energy-conservation techniques and provide the patient with assistive devices as needed. QSEN: Patient-centered care.

The use of assistive devices can minimize energy expenditure and prevent injury with activities.

Setting priorities is one example of an energy-conservation technique that allows the patient to use available energy to accomplish important activities. Achieving desired goals can improve the patient's mood and sense of emotional well-being.

The patient will need properly balanced intake of fats, carbohydrates, protein, vitamins, and minerals to provide energy resources.

Actions/Interventions

- Encourage an exercise conditioning program as appropriate.

- Encourage the patient and family to verbalize feelings about the impact of fatigue.

Rationales

Fatigue caused by deconditioning and prolonged bed rest can be reduced through improved functional capacity using aerobic and muscle-strengthening exercise.

Acknowledgment that living with fatigue is both physically and emotionally difficult aids in coping. Fatigue can have a profound negative influence on family processes and social interaction. The type or duration of the fatigue experience (acute/temporary versus more chronic fatigue syndrome) affects the significance of any changing roles and responsibilities within the family unit.

Education/Continuity of Care

Actions/Interventions

- Teach the patient and family energy-conservation techniques and time-management strategies.
- Help the patient engage in increasing levels of physical activity and exercise.
- Teach the patient signs and symptoms of overexertion with activity.
- Help the patient develop habits to promote effective rest/sleep patterns.

Rationales

Organization and time management can help the patient conserve energy and prevent fatigue.

Exercise can help the patient build endurance for physical activity and subsequently reduce fatigue.

Changes in heart rate, oxygen saturation, and respiratory rate will reflect the patient's tolerance for activity.

Promoting relaxation before sleep and providing for several hours of uninterrupted sleep can contribute to energy restoration.

Related Care Plans

Insomnia, Chapter 2
Obstructive sleep apnea, Chapter 6

Fear

Definition: Response to perceived threat that is consciously recognized as a danger

Fear is a strong and unpleasant emotion caused by the awareness or anticipation of pain or danger. This emotion is primarily externally motivated and source-specific; that is, the individual experiencing the fear can identify the person, place, or thing precipitating this feeling. The factors that precipitate fear are, to some extent, universal; fears of death, pain, and bodily injury are common to most people. Other fears are derived from the life experiences of the individual person. How fear is expressed may be strongly influenced by the culture, age, or gender of the person under consideration. In some cultures it may be unacceptable to express fear regardless of the precipitating factors. Rather than manifesting outward signs of fear as described in the defining characteristics, responses may range from risk-taking behavior to expressions of bravado and defiance of fear as a legitimate feeling. In other cultures fear may be freely expressed and manifestations may

be universally accepted. In addition to one's own individual ways of coping with the feeling of fear, there are aspects of coping that are cultural as well. Some cultures control fear through the use of magic, mysticism, or religiosity. Whatever one's mechanism for controlling and coping with fear, it is a normal part of everyone's life. The nurse may encounter the fearful patient in the community, during the performance of diagnostic testing in an outpatient setting, or during hospitalization. The nurse must learn to identify when patients are experiencing fear and must find ways to assist them in a respectful way to negotiate these feelings. The nurse must also learn to identify when fear becomes so persistent and pervasive that it impairs an individual's ability to carry on his or her activities of daily living. Under these circumstances, referral can be made to programs designed to assist the patient in overcoming phobias and other truly debilitating fears.

■ = Independent   ▲ = Interprofessional Collaboration

Nursing Diagnosis Care Plans

Common Related Factors

Unfamiliar setting
Separation from support system
Learned response
Language barrier
Sensory deficit (e.g., visual, hearing)
Phobic stimulus
Anticipation of pain
Anticipation or perceived physical threat or danger

Defining Characteristics

Identifies object of fear
Focus narrowed to the source of the fear
Change in physiological response (increased BP, HR, and respiratory rate)
Dry mouth
Nausea
Increase in tension
Jitteriness
Apprehensiveness
Impulsiveness
Increase in alertness
Avoidance behavior

Common Expected Outcomes

Patient avoids source of fear if possible.
Patient uses effective coping strategies to reduce fear response.
Patient verbalizes or manifests a reduction or absence of fear.

NOC Outcomes
Fear Self-Control; Coping
NIC Interventions
Anxiety Reduction; Emotional Support

Ongoing Assessment

Actions/Interventions	Rationales
■ Assess the nature of the patient's fear by careful, thoughtful questioning and active listening.	The external source of fear can be identified. Patients who find it unacceptable to express fear may find it helpful to know that someone is willing to listen if they decide to share their feelings at some time in the future. QSEN: Patient-centered care.
■ Assess the measures the patient uses to cope with that fear.	This information helps determine the effectiveness of coping strategies used by the patient.
■ Assess the behavioral and verbal expression of fear.	The nurse interprets behavioral and verbal cues from the patient to determine the patient's fears. Physiological symptoms/complaints intensify as the level of fear increases. Manifestations of fear are similar to those of anxiety. This information provides a basis for planning interventions to support the patient's coping strategies.
■ Determine to what degree the patient's fears may be affecting his or her ability to perform ADLs.	Persistent, immobilizing fears may require treatment with anti-anxiety medications or referral to specially designed treatment programs. Patient safety must always be a priority.

Therapeutic Interventions

Actions/Interventions	Rationales
■ Acknowledge awareness of the patient's fear.	This approach validates the feelings the patient is having and communicates an acceptance of those feelings.
■ Confirm that fear is a normal and appropriate response to situations in which pain, danger, or loss of control is anticipated or experienced.	This reassurance places fear within the scope of normal human experiences.
■ Stay with the patient to promote safety, especially during frightening procedures or treatments.	The presence of a trusted person increases the patient's sense of security and safety during a period of fear.

Actions/Interventions

- Maintain a calm and accepting manner while interacting with the patient.
- Orient the patient to the environment as needed.

- Use simple language and brief statements when instructing the patient regarding diagnostic and surgical procedures. Explain what physical or sensory sensations will be experienced.
- Reduce sensory stimulation by maintaining a quiet environment, whether in the hospital or home situation. Remove unnecessary threatening equipment.

- Provide safety measures within the home when indicated (e.g., alarm system, safety devices in showers or bathtubs).
- Assist the patient in identifying strategies used in the past to deal with fearful situations.

- As the patient's fear subsides, encourage him or her to explore specific events preceding the onset of the fear.
- Encourage rest periods.

- When the patient must be hospitalized or away from home, suggest bringing in comforting objects from home (e.g., music, pillow, blanket, pictures).
- ▲ Refer the patient/family to the interprofessional health team (e.g., spiritual counselor, social worker).

Rationales

The patient's feeling of stability increases in a calm and non-threatening atmosphere.
Orientation to and familiarity with the environment promote comfort and may decrease fear experienced by the patient.
When experiencing excessive fear or dread, the patient may be unable to comprehend more than simple, clear, and brief instructions. Repetition may be necessary.

Fear may escalate with excessive conversation, noise, and equipment around the patient. Even though the staff or caregiver may be comfortable around high-tech or medical equipment, the patient may not be. QSEN: Safety.
If the home environment is unsafe, the patient's fears are not resolved and fear may become disabling.
This measure helps the patient focus on fear as a real and natural part of life that has been and can continue to be dealt with successfully.
Recognition and explanation of factors leading to fear are significant in developing alternative responses.
Rest improves ability to cope. The interprofessional health care team will need to pace activities (especially for older adults) in order to conserve the patient's energy and offset fatigue.
Familiar objects in a new environment can enhance feelings of security.

Integrating the contributions of members of the interprofessional team helps the patient and family achieve health goals and allows for shared decision-making to achieve quality patient care. QSEN: Teamwork and collaboration.

Education/Continuity of Care

Actions/Interventions

- Teach the patient about using the following self-calming measures to reduce fear or make it more manageable:

  - Breathing modifications

  - Progressive relaxation, meditation, or guided imagery

  - Positive self-affirmations and calming self-talk

- Instruct the patient in the use of physician-ordered antianxiety medications.

- ▲ Initiate alternative therapies.

- Caution the patient against the use of illicit drugs or the overuse of alcohol to deal with fearful feelings.

Rationales

Educating the patient and significant others about anticipatory coping mechanisms will focus energy on prevention with opportunity for growth rather than reaction to the identified fear.
Controlled, rhythmic breathing can promote relaxation and feelings of being in control.
These activities reduce the physiological response to fear (i.e., increased BP, pulse, respiration).
These enhance the patient's sense of confidence and reassurance.
Short-term use of antianxiety medications can enhance patient coping and reduce physiological manifestations of fear.
Measures such as meditation, prayer, music, and Therapeutic Touch may help alleviate fear and promote calm.
Abuse of drugs and alcohol limits the effectiveness of the patient's coping ability.

■ = Independent   ▲ = Interprofessional Collaboration

Actions/Interventions

■ Encourage an increase in patient and family participation in care.

Rationales

Participation in care assists in coping and may increase a sense of control.

Related Care Plan

Anxiety, Chapter 2

NANDA-I
NDx **Deficient Fluid Volume**

Definition: Decreased intravascular, interstitial, and/or intracellular fluid. This refers to dehydration, water loss alone without change in sodium

Fluid volume deficit, or hypovolemia, occurs from a loss of body fluid or the shift of fluids into the third space, or from a reduced fluid intake. Common sources for fluid loss are the gastrointestinal tract, polyuria, and increased perspiration. Fluid volume deficit may be an acute or chronic condition managed in the hospital, outpatient center, or home setting. The therapeutic goal is to treat the underlying disorder and return the extracellular fluid compartment to normal. Treatment consists of restoring fluid volume and correcting any electrolyte imbalances. Early recognition and treatment are paramount to prevent potentially life-threatening hypovolemic shock. Older patients are more likely to develop fluid imbalances.

Common Related Factors

Active fluid loss (diuresis, abnormal drainage or bleeding, diarrhea)
Compromised regulatory mechanisms
Inadequate fluid intake
Increased metabolic rate (fever, infection)
Fluid shifts (edema or effusions)

Defining Characteristics

Decrease in urine output (less than 30 mL/hr)
Increase in urine concentration (specific gravity > 0.125)
Sudden weight loss
Decrease venous filling
Increase in hemoglobin
Decrease in BP/orthostasis
Thirst
Tachycardia/weak, rapid HR
Alteration in skin turgor
Dry mucous membranes
Weakness
Alteration in mental state

Common Expected Outcome

Patient is normovolemic as evidenced by systolic BP greater than or equal to 90 mm Hg (or patient's baseline), absence of orthostasis, HR 60 to 100 beats/min, urine output greater than 30 mL/hr, and normal skin turgor.

NOC Outcomes
Fluid Balance; Hydration
NIC Interventions
Fluid Monitoring; Fluid Management; Fluid Resuscitation

Ongoing Assessment

| **Actions/Interventions** | **Rationales** |

Actions/Interventions

■ Obtain a patient history to ascertain the probable cause of the fluid disturbance.

■ Assess, or instruct the patient to monitor weight daily and consistently, with the same scale and preferably at the same time of day (before breakfast) and wearing the same amount of clothing.

■ Evaluate fluid status in relation to dietary intake. Determine whether the patient has been on fluid restriction.

■ Monitor and document BP and HR.

■ Monitor BP for orthostatic changes (changes seen when changing from supine to standing position). Monitor HR for orthostatic changes as reflected by a 20-mm Hg drop in systolic BP and a 10 mm Hg drop in diastolic BP.

■ Assess skin turgor and oral mucous membranes for signs of dehydration.

■ Assess the color and amount of urine. Report urine output less than 30 mL/hr for 2 consecutive hours.

■ Monitor temperature.

■ Monitor active fluid loss from wound drainage, tubes, diarrhea, bleeding, and vomiting; maintain accurate input and output record.

▲ Monitor serum electrolytes and urine osmolality, and report abnormal values.

■ Monitor for changes in mental status.

■ Evaluate whether the patient has any related heart problem before initiating parenteral therapy.

Rationales

Such information can help guide interventions. Causes may include acute trauma and bleeding, reduced fluid intake from changes in cognition, large amount of drainage after surgery, or persistent diarrhea. QSEN: Patient-centered care.

Instruction facilitates accurate measurement and assessment provides useful data for comparisons and helps in following trends.

Most fluid enters the body through drinking, water in foods, and water formed by oxidation of foods. For some older adult patients fluids may be purposely restricted to avoid problems with incontinence.

Reduction in circulating blood volume can cause hypotension and tachycardia. The change in HR is a compensatory mechanism to maintain cardiac output. Usually the pulse is weak and may be irregular if electrolyte imbalance also occurs. Hypotension is evident in hypovolemia.

Effective attention to these assessments reduces the risk of harm to the patient. Postural hypotension is a common manifestation in fluid loss. The incidence increases with age. Note the following orthostatic hypotension significance:
- Greater than 10 mm Hg drop: circulating blood volume is decreased by 20%.
- Greater than 20 to 30 mm Hg drop: circulating blood volume is decreased by 40%.
- Orthostatic hypotension caused by volume depletion is associated with a compensatory increase in HR (more than 20 beats/min). QSEN: Safety.

Loss of interstitial fluid causes loss of skin turgor. Assessment of skin turgor in older adults is less accurate because the skin normally loses its elasticity. Therefore skin turgor assessed over the sternum or the forehead is best. Several longitudinal furrows and coating may be noted along the tongue.

Concentrated urine denotes fluid deficit.

Febrile states further decrease body fluids through perspiration and increased respiration.

Fluid loss from wound drainage, diarrhea, bleeding, and vomiting causes decreased fluid volume and can lead to dehydration.

Elevated blood urea nitrogen suggests fluid deficit. Urine specific gravity is likewise increased (>0.125).

Dehydration may alter mental status, especially among older adults. Manifestations may include restlessness, anxiety, lethargy, and confusion.

Cardiac and older patients are often susceptible to fluid volume deficit and dehydration as a result of minor changes in fluid volume. They also are susceptible to the development of pulmonary edema.

■ = Independent ▲ = Interprofessional Collaboration

Actions/Interventions

- Determine the patient's fluid preferences: type, temperature (hot or cold).

- During treatment, monitor closely for signs of circulatory overload (headache, flushed skin, tachycardia, venous distention, elevated CVP, shortness of breath, increased BP, tachypnea, cough).

▲ If hospitalized, monitor hemodynamic status, including CVP, pulmonary artery diastolic pressure, pulmonary capillary wedge pressure, and cardiac output/cardiac index if available.

Rationales

Selecting those fluids that the patient enjoys drinking can facilitate replacement therapy. QSEN: Patient-centered care.

Close monitoring for responses during therapy reduces complications associated with fluid replacement. QSEN: Safety.

These direct measurements serve as optimal guides for therapy. Attention to these parameters reduces the risk of harm to the patient. QSEN: Safety

---

Therapeutic Interventions

Actions/Interventions

▲ Encourage the patient to drink prescribed fluid amounts.

- Assist the patient if unable to eat without assistance, and encourage the caregiver to assist with feedings, as appropriate.
- Provide oral hygiene.

For more severe hypovolemia:

▲ Insert an IV catheter to maintain IV access.

▲ Administer parenteral fluids as ordered. Anticipate the need for an IV fluid challenge with immediate infusion of fluids for patients with abnormal vital signs.

▲ Administer blood products as prescribed.

▲ Assist the physician with insertion of a central venous line and arterial line, as indicated.

▲ Maintain IV flow rate. If signs of fluid overload occur, stop the infusion and have the patient sit up or dangle the legs.

▲ Institute measures to control excessive electrolyte loss (e.g., resting the gastrointestinal tract, administering antipyretics, as ordered). For hypovolemia resulting from severe diarrhea or vomiting, administer antidiarrheal or antiemetic medications as prescribed, in addition to IV fluids.

▲ Once ongoing fluid losses have stopped, begin to advance the diet in volume and composition.

Rationales

Oral fluid replacement is indicated for mild fluid deficit and is a cost-effective method for replacement treatment. Older patients have a decreased sense of thirst and may need ongoing reminders to drink. Being creative in selecting fluid sources (e.g., flavored gelatin, frozen juice bars, sports drink) can facilitate fluid replacement. Oral rehydration solutions (e.g., Rehydralyte, Gatorade, Pedialyte) can be considered as needed.

Dehydrated patients may be weak and unable to meet prescribed intake independently.

Fluid deficit can cause a dry, sticky mouth. Attention to mouth care promotes interest in drinking and reduces discomfort of dry mucous membranes.

Parenteral fluid replacement is indicated to prevent or treat hypovolemic complications.

Fluids are needed to maintain hydration states. Determination of the type and amount of fluid to be replaced and infusion rates will vary depending on clinical status.

Blood transfusions may be required to correct fluid loss from active gastrointestinal bleeding.

A central venous line allows fluids to be infused centrally and for the monitoring of CVP and fluid status. An arterial line allows for the continuous monitoring of BP.

Close monitoring of fluid prevents iatrogenic volume overload. Older patients are especially susceptible to fluid overload. Upright positioning decreases venous return and optimizes breathing. QSEN: Safety.

Fluid losses from diarrhea should be concomitantly treated with antidiarrheal medications, as indicated. Antipyretics can reduce fever and associated fluid losses from diaphoresis.

Addition of fluid-rich foods can enhance continued interest in eating.

Education/Continuity of Care

Actions/Interventions

- Describe or teach causes of fluid losses or decreased fluid intake.
- Explain or reinforce the rationale for and intended effect of the treatment program. Inform the patient or caregiver of the importance of maintaining the prescribed fluid intake and special diet.
- Teach interventions to prevent future episodes of inadequate intake.

- If patients are to receive IV fluids at home, instruct the caregiver in managing IV equipment. Allow sufficient time for return demonstration.

- ▲ Refer to a home health agency as appropriate.

Rationales

Increasing the patient's knowledge level will assist in preventing and managing the problem.

Follow-up care will be the patient's/caregiver's responsibility. Information is needed for making correct choices. QSEN: Patient-centered care.

Patients need to understand the importance of drinking extra fluid during bouts of diarrhea, fever, and other conditions causing fluid deficits.

Responsibility for maintaining venous access sites and IV supplies may be overwhelming for the caregiver. In addition, older caregivers may not have the cognitive ability or manual dexterity required for this therapy.

Continuity of care is facilitated through the use of community resources.

Related Care Plan

Shock, hypovolemic, Chapter 5

NANDA-I

Excess Fluid Volume

Definition: Increased isotonic fluid retention

Fluid volume excess, or hypervolemia, occurs from an increase in total body sodium content and an increase in total body water. This fluid excess usually results from compromised regulatory mechanisms for sodium and water as seen in heart failure (HF), kidney failure, and liver failure. It may also be caused by excessive intake of sodium from foods, IV solutions, medications, or diagnostic contrast dyes. Hypervolemia may be an acute or chronic condition managed in the hospital, outpatient center, or home setting. The therapeutic goal is to treat the underlying disorder and return the extracellular fluid compartment to normal. Treatment consists of fluid and sodium restriction and the use of diuretics. For acute cases, ultrafiltration or dialysis may be required.

■ = Independent   ▲ = Interprofessional Collaboration

Common Related Factors

Excessive fluid intake
Excessive sodium intake
Compromised regulatory mechanisms (e.g., renal insufficiency or failure, systemic and metabolic abnormalities, endocrine abnormalities)
Low protein intake or malnutrition

Defining Characteristics

Weight gain over a short period of time
Edema
Intake exceeds output
Changes in urine specific gravity (<1.010)
Tachycardia
Oliguria
Orthopnea/dyspnea
Adventitious breath sounds: crackles
Alteration in respiratory pattern
Presence of third heart sound (S₃)
Alteration in BP
Jugular vein distention
Increased CVP
Increased pulmonary artery diastolic pressure
Alteration in mental status
Azotemia
Electrolyte imbalance
Decreased Hgb or Hct
Restlessness and anxiety

Common Expected Outcome

Patient is normovolemic as evidenced by urine output greater than or equal to 30 mL/hr, balanced intake and output, stable weight (or loss attributed to fluid loss), absence or reduction of edema, HR 60 to 100 beats/min, and absence of pulmonary crackles.

NOC Outcomes
Fluid Balance; Cardiopulmonary Status
NIC Interventions
Fluid Monitoring; Fluid Management

Ongoing Assessment

Actions/Interventions	Rationales
■ Obtain a patient history to ascertain the probable cause of the fluid disturbance.	History may include increased fluids or sodium intake, medical conditions that cause the abnormal retention of fluids (e.g., heart failure, renal failure), or shifts between the interstitial space and plasma. QSEN: Patient-centered care.
■ Assess, or instruct the patient to monitor weight daily and consistently with the same scale, preferably at the same time of day and wearing the same amount of clothing.	Instruction facilitates accurate measurement and helps follow trends. Sudden weight gain may indicate fluid retention. Different scales or heavier/lighter clothing may show false weight fluctuations.
■ Monitor for a significant weight change (2 pounds in 1 day).	Body weight is a more sensitive indicator of fluid or sodium retention than intake and output. A 2- to 3-pound increase in weight normally indicates a need to adjust fluid or diuretic therapy; 2.2 pounds (1 kg) is equivalent to 1 L of fluid.
■ Monitor input and output closely.	Although overall fluid intake may be adequate, shifting of fluid out of the intravascular to the extravascular spaces may result in dehydration. The risk for this occurring increases when diuretics are given. Patients may use diaries for home assessment.

Actions/Interventions	Rationales
■ Evaluate weight in relation to nutritional status.	In some patients with heart failure, weight may be a poor indicator of fluid volume status. Poor nutrition and decreased appetite over time result in a decrease in weight, which may be accompanied by fluid retention even though the net weight remains unchanged.
■ If the patient is on fluid restriction, review the daily log or chart for recorded intake.	Patients should be reminded to include items that are liquid at room temperature such as gelatin, sherbet, soup, and frozen juice pops.
■ Monitor and document BP and HR.	Sinus tachycardia and increased BP are seen in early stages. Older patients have a reduced response to catecholamines; thus their response to fluid overload may be blunted, with less increase in HR.
■ Monitor for distended neck veins and ascites. Monitor abdominal girth to follow any ascites accurately.	Distended neck veins are caused by elevated CVP pressure. Ascites occurs when fluid accumulates in extravascular spaces.
■ Auscultate for S_3, and assess for bounding peripheral pulses.	These assessment findings are signs of fluid overload.
■ Assess for crackles in the lungs, changes in respiratory pattern, shortness of breath, and orthopnea.	These signs are caused by accumulation of fluid in the lungs.
■ Assess for the presence of edema by palpating over the tibia, ankles, feet, and sacrum.	Edema occurs when fluid accumulates in the extravascular spaces. Dependent areas more readily exhibit signs of edema formation. Edema is graded from trace (indicating barely perceptible) to 4 (severe edema). Pitting edema is manifested by a depression that remains after one's finger is pressed over an edematous area and then removed. Measurement of an extremity with a measuring tape is another method of following edema.
▲ Monitor chest x-ray reports.	As interstitial edema accumulates, the x-ray studies show cloudy white lung fields.
■ Evaluate urine output in response to diuretic therapy.	At home, the focus is on monitoring the response to the diuretics, rather than the actual amount voided. It is unrealistic to expect patients to measure each void. Therefore recording two voids versus six voids after a diuretic medication may provide more useful information. Fluid volume excess in the abdomen may interfere with absorption of oral diuretic medications. Medications may need to be given intravenously by a nurse in the home or outpatient setting.
■ Monitor for an excessive response to diuretics: 2-pound loss in 1 day, hypotension, weakness, blood urea nitrogen elevated out of proportion to serum creatinine level.	Significantly increased response to diuretic therapy can result in fluid deficit and electrolyte imbalances.
▲ Monitor serum electrolytes, urine osmolality, and urine specific gravity.	All are indicators of fluid status and guide therapy. Urine specific gravity readings of less than 1.010 indicate dilute urine.
■ Assess the need for an external or indwelling urinary catheter.	Treatment focuses on diuresis of excess fluid. Urinary catheters provide a more accurate measurement of the response to diuretics.
▲ If hospitalized, monitor hemodynamic status, including CVP, pulmonary artery diastolic pressure, and pulmonary capillary wedge pressure, if available.	Attention to these parameters reduces the risk of harm to the patient. QSEN: Safety.

■ = Independent   ▲ = Interprofessional Collaboration

Therapeutic Interventions

Actions/Interventions	Rationales
▲ Institute and instruct the patient/caregiver regarding fluid restrictions, as appropriate.	Fluid restrictions help reduce extracellular volume. For some patients, fluids may need to be restricted to 1000 mL/day. Information is key for patients who will be co-managing fluids.
■ Provide innovative techniques for monitoring fluid allotment at home. For example, suggest that patients measure out and pour into a large pitcher the prescribed daily fluid allowance (e.g., 1000 mL).	This will provide a visual guide for how much fluid is still allowed throughout the day, enhancing compliance with the regimen.
▲ Restrict sodium intake as prescribed.	Restriction of sodium intake assists in decreasing fluid retention. Diets containing 2 to 3 g of sodium are usually prescribed.
▲ Administer or instruct the patient to take diuretics as prescribed.	Diuretics aid in the excretion of excess body fluids. Diuretic therapy may include several different types of agents for optimal therapy, depending on the acuteness or chronicity of the patient's problem.
■ Elevate edematous extremities, and handle with care.	Elevation increases venous return to the heart and, in turn, decreases edema. Edematous skin is more susceptible to injury.
■ Anticipate interventions related to specific etiological factors (e.g., inotropic medications for heart failure, paracentesis for liver disease).	Knowledge of etiological factors provides direction for subsequent interventions.

For acute cases:

Actions/Interventions	Rationales
▲ Consider admission to an acute care setting for hemofiltration or ultrafiltration.	These therapies are very effective methods to draw off excess fluid.
▲ Collaborate with the pharmacist to maximally concentrate IV fluids and medications.	Concentration decreases unnecessary fluids. QSEN: Teamwork and collaboration.
■ Apply a heparin lock device.	This device maintains IV access and patency but decreases fluid delivered to the patient in a 24-hour period.
▲ Administer IV fluids through an infusion pump, if possible.	Pumps ensure accurate delivery of IV fluids. Effective use of this strategy reduces the risk of harm to the patient. QSEN: Safety.
■ Position the patient in a semi-Fowler's or high-Fowler's position.	Elevating the head of the bed allows for ease in breathing.
■ Assist with repositioning every 2 hours if the patient is not mobile.	Repositioning prevents fluid accumulation in dependent areas.

Education/Continuity of Care

Actions/Interventions	Rationale
■ Teach causes of fluid volume excess to the patient or caregiver.	Information is key to managing problems.
■ Provide information as needed regarding the patient's medical diagnosis (e.g., heart failure, renal failure).	Patients are better able to ask questions and seek assistance when they know basic information about their condition.
■ Explain or reinforce the rationale and intended effect of the treatment program.	Follow-up care will be the patient's and/or caregiver's responsibility. Information is needed for making correct choices. QSEN: Patient-centered care.
■ Teach signs and symptoms of fluid volume excess and symptoms to report.	Patients must have information to make correct choices regarding future treatments. QSEN: Safety.
■ Instruct the patient to avoid medications that may cause fluid retention, such as over-the-counter NSAIDs, certain vasodilators, and steroids.	Thorough understanding of specific causes, such as medication side effects, is necessary for appropriate follow-up of treatment.

Actions/Interventions

- Instruct in the need for antiembolic stockings or bandages, as ordered.
- Explain the importance of maintaining proper nutrition, hydration, and diet modifications.

Rationale

These aids help promote venous return and minimize fluid accumulation in the extremities.

Knowledge enhances compliance with the treatment plan.

NANDA-I

NDx Frail Elderly Syndrome

Definition: Dynamic state of unstable equilibrium that affects the older individual experiencing deterioration in one or more domain of health (physical, functional, psychological, or social) and leads to increased susceptibility to adverse health effects, in particular disability

Frail elderly syndrome is a progressive condition that has both biological and psychosocial contributing factors. The biological factors include weight loss, decreased physical activity, impaired mobility, and fatigue/weakness. The psychosocial factors associated with frail elderly syndrome are a decrease in the patient's social support network, reduced effectiveness of coping skills, and an increase in psychological stressors. When the deficits associated with frail elderly syndrome are combined with the normal physiological processes of aging, the older adult has an increased risk for disability and mortality. This increased disability risk is manifested as increased falls, decreased self-care ability with ADLs, institutionalization, and reduced life span. Frail elderly syndrome is considered a reversible condition that exists on a continuum of hardiness (nonfrail) to frailness. The older adult may experience variability on this continuum on a day-to-day basis. The goal of nursing interventions for frail elderly syndrome is to help the older adult minimize the loss of independence, promote health, and prevent disability.

Common Related Factors

Alteration in cognitive functioning
Chronic illness
History of falls
Living alone
Malnutrition
Prolonged hospitalization
Psychiatric disorder
Sarcopenia
Sarcopenic obesity
Sedentary lifestyle

Defining Characteristics

Activity intolerance
Self-care deficits: bathing, dressing, feeding, toileting
Decreased cardiac output
Fatigue
Hopelessness
Imbalanced nutrition: less than body requirements
Impaired memory
Impaired physical mobility
Impaired walking
Social isolation

Common Expected Outcomes

Patient achieves an extended time of independence in his/her preferred home/care setting.
Patient uses appropriate adaptive resources and environmental modifications to maintain safety and independence with ADLs and ambulation.

NOC Outcomes

Personal Health Status; Self-Management: Chronic Illness; Nutritional Status: Nutrient Intake; Weight Maintenance Behavior; Exercise Participation

NIC Interventions

Nutrition Management; Energy Management; Self-Care Assistance; Exercise Promotion: Strength Training

■ = Independent   ▲ = Interprofessional Collaboration

Nursing Diagnosis Care Plans

Ongoing Assessment

Actions/Interventions	Rationales
■ Review the patient's health history for risk factors of frailty.	Multiple chronic illnesses, especially those that include cognitive impairment and depression, falls, or polypharmacy are associated with an increased risk for frailty.
■ Assess the patient's response to medications including side effects and therapeutic effects.	Frailty alters drug pharmacokinetics and pharmacodynamics associated with decreased serum albumin, decreased cellular drug receptors, and a compromised blood-brain barrier. The distribution of fat-soluble drugs increases and results in a diminished drug effect because of a wider volume of distribution. The distribution of water-soluble drugs will be decreased. A decrease in serum albumin leads to more availability of unbound drug with an increased risk of adverse reactions and toxicity. Changes in the blood-brain barrier put the patient at risk for central nervous system side effects. Polypharmacy can be a major contributor to the manifestations of frailty in the older adult.
■ Assess the adequacy of the patient's nutritional intake of the following:	
• Carotenoids	Low levels of serum carotenoids are associated with increased risk for frailty in women.
• Protein	Protein intake may decrease with aging, especially in women. Many elderly patients do not consume an adequate amount of protein and are affected by a deficiency as evidenced by decreased immunity, decreased muscle function, decreased facilitation of biochemical reactions, decreased availability and action of hormonal proteins, and inability to maintain structure of the body.
• Folate	A decreased folate intake contributes to anemia as a risk for frailty.
• Vitamins C, D, and E	The risk for frailty increases with decreased intake of vitamins C, D, and E.
■ Assess the patient's mouth, teeth, facial muscles, and taste sensitivity.	Problems with chewing ability may contribute to a decreased intake of foods high in protein. The older adult may select foods easily chewed but with decreased amino acid content. Changes in taste sensitivity may lead the older adult to select sweet foods with minimal protein content.
■ Assess the patient's body weight.	A self-reported unintentional weight loss of more than 10 pounds in 1 year is considered a significant early indicator of the risk for frailty, especially in women.
■ Assess muscle size and grip strength.	Sarcopenia is an age-related decrease in muscle mass and increase in fat accumulation associated with the development of frailty in the elderly. Decreased grip strength is a moderately reliable indicator of decreased muscle mass and strength. Using a dynamometer, the average grip strength of an elderly woman is 18 to 25 kg and 27 to 39 kg for an elderly man. Loss of muscle mass and strength accounts for a reduction in mobility and an increased risk for falls and associated injuries such as fractures. QSEN: Patient-centered care.

Actions/Interventions

- Ask the patient about weakness or feeling exhausted with activity.

- Assess walking speed using the "Timed Get Up and Go" test.

- Ask the patient about his or her perception of the adequacy of a social support network and effectiveness of personal coping skills.

▲ Monitor RBC count, Hgb, and Hct.

▲ Monitor for the presence of serum inflammatory mediators such as interleukin 6 (IL-6), tumor necrosis factor-alpha (TNF-alpha), and/or C-reactive protein (CRP).

Rationales

Self-reports of exhaustion three to four times per week or most of the time are considered moderately reliable indicators of frailty. Low physical activity levels predispose the older adult to muscle atrophy and weakness. QSEN: Patient-centered care.

This test is considered an objective measure of functional status and fall risk compared to self-report scales of ADLs and instrumental activities of daily living (IADLs). The test measures the older adult's speed, agility, and balance when moving. The test begins with the patient seated in a chair. The patient wears normal footwear and may use the arms of the chair to get up and any support device (e.g., cane, walker, another person) normally used for walking. The nurse tells the patient to begin and starts a timer. The patient gets up from the chair, walks a distance of 10 feet, turns around, returns to the chair, and sits down. The timer is stopped when the patient sits down. A normal, healthy older adult usually completes this test in 10 seconds or less. Times within 11 to 20 seconds are appropriate for frail elderly. Older adults who take longer than 20 seconds to complete the test indicate a need for more mobility assistance and may be at higher risk for falls. QSEN: Evidence-based practice.

A decrease in the patient's social support network and coping effectiveness contributes to the development of frailty. The older adult who feels unable to cope effectively with psychological stressors is more likely to experience diminished self-esteem and less inner strength. QSEN: Patient-centered care.

Low RBC count, low Hgb, and low Hct indicate anemia. The Women's Health and Aging Study (WHAS) identified anemia as a risk for frailty. QSEN: Evidence-based practice.

An increase in these inflammatory mediators is predictive of sarcopenia. Research indicates a strong association with IL-6 and CRP as predictors of frailty and fatality in the elderly. Increased levels of IL-6 and TNF-alpha indicate an increase in catabolic activity. Sarcopenia develops when this catabolic change is combined with a reduction in anabolic activity from a decreased dietary protein intake. QSEN: Evidence-based practice.

Therapeutic Interventions

Actions/Interventions

- Provide the patient with 25 to 30 g of high-quality animal or plant-based protein with each meal.

Rationales

Essential amino acids (EAAs) from dietary protein stimulate muscle protein synthesis even without exercise. This serving size (about 3 oz of animal meat or fish) contains about 10 g of EAAs. Aging muscles are less able to synthesize protein with EAA intake less than 10 g.

■ = Independent   ▲ = Interprofessional Collaboration

Actions/Interventions

- Encourage the patient to maintain an oral hygiene regimen.

- Support the patient's use of adaptive devices for mobility and ADLs.

- Encourage the patient to develop a regular routine of exercise that includes:

  • Tai chi

  • Resistance training three times a week

- Encourage rest periods, especially before meals, ADLs, exercise sessions, and ambulation.

Rationales

Brushing and flossing twice a day promote integrity of the oral mucous membranes, gums, and teeth. Healthy dentition will contribute to improved nutritional intake, especially of protein.

The use of adaptive devices for mobility will minimize the impact of diminished physiological reserve. These devices help preserve the patient's mobility in his or her preferred living setting. The use of adaptive devices for ADLs promotes the older adult's independence with self-care activities for bathing, dressing, feeding, and toileting.

Exercises that involve strength and balance training can increase muscle strength and functional ability for the older adult. Increased physical activity helps the patient experience well-being and contributes to a sense of inner strength.

Tai chi involves slow, rhythmic movements. Research supports tai chi as a beneficial activity for older adults to improve balance and strength. QSEN: Evidence-based practice.

Resistance training exercises stimulate muscle growth of both type 1 muscle fibers for endurance and type 2 muscle fibers for strength. This type of activity reduces sarcopenia by increasing muscle mass. Resistance training includes weight lifting and weight-bearing exercises of the large skeletal muscle groups.

Weakness and fatigue are major biological factors for frailty. Rest between activities provides time for energy conservation and recovery.

Education/Continuity of Care

Actions/Interventions

- ▲ Refer patient and family members to the interprofessional health team for assistance with:

  • Case management

  • Financial resources

  • Legal resources

Rationales

The patient's loss of independence in managing needs places a burden on caregivers. QSEN: Teamwork and collaboration.

Family members often need to assume responsibility for coordination among multiple providers. Caregivers may begin to experience anger, depression, and a decreased quality of life.

Case management by a member of the interprofessional team helps the patient and family achieve health goals and allows for shared decision-making to achieve quality patient care.

The management of complex health needs may create an increased economic strain for the patient and family members. The family may need assistance coordinating health insurance resources to cover the cost of frequent hospitalizations and in-home care.

The patient and family members may need help creating legal documents for durable powers of attorney and advance directives.

ⓔvolve   **For additional care plans, go to http://evolve.elsevier.com/Gulanick/.**

Actions/Interventions

- Polypharmacy reduction

■ Teach the patient and family about modifications in the patient's living environment to promote safety, especially with mobility.

■ Teach the patient and family about assistive devices to promote independence with ADLs.

■ Teach the patient and family about activities that support the patient's inner strength such as interactions with others, setting one's own goals, and feeling useful to others.

Rationales

The updated Beers Criteria from the American Geriatrics Society provides evidence-based guidelines for making decisions about safe and appropriate use of medications in care of the older adult. Collaboration among members of the interprofessional team can reduce unnecessary or inappropriate medications used by the older adult. These changes in medications not only decrease costs but also decrease medication side effects that contribute to frailty. QSEN: Evidence-based practice; Teamwork and collaboration.

A variety of modifications can be made to the patient's environment that will promote increased physical activity and reduce the risk for falls. These modifications may include installing brighter lighting, adding handrails for stairs, putting nonslip surfaces in tubs/showers, and keeping pathways clear of clutter and obstacles. QSEN: Safety.

The use of assistive devices for that allow independence with ADLs promotes self-esteem for the older adult. These devices may minimize the weakness and fatigue that occurs with frailty. These assistive devices may include grab bars in the bathroom, a raised toilet seat, shower chair, hand held showerhead, wide-grip eating utensils and toothbrush, and clothing that is easy to put on and remove.

These activities provide the patient with a resource for focusing on his or her capacities despite the factors that contribute to frailty. Older adults who have meaningful interactions with others, especially at mealtimes, can improve their socialization and may have increased nutritional intake. When older adults are able to set goals for themselves they feel a sense of purpose and independence in being able to carry out what they have set out to do. Feeling needed by others helps the older adult build self-esteem. QSEN: Patient-centered care.

Related Care Plans

Activity intolerance, Chapter 2
Caregiver role strain, Chapter 2
Risk for falls, Chapter 2
Impaired physical mobility, Chapter 2
Impaired nutrition: less than body requirements,
    Chapter 2
Relocation stress syndrome, Chapter 2

■ = Independent ▲ = Interprofessional Collaboration

Nursing Diagnosis Care Plans

Impaired Gas Exchange

Definition: Excess or deficit in oxygenation and/or carbon dioxide elimination at the alveolar-capillary membrane

By the process of diffusion, the exchange of oxygen and carbon dioxide occurs in the alveolar-capillary membrane area. The relationship between ventilation (airflow) and perfusion (blood flow) affects the efficiency of the gas exchange. Normally a balance exists between ventilation and perfusion; however, certain conditions can offset this balance, resulting in impaired gas exchange. Altered blood flow from a pulmonary embolus, decreased cardiac output, or shock can cause ventilation without perfusion. Conditions that cause changes or collapse of the alveoli (e.g., atelectasis, pneumonia, pulmonary edema, and acute respiratory distress syndrome) impair ventilation. Other factors affecting gas exchange include high altitudes, hypoventilation, and altered oxygen-carrying capacity of the blood from reduced hemoglobin. Older patients have a decrease in pulmonary blood flow and diffusion as well as reduced ventilation in the dependent regions of the lung, where perfusion is greatest. Chronic conditions (e.g., COPD) put these patients at greater risk for hypoxia. Other patients at risk for impaired gas exchange include those with a history of smoking or pulmonary problems, obesity, prolonged periods of immobility, and chest or upper abdominal incisions.

Common Related Factors

Alveolar-capillary membrane changes
Ventilation-perfusion imbalance
Altered oxygen supply
Altered oxygen-carrying capacity of blood

Defining Characteristics

Confusion
Somnolence
Restlessness/irritability
Hypoxia/hypoxemia
Dyspnea
Abnormal ABG values
Abnormal breathing pattern (rate, depth, rhythm)
Tachycardia
Abnormal skin color (pale, dusky)

Common Expected Outcome

Patient maintains optimal gas exchange as evidenced by ABGs within the patient's usual range, alert responsive mentation or no further reduction in level of consciousness, relaxed breathing, and baseline HR for patient.

NOC Outcomes

Respiratory Status: Gas Exchange;
Cardiopulmonary Status

NIC Interventions

Respiratory Monitoring; Oxygen Therapy; Airway Management

Ongoing Assessment

Actions/Interventions

■ Assess respirations, noting the quality, rate, rhythm, depth, breathing effort, and use of accessory muscles.

■ Assess the lungs for areas of decreased ventilation and the presence of adventitious sounds.

Rationales

Patients will adapt their breathing patterns over time to facilitate gas exchange. Both rapid, shallow breathing patterns and hypoventilation affect gas exchange. Shallow, "sighless" breathing patterns after surgery (as a result of the effect of anesthesia, pain, and immobility) reduce lung volume and decrease ventilation. Hypoxia is associated with signs of increased breathing effort.

Changes in breath sounds may reveal the cause of impaired gas exchange. Diminished breath sounds are associated with poor ventilation.

 For additional care plans, go to http://evolve.elsevier.com/Gulanick/.

Nursing Diagnosis Care Plans

Actions/Interventions	**Rationales**
■ Assess for restlessness and changes in level of consciousness.	Restlessness and irritability are early indicators of development of further hypoxia and decreased perfusion to the brain; lethargy and somnolence are late signs. Cognitive changes may occur with chronic hypoxia.
■ Assess for signs and symptoms of atelectasis: diminished chest excursion, limited diaphragm excursion, bronchial or tubular breath sounds, crackles, and tracheal shift to affected side.	Collapse of alveoli increases shunting (perfusion without ventilation), resulting in hypoxemia.
■ Assess for signs and symptoms of pulmonary infarction: cough, hemoptysis, pleuritic pain, consolidation, pleural effusion, bronchial breath sounds, pleural friction rub, and fever.	Hypoxia results from increased dead space ventilation (ventilation without perfusion) and reflex bronchoconstriction in areas adjacent to the pulmonary infarct.
■ Monitor for changes in BP and HR.	With initial hypoxia and hypercapnia, BP, HR, and respiratory rate all increase. As the hypoxia and/or hypercapnia becomes severe, BP and HR decrease, and dysrhythmias may occur. Respiratory failure may ensue when the patient is unable to maintain the rapid respiratory rate.
■ Assess for headache, dizziness, lethargy, reduced ability to follow instructions, disorientation, and coma.	These are signs of hypercapnia as seen with elevated carbon dioxide levels in the blood. QSEN: Safety.
▲ Monitor ABGs, and note changes.	Increasing $Paco_2$ and decreasing Pao_2 are signs of respiratory acidosis and hypoxemia. As the patient's condition deteriorates, the respiratory rate will decrease and $Paco_2$ will begin to increase. Some patients, such as those with COPD, have a significant decrease in pulmonary reserves, and additional physiological stress may result in acute respiratory failure. QSEN: Safety.
▲ Use pulse oximetry to monitor oxygen saturation.	Pulse oximetry is a useful tool to detect changes in oxygenation. Oxygen saturation should be maintained at 90% or greater.
▲ Monitor the effects of position changes on oxygenation (ABGs, venous oxygen saturation [Svo_2], and pulse oximetry).	Upright and sitting positions optimize diaphragmatic excursions and lung perfusion. When the patient is positioned on one side, the affected area should not be dependent. Putting the most compromised lung areas in the dependent position (where perfusion is greatest) further increases ventilation and perfusion imbalances.
■ Assess the patient's nutritional status.	Obesity may restrict downward movement of the diaphragm, increasing the risk for atelectasis, hypoventilation, and respiratory infections. Work of breathing is increased in severe obesity as a result of the excessive weight of the chest wall. Hypercapnia and hypoxia result. Malnutrition may reduce respiratory mass and strength, affecting muscle function.
▲ Monitor Hgb levels.	Low levels reduce the uptake of oxygen at the alveolar-capillary membrane and oxygen delivery to the tissues.
■ Assess the skin, nail beds, and mucous membranes for pallor or cyanosis.	Cool, pale skin may be secondary to a compensatory vasoconstrictive response to hypoxemia. As oxygenation and perfusion become impaired, peripheral tissues become cyanotic.
▲ Monitor chest x-ray reports.	Chest x-ray studies reveal the etiological factors of the impaired gas exchange.
■ Assess the patient's ability to cough effectively to clear secretions. Note the quantity, color, and consistency of sputum.	Productive coughing is the most effective way to remove most secretions. Retained secretions impair gas exchange.

■ = Independent   ▲ = Interprofessional Collaboration

Actions/Interventions

■ Evaluate the patient's hydration status.

Rationales

Gas exchange may be impaired by overhydration (in conditions such as heart failure). In conditions associated with increased sputum production (e.g., pneumonia, COPD), insufficient hydration may reduce the ability to clear secretions.

Therapeutic Interventions

Actions/Interventions

■ Position the patient with proper body alignment for optimal respiratory excursion (if tolerated, head of bed at 45 degrees when supine).

■ Routinely check the patient's position so that he or she does not slump down in bed.
■ Position the patient to facilitate ventilation-perfusion matching when a side-lying position is used.

■ Change the patient's position every 2 hours.

■ Encourage or assist with ambulation as indicated.

▲ Maintain an oxygen administration device as ordered, attempting to maintain oxygen saturation at 90% or greater.
■ Avoid a high concentration of oxygen in patients with COPD unless ordered.

■ If the patient is allowed to eat, give oxygen to the patient but in a different manner (e.g., changing from mask to a nasal cannula).
▲ For patients who should be ambulatory, provide extension tubing or a portable oxygen apparatus.
■ Encourage slow deep breathing, using an incentive spirometer as indicated.
■ For postoperative patients, assist with splinting the chest.
■ Assist with coughing or suction as needed.

■ Provide reassurance and allay anxiety.

■ Pace activities and schedule rest periods to prevent fatigue. Assist with ADLs.

Rationales

Upright position allows for increased thoracic capacity and full descent of diaphragm, preventing the abdominal contents from crowding the lungs and preventing their full expansion.
Slumped positioning causes the abdomen to compress the diaphragm and limits full lung expansion.
When the patient is positioned on the side, the good side should be down (e.g., lung with pulmonary embolus or atelectasis should be up). When lung hemorrhage or abscess is present, the affected lung should be placed downward to avoid drainage to the healthy lung.
Repositioning facilitates secretion movement and drainage and decreases atelectasis.
Ambulation promotes lung expansion, facilitates secretion clearance, and stimulates deep breathing.
Supplemental oxygen may be required to maintain Pao_2 at an acceptable level.

Hypoxia stimulates the drive to breathe in the patient who chronically retains carbon dioxide. When administering oxygen, close monitoring is imperative to prevent unsafe increases in the patient's Pao_2, which could result in apnea. QSEN: Safety.
Eating is an activity, and more oxygen will be consumed than when the patient is at rest. Immediately after the meal, the original oxygen delivery system should be returned.
These measures may improve exercise tolerance by maintaining adequate oxygen levels during activity.
These techniques promote deep inspiration, which increases oxygenation and prevents atelectasis.
Splinting optimizes deep breathing and coughing efforts.
Coughing is an effective way to clear secretions. Suctioning removes secretions to maintain a patent airway, thereby enhancing oxygenation. However, excessive suctioning may lead to desaturation of the blood and impair gas exchange.
The presence of a trusted person may help the patient feel less threatened and can reduce anxiety, thereby reducing oxygen requirements. Anxiety increases dyspnea, respiratory rate, and work of breathing.
Activities will increase oxygen consumption and should be planned so the patient does not become hypoxic. Rest helps mobilize energy for more effective breathing and coughing efforts.

Actions/Interventions

▲ Administer medications as prescribed.

■ Anticipate the need for intubation and mechanical ventilation.

Rationales

The type depends on the etiological factors of the problem (e.g., antibiotics for pneumonia, bronchodilators for COPD, anticoagulants and thrombolytics for pulmonary embolus, analgesics for thoracic pain).

Early intubation and mechanical ventilation are recommended to prevent full decompensation of the patient. Mechanical ventilation provides supportive care to maintain adequate oxygenation and ventilation. QSEN: Safety.

Education/Continuity of Care

Actions/Interventions

■ Explain the need to pace activities and to avoid unnecessary tasks during the acute episode.
■ Teach the patient appropriate breathing and coughing techniques.
■ Instruct about medications: indications, dosage, frequency, side effects, and administration requirements. Include a review of metered-dose inhalers if applicable.
■ Explain the type of oxygen therapy being used and why its maintenance is important.
■ Teach the patient or caregivers the signs of early respiratory compromise and their appropriate management.

▲ Refer to home health services for nursing care or oxygen management as appropriate.
▲ For chronic respiratory disorders, refer for pulmonary rehabilitation.

Rationales

Energy conservation methods reduce fatigue, dyspnea, and oxygen consumption.
These techniques facilitate adequate air exchange and clearance of secretions.
Knowledge promotes safe and effective medication administration.

Issues related to home oxygen use, storage, or precautions need to be addressed for safe and effective treatment.
Early detection and treatment may reduce emergency department visits, hospitalizations, and mortality. Such instruction prevents delays in seeking help and facilitates appropriate management in life-threatening situations. QSEN: Safety.
Referral facilitates continuation of needed services.

Rehabilitation training decreases dyspnea and fatigue, and it increases exercise capacity and perception of control over condition. QSEN: Teamwork and collaboration.

NANDA-I NDx Grieving

Definition: A normal complex process that includes emotional, physical, spiritual, social, and intellectual responses and behaviors by which individuals, families, and communities incorporate an actual, anticipated, or perceived loss into their daily lives

Grieving is an individual's emotional response to a perceived or actual loss. Patients may experience grieving associated with the death of a loved one or loss of a body part. People grieve when they learn of a terminal diagnosis for themselves or a loved one. Patients and families may experience grieving as they face long-term illness or disability, divorce, loss of employment, or loss of home or personal possessions. Grief is an aspect of the human condition that touches every individual, but how an individual or a family system responds to loss and how grief is expressed vary widely. That process is strongly influenced by factors such as age, gender, and culture, as well as personal and intrafamilial reserves and strengths. The nurse will encounter the patient and family experiencing grief in the hospital setting, but increasingly, with more hospice and palliative care services provided in the community, the nurse will find patients struggling with these issues in their own homes, where professional help may be limited or fragmented. This care plan discusses measures the nurse can use to help the patient and family members begin the process of grieving. Additional interventions related to death and dying can be found in Chapter 4.

■ = Independent ▲ = Interprofessional Collaboration

Nursing Diagnosis Care Plans

Common Related Factors

Anticipatory loss of significant object (e.g., possession, job, status)
Anticipatory loss of significant other
Death of a significant other
Loss of significant object (e.g., possession, job, status, home, body part)

Defining Characteristics

Psychological distress
Anger/blaming
Alterations in sleep or dream patterns
Detachment/despair
Disorganization
Suffering
Finding meaning in a loss
Personal growth
Alteration in activity level
Alteration in immune functioning
Alteration in neuroendocrine functioning

Common Expected Outcome

Patient or family verbalizes feelings and establishes and maintains functional support systems.

NOC Outcomes

Psychosocial Adjustment: Life Change; Family Resiliency; Grief Resolution; Hope

NIC Interventions

Coping Enhancement; Grief Work Facilitation; Presence; Emotional Support

Ongoing Assessment

Actions/Interventions	Rationales
■ Identify behaviors suggestive of the grieving process.	Mourning is associated with the behavioral manifestation of grief. These behaviors, such as crying, loud vocalizations, or wide gestures of the hands or body are strongly influenced by factors such as age, gender, and culture. Bereavement is a broader concept that describes both the inner emotional and outward behavioral components of the grieving process. Grief is an individual and exquisitely personal experience. Identification of normal bereavement occurs within the context of a variety of cultural norms and spiritual beliefs for the patient and family. QSEN: Patient-centered care.
■ Assess the phase of grieving being experienced by the patient and significant others.	Although the process of grieving has been described as clearly defined phases, grief rarely manifests in a prescribed sequencing of feelings and experiences. Many theories offer explanations of the phases of grief. The commonalities among these theories include notification and shock, experience of the loss emotionally and cognitively, and reintegration. QSEN: Evidence-based practice.
	Initially, the patient may express surprise and disbelief with awareness of a loss. Sadness, despair, and other manifestations of emotional pain may develop as the patient experiences loss. The patient may take several months to adjust to the loss and return to normal daily functioning. Patients and their families revisit the phases of the grief process repeatedly.

Actions/Interventions	Rationales
■ Assess whether the patient and significant others differ in their stages of grieving.	Patients and family members may experience turbulent relationships, conflicts, and differences in expectations if they are at different phases of the grief process. People within the same family system may become impatient when others do not reconcile their feelings as quickly as they do. Older adults may take longer to reintegrate the loss and reconcile their grief.
■ Assess the patient's ability to make decisions.	Grief may limit cognitive skills needed for problem-solving and decision-making.
■ Identify the availability of support systems for the patient.	If the patient's main support is the object of perceived loss, the patient may need help in identifying other sources of support.
■ Identify the potential for a complicated grieving response.	Complicated grieving is more likely to occur in situations such as multiple losses, lack of social support, unresolved family relationships and issues, or losses as a result of violence (e.g., homicide, suicide, loss of home or job).
■ Evaluate the need for referral to social services, legal consultants, or support groups.	It may be helpful to have patients and family members associated with these supports as early as possible so that financial considerations and other special needs are taken care of before the anticipated loss occurs. For example, a person facing loss of home from mortgage foreclosure or bankruptcy may need help mobilizing legal and financial resources. QSEN: Teamwork and collaboration.

Therapeutic Interventions

Actions/Interventions	Rationales
■ Listen and encourage the patient or significant others to verbalize feelings.	Exploring issues in a nonthreatening manner will lead to informed decision-making and assist the patient and family in verbalization of the anticipated loss. Sharing feelings with a caring professional may help the patient find meaning in the experience of loss.
■ Help the patient and significant others share mutual fears, concerns, plans, and hopes for each other, including the patient.	Secrets are rarely helpful during these times of crisis. An open sharing and exchange of information makes it easier to address important issues and facilitates effective family process. They can be important and sometimes final opportunities for resolving conflict and issues. They can also be used as times for potential personal and intrafamilial growth.
■ Anticipate increased affective behavior.	All affective behavior may seem increased or exaggerated during this time. Older adults may exhibit a preoccupation with thoughts of the impending death and confusion, especially if multiple losses are anticipated. Defense mechanisms support coping until the patient is ready to acknowledge the pain of the loss. Displaced anger and hostility may occur when the loss does not occur as anticipated by those grieving. Regression may be an adaptive mechanism during this time.

■ = Independent ▲ = Interprofessional Collaboration

Actions/Interventions

- Reinforce the patient's efforts to go on with his or her life and normal ADLs.

- Offer encouragement; point out strengths and progress to date.

- Accept the need of the patient or family to deny loss as part of the normal grief process. Recognize the need of the patient or family to maintain hope for the future.

- Encourage significant others to maintain their own self-care needs for rest, sleep, nutrition, leisure activities, and time away from the patient.

- Recognize the patient's need to review (relive) the loss experience.

Rationales

Support from the nurse helps the patient and family understand the strength and the reserves that must be present for them to feel enabled to do this. This behavior is the same strength and reserve each of them will use to reconstitute their lives after the loss.

Patients often lose sight of their achievements while engaged in grief. When seen as a whole, the process of reorganization after a loss seems enormous, but reviewing the patient's progress toward that end is very helpful and provides perspective on the whole process.

The nurse needs to see these events as a time during which the individual or family member consolidates his or her strength to go on to the next stage of grief. Grief remains a highly dynamic and individualized process. They may continue to deny the inevitability of the loss as a means of maintaining some degree of hope. As the loss begins to manifest, the mourners start accepting aspects of the loss, piece by piece, until the whole is actually grasped. QSEN: Patient-centered care.

Somatic complaints often accompany mourning; changes in sleep and eating patterns and interruption of normal routines are a usual occurrence. Care should be taken to treat these symptoms so that emotional reconstitution is not complicated by illness.

Telling the event allows them an opportunity to hear it described and gain some perspective on the event. This is one way in which the patient or the family integrates the event into their experience.

Education/Continuity of Care

Actions/Interventions

- ▲ Refer the patient and family to community grief support groups.

- ▲ Refer the patient and family to the interprofessional team.

Rationales

Grief is a universal experience. Support in the grieving process will come in many forms. Patients and family members often find the support of others encountering the same experiences helpful.

The contributions of members of the interprofessional team helps the patient and family achieve health goals and allows for shared decision-making to move toward grief resolution. QSEN: Teamwork and collaboration.

Related Care Plans

Death and dying: end-of-life issues, Chapter 4
Complicated grieving, ⊖volve

Ineffective Health Maintenance

Definition: Inability to identify, manage, and/or seek help to maintain health

Ineffective health maintenance reflects a change in an individual's ability to perform the functions necessary to maintain health or wellness. That individual may already manifest symptoms of existing or impending physical ailment or display behaviors that are strongly or certainly linked to disease. The nurse's role is to identify factors that contribute to an individual's inability to maintain healthy behavior and implement measures that will result in improved health maintenance activities. The nurse may encounter these patients either in the hospital or in the community; the increased presence of the nurse in the community and home health settings improves the ability to assess patients in their own environment. Patients most likely to experience more than transient alterations in their ability to maintain their health are those whose age or infirmity (either physical or emotional) absorb much of their resources or those for whom the economic challenges of daily life negate an interest in personal health. The task before the nurse is to identify measures that will be successful in empowering patients to maintain their own health within the limits of their ability.

Common Related Factors

Alteration in cognitive functioning
Impaired decision-making
Ineffective coping strategies
Ineffective communication skills

Defining Characteristics

Insufficient knowledge about basic health practices
Absence of interest in improving health behaviors
Inability to take responsibility for meeting basic health practices
Insufficient social support
Pattern of lack of health-seeking behavior

Common Expected Outcomes

Patient demonstrates positive health maintenance behaviors as evidenced by keeping scheduled appointments, participating in smoking and substance abuse programs, making diet and exercise changes, improving home environment, and following treatment regimen.
Patient identifies available resources.
Patient uses available resources.

NOC Outcomes

Health Promoting Behavior; Health-Seeking Behavior; Social Support

NIC Interventions

Health System Guidance; Support System Enhancement; Discharge Planning; Health Screening; Risk Identification

Ongoing Assessment

Actions/Interventions	Rationales
■ Assess the patient's knowledge of health maintenance behaviors.	The health care provider needs to ensure that the patient has all of the information needed to make good lifestyle choices. Some patients may know that certain unhealthy behaviors can result in poor health outcomes but continue the behavior despite this knowledge. QSEN: Patient-centered care.
■ Assess the patient's health history over the past 5 years.	Assessment may give some perspective on whether poor health habits are recent or chronic in nature. History may also reflect multiple risk factors for health problems.
■ Assess to what degree environmental, social, intrafamilial disruptions, or changes have correlated with poor health behaviors.	These changes may be precipitating factors or may be early fallout from a generalized condition reflecting decline.

■ = Independent   ▲ = Interprofessional Collaboration

Actions/Interventions	Rationales
■ Determine the patient's specific questions related to health maintenance.	Patients may have health education needs; meeting these needs may be helpful in mobilizing the patient.
■ Determine the patient's motives for failing to report symptoms reflecting changes in health status.	The patient may not want to "bother" the provider, may minimize the importance of the symptoms, or may fear what may be discovered. Language barriers and poor access to care are other common reasons.
■ Discuss noncompliance with instructions or programs with the patient to determine the rationale for failure.	The patient may experience obstacles in compliance that can be resolved.
■ Assess the patient's educational preparation and ability to integrate and relate to information.	Patients may not have understood information because of a sensory impairment or the inability to read or understand information. Culture, literacy, language barriers, or age may impair a patient's ability to comply with the established treatment plan. Health literacy has become a patient safety issue.
■ Assess the history of other adverse personal habits, including smoking, obesity, lack of exercise, and alcohol or substance abuse.	Long-standing habits may be difficult to break; once they have been established, patients may feel that nothing positive can come from a change in behavior.
■ Determine whether the patient's manual dexterity or lack of mobility is a factor in the patient's altered capacity for health maintenance.	Patients may need assistive devices for ambulation or to complete tasks of daily living.
■ Determine to what degree the patient's cultural beliefs and personality contribute to altered health habits.	Health teaching may need to be modified to be consistent with cultural or religious beliefs.
■ Determine whether the required health maintenance facilities/equipment (e.g., access ramps, motor vehicle modifications, shower bar or chair) are available to the patient.	With adequate assistive devices, the patient may be able to effect enormous changes in maintaining his or her personal health.
■ Assess whether economic problems present a barrier to maintaining health behaviors.	Decreasing the number of uninsured is a key goal of the Affordable Care Act (2014) through the expansion of Medicaid eligibility and the establishment of health insurance Marketplaces to many low-income individuals. However, too many low-income working families remain uninsured, citing the high cost of insurance as a key reason for lack of coverage. Many people do not have access to coverage through a job, and some people live in states that did not expand Medicaid and remain ineligible for public and private coverage. Likewise, undocumented immigrants are ineligible for Medicaid or Marketplace coverage. QSEN: Patient-centered care.
■ Assess hearing and orientation to time, place, and person to determine the patient's perceptual abilities.	Perceptual handicaps may impair a patient's ability to maintain healthy behaviors.
■ Make a home visit to determine safety, accessibility, and quality of living conditions.	Home visits can help identify and solve problems that complicate health maintenance.
■ Assess the patient's experience of stress and disruptors as they relate to health habits.	If stressors can be relieved, patients may again be able to resume their self-care activities.

Therapeutic Interventions

Actions/Interventions	Rationales
■ Assist the patient with problem-solving–specific related factors as able.	Health maintenance is complicated because of the complexities of each individual's circumstance. A "one size fits all" approach will not work. QSEN: Patient-centered care.
■ Define your role as patient advocate.	The nurse is in an ideal position to guide the patient through the health care system.

Actions/Interventions

- Provide the patient with a means of contacting health care providers.

- Involve family and friends in health-planning conferences.

- Compliment the patient on positive accomplishments.

Rationales

Guidance will add available resources for questions or problem resolution. An ongoing relationship can establish trust and facilitate change.

Family members need to understand that care is planned to focus on what is most important to the patient. This enables the patient to maintain a sense of autonomy.

Positive reinforcement enhances behavior change. Patients with stronger self-efficacy are more likely to engage in positive behaviors.

Education/Continuity of Care

Actions/Interventions

- Provide the patient with a rationale for the importance of behaviors such as the following:
  - Proper nutrition

  - Regular exercise

  - Proper hygiene

  - Smoking cessation

  - Cessation of alcohol and drug abuse

  - Stress management

  - Regular physical and dental checkups and screenings

  - Regular inoculations and immunizations

  - Early and regular prenatal care
  - Reporting of unusual symptoms to a health professional
- ▲ Ensure that other agencies (e.g., Department of Children and Family Services, Social Services, Visiting Nurse Association, Meals On Wheels) are following through with plans.

Rationales

The FDA provides a variety of tools on recommended food groups across a variety of populations. Cardiovascular disease, cancer, type 2 diabetes, and osteoporosis are but a few of the many medical diseases related to nutrition.

Exercise promotes weight loss and increases agility and stamina. The Surgeon General recommends at least 150 minutes of moderate exercise each week.

Hygiene decreases risk for infection and promotes maintenance and integrity of skin and teeth.

Smoking has been directly linked to cancer, heart disease, and respiratory disease.

In addition to physical addictions and the social consequences, the physical consequences of substance abuse mitigate against it.

Stress management can be considered a cornerstone to a healthy lifestyle.

Checkups identify and treat problems early. Screening procedures are based on age and prior history (e.g., Papanicolaou, cholesterol, mammogram, BP, prostate, colonoscopy screening).

These include immunizations for tetanus, diphtheria, hepatitis B (as appropriate), pneumonia, and influenza, among others.

These checkups identify and treat problems early.

Early contact facilitates early treatment.

These services may be necessary to provide care. Coordinated efforts are more meaningful and effective.

■ = Independent   ▲ = Interprofessional Collaboration

Nursing Diagnosis Care Plans

Ineffective Health Management

Definition: Pattern of regulating and integrating into daily living a therapeutic regimen for the treatment of illness and its sequelae that is unsatisfactory for meeting specific health goals

With the ongoing changes in health care, patients are being expected to be co-managers of their care. They are being discharged from hospitals earlier and are faced with increasingly complex therapeutic regimens to be handled in the home environment. Likewise, patients with chronic illness often have limited access to health care providers and are expected to assume responsibility for managing the nuances of their disease (e.g., heart failure patients taking an extra furosemide [Lasix] tablet for a 2-pound weight gain).

Patients with sensory perception deficits, altered cognition, or financial limitations and those who lack support systems may find themselves overwhelmed and unable to follow the treatment plan. Older patients, who often experience most of these problems, are especially at high risk for ineffective management of the therapeutic plan. Other vulnerable populations include patients living in adverse social conditions (e.g., poverty, unemployment, little education); patients with emotional problems (e.g., depression over the illness being treated or other life crises or problems); and patients with substance abuse problems. Culture, ethnicity, and religion may influence one's health beliefs, health practices (e.g., folk medicine, alternative therapies), access to health services, and assertiveness in pursuing specific health care services.

Common Related Factors

Complexity of health care system
Complex therapeutic regimen
Economically disadvantaged
Excessive demands made on individual or family
Decisional conflicts
Family pattern of health care
Inadequate number of cues to action
Insufficient knowledge of therapeutic regimen
Perceived barriers
Insufficient social support

Defining Characteristics

Ineffective choices of daily living for meeting heath goals
Failure to take action to reduce risk factor
Difficulty with prescribed regimen
Failure to include the treatment regimen in daily living

Common Expected Outcomes

Patient verbalizes intention to follow prescribed regimen.
Patient describes or demonstrates required competencies.
Patient identifies appropriate resources.
Patient demonstrates ongoing adherence to treatment plan.

NOC Outcomes

Compliance Behavior; Knowledge: Treatment Regimen

NIC Interventions

Self-Modification Assistance; Teaching: Individual; Health System Guidance

Ongoing Assessment

Actions/Interventions

■ Assess prior efforts to follow a regimen.

■ Assess for related factors that may negatively affect success with following the regimen.

Rationales

This knowledge provides an important starting point in understanding any complexities in implementation of the treatment plan.
Knowledge of causative factors provides direction for subsequent intervention. These factors may range from financial constraints to physical limitations.

Actions/Interventions

- Assess the patient's individual perceptions of health problems.

- Assess the patient's confidence in his or her ability to perform the desired behavior.

- Assess the patient's ability to learn or remember the desired health-related activity.

- Assess the patient's ability to perform the desired activity.

Rationales

According to the Health Belief Model, the patient's perceived susceptibility to and perceived seriousness and threat of disease, along with perceived benefits from adhering to treatment plan, affect compliance. In addition, factors such as cultural phenomena and heritage can affect how people view their health. QSEN: Evidence-based practice; Patient-centered care.

According to the self-efficacy theory, positive conviction that one can successfully execute a behavior is correlated with performance and a successful outcome.

Cognitive impairments need to be identified so an appropriate alternative plan can be devised. For example, the Mini-Mental State Examination (MMSE) can be used to identify memory problems that could interfere with accurate pill taking. Once these problems are identified, alternative actions, such as using egg cartons to dispense medications or receiving daily phone reminders, can be instituted. QSEN: Evidence-based practice; Patient-centered care.

The patient's ability to perform the activity determines the amount and type of education that needs to be provided. For example, patients with limited financial resources may be unable to purchase special diet foods such as those low in fat or low in salt. Patients with arthritis may be unable to open childproof pill containers.

Therapeutic Interventions

Actions/Interventions

- Include the patient in planning the treatment regimen.

- Inform the patient of the benefits of adhering to the prescribed regimen.

- Tailor the therapy to the patient's lifestyle (e.g., taking diuretics at dinner if working outside the home during the day) and culture (incorporate herbal medicinal massage or prayer, as appropriate).
- Simplify the regimen. Suggest long-acting forms of medications, and eliminate unnecessary medication.

- Eliminate unnecessary clinic visits.

Rationales

Patients who become co-managers of their care have a greater stake in achieving a positive outcome. They know best their personal and environmental barriers to success. QSEN: Patient-centered care.

Patients who believe in the efficacy of the recommended treatment to reduce risk or to promote health are more likely to engage in it.

Tailoring the therapy will foster a patient-centered focus and promote compliance. A "one size fits all" approach is usually ineffective.

The greater the number of times during the day that patients need to take medications, the greater the risk for not following through. Polypharmacy is a significant problem with older patients. Attempt to reduce nonessential drug usage.

The physical demands of traveling to an appointment, the financial costs incurred (loss of day's work, need for child care), the negative feelings of being "talked down to" by health care providers not fluent in the patient's language, as well as the commonly long waits can cause patients to avoid follow-ups when they are required. Telephone follow-up may be substituted as appropriate.

■ = Independent   ▲ = Interprofessional Collaboration

Actions/Interventions

- Develop a system for the patient to monitor his or her own progress.

- Develop with the patient a system of rewards that follow successful follow-through.

- Concentrate on the behaviors that will make the greatest contribution to the therapeutic effect.

- If negative side effects of the prescribed treatment are a problem, explain that many side effects can be controlled or eliminated.

- If the patient lacks adequate support in following the prescribed treatment plan, initiate referral to a support group (e.g., AARP, American Diabetes Association, senior groups, weight loss programs, Breast Cancer Network of Strength, smoking cessation clinics, stress management classes, social services).

Rationales

Self-monitoring is a key component of a successful change in behavior. Gadgets such as exercise monitors (e.g., Fitbits) and calorie counters and software programs to track performance can have a positive influence on health outcomes.

Rewards may consist of verbal praise, monetary rewards, special privileges (e.g., earlier office appointment, free parking), or telephone calls.

Behavior change is never easy. Efforts should be directed to activities known to result in specific benefits (e.g., smoking cessation, fluid control in heart failure patients).

Nonadherence because of medication side effects is a commonly reported problem. Health care providers need to determine actual etiological factors for side effects and possible interplay with over-the-counter medications. Similarly, patients may report fatigue or muscle cramps with exercise. If so, the exercise prescription may need to be revised.

Groups that come together for mutual support and information can be beneficial, especially to patients coping with chronic illness. Social media support groups have long been a vital part of therapy for those living with health challenges.

Education/Continuity of Care

Actions/Interventions

- Use a variety of teaching methods to match the patient's preferred learning style.

- Introduce complicated therapy one step at a time.

- Instruct the patient in the importance of reordering medications 2 to 3 days before running out. Consider 90-day refills for long-term chronic conditions.

- Include significant others in explanations and teaching. Encourage their support and assistance in following plans.

- Allow the learner to practice new skills; provide immediate feedback on performance.

Rationales

Different people learn in different ways. Match the learning style with the educational approach. For some patients this may require grocery shopping for "healthy foods" with a dietitian or a home visit by the nurse to review a psychomotor skill. QSEN: Patient-centered care.

This format allows the learner to concentrate more completely on one topic at a time.

A percentage of medication nonadherence is caused by patients simply being too late to get a pharmacy refill. This may be due to cultural issues whereby patients are more time-oriented to the present versus future needs or to insurance company restrictions on early refills, or to preferences for the standard 30-day refill. The 90-day supplies require refills only 4 times a year versus the typical 12 times.

Inclusion of significant others encourages support and assistance in reinforcing appropriate behaviors and facilitating lifestyle modification.

Practice allows the patient to use new information immediately, thus enhancing retention. Immediate feedback allows the learner to make corrections rather than practice the skill incorrectly.

Actions/Interventions

- Role-play scenarios when nonadherence to the plan may easily occur. Demonstrate appropriate behaviors.

Rationales

Relapse prevention needs to be addressed early in the treatment plan. Helping the patient expand his or her repertoire of responses to difficult situations assists in meeting treatment goals.

NANDA-I NDx Hopelessness

Definition: Subjective state in which an individual sees limited or no alternatives or personal choices available and is unable to mobilize energy on own behalf

A person may experience hopelessness in response to a sudden event, such as spinal cord injury that leaves the patient with permanent paralysis. Hopelessness may be the result of a lifetime of multiple stresses and losses that leave the patient no longer able to mobilize the energy needed to act in his or her own behalf. Chronic diseases associated with progressive loss of functional ability may contribute to the patient's sense of hopelessness, especially if the person sees no chance for improvement with continued treatment. Hopelessness is evident in patients living in social isolation, who are lonely and have no social support system or resources. Patients living in poverty, the homeless, and those with limited access to health care all may feel hopeless about changing their health care status and being able to cope with life events. Loss of trust in prior spiritual beliefs may foster a sense of hopelessness.

Common Related Factors

Chronic stress
Prolonged activity restriction
Social isolation
Loss of belief in transcendent values
Loss of belief in spiritual power
Deterioration in physiological condition
History of abandonment

Defining Characteristics

Passivity
Decrease in affect
Decrease in verbalization
Decrease in initiative
Decrease in response to stimuli
Despondent verbal cues
Alteration in sleep pattern
Decrease in appetite

Common Expected Outcomes

Patient expresses positive expectations about the future.
Patient mobilizes energy in own behalf (e.g., making decisions).
Patient sets goals consistent with optimism, meaning in life, and belief in self and others

NOC Outcomes

Hope; Coping; Mood Equilibrium

NIC Interventions

Hope Inspiration; Coping Enhancement; Mood Management

Ongoing Assessment

Actions/Interventions

- Assess the role that illness plays in the patient's hopelessness.

- Assess physical appearance (e.g., grooming, posture, hygiene).

Rationales

Changes in the patient's level of physical functioning, endurance for activities, duration and course of illness, prognosis, and treatments can contribute to hopelessness. Certain misconceptions (e.g., patients with cancer always die) may be part of the patient's perception of the situation.
Hopeless patients may not have the energy or interest to engage in self-care activities.

■ = Independent   ▲ = Interprofessional Collaboration

Actions/Interventions	Rationales
■ Assess appetite, exercise, and sleep patterns.	Deviations from normal patterns are evident during periods of hopelessness. Patients may have a decreased appetite and limited activity level. Patients may sleep more or experience insomnia.
■ Assess the patient's belief in self and his or her own abilities. Identify the patient's values and satisfaction with his or her role or purpose in life.	Patients may feel that the threat is greater than their resources to handle it, and feel a loss of control over solving the threat or problem. Eliciting the patient's values, preferences, and expressed needs allows the patient to be a full partner in providing care. QSEN: Patient-centered care.
■ Evaluate the patient's ability to set goals, make decisions, and solve problems.	Patients who feel hopeless will feel that goal setting is futile and that goals cannot be met. They may be unable to make decisions or solve problems.
■ Assess the patient's perceptions of unachieved outcomes as failures or persistent focus on failures instead of accomplishments.	Repeated perceptions of failure will reinforce the patient's feelings of hopelessness. The patient may express loss of control or an inability to change the situation.
■ Listen for verbalizations of hopelessness, lack of self-worth, giving up, and suicidal ideas.	Hopelessness is associated with dysfunctional personality characteristics as well as suicidal ideation and behaviors.
■ Assess previous coping strategies used and their effectiveness.	Successful coping is influenced by past experiences. Patients with a history of maladaptive coping may require additional resources. Past strategies may not be sufficient in the present situation.
■ Assess the patient's expectations for the future.	Uncertainty about events, duration and course of illness, prognosis, and dependence on others for help and treatments involved can contribute to a feeling of hopelessness. QSEN: Patient-centered care.
■ Assess the patient's social support network and potential source of hope (e.g., self, significant others, religion).	Patients in social isolation find it difficult to change their condition. Evaluation of supportive people from the past may provide the assistance the patient requires at this time. Trusted others (e.g., clergy, family, health team) can support the patient's basic belief system that enhances hope. Community groups, church groups, and self-help groups may also be available for assistance.

Therapeutic Interventions

Actions/Interventions	Rationales
■ Provide opportunities for the patient to express feelings of pessimism.	The nurse creates a supportive environment by listening to the patient in a nonjudgmental manner.
■ Maintain consistency in personnel assigned to care for the patient.	An ongoing, consistent relationship establishes trust, reduces the patient's feeling of isolation, eases fear of abandonment, and may facilitate coping and restore hope. QSEN: Patient-centered care.
■ Encourage the patient to identify his or her own strengths and abilities.	During a period of hopelessness, patients may not be able to recognize their strengths. Fostering awareness can expedite use of these strengths.
■ Provide the physical care that the patient is unable to provide for self in a manner that communicates warmth, respect, and acceptance of the patient's abilities.	This approach to providing care reduces guilt and other negative feelings the patient may experience when unable to care for self. QSEN: Patient-centered care.
■ Assist the patient in developing a realistic appraisal of the situation.	Patients may not be aware of all the support services available that can help them move through this stressful situation (e.g., home care aides, financial assistance, free medications, community counseling programs, legal services, companion services).

Actions/Interventions	Rationales
■ Help the patient set realistic goals by identifying short-term goals and revising them as needed.	Patients may feel overwhelmed when viewing the situation from a "big picture" perspective. Guiding the patient to view the situation in smaller parts may make the problem more manageable. It is important that the patient set truly realistic goals so as not to be frustrated with the inability to accomplish them.
■ Convey feelings of acceptance and understanding. Avoid false reassurances.	An honest relationship facilitates problem-solving. False reassurances are never helpful to the patient and only may serve to relieve the discomfort of the care provider.
■ Encourage an attitude of realistic hope.	Emphasizing the patient's intrinsic worth and viewing the immediate problem as manageable in time may provide support. Fostering unrealistic hope is not helpful and may significantly worsen the trust the patient places in the health care provider. Belief in the nurse-patient relationship as a partnership in the journey toward hope is key to fostering hope.
■ Assure the patient and family that they will not be abandoned and that every effort will be made to optimize the highest quality of care.	Compassionate assurance gives patients and families an increased sense of feeling cared for and understood. This approach to care plays a role in restoring the patient's sense of hope.
■ Support the patient's relationships with significant others; involve them in the patient's care as appropriate.	Interest from others may help change the patient's focus from self. Enhancing a sense of connectedness to a caring relationship fosters hope.
■ Provide opportunities for the patient to control the care environment.	Hopeless patients may feel they have no control. Yet when given opportunities to make choices, their perception of hopelessness may be reduced.
■ Encourage the patient to reminisce about the past (self-validation).	Older patients especially find a renewed sense of hope when reviewing life's events and accomplishments.
■ Facilitate problem-solving by identifying the problem and appropriate steps.	Small steps that are successful will foster confidence in oneself and may promote a more hopeful outlook. This approach may help the patient experience a gradual mastery of the situation. QSEN: Patient-centered care.
■ Expand the patient's repertoire of coping skills.	The patient may benefit from learning new techniques for coping with stressful situations. These skills may foster a renewed sense of control and restore hope.
■ Encourage the use of spiritual resources as desired.	Religious practices may provide strength and inspiration.

Education/Continuity of Care

Actions/Interventions	Rationales
■ Provide accurate and ongoing information about illness, treatment effects, and care needed.	Misconceptions about diagnosis and prognosis may be contributing to hopelessness. Patients may not recognize that the situation is temporary rather than permanent. Accurate information helps the patient develop a realistic frame of reference for the experience.
■ Educate the patient or family on using a combination of problem-solving and emotional coping skills.	These skills can enhance the coping ability of the patient and family members.
■ Ensure that strategies to maintain hope within the patient are also used to support family caregivers.	Family caregivers are an integral component to instilling and supporting a sense of hope in their loved one.

■ = Independent ▲ = Interprofessional Collaboration

Nursing Diagnosis Care Plans

NDx Functional Urinary Incontinence

Definition: Inability of usually continent person to reach the toilet in time to avoid unintentional loss of urine

The person with functional urinary incontinence has normal function of the neurological control mechanisms for urination. The bladder is able to fill and store urine appropriately. The person is able to recognize the urge to void. The most common problem is environmental barriers that make it difficult for the person to reach an appropriate receptacle for voiding. This type of incontinence occurs more often in older adults, who have mobility limitations. People with arthritis of the hands may have difficulty undoing clothing buttons or zippers to prepare for voiding. The patient with limited mobility may be dependent on others for help transferring to a bedside commode or ambulating to the bathroom. If mobility assistance is not readily available, the person is not able to suppress the urge to void and becomes incontinent. Wet clothing, urine odor, and the loss of independence for toileting contribute to the person's feelings of embarrassment in this situation. Over time the person may have changes in body image and self-concept.

Common Related Factors

Alteration in environmental factors
Neuromuscular impairment
Alteration in cognitive function

Defining Characteristics

Sensation of need to void
Early morning urinary incontinence
Completely empties bladder
Voiding prior to reaching toilet

Common Expected Outcomes

Patient receives assistance for toileting in a timely manner.
Patient has no episodes of incontinence.

NOC Outcomes

Urinary Continence; Urinary Elimination; Self-Care: Toileting

NIC Interventions

Urinary Habit Training; Urinary Incontinence Care

Ongoing Assessment

Actions/Interventions

- Assess the patient's recognition of the need to urinate.

- Assess the availability of functional toileting facilities (working toilet, bedside commode).
- Assess the patient's ability to reach a toileting facility, both independently and with help.

- Assess the patient's usual pattern of urination and occurrence of incontinence.

Rationales

Patients with functional incontinence are incontinent because they cannot get to an appropriate place to void. Institutionalized patients are often labeled "incontinent" because their requests for toileting are unmet. Older patients with cognitive impairment may recognize the need to void but may be unable to express the need.

Patients may need a bedside commode if mobility limitations interfere with getting to the bathroom.

This information allows the nurse to plan for assistance with transfer to a toilet or bedside commode. Functional continence requires that the patient be able to get to a toilet either independently or with assistance.

This assessment provides a basis for an individualized toileting program. Many patients are incontinent only in the early morning when the bladder has stored a large urine volume during sleep. QSEN: Patient-centered care.

Therapeutic Interventions

Actions/Interventions

- Establish a toileting schedule.

- Place a bedside commode near the patient's bed. Ensure privacy.

- Place mobility assistive devices within easy reach of the patient.
- Encourage use of clothing that can be easily and quickly removed.

- Encourage the patient to limit fluid intake 2 to 3 hours before bedtime and to void just before bedtime.
- Treat any existing perineal skin excoriation with a vitamin-enriched cream, followed by a moisture barrier.

Rationales

A toileting schedule assures the patient of a specified time for voiding and reduces episodes of functional incontinence. QSEN: Patient-centered care.

The patient needs to accept this alternative toileting facility. Some people may be embarrassed when using a toilet in a more open area.

The patient needs to have ready access to canes or walkers needed to support ambulation to the toilet.

Clothing can be a barrier to functional continence if it takes time to remove before voiding. Women may find skirts or dresses easier to wear while implementing a toileting program. Pants with an elastic waistband may be easier for men and women to remove for toileting.

Limiting fluid intake and voiding before bedtime reduce the need to disrupt sleep for voiding.

Moisture-barrier ointments are useful in protecting perineal skin from urine. QSEN: Safety.

Education/Continuity of Care

Actions/Interventions

- Teach the patient or caregiver the rationale behind and implementation of a toileting program.
- Teach family members and other caregivers to respond immediately to the patient's request for assistance with voiding.

Rationales

Successful functional continence requires consistency in use of a toileting program.

Functional continence is promoted when caregivers respond promptly to the patient's request for help with voiding.

NANDA-I

Reflex Urinary Incontinence

Definition: Involuntary loss of urine at somewhat predictable intervals when a specific bladder volume is reached

Reflex urinary incontinence represents dysfunction of the normal neurological control mechanisms for coordination of detrusor contraction and sphincter relaxation. Neurological disorders in the detrusor motor area of the brain result in detrusor hyperreflexia. Examples of such disorders include strokes, traumatic brain injury, hydrocephalus, tumors, Alzheimer's disease, and multiple sclerosis. Cervical and thoracic spinal cord injuries and Guillain-Barré syndrome may cause detrusor hyperreflexia with sphincter dyssynergia. The patient with reflex incontinence experiences periodic urination without an awareness of needing to void. Urination is frequent throughout the day and night. Urine volume is consistent with each voiding. Residual urine volumes are usually less than 50 mL. Urodynamic studies will indicate detrusor contraction when bladder volume reaches a specific amount.

Common Related Factors

Neurological impairment above level of sacral micturition center
Neurological impairment above level of pontine micturition center

Defining Characteristics

Absence of sensation of bladder fullness
Absence of urge to void
Inability to voluntarily initiate or inhibit voiding
Predictable pattern of voiding

■ = Independent   ▲ = Interprofessional Collaboration

Common Expected Outcomes

Patient establishes a regular voiding pattern.
Patient has no episodes of incontinence.

NOC Outcomes
Urinary Continence; Urinary Elimination
NIC Interventions
Urinary Catheterization; Urinary Catheterization: Intermittent; Urinary Incontinence Care

Ongoing Assessment

Actions/Interventions	Rationales
■ Assess the patient's recognition of the need to void.	Patients with neurological disorders may have damaged sensory fibers, and may not have the sensation of the need to void.
■ Measure urine volume with each voiding.	Urine volumes are usually consistent with reflex incontinence.
■ Encourage the patient to maintain a "bladder diary."	Information about fluid intake and voiding patterns provides a basis for planning bladder management techniques. QSEN: Patient-centered care.
▲ Monitor the results of urodynamic studies.	A cystometrogram will measure bladder pressures and fluid volumes during filling, storage, and urination. Electromyography will record detrusor activity during voiding. Test results will indicate the degree of coordination between detrusor muscle and sphincter activity. QSEN: Evidence-based practice.

Therapeutic Interventions

Actions/Interventions	Rationales
■ Encourage voiding at scheduled intervals before predictable voiding.	Voiding at regular intervals, based on knowledge of the patient's voiding pattern, decreases the chance of uncontrolled incontinence. QSEN: Patient-centered care.
■ Encourage the patient to limit fluid intake 2 to 3 hours before bedtime and to void just before bedtime.	Limiting fluid intake and voiding before bedtime reduce the need to disrupt sleep for voiding.
■ Consider the use of an external catheter for the male patient.	An external catheter connected to a gravity drainage device allows the patient to remain dry.
▲ Catheterize the patient at regular intervals if spontaneous voiding is not possible. Use an indwelling catheter as a last resort.	Emptying the bladder at regular intervals will reduce incontinence episodes. The risk for infection is considerable with indwelling catheters. QSEN: Safety.

Education/Continuity of Care

Actions/Interventions	Rationales
■ Teach the patient or caregiver (or perform for patient) intermittent (self-) catheterization.	This technique empties the bladder at specified intervals.
■ Discuss the use of absorbent pads or incontinence briefs in social situations.	Absorbent pads and incontinence briefs will protect clothing when the patient is in public. The patient needs to understand about changing the pads and briefs at regular intervals to prevent skin irritation from exposure to urine and moisture.

NANDA-I NDx **Stress Urinary Incontinence**

Definition: Sudden leakage of urine with activities that increase intra-abdominal pressure

Stress incontinence occurs more often in women than men. The predisposing factors for women include pregnancy, obesity, decreased estrogen levels associated with menopause, and surgery involving the lower abdominal area. Men may develop stress incontinence following surgical treatment for benign prostatic hyperplasia or prostate cancer. These factors contribute to a decrease in muscle tone at the urethrovesical junction. When the muscles of the abdomen and pelvic floor are weak, they no longer provide support for the urinary sphincter. The urinary sphincter cannot remain constricted with increasing abdominal pressure. Straining with defecation, laughing, sneezing, coughing, heavy lifting, jumping, or running are examples of activities that increase intra-abdominal pressure and lead to stress incontinence. The amount of urine lost may vary from a few drops to 100 mL or more. Regardless of the amount of urine lost during a stress incontinence episode, the person may experience embarrassment and changes in body image and self-concept. As a result, the person may decrease social interactions and physical activities to minimize the risks of incontinence occurring in public situations.

Common Related Factors
Weak pelvic muscles
Increase in intra-abdominal pressure
Degenerative changes in pelvic muscles
Intrinsic urethral sphincter deficiency

Common Expected Outcomes
Patient has no episodes of incontinence.
Patient implements activities to increase abdominal and pelvic floor muscle tone.

Defining Characteristics
Involuntary leakage of small volume of urine (e.g., with coughing, laughing, sneezing, on exertion)
Involuntary leakage of small volume of urine in the absence of detrusor contraction or an overdistended bladder

NOC Outcomes
Urinary Continence; Urinary Elimination
NIC Interventions
Pelvic Muscle Exercise; Urinary Incontinence Care

Ongoing Assessment

Actions/Interventions

- Ask about involuntary urine loss during coughing, laughing, sneezing, lifting, or exercising.

- Examine the perineal area for evidence of pelvic relaxation:
  - Cystourethrocele (sagging bladder or urethra)
  - Rectocele (relaxed, sagging rectal mucosa)
  - Uterine prolapse (relaxed uterus)
- Determine the patient's parity.

- Explore the patient's menstrual history.

- Ask about previous surgical procedures.

Rationales

Whenever intra-abdominal pressure increases, a weak sphincter and relaxed pelvic floor muscles allow urine to escape involuntarily.
The presence of these conditions can lead to incontinence because of poor muscular control.

Pregnancy and vaginal births weaken pelvic muscles. The weakness increases with multiple pregnancies.
Postmenopausal hypoestrogenism contributes to relaxation of the urethra.
In men, transurethral resection of the prostate gland can result in urinary incontinence.

■ = Independent   ▲ = Interprofessional Collaboration

Nursing Diagnosis Care Plans

Therapeutic Interventions

Actions/Interventions	Rationales
■ Encourage weight loss if the patient is obese.	Obesity is associated with increased intra-abdominal pressure on the urinary bladder.
■ Encourage the patient to maintain adequate fluid intake.	Patients often restrict fluid intake to reduce incontinence episodes.
▲ Administer or encourage the use of medication as ordered: • Pseudoephedrine • Vaginal estrogen	These medications increase bladder sphincter tone and improve pelvic muscle tone.
■ Prepare the patient for surgery (Marshall-Marchetti-Krantz, Burch's colposuspension, and sling procedures) as indicated.	Many surgical procedures are done to control stress incontinence. These procedures provide support to the bladder and urinary sphincter.

Education/Continuity of Care

Actions/Interventions	Rationales
■ Teach the patient to perform Kegel exercises.	Kegel exercises are used to strengthen the muscles of the pelvic floor and can be practiced with a minimum of exertion. The repetitious tightening and relaxation of these muscles (10 repetitions four or five times per day) helps some patients regain continence. Kegel exercises may be used in combination with biofeedback to enhance a positive outcome.
■ Teach the patient about appropriate use of absorption pads.	Disposable pads or briefs may be worn to absorb urine and increase the patient's social activities. The patient needs to change the pads at regular intervals to prevent skin irritation from contact with urine and moisture.
■ Teach the patient to use transcutaneous electrical nerve stimulation (TENS), as indicated.	This device improves pelvic floor tone and inhibits the micturition reflex.
■ Teach female patients the use of a vaginal pessary (a device reserved for nonsurgical candidates).	A pessary works by elevating the bladder neck, thereby increasing urethral resistance.
▲ Refer the patient for biofeedback training.	Biofeedback techniques combined with electromyography or pressure manometry help the patient learn to contract pelvic floor muscles and control incontinence. QSEN: Teamwork and collaboration.
■ Refer to the stress urinary incontinence website (www.nafc.org; National Association for Continence).	The site provides additional resources, support, and information.

NANDA-I
NDx Urge Urinary Incontinence

Definition: Involuntary passage of urine occurring soon after a strong sense of urgency to void

Urge urinary incontinence is associated with overactivity or uncontrolled contraction of the detrusor muscle. The person has uncontrolled passage of urine within a few seconds to a few minutes after feeling a strong sense of urgency to void. The person is unable to voluntarily suppress voiding once the urge is felt. Urge incontinence may develop as a result of spinal cord lesions or following pelvic surgery. Central nervous system disorders such as Alzheimer's disease, multiple sclerosis, and Parkinson's disease may contribute to urge incontinence. Overactivity of the detrusor may be the result of interstitial cystitis, urinary tract infection, or pelvic radiation. Excessive alcohol or caffeine intake may stimulate urge incontinence. As with other types of urinary incontinence, the person with urge incontinence may experience embarrassment with loss of control of urinary elimination. The person begins to plan activities to be close to a toilet at all times. This change in behavior may affect the person's social interaction and work performance.

Common Related Factors
Alcohol consumption
Caffeine intake
Bladder infection
Detrusor hyperactivity with impaired bladder contractility
Treatment regimen
Atrophic vaginitis/urethritis

Defining Characteristics
Inability to reach toilet in time to avoid urine loss
Involuntary loss of urine with bladder contractions/spasms
Urinary urgency

Common Expected Outcomes
Patient maintains a pattern of predictable voiding.
Patient has no periods of incontinence.

NOC Outcomes
Urinary Continence; Urinary Elimination; Self-Care: Toileting
NIC Interventions
Urinary Bladder Training; Urinary Habit Training; Urinary Incontinence Care

Ongoing Assessment

Actions/Interventions	Rationales
■ Ask the patient to describe episodes of incontinence.	Urge incontinence occurs when the bladder muscle suddenly contracts. The patient may describe feeling the need suddenly to urinate but being unable to get to the bathroom in time.
■ Instruct the patient to keep a daily bladder diary indicating voiding frequency and patterns.	This assessment allows for an individualized treatment plan. The patient may be voiding as often as every 2 hours. QSEN: Patient-centered care.
▲ Obtain a specimen of urine for culture.	Bladder infection can result in a strong urge to urinate; successful management of a urinary tract infection may eliminate or improve incontinence.
▲ Monitor the results of cystometry.	Diagnostic testing is used to measure bladder pressures and fluid volume during filling, storage, and urination. The results of this test may indicate the underlying problem leading to urge incontinence.

■ = Independent ▲ = Interprofessional Collaboration

Nursing Diagnosis Care Plans

Therapeutic Interventions

Actions/Interventions	Rationales
■ Facilitate access to toileting facilities, and teach the patient to make scheduled trips to the bathroom.	Scheduled voiding allows for frequent bladder emptying.
■ Administer or encourage the use of medications as ordered: • Anticholinergics • Tricyclic antidepressants	Anticholinergics reduce or block detrusor contractions, thereby reducing episodes of incontinence. The tricyclics increase serotonin or norepinephrine, which results in relaxation of the bladder wall and increased bladder capacity.

Education/Continuity of Care

Actions/Interventions	Rationales
■ Teach the patient to limit intake of alcohol and caffeine.	These chemicals are known to be bladder irritants. They can increase detrusor overactivity.
■ Assist the patient with developing a bladder training program that includes voiding at scheduled intervals, and gradually increasing the time between voidings.	A bladder training program helps the patient increase bladder capacity through regulation of fluid intake, pelvic exercises, and scheduled voiding. A regular schedule of voiding helps decrease detrusor overactivity and increase bladder fluid volume capacity. QSEN: Patient-centered care.
■ Teach Kegel exercises.	These exercises improve pelvic floor muscle tone and urethrovesical junction sphincter tone.

NANDA-I NDx **Risk for Infection**

Definition: Vulnerable to invasion and multiplication of pathogenic organisms, which may compromise health

People at risk for infection are those whose natural defense mechanisms are inadequate to protect them from the inevitable injuries and exposures that occur throughout the course of living. Infections occur when an organism (e.g., bacterium, virus, fungus, or other parasite) invades a susceptible host. Breaks in the integument and/or the mucous membranes, the body's first line of defense, allow for invasion by pathogens. If the patient's immune system cannot combat the invading organism adequately, an infection occurs. Open wounds, traumatic or surgical, can be sites for infection; soft tissues (cells, fat, muscle) and organs (kidneys, lungs) can also be sites for infection after trauma, invasive procedures, or invasion of pathogens carried through the bloodstream or lymphatic system. Infections can be transmitted by contact or through airborne transmission, sexual contact, or sharing of IV drug paraphernalia. Being malnourished, having inadequate resources for sanitary living conditions, and lacking knowledge about disease transmission place individuals at risk for infection. Inadequate vaccination of at-risk individuals increases the spread of infection. Health care workers, to protect themselves and others from disease transmission, must understand how to take precautions to prevent transmission. Because identification of infected individuals is not always apparent, standard precautions recommended by the Centers for Disease Control and Prevention (CDC) are widely practiced. The Agency for Healthcare Research and Quality (AHRQ) published important guidelines and recommendations in this resource: *Patient Safety and Quality: An Evidence-Based Handbook for Nurses.* In addition, the Occupational Safety and Health Administration (OSHA) set forth the Bloodborne Pathogens Standard, developed to protect workers and the public from infection. Ease of and increase in world travel also have increased opportunities for transmission of disease from abroad such as Ebola virus or Middle East respiratory syndrome. Infections prolong healing and can result in death if untreated. Antimicrobial drugs are used to treat infections when susceptibility is present. Organisms may become resistant to antimicrobial agents. The overuse of antimicrobials to treat infections and in agricultural settings has led to an increase in strains of drug-resistant microorganisms including methicillin-resistant *Staphylococcus aureus* (MRSA), vancomycin-resistant *Enterococcus* (VRE), and multidrug-resistant tuberculosis (MDRTB). Infections with these drug-resistant microorganisms present challenges for safe and effective treatment of patients. For some organisms no antimicrobial treatment is effective, such as the human immunodeficiency virus (HIV).

Common Risk Factors

Inadequate primary defenses: altered skin integrity; smoking; stasis of body fluids

Inadequate secondary defenses: immunosuppression; leukopenia; suppressed inflammatory response

Insufficient knowledge to avoid exposure to pathogens

Malnutrition

Invasive procedures

Chronic disease

Inadequate vaccination

Common Expected Outcomes

Patient remains free of infection, as evidenced by normal vital signs and absence of purulent drainage from wounds, incisions, and tubes.

Infection is recognized early to allow for prompt treatment.

NOC Outcomes
Immune Status; Infection Severity

NIC Interventions
Infection Control; Infection Protection; Immunization/Vaccination Management

Ongoing Assessment

Actions/Interventions	Rationales
■ Assess for the presence, existence, and history of risk factors such as open wounds and abrasions; indwelling catheters (Foley, peritoneal); wound drainage tubes (T-tubes, Penrose drain, Jackson-Pratt drain); endotracheal or tracheostomy tubes; venous or arterial access devices; and orthopedic fixator pins.	Each of these examples represents a break in the body's normal first line of defense.
▲ Monitor white blood cell (WBC) count.	An increasing WBC count indicates the body's efforts to combat pathogens. Normal values are 4000 to 11,000/mm^3. Very low WBC count (less than 1000/mm^3) indicates severe risk for infection because the patient does not have sufficient WBCs to fight infection. In older patients, infection may be present without an increased WBC count. QSEN: Evidence-based practice.
■ Assess nutritional status, including weight, history of weight loss, and serum albumin.	Patients with poor nutritional status may be anergic or unable to muster a cellular immune response to pathogens and are therefore more susceptible to infection.
■ Assess for exposure to individuals with active infections.	This information provides warning for potential infection. This exposure may be direct contact with the individual or through indirect contact with objects used by the individual. QSEN: Safety.
■ Assess for the use of medications or treatment modalities that may cause immunosuppression.	Antineoplastic agents and corticosteroids reduce immunocompetence.
■ Assess immunization status.	Older patients and those not raised in the United States may not have completed immunizations and therefore may not have sufficient acquired active immunity. Some patients may not be vaccinated owing to fear, lack of knowledge, or cultural/religious beliefs. QSEN: Patient-centered care.
■ For patients at risk, monitor the following for signs of actual infection:	Early identification of the signs of infection allows for prompt treatment. QSEN: Safety.

■ = Independent   ▲ = Interprofessional Collaboration

Nursing Diagnosis Care Plans

Actions/Interventions

- Redness, swelling; increased pain; purulent drainage from incisions, injury, and exit sites of tubes, drains, or catheters

- Elevated temperature

- Color of respiratory secretions

- Appearance of urine

Rationales

Classic signs of any infection are localized redness, heat, swelling, and pain. Any suspicious drainage should be cultured; antibiotic therapy is determined by pathogens identified at culture.

Temperature of up to 38°C (100.4°F) for 48 hours after surgery is related to surgical stress; after 48 hours, temperature greater than 37.7°C (99.8°F) suggests infection; fever spikes that occur and subside are indicative of wound infection; very high temperature accompanied by sweating and chills may indicate septicemia.

Yellow or yellow-green sputum is indicative of respiratory infection.

Cloudy, foul-smelling urine with visible sediment is indicative of urinary tract or bladder infection.

Therapeutic Interventions

Actions/Interventions

- Maintain or teach asepsis for dressing changes and wound care, catheter care and handling, and peripheral IV and central venous access management.

- Wash hands and teach other caregivers to wash hands before contact with patients and between procedures with the patient.

- Encourage intake of protein- and calorie-rich foods.

- Encourage a fluid intake of 2000 to 3000 mL of water per day (unless contraindicated).

- Encourage coughing and deep breathing; consider the use of an incentive spirometer.

- Recommend the use of soft-bristled toothbrushes and stool softeners to protect mucous membranes.

Rationales

Use of aseptic technique decreases the chances of transmitting or spreading pathogens to the patient. A basic tenet of any infection prevention–related intervention is to interrupt the transmission of infection along the various steps that compromise the chain of infection. For example, central line–associated bloodstream infection (CLABSI) reduction interventions are effective when they target the microbes on the skin surface that enter the catheter tract (agent, reservoir, host, portal of entry), contaminated hands (mode of transmission), contamination of the catheter hub (reservoir), seeding from another site (host), and infusate (reservoir). QSEN: Evidence-based practice; Safety.

Friction and running water effectively remove microorganisms from hands. Washing between procedures reduces the risk for transmitting pathogens from one area of the body to another (e.g., perineal care or central line care). Alcohol-based hand sanitizers can be used between handwashing episodes if the hands are not visibly soiled. Use of disposable gloves does not reduce the need for hand washing. The CDC provides guidelines for hand hygiene in health care settings. QSEN: Evidence-based practice.

Optimal nutritional status supports immune system responsiveness.

Fluids promote diluted urine and frequent emptying of bladder; reducing stasis of urine, in turn, reduces risk for bladder infection or urinary tract infection.

These measures reduce stasis of secretions in the lungs and bronchial tree. When stasis occurs, pathogens can cause upper respiratory tract infections, including pneumonia.

Hard-bristled toothbrushes and constipation may compromise the integrity of the mucous membranes and provide a port of entry for pathogens.

⊖volve **For additional care plans, go to http://evolve.elsevier.com/Gulanick/.**

Actions/Interventions

■ Limit visitors.

▲ Place the patient in protective isolation if he or she is at very high risk.

▲ Administer or teach the use of antimicrobial (antibiotic) drugs, as ordered.

Rationales

Restricting visitation by individuals with any type of infection reduces the transmission of pathogens to the patient at risk for infection. The most common modes of transmission are by direct contact (touching) and by droplet (airborne). QSEN: Safety.

Protective isolation is established when WBC counts indicate neutropenia (less than 500 to 1000/mm^3). Institutional protocols may vary. National guidelines, such as those published by the CDC, provide general recommendations.

Antimicrobial drugs include antibacterial, antifungal, antiparasitic, and antiviral agents. All of these agents are either toxic to the pathogen or retard the pathogen's growth. Ideally, the selection of the drug is based on cultures from the infected area; this is often impossible or impractical, and, in these cases, empirical management usually is undertaken with a broad-spectrum drug. QSEN: Evidence-based practice.

Education/Continuity of Care

Actions/Interventions

■ Teach the patient or caregiver to wash hands often, especially after toileting, before meals, and before and after administering self-care.

■ Teach the patient the importance of avoiding contact with those who have infections or colds. Teach family members and caregivers about protecting susceptible patients from themselves and others with infections or colds.

■ Teach the patient, family members, and caregivers about obtaining appropriate vaccinations

■ Demonstrate and allow return demonstration of all high-risk procedures that the patient or caregiver will do after discharge, such as dressing changes, peripheral or central IV site care, peritoneal dialysis, and self-catheterization (may use clean technique).

■ Teach the patient, family, and caregivers the purpose and proper technique for maintaining isolation.

■ Teach the patient and caregiver the signs and symptoms of infection, and when to report them to the physician or nurse.

■ If infection occurs, teach the patient to take antibiotics as prescribed.

■ Instruct the patient to take the full course of antibiotics even if symptoms improve or disappear.

Rationales

Patients and caregivers can spread infection from one part of the body to another, as well as pick up surface pathogens; hand washing reduces these risks. QSEN: Safety.

Family members or others can spread infections or colds to a susceptible patient through direct contact, contaminated inanimate objects (indirect contact), or through air currents.

Vaccinations provide protection for a wide range of diseases spread by microorganisms. QSEN: Safety.

Patient and caregivers need opportunities to master new skills to reduce risk for infection.

Knowledge about isolation can help patients and family members cooperate with specific precautions.

Patients need to be able to recognize important signs and changes in their condition so early treatment can be initiated. QSEN: Safety.

Most antibiotics work best when a constant blood level is maintained; a constant blood level is maintained when medications are taken as prescribed. The absorption of some antibiotics is hindered by certain foods; patients should be instructed accordingly.

Not completing the entire course of the prescribed antibiotic regimen can lead to drug resistance in the pathogens and reactivation of symptoms.

Related Care Plan

Readiness for enhanced immunization status, Chapter 3

■ = Independent   ▲ = Interprofessional Collaboration

Nursing Diagnosis Care Plans

NANDA-I

NDx Insomnia

Definition: A disruption in amount and quality of sleep that impairs functioning

Sleep is required to provide energy for physical and mental activities. The disruption in the individual's usual diurnal pattern of sleep and wakefulness may be temporary or chronic. Short-term insomnia may occur in response to changes in work schedules, temporary stressors, or travel across several time zones. Long-term insomnia is associated with alcohol and drug abuse, chronic pain, chronic depression, obesity, and aging. Such disruptions may result in both subjective distress and apparent impairment in functional abilities. Sleep patterns can be affected by environment, especially in hospital critical care units. These patients experience insomnia secondary to the noisy, bright environment and frequent monitoring and treatments. Such sleep disturbance is a significant stressor in the intensive care unit and can affect recovery. The care plan focuses on nursing care to manage insomnia in the acute care and home setting.

Common Related Factors

Physical discomfort
Environmental barrier (e.g., ambient noise, daylight/darkness exposure, ambient temperature/humidity, unfamiliar setting)
Anxiety/fear
Depression
Pharmaceutical agent
Inadequate sleep hygiene
Frequent naps
Alcohol consumption

Defining Characteristics

Difficulty initiating sleep
Early awakening
Difficulty maintaining sleep
Dissatisfaction with sleep
Insufficient energy
Increase in absenteeism/accidents
Decrease in quality of life
Alteration in concentration

Common Expected Outcome

Patient achieves optimal amounts of sleep as evidenced by rested appearance, verbalization of feeling rested, and improvement in sleep pattern.

NOC Outcome
Sleep
NIC Intervention
Sleep Enhancement

Ongoing Assessment

Actions/Interventions

- Document nursing or caregiver observations of sleeping and wakeful behaviors. Record number of sleep hours. Note physical (e.g., noise, pain or discomfort, urinary frequency) and/or psychological (e.g., fear, anxiety) circumstances that interrupt sleep.
- Evaluate the timing or effects of medications that can disrupt sleep.

Rationales

Often the patient's perception of the problem may differ from objective evaluation. QSEN: Patient-centered care.

In both the hospital and home care settings, patients may be following medication schedules that require awakening in the early morning hours. Some medications may have insomnia as a side effect. Attention to changes in the schedule or changes to once-a-day medication may solve the problem.

Therapeutic Interventions

Actions/Interventions	Rationales
■ Instruct the patient to follow as consistent a daily schedule for retiring and arising as possible.	Consistent schedules promote regulation of the circadian rhythm and reduce the energy required for adaptation to changes.
■ Instruct the patient to avoid heavy meals, alcohol, caffeine, or smoking before retiring.	Full meals close to bedtime may produce gastrointestinal upsets and hinder sleep onset. Caffeine, found in food and fluids (coffee, tea, colas, and chocolate), and nicotine stimulate the central nervous system. This stimulation may interfere with the patient's ability to relax and fall asleep. Alcohol produces drowsiness and may facilitate the onset of sleep but interferes with REM sleep.
■ Instruct the patient to avoid large fluid intake before bedtime.	Evening fluid restriction helps the patient who otherwise may need to get up to go to the bathroom during the night.
■ Increase daytime physical activities as indicated, but instruct the patient to avoid strenuous activity before bedtime.	Activity reduces stress and promotes sleep. However, overfatigue may cause insomnia.
■ Discourage a pattern of daytime naps unless deemed necessary to meet sleep requirements or if part of one's usual pattern.	Napping can disrupt normal sleep patterns; however, older patients do better with frequent naps during the day to counter their shorter nighttime sleep schedules. QSEN: Evidence-based practice.
■ Suggest the use of soporifics such as milk.	Milk contains L-tryptophan, which facilitates sleep.
■ Recommend an environment conducive to sleep or rest (e.g., quiet, comfortable temperature, ventilation, darkness, closed door). Suggest the use of earplugs or eye shades as appropriate.	Many people sleep better in cool, dark, quiet environments.
■ Encourage the patient to limit use of electronic devices 2 to 3 hours before retiring (e.g., mobile phone, tablets, computers).	Melatonin is a hormone from the pineal gland that helps regulate the person's sleep-wake cycle. Blue-spectrum light from the screens of these devices has been found to decrease secretion of melatonin. Energy-efficient light bulbs (LED) also produce blue-spectrum light that may disrupt sleep. QSEN: Evidence-based practice.
■ Suggest engaging in a relaxing activity before retiring (e.g., warm bath, calm music, reading an enjoyable book, relaxation exercises).	These activities provide relaxation and distraction to prepare the body and mind for sleep.
■ Explain the need to avoid concentrating on the next day's activities or on one's problems at bedtime.	Planning a designated time during the next day to address these concerns may provide permission to "let go" of the worries at bedtime.
■ Encourage patients to journal or write down their problems or activities before going to sleep.	Journaling allows the patient to "put aside" the mental activities until the morning.
■ If unable to fall asleep after about 30 to 45 minutes, suggest getting out of bed and engaging in a relaxing activity.	The bed should not be associated with wakefulness, TV watching, or work.
■ Discuss the use of over-the-counter, herbal, and prescription sleep aids:	Short-term use of pharmacological sleep aids may be beneficial when the patient experiences temporary sleep disturbances. QSEN: Evidence-based practice.
• Melatonin	This nutritional supplement acts as a neurotransmitter to promote sleep onset. Older adults seem to tolerate melatonin with minimal side effects.
• Valerian, chamomile, lavender, kava	These herbal preparations are known to have mild sedating effects that promote sleep onset. The patient needs to be careful in selecting herbal products from reputable sources, because the FDA does not regulate these supplements. Some herbal products used for sedation may have significant interactions with other medications taken by the patient.

■ = Independent   ▲ = Interprofessional Collaboration

Actions/Interventions	**Rationales**
• Antihistamines	Many over-the-counter sleep aids contain antihistamines as the active ingredient that promotes sedation. These drugs produce anticholinergic side effects that may be especially troublesome for the older adult.
• Prescription sedative-hypnotics, antianxiety drugs	These drugs are associated with physical tolerance and dependence with long-term use. Many drugs in this class act through general central nervous system depression and disrupt the normal stages of non-REM (NREM) and REM sleep. With long-term use, side effects include daytime drowsiness, rebound insomnia, and increased dreaming when discontinued.

For patients who are hospitalized:

■ Provide bedtime nursing care (e.g., back rub, pain relief, comfortable position, relaxation techniques).	These activities promote relaxation and enhance the onset of sleep.
■ Eliminate nonessential nursing activities.	This approach to care promotes minimal interruption in sleep or rest.
■ Attempt to allow for sleep cycles of at least 90 minutes.	Research studies indicate that 60 to 90 minutes are needed to complete one sleep cycle and that the completion of an entire cycle is necessary to benefit from sleep. QSEN: Evidence-based practice.
■ Move the patient to a room farther from the nursing station if noise is a contributing factor.	The nursing station is often the center of noise and activity.
■ Post a "do not disturb" sign on the door.	It is important to alert people to avoid entering the room and interrupting sleep.

Education/Continuity of Care

Actions/Interventions	**Rationales**
■ Teach about possible causes of sleeping difficulties and optimal ways to treat them.	Considerable confusion and myths about sleep exist. Knowledge of its role in health and wellness and the wide variation among individuals may allay anxiety, thereby promoting rest and sleep.
■ Instruct in nonpharmacological sleep-enhancement techniques.	Nonpharmacological sleep-enhancement techniques can be used throughout a lifetime. Pharmacological sleep agents should be used only for a limited time.

NANDA-I
NDx Decreased Intracranial Adaptive Capacity

Definition: Intracranial fluid dynamic mechanisms that normally compensate for increases in intracranial volumes are compromised, resulting in repeated disproportionate increases in intracranial pressure (ICP) in response to a variety of noxious and non-noxious stimuli.

Intracranial pressure reflects the pressure exerted by the intracranial components of blood, brain, and cerebrospinal fluid (CSF), each ordinarily remaining at a constant volume within the rigid skull structure. Any additional fluid or mass (e.g., cerebral edema, subdural hematoma, tumor, abscess) increases the pressure within the cranial vault. Because the total volume cannot change (Monro-Kellie hypothesis), blood, CSF, and ultimately brain tissue are forced out of the vault. The normal range of ICP is 5 to 15 mm Hg; elevations above that level occur normally but readily return to baseline parameters as a result of the adaptive capacity or compensatory mechanisms of the brain, blood, and CSF, such as vasoconstriction and increased venous outflow. In the event of disease, trauma, or a pathological condition, disturbances in autoregulation occur, and ICP is increased and sustained. Exceptions include people with unfused skull fractures (the skull is no longer rigid at the fracture site), infants whose suture lines are not yet fused (this is normal to accommodate growth), and older patients whose brain tissues have shrunk, taking up less volume in the skull (allowing for abnormal tissue growth or intracranial bleeding to occur for a longer period before ICP increases).

Common Related Factors

Brain injury (e.g., cerebrovascular impairment, neurological illness, trauma, tumor)
Decreased cerebral perfusion

Defining Characteristics

Repeated increase in ICP ≥ 10 mm Hg for more than 5 minutes following external stimuli
Baseline ICP greater than 10 mm Hg
Wide amplitude ICP waveform

Common Expected Outcome

Patient maintains optimal cerebral tissue perfusion, as evidenced by stable neurological status, ICP less than 10 mm Hg, and cerebral perfusion pressure (CPP) from 60 to 90 mm Hg.

NOC Outcomes

Neurological Status: Consciousness; Neurological Status: Autonomic; Tissue Perfusion: Cerebral; Fluid Balance

NIC Interventions

ICP Monitoring; Neurologic Monitoring; Cerebral Edema Management; Cerebral Perfusion Promotion

Ongoing Assessment

Actions/Interventions

■ Assess the patient's neurological status, including level of consciousness (LOC); pupil size, symmetry, and reaction to light; extraocular movement; gaze preference; motor function abnormal Babinski reflex; and postural rigidity.

■ Evaluate the presence or absence of protective reflexes (e.g., swallowing, gagging, blinking, coughing).

■ Monitor vital signs.

Rationales

Deteriorating neurological signs indicate increased cerebral ischemia. A decreased LOC is the first sign of increased ICP. This change usually presents as increasing restlessness, irritability, or agitation. The patient may become disoriented and confused. Changes in pupil size, symmetry, and reactivity to light will occur with increased ICP. When the patient's head is turned there will be lack of conjugate gaze and absence of the oculocephalic reflex response (doll's eyes). The patient may exhibit postural rigidity as ICP rises. These postural changes may be flexion (decorticate) or extension (decerebrate). As ICP increases the patient will exhibit fanning of the toes with dorsiflexion of the great toe when testing the Babinski reflex.

Loss of protective reflexes occurs with increasing ICP and puts the patient at risk for injuries such as aspiration or corneal abrasions. QSEN: Safety.

Continually increasing ICP results in life-threatening hemodynamic changes; early recognition is essential to survival. As compensatory mechanisms fail to regulate ICP the patient may exhibit a full, bounding pulse with a gradually slowing rate. The BP begins to show a widening pulse pressure. The respiratory rate begins to slow and the patient may develop breathing pattern changes such as Cheyne-Stokes breathing. Core body temperature may be unstable as increasing ICP exerts pressure on the hypothalamus. QSEN: Safety.

■ = Independent   ▲ = Interprofessional Collaboration

Actions/Interventions

- Assess for headache and vomiting.

- ▲ Monitor arterial blood gases and/or pulse oximetry (recommended parameters: Pao_2 greater than 80 mm Hg and $Paco_2$ less than 35 mm Hg with normal ICP). If the patient's lungs are being hyperventilated to decrease ICP, $Paco_2$ should be between 25 and 30 mm Hg.
- ▲ Monitor ICP with an appropriate measurement device. Report ICP greater than 10 mm Hg for 5 minutes. Serially monitor ICP pressure and waveforms.

- Analyze changes in ICP waveforms.

- Calculate CPP by subtracting ICP from the mean arterial pressure (MAP):

$$CPP = MAP - ICP$$

Determine MAP using the following formula:

$$\frac{Systolic\ BP - Diastolic\ BP}{3} + Diastolic\ BP$$

Rationales

Pressures on brain tissue and blood vessels with increasing ICP causes pain. Vomiting, sometimes projectile, may occur suddenly without a sensation of nausea beforehand as increased ICP exerts pressure on the medulla oblongata.

A $Paco_2$ less than 20 mm Hg may decrease cerebral blood flow (CBF) because of profound vasoconstriction that produces hypoxia. $Paco_2$ greater than 45 mm Hg induces vasodilation with increase in CBF, which may trigger increase in ICP.

Insertion of a ventriculostomy catheter is the traditional method for monitoring ICP. Newer methods use fiberoptic catheters that measure not only ICP but also cerebral oxygenation. QSEN: Evidence-based practice.

Waveform analysis provides information to identify patient experiencing changes in brain compliance and decreased intracranial adaptive capacity. Changes in the pulse component (P_1, P_2, P_3) of the ICP waveform are associated with alterations in arterial pulsations in the large cerebral vessels. Increased ICP and decreased intracranial compliance produce elevations in the amplitude of the pulse component waveforms.

Pressure should be approximately 90 to 100 mm Hg and not less than 50 mm Hg to ensure blood flow to brain.

Therapeutic Interventions

Actions/Interventions

- Elevate the head of bed 30 degrees, and keep the head in a neutral alignment.

- Avoid the Valsalva maneuver.

- Limit nursing and medical procedures to those absolutely necessary.
- ▲ Maintain normothermia with antipyretics, antibiotics, and a cooling blanket.
- ▲ If ICP increases and fails to respond to repositioning of the head in neutral alignment and head elevation, one or more of the following may be prescribed by the physician:
  - Hyperventilate the patient.

Rationales

Elevation promotes venous outflow and contributes to a decrease in cerebral blood volume and ICP. Exceptions to this positioning may include shock and cervical spine injuries. A neutral head position prevents venous obstruction.

Valsalva maneuvers, as occurs with straining, increase intrathoracic pressure and CBF, thereby increasing ICP. QSEN: Safety.

Both prescribed and unnecessary procedures can serve as a noxious stimulus that can further increase ICP.

Fever increases cerebral metabolic demand and may increase CBF and ICP.

Hyperventilation can decrease $Paco_2$ to between 25 and 30 mm Hg and induce vasoconstriction and a decrease in CBF and ICP. Hyperventilation is often reserved for brain-injured patients exhibiting signs of herniation.

Actions/Interventions

- Administer mannitol over 30 to 60 minutes.

- Administer barbiturates as needed.

- If the patient is intubated, administer a neuromuscular blocking agent.

- Administer a short-acting pain reliever (e.g., morphine, meperidine [Demerol], or midazolam [Versed]) before painful stimulation or stress-related care such as suctioning or IV line changes.
- ▲ Drain CSF at the ordered rate and amount.

- ▲ Consult with the dietitian about providing appropriate nutritional support.

Rationales

Mannitol is a hyperosmotic agent that should be used carefully because it can induce cerebral ischemia. It is contraindicated with hypovolemic symptoms. A diuretic response can be anticipated within 30 to 60 minutes. A Foley catheter should be in place. An IV filter should be used when mannitol is infused. Electrolytes, osmolality, and serum glucose must be monitored during mannitol infusion.
Barbiturates reduce cerebral metabolism, cerebral oxygen demand, and ICP.
Neuromuscular blockers reduce shivering, coughing, and Valsalva maneuver. However, neuromuscular blocking agents have no effect on cerebration; therefore the patient should receive short-acting sedation before noxious stimulation.
Pain and agitated body movements cause further increases in ICP.

Removal of a small amount of CSF through a pressure monitoring system can significantly lower ICP. This can be accomplished intermittently or, as in patients with hydrocephalus, continuously.
Increased ICP is associated with a hypermetabolic state in brain tissue. Inadequate glucose levels will contribute to cerebral edema and therefore increase ICP. QSEN: Teamwork and collaboration.

Education/Continuity of Care

Actions/Interventions

- ■ Teach the patient and family about causes, treatment, and expected outcome. Offer the family frequent feedback regarding the patient's status.
- ■ Reinforce discussions related to treatment (e.g., head of bed elevated, medication).

- ■ Encourage the family's presence and participation in comfort measures.

Rationales

Knowledge about increased ICP can calm anxieties about this condition.

The patient and family will be able to cooperate with care when they understand the purpose of specific interventions.
The presence of familiar people may calm the patient and decrease ICP.

Deficient Knowledge

Definition: Absence or deficiency of cognitive information related to a specific topic

Knowledge deficit is a lack of cognitive information or psychomotor skills required for health recovery, maintenance, or health promotion. Teaching may take place in a hospital, ambulatory care, or home setting. The learner may be the patient, a family member, a significant other, or a caregiver unrelated to the patient. Learning may involve any of the three domains: cognitive domain (intellectual activities, problem-solving, and others); affective domain (feelings, attitudes, belief); and psychomotor

domain (physical skills or procedures). The nurse must decide with the learner what to teach, when to teach, and how to teach the mutually agreed-upon content. Adult learning principles guide the teaching-learning process. Information should be made available when the patient wants and needs it, at the pace the patient determines, and using the teaching strategy the patient deems most effective. Many factors influence patient education, including age, cognitive level, developmental stage, physical

■ = Independent ▲ = Interprofessional Collaboration

limitations (e.g., visual, hearing, balance, hand coordination, strength), the primary disease process and comorbid conditions, and sociocultural factors. Older patients need more time for teaching and may have sensory-perceptual deficits/cognitive changes that may require a modification in teaching techniques. Certain ethnic and religious groups hold unique beliefs and health practices that must be considered when designing a teaching plan. These practices may vary from home remedies (e.g., special soups, poultices) and alternative therapies (e.g., massage, biofeedback, energy healing, macrobiotics, or megavitamins in place of prescribed medications) to reliance on an elder in the family to coordinate the care plan. Patients with low literacy skills will require educational programs that include more simplified treatment regimens, simplified teaching tools (e.g., cartoons, lower readability levels), a slower presentation pace, and techniques for cueing patients to initiate certain behaviors (e.g., pill schedule posted on refrigerator, timer for taking medications). The National Patient Safety Foundation has identified the pervasiveness of low health literacy and its implications for poorer health outcomes. It has launched the *Ask Me 3* initiative to improve health communication between patients and providers.

Although the acute hospital setting provides challenges for patient education because of the high acuity and emotional stress inherent in this environment, the home setting can be similarly challenging because of the high expectations for patients or caregivers to self-manage complex procedures such as IV therapy, dialysis, or even ventilator care in the home. Caregivers are often overwhelmed by the responsibility delegated to them by the interprofessional health care teams. Many caregivers have their own health problems and may be unable to perform all the behaviors assigned to them because of visual limitations, generalized weakness, or feelings of inadequacy or exhaustion.

This care plan describes adult learning principles that can be incorporated into a teaching plan for use in any health care setting.

Common Related Factors
Alteration in cognitive functioning
Insufficient information
Insufficient interest in learning
Insufficient knowledge of resources
Alteration in memory
Misinformation presented by others

Defining Characteristics
Insufficient knowledge
Inaccurate follow-through of instruction
Inaccurate performance on a test
Inappropriate behavior

Common Expected Outcomes
Patient demonstrates motivation to learn.
Patient identifies perceived learning needs.
Patient verbalizes understanding of desired content/performs desired skill.

NOC Outcomes
Knowledge: (Specify Type); Information Processing
NIC Interventions
Health Literacy Enhancement; Learning Facilitation; Teaching: Individual

Ongoing Assessment

Actions/Interventions	Rationales
■ Determine who will be the learner: the patient, family, significant other, or caregiver.	Many older or terminal patients may view themselves as dependent on their caregiver and therefore will not want to be part of the educational process.
■ Assess the motivation and willingness of the patient and caregivers to learn.	Adults must see a need or purpose for learning. Some patients are ready to learn soon after they are diagnosed; others cope better by denying or delaying the need for instruction. Learning also requires energy, which patients may not be ready to use. Patients also have a right to refuse educational services.

Actions/Interventions

- Assess the ability to learn, remember, or perform desired health-related care.

- Identify the priority of learning needs within the overall care plan.

- Question the patient regarding previous experience and health teaching.

- Identify any existing misconceptions regarding material to be taught.
- Determine cultural influences on health teaching.

- Determine the patient's learning style, especially if the patient has learned and retained new information in the past.

- Determine the patient's or caregiver's self-efficacy to learn and apply new knowledge.

Rationales

Cognitive impairments need to be identified so an appropriate teaching plan can be designed. For example, the Mini-Mental State Examination (MMSE) can be used to identify memory problems that would interfere with learning. Physical limitations (e.g., impaired hearing or vision, poor hand coordination) can likewise compromise learning and must be considered when designing the educational approach. Patients with decreased lens accommodation may require bolder, larger fonts or magnifying lenses for written material. QSEN: Evidence-based practice.

This information provides the starting base for educational sessions. Teaching standardized content that the patient already knows wastes valuable time and hinders critical learning. Adults learn material that is important to them. During the acute stages, the family or significant others may require the most teaching. QSEN: Patient-centered care.

Adults bring many life experiences to each learning session. Adults learn best when teaching builds on previous knowledge or experience. This experience is the foundation for an individualized teaching plan.

Assessment provides an important starting point in education. Knowledge serves to correct faulty ideas.

To be effective, interventions need to be specific to the patient and address individual differences. Providing a climate of acceptance allows patients to be themselves and to hold their own beliefs as appropriate. Language problems can pose significant barriers to learning.

Each patient has his or her own learning style, which must be considered when designing a teaching program. Some people may prefer written over visual materials, or they may prefer group versus individual instruction. Matching the learner's preferred style with the educational method will facilitate success in mastery of knowledge.

Self-efficacy refers to a person's confidence in his or her ability to perform a behavior. A first step in teaching may be to foster increased self-efficacy in the learner's ability to learn the desired information or skills. Some lifestyle changes can be difficult to make.

Therapeutic Interventions

Actions/Interventions

- Provide physical comfort for the learner.

- Provide a quiet atmosphere without interruption.

- Provide an atmosphere of respect, openness, trust, and collaboration.

Rationales

According to Maslow's theory, basic physiological needs must be addressed before patient education. Ensuring physical comfort allows the patient to concentrate on what is being discussed or demonstrated.

A calm quiet environment assists the patient with concentrating more completely.

Conveying respect is especially important when providing education to patients with different values and beliefs about health and illness.

■ = Independent   ▲ = Interprofessional Collaboration

Actions/Interventions

- Involve the patient in developing the teaching plan, beginning with establishing objectives and goals for learning at the beginning of the session.
- Allow the learner to identify what is most important to him or her.

- Explore attitudes and feelings about changes.

- Allow for and support self-directed, self-designed learning.

- Assist the learner in integrating information into daily life.

- Allow adequate time for integration that is in direct conflict with existing values or beliefs.

- Give clear, thorough explanations and demonstrations.

- Provide information using various media (e.g., explanations, discussions, demonstrations, pictures, written instructions, computer-assisted programs, and videotapes).
- Ensure that required supplies and equipment are available so that the environment is conducive to learning.
- When presenting material, move from familiar, simple, and concrete information to less familiar, complex, or more abstract concepts.
- Focus teaching sessions on a single concept or idea.

- Pace the instruction and keep sessions short.

Rationales

Goal setting allows the learner to know what will be discussed and expected during the session. Adults tend to focus on here-and-now, problem-centered education.

Adult learning is problem-oriented. Priority setting is key. Allowing the patient to determine the most significant content to be presented first is most effective (i.e., what the patient needs to know now versus later). Patients may want to focus only on self-care techniques that facilitate discharge from the hospital or enhance survival at home (e.g., how to take medications, emergency side effects, suctioning a tracheal tube) and are less interested in specifics of the disease process. The *Ask Me 3* program for health literacy stresses the importance of focusing on three questions: What is my main problem? What do I need to do? Why is it important for me to do this? QSEN: Patient-centered care.

Assessment assists the nurse in understanding how the learner may respond to the information and possibly how successful the patient may be with the expected changes.

Adults learn when they feel they are personally involved in the learning process. Patients know what difficulties will be encountered in their own environments, and they must be encouraged to approach learning activities from their priority needs.

This technique helps the learner make adjustments in daily life that will result in the desired change in behavior (or learning).

Information that is in direct conflict with what is already held to be true forces a reevaluation of the old material and is thus integrated more slowly.

Patients are better able to ask questions when they have basic information about what to expect. Accurate, clear information provides rationale for treatment and aids the patient in assuming responsibility for care at a later time.

Different people take in information in different ways. Match the learning style with the educational approach.

Adequate preparation is especially important when teaching in the home setting.

This technique provides the patient with the opportunity to understand new material in relation to familiar material.

Clearly focused teaching allows the learner to concentrate more completely on material being discussed. Highly anxious and older patients have reduced short-term memory and benefit from mastery of one concept at a time.

Learning requires energy, so shorter, well-paced sessions reduce fatigue.

Actions/Interventions

- Use the teach-back technique to determine the patient's understanding of what was taught:
  - The nurse gives information in a caring manner, using plain language.
  - Ask the patient to explain in his or her own words.
  - Rephrase the information if unable to repeat it accurately.
  - Again ask the patient to teach-back the information using his or her own words until the nurse is comfortable that it is understood.
  - If the patient still does not understand, consider other strategies.
- Encourage questions.

- Allow the learner to practice new skills; provide immediate feedback on performance.

- Encourage repetition of the information or new skill.

- Provide positive, constructive reinforcement of learning. Incorporate rewards into the learning process.

- Document the progress of teaching and learning.

Rationales

The teach-back technique consists of specific steps in a repetitive order to evaluate the recipient's knowledge of the content discussed. It is not a test of the patient, but of how well the nurse explained the content. It provides a check for understanding and if necessary, for reteaching the information. Patients who are not able to accurately "teach-back" content after multiple cycles are usually identified as cognitively impaired. QSEN: Evidence-based practice.

Questions facilitate open communication between patient and health care professionals and allow verification of understanding of given information and the opportunity to correct misconceptions. Learners often feel shy or embarrassed about asking questions and often want permission to ask them. Patients must have correct information to make valid choices.

Assisting allows the patient to use new information immediately and enhances retention. Immediate feedback allows the learner to make corrections rather than practicing the skill incorrectly.

Repeated practice by the patient will help him or her gain confidence in self-care ability.

A positive approach allows the learner to feel good about learning accomplishments, gain confidence, and maintain self-esteem while correcting mistakes. Rewards help to make learning fun.

Documentation allows additional teaching to be based on what the learner has completed, thus enhancing the learner's self-efficacy and encouraging the most cost-effective teaching.

Education/Continuity of Care

Actions/Interventions

- Provide instruction for specific topics.

- ▲ Refer the patient to community resources or support groups, as needed.

- Include significant others whenever possible.

Rationales

Patients must have correct information to make informed choices in their treatment, identify when therapy adjustments are needed, and recognize important changes in their condition that could lead to serious outcomes. Long-term care will be the patient's responsibility.

Patients may be unaware of services available for questions or problem-solving. These resources allow the patient to interact with others who have similar problems, learning needs, or specialty resources.

One's partner usually assumes a crucial supportive role when the patient is gathering information and initiating new treatments.

■ = Independent   ▲ = Interprofessional Collaboration

Nursing Diagnosis Care Plans

NDx Sedentary Lifestyle

Definition: Reports a habit of life that is characterized by a low physical activity level

Today's social changes have shifted lifestyles of once high physical effort to more sedentary ways of life, making physical inactivity a national health problem. An inactive person takes about 3000 steps or less in carrying out the daily activity of moving around their house. Unfortunately, many individuals do not actively seek out regular exercise routines, with more than 60% of Americans not exercising on a regular basis and 25% not exercising at all.

Lack of physical activity can lead to many chronic conditions, including diabetes, heart disease, obesity, and various cancers. The *2008 Physical Activity Guidelines for* *Americans* provides a science-based prescription for assisting individuals with improving their health through regular physical activity. Health benefits are attainable by individuals of all ages and even those with chronic medical problems. Stressful and busy lifestyles, socioeconomic factors, physical constraints, and lack of motivation are all barriers that can contribute to low physical activity. Nursing objectives are to educate patients on the importance of adopting an active lifestyle and to assist patients in finding ways to personalize the recommended exercise prescription.

Common Related Factors

Insufficient knowledge of health benefits associated with physical exercise
Insufficient interest in physical activity
Insufficient motivation for physical activity
Insufficient resources for physical activity (time, money, companionship, facilities)
Insufficient training for physical exercise
Cultural habits or beliefs

Defining Characteristics

Average daily physical activity is less than recommended for gender and age
Physical deconditioning
Preference for activity low in physical activity

Common Expected Outcomes

Patient verbalizes accurate information about benefits of increasing physical activity.
Patient verbalizes strategies to develop a personal program of increased lifestyle activity.
Patient engages in an increased level of lifestyle physical activity.

NOC Outcomes
Knowledge: Prescribed Activity; Physical Fitness
NIC Interventions
Exercise Promotion; Teaching: Prescribed Exercise

Ongoing Assessment

Actions/Interventions

- Assess the patient's current level of physical activity, including both lifestyle activity and structured exercise.
- Assess the patient's past experiences with structured physical activity.

Rationales

This assessment provides a basis for increasing activity. Some physical activity is always better than none.
Adults bring many life experiences to learning sessions. Many patients have had positive experiences in the past that can serve as a base on which to build. Similarly, often patients have previously tried unsuccessfully to become more active. Reasons for difficulties need to be explored.

Actions/Interventions

- Assess the patient's views on physical activity by asking questions, including the following: How do you feel about physical activity or exercise? Do you find exercise important to your health?

- Assess the patient's readiness to initiate a physical activity regimen by asking questions such as the following: How do you feel about starting an exercise routine? Are you ready to choose a time to start being more active?

- Assess the patient's confidence in his or her ability to increase physical activity using a scale of 0 to 10.

- Assess the patient's level of mobility and physical status before prescribing an activity plan.

- Assess any possible barriers to increasing physical activity, such as lack of motivation, interpersonal support, skills, knowledge, or resources.

Rationales

Insight into the patient's priorities and values regarding physical activity will provide a basis for developing a physical activity program. Patients learn material and engage in activities most important to them. QSEN: Patient-centered care.

The Transtheoretical Model emphasizes that interventions for change should be matched with the stage of change at which patients are situated. For example, if the patient is only contemplating starting an exercise program, efforts may be directed toward emphasizing the health benefits of exercise, whereas if the patient is in the preparation or action stages, more specific directions regarding exercise (e.g., walking is a great way to start, moderate versus vigorous activity, places to exercise) can be addressed. QSEN: Evidence-based practice.

If patients have strong self-efficacy, they are more likely to welcome the challenge and begin to initiate an exercise program, whereas patients with low self-efficacy tend to shy away from the challenges of making a change.

Many sedentary patients will have evidence of deconditioning. A baseline assessment of physical status will allow the nurse to safely initiate an exercise regimen specific to patient needs and abilities. Screening tools such as the Physical Activity Readiness Questionnaire (PAR-Q) provide guidance as to when a medical examination may be required before initiating a program. Older adults with chronic conditions may need personalized assessments. QSEN: Safety.

If the patient is aware of possible barriers and has formulated plans for dealing with them, successful change is more likely to occur. For example, when trying to engage in a walking program, walking in a shopping mall can be substituted for outdoor activity during periods of inclement weather.

Therapeutic Interventions

Actions/Interventions

- Guide the patient in setting realistic short-term and long-term goals for increasing physical activity.

- Discuss ways to incorporate exercise into one's daily life by suggesting parking further away from the store, taking the stairs instead of the elevator, and taking walks during lunch breaks.
- Explain to the patient how to make sedentary activities more active (e.g., pacing or walking while on the telephone, stretching while watching television, dancing while listening to favorite music).

Rationales

Adults have many options for increasing their current level of activity. Setting realistic achievable goals helps maintain motivation and eventual success of the exercise regimen. Walking is a great way to get physically active. Some patients may start with simply walking for 10 minutes a day, whereas others may be ready to commit to 30 minutes. Patients may need assistance in selecting safer activities that are appropriate to their current fitness level.

Lifestyle activities are an easy starting point. Even brief episodes of activity, as little as 10 minutes each, can add up to the 150 minutes of recommended exercise per week.

Exercise can easily be incorporated into many sedentary activities and may get patients in the habit of choosing active behaviors. Some activity is always better than none.

■ = Independent ▲ = Interprofessional Collaboration

Actions/Interventions	Rationales
■ Suggest purposeful physical activities.	Patients are more likely to begin and maintain activities when they perceive that the activity is beneficial and has a purpose. For example, patients may select an exercise class for the socialization, not just for the exercise, or they may focus more on lifestyle activities carried out during the course of a day, such as walking the dog, using a bathroom on another floor, or getting off a bus one stop earlier. The best activity is the one that the patient enjoys and will continue to do.
■ For patients with decreased mobility or chronic conditions such as arthritis and COPD, stress the importance of starting slow and gradually increasing activity.	Too much exercise initially can cause injury or exacerbation of symptoms and discourage patients from continuing the exercise routine. Patients with chronic medical conditions should increase their physical activity under the supervision of their health care professional.
■ Introduce the use of a pedometer/step counter to track steps per day. Determine the number of steps needed to accomplish at least a 10-minute walk.	Pedometers can be a useful tool to quantify activity level as well as provide tangible goals. A key to successful use is to focus on number of steps walked per 10 minutes, with the idea of moving toward the 150 minutes per week goal. Patients with low fitness levels tend to walk slower, so they will complete fewer steps in 10 minutes than someone with a higher fitness level. However, each patient will have his or her own goal to work toward.
■ Introduce an activity calendar, so patients can monitor their physical activity on a daily basis.	Such tracking devices serve as a visual reminder of exercise achievement as well as a self-monitoring technique.
■ Suggest the patient find an activity/exercise partner.	Recruiting a support person to share in the activity can increase motivation and compliance with the regimen.
■ Provide emotional support while increasing activity.	Patients may be fearful of starting an exercise regimen. Ongoing support and coaching can encourage compliance and enjoyment of physical activity.
■ Assist in developing a time frame for achievement of the goals.	Depending on one's starting point, previously inactive people need to "start low and go slow" by gradually increasing the amount of activity they do. Maintaining an active lifestyle is a lifetime goal, thus starting too fast may not result in the best outcome.
■ For patients ready to engage in a more active physical activity program, see care plan: Readiness for Engaging in a Regular Physical Activity Program, Chapter 3	This care plan provides information based on the *2008 Physical Activity Guidelines for Americans,* which is a science-based prescription for assisting individuals with improving their health through regular physical activity. QSEN: Evidence-based practice.

Education/Continuity of Care

Actions/Interventions	Rationales
■ Provide ongoing education about the benefits of physical activity to both the patient and significant others.	Patients and families need information on the many health benefits of exercise and the potential health risks of being sedentary. This will need to be reinforced over time.
■ Refer patients to community resources such as the YMCA, park districts, or other community activity centers.	Patients may not be aware of resources that can be a basis of support and success.
■ Teach patients to reward themselves for the accomplishment of short-term and long-term goals.	Rewards are motivational and can give a sense of satisfaction for a job well done.

Related Care Plans

Activity intolerance, Chapter 2
Readiness for engaging in a regular physical activity
    program, Chapter 3

NANDA-I NDx **Impaired Memory**

Definition: Inability to remember or recall bits of information or behavioral skills

Memory is the result of a complicated cognitive process used by an individual for learning, storing, and retrieving information. Cognitive abilities for reasoning, problem-solving, interpreting information, and communication are dependent on the diverse and complex neural network that supports information processing. Structurally, memories are formed by the complex interactions of the hippocampus, thalamus, hypothalamus, and temporal lobes. Any change that disrupts these neural networks may result in problems with transferring information between immediate, short-term, and long-term memory. Amnesia is the complete loss of memory ability. This type of memory impairment represents an inability to recall previously learned information and an inability to learn new information. Memory impairment may be temporary or permanent. Situations that are associated with impaired memory include seizures, head trauma, strokes, cerebral infections, brain tumors, vitamin B_1 deficiency with alcohol abuse, personality disorders, and progressive degenerative dementias. Any clinical condition associated with decreased cardiac output or general hypoperfusion may contribute to impaired memory. Changes in recent memory often occur with organic disorders such as delirium, dementia, or chronic alcohol abuse. Diminished long-term or remote memory is associated with damage to the area of the cerebral cortex used for storage of that memory. This type of memory loss is seen in Alzheimer's disease. Post-traumatic amnesia is an indicator of the severity of a closed head injury. Slowing of information processing and impaired episodic memory are common problems with head trauma. This care plan focuses on general care to support memory for the patient in the acute care or home setting.

Common Related Factors

Alteration in fluid volume
Electrolyte imbalance
Neurological impairment (e.g., positive EEG, head trauma,
    seizure disorder)
Distractions in the environment
Anemia
Hypoxia
Decrease in cardiac output

Defining Characteristics

Forgetfulness
Inability to recall factual information
Inability to recall events
Inability to perform a previously learned skill
Inability to retain new information
Inability to learn a new skill
Inability to determine if a behavior was performed
Forgets to perform a behavior at a scheduled time

Common Expected Outcomes

Patient is able to recall immediate, recent, and remote information accurately within limits of disease.
Patient is able to maintain attention and respond appropriately to environmental cues within limits of disease.
Patient is oriented to time, person, place, and self within limits of disease.
Patient uses techniques to promote retention and recall of information.

NOC Outcomes
Memory; Cognitive Orientation; Concentration
NIC Interventions
Memory Training; Reality Orientation

■ = Independent   ▲ = Interprofessional Collaboration

Nursing Diagnosis Care Plans

Ongoing Assessment

Actions/Interventions	Rationales
■ Assess neurological function with special attention to the mental status portion of the examination (e.g., Mini-Mental State Examination [MMSE]): • Orientation to time (e.g., "What is the year, season, month, day, and date?") • Orientation to place (e.g., "Where are we now [state, city, and building]?") • Registration and recall of three words • Serial 7s subtraction • Naming familiar objects • Repetition of a phrase • Following a two-step direction • Reading • Writing a sentence • Copying a figure	Memory is associated with cognitive information processing. Changes in memory will be most evident during the mental status examination of the patient. The MMSE is a simplified scoring tool for assessing changes in cognitive function. The tool will provide information about immediate, recent, and long-term memory function. The MMSE can help differentiate memory loss as an isolated problem from delirium or dementia. Modifications in the MMSE may be made based on the patient's heritage. QSEN: Evidence-based practice.
■ Assess the patient's use of alcohol.	Excessive and long-term alcohol use is associated with development of Korsakoff's syndrome and memory loss.
■ Assess the patient's use of prescription medications, over-the-counter medications, and herbal supplements. Ask about use of illegal drugs.	Memory loss may be a drug side effect or a sign of drug interactions. Benzodiazepines, H_2-histamine antagonists, beta-blockers, digoxin, and glucocorticosteroids may contribute to decreases in both short-term and long-term memory function. Illegal drugs, such as marijuana, cocaine, and ecstasy, produce impaired memory as a side effect.
■ Assess the patient's nutritional status and dietary intake.	A persistent elevation of blood glucose is associated with decline in memory. Long-term nutritional deficiencies, especially vitamin deficiencies, contribute to memory loss.
■ Assess for behavioral changes such as anxiety, combativeness, or withdrawal.	The patient with memory loss and diminished orientation may exhibit restlessness, anxiety, agitation, aggressiveness, and combativeness. Depression may contribute to impaired memory, especially in the older adult.
■ Include family members and caregivers in the assessment of the patient.	Patients with impaired memory may not be able to provide detailed information about their past history or health status.
■ Assess the impact of memory loss on the patient and family members. Give special attention to assessing safety issues in the patient's living situation.	Memory loss can limit the patient's day-to-day functioning. The patient may be unable to effectively manage family and occupational responsibilities. The patient's safety may be impaired because memory loss interferes with other cognitive abilities to problem solve and make judgments. Patients may forget to turn off stoves or water faucets. Family members may experience increased frustration and stress as they cope with the patient's memory loss and safety concerns. QSEN: Patient-centered care; Safety.
■ Assess the quality of sleep.	Normal sleep plays a role in the consolidation of memories. Inadequate sleep can limit cognitive functions such as formation of memories and new learning.

Actions/Interventions

▲ Refer the patient for diagnostic testing.

Rationales

Neurological and laboratory testing are indicated to rule out problems that may account for memory loss. Blood tests provide information on electrolyte imbalances or anemia. Hemodynamic assessments provide information on oxygen saturation and cardiac output. Diagnostic testing may include computed tomography scan, magnetic resonance imaging, lumbar puncture, and electroencephalogram. Psychoneurological evaluation by a trained specialist is important to arrive at a diagnosis of conditions such as Alzheimer's disease. QSEN: Teamwork and collaboration.

Therapeutic Interventions

Actions/Interventions

■ Provide reality orientation for the patient at every contact. For example, address the patient by name, introduce yourself, and review the day, time, location, and activity being completed.

■ Provide a low-stimulation environment.

■ Ask the patient about recent events.

■ Encourage the patient to reminisce about past experiences.

■ Provide opportunities for repeated practice of new information using an errorless learning approach.

■ Encourage the use of games and puzzles as appropriate.

▲ Refer the patient to a professional counselor, as needed.

▲ Administer medications as prescribed.

Rationales

The patient with impaired memory will have difficulty maintaining orientation to the immediate environment. Reality orientation helps the patient remain mentally integrated with the immediate environment. Misinterpretations by the patient can be clarified immediately. QSEN: Patient-centered care.

Excessive auditory and visual stimulation can add to disorientation and confusion. The patient needs a setting with limited distractions to enhance accurate information processing.

Review of events in response to questions assists the patient in encoding information for retrieval at a later time.

The mental stimulation that occurs with recall and review of life events can enhance information retrieval from remote memory.

An errorless learning approach provides the patient with the correct information each time it is needed. The patient then records the information in a memory aid such as a notebook or computer. When errors occur in learning new information, this impedes memory development of correct information. QSEN: Patient-centered care.

Games such as crossword puzzles, jigsaw puzzles, or chess have been shown to aid in stimulating important neural centers that enhance memory function.

The patient with memory loss associated with psychogenic problems may benefit from talk therapy. QSEN: Teamwork and collaboration.

Thiamine may be given to patients with memory loss associated with Wernicke encephalopathy from alcohol abuse. Improvement in memory has been seen in patients treated with clonidine and vasopressin. Patients with Alzheimer's disease may receive medications that slow the progression of the disorder and preserve memory function for a short period of time. Acetylcholinesterase inhibitors such as tacrine (Cognex), donepezil (Aricept), and rivastigmine (Exelon) increase acetylcholine at neuron receptors. This action improves cholinergic transmission and slows decline in memory and cognitive function. QSEN: Evidence-based practice.

■ = Independent ▲ = Interprofessional Collaboration

Nursing Diagnosis Care Plans

Education/Continuity of Care

Actions/Interventions	Rationales
■ Educate the patient and family about using memory techniques:	Learning to use memory aids is a memory task itself. The patient may need extended time and reinforcement to become successful in using these techniques.
• Mnemonic devices	This internal approach to memory rehabilitation uses a variety of verbal and visual techniques to facilitate the encoding and retrieval of information.
• Imagery	Visual imagery techniques can be used to assist the patient in organizing and retrieving information.
• External memory aids such as calendars, alarms, timers, posted notes, lists, computers, and memory notebooks	These external strategies rely on environmental approaches to assist the patient in developing behavioral consistency to compensate for memory loss. Research indicates that external memory aids have more value than internal techniques. Learning to use them can be challenging for the patient. QSEN: Evidence-based practice.
■ Provide family members and caregivers with information about impaired memory and the patient's behavior.	Knowledge about impaired memory may help family members and caregivers understand the meaning of a patient's behavior. This information may help the family support the patient and provide a safer environment.
■ Allow family members and caregivers to express feelings about the patient's impaired memory and behavior.	The demands of caring for the patient with impaired memory may have a significant impact on the family's lifestyle and interactions. Unresolved stress and frustration may lead to angry verbal or physical outbursts directed toward the patient. These strategies help the family resolve stress associated with the burden of caregiving and reduce the risk of harm directed toward the patient. QSEN: Safety.
▲ Refer the patient and family to the interprofessional health team and community resources to assist in creating safe living environments.	Patients with impaired memory may no longer be able to live alone or with family members because of safety issues. The family may need help in finding alternative living arrangements for the patient such as supervised group homes or assisted living. QSEN: Teamwork and collaboration.

Related Care Plans

Chronic confusion, Chapter 2
Alzheimer's disease/dementia, Chapter 7

NANDA-I NDx Impaired Physical Mobility

Definition: Limitation in independent, purposeful physical movement of the body or of one or more extremities

Alteration in mobility may be a temporary or more permanent problem. Most disease and rehabilitative states involve some degree of immobility (e.g., as seen in strokes, leg fracture, trauma, morbid obesity, neurologic disease). With the longer life expectancy for most Americans, the incidence of disease and disability continues to grow. With shorter hospital stays, patients are being transferred to rehabilitation facilities or sent home for physical therapy in the home environment.

Mobility is also related to body changes from aging. Loss of muscle mass, reduction in muscle strength and function, stiffer and less mobile joints, and gait changes affecting balance can significantly compromise the mobility of older patients. Mobility is paramount if older patients are to maintain any independent living. Restricted movement affects the performance of most ADLs. Patients are also at increased risk for the complications of immobility. Physical and occupational therapists are key members of the interprofessional team working with nurses to care for these patients. Goals are to maintain functional ability, prevent additional impairment of physical activity, and ensure a safe environment.

Patients with decreased physical mobility often need assistance with repositioning in bed and transfer from bed to chair, commode, or wheelchair. Traditionally nurses have relied on the use of body mechanics to prevent personal injury to their back and shoulders. However, research shows that body mechanics alone is not sufficient to protect the nurse from the physical demands of manual patient handling and movement. The high incidence of work-related musculoskeletal disorders (MSDs) prompted the National Institute for Occupational Safety and Health (NIOSH) to establish evidence-based guidelines for safe patient handling (SPH). The American Nurses Association, in partnership with NIOSH and the Veterans Health Administration, has established an SPH curriculum and training program that encourages the use of safe approaches to handling patients and contributes to the prevention of MSDs.

Common Related Factors

Physical deconditioning
Alteration in cognitive function
Musculoskeletal impairment
Neuromuscular impairment
Insufficient muscle strength
Imposed restrictions of movement, including mechanical and medical protocol
Insufficient knowledge of mobility strategies
Pain/discomfort
Pharmacological agent
Obesity

Defining Characteristics

Impaired ability to reposition self in bed
Impaired ability to turn from side to side
Impaired ability to move between sitting and supine positions
Impaired ability to move between long sitting and supine positions
Impaired ability to move between prone and supine positions

Common Expected Outcomes

Patient performs physical activity independently or within limits of disease.
Patient demonstrates use of adaptive techniques that promote ambulation and transferring.
Patient is free of complications of immobility, as evidenced by intact skin, absence of thrombophlebitis, normal bowel pattern, and clear breath sounds.

NOC Outcomes
Ambulation; Joint Movement; Mobility; Transfer Performance
NIC Interventions
Exercise Therapy: Ambulation; Exercise Therapy: Joint Mobility; Fall Prevention; Positioning; Bed Rest Care; Self-Care Assistance: Transfer

Ongoing Assessment

Actions/Interventions	Rationales
■ Assess for impediments to mobility.	Identifying barriers to mobility (e.g., chronic arthritis versus stroke versus pain) guides design of an optimal treatment plan.
■ Assess the patient's ability to perform ADLs effectively and safely on a daily basis using an appropriate assessment tool, such as the Functional Independence Measures (FIM).	Restricted movement affects the ability to perform most ADLs. A variety of assessment tools are available, depending on the clinical setting. Such tools provide objective data for baselines. For example, the FIM assesses 18 self-care items related to eating, bathing, grooming, dressing, toileting, bladder and bowel management, transfer, ambulation, and stair climbing. QSEN: Patient-centered care.

■ = Independent　▲ = Interprofessional Collaboration

Actions/Interventions

- Assess the ability to perform ROM to all joints.

- Assess the emotional response to the limitation or disability.

- Assess the patient's or caregiver's knowledge of immobility and its implications.

- Assess for developing thrombophlebitis (e.g., calf pain, Homans' sign, redness, localized swelling, rise in temperature).
- Assess skin integrity for signs of redness and tissue ischemia (especially over ears, shoulders, elbows, sacrum, hips, heels, ankles, and toes).
- Monitor nutritional status.

- Assess elimination status (e.g., usual pattern, present patterns, signs of constipation).
- Evaluate the patient for safe patient handling and movement, using a standardized tool if available.
  - Ability of patient to provide assistance (independent; partial assist; dependent)
  - Weight-bearing capability (full, partial, none)
  - Upper-extremity strength (yes/no)
  - Ability of patient to cooperate and follow instructions (cooperative; unpredictable)
  - Height/weight/body mass index (BMI)
  - Special circumstances likely to affect transfer or repositioning tasks (e.g., amputation, abdominal wound, history of falls, fractures, tube insertion)
  - Specific physician orders or physical therapy recommendations that relate to transferring or repositioning patients (e.g., hip abduction during transfer)
- Refer to a safe patient handling and movement algorithm if available. For example:
  - Transfer to and from bed to chair, toilet
  - Lateral transfer to and from bed to stretcher
  - Reposition in bed: side to side, up in bed
  - Reposition in chair
  - Transfer a patient up from floor
  - Bariatric (BMI > 50) handling of preceding examples

- Evaluate the need for ambulatory aids (e.g., single point cane, quad cane, crutches, walker).

Rationales

This assessment provides data on extent of any physical problems and guides therapy. Testing by a physical therapist may be needed. QSEN: Teamwork and collaboration.

Acceptance of temporary or more permanent limitations can vary widely among individuals. Each person has his or her own definition of acceptable quality of life.

Even patients who are temporarily immobile are at risk for effects of immobility such as skin breakdown, muscle weakness, thrombophlebitis, constipation, pneumonia, and depression. The hazards of bed rest, especially in older adults, are serious. Deconditioning of the cardiovascular system can occur in days.

Reduced activity or immobility affects peripheral circulation and can promote clot formation.

Regular examination of the skin (especially over bony prominences) will allow for prevention or early recognition and treatment of pressure ulcers.

Proper nutrition provides needed energy for ambulation, transfer techniques, and participating in an exercise or rehabilitative program. Moreover, pressure ulcers develop more quickly in patients with a nutritional deficit.

Reduced activity and immobility decrease gastrointestinal motility.

Patient handling and movement activities are a basic part of nursing care. Use of a patient assessment tool can provide a standardized way to assess patients and make appropriate decisions about how to safely perform high risk tasks. Attention to these assessments reduces the risk for harm to the patient. QSEN: Safety.

Best practices algorithms and decision tools help nurses assess patient needs to determine the technique, equipment, and number of staff required for performing high-risk patient handling tasks. The Veterans Health Administration provides algorithms for selecting the right combination of equipment and personnel needed to handle or move patients safely. A sample algorithm is available at www.visn8.med.va.gov/visn8/patientsafety center/safePtHandling/default.asp. QSEN: Evidence-based practice.

Proper use of canes and walkers and other assistance can promote activity and reduce dangers of falls. The specific aid required depends on the amount of weight bearing that is tolerated, and the ability of the patient to balance safely.

Actions/Interventions

- Evaluate the safety of the immediate environment.

- Evaluate the need for home assistance (e.g., physical therapy, home care nurse).

Rationales

Obstacles such as throw rugs and children's toys, wet floors, and uneven surfaces can impede one's ability to ambulate safely. Moveable chairs need to be locked. QSEN: Safety.

Obtaining appropriate assistance for the patient can ensure safe and proper progression of activity. QSEN: Teamwork and collaboration.

Therapeutic Interventions

Actions/Interventions

- Provide a safe environment: bed rails up per protocol, bed in down position, necessary items close by.
- Perform passive or active assistive ROM exercises to all extremities.

- For more independent patients, encourage and facilitate early ambulation when possible. Assist with each initial change: dangling legs, sitting in chair, ambulation.

- Encourage the appropriate use of assistive devices. Use gait belts for safety as indicated.

- For high-risk tasks associated with safe patient handling and movement, gather the appropriate equipment and other staff members as needed, for example:
  - Powered, mechanical full-body lifts (either mobile or ceiling-mounted)
  - Powered, mobile sit-to-stand lifts
  - Friction-reducing devices
  - Patient lift teams

Rationales

These measures promote a safe, secure environment and may reduce risk for falls. QSEN: Safety.

Exercise promotes increased venous return, prevents stiffness, and maintains muscle strength and endurance. To be most effective, all joints should be exercised to prevent contractures.

These activities keep the patient as functionally active as possible. Early mobility promotes confidence about regaining independence and reduces the chance that debilitation will occur.

Crutches, canes, or walkers may be provided to assist the patient with mobility. These aids can compensate for impaired function and increase level of activity. Patients should wear a gait belt for safety so the nurse or physical therapist can guide them to reduce the risk for falling. The goal for using assistive devices is to promote safety, increase mobility, prevent falls, and conserve energy. However, some patients may refuse to use assistive devices because they attract attention to a disability. Additional home evaluation may be needed to promote a safe environment. QSEN: Safety.

Depending on the patient's needs, the use of mechanical equipment or other SPH aids (ergonomic interventions) may be required to modify the positioning or transfer activity to protect the worker. These aids work by bearing most of the load, reducing the load by lowering the friction between skin against cloth. Examples include lifting fully dependent patient out of bed and into chair using powered full-body sling lift (overhead or mobile); assisting a cooperative patient with minimal lower body strength from sitting position to standing position using powered sit to stand lift; transferring a fully dependent patient to stretcher from bed using lateral transfer aid such as a friction-reducing device; repositioning a patient in bed (side to side, up in bed) using a friction-reducing device. Staff training in the proper use of lifting equipment and devices is required. In some institutions, patient lift teams have been created composed of two or more physically fit people competent in lifting techniques, who work to perform high-risk patient transfers. They are trained in use of mechanical lifting devices. QSEN: Safety.

■ = Independent ▲ = Interprofessional Collaboration

Nursing Diagnosis Care Plans

Actions/Interventions	Rationales
■ Use the following manual principles of body mechanics: • Maintain a wide, stable base with your feet. • Put the bed at the correct height (waist level when providing care; hip level when moving a patient). • Try to keep the work directly in front of you to avoid rotating the spine. • Keep the patient as close to your body as possible to minimize reaching.	These principles should be used in conjunction with SPH measures when handling and moving patients to reduce potential for injury to patient and staff. QSEN: Evidence-based practice; Safety.
■ Allow the patient to perform tasks at his or her own rate. Do not rush the patient. Encourage independent activity as able and safe.	Hospital workers and family caregivers are often in a hurry and do more for patients than needed, thereby slowing the patient's recovery and reducing his or her self-esteem.
■ Encourage the patient to rest between activities that are tiring. Teach energy-saving techniques.	Rest periods are necessary to conserve energy. The patient must learn to respect the limitations of his or her restrictions.
■ Provide positive reinforcement during activity.	Patients may be reluctant to move or initiate new activity because of a fear of falling. A positive approach allows the learner to feel good about learning accomplishments.
■ Administer medications as appropriate.	Antispasmodic medications may reduce muscle spasms or spasticity that interferes with mobility; analgesics may reduce pain that impedes movement.
■ Assist the patient in accepting limitations. Emphasize abilities.	Quality of life is influenced by a variety of factors that can extend beyond only physical function. Help may be required for safety and comfort, but assistance needs to be balanced to avoid making the patient unnecessarily dependent.
■ Encourage resistance-training exercises using light weights when appropriate.	Research supports that strength training and other forms of exercise in older adults can preserve the ability to maintain independent living status and reduce risk for falling.
■ Institute measures to prevent skin breakdown and thrombophlebitis from prolonged immobility: • Clean, dry, and moisturize skin as needed. • Use antiembolic stockings or sequential compression devices if appropriate. • Use pressure-relieving devices as indicated (gel mattress).	These measures reduce skin breakdown, and the compression devices promote increased venous return to prevent venous stasis and possible thrombophlebitis in the legs. QSEN: Safety.
▲ Provide recommendations for nutritional intake for adequate energy resources and metabolic requirements.	The patient will need adequate, properly balanced intake of carbohydrate, fats, protein, vitamins, and minerals to provide energy resources.
▲ Set up a bowel program (e.g., adequate fluid, foods high in bulk, physical activity, stool softeners, laxatives) as needed. Record bowel activity levels.	Prolonged bed rest, lack of exercise, and physical inactivity contribute to constipation. A variety of interventions will promote normal elimination.
■ Encourage coughing and deep-breathing exercises. Use suction as needed. Use an incentive spirometer.	Decreased chest excursions and stasis of secretions are associated with immobility. Coughing and deep breathing prevent buildup of secretions. Incentive spirometry increases lung expansion.

Education/Continuity of Care

Actions/Interventions	Rationales
■ Explain progressive activity to the patient. Help the patient or caregivers establish reasonable and obtainable goals.	Information promotes awareness of the treatment plan. Setting small, attainable goals helps increase self-confidence and reduces frustration.
■ Instruct the patient or caregivers regarding hazards of immobility. Emphasize the importance of measures such as position changes, ROM, coughing, and exercises.	Information enables the patient to assume some control over the rehabilitative process.

⊖volve **For additional care plans, go to http://evolve.elsevier.com/Gulanick/.**

Actions/Interventions

- Reinforce principles of progressive exercise, emphasizing that joints are to be exercised to the point of pain, not beyond.

- Instruct the patient and family regarding the need to make the home environment safe and easier to navigate.

▲ Refer the patient to the interprofessional health team as appropriate.

Rationales

"No pain, no gain" is not always true! Pain occurs as a result of joint or muscle injury. Continued stress on joints or muscles may lead to more serious damage and limit ability to move.

A safe environment will help prevent injury related to falls. Home modification can help the patient maintain a desired level of functional independence and reduce fatigue with activity. QSEN: Safety.

Physical and occupational therapists can provide specialized services to promote effective mobility. QSEN: Teamwork and collaboration.

Related Care Plans

Risk for falls, Chapter 2
Risk for impaired skin integrity, Chapter 2

Nausea

Definition: A subjective phenomenon of an unpleasant feeling in the back of the throat and stomach, which may or may not result in vomiting

Nausea is a common and distressing symptom with a myriad of causes, including intracranial or labyrinthine lesions, chemical stimulation of the vomiting center by most medications, ingestion of toxins (chemotherapy), inhalation of anesthetic gases, microorganisms in the gastrointestinal tract, gastrointestinal obstruction, or mucosal diseases. Decreased motility and delayed emptying of the stomach are the underlying physiological factors for most causes of nausea. Decreased peristalsis in the intestines may also contribute to nausea. Nausea may have psychogenic

origins, which should be considered in cases of chronic nausea or gastroparesis. Nausea can also be associated with severe pain or aberrant motion such as in carsickness or seasickness. During the first trimester of pregnancy, nausea is common and may be related to excessive hormone production. For most women, this subsides by their second trimester; for other women, mild nausea may persist throughout the pregnancy. Because nausea is a subjective experience, the patient may find others are not supportive of their symptom if it is not associated with vomiting.

Common Related Factors

Biophysical:
- Gastrointestinal irritation
- Gastriointestinal distention
- Biochemical dyfunction (e.g., uremia, diabetic ketoacidosis)
- Pancreatic disease
- Liver/splenic capsule stretch
- Intra-abdominal tumors
- Motion sickness
- Increased intracranial pressure (ICP)
- Exposure to toxin
Situational:
- Anxiety
- Fear
- Noxious environmental stimuli
- Psychological disorder

Defining Characteristics

Reports "nausea" or "sick to stomach"
Increased salivation
Increased swallowing
Gagging sensation
Sour taste in mouth
Aversion to food

■ = Independent ▲ = Interprofessional Collaboration

Common Expected Outcome

Patient reports diminished severity or elimination of nausea.

NOC Outcomes
Comfort Status: Physical; Appetite; Nausea & Vomiting Control; Nutritional Status: Food and Fluid Intake

NIC Interventions
Nausea Management; Medication Management; Fluid Monitoring

Ongoing Assessment

Actions/Interventions

- Assess for the cause of nausea.

- Assess nausea characteristics:
  - History
  - Duration
  - Frequency
  - Severity
  - Precipitating factors
  - Medications
  - Measures used to alleviate the problem
- Assess the patient's hydration status such as measuring daily weights, BP, fluid intake and output, and skin turgor.

Rationales

Determining the cause of the nausea will guide the choice of interventions to be used. Sometimes removing the stimulus will resolve the nausea without additional treatment. Surgery may even be required to treat some causes.

A comprehensive assessment of the nausea can help determine interventions to minimize or alleviate the problem. QSEN: Patient-centered care.

Nausea is often associated with vomiting that can alter a patient's hydration status because of fluid loss. QSEN: Safety.

Therapeutic Interventions

Actions/Interventions

- Assist the patient in preparing for diagnostic testing as ordered.

- Keep an emesis basin within easy reach of the patient.

- Offer and/or assist with oral hygiene every 2 to 4 hours if tolerated.
- Remove noxious odors from the room (e.g., perfumes, dressings, emesis).
- Offer cold water, ice chips, ginger products, and room-temperature broth or bouillon if tolerated and appropriate to the patient's diet.

- Maintain fluid balance in patients at risk for nausea.

- Offer frequent, small amounts of foods that appeal to the patient:

Rationales

A variety of tests may be used to determine the cause of the nausea (e.g., upper gastrointestinal tract study, abdominal computed tomography scan, ultrasonography).
Nausea is often associated with vomiting. Keep emesis basin out of sight but in easy reach if nausea has a psychogenic component.
Nausea is often associated with anorexia and increased salivation. Oral hygiene will help promote comfort.
Strong or noxious odors can contribute to nausea.

These fluids help with hydration. For some patients, ginger helps relieve nausea whether in ginger ale, ginger tea, or chewed as crystallized ginger. Fluids with extreme temperatures may be difficult to tolerate.
Adequate hydration before surgery or chemotherapy has been shown to reduce the risk of nausea in these situations.
For some patients, an empty stomach exacerbates the nausea. QSEN: Patient-centered care.

Actions/Interventions

- Dry foods such as toast or crackers

- Bland, simple foods such as broth, rice, bananas, or Jell-O
- ■ Avoid greasy or fried foods.
- ■ Encourage the patient to use nonpharmacological nausea control techniques such as relaxation, guided imagery, music therapy, distraction, or deep breathing.
- ▲ Administer antiemetics as ordered.

- ▲ Apply acustimulation bands as ordered, or apply acupressure.

Rationales

Dry toast or crackers before rising are especially known to be effective for pregnancy-related nausea.
Patients may tolerate these types of foods. They should try to eat more when nausea is absent.
Fats are difficult to digest and may exacerbate the nausea.
These techniques have helped patients manage their nausea, but they need to be used before nausea occurs or increases, as well as with other nausea control measures.
Most antiemetics act by raising the threshold of the chemoreceptor trigger zone to stimulation. Drugs with antiemetic actions include antihistamines, anticholinergics, dopamine antagonists, serotonin (5-HT3) receptor antagonists, and benzodiazepines. Glucocorticosteroids and cannabinoids are effective to treat chemotherapy-induced nausea and vomiting. For the preoperative patient, administration of antiemetics before surgery has been shown to reduce postoperative nausea and vomiting. QSEN: Evidence-based practice.
Stimulation of the Neiguan P6 acupuncture point on the ventral surface of the wrist has been found to control nausea in some patients. This technique has been found to be especially helpful for patients who experience motion-related nausea. QSEN: Evidence-based practice.

Education/Continuity of Care

Actions/Interventions

- ■ Teach the patient to change positions slowly.
- ■ Teach the patient or caregiver about appropriate fluid and dietary choices for nausea.

- ■ Teach the patient or caregiver nonpharmacological nausea control techniques such as relaxation, guided imagery, music therapy, distraction, or deep breathing.
- ■ Teach the patient to take prescribed medications as ordered.
- ■ Evaluate the patient's response to antiemetics or interventions to alleviate nausea.

- ■ Teach the patient or caregiver how to apply acustimulation bands or acupressure.
- ■ Teach the patient or caregiver to seek medical care if vomiting develops or persists longer than 24 hours.

Rationales

Sudden or gross movement may increase nausea.
Patients and caregivers can promote adequate hydration and nutritional status by knowing dietary considerations to follow when nauseated.
Teaching the patient and caregiver methods to control nausea increases the sense of personal efficacy in managing the nausea. QSEN: Patient-centered care.
Appropriate timing for medications reduces episodes of nausea.
It is important to evaluate the interventions used to determine their effectiveness or to find other interventions that may be more effective for the patient.
Patients and caregivers may want to continue with this intervention if it was found effective in controlling nausea.
Persistent vomiting can lead to dehydration, electrolyte imbalance, and nutritional deficiencies. QSEN: Safety.

■ = Independent ▲ = Interprofessional Collaboration

Nursing Diagnosis Care Plans

NANDA-I NDx **Noncompliance**

Definition: Behavior of person and/or caregiver that fails to coincide with a health-promoting or therapeutic plan agreed on by the person (and/or family and/or community) and health care professional. In the presence of an agreed-on health-promoting or therapeutic plan, a person's or caregiver's behavior is fully or partially nonadherent and may lead to clinically ineffective or partially ineffective outcomes.

The fact that a patient has attained knowledge regarding the treatment plan does not guarantee compliance. Failure to follow the prescribed plan may be related to a number of factors. Much research has been conducted in this area to identify key predictive factors. Several theoretical models, such as the Health Belief Model, Theory of Reasoned Decision Making, and Theory of Planned Behavior, serve to explain those factors that influence patient compliance. Patients are more likely to comply when they believe that they are susceptible to an illness or disease that could seriously affect their health, that certain behaviors will reduce the likelihood of contracting the disease, that the prescribed actions are less threatening than the disease itself, and when normative groups support the change. Factors that may predict noncompliance include past history of noncompliance, stressful lifestyles, contrary cultural or religious beliefs and values, lack of social support, lack of financial resources, and compromised emotional state. People living in adverse social situations (e.g., battered women, homeless individuals, those living amid street violence, the unemployed, or those in poverty) may purposefully defer following medical recommendations until their acute socioeconomic situation is improved. The rising costs of health care and the growing number of uninsured and underinsured patients often force patients with limited incomes to choose between food and medications. The problem is especially complex for older patients living on fixed incomes but requiring complex and costly medical therapies.

Common Related Factors

Values incongruent with plan
Health beliefs incongruent with plan
Cultural incongruence
Difficulty in patient-provider relationship
Health care system barriers
Complex treatment regimen
Intensity of regimen
Insufficient knowledge about the regimen
Financial barriers

Defining Characteristics

Failure to meet outcomes
Nonadherence behavior
Development of complications
Exacerbation of symptoms
"Revolving-door" hospital admissions
Missing appointments

Common Expected Outcomes

Patient/significant other reports compliance with therapeutic plan.
Patient complies with therapeutic plan, as evidenced by appropriate pill count, appropriate amount of drug in blood or urine, evidence of therapeutic effect, maintained appointments, and/or fewer hospital admissions.

NOC Outcomes

Adherence Behavior; Compliance Behavior; Knowledge: Treatment Regimen; Participation in Health Care Decisions

NIC Interventions

Behavior Modification; Decision-Making Support; Patient Contracting; Health Education

 evolve **For additional care plans, go to http://evolve.elsevier.com/Gulanick/.**

Ongoing Assessment

Actions/Interventions	Rationales
■ Compare the actual therapeutic effect with the expected effect.	These data provide information on compliance; however, if therapy is ineffective or based on a faulty diagnosis, even perfect compliance will not result in the expected therapeutic effect.
■ Ask the patient to bring prescription drugs to appointments; count remaining pills.	This technique provides some objective evidence of compliance. It is commonly used in drug research protocols.
■ Assess serum or urine drug levels.	Therapeutic blood levels will not be achieved without consistent ingestion of medication; overdosing or overtreatment can likewise be assessed. Information may also help distinguish between patients not using recommended treatment and those not responding to a prescribed treatment.
■ Plot the pattern of hospitalizations and clinic appointments.	These data provide objective information regarding follow-up, but do not necessarily mean that the patient is not complying with other prescribed therapies.
■ Assess the factors that the patient thinks interfere with compliance.	Identifying barriers unique to each patient allows for individualizing the corrective plan. Such barriers may include cognitive impairment, fear of actually experiencing medication side effects, failure to understand instructions regarding the plan (e.g., difficulty understanding a low-sodium diet), impaired manual dexterity (e.g., pill container is too difficult to open), sensory deficit (e.g., unable to read written instructions), costly therapies, and regard for nontraditional treatments (e.g., herbs, liniments, prayer, acupuncture). QSEN: Patient-centered care.
■ Assess the patient's individual perceptions of health problems and interest in following the treatment plan.	According to the Health Belief Model, a patient's perceived susceptibility to and perceived seriousness and threat of disease, along with perceived benefits from adhering to treatment plan, affect compliance. Some patients may not understand the chronicity of their disease or their ability to manage some of the ongoing symptoms. QSEN: Evidence-based practice; Patient-centered care.
■ Assess the patient's beliefs about his or her current illness and the importance of health care.	Not all people view maintenance of health the same. For example, some may place trust in God for treatment and refuse pills, blood transfusions, or surgery. Others may only want to follow a "natural" or "health food" regimen. Determining what the patient thinks is causing his or her symptoms or disease, how likely it is that the symptoms may return, and any concerns about the diagnosis or symptoms will provide a basis for planning future care. QSEN: Patient-centered care.
■ Assess the patient's religious beliefs or practices that affect health and disease management.	People of other cultures and religious heritages may hold differing views regarding health and illness. For some cultures the causative agent may be a person, not a microbe. Many people view illness as a punishment from God that must be treated through spiritual healing practices (e.g., prayer, pilgrimage), not medications.
■ Assess the patient's beliefs about the treatment plan.	Understanding any worries or misconceptions that the patient may have about the plan or side effects will guide future interventions.

■ = Independent ▲ = Interprofessional Collaboration

Therapeutic Interventions

Actions/Interventions	Rationales
■ Develop a therapeutic relationship with the patient and family.	Compliance increases when there is a trusting relationship and a consistent caregiver. Use of a skilled interpreter is necessary for patients who do not speak the dominant language.
■ Include the patient in planning the treatment regimen.	Patients who become co-managers of their care have a greater stake in achieving a positive outcome. They know best their personal and environmental barriers to success.
■ Remove disincentives to compliance.	Actions to increase compliance include such examples as decreasing waiting time in the clinic, finding ways to reduce the cost of therapies (e.g., prescribing generic medications, refilling for 90 vs. 30 days), or suggesting medications with fewer side effects.
▲ Simplify therapy. Suggest long-acting forms of medications, and eliminate unnecessary medication.	Compliance increases when therapy is short and includes as few treatments as possible. Polypharmacy is a significant problem with older patients.
■ Eliminate unnecessary clinic visits.	The physical demands of traveling to an appointment, the financial costs incurred (loss of day's work, child care), the negative feelings of being "talked down to" by health care providers not fluent in the patient's language, as well as the commonly long waits can cause patients to avoid follow-ups when they are required. Telephone follow-up may be substituted as appropriate.
■ Tailor the therapy to the patient's lifestyle (e.g., diuretics may be taken with the evening meal for patients who work outside the home) and culture (incorporate herbal medicinal massage or prayer, as appropriate).	Individualization will ensure a patient-centered focus and promote compliance. A "one size fits all" approach is usually ineffective. QSEN: Patient-centered care.
■ If negative side effects of prescribed treatment are a problem, explain that many side effects can be controlled or eliminated.	Nonadherence because of medication side effects is a commonly reported problem. Health care providers need to determine actual etiological factors for side effects and possible interplay with over-the-counter medications. Similarly, patients may report fatigue or muscle cramps with exercise. If so, the exercise prescription may need to be revised.
■ Increase the amount of supervision provided; as compliance improves, gradually reduce the amount of professional supervision and reinforcement.	Home health nurses, telephone monitoring, and frequent return visits or appointments can provide increased supervision as needed that can be tapered as appropriate.
■ Develop a behavioral contract.	A contract helps the patient understand and accept his or her role in the care plan and clarifies what the patient can expect from the health care worker or system.
■ Develop with the patient a system of rewards that follow successful compliance.	Rewards provide positive reinforcement for compliant behavior. They may consist of verbal praise, monetary rewards, special privileges, or telephone calls by health care providers.

Education/Continuity of Care

Actions/Interventions	Rationales
■ Provide specific instruction as indicated.	Information enables the patient to better take control in selecting and implementing required changes in behavior.
■ Tailor the information in terms of what the patient feels is the cause of his or her health problem and his or her concerns about therapy.	Adult learning is problem-oriented. Focus should be on strategies that reduce barriers to treatment and enhance desired outcome.

⊖volve **For additional care plans, go to http://evolve.elsevier.com/Gulanick/.**

Actions/Interventions

- Instruct the patient in the importance of reordering medications 2 to 3 days before running out. Consider 90-day refills for long-term chronic conditions.

- For long-term medications, explore the benefits of home-delivery pharmacy services.
- Teach significant others to eliminate disincentives/increase rewards to the patient for compliance.
- Provide social support through the patient's family and self-help groups.

Rationales

A percentage of medication nonadherence is caused by patients simply being late to get a pharmacy refill. This may be due to cultural issues whereby patients are more time-oriented to the present rather than future needs, to insurance company restrictions on early refills to the standard 30-day fill, or to simple forgetfulness and procrastination. The 90-day supplies require refills only 4 times a year instead of the typical 12 times.

Patients can be more adherent to their therapy with easier access.

Nagging is never effective in promoting change. Incorporating rewards for positive accomplishments is more effective.

Such groups may assist the patient in gaining greater understanding of the benefits of treatment.

 NANDA-I
NDx

Imbalanced Nutrition: Less Than Body Requirements

Definition: Intake of nutrients insufficient to meet metabolic needs

Adequate nutrition is necessary to meet the body's demands. Nutritional status can be affected by disease or injury states (e.g., gastrointestinal malabsorption, cancer, burns); physical factors (e.g., muscle weakness, poor dentition, activity intolerance, pain, substance abuse); social factors (e.g., lack of financial resources to obtain nutritious foods); or psychological factors (e.g., depression, boredom, dementia). During times of illness (e.g., trauma, surgery, sepsis, burns), adequate nutrition plays an important role in healing and recovery. Cultural and religious factors strongly affect the food habits of patients. Women exhibit a higher incidence of voluntary restriction of food intake secondary to anorexia, bulimia, and self-constructed fad dieting. Patients who are older experience problems in nutrition related to lack of financial resources, cognitive impairments causing them to forget to eat, physical limitations that interfere with preparing food, deterioration of their sense of taste and smell, reduction of gastric secretion that accompanies aging and interferes with digestion, and social isolation and boredom that cause a lack of interest in eating. This care plan addresses general concerns related to nutritional deficits for the hospital or home setting.

Common Related Factors

Inability to ingest foods
Inability to digest foods
Inability to absorb nutrients
Economically disadvantaged
Biological factors
Psychological disorders
Insufficient dietary intake

Defining Characteristics

Weight loss with adequate food intake
Body weight 20% or more below ideal weight range
Food intake less than recommended dietary allowance (RDA)
Excessive hair loss
Pale mucous membranes
Insufficient interest in food
Sore buccal cavity
Weakness of muscles needed for mastication and/or swallowing

Common Expected Outcomes

Patient or caregiver verbalizes and demonstrates selection of foods or meals that will achieve a cessation of weight loss.
Patient weighs within 10% of ideal body weight range.

NOC Outcomes
Nutritional Status: Food and Fluid Intake;
  Nutritional Status: Nutrient Intake; Knowledge:
  Healthy Diet
NIC Interventions
Nutritional Monitoring; Nutrition Therapy;
  Nutrition Management

■ = Independent ▲ = Interprofessional Collaboration

Ongoing Assessment

Actions/Interventions	Rationales
■ Measure weight and height; do not estimate.	A patient's estimate of his or her actual weight and height or weight loss may be inaccurate. These anthropomorphic assessments are used to determine the patient's caloric and nutrient requirements. QSEN: Evidence-based practice.
■ Obtain a nutritional history; include the family, significant others, or the caregiver in the assessment.	The patient's perception of actual intake may differ from his or her actual intake. Family members may provide a more accurate estimate of the patient's eating habits and food intake.
■ Determine the etiological factors for reduced nutritional intake.	Proper assessment guides intervention. For example, patients with dentition problems require referral to a dentist, whereas patients with memory losses may require services such as Meals On Wheels. The patient may be taking medications that suppress appetite as a side effect.
■ Assess the patient's attitudes and beliefs toward eating and food.	Many psychological, social, religious, and cultural factors determine the type, amount, and appropriateness of food consumed by the patient. The nurse incorporates this information in the planning and evaluation of care and communicates the information to the interprofessional team. QSEN: Patient-centered care.
■ Assess the environment in which eating occurs.	Many adults find themselves "eating on the run" (e.g., at their desk, in the car) or relying heavily on fast foods with reduced nutritional components. Older adults living alone may not have the motivation to prepare a meal for themselves.
▲ Monitor laboratory values that indicate nutritional well-being or deterioration:	A variety of laboratory tests may be used to monitor the patient's nutritional status. QSEN: Evidence-based practice.
• Serum albumin	This test indicates degree of protein depletion (2.5 g/dL indicates severe depletion; 3.8 to 4.5 g/dL is normal).
• Transferrin	Transferrin is a plasma protein that is important for iron transfer and typically decreases as serum protein decreases.
• RBC and WBC counts	Anemia and leukopenia occur in malnutrition, leading to weakness, and are usually decreased in malnutrition.
• Serum electrolyte values	Potassium is typically increased and sodium is typically decreased in malnutrition.
■ Assess for physical signs of poor nutritional intake.	The patient experiencing nutritional deficiencies may appear listless and fatigued. The patient may have a decreased attention span and episodes of confusion. The skin may be pale and dry, with loss of subcutaneous tissue. Hair will be dull, brittle, and easily plucked from the scalp. The tongue and oral mucous membranes may be pale and sore. Vital signs may show tachycardia and elevated BP.

Therapeutic Interventions

Actions/Interventions	Rationales
▲ Consult a dietitian for further assessment and recommendations regarding nutritional status and methods for nutritional support.	The dietitian can determine nitrogen balance as a measure of the patient's nutritional status. Protein malnutrition leads to a negative nitrogen balance. The dietitian can calculate the patient's daily requirements of specific nutrients to promote adequate nutritional intake. Based on the patient's nutritional requirements, the dietitian will recommend the most appropriate method to increase nutritional intake that is consistent with the patient's food and eating preferences. QSEN: Teamwork and collaboration.
■ Establish appropriate short-term and long-term goals.	Depending on the etiological factors of the problem, improvement in nutritional status may take several months. Without realistic short-term goals to provide tangible rewards, patients may lose interest in addressing this problem.
■ Ensure a pleasant environment, facilitate proper positioning, and provide good oral hygiene and dentition.	The patient is more likely to eat in a setting that is free of unpleasant odors and noisy distractions. Oral hygiene before meals has a positive effect on appetite and the taste of food. Dentures need to be clean, fit comfortably, and be in the patient's mouth to encourage eating. Elevating the head of bed 30 degrees aids in swallowing and reduces risk for aspiration with eating. QSEN: Patient-centered care; Safety.
■ Provide companionship during mealtime.	Attention to the social aspects of eating is important in both the hospital and home settings.
■ For patients with changes in their sense of taste, encourage the use of seasoning.	Seasoning may enhance the flavor of foods and entice eating.
▲ For patients with physical impairments, refer to an occupational therapist for adaptive devices.	The occupational therapist can offer devices such as plate guards and strap-on utensils that can help patients feed themselves. QSEN: Teamwork and collaboration.
▲ For patients with impaired swallowing, refer to a speech therapist for evaluation and recommendations.	The speech therapist can evaluate the degree of swallowing impairment and make recommendations about adjusting the thickness and consistency of foods to increase nutritional intake. QSEN: Teamwork and collaboration.
■ For hospitalized patients, encourage the family to bring food from home as appropriate.	Patients with specific ethnic or religious preferences or restrictions may not be able to eat hospital foods.
■ Suggest the use of nutritional supplements between meals.	Such supplements can be used to increase calories and protein without interfering with voluntary food intake.
■ Discourage beverages that are caffeinated or carbonated.	These beverages may decrease appetite and lead to early satiety.
■ Discuss the possible need for enteral or parenteral nutritional support with the patient, family, and caregiver, as appropriate.	For patients who are unable to maintain nutritional intake by the oral route, other means of nutritional support may be indicated. Enteral tube feedings are preferred for patients with a functioning gastrointestinal tract. Parenteral nutrition may be indicated for patients who cannot tolerate enteral feedings. Enteral and parenteral feeding formulas can be modified to provide required glucose, protein, essential fatty acids, electrolytes, vitamins, minerals, and trace elements. These feedings may be used with in-hospital, long-term care, and subacute care settings, as well as in the home.
■ Encourage exercise.	Metabolism and utilization of nutrients are enhanced by activity.

■ = Independent   ▲ = Interprofessional Collaboration

Nursing Diagnosis Care Plans

Education/Continuity of Care

Actions/Interventions

■ Review and reinforce the following to the patient or caregivers:
  • The basic four food groups, MyPyramid/MyPlate food guides, and the need for specific minerals or vitamins
  • Importance of maintaining adequate caloric intake; an average adult (70 kg) needs 1800 to 2200 kcal/day; patients with burns, severe infections, or draining wounds may require 3000 to 4000 kcal/day
  • Foods high in calories and protein that will promote weight gain and nitrogen balance (e.g., small frequent meals of foods high in calories and protein)
■ Provide referral to community nutritional resources such as Meals On Wheels or hot lunch programs for seniors as indicated.

Rationales

Patients may not understand what is involved in a balanced diet. They are better able to ask questions and seek assistance when they know basic information.

Many seniors (especially those living alone) do not take the time or effort to cook for themselves.

NANDA-i NDx Overweight/Obesity

Definitions: *Overweight:* A condition in which an individual accumulates abnormal or excessive fat for age and gender. *Obesity:* A condition in which an individual accumulates abnormal or excessive fat for age and gender that exceeds overweight.

Overweight and obesity are common health problems in the United States, and their prevalence is growing globally, accounting for significant other health problems, including cardiovascular disease, type 2 diabetes mellitus, sleep disorders, infertility in women, aggravated musculoskeletal problems, and shortened life expectancy. Women are more likely to be overweight than men. African Americans and Hispanic individuals are more likely to be overweight than Caucasians. Although multiple factors contribute to overweight/obesity (genetics, the biology of one's regulatory systems, environment, medications, psychological state), the fact remains that most people gain weight because they consume more calories than they expend.

Overall nutritional requirements of older patients are similar to those of younger individuals, except calories should be reduced for older adults who have a sedentary lifestyle and reduced metabolic rate. The care of the overweight and obese patient is combined in this one care plan because there is so much overlap in assessments and interventions. The nurse is directed to the additional care plan: Readiness for Weight Management in Chapter 3, as needed.

Common Related Factors

Obesity in childhood
Parental obesity
Portion sizes larger than recommended
High frequency of restaurant or fried food
Consumption of sugar-sweetened beverages
Frequent snacking
Disordered eating behaviors
Average daily physical activity is less than recommended for gender and age
Economically disadvantaged
Genetic disorder

Defining Characteristics

Overweight: BMI > 25 kg/m^2
Obesity: BMI > 30 kg/m^2

Common Expected Outcomes

Patient verbalizes accurate information about benefits of weight loss.

Patient verbalizes measures necessary to achieve beginning weight reduction.

Patient demonstrates appropriate selection of meals or menu planning toward the goal of weight reduction.

NOC Outcomes
Nutritional Status: Food and Fluid Intake; Weight Loss Behavior; Knowledge: Weight Management

NIC Interventions
Nutritional Monitoring; Nutritional Counseling; Weight Reduction Assistance; Knowledge: Healthy Diet; Knowledge: Weight Management

Ongoing Assessment

Actions/Interventions	Rationales
■ Determine weight, waist circumference, and BMI.	Weight needs to be documented objectively, as patient may have been only estimating over time. Men with waist circumference greater than 40 inches and women with greater than 35 inches are at higher risk for obesity-related complications. BMI describes relative weight for height and is significantly correlated with total body fat content. BMI is calculated as the patient's weight (in kilograms) divided by the height squared (in meters squared). A BMI between 20 and 24 is associated with healthier outcomes. A BMI greater than 25 is associated with increased risk of morbidity and mortality. A BMI of >30 should be referred for intensive multicomponent behavioral interventions.
■ Assess the effects or complications of being overweight.	Medical complications include cardiovascular and respiratory dysfunction, sleep-disordered breathing, higher incidence of diabetes mellitus, and aggravation of musculoskeletal disorders. Social complications and poor self-esteem may also result from obesity.
■ Assess the patient's readiness to initiate a weight loss regimen by asking questions such as the following: How do you feel about starting a weight loss program? Are you ready to choose a time to start changing your eating habits?	The Transtheoretical Model emphasizes that interventions for change should be matched with the stage of change at which patients are situated. For example, if the patient is only contemplating starting a weight loss program, efforts may be directed toward emphasizing the health benefits of healthy eating, whereas if the patient is in the preparation or action stages, more specific directions regarding weight loss (e.g., calorie counting, portion sizes) can be addressed. QSEN: Evidence-based practice; Patient-centered care.
■ Perform a nutritional assessment to include: • Daily food intake—type and amount • Approximate caloric intake • Activity at time of eating • Feelings at time of eating • Location of meals • Meals skipped • Snacking patterns • Social/familial considerations	Environmental factors contribute to obesity more than genetics or biological vulnerability. Assessment of current eating patterns provides a baseline for change. Assessment methods may include a 24-hour recall of foods eaten, food diaries/records, or food frequency recording using typical food groups. QSEN: Patient-centered care.
■ Determine the behavioral factors that contribute to overeating.	Overeating may be triggered by environmental cues and behavioral factors unrelated to physiological hunger sensations.

■ = Independent ▲ = Interprofessional Collaboration

Actions/Interventions

- Assess any possible barriers to initiating a weight loss program, such as lack of motivation, interpersonal support, skills, knowledge, or resources.
- Assess the patient's ability to read food labels.

- Assess the patient's ability to plan a menu and make appropriate food selections.

- Assess the patient's ability to accurately identify appropriate food portions.

Rationales

If the patient is aware of possible barriers and has formulated plans for dealing with them, successful change is more likely to occur.

Food labels contain information necessary in making appropriate selections, but can be misleading. Patients need to understand that "low-fat" or "fat-free" does not mean that a food item is calorie free. In addition, attention should be paid to serving size and the number of servings in the food item.

This information provides the starting point for the educational sessions. Teaching content the patient already knows wastes valuable time and hinders critical learning.

Serving sizes must be understood to limit intake according to a planned diet.

Therapeutic Interventions

Actions/Interventions

- Establish appropriate short-term and long-term goals.

- Encourage the patient to keep a daily log of food or liquid ingestion and caloric intake.

▲ Consult a dietitian for further assessment and recommendations regarding a weight loss program.

- For patients ready to engage in a serious weight management program, refer to care plan: Readiness for Weight Management, in Chapter 3 as appropriate. For significantly obese patients, refer to care plan for Bariatric Surgery, in Chapter 8.

Rationales

Depending on the etiological factors of the problem, improvement in nutritional status may take a long time. Without realistic short-term goals to provide tangible rewards, patients may lose interest in addressing this problem. QSEN: Patient-centered care.

Memory is inadequate for quantification of intake, and a visual record may also help the patient make more appropriate food choices and serving sizes.

Changes in eating patterns are required for weight loss. The type of program may vary (e.g., three balanced meals a day, avoidance of certain high-fat foods). Dietitians have a greater understanding of the nutritional value of foods and may be helpful in assessing or substituting specific high-fat cultural or ethnic foods. QSEN: Teamwork and collaboration.

This care plan provides information on strategies for engaging in a successful weight management program.

Education/Continuity of Care

Actions/Interventions

- Provide ongoing education about the benefits of weight loss to both the patient and significant others.

- Review and reinforce teaching regarding the four major food groups, proper serving size, caloric content of food, and methods of food preparation to avoid additional calories.

Rationales

Patients and families need information on the many health benefits of weight loss and the potential health risks of being overweight. This will need to be reinforced over time.

The key principle of weight loss therapy is to eat fewer calories than are expended in order to consume fat stores as fuel. Patients need to learn to eat a variety of foods in appropriate portion sizes when changing their eating pattern to ensure lifelong success at weight maintenance. See related care plans for additional information.

Actions/Interventions

■ Include the family, caregiver, or food preparer in nutrition counseling.

■ Review the complications associated with obesity.

Rationales

The patient will be more likely to adhere to changes in food intake when family members are involved in the changes. Research has documented that men whose wives diet with them are more likely to achieve goals than those for whom special food is prepared.

Patients need to be aware of long-term health problems as stimulus for change. Medical complications include cardiovascular and respiratory dysfunction, higher incidence of diabetes mellitus, and aggravation of musculoskeletal disorders. Social complications and poor self-esteem may also result from obesity.

Related Care Plans

Readiness for enhanced nutrition, Chapter 3
Readiness for weight management, Chapter 3

Impaired Oral Mucous Membrane

Definition: Injury to the lips, soft tissue, buccal cavity, and/or oropharynx

Minor irritations of the oral mucous membrane occur occasionally in all people and are usually viral-related, self-limiting, and easily treated. Patients who have severe stomatitis often have an underlying illness. Patients who are immunocompromised, such as the oncology patient receiving chemotherapy, are often affected with severe tissue disruption and pain. Infections such as candidiasis, if left untreated, can spread through the entire gastrointestinal tract, causing further complications and sometimes perineal pain. Oral mucous membrane problems can be encountered in any setting, especially in home care and hospice settings.

Common Related Factors

Dehydration
NPO for more than 24 hours
Mouth breathing
Decrease in salivation
Insufficient knowledge of appropriate oral hygiene
Insufficient oral hygiene
Infection
Malnutrition
Treatment regimen
Chemical injury
Mechanical factors (e.g., ill-fitting dentures, braces, tubes [endotracheal or nasogastric]); oral surgery

Defining Characteristics

Oral pain or discomfort
Xerostomia (dry mouth)
Coated tongue
Stomatitis
Oral lesions or ulcers
Spongy patches in mouth
Hyperemia
Oral vesicles
Desquamation
Oral edema
Gingival pocketing
Halitosis
Impaired ability to swallow

■ = Independent ▲ = Interprofessional Collaboration

Common Expected Outcomes

Patient has healthy oral cavity as evidenced by intact, pink, moist mucous membranes.
Patient demonstrates appropriate oral hygiene practices.
Patient verbalizes absence of discomfort or inflammation of oral mucous membranes.

NOC Outcomes
Oral Health; Tissue Integrity: Skin and Mucous Membranes; Self-Care: Oral Hygiene
NIC Interventions
Oral Health Restoration; Oral Health Maintenance

Ongoing Assessment

Actions/Interventions	Rationales
■ Assess the patient's oral hygiene practices.	Information provides direction on possible causative factors and guidance for subsequent education. QSEN: Patient-centered care.
■ Assess the status of the oral mucosa; include the tongue, lips, mucous membranes, gums, saliva, and teeth. Use adequate light. Examine after removal of dental appliances. Use a moist, padded tongue blade to gently pull back the cheeks and tongue.	A systematic inspection should be performed of listed sites using a tongue blade to expose areas of the oral cavity. Denture removal is important because lesions may be underlying and further irritated by the appliance. Caregivers also need to be informed of the importance of these assessments.
■ Assess for the extensiveness of ulcerations involving the intraoral soft tissues, including the palate, tongue, gums, and lips.	Sloughing of mucosal membrane can progress to ulceration.
▲ Observe for any evidence of infection, and culture lesions as needed. Report to the physician or home health nurse. Severe mucositis may manifest as any of the following: • Candidiasis: cottage cheese-like white or pale yellowish patches on tongue, buccal mucosa, and palate • Herpes simplex: painful itching vesicle (typically on upper lips) that ruptures within 12 hours and becomes encrusted with a dried exudate • Gram-positive bacterial infection, specifically staphylococcal and streptococcal infections: dry, raised, wartlike yellowish brown, round plaques on buccal mucosa • Gram-negative bacterial infections: creamy to yellow-white, shiny, nonpurulent patches often seated on painful, red, superficial mucosal ulcers and erosions • Fevers, chills, rigors	Early assessment facilitates prompt treatment. Specific manifestations guide accurate treatment.
■ Assess nutritional status.	Malnutrition can be a contributing cause. Oral fluids are needed for moisture to membranes.
■ Assess for the ability to eat and drink.	Inability to chew and swallow may occur secondary to pain of inflamed or ulcerated oral and/or oropharyngeal mucous membranes.

Therapeutic Interventions

Actions/Interventions	Rationales
For hospitalized or home care patients: ■ Implement a meticulous mouth care regimen after each meal and every 4 hours while awake. Caregivers need to be taught these procedures. (See the Education/Continuity of Care section for a description of oral care.)	Mouth care prevents buildup of oral plaque and bacteria. Patients with oral catheters and oxygen may require additional care.

Actions/Interventions

▲ If signs of mild stomatitis occur (sensation of dryness and burning; mild erythema and edema along the mucocutaneous junction):
- Increase the frequency of oral hygiene by rinsing with one of the suggested solutions between brushings and once during the night.
- Discontinue flossing if it causes pain.
- Provide systemic or topical analgesics as ordered.

■ Instruct the patient that topical analgesics can be administered as "swish and swallow" or "swish and spit" 15 to 20 minutes before meals, or painted on each lesion immediately before mealtime.

■ Instruct the patient to hold the solution for several minutes before expectorating and not to use the solution if the mucosa is severely ulcerated or if drug sensitivity exists.

■ Explain the use of topical protective agents:

- Zilactin or Zilactin-B

- Gelclair

- Substrate of an antacid and kaolin preparation

- Palifermin

▲ For severe mucositis infection:
- Administer local antimicrobial agents as ordered.

- Discontinue the use of a toothbrush and flossing.

■ Continue the use of lubricating ointment on the lips.
■ For eating problems:
- Encourage a diet high in protein and vitamins.
- Serve foods and fluids lukewarm or cold.
- Serve frequent small meals or snacks spaced throughout the day.
- Encourage soft foods (e.g., mashed potatoes, puddings, custards, creamy cereals).
- Encourage the use of a straw.
- Encourage peach, pear, or apricot nectars and fruit drinks instead of citrus juices.

▲ Refer the patient to the dietitian for instructions on the maintenance of a well-balanced diet.

Rationales

These safety measures reduce further damage and may promote comfort. Increased sensitivity to pain is a result of thinning of oral mucosal lining and may require analgesia. QSEN: Safety.

A variety of options are available to patients, such as viscous lidocaine gel (2%). Each must be performed as prescribed for optimal results. These topical analgesics provide a "numbing" feeling to ease discomfort. They may be used alone or combined with a liquid antacid or antihistamine for greater comfort.

This technique enhances full therapeutic effect.

A variety of more protective topical agents are available to coat the lesions and promote healing as prescribed.

This medicated gel contains benzocaine for pain and is painted on the lesion and allowed to dry to form a protective seal and promote healing of mouth sores.

This bioadherent oral gel coats the oral cavity and forms a protective barrier to soothe pain.

This mucosal coating agent is prepared by allowing antacid to settle. The pasty residue is swabbed onto the inflamed areas and, after 15 to 20 minutes, is rinsed with saline or water. The residue remains as a protectant on the lesion.

This agent decreases the incidence and duration of severe oral mucositis in patients with hematological cancers undergoing high-dose chemotherapy followed by bone marrow transplantation.

Mycostatin, nystatin, and Mycelex Troche are commonly prescribed.

Brushing could increase damage to ulcerated tissues. A disposable foam stick (Toothette) or sterile cotton swab is a way to gently apply cleansing solutions.

Lubrication prevents drying and cracking.

Dietary modifications may be necessary to promote healing and tissue integrity. The patient may need to select food and fluids that are less irritating to oral tissues. Soft, bland foods served at lukewarm or cool temperatures may feel soothing on oral tissues.

Nutritional expertise may be required to optimize the therapeutic diet needed to promote healing. QSEN: Teamwork and collaboration.

■ = Independent   ▲ = Interprofessional Collaboration

Education/Continuity of Care

Actions/Interventions	Rationales
■ Instruct the patient or caregiver to perform the following:	
• Gently brush all surfaces of the teeth, gums, and tongue with a soft-bristled nylon or foam brush. Floss gently.	Careful mechanical cleansing and flossing loosens debris, stimulates circulation, and reduces risk for infection. Toothbrushes should be replaced every few months.
• Brush with a nonabrasive dentifrice such as baking soda.	Baking soda promotes further cleaning of teeth.
• Remove and brush dentures thoroughly during and after meals and as needed.	Dental care is key to reducing risk for infection and improving appetite.
• Have loose-fitting dentures adjusted.	Rubbing and irritation from ill-fitting dentures promotes disruption of the oral mucous membrane.
• Rinse the mouth thoroughly during and after brushing.	Removing food particles decreases risk for infection related to trapped decaying food.
• Avoid alcohol-containing mouthwashes and lemon/glycerin types of swabs.	Alcohol and lemon/glycerin actually dry oral mucous membranes, increasing risk for disruption of mucous membrane.
• Use the following recommended mouth rinses: • Baking soda (1 teaspoon) and water (8 oz) • Salt (½ teaspoon), baking soda (1 teaspoon), and water (8 oz)	Commercial mouthwashes can be irritating; special formulas are better tolerated and may reduce irritation and promote healing. Antiplaque mouthwashes are indicated for preventive care. Saline solutions can enhance oral lubrication directly as well as stimulating salivary glands to increase salivary flow.
• Keep lips moist. Use a lip product or a water-soluble lubricant (e.g., K-Y jelly, Aquaphor Cream).	Lubrication prevents drying and cracking of lips. These products minimize risk for aspirating a non–water-soluble agent.
• Encourage the use of commercial saliva products as indicated.	A variety of synthetic saliva-producing products are available to treat dry mouth.
• Include food items with each meal that require chewing.	Chewing stimulates gingival tissue and promotes circulation.
• Avoid the use of tobacco and alcohol, extremely hot or cold foods, and acidic or highly spiced foods.	These products are irritating and drying to the mucosa, and can aggravate xerostomia.

NANDA-I NDx Acute Pain

Definition: An unpleasant sensory and emotional experience associated with actual or potential tissue damage or described in terms of such damage (International Association for the Study of Pain); sudden or slow onset of any intensity from mild to severe with an anticipated or predictable end

Pain is a highly subjective state in which a variety of unpleasant sensations and a wide range of distressing factors may be experienced by the patient. Acute pain serves a protective function to make the patient aware of an injury or illness. The sudden onset of acute pain prompts the patient to seek relief. The physiological manifestations that occur with acute pain result from the body's response to pain as a stressor. The patient's cultural background, emotions, and psychological or spiritual distress may contribute to the suffering with acute pain. Pain assessment can be challenging, especially in older patients, in whom cognitive impairment and sensory-perceptual deficits are more common. This care plan focuses on the assessment and management of acute pain in the hospital or home care settings.

Common Related Factors

Biological injury agent (e.g., infection, ischemia, neoplasm)
Chemical injury agent (e.g., burn, capsaicin, methylene chloride, mustard agent)
Physical injury agent (e.g., abscess, amputation, burn, cut, heavy lifting, operative procedure, trauma, overtraining)

Defining Characteristics

Self-report of intensity using standardized pain scale (e.g., Wong-Baker FACES scale, visual analog scale, numeric rating scale)
Self-report of pain characteristics using standardized pain instrument (e.g., McGill Pain Questionnaire, Brief Pain Inventory)
Guarding behavior
Protective behavior
Diaphoresis
Self-focused
Narrowed focus (e.g., time perception, interaction with people and environment)
Distraction behavior
Expressive behavior (e.g., crying, restlessness, vigilance)
Facial expression of pain (e.g., eyes lack luster, beaten look, fixed or scattered movement, grimace)
Positioning to ease pain
Change in physiological parameter (e.g., blood pressure, heart rate, respiratory rate, and oxygen saturation)

Common Expected Outcomes

Patient reports satisfactory pain control and a decreased intensity using a standardized pain scale.
Patient uses pharmacological and nonpharmacological pain management strategies.
Patient exhibits increased comfort such as baseline levels for pulse, BP, respirations, and relaxed muscle tone or body posture.

NOC Outcomes

Comfort Status; Medication Response; Pain Control; Pain Level

NIC Interventions

Analgesic Administration; Pain Management; Patient-Controlled Analgesia (PCA) Assistance; Sedation Management

Ongoing Assessment

Actions/Interventions

- Assess pain characteristics:

  - Quality (e.g., sharp, burning, shooting)
  - Intensity (scale of 0 [meaning no pain] to 10 [meaning the most severe pain])
  - Location (anatomical description)
  - Onset (gradual or sudden)
  - Duration (how long; intermittent or continuous)
  - Precipitating or relieving factors
- Assess for signs and symptoms associated with pain.

Rationales

Assessment of the pain experience is the first step in planning pain management strategies. The patient is the most reliable source of information about his or her pain. Eliciting the patient's expressed needs allows the patient to be a full partner in providing pain management care. QSEN: Patient-centered care.

A numeric rating scale or other descriptive scales can be used to identify the intensity of pain.

Some people deny the experience of pain when it is present. Attention to associated signs may help the nurse in evaluating pain. The patient in acute pain may have an elevated BP, HR, and temperature. The patient's skin may be pale and cool to touch. The patient may be restless and have difficulty concentrating.

■ = Independent ▲ = Interprofessional Collaboration

Actions/Interventions	Rationales
■ Evaluate the patient's response to pain and pain management strategies.	It is important to help patients express as factually as possible (i.e., without the effect of mood, emotion, or anxiety) the effect of pain relief measures. Discrepancies between behavior or appearance and what the patient says about pain relief (or lack of it) may be more a reflection of other methods the patient is using to cope with the pain rather than pain relief itself. QSEN: Patient-centered care.
■ Assess to what degree cultural, environmental, intrapersonal, and intrapsychic factors may contribute to pain or pain relief.	These variables may modify the patient's expression of his or her experience. For example, some cultures openly express feelings, whereas others restrain such expression. However, health care providers should not stereotype any patient response but rather evaluate the unique response of each patient. QSEN: Patient-centered care.
■ Evaluate what the pain means to the patient.	The meaning of the pain will directly influence the patient's response. Some patients, especially the dying, may feel that the "act of suffering" meets a spiritual need.
■ Assess the patient's expectations for pain relief.	Some patients may be content to have pain decreased; others will expect complete elimination of pain. This affects their perceptions of the effectiveness of the treatment modality and their willingness to participate in additional treatments. QSEN: Patient-centered care.
■ Assess the patient's willingness or ability to explore a range of techniques aimed at controlling pain.	Some patients may be unaware of the effectiveness of non-pharmacological methods and may be willing to try them, either with or instead of traditional analgesic medications. Often a combination of therapies (e.g., mild analgesics with distraction or heat) may be more effective. Some patients will feel uncomfortable exploring alternative methods of pain relief. However, patients need to be informed that there are multiple ways to manage pain.
■ Assess the appropriateness of the patient as a PCA candidate.	PCA is the IV infusion of an opioid (usually morphine or hydromorphone) through an infusion pump that is controlled by the patient. This allows the patient to manage pain relief within prescribed limits. The criteria for implementing PCA include no history of substance abuse; no allergy to opioid analgesics; clear sensorium; cooperative and motivated about use; no history of renal, hepatic, or respiratory disease; manual dexterity; and no history of major psychiatric disorder. In the hospice or home setting, a nurse or caregiver may be needed to assist the patient in managing the infusion.
If the patient is on PCA, assess the following:	
■ Compare the amount of pain medication the patient is using to his or her reports of pain.	If demands for medication are quite frequent, the patient's dosage may need to be increased to promote pain relief. If demands are very low, the patient may require further instruction to properly use PCA.
■ Consider possible PCA complications such as excessive sedation; respiratory distress; urinary retention; nausea and vomiting; constipation; and IV site pain, redness, or swelling	Early assessment of complications is necessary to prevent serious adverse reactions to opioid analgesics. QSEN: Safety.

Actions/Interventions

If the patient is receiving epidural analgesia, assess the following:

- Numbness, tingling in the extremities, a metallic taste in the mouth

- Possible epidural analgesia complications such as excessive sedation, respiratory distress, urinary retention, or catheter migration

Rationales

These symptoms may be indicators of an allergic response to the anesthesia agent or of improper catheter placement. QSEN: Safety.

Respiratory depression and intravascular infusion of anesthesia (resulting from catheter migration) can be potentially life threatening. QSEN: Safety.

Therapeutic Interventions

Actions/Interventions

- Anticipate the need for pain relief.

- Respond immediately to reports of pain.

- Eliminate additional stressors or sources of discomfort whenever possible.

- Provide rest periods to facilitate comfort, sleep, and relaxation.

▲ Determine the appropriate pain relief method.

Pharmacological methods include the following:
- Nonopioids (acetaminophen), a nonselective NSAID, or a selective NSAID (e.g., COX-2 inhibitor)

- Opioid analgesics

- Local anesthetic agents

Nonpharmacological methods include the following:
- Cognitive-behavioral strategies as follows:
  - Imagery

Rationales

One can most effectively deal with pain by preventing it. Early intervention may decrease the total amount of analgesic required.

In the midst of painful experiences, a patient's perception of time may become distorted. Anxiety and fear about delayed pain relief can exacerbate the pain experience. Prompt responses to reports of pain may result in decreased anxiety in the patient. Demonstrated concern for the patient's welfare and comfort fosters the development of a trusting relationship. QSEN: Patient-centered care.

Patients may experience an exaggeration in pain or a decreased ability to tolerate painful stimuli if environmental, intrapersonal, or intrapsychic factors are further stressing them.

The patient's experiences of pain may become exaggerated as the result of fatigue. In a cyclic fashion, pain may result in fatigue, which may result in exaggerated pain and exhaustion. A quiet environment, a darkened room, and a disconnected phone are all measures geared toward facilitating rest.

Unless contraindicated, all patients with acute pain should receive a nonopioid analgesic around-the-clock.

NSAIDs work in peripheral tissues. Some block the synthesis of prostaglandins, which stimulate nociceptors. They are effective in managing mild to moderate pain. QSEN: Evidence-based practice.

Opioids may be administered orally, intravenously, systemically by PCA systems, or epidurally (either by bolus or continuous infusion). Intramuscular injections are not reliably absorbed. Opioids are indicated for severe pain, especially in the hospice or home setting. QSEN: Evidence-based practice.

Local anesthetics block pain transmission and are used for pain in specific areas of nerve distribution.

The use of a mental picture or an imagined event involves use of the five senses to distract oneself from painful stimuli.

Nursing Diagnosis Care Plans

Actions/Interventions

- Distraction techniques

- Relaxation exercises, biofeedback, breathing exercises, music therapy

- Cutaneous stimulation as follows:
  - Massage of the affected area when appropriate

  - Transcutaneous electrical nerve stimulation (TENS) units

  - Hot or cold compress

▲ Give analgesics as ordered, evaluating their effectiveness and observing for any signs and symptoms of untoward effects.

■ Consult with the physician if interventions are unsuccessful or if the current complaint is a significant change from the patient's past experience of pain.

■ Whenever possible, reassure the patient that pain is time limited and that there is more than one approach to easing pain.

If the patient is on PCA:
▲ Dedicate the use of an IV line for PCA only; consult a pharmacist before mixing other drugs with opioids being infused.

If the patient is receiving epidural analgesia:
■ Label all tubing (e.g., epidural catheter, IV tubing to epidural catheter) clearly to prevent the inadvertent administration of inappropriate fluids or drugs into the epidural space.

For the patient with PCA or epidural analgesia:
■ Keep Narcan or other opioid-reversing agents readily available.
■ Post a "no additional analgesia" sign over the bed.

Rationales

These techniques heighten one's concentration upon non-painful stimuli to decrease one's awareness and experience of pain. Some methods are breathing modifications and nerve stimulation.

Techniques are used to bring about a state of physical and mental awareness and tranquility. The goal of these techniques is to reduce tension, subsequently reducing pain.

Massage interrupts pain transmission, increases endorphin levels, and decreases tissue edema. This intervention may require another person to provide the massage.

TENS requires the application of two to four skin electrodes. Pain reduction occurs through a mild electrical current. The patient is able to regulate the intensity and frequency of the electrical stimulation.

Heat reduces pain through improved blood flow to the area and through reduction of pain reflexes. Cold reduces pain, inflammation, and muscle spasticity by decreasing the release of pain-inducing chemicals and slowing the conduction of pain impulses.

Pain medications are absorbed and metabolized differently by patients. Therefore the effectiveness of the analgesics must be evaluated individually for each patient. Analgesics may cause side effects that range from mild to life threatening. QSEN: Safety.

Patients who request pain medications at more frequent intervals than prescribed may actually require higher doses or more potent analgesics. QSEN: Teamwork and collaboration.

When pain is perceived as everlasting and unresolvable, the patient may give up trying to cope with it or experience a sense of hopelessness and loss of control.

IV incompatibilities are possible.

Inappropriate use of an epidural catheter can cause neurological injury or infection. QSEN: Safety.

In case of respiratory depression, these drugs reverse the opioid effect. QSEN: Safety.

This signage prevents inadvertent analgesic overdosing. QSEN: Safety.

Education/Continuity of Care

Actions/Interventions

■ Provide anticipatory instruction on pain causes, appropriate prevention, and relief measures.

Rationales

Knowledge about what to expect can help the patient develop effective coping strategies for pain management. Patients need to learn the importance of reporting pain early to achieve more effective pain relief.

⊖volve **For additional care plans, go to http://evolve.elsevier.com/Gulanick/.**

Actions/Interventions

- Instruct the patient to evaluate and report the effectiveness of measures used.
- Teach the patient effective timing of the medication dose in relation to potentially uncomfortable activities and the prevention of peak pain periods.

For patients on PCA or those receiving epidural analgesia:

- Teach the patient preoperatively about postoperative pain management with PCA. Information given to the patient includes the purpose, benefits, techniques of use and action, need for IV line (PCA only), other alternatives for pain control, and the need to notify the nurse of machine alarm and occurrence of untoward effects.

Rationales

Pain relief strategies can be modified to promote more satisfactory comfort levels.

Patients need to learn to use pain relief strategies to minimize the pain experience.

Effective pain management with PCA requires patient knowledge of how to use the equipment. Anesthesia effects should not obscure teaching.

NANDA-I NDx Chronic Pain

Definition: Unpleasant sensory and emotional experience arising from actual or potential tissue damage or described in terms of such damage (International Association for the Study of Pain); sudden or slow onset of any intensity from mild to severe, constant or recurring without an anticipated or predictable end and a duration of greater than 3 months

Chronic pain may be classified as chronic malignant pain or chronic nonmalignant pain. In the former, the pain is associated with a specific cause such as cancer. With chronic nonmalignant pain, the original tissue injury is not progressive or has been healed but the patient continues to experience pain. Identifying an organic cause for this type of chronic pain is more difficult.

Chronic pain differs from acute pain in that it is harder for the patient to provide specific information about the location and the intensity of the pain. Over time it becomes more difficult for the patient to differentiate the exact location of the pain and clearly identify the intensity of the pain. The patient with chronic pain often does not present with behaviors and physiological changes characteristic of acute pain. Family members, friends, co-workers, employers, and health care providers may question the legitimacy of the patient's pain reports because the patient may not look like someone in pain. The patient may be accused of using pain to gain attention or to avoid work and family responsibilities. With chronic pain, the patient's level of suffering usually increases over time. Chronic pain can have a profound impact on the patient's activities of daily living, mobility, activity tolerance, ability to work, role performance, financial status, mood, emotional status, spirituality, family interactions, and social interactions.

Common Related Factors

Alteration in sleep pattern
Chronic musculoskeletal condition
Damage to nervous system
Emotional distress
History of static work postures
History of vigorous exercise
Imbalance of neurotransmitters, neuromodulators, and receptors
Immune disorder (e.g., HIV-associated neuropathy, varicella-zoster virus)
Impaired metabolic functioning
Prolonged computer use (>20 hours/week)
Repeated handling of heavy loads
Tumor infiltration
Whole-body vibration

Defining Characteristics

Self-report of intensity using standardized pain scale (e.g. Wong-Baker FACES scale, visual analog scale, numeric rating scale)
Self-report of pain characteristics using standardized pain instrument (e.g., McGill Pain Questionnaire, Brief Pain Inventory)
Self-focused
Anorexia
Alteration in sleep pattern
Altered ability to continue previous activities

■ = Independent   ▲ = Interprofessional Collaboration

Common Expected Outcomes

Patient reports satisfactory pain control at a decreased intensity using a standardized pain scale.

Patient uses pharmacological and nonpharmacological pain management strategies.

Patient engages in desired activities without an increase in pain intensity.

NOC Outcomes
Pain Control; Pain: Disruptive Effects; Pain: Adverse Psychological Response

NIC Interventions
Pain Management; Medication Management; Acupressure; Heat/Cold Application; Progressive Muscle Relaxation; Transcutaneous Electrical Nerve Stimulation (TENS); Massage

Ongoing Assessment

Actions/Interventions	Rationales
■ Assess pain characteristics: • Quality (e.g., sharp, burning) • Severity (scale of 0 [meaning no pain] to 10 [meaning the most severe pain]) • Location (anatomical description) • Onset (gradual or sudden) • Duration (e.g., continuous, intermittent) • Precipitating factors • Relieving factors	The most reliable source of information about the chronic pain experience is the patient's self-report. Systematic assessment and documentation of the chronic pain experience provides direction for a pain management plan. QSEN: Patient-centered care.
■ Assess for signs and symptoms associated with chronic pain such as fatigue, decreased appetite, weight loss, changes in body posture, sleep pattern disturbance, anxiety, irritability, restlessness, or depression.	Patients with chronic pain may not exhibit the physiological changes and behaviors associated with acute pain. Pulse and BP are usually within normal ranges. The guarding behavior of acute pain may become a persistent change in body posture for the patient with chronic pain. Coping with chronic pain can deplete the patient's energy for other activities. The patient often looks tired, with a drawn facial expression that lacks animation.
■ Assess the patient's perception of the effectiveness of methods used for pain relief in the past.	Patients with chronic pain have a long history of using many pharmacological and nonpharmacological methods to control their pain. An effective pain management plan will be based on the patient's previous experience with pain relief measures. QSEN: Patient-centered care.
■ Evaluate the gender, cultural, societal, and religious factors that may influence the patient's pain experience and response to pain relief.	Understanding the variables that affect the patient's pain experience can be useful in developing a care plan that is acceptable to the patient. The patient's heritage will influence the meaning of pain, expressions of suffering associated with pain, and selection of pain management strategies. QSEN: Patient-centered care.
■ Assess the patient's expectations about pain relief.	The patient with chronic pain may not expect complete absence of pain but may be satisfied with decreasing the intensity of the pain and increasing activity level. QSEN: Patient-centered care.
■ Assess the patient's attitudes toward pharmacological and nonpharmacological methods of pain management.	Patients may question the effectiveness of nonpharmacological interventions and see medications as the only treatment for pain. Patients may have misconceptions regarding alternative and complementary therapies for pain relief. This information provides a basis for teaching the patient about pain management strategies.

Actions/Interventions

- For patients taking opioid analgesics, assess for side effects, dependency, and tolerance.

- Assess the patient's ability to accomplish activities of daily living, instrumental activities of daily living, and demands of daily living.

Rationales

Drug dependence and tolerance to opioid analgesics are concerns in the long-term management of chronic pain. The patient and family may have misconceptions and fears about drug tolerance, dependence, and addiction.

Fatigue, anxiety, and depression associated with chronic pain can limit the person's ability to complete self-care activities and fulfill role responsibilities.

Therapeutic Interventions

Actions/Interventions

- Encourage the patient to keep a pain diary to help in identifying aggravating and relieving factors of chronic pain.

- Acknowledge and convey acceptance of the patient's pain experience.

- Assist the patient in making decisions about selecting a particular pain management strategy.

- ▲ Refer the patient to a physical therapist for evaluation.

Rationales

Knowledge about factors that influence the pain experience can guide the patient in making decisions about lifestyle modifications that promote more effective pain management. QSEN: Patient-centered care.

The patient may have had negative experiences in the past with attitudes of health care providers toward the patient's pain experience. Conveying acceptance of the patient's pain promotes a more cooperative nurse-patient relationship.

Guidance and support from the nurse can increase the patient's willingness to choose new interventions to promote pain management. A combination of nonpharmacological therapies and analgesic medications may be most effective. Nonopioid medications are preferred medications because of their low side-effect profile, especially among older patients. Medications should be given around-the-clock to achieve a consistent level of pain relief and comfort. The oral route is preferred.

The physical therapist can help the patient with exercises to promote muscle strength and joint mobility and therapies to promote relaxation of tense muscles. QSEN: Teamwork and collaboration.

Education/Continuity of Care

Actions/Interventions

- Teach the patient and family about chronic pain and options available for pain management.

- Teach the patient and family about using nonpharmacological pain management strategies:

  • Cold applications

Rationales

Lack of knowledge about the characteristics of chronic pain and pain management strategies can add to the burden of pain in the patient's life.

Knowledge about how to implement nonpharmacological pain management strategies can help the patient and family gain maximum benefit from these interventions. QSEN: Evidence-based practice.

Cold reduces pain, inflammation, and muscle spasticity by decreasing the release of pain-inducing chemicals and slowing the conduction of pain impulses. This intervention requires no special equipment and can be cost-effective. Cold applications should last about 20 to 30 minutes per hour.

■ = Independent   ▲ = Interprofessional Collaboration

Actions/Interventions	**Rationales**
• Heat applications	Heat reduces pain through improved blood flow to the area and through reduction of pain reflexes. This is a cost-effective intervention that requires no special equipment. Heat applications should last no more than 20 minutes per hour. Special attention needs to be given to preventing burns with this intervention. QSEN: Safety.
• Massage of the painful area	Massage interrupts pain transmission, increases endorphin levels, and decreases tissue edema. This intervention may require another person to provide the massage. Many health insurance programs will not reimburse for the cost of therapeutic massage.
• Progressive relaxation, imagery, and music	These centrally acting techniques for pain management work through reducing muscle tension and stress. The patient may feel an increased sense of control over his or her pain. Guided imagery can help the patient explore images about pain, pain relief, and healing. These techniques require practice to be effective.
• Distraction	Distraction is a temporary pain management strategy that works by increasing the pain threshold. It should be used for a short duration, usually less than 2 hours at a time. Prolonged use can add to fatigue and increased pain when the distraction is no longer present.
• Acupressure	Acupressure involves finger pressure applied to acupressure points on the body. Using the gate control theory, the technique works to interrupt pain transmission by "closing the gate." This approach requires training and practice.
• Transcutaneous electrical nerve stimulation (TENS)	TENS requires the application of two to four skin electrodes. Pain reduction occurs through a mild electrical current. The patient is able to regulate the intensity and frequency of the electrical stimulation.
■ Teach the patient and family about the use of pharmacological interventions for pain management:	
• Nonopioids (acetaminophen); nonselective NSAIDs; and selective NSAIDs (COX-2 inhibitor)	These drugs are the first step in an analgesic ladder. They work in peripheral tissues by inhibiting the synthesis of prostaglandins that cause pain, inflammation, and edema. The advantages of these drugs are that they can be taken orally and are not associated with dependency and addiction. They should be given around-the-clock to provide a consistent level of pain relief. QSEN: Evidence-based practice.
• Opioid analgesics (narcotics)	These drugs act on the central nervous system to reduce pain by binding with opiate receptors throughout the body. The side effects associated with this group of drugs tend to be more significant than those with the NSAIDs. Nausea, vomiting, constipation, sedation, respiratory depression, tolerance, and dependency are of concern in patients using these drugs for chronic pain management.
• Antidepressants • Anticonvulsants	Antidepressants and anticonvulsants may be useful adjuncts in a total program of pain management, especially for those with chronic neuropathic pain. In addition to their effects on the patient's mood, the antidepressants may have analgesic properties apart from their antidepressant actions.

Actions/Interventions

- Assist the patient and family in identifying lifestyle modifications that may contribute to effective pain management. Guide the patient to plan activities during periods of greatest relief from pain.

- Refer the patient and family to community support groups and self-help groups for people coping with chronic pain.

Rationales

Changes in work routines, household responsibilities, and the home physical environment may be needed to promote more effective pain management. Providing the patient and family with ongoing support and guidance will increase the success of these strategies.

Adding to the patient's network of social support can reduce the burden of suffering associated with chronic pain and provide additional resources.

Related Care Plans

Fatigue, Chapter 2
Acute pain, Chapter 2

NANDA-I

Post-Trauma Syndrome

Definition: Sustained maladaptive response to a traumatic, overwhelming event

Post-trauma syndrome, also called post-traumatic stress disorder (PTSD), occurs in individuals who have experienced, witnessed, or been confronted by an event or events that have involved actual or threatened death or serious injury or a threat to the physical integrity of self or others. New evidence suggests that patients who sustain traumatic brain injury, especially concussion force injury, develop PTSD. The individual's response with PTSD involves intense fear, helplessness, or horror. Typically the maladaptive response(s) continue beyond 1 month, causing significant distress or impairment in social, occupational, physical, spiritual, or psychological functioning. These maladaptive responses may be acute or chronic.

Common Related Factors

History of abuse (physical, psychosocial, sexual)
History of being held prisoner of war
History of criminal victimization
Events outside the range of usual human experience
Destruction of one's home or community
Serious injury, accidents, or threat to self or loved one
History of torture
Exposure to event involving multiple deaths
Witnessing mutilation or violent death
Exposure to war, epidemic, disaster (natural or man-made)

Defining Characteristics

Aggression, anger, rage
Alienation, avoidance behaviors
Anxiety
Compulsive behavior
Denial
Depression
Alteration in concentration
Exaggerated startle response
Hypervigilance
Fear
Flashbacks, intrusive thoughts and dreams, nightmares
Guilt, shame
Headache
Panic attacks
Dissociative amnesia
Reports feeling numb
Substance abuse

■ = Independent   ▲ = Interprofessional Collaboration

Common Expected Outcomes

Patient experiences fewer flashbacks, intrusive recollections, and nightmares.

Patient demonstrates increased concentration.

Patient contacts nurse/therapist/physician for appointment when symptoms reappear or increase.

Patient verbalizes reduction of depressed mood, anxiety, physical symptoms, and physical aggression.

Patient verbalizes hopefulness and empowerment.

NOC Outcomes
Aggression Self-Restraint; Coping; Mood Equilibrium; Personal Resiliency

NIC Interventions
Active Listening; Anger Control Assistance; Emotional Support; Guilt Work Facilitation; Hope Inspiration; Mood Management; Support Group; Counseling

Ongoing Assessments

Actions/Interventions	Rationales
Review the patient's history for traumatic events.	PTSD may develop months or years following a traumatic event. Childhood losses, exposure to violence, or trauma may manifest as PTSD in adulthood. People who faced combat in wars are more likely to have delayed onset and prolonged duration of PTSD.
■ Assess for the presence and degree of depression and anxiety.	A thorough assessment results in early identification and intervention to prevent escalation of symptoms. The patient with PTSD may withdraw from interactions with family, friends, and co-workers. QSEN: Patient-centered care.
■ Assess for statements of guilt or self-blame for the traumatic event or the patient's own survival.	The patient may feel responsible for the event or the deaths of others. The patient's religious or cultural heritage may support feelings of guilt or shame related to behavior during the traumatic event. The patient may make statements about not having done enough in the event or not deserving to survive the event. QSEN: Patient-centered care.
■ Identify fearful reactions or hypervigilance to ordinary objects or situations.	Ordinary objects and situations (e.g. walking in crowded areas, sudden loud noises, driving in heavy traffic, approaching strangers) may cause the person to experience feelings from the original traumatic event. The patient may startle easily or respond aggressively in response to these situations.
■ Assess for the presence and degree of suicidal ideation, including a plan, means, past attempts, family history, and ability to agree to a contract for safety.	Feelings of guilt, low self-worth as a survivor, or depression may lead to thoughts of suicide. QSEN: Safety.
■ Assess for the presence and degree of homicidal ideation, including a plan, identified target/person, history of violence toward others, intended means, and availability of means.	Disorganized thinking and increasing anxiety may lead to aggression and violence directed toward others. Domestic violence may develop as part of PTSD. QSEN: Safety.
■ Assess the effectiveness of relationships with family, friends, and co-workers.	The patient experiencing PTSD is more likely to react aggressively with family members, leading to domestic violence. Family members, friends, and co-workers may not know how to effectively provide support. Family and friends may be overly attentive or withdrawn. Either type of reaction is not supportive to the patient with PTSD. Inability to function in the workplace may lead to being fired and unemployment.
■ Assess for adherence to the prescribed medication regimen.	Adherence to drug therapy can lessen the symptoms or prevent relapse. Antidepressants (e.g., SSRIs) have been used effectively in the management of PTSD. QSEN: Evidence-based practice.

Actions/Interventions	**Rationales**
■ Assess for active substance abuse.	The patient may abuse alcohol or drugs to blunt the painful feelings associated with the trauma. These behaviors will interfere with and delay the recovery process.
■ Monitor sleep and activity patterns.	Sleep disturbance is a common manifestation of PTSD. The patient may experience excessive fatigue that limits participation in work or family activities.

Therapeutic Interventions

Actions/Interventions	**Rationales**
■ Establish trust by being nonjudgmental and honest; offer empathy and support; allow the patient to feel a sense of control.	Developing trust following trauma may be difficult for patients. The patient who feels a sense of control may be less likely to exhibit aggressive responses.
■ Assure the patient that his or her feelings and behaviors are typical following a traumatic event.	Patients often believe they are guilty for the event and that they are going crazy. The patient needs to understand that his or her feelings are a normal response to an extraordinary event. QSEN: Patient-centered care.
■ Maintain safety for the patient and his or her environment.	A patient's anxiety can escalate to panic, and he or she may become suicidal or outwardly violent. QSEN: Safety.
■ Provide the patient with a safe means for expressing feelings, especially those of anger and aggression.	Physical activities, journaling, or drawing give the patient an outlet for intense emotions. These activities provide opportunities to dissipate the energy associated with these emotions. The energy is directed to the activity rather than toward self or others. Creative expression of emotions may facilitate coping with the traumatic event.
■ Assist patients in recognizing the connection between the trauma experience and their current feelings.	Patients are often unaware of this connection.
■ Assist patients in evaluating past behaviors in the context of the traumatic event, not in the context of current values.	Patients are often guilty about past behaviors and judgmental toward themselves.
■ Encourage adaptive coping behaviors based on past successes.	Patients might be using maladaptive or dysfunctional coping to avoid dealing with feelings and issues.
■ Encourage the establishment or reestablishment of healthy relationships.	Relationships may have been negatively affected by the patient's feelings of detachment.
■ Monitor adherence to the prescribed medication regimen.	Adherence to the prescribed medication regimen can prevent or lessen exacerbation of symptoms.
▲ Refer the patient to resources for professional counseling.	Evidence supports the effectiveness of a variety of cognitive and behavior therapies in the management of the patient with PTSD. QSEN: Teamwork and collaboration; Evidence-based practice.

Education/Continuity of Care

Actions/Interventions	**Rationales**
■ Teach the distinction between anxiety that is connected to identifiable sources/objects and anxiety for which there is no identifiable object or source.	Knowledge of anxiety and its related components increases the patient's feelings of control. QSEN: Patient-centered practice.
■ Teach anxiety-reducing strategies: • Progressive relaxation • Mindful meditation • Slow deep-breathing exercises • Focusing on single object in the room • Listening to soothing music or relaxation tapes • Visual imagery	These activities assist in lessening anxiety and its related components. Knowledge and use of them increases the patient's control over the disorder.

■ = Independent ▲ = Interprofessional Collaboration

Nursing Diagnosis Care Plans

Actions/Interventions

- Encourage the patient to seek support people/groups to assist with performing personal tasks and activities that are currently difficult to perform.
- Educate the patient on the actions, benefits, and side effects of prescribed medications.

- Educate the patient on the importance of limiting caffeine, nicotine, and other central nervous system stimulants.
- Teach family members about post-trauma syndrome and methods to provide helpful support.

Rationales

A strong support system will assist the patient in avoiding anxiety-provoking situations/activities.

Knowledge can lessen the seriousness of potential side effects and increase the likelihood of patient adherence to prescribed regimen. QSEN: Safety.

Limiting these substances prevents/minimizes the physical symptoms of anxiety.

Family members who did not experience the traumatic event may have unrealistic expectations about the patient's response to and recovery from the trauma. When family members can provide effective support, they may feel less helpless.

Related Care Plans

Rape-trauma syndrome, Chapter 2
Risk for suicide, Chapter 2

NANDA-I
NDx Powerlessness

Definition: The lived experience of lack of control over a situation, including a perception that one's actions do not significantly affect an outcome.

Powerlessness may be expressed at any time during a patient's illness. During an acute episode, people used to being in control may temporarily find themselves unable to navigate the health care system and environment. The medical jargon, the swiftness with which decisions are made, and the vast array of health care providers to which the patient has to relate can all cause a feeling of powerlessness. This response is compounded by patients of cultural, religious, or ethnic backgrounds that differ from those of the dominant health care providers. Patients with chronic, debilitating, or terminal illnesses may have long-term feelings of powerlessness because they are unable to change their inevitable outcomes. Older patients are especially susceptible to the threat of loss of control and increasing dependence that comes with aging, as well as the consequences of illness and disease. Patients suffering from feelings of powerlessness may be seen in the hospital, ambulatory care, rehabilitation, or home care environment.

Common Related Factors

Dysfunctional institutional environment
Complex treatment regimen
Insufficient interpersonal interactions

Defining Characteristics

Insufficient sense of control
Inadequate participation in care
Alienation
Dependency
Depression
Doubt about role performance
Frustration about inability to perform previous activities

Common Expected Outcomes

Patient identifies ways to achieve control over personal situation.
Patient expresses sense of personal control.
Patient makes decisions free from undue pressure from others.
Patient expresses satisfaction with life choices.

NOC Outcomes

Health Beliefs: Perceived Ability to Perform; Health Beliefs: Perceived Control; Participation in Health Care Decisions

NIC Interventions

Decision-Making Support; Self-Efficacy Enhancement

Ongoing Assessment

Actions/Interventions	Rationales
■ Assess the patient's power needs or need for control.	Patients are usually able to identify those aspects of self-governance that they miss most and that are most important to them. QSEN: Patient-centered care.
■ Assess for feelings of hopelessness, depression, and apathy.	These feelings may be a component of powerlessness.
■ Identify the patient's locus of control.	The degree to which people attribute responsibility to themselves (internal control) versus other forces (external control) determines the locus of control. Patients with a predominantly external locus of control may be more susceptible to feelings of powerlessness. QSEN: Patient-centered care.
■ Identify situations/interactions that may add to the patient's sense of powerlessness.	Many medical routines are superimposed on patients without ever receiving their permission, fostering a sense of powerlessness. It is important for health care providers to recognize the patient's right to refuse procedures such as feeding tubes and intubation.
■ Assess the patient's decision-making ability.	Powerlessness is the feeling that one has lost the implicit power for self-governance. It is not the same as the inability to make a decision.
■ Assess the role the illness plays in the patient's sense of powerlessness.	Uncertainty about events, duration and course of illness, prognosis, and dependence on others for help and treatments can contribute to powerlessness.
■ Assess the impact of powerlessness on the patient's physical condition (e.g., appearance, oral intake, hygiene, sleep habits).	Individuals may feel as though they are unable to control very basic aspects of life and self-care activities. Patients most vulnerable to powerlessness are those who are increasingly susceptible to stressful events (e.g., illness with impaired mobility, older age). QSEN: Patient-centered care.
■ Assess the effects of the information about illness and treatment provided on the patient's behavior and feelings.	This assessment approach will help the nurse differentiate powerlessness from knowledge deficit. A patient experiencing powerlessness may ignore information. Too much information may overwhelm the patient and add to feelings of powerlessness. A patient simply experiencing a knowledge deficit may be mobilized to act in his or her own best interest after information is given and options are explored. The act of providing information may heighten a patient's sense of autonomy. QSEN: Patient-centered care.

Therapeutic Interventions

Actions/Interventions	Rationales
■ Encourage the verbalization of feelings, perceptions, and fears about making decisions.	This nursing action creates a supportive climate and sends a message of caring. The verbalization of feelings and perceptions helps the patient develop a more realistic appraisal of the stressful situation. QSEN: Patient-centered care.

■ = Independent   ▲ = Interprofessional Collaboration

Actions/Interventions	Rationales
■ Consult with the patient regarding his or her care (e.g., treatment options, convenience of visits, or time of ADLs).	Allowing the patient to participate in deciding when and how these things are to be accomplished will increase the patient's sense of autonomy through shared decision-making. Patients may become overwhelmed by the high-tech medical environment and may relegate decision-making to the health care providers. This behavior may be especially evident in patients whose cultural heritage differs from that of the dominant health care providers. QSEN: Patient-centered care.
■ Encourage the patient to identify strengths.	Review of past coping experiences and prior decision-making skills may assist the patient in recognizing inner strengths. Self-confidence and security come with a sense of control.
■ Assist the patient in reexamining negative perceptions of the situation.	The patient may have misconceptions or unrealistic expectations for the situation.
■ Eliminate the unpredictability of events by allowing adequate preparation for tests or procedures.	Information in advance of a procedure can provide the patient with a sense of control.
■ Encourage an increased responsibility for self.	The perception of powerlessness may negate the patient's attention to areas in which self-care is attainable; however, the patient may require significant support systems and resources to accomplish goals.
■ Give the patient control over his or her environment. Encourage the patient to furnish the environment with those things that he or she finds comforting.	This technique enhances the patient's sense of autonomy and acknowledges his or her right to have dominion over controllable aspects of life. It applies to the hospital as well as the extended care or home care environment.
■ Assist with creating a timetable to guide increased responsibility in the future.	With short hospital stays, patients may find themselves helpless and dependent on discharge, and they may unrealistically perceive their situation as unchangeable. Use of realistic short-term goals for resuming aspects of self-care may foster confidence in one's abilities.
■ Provide positive feedback for making decisions and participating in self-care.	Success fosters confidence in abilities and a sense of control. Praise and positive reinforcement for self-care are profound motivators for enhancing self-esteem and feelings of self-governance.
■ Assist the patient in identifying the significance of culture, religion, race, gender, and age on his or her sense of powerlessness.	Especially in the hospital environment when the patient does not speak the dominant language, food is different, and customs such as bathing, personal space, and privacy differ, patients may retreat and develop a sense of powerlessness. The use of patient advocates and outreach workers from a given ethnic community may provide a bridge to the health care providers. QSEN: Patient-centered care.
■ Avoid using coercive power when approaching the patient.	This approach may intensify the patient's feelings of powerlessness and result in decreased self-esteem.

Education/Continuity of Care

Actions/Interventions	Rationales
■ Assist family members or caregivers in allowing the patient to be independent with activities within his or her abilities.	Caregivers may foster a sense of dependence in their efforts to be helpful and caring.
■ Refer to support groups or self-help groups and community resources as appropriate.	People who have "been there" may be most helpful in providing the supportive empathy necessary to move the patient to the next level of independence and control.

⊖volve **For additional care plans, go to http://evolve.elsevier.com/Gulanick/.**

NANDA-I
NDx Rape-Trauma Syndrome

Definition: Sustained maladaptive response to a forced, violent, sexual penetration against the victim's will and consent

Rape-trauma syndrome refers to the immediate period of psychological disorganization and the long-term process of reorganization that occur as a result of attempted or actual sexual assault. Every survivor of sexual assault will express unique emotional needs and may respond differently to rape. However, almost all survivors, male and female, experience elements of the syndrome as a response to the extreme stress, profound fear of death, and sense of violation and vulnerability. Sexual assault survivors may suffer various effects of this violent crime for the remainder of their lives. Recovery from the physical trauma associated with the rape may prolong and complicate the survivor's response to and recovery from the psychological trauma. Cultural bias, social attitudes, and preconceived ideas about rape victims may make it difficult for victims to report the crime. Male victims of sexual assault tend to be more stigmatized, experience more guilt and difficulty reconciling their masculine identity with their experience of being an assault victim, and are even less likely to report the offense than females. These biases and attitudes also make effective recovery more difficult for survivors. Improved education about the impact of rape on survivors has led to more supportive responses by law enforcement officers, emergency care first responders, and emergency department care providers.

Common Related Factors

Rape
Sexual assault trauma

Defining Characteristics

Aggression and anger
Agitation, anxiety, hyperalertness
Change in relationships
Confusion
Denial
Disorganization
Embarrassment, guilt, humiliation, self-blame, shame
Fear, paranoia, phobias
Impaired decision-making, helplessness, powerlessness
Mood swings
Muscles spasms and tension

Common Expected Outcomes

Patient verbalizes relief or reduction of discomfort from physical injuries.
Patient adopts healthy coping behaviors.
Patient refers to self as a victim or survivor, not as being responsible for the rape.

NOC Outcomes
Abuse Recovery: Emotional; Abuse Recovery: Sexual; Sexual Functioning
NIC Interventions
Rape-Trauma Treatment; Counseling; Crisis Intervention

Ongoing Assessment

Actions/Interventions

■ Assess the degree of injury sustained during the assault: bruises; lacerations; abrasions; scratches; vaginal, oral, and rectal trauma; knife wounds; gunshot wounds; strangulation marks.

Rationales

Injuries range from minor to disabling and life threatening. Serious genital injury is a common component of sexual assault. All injuries, regardless of the extent, may have a strong emotional impact on the victim. The patient may have been unconscious or psychologically guarded during the assault and may not remember details to be able to report injuries.

■ = Independent   ▲ = Interprofessional Collaboration

Actions/Interventions
- Assess for emotional and behavioral responses.

- Identify the patient's previous coping mechanisms, including cultural, religious, and personal beliefs about assault.

- Assess the patient's readiness for a physical, genital, and/or pelvic examination.

- Listen for the language the patient uses to describe himself or herself and his or her feelings about the assault.

- Assess the response of family members and significant others toward the patient.

Rationales

Defensive coping behaviors that seem normal after sexual assault may become ineffective if they persist and interfere with recovery.

In a crisis, individuals fall back on old coping mechanisms that may or may not be effective in the present situation. Beliefs about sexual assault may influence the patient's ability to come to terms with the event and whether family and friends will be effective support systems. QSEN: Patient-centered care.

The patient may respond to the intrusiveness of the examination as a continuation of the sexual assault. The patient may not understand the need to determine the extent of physical trauma and collect forensic evidence.

It is considered a normal initial response for survivors to express feelings of shame or guilt about the assault. The patient may describe himself or herself as dirty and unclean. The patient may need anticipatory guidance to reframe these feelings and view himself or herself as a victim and survivor of the assault. When extremely negative feelings persist for a prolonged time, they pose a substantial threat to the recovery of the survivor. QSEN: Patient-centered care.

Family members and significant others may struggle with their own feelings about the patient and the rape. They may experience feelings and reactions similar to the patient including guilt, anger, embarrassment, or humiliation. They may blame the victim based on cultural, religious, or personal beliefs about rape. They may be hesitant to talk with the survivor or listen to the survivor talk about the incident. Their responses may interfere with the survivor's recovery.

Therapeutic Interventions

Actions/Interventions
- Assure the survivor of immediate safety.

- Provide access to sexual assault advocate, crisis intervention specialist, or social services counselor.

- Assist the survivor in identifying and contacting family or significant others.

Rationales

Predominant emotions experienced by the survivor include horror, terror, fear of death, humiliation, and anger. They may feel vulnerable and threatened in unfamiliar surroundings. Survivors need to know that they are in a safe place and protected from further harm. QSEN: Safety.

Integrating the contributions of specially trained sexual assault response team members provide effective support and immediate crisis intervention to patients and family members. QSEN: Teamwork and collaboration.

The survivor may need help identifying the person who is likely to be the most supportive at this time. Male victims of sexual assault experience difficulty reconciling their masculine identity with their experience of being an assault victim.

Actions/Interventions

- Facilitate the survivor's expression of feelings and need to talk about the sexual assault. Show interest, respect, and caring without judgment. Avoid statements and questions that may be interpreted as accusing or blaming the survivor.

  - Acknowledge the survivor's mixed feelings about the assault.
  - Encourage the survivor to direct anger and hostility toward the assailant not himself or herself.
- Prepare the patient for the physical, genital, and/or pelvic examination:
  - Obtain written consent.
  - Explain each step of the procedure in advance, and ask permission.

  - Collect and prepare evidence in accordance with procedures required by law

- ▲ Provide appropriate care for wounds and physical symptoms.
  - Administer tetanus toxoid.
  - Provide wound care.
  - Administer medications for pain, nausea, and muscle tension.
  - Administer medications to prevent sexually transmitted infections.
  - Offer the survivor medication to prevent pregnancy.
- Make sure the survivor does not go home alone on discharge. If no family or significant other is available, the sexual assault response team may arrange for someone to accompany the patient home.

Rationales

The patient may be experiencing a state of emotional or psychological shock and require time to process reactions to the sexual assault. Survivors need help understanding that they did what was necessary to survive the assault, regardless of how others may interpret their behavior during the assault. QSEN: Patient-centered care.

The survivor may be feeling guilt and shame, as well as anger, aggression, and hostility.

Feelings of anger toward the offender need to be expressed to promote effective coping.

Survivors may experience a profound loss of control over their bodies. Obtaining consent and asking permission during the examination helps the survivor regain a sense of control. The survivor needs to understand that some specimens collected during the examination will be sent to the hospital laboratory for analysis. Other specimens will be sent to a forensic laboratory and considered legal evidence if the offender is caught and faces criminal charges. QSEN: Patient-centered care.

Evidence must be collected and protected until it can be given to the proper law enforcement officials. Deviation from procedures may result in evidence being disallowed in future court proceedings.

The extent of physical injury sustained during the assault will determine priorities for physical care. Tetanus toxoid is given as prophylaxis if the patient has not had a booster immunization in the previous 10 years. The patient needs to know that medication is available to prevent pregnancy that might occur from the rape. The survivor's cultural and religious beliefs may influence a decision to accept this type of medication.

The patient needs to feel safe and protected during the transition from hospital to home. Feelings of vulnerability and fear of strangers may continue for an extended period. QSEN: Safety.

Education/Continuity of Care

Actions/Interventions

- ▲ Refer the survivor, family, and significant others for individual and/or family counseling to begin within 1 to 2 days of the assault.
- Educate the survivor, family, and significant others about the potential long-term effects of rape-trauma syndrome.

Rationales

Professional counseling provides the survivor and family members with a mechanism of support during this phase of crisis recovery. QSEN: Teamwork and collaboration.

The survivor needs to understand that anger, fear, sadness, hyperalertness, insomnia, depression, and nightmares are some of the symptoms that may be experienced for months and years after the assault. The survivor may experience mood swings. The survivor may be hesitant or fearful to resume intimate relationships and sexual activity. These symptoms may be triggered by new situational crises later in life. Many long-term symptoms reflect the survivor's struggle to reorganize his or her life. QSEN: Patient-centered care.

■ = Independent   ▲ = Interprofessional Collaboration

Actions/Interventions

- Discuss with the family and significant others ways to provide support for the survivor.

▲ Refer the survivor for follow-up care to assess for complications from the physical trauma of the assault.

Rationales

The type of support and caring relationships the survivor experiences during crisis recovery will have a direct effect on long-term efforts to reorganize his or her life. The family and significant others may provide support by encouraging verbalization of feelings, helping the survivor resume usual activities, avoiding overprotection of the survivor, directing feelings of anger toward the assailant, holding and touching the survivor so as not to reinforce feelings of shame and being unclean, being nonjudgmental.

The survivor may need assessment for sexually transmitted infections, pregnancy, and HIV infection at appropriate intervals after the assault. QSEN: Teamwork and collaboration.

NANDA-I
NDx Relocation Stress Syndrome

Definition: Physiological and/or psychological disturbance following transfer from one environment to another

The physiological and psychological stress associated with relocation is now recognized as so extreme that it is associated with the stress of divorce or the death of a loved one. Adjustment to moving from what was once familiar to what is a new environment can last for several months to several years and longer. Current evidence suggests that recovery from a significant move leads to significant decline in the person's health and many times leads to death. The degree of severity depends on many variables such as age, stage of life, personality, number of concurrent losses, amount of preparation, and the degree and type of support before, during, and after the move. Older adults, in particular, are at high risk for experiencing the negative impact of relocation. This syndrome may also be seen in the hospitalized patient who experiences several hospital locations within one hospital stay.

Common Related Factors

Compromised health status
Powerlessness
Impaired psychosocial functioning
Social isolation
Insufficient support systems
Insufficient predeparture counseling
Language barrier
History of loss
Unpredictability of experience
Ineffective coping strategies

Defining Characteristics

Alienation
Aloneness; loneliness
Anger
Anxiety
Concern about relocation
Depression
Dependency
Fear
Frustration
Loss of identity, self-worth, or self-esteem
Increased physical symptoms or illness
Increased verbalization of needs
Insecurity
Pessimism
Unwillingness to move
Withdrawal
Worried

Common Expected Outcomes

The patient maintains orientation and safety in new environment.

The patient verbalizes acceptance of recent relocation.

The patient expresses satisfaction with new living arrangements.

NOC Outcomes

Relocation Adaptation; Anxiety Level; Coping; Personal Resiliency; Psychosocial Adjustment: Life Change; Caregiver Adaptation to Patient Institutionalization

NIC Interventions

Relocation Stress Reduction; Coping Enhancement; Discharge Planning

Ongoing Assessments

Actions/Interventions	Rationales
■ Determine the reason for the relocation and the patient's degree of participation in the relocation decision.	An anticipated and planned move is often less stressful for the patient than a move that is forced on the patient. This option is not usually available in acute care settings.
■ Assess the patient's orientation.	Loss of familiar surroundings and changes in daily routines may lead to disorientation and acute confusion, especially in the older adult.
■ Assess the presence and degree of anxiety.	A thorough assessment results in early identification and intervention to prevent escalation of symptoms. Anxiety is a common emotional response to relocation. The interaction of anxiety with the stress of relocation can become a vicious cycle for the patient.
■ Obtain a history of recent losses and life changes.	A patient's ability to adjust to a move may be compromised when he or she is coping with other losses and significant life changes. Grief is a common reaction to the loss of familiar surroundings. Other life changes such as decreased health status and loss of independence contribute to the stress of relocation. QSEN: Patient-centered care.
■ Assess the patient's physiological status and level of functioning.	The stress associated with relocation may contribute to an exacerbation of physiological symptoms and a decline in the patient's level of function.
■ Explore what is most important to the patient.	The impact of relocation on the patient is related to the loss of things the patient values, such as closeness to family and friends or loss of personal belongings. QSEN: Patient-centered care.
■ Determine previous coping strategies.	Previous coping strategies may not support adjustment to the current move.
■ Assess the patient's level of social support.	The patient's adjustment to the move may be compromised if he or she is unable to maintain desired contact with family and friends.

Therapeutic Interventions

Actions/Interventions	Rationales
■ Include the patient in making decisions about the move, when possible.	The patient's adjustment to the move will be less stressful when he or she participates in planning the change. QSEN: Patient-centered care.
■ Include significant others in discussions and decisions as appropriate.	Decisions following acute stress can be detrimental for the patient. Significant others are trusted individuals with whom the patient can share the process of making decisions about the relocation. QSEN: Patient-centered care.

■ = Independent   ▲ = Interprofessional Collaboration

Actions/Interventions	Rationales
■ Avoid referring to the new location as "home."	Referring to the new location as "home" may lead the patient to believe that he or she is going back to the previous home. This misconception may lead to disorientation, confusion, or even anger about the new location.
■ Avoid unplanned or abrupt transfers, especially at night or change of shift.	Unplanned or abrupt moves disrupt feelings of safety and increase the risk for acute confusion in the institutionalized patient. QSEN: Safety.
■ Allow personal belongings to be arranged in the room before the patient arrives.	Seeing familiar and valued objects can help the patient feel less disoriented in the new surroundings.
■ Assign a current resident to be a "buddy" to the patient. Encourage participation in social activities.	The patient may need help establishing friendships in the new location. The use of a buddy may reduce the patient's anxiety level by providing orientation to the new surroundings. This relationship helps the patient establish interpersonal relationships and a support system in the new location.
■ Arrange for the maintenance of familiar routines and consistency in contact with care providers.	Maintaining familiar daily routines provides the patient with a sense of normalcy. Interactions with the same people each day builds a sense of safety in the new location. Frequent changes in routines and care providers may contribute to anxiety and disorientation.
■ Encourage the expression of feelings.	Exploration of feelings assists in perceiving the situation more realistically and assists with adaptability. Active listening can facilitate grief work related to losses of home, friends, and independence.
■ Reorient the patient to the new environment as often as needed.	Knowing where a person is, how he or she came to be here, and why he or she is here assists the patient in feeling safe. This orientation needs to be repeated frequently for acutely ill patients in intensive care settings, where environmental stimuli can overtax their coping abilities.
■ Use a calm, reassuring approach.	Anxiety may be reduced in a calm environment.
■ Seek to understand the patient's perspective of the event.	Demonstration of understanding is part of building trusting relationships in the new location.
■ Arrange situations to encourage the patient's autonomy and participation in decisions about his or her own care.	Autonomy reinforces self-worth and feelings of value. Taking responsibility for making choices will increase feelings of control and decrease feelings of powerlessness. QSEN: Patient-centered care.

Education/Continuity of Care

Actions/Interventions	Rationales
■ Allow family members to discuss their concerns and feelings related to the move.	Family members may feel a mixture of relief and guilt related to the move of the patient. They may have unresolved issues with the patient that come to the surface as a result of the move.
■ Teach the patient the characteristics of normal grief.	Knowing what is normal can provide reassurance and decrease anxiety. The patient needs to understand that grief is part of any loss or significant life change. Many people limit their understanding of grief to death.
■ Discuss with the patient and significant others the differences in patterns of adjustment.	The patient and family members need to understand that people adjust to change in different ways. Identification of differences assists in normalizing the patient's feelings.

Actions/Interventions

▲ Refer family members to counseling and social services, as appropriate.

Rationales

Family members may benefit from interprofessional support services to facilitate the relocation of the patient. The family may need help adjusting to changes in responsibilities and roles as a result of the relocation. QSEN: Teamwork and collaboration.

NANDA-I NDx Self-Care Deficit: Bathing, Dressing, Feeding, Toileting, Transfer/Ambulation

Definition: Impaired ability to perform or complete activities of daily living for oneself, such as bathing, dressing, feeding, toileting, transfer/ambulation

The nurse may encounter the patient with a self-care deficit in the hospital or in the community. The deficit may be the result of transient limitations, such as those one might experience while recuperating from surgery, or the result of progressive deterioration that erodes the individual's ability or willingness to perform the activities required to care for himself or herself. Patients who are depressed or those with low levels of motivation may not have the interest to engage in self-care activities. Careful examination of the patient's deficiency is required to be certain that the patient is not failing at self-care because of a lack of material resources or a problem with arranging the environment to suit the patient's physical limitations. The nurse coordinates services to maximize the independence of the patient and to ensure that the environment the patient lives in is safe and supportive of his or her special needs. This care plan combines a variety of self-care deficits into one comprehensive plan.

Patients with reduced physical mobility often need assistance with transfer from bed to chair, commode, or wheelchair. Traditionally nurses have relied on the use of body mechanics to prevent personal injury to their back and shoulders. However, research shows that body mechanics alone is not sufficient to protect the nurse from the physical demands of manual patient handling and movement. The high incidence of work-related musculoskeletal disorders (MSDs) prompted the National Institute for Occupational Safety and Health (NIOSH) to establish evidence-based guidelines for safe patient handling (SPH). The American Nurses Association, in partnership with NIOSH and the Veterans Health Administration, has established a SPH curriculum and training program that encourages the use of safe approaches to handling patients and contributes to the prevention of MSDs.

Common Related Factors

Neuromuscular impairment
Musculoskeletal impairment
Alteration in cognitive functioning
Perceptual impairment
Fatigue, weakness
Pain
Anxiety
Decrease in motivation
Environmental barrier

Defining Characteristics

Impaired ability to bathe and groom self independently
Impaired ability to dress/undress self independently
Impaired ability to feed self independently
Impaired ability to perform toileting tasks independently
Impaired ability to transfer from bed to wheelchair
Impaired ability to ambulate independently

■ = Independent   ▲ = Interprofessional Collaboration

Common Expected Outcomes

Patient safely performs (to maximum ability) self-care activities.

Patient identifies resources that are useful in optimizing autonomy and independence.

NOC Outcomes

Self-Care: Eating; Self-Care: Bathing; Self-Care: Dressing; Self-Care: Hygiene; Self-Care: Toileting; Transfer Performance; Ambulation

NIC Interventions

Self-Care Assistance: Bathing/Hygiene; Self-Care Assistance: Dressing/Grooming; Self-Care Assistance: Feeding; Self-Care Assistance: Toileting; Self-Care Assistance: Transfer; Environmental Management

Ongoing Assessment

Actions/Interventions

■ Assess the patient's ability to perform ADLs effectively and safely on a daily basis using an appropriate assessment tool, such as the Functional Independence Measures (FIM).

■ Assess the specific cause of each deficit (e.g., weakness, visual problems, cognitive impairment).

■ Assess the patient's need for assistive devices (e.g., shower chair, grab bars, wide grip utensils, cane, walker). Assess the need for home health care after discharge.

■ Identify preferences for food, personal care items, and other things.

■ If indicated, assess for a gag reflex or the need for swallowing evaluation by a speech therapist/pathologist before the initial oral feeding.

■ For more complex, high-risk patients, evaluate the patient for safe patient handling and movement, using a standardized tool if available, as follows:
  • Ability of patient to provide assistance (independent; partial assist; dependent)
  • Weight-bearing capability (full, partial, none)
  • Upper-extremity strength (yes/no)
  • Ability of patient to cooperate and follow instructions (cooperative; unpredictable)
  • Height/weight/BMI
  • Special circumstances likely to affect transfer or repositioning tasks (e.g., amputation, abdominal wound, history of falls, fractures, tube insertion)
  • Specific physician orders or physical therapy recommendations that relate to transferring or repositioning patients (e.g., hip abduction during transfer)

Rationales

The patient may only require assistance with some self-care measures. A variety of tools are available, depending on the clinical setting. Such tools provide objective data for baselines. For example, the FIM assesses 18 self-care items related to eating, bathing, grooming, dressing, toileting, bladder and bowel management, transfer, ambulation, and stair climbing. QSEN: Evidence-based practice: Patient-centered care.

Different etiological factors may require more specific interventions to enable self-care.

Assistive devices increase independence in performance of ADLs. Shortened hospital stays have resulted in patients being more debilitated on discharge and therefore requiring more assistance at home. Occupational therapists have access to a wide range of self-help devices. QSEN: Teamwork and collaboration.

The patient is more likely to participate in self-care that supports his or her individual and personal preferences. QSEN: Patient-centered care.

Absence of gag reflex or inability to chew or swallow properly may lead to choking or aspiration. QSEN: Teamwork and collaboration.

Patient handling and movement activities are a basic part of nursing care. Use of a patient assessment tool can provide a standardized way to assess patients and make appropriate decisions about how to safely perform high risk tasks. QSEN: Evidence-based practice; Safety.

Actions/Interventions

- Refer to a safe patient handling and movement algorithm if available. For example:
  - Transfer to and from bed to chair, toilet
  - Lateral transfer to and from bed to stretcher
  - Reposition in bed: side to side, up in bed
  - Reposition in chair
  - Transfer a patient up from floor
  - Bariatric (BMI > 50) handling of preceding examples

Rationales

Best practices algorithms or decision tools help nurses assess patient needs to determine the technique, equipment, and number of staff required for performing high-risk patient handling tasks. The Veterans Health Administration provides algorithms for selecting the right combination of equipment and personnel needed to handle or move patients safely. A sample algorithm is available at www.visn8.med.va.gov/visn8/patientsafetycenter/safePtHandling/default.asp. QSEN: Evidence-based practice; Safety.

Therapeutic Interventions

Actions/Interventions

- Assist the patient in accepting the necessary amount of dependence.

- Set short-term goals with the patient.

- Implement measures to facilitate independence, but intervene when the patient cannot perform.

- Use consistent routines, and allow adequate time for the patient to complete tasks.

- Provide positive reinforcement for all activities attempted; note partial achievements.

- Provide supervision for each activity until the patient performs the skill competently and is safe in independent care; reevaluate regularly to be certain that the patient is maintaining the skill level and remains safe in the environment.
- Encourage maximum independence.

Feeding:
- Place the patient in an optimal position for feeding, preferably sitting up in a chair; support the arms, elbows, and wrists, as needed.
- Encourage the patient to feed himself or herself as soon as possible (using the unaffected hand, if appropriate). Assist with setup as needed.
- Ensure that the patient wears dentures and eyeglasses if needed.
- ▲ Ensure that the consistency of diet is appropriate for the patient's ability to chew and swallow, as assessed by the speech therapist/pathologist.
- Provide the patient with appropriate utensils (e.g., drinking straw, plate guard, rocking knife, wide-grip utensils, nonskid placemat) to aid in self-feeding.

Rationales

If disease, injury, or illness resulting in self-care deficit is recent, the patient may need to grieve before accepting that dependence is necessary. Patients may need help in determining the safe limits of trying to be independent versus asking for help when needed.

Assisting the patient with setting realistic goals will decrease frustration. QSEN: Patient-centered care.

An appropriate level of assistive care can prevent injury from activities without causing frustration. Nurses can be key in helping patients accept both temporary and permanent dependence.

An established routine becomes rote and requires less effort. This helps the patient organize and carry out self-care skills.

External sources of positive reinforcement may promote ongoing efforts. Patients often have difficulty seeing progress.

The patient's ability to perform self-care measures may change often over time and will need to be assessed regularly.

The goal of rehabilitation is one of achieving the highest level of independence possible.

Proper positioning can make the task easier while also reducing risk for aspiration.

It is probable that the dominant hand will also be the affected hand if there is upper extremity involvement.

Deficits may be exaggerated if other senses or strengths are not functioning optimally.

Thickened semisolid foods such as pudding and hot cereal are most easily swallowed and less likely to be aspirated. QSEN: Safety; Teamwork and collaboration.

These items increase opportunities for success.

■ = Independent ▲ = Interprofessional Collaboration

Actions/Interventions	**Rationales**
■ Consider an appropriate setting for feeding where the patient has supportive assistance yet is not embarrassed.	Embarrassment or fear of spilling food on self may hinder the patient's attempts to feed self.
■ If the patient has visual problems, advise the patient of the placement of food on the plate.	After a CVA, patients may have unilateral neglect and may ignore half the plate.
Dressing/grooming:	
■ Provide privacy during dressing.	The need for privacy is fundamental for most patients. Patients may take longer to dress and may be fearful of breaches in privacy.
■ Provide frequent encouragement and assistance with dressing as needed.	Assistance can reduce energy expenditure and frustration. However, care needs to be taken so the care provider does not rush through tasks, negating the patient's attempts.
■ Plan daily activities so the patient is rested before activity.	A plan that balances periods of activity with periods of rest can help the patient complete the desired activity without undue fatigue and frustration.
▲ Provide appropriate assistive devices for dressing as assessed by the nurse and occupational therapist.	The use of a buttonhook or of loop-and-pile closures on clothes may make it possible for a patient to continue independence in this self-care activity. QSEN: Teamwork and collaboration.
■ Place the patient in a wheelchair or stationary chair.	Dressing can be fatiguing. A chair that provides more support for the body than sitting on the side of the bed conserves energy when dressing.
■ Encourage the use of clothing one size larger.	A larger size ensures easier dressing and comfort.
■ Suggest a front-opening brassiere and half-slips.	Clothing that is easier to put on and remove enhances self-care with dressing.
■ Suggest elastic shoelaces or Velcro closures on shoes.	These closures eliminate tying, which can add to frustration.
■ Provide makeup and a mirror; assist as needed.	Fine motor activities may take more coordinated actions and may be beyond the abilities of the patient.
■ Encourage the patient to comb his or her own hair (a one-handed task). Suggest hairstyles that are low maintenance.	Simplified hairstyles enable the patient to maintain autonomy for as long as possible.
Bathing/hygiene:	
■ Maintain privacy during bathing as appropriate.	The need for privacy is fundamental for most patients.
■ Ensure that needed utensils are close by.	Nearby placement of items such as washcloth, soap, and towel conserves energy and optimizes safety.
■ Instruct the patient to select the bath time when he or she is rested and unhurried.	Hurrying may result in accidents, and the energy required for these activities may be substantial.
■ Provide the patient with the appropriate assistive devices (e.g., long-handled bath sponge, shower chair, safety mats for floor, grab bars for bath or shower).	Assistive devices aid in the ability to bathe self and increase safety.
■ Encourage the patient to bathe himself or herself as much as he or she is capable of. Assist with completion of the bath, brushing teeth, shaving, and so on, only as needed.	Hospital workers and family caregivers are often in a hurry and do more for patients than needed, thereby slowing the patient's efforts at regaining independence.
■ Assist the patient with care of the fingernails and toenails as required.	Patients may require podiatric care to prevent injury to feet during nail trimming or because special implements are required to cut nails.
Toileting:	
■ Evaluate or document previous and current patterns for toileting; institute a toileting schedule that factors these habits into the program.	The effectiveness of the bowel or bladder program will be enhanced if the natural and personal patterns of the patient are respected.
■ Encourage the use of a commode or toilet as soon as possible.	Patients are more effective in evacuating the bowel and bladder when sitting on a commode. Some patients find it impossible to toilet on a bedpan.

Actions/Interventions	Rationales
■ Provide appropriate assistive devices (e.g., raised toilet seat and grab bar near toilet).	These devices facilitate ease in sitting down and getting up.
■ Assist the patient in removing or replacing necessary clothing.	Clothing that is difficult to get into and out of may compromise a patient's ability to be continent.
■ Provide privacy while the patient is toileting.	Lack of privacy may inhibit the patient's ability to evacuate bowel and bladder.
■ Keep the call light within reach, and instruct the patient to call as early as possible.	Staff members need time to reach patient's room to assist with transfer to commode or toilet.
Transferring/ambulation:	
■ Plan a teaching session for transferring/walking when the patient is rested.	Tasks require energy. Fatigued patients may have more difficulty and may become unnecessarily frustrated.
■ Assist with bed mobility by doing the following:	Bed mobility prevents disabling contractures, pressure ulcers, and muscle weakness from disuse.
• Allow the patient to work at his or her own rate of speed.	Many factors may influence a patient's ability to move freely, and each of these factors must be considered when developing or teaching a patient a new system for self-care.
• Encourage the patient to use the stronger side (if appropriate) as much as possible.	If patients who have had a stroke experience weakness in their dominant side, it will be necessary for them to develop muscle strength and coordination on the nondominant side.
■ When transferring to wheelchair, always place the chair on the patient's stronger side at a slight angle to the bed and lock the brakes.	The patient will bear weight on the stronger side. Physical or occupational therapists can provide additional guidelines. QSEN: Teamwork and collaboration.
■ When minimal assistance is needed, use the following manual principles of body mechanics:	These principles should be used in conjunction with safe patient handling measures when assisting patients to reduce potential for injury to patient and staff. QSEN: Evidence-based practice; Safety.
• Maintain a wide, stable base with your feet.	
• Keep the patient as close to your body as possible to minimize reaching.	
• Use a gait belt to assist patient who can stand with minimal assistance.	
■ For high-risk patients associated with safe patient handling and movement, gather the appropriate equipment and other staff members as needed: For example:	Depending on the patient's needs, the use of mechanical equipment or other SPH aids (ergonomic interventions) may be required to modify the transfer activity to protect the worker. These aids work by bearing most of the load, reducing the load by lowering the friction between skin against cloth. Examples include assisting a cooperative patient with minimal lower-body strength from sitting position to standing position using powered sit to stand lift. Staff training in the proper use of lifting equipment and devices is required. In some institutions, patient lift teams have been created composed of two or more physically fit people competent in lifting techniques, who work to perform high-risk patient transfers. They are trained in use of mechanical lifting devices.
• Powered, mechanical full-body lifts (either mobile or ceiling-mounted)	
• Powered, mobile sit-to-stand lifts	
• Friction-reducing devices	
• Patient lift teams	
■ Assist with ambulation; teach the use of ambulation devices such as canes, walkers, and crutches:	These techniques enhance patient safety and assist with balance and support. QSEN: Safety.
• Stand on the patient's weak side.	
• If using a cane, place the cane in the patient's strong hand and ensure proper foot-cane sequence.	

Education/Continuity of Care

Actions/Interventions	Rationales
■ Plan teaching sessions so the patient has time to practice tasks.	This allows the patient to use new information immediately, thus enhancing retention.
■ Instruct the patient in the use of assistive devices as appropriate.	Information enables the patient to take some control.
■ Teach the family and caregivers to foster independence and to intervene if the patient becomes fatigued, is unable to perform tasks, or becomes excessively frustrated.	This demonstrates caring and concern but does not interfere with the patient's efforts to achieve independence.

NANDA-I NDx

Situational Low Self-Esteem

Definition: Development of a negative perception of self-worth in response to a current situation

Self-esteem is a component of an individual's self-concept. Positive self-esteem is based on the person's feeling worthwhile and capable of responding to challenges and stressors. Low self-esteem represents a mild to marked alteration in an individual's view of himself or herself, including negative self-evaluation or negative feelings about self or capabilities. This change in self-esteem is a temporary state in response to feeling unable to manage the current situation. A person's self-esteem is affected by (and may also affect) his or her ability to function in the larger world and relate to others within it. Self-esteem disturbance may be expressed directly or indirectly. Cultural norms, gender, and age are variables that influence how an individual perceives himself or herself. The emotional work that patients do to enhance self-esteem takes weeks, months, or even years and may require professional help beyond the scope of the bedside or community nurse. A caring individual, who is able to identify the special needs of the patient struggling with self-esteem issues, is in a unique position to provide support and compassion, enhancing the work the patient must do.

Common Related Factors

Alteration in body image
History of loss
Alteration in social role
Behavior inconsistent with values
Functional impairment
Inadequate recognition
History of rejection

Defining Characteristics

Situational challenge to self-worth
Self-negating verbalizations
Indecisive, nonassertive behavior
Underestimates ability to deal with situation
Helplessness

Common Expected Outcomes

Patient verbalizes positive self-acceptance.
Patient describes successes in current situations.

NOC Outcomes
Self-Esteem; Personal Resiliency; Body Image
NIC Interventions
Self-Esteem Enhancement; Body Image Enhancement; Coping Enhancement

Ongoing Assessment

Actions/Interventions	Rationales
■ Review with the patient past and current accomplishments: emotional, social, interpersonal, intellectual, vocational, and physical.	Patients experiencing situational stress often lose sight of their past successes in managing similar situations. QSEN: Patient-centered care.
■ Listen to statements the patient makes about himself or herself.	Low self-esteem is often expressed as feeling unloved, unworthy, or incompetent. The patient may be self-critical especially about his or her ability to manage the current situation.
■ Ask the patient if he or she is able to relate these changes to a specific event.	The patient may be aware of recent events that negatively affect his or her self-concept.
■ Assess for recent changes in the patient's behavior.	Patients may be able to compensate for low self-esteem through extraordinary performance in work or areas of special interest while still having problems with how he or she envisions self. Some patients may withdraw from engagement in work or family situations in an attempt to diminish the impact of the situation on self-esteem. Low self-esteem will not be resolved without considering these issues into the care plan. QSEN: Patient-centered care.
■ Assess the degree to which the patient feels "in control" of his or her own behavior.	Patients may be caught in a vicious cycle of behaviors designed to camouflage the primary self-esteem problem. The acting-out feeds a sense of unworthiness and sabotages attempts at esteem-building.
■ Assess the degree to which the patient feels loved and respected by others.	Rejection by others or lack of recognition of accomplishments may contribute to feelings of unworthiness. The patient's ability to establish and maintain meaningful relationships is a positive indicator for developing self-esteem. The care and support of others will be helpful in building the patient's self-esteem.
■ Assess the patient's feelings of satisfaction with his or her own behavior.	Patients with self-esteem disturbance may feel as though their behaviors are not in keeping with their own personal, moral, or ethical values; they may also deny these behaviors, project blame, and rationalize personal failures.
■ Assess how competent patients feel about their ability to perform and/or carry out their own and others' expectations.	The patient may have developed the ability to carry out personal responsibilities despite low self-esteem. This may be a positive indicator of the patient's potential for successful enhancement of self-esteem. QSEN: Patient-centered care.
■ Assess for unresolved grief.	Unresolved grief may inhibit patients' ability to move beyond the loss or disability and to accept themselves as they are now.

Therapeutic Interventions

Actions/Interventions	Rationales
■ Provide an environment conducive to the expression of feelings:	The nurse creates a caring and supportive environment to help the patient begin the work of restoring self-esteem in the current situation. QSEN: Patient-centered care.
• Spend time with the patient; set aside sufficient time so that the encounter is unhurried.	The patient needs time to express concerns. Spending time with the patient conveys the nurse's interest in and acceptance of the patient's feelings. These issues are deserving of the patient and the nurse's complete attention. The work of building self-esteem requires problem-solving and reality testing that is best accomplished within the context of a trusting relationship.

■ = Independent   ▲ = Interprofessional Collaboration

Actions/Interventions

- Use active listening and open-ended questions.

- Provide privacy.

■ Serve as role model for the patient or significant others in healthy expression of feelings or concerns. Assume responsibility for own thoughts and actions by using "I think" language in discussions.

■ Discuss the "normal" impact of change on self-esteem. Reassure the patient that such changes often result in a variety of emotional or behavioral responses.

■ Provide anticipatory guidance to minimize anxiety and fear if disturbances in self-esteem are an expected part of the process of adjustment to changes in health status.

■ Assist the patient in his or her efforts to maintain independence, reality, positive self-esteem, sense of capability, and problem-solving.

Rationales

These communication techniques allow the patient to express concerns, fears, and ideas without interruption. This approach to the patient will convey a sense of respect for the patient's abilities and strengths in addition to recognizing problems and concerns.

Sensitive discussions need to take place in a setting where the patient is free to express self without being overheard.

Patients may need an example of positive ways to express feelings. Self-awareness allows the nurse to demonstrate authentic behavior.

Disturbances in self-esteem are natural responses to significant changes. Reconstitution of the patient's self-esteem occurs as part of the patient's adjustment to change.

The patient needs a perspective that places the shift in self-esteem within the context of the normal recuperative process.

The patient needs ongoing positive feedback and reinforcement to maintain behaviors to promote self-esteem. The patient will benefit from feedback that provides a realistic appraisal of his or her progress and reinforces the constructive changes made by the patient. QSEN: Patient-centered care.

Education/Continuity of Care

Actions/Interventions

■ Teach the patient the harmful effects of negative self-talk.

■ Teach the patient to engage in activities likely to result in a healthy self-esteem.

▲ Refer the patient to members of the interprofessional team for professional counseling and to community resources such as self-help groups.

Rationales

Awareness of destructive thoughts can help the patient develop new approaches to coping. The patient needs to replace negative thoughts with positive thoughts about self.

The patient needs to explore alternatives to promote self-esteem by replacing destructive behaviors with positive actions.

Professional and community sources of support provide the patient with more resources to continue the work of restoring positive self-esteem. QSEN: Teamwork and collaboration.

NANDA-I
NDx # Ineffective Sexuality Pattern

Definition: Expressions of concern regarding own sexuality

A patient or significant other may express concern regarding the means or manner of sexual expression or physical intimacy within their relationship. Alterations in human sexual response may be related to genetic, physiological, emotional, cognitive, religious, and/or sociocultural factors or to a combination of these factors. All of these factors play a role in determining what is normative for each individual within a relationship. The problem of altered patterns of sexuality is not limited to a single gender, age, sexual orientation, or cultural group. People who identify themselves as lesbian, gay, bisexual, or transgender (LGBT) may be fearful of seeking health care for sexual issues. They may have experienced discrimination by health care providers. It is probable that most couples encounter some point in their relationship where patterns of sexual expression become altered to the dissatisfaction of one or both members. The ability to communicate effectively, to seek professional help whenever necessary, and to modify existing patterns to the mutual satisfaction of both members are skills that enable the couple to grow and evolve in this aspect of their relationship. The nurse is in a unique position to provide anticipatory guidance relative to altered patterns of sexual function when the problem is an inevitable or probable result of illness or disability. The ability to discuss these issues openly when the patient raises concerns about sexual expression highlights the legitimacy of the couple's feelings and the normalcy of sexual expression as a part of intimacy, as well as emotional and physical well-being.

Common Related Factors

Inadequate role model
Conflict about sexual orientation or variant preferences
Fear of sexually transmitted infections
Fear of pregnancy
Impaired relationship with a significant other
Insufficient knowledge about alternatives related to sexuality
Absence of privacy
Absence of significant other

Defining Characteristics

Alteration in relationship with significant other
Values conflict
Change in sexual role
Difficulty with sexual activity or behavior
Alteration in sexual activity or behavior

Common Expected Outcomes

Patient or couple verbalizes satisfaction with the way physical intimacy is expressed.
Both members of the couple exhibit behavior that is acceptable to his or her partner.

NOC Outcomes

Role Performance; Body Image; Sexual Identity; Knowledge: Sexual Functioning

NIC Interventions

Sexual Counseling; Anticipatory Guidance; Teaching: Sexuality; Teaching: Safe Sex

Ongoing Assessment

Actions/Interventions

- Identify the level of comfort in the discussion for the patient/significant other.

- Assess the level of understanding regarding human sexuality and functioning.
- Explore current and past sexual patterns, practices, and the degree of satisfaction.
- Solicit information from the patient about the nature, onset, and duration of sexual difficulty.

- Identify factors that may contribute to the current alteration in sexual functioning.

Rationales

It is important for the nurse to create an environment where the couple or patient feels safe and comfortable in discussing feelings.
Many people have misconceptions about sexual intimacy.

This information determines a realistic approach to planning appropriate care for the patient or the couple.
Problems with sexuality may be long-standing or of short duration. The patient may have some understanding of reason for the sexual dysfunction. QSEN: Patient-centered care.
A plan of care will be developed in the context of the patient's overall health status. Different interventions will address specific contributing factors. For example, patients may be taking medications that suppress libido as a side effect. An adjustment in the dosage or a change to a different medication may help resolve the problem with sexual function. A patient with erectile dysfunction may benefit from taking an erectogenic drug such as sildenafil (Viagra). QSEN: Evidence-based practice.

■ = Independent   ▲ = Interprofessional Collaboration

Nursing Diagnosis Care Plans

Therapeutic Interventions

Actions/Interventions	Rationales
■ Use a relaxed, accepting manner in discussing sexual issues. Convey acceptance and respect for the patient's concerns.	Patients are often hesitant to report such concerns/difficulties because sexuality remains a private matter within many cultures, and it is uncomfortable to discuss. LGBT patients may have experienced disrespectful behavior by health care providers because of their sexual orientation or gender expression. QSEN: Patient-centered care.
■ Provide privacy and adequate time to discuss sexuality.	The patient is more likely to discuss sexual concerns in a private setting without feeling rushed.
■ Encourage the sharing of concerns, feelings, and information between the patient and current or future partner. Whenever possible, involve both in sexual health education and counseling efforts.	Respecting the individual and treating his or her concerns and questions as normal and important may foster greater self-acceptance and decrease anxiety. For some sexual problems, it is the couple's relationship that provides the focus for intervention. QSEN: Patient-centered care.
■ Discuss the multiplicity of influences on sexual functioning (both physiological and emotional). Offer opportunities to ask questions and express feelings.	Patients and couples may have limited knowledge of sexual function and factors that influence sexuality. Open discussion can relieve feelings of guilt or shame.
■ Explore the awareness of and comfort with a range of sexual expression and activities (not just sexual intercourse).	Patients and couples may have limited knowledge of ways to express their sexuality. They may be uncomfortable with some types of sexual expression based on cultural, social, or religious beliefs. QSEN: Patient-centered care.
■ Assist the patient and significant other in identifying possible options to overcome situational, temporary, or long-term influences on sexual functioning.	The nurse can facilitate open discussion by the couple of possible ways to adapt to changes in sexual function. The couple needs to share responsibility for exploring options. QSEN: Patient-centered care.

Education/Continuity of Care

Actions/Interventions	Rationales
■ Provide accurate information regarding the "normal" range of possibilities for sexual expression and sexual practices.	Information is necessary to support the couple or the individual patient making decisions about sexual activity. Satisfying sexual functioning and practice are not automatic and need to be learned.
■ Offer information regarding birth control methods and "safe sex" practices.	The patient and significant other need accurate information about preventing unintended pregnancy or transmission of infections through sexual contact.
■ Teach the patient and sexual partner about alternative means or forms of expressing intimacy/sexual expression (e.g., alternative positions for intercourse) that decrease discomfort or degree of physical exertion for those with impaired mobility or cardiopulmonary disease.	The patient needs to understand the relationship between illness, treatment methods, and sexuality. The amount and type of information provided should match the patient's or couple's level of interest and comfort. Alternative ways of sexual expression should be mutually pleasing and acceptable to the patient and the significant other. QSEN: Patient-centered care.
▲ Refer the patient to members of the interprofessional team for further care.	Members of the interprofessional health team (e.g., primary health care provider, mental health consultant, substance abuse treatment program, or sexual dysfunction clinic) can assist the patient and significant other in finding acceptable solutions to problems with sexual function and expression. QSEN: Teamwork and collaboration.

Actions/Interventions

■ Refer the patient or couple to self-help/support groups (e.g., Reach for Recovery, ostomy support groups, Mended Hearts, Huff and Puff, Sexual Impotence Resolved, Us TOO, HIV support groups, Breast Cancer Network of Strength, Survivors of Abuse, or Resolve).

Rationales

Self-help support groups are unique sources of empathy, information, and successful role models. These organizations can provide information about sexuality and specific health problems.

Related Care Plans

Gender dysphoria, Chapter 12
Erectile dysfunction, ⊖*volve*

Risk for Impaired Skin Integrity

Definition: Vulnerable to alteration in epidermis and/or dermis, which may compromise health

Maintenance of skin integrity and prevention of pressure ulcers have been identified as a key marker of quality care. The Centers for Medicare and Medicaid Services (CMS) and The Joint Commission (TJC) have identified pressure ulcer prevention as one of the first major nursing-sensitive outcomes. Although the literature suggests that not all pressure ulcers can be prevented, the nurse is in a key role to implement comprehensive guidelines to aid in the prevention and early detection of impaired skin integrity. Nurses must be aware of the myriad factors that place patients at risk for skin breakdown. The literature reports that pressure ulcers can develop in 2 to 6 hours; thus, identifying at-risk individuals is key.

Immobility, which leads to pressure, shear, and friction, is the factor most likely to put an individual at risk for altered skin integrity. Advanced age, the normal loss of elasticity, inadequate nutrition, environmental moisture (especially from incontinence), and vascular insufficiency potentiate the effects of pressure and hasten the development of skin breakdown. Groups of people with the highest risk for altered skin integrity are those with spinal injuries, those who are confined to bed or wheelchair for prolonged periods of time, those with edema, and those who have altered sensation that triggers the normal protective weight shifting. Pressure relief and pressure redistribution devices for the prevention of skin breakdown include a wide range of surfaces, specialty beds and mattresses, and other devices. Preventive measures are usually not reimbursable, even though costs related to treatment once breakdown occurs are greater.

Evidence is accumulating to support the significant reductions in the prevalence of pressure ulcers when a standardized program for prevention is implemented. Several guidelines can be found in the literature. This care plan is based on recommendations from the National Pressure Ulcer Advisory Panel (NPUAC), the National Guideline Clearinghouse, and the Agency for Healthcare Research and Quality (AHRQ).

Common Risk Factors

External
- Extremes of age
- Mechanical factors (e.g., shearing forces, pressure)
- Excretions
- Secretions
- Humidity
- Moisture
- Radiation therapy
- Hyperthermia or hypothermia
- Chemical injury agent

Internal
- Inadequate nutrition
- Pressure over bony prominence
- Impaired circulation
- Alteration in sensation (resulting from spinal cord injury, diabetes mellitus, etc.)
- Immunodeficiency
- Alteration in metabolism
- Alteration in pigmentation
- Alteration in skin turgor
- Hormonal change
- Pharmaceutical agent

Common Expected Outcome

Patient's skin remains intact, as evidenced by no redness over bony prominences and capillary refill less than 6 seconds over areas of redness.

NOC Outcomes
Risk Control; Risk Detection; Tissue Integrity: Skin and Mucous Membranes

NIC Interventions
Pressure Ulcer Prevention; Skin Surveillance; Pressure Management

Ongoing Assessment

Actions/Interventions	Rationales
▪ Assess the general condition of the skin.	Assessment provides a basis for interventions. Healthy skin varies among individuals but should have good turgor (an indication of moisture), feel warm and dry to the touch, be free of impairment (scratches, bruises, excoriation, rashes), and have quick capillary refill (less than 6 seconds). Older patients' skin is normally less elastic, has less moisture, and has thinning of the epidermis, making for higher risk for skin impairment. QSEN: Patient-centered care.
▪ Specifically assess the skin over bony prominences (e.g., sacrum, trochanters, scapulae, elbows, heels, inner and outer malleoli, inner and outer knees, back of head).	Areas where skin is stretched tautly over bony prominences are at higher risk for breakdown because the possibility of ischemia to skin is high as a result of compression of skin capillaries between a hard surface (e.g., mattress, chair, or table) and the bone. Pressure areas initially appear as persistent reddened areas in light pigmented skin. In darker skin tones, the area may appear as red, blue, or purple hue spots.

Actions/Interventions

- Assess the patient's awareness of the sensation of pressure.

- Use an objective tool for pressure ulcer risk assessment.
  - Braden Scale
  - Norton Scale

- Assess the patient's ability to move (e.g., shift weight while sitting, turn over in bed, move from bed to chair).
- Assess the patient's nutritional status, including weight, weight loss, and serum albumin levels.

- Assess for edema.

- Assess for a history of radiation therapy.

- Assess for a history or presence of AIDS or other immunological problems.

- Assess for fecal/urinary incontinence.

- Assess for environmental moisture (e.g., wound drainage, high humidity).
- Assess the surface that the patient spends a majority of time on (e.g., mattress for bedridden patient, cushion for people in wheelchairs).

- Assess the amount of shear (pressure exerted laterally) and friction (rubbing) on the patient's skin.

Rationales

Normally, individuals shift their weight off pressure areas every few minutes; this occurs more or less automatically, even during sleep. Patients with decreased sensation are unaware of unpleasant stimuli (pressure) and do not shift weight. This results in prolonged pressure on skin capillaries and ultimately in skin ischemia. QSEN: Patient-centered care.

These assessment tools have been validated for risk assessment through extensive research. The Braden Scale is the most widely used. It consists of six subscales: sensory, perception, moisture, activity and mobility, nutrition, and fraction/sheer. QSEN: Evidence-based practice.
- Acute care: Assessment should be carried out on all patients on admission and every 24 to 48 hours or sooner if the patient's condition changes.
- Long-term care: Assess on admission, weekly for 4 weeks, and then quarterly and whenever resident's condition changes.
- Home care: Assess on admission and at every visit (see http://www.NPUAP.org).

Immobility is the greatest risk factor in skin breakdown.

An albumin level less than 2.5 g/dL is a grave sign, indicating severe protein depletion. Research has shown that patients whose serum albumin level is less than 2.5 g/dL are at high risk for skin breakdown, all other factors being equal. QSEN: Evidence-based practice.

Skin stretched tautly over edematous tissue is at risk for impairment.

Radiated skin becomes thin and friable, may have less blood supply, and is at higher risk for breakdown.

Early manifestations of diseases related to HIV may include skin lesions (e.g., Kaposi's sarcoma); in addition, because of their immunocompromised state, patients with AIDS often have skin breakdown.

The urea in urine turns into ammonia within minutes and is caustic to the skin. Stool may contain enzymes that cause skin breakdown. Use of diapers and incontinence pads with plastic liners traps moisture and hastens breakdown.

Moisture may contribute to skin maceration.

Patients who spend the majority of time on one surface need a pressure reduction or pressure relief device to distribute pressure more evenly and lessen the risk for breakdown. QSEN: Safety.

A common cause of shear is elevating the head of the patient's bed: the body's weight is shifted downward onto the patient's sacrum. Common causes of friction include the patient rubbing heels or elbows against bed linen, and moving the patient up in bed without the use of a lift sheet.

■ = Independent ▲ = Interprofessional Collaboration

Actions/Interventions

- Reassess the skin often and whenever the patient's condition or treatment plan results in an increased number of risk factors.
- Assess the skin for:
  - Dermatitis or exposure to chemical irritants

  - Pruritus (itching) or mechanical trauma

  - Long-term steroid use

Rationales

The incidence and onset of skin breakdown are directly related to the number of risk factors present.

These conditions can cause inflammation, resulting in redness and itching, and may cause blisters.

Itching or mechanical traumas can result in disruptions to skin integrity and reduce its barrier function.

Long-term steroid use may leave skin papery thin and prone to injury.

Therapeutic Interventions

Actions/Interventions

- If the patient is restricted to bed, encourage the implementation and posting of a turning schedule, restricting time in one position to 2 hours or less, and customizing the schedule to the patient's routine and caregiver's needs.

- Encourage the use of lifting devices (bed linen or trapeze) to move the patient in bed, and discourage the patient or caregiver from elevating the head of bed repeatedly.

- Use pillows or foam wedges to keep bony prominences from direct contact with each other. Keep pillows under the heels to raise off the bed.

- Change chair-bound positions every hour and encourage the patient to shift weight every 15 minutes.

- Encourage ambulation if the patient is able.

- Encourage the implementation of pressure-relieving devices commensurate with degree of risk for skin impairment:
  - For low-risk patients: good-quality (dense, at least 5 inches thick) foam mattress overlay

  - For moderate-risk patients: water mattress, static or dynamic air mattress

  - For high-risk patients or those with existing stage III or IV pressure ulcers (or with stage II pressure ulcers and multiple risk factors): low–air-loss beds (Mediscus, Flexicare, KinAir) or air-fluidized therapy (Clinitron, Skytron)

Rationales

This nursing action is part of the QSEN competency for patient-centered care. A schedule that does not interfere with the patient's and caregiver's activities is most likely to be followed. Use of a written schedule may be effective. Turning every 2 hours is key. The head of the bed should be kept at 30 degrees or less (or as condition allows) to avoid sliding down in bed. QSEN: Patient-centered care.

A common cause of shear is elevating the head of the patient's bed: the body's weight is shifted downward onto the patient's sacrum. Common causes of friction include the patient rubbing heels or elbows against bed linen, and moving the patient up in bed without the use of a lift sheet.

These measures reduce shearing forces on the skin. QSEN: Safety.

Pressure over the sacrum may exceed 100 mm Hg during sitting. The pressure necessary to close skin capillaries is around 32 mm Hg; any pressure greater than 32 mm Hg results in skin ischemia. QSEN: Evidence-based practice.

Ambulation reduces pressure on the skin from immobility. QSEN: Safety.

Egg crate–type mattresses less than 4 to 5 inches thick do not relieve pressure. Because they are made of foam, moisture can be trapped. A false sense of security with the use of these mattresses can delay initiation of devices useful in relieving pressure.

Dynamic devices electronically alternate inflation and deflation of the device. Static devices consist of gel, foam, water, or air that remains in a constant state of inflation. In the home, a waterbed is a good alternative.

Low–air-loss beds allow elevated head of bed and patient transfer. They should be used when pulmonary concerns necessitate elevating the head of bed or when getting the patient up is feasible. Air-fluidized therapy supports the patient's weight at well below capillary closing pressure but restricts getting the patient out of bed easily. QSEN: Evidence-based practice; Safety.

Actions/Interventions

▲ Encourage adequate nutrition and hydration:
- 2000 to 3000 kcal/day (more if increased metabolic demands)
- Fluid intake of 2000 mL/day unless medically restricted

■ Increase tissue perfusion by massaging *around* the affected area.

■ Clean, dry, and moisturize skin, especially over bony prominences, twice daily or as indicated by incontinence or sweating. Avoid hot water. If powder is desirable, use medical grade cornstarch; avoid talc.

▲ Leave blisters intact by wrapping them in gauze or applying a hydrocolloid or a vapor-permeable membrane dressing.

Rationales

Adequate hydration and nutrition help maintain skin turgor, moisture, and suppleness, which provide resilience to damage caused by pressure. Patients with limited cardiovascular reserve may not be able to tolerate this much fluid.

Massaging the actual reddened area may damage the skin further.

Smooth, supple skin is more resistant to injury. Use a mild cleansing agent. Moisturizers or emollients should contain lipids that help to trap water and prevent evaporation away from skin. Emollients also attract water from the dermis and retain it in the epidermis. Avoid talc, which can be inhaled and cause lung injury.

Blisters are sterile natural dressings. Leaving them intact maintains the skin's natural function as a barrier to pathogens while the impaired area below the blister heals. QSEN: Safety.

Education/Continuity of Care

Actions/Interventions

▲ Consult a dietitian as appropriate.

■ Teach the patient and caregiver the causes of pressure ulcer development:
- Pressure on skin, especially over bony prominences
- Incontinence
- Poor nutrition
- Shearing or friction against skin

■ Reinforce the importance of mobility, turning, or ambulation in the prevention of pressure ulcers.

■ Teach the patient or caregiver the proper use and maintenance of pressure-redistribution devices to be used at home.

■ Teach patients and caregivers about proper skin care to prevent skin breakdown:

- Avoid bar soaps. Use soap substitutes such as aqueous creams.

- Moisturize skin with creams and lotions or emollients.
- Avoid soaps or lotions with perfumes/dyes or alcohol.

▲ Consult a wound, ostomy, and continence nurse (WOCN).

Rationales

The dietitian can assist the patient and family in food choices to meet adequate nutritional and hydration goals to support skin integrity. QSEN: Teamwork and collaboration.

This information can assist the patient or caregiver in finding methods to prevent skin breakdown.

Teaching the patient or caregiver methods to prevent pressure ulcers will enhance their sense of self-efficacy and can improve compliance with the prescribed interventions. QSEN: Patient-centered care.

Care and maintenance of pressure-redistribution devices will promote their ongoing effectiveness.

Teaching patients and caregivers methods to maintain skin integrity enhances their sense of self-efficacy and prevents skin breakdown. QSEN: Patient-centered care.

Bar soaps can strip skin of natural oils needed for elasticity and hydration. Soaps change the acidity of the skin, which can lead to breakdown.

Moisturizers rehydrate the skin and optimize skin integrity. Drier skin may need emollients (greasier moisturizers).

The perfumes or dyes may cause skin irritation, and the alcohol can lead to skin dryness.

The WOCN can assist staff, patient, and family in product selection, education, and development of a prevention plan. QSEN: Teamwork and collaboration.

Related Care Plan

Pressure ulcers (impaired skin integrity), Chapter 14

■ = Independent　▲ = Interprofessional Collaboration

Nursing Diagnosis Care Plans

NDx **Spiritual Distress**

Definition: A state of suffering related to impaired ability to experience meaning in life through connections with self, others, the world, or a superior being

Spiritual distress is an experience of profound disharmony in the person's belief or value system that threatens the meaning of his or her life. During spiritual distress the patient may lose hope, question his or her belief system, or feel separated from his or her personal source of comfort and strength. Pain, chronic or terminal illness, impending surgery, and the death of a loved one are crises that may cause spiritual distress. Prescribed treatments may present conflicts with the person's values, beliefs, or faith traditions. The health care environment may limit the person's ability to engage in practices or rituals that support spiritual well-being and a sense of connectedness. Being physically separated from family and familiar culture contributes to feeling alone and abandoned. Nurses in the hospital, home care, and ambulatory settings can assist the patient in reestablishing a sense of spiritual well-being.

Common Related Factors

Actively dying
Illness
Death of a significant other
Life transitions
Self-alienation
Social alienation
Increasing dependence on another
Loneliness
Perception of having unfinished business
Sociocultural deprivation
Unexpected life event

Defining Characteristics

Anxiety
Crying
Fatigue
Questioning identity
Questioning meaning of life
Questioning meaning of suffering
Connections to self
  • Anger
  • Inadequate acceptance
  • Insufficient courage
  • Perceived insufficient meaning in life
  • Decrease in serenity
Connections with others
  • Alienation
  • Separation from support system
  • Refusal to interact with significant other or spiritual leader
Connections with art, music, literature, and nature
  • Decrease in expression of previous pattern of creativity
Connections with power greater than self
  • Feeling abandoned
  • Hopelessness
  • Anger toward a power greater than self
  • Inability to experience the transcendent or to be introspective
  • Inability to participate in religious activities
  • Inability to pray
  • Request for a spiritual leader
  • Sudden change in spiritual practice

 For additional care plans, go to http://evolve.elsevier.com/Gulanick/.

Common Expected Outcomes

Patient expresses hope in and value of his or her own belief system and inner resources.

Patient expresses a sense of well-being through art, music, or writing.

Patient participates in spiritual activities.

Patient expresses connectedness with self, others, or a power greater than self.

NOC Outcomes
Hope; Spiritual Health
NIC Interventions
Spiritual Support; Spiritual Growth Facilitation; Coping Enhancement

Ongoing Assessment

Actions/Interventions	Rationales
■ Assess the patient's history of formal religious affiliation, perceived spiritual needs, and desire to engage in spiritual practices.	Eliciting information regarding religious affiliation, spiritual practices and perceived spiritual needs allows the patient to be a full partner in providing care. QSEN: Patient-centered care.
■ Assess the patient's cultural heritage.	All people have a spiritual dimension even if they do not express association with a specific religion or faith tradition. The patient's cultural heritage may be a source of important beliefs besides religion that provide strength and inspiration. QSEN: Patient-centered care.
■ Assess the spiritual meaning of illness or treatment. Questions such as the following provide a basis for future care planning: • "What is the meaning of your illness?" • "How does your illness or treatment affect your relationship with God, your beliefs, or other sources of strength?" • "Does your illness or treatment interfere with expressing your spiritual beliefs?"	Level of physical functioning, duration and course of illness, prognosis, and treatments involved can contribute to spiritual distress. Physical impairments or suffering may be seen as "punishment from God." Proposed treatments may present a conflict with the patient's beliefs or faith tradition.
■ Assess for expressions of hope.	Patients with a positive sense of connectedness or spirituality will express having something to live for or look forward to, even in the face of illness or situational crisis. Hope allows the patient to face the seriousness of the situation.
■ Assess whether the patient has any unfinished business.	Patients may not find peace or harmony until business is completed, such as resolving strained family relations. QSEN: Patient-centered care.

Therapeutic Interventions

Actions/Interventions	Rationales
■ Encourage the verbalization of feelings of anger or loneliness.	Evidence suggests that the nurse's listening to concerns is important to support a patient's sense of spiritual well-being. QSEN: Evidence-based practice.
■ Acknowledge understanding of the patient's spiritual beliefs and practices.	The patient needs to feel that the nurse accepts his or her beliefs. Patients have a right to their beliefs and practices, even if they conflict with the nurse's beliefs. QSEN: Patient-centered care.
■ Develop an ongoing relationship with the patient.	An ongoing relationship establishes trust, reduces the feeling of isolation, and may facilitate resolution of spiritual distress.
■ Facilitate decision-making consistent with the patient's beliefs and values.	The nurse may advocate and support a patient's decision to accept or refuse health care treatment consistent with his or her spiritual beliefs. QSEN: Patient-centered care.

■ = Independent   ▲ = Interprofessional Collaboration

Actions/Interventions

- When requested by the patient or family, arrange for visits from spiritual leaders, spiritual practices, or the display of religious objects, especially when the patient is hospitalized.

- Assist the patient with spiritual rituals. If requested, pray with the patient.

- Do not provide logical solutions for spiritual dilemmas.

- Facilitate communication between the patient and family, spiritual leaders, and other caregivers.

Rationales

Spiritual rituals and religious objects help lessen feelings of separation and provide strength and inspiration. If the patient belongs to a highly codified or ritualized religion, the presence of spiritual leaders are important at times of passage, such as birth or death. In times of crisis the patient may not have the inner strength to contact spiritual leaders without assistance. QSEN: Teamwork and collaboration.

Spiritual rituals and prayer provide a sense of connectedness to others and a power greater than self. Prayer combined with authentic empathy from the nurse can help patients meet their spiritual needs. Some faith traditions may require the patient to face a specific direction during prayer. The patient may need assistance to change positions for prayer. QSEN: Patient-centered care.

Spiritual beliefs are based on faith and are independent of logic.

The patient may desire privacy or rest or may not want spiritual leaders present, but may find it difficult to express.

Education/Continuity of Care

Actions/Interventions

- Provide information in a way that does not interfere with the patient's beliefs, faith, or hopes.

- Inform the patient and family of how to obtain help implementing spiritual practices or seek spiritual guidance.

Rationales

This nursing action demonstrates respect for the patient's individuality and spiritual beliefs. QSEN: Patient-centered care.

Religious rites or spiritual guidance may be essential when patients and families are faced with decisions about prolonging life, organ donation, or medical therapy (e.g., blood transfusion).

Related Care Plans

Ineffective coping, Chapter 2
Hopelessness, Chapter 2
Powerlessness, Chapter 2

NANDA-I
NDx   Risk for Suicide

Definition: Vulnerable to self-inflicted, life-threatening injury

The overwhelming majority of patients who attempt suicide have a psychiatric disorder. However, suicide is not a mental health disorder. The patient who is depressed or who has a bipolar disorder may attempt suicide in response to acute symptoms. The patient with schizophrenia or an organic brain disorder that includes psychosis may respond to voices that tell the patient to hurt himself or herself. Other diagnoses in which suicide is observed as a behavior include personality disorders, in which patients may establish a pattern of self-injury as a response to substance abuse or feelings of anger and anxiety.

A variety of theories have been proposed to explain factors that lead a person to attempt suicide. Patients may use suicide to end prolonged distress, suffering, pain, or disability. Suicide is seen by some as a means of dealing with a sense of utter hopelessness, feelings of desperation or rage, a cry for help, or a means to punish someone. Suicide may be a carefully planned event that the patient has prepared as a final choice or an impulsive act in response to a specific precipitating event perceived as overwhelming. The causes and effects of suicide are the focus of widespread debate in the popular press, among health professionals, and in the courts. Whatever the circumstances, the effects of suicide may resonate in the lives of family members and friends as well as the larger community for years afterward.

Common Risk Factors

Behavioral
- Changing a will
- Giving away possessions
- History of suicide attempt
- Marked change in attitude and/or behavior
- Purchase of a gun
- Stockpiling medication
- Sudden euphoric recovery from major depression

Verbal
- Reports desire to die
- Threat of killing self

Psychological
- Family history of suicide
- Guilt
- Psychiatric disorder
- History of childhood abuse
- Substance abuse
- Homosexual youth

Physical
- Chronic pain
- Physical illness
- Terminal illness

Situational
- Access to weapon
- Economically disadvantaged
- Living alone
- Loss of autonomy
- Loss of independence
- Retired

Social
- Cluster suicides
- Disruptive family life
- Hopelessness
- Insufficient social support
- Loneliness
- Loss of important relationship
- Social isolation

Common Expected Outcomes

Patient discloses suicidal thoughts and feelings.
Patient agrees to treatment plan to reduce risk for suicidal behaviors.
Patient discloses all impulses to harm self and talks to staff immediately.

NOC Outcomes
Suicide Self-Restraint; Impulse Self-Control; Risk Control
NIC Interventions
Suicide Prevention; Mood Management; Environmental Management: Safety; Counseling; Behavior Management: Self-Harm; Patient Contracting

■ = Independent ▲ = Interprofessional Collaboration

Ongoing Assessment

Actions/Interventions	Rationales
■ Interview the patient to assess the potential for self-harm. Ask the following questions:	People who are suicidal often are ambivalent about wanting to end their lives. Patients contemplating suicide may exhibit verbal and behavioral cues about their intent to end their life. QSEN: Patient-centered care; Evidence-based practice; Safety.
• "Have you ever felt like hurting yourself?"	Suicide ideation is the process of thinking about killing oneself. The patient's risk for suicide increases as these thoughts become more frequent.
• "Have you ever attempted suicide?"	The patient's degree of suicide risk is higher if there is a history of previous suicide attempts.
• "Do you currently feel like killing yourself?"	This question needs to be asked directly to assure the patient of the nurse's comfort in hearing his or her response. The patient's response allows the nurse to create a safe environment for the person to discuss feelings and issues openly.
• "Do you have a plan to kill yourself?" "What is your plan?" "What means do you have to carry out your plan?"	Development of a plan and the ability to carry it out greatly increase the risk for suicide. The more lethal the plan or the more detailed and specific the plan, the more serious the risk for suicide. The person who has direct access to the means for suicide is at highest risk.
• "Do you trust yourself to maintain control over your thoughts, feelings, and impulses?"	Patients with strong suicidal thoughts may sense their control of suicidal thoughts slipping away, or they may feel themselves surrender to an impulse to end their life.
■ Assess for risk factors that may increase the potential for a suicide attempt:	It is a myth that suicide occurs without forewarning. It is also a myth that there is a typical type of person who commits suicide. The potential for suicide exists in all people. QSEN: Evidence-based practice; Safety.
• History of suicidal attempts by self or by people who are important in the patient's life	Prior experience removes the prohibitions against suicide. Suicide by a close family member or friend increases the patient's risk for suicide.
• Suicidal statements	The majority of patients who attempt suicide give verbal cues of their intentions to do so. The patient may make statements about suicide or feelings of hopelessness. The person may talk idealistically about release from his or her life and the resolution of problems.
• Unexplained euphoria or energy	This behavioral cue may represent the person's decision to carry out a suicide plan.
• Giving away personal possessions	This behavioral cue may indicate that the person is contemplating suicide. This action represents the person's detachment and disengagement from life.
• Male gender	Men die by suicide almost four times more often than women, whereas women attempt suicide two to three times more often than men. Men are more likely to use firearms; women are more likely to use drug overdoses.
• History of mood disorders or other psychiatric diagnoses	Depression is a common diagnosis among patients who attempt suicide. Improvement in the mood of the patient with depression provides him or her with sufficient energy to act on suicidal thoughts. Patients who have a history of hallucinations or delusions may respond to internal cues that compel them to hurt themselves with little or no warning. Impulsivity may be a component of mood and bipolar disorders.
• Sleep habits	Suicide risk is higher among people who have a history of severe insomnia.

Actions/Interventions	Rationales
• Use of alcohol and drugs	The risk for suicide increases with use of alcohol and drugs such as barbiturates. The highest risk is among patients who continually abuse substances. The patient considering suicide may save prescription drugs to use later as an overdose.
■ Assess all support resources available to the patient.	Patients who are depressed and whose lives are pervaded with a sense of hopelessness may isolate themselves or be unable to access available supports. The patient contemplating suicide often has few contacts with a meaningful social support system.
■ Assess decision-making and problem-solving ability.	Suicide seems an acceptable solution when an individual is no longer able to effectively solve problems solve or make decisions. The patient may need guidance in decision-making.
■ Assess all available and useful coping methods.	Patients with a history of ineffective coping may need new resources. A discussion of what has been useful or ineffective is important information. QSEN: Patient-centered care.
■ Assess the need for hospitalization and safety precautions.	Maintaining patient safety is a priority. The patient who presents a high risk for suicide needs to be in a setting where direct supervision is provided to reduce suicidal actions. QSEN: Safety.

Therapeutic Interventions

Actions/Interventions	Rationales
■ Provide a safe environment.	Suicide precautions are used to prevent the patient from acting on sudden self-destructive impulses. These measures include removing potentially harmful objects (e.g., electrical appliances, sharp instruments, belts and ties, glass items, and medications) and maintaining visual contact with the patient at all times. QSEN: Safety.
■ Provide close patient supervision by maintaining observation or awareness of the patient at all times.	The degree of supervision is defined by the degree of risk. Suicide may be an impulsive act with little or no warning. The patient may need direct observation by health care staff at frequent intervals as often as 30 minutes or less. QSEN: Safety.
■ Develop a verbal or written contract stating that the patient will not act on impulse to do self-harm. Review and update the contract as needed.	A written or verbal agreement establishes permission to discuss the subject, makes a commitment not to act on impulse, and defines a plan of action in case impulse occurs. QSEN: Safety; Patient-centered care.
■ Provide opportunities for the patient to express concerns, fears, feelings, and expectations in a nonjudgmental environment.	The patient benefits from talking about suicidal thoughts with trusted staff. Patients need the opportunity to discuss suicidal thoughts and intentions to harm themselves. Verbalization of these feelings may lessen their intensity. Patients also need to see that staff members are open to discussion of suicidal thoughts. QSEN: Patient-centered care.
■ Spend time with the patient.	The trusting relationship with the nurse provides the patient with a sense of security and reinforces self-worth.
■ Assist the patient with problem-solving in a constructive manner.	Patients learn to recognize situational, interpersonal, or emotional triggers and learn to assess a problem and implement problem-solving measures before reacting.

■ = Independent   ▲ = Interprofessional Collaboration

Actions/Interventions	Rationales
■ Discourage the patient from making decisions when under severe stress.	Patients can learn to identify mood changes that signal problems with impulsivity or signal a deepening depressive state. At these times, deciding not to make a decision may be best.

Education/Continuity of Care

Actions/Interventions	Rationales
▲ Refer the patient to other members of the interprofessional team for additional and ongoing support.	Recovery from a suicide attempt will likely require involvement from many sources, including community-based mental health resources, crisis lines, spiritual support, financial aid, housing, and welfare resources. Recovery may require psychological insight that builds slowly. QSEN: Teamwork and collaboration.
■ Instruct the patient in the appropriate use of medications to facilitate his or her ability to cope.	Drug therapy may help the patient manage underlying health problems such as depression.
■ Contact the patient daily (every 24 hours) to assess recurrent suicide ideation as indicated by the patient's symptoms.	The intermittently suicidal patient is difficult to manage in an outpatient setting. Risks are implicit. The most critical skills include keeping a good therapeutic relationship, regular therapy appointments, and careful assessment of level of consciousness. QSEN: Safety.
■ Teach the patient cognitive-behavioral self-management responses to suicidal thoughts.	Patients are better able to recognize and respond to early thoughts of suicide. The patient can be taught to identify negative self-talk or automatic thoughts that lead to suicidal ideas. Then the patient learns how to develop positive approaches and positive self-talk to counter those negative ideas. QSEN: Patient-centered care.
■ Teach patients to use self-expression methods to self-manage suicidal feelings.	Patients are better able to recognize and safely manage suicidal feelings by methods such as keeping journals and calling hotlines.

Related Care Plans

Ineffective coping, Chapter 2
Hopelessness, Chapter 2

NANDA-I
NDx **Impaired Swallowing**

Definition: Abnormal functioning of the swallowing mechanism associated with deficits in oral, pharyngeal, or esophageal structure or function

Impaired swallowing can be a temporary or permanent complication that can be life threatening. Aspiration of food or fluid is the most serious complication. Impaired swallowing can be caused by a structural problem, interruption or dysfunction of neural pathways, decreased strength or excursion of muscles involved in mastication, facial paralysis, or perceptual impairment. Swallowing difficulties are a common complaint among older adults, in those individuals who have had a stroke, suffered head trauma, have head or neck cancer, or experience progressive neurological diseases like Parkinson's disease, multiple sclerosis, and amyotrophic lateral sclerosis. Dysphagia severity rating scales are available to guide extent of modification in diet plan. The speech pathologist and dietitian are key members of the interprofessional team to guide the treatment plan. Many of the nursing actions reflect the QSEN competencies for safety.

 For additional care plans, go to http://evolve.elsevier.com/Gulanick/.

Common Related Factors

Cranial nerve involvement
Neuromuscular impairment
Neurological problems
Respiratory condition
Esophageal reflux disease
Laryngeal abnormality
Mechanical obstruction

Defining Characteristics

Observed evidence of difficulty in swallowing (coughing, choking, gagging prior to swallowing, delayed swallowing, inability to clear oral cavity)
Reports of "something stuck" in throat

Common Expected Outcomes

Patient demonstrates effective swallowing, as evidenced by absence of aspiration, no evidence of coughing or choking during eating/drinking, no stasis of food in oral cavity after eating, and ability to ingest foods/fluid.
Patient verbalizes appropriate maneuvers to prevent choking and aspiration: positioning during eating, type of food tolerated, and safe environment.
Patient and caregiver verbalize emergency measures to be enacted should choking occur.

NOC Outcomes
Swallowing Status; Risk Control; Self-Care: Eating
NIC Interventions
Aspiration Precautions; Swallowing Therapy

Ongoing Assessment

Actions/Interventions	Rationales
■ Assess for the presence of gag and cough reflexes.	The lungs are normally protected against aspiration by reflexes such as cough or gag. When reflexes are depressed, the patient is at increased risk for aspiration. QSEN: Safety.
■ Assess the strength of facial muscles.	Cranial nerves VII, IX, X, and XII regulate motor function in the mouth and pharynx. Coordinated function of muscles innervated by these nerves is necessary to move a bolus of food from the front of the mouth to the posterior pharynx for controlled swallowing. QSEN: Safety.
■ Assess for coughing or choking during eating and drinking.	These signs indicate an aspiration risk. QSEN: Safety.
■ Assess the ability to swallow a small amount of water.	If water is aspirated, little or no harm to the patient occurs.
■ Assess for residual food in the mouth after eating.	Pocketed food may be easily aspirated at a later time.
■ Assess for the regurgitation of food or fluid through the nares.	Regurgitation indicates a decreased ability to swallow food or fluids and an increased risk for aspiration.
▲ Assess the results of swallowing studies as ordered.	A videofluoroscopic swallowing study may be indicated to determine the nature and extent of any oropharyngeal swallowing abnormality, which aids in designing interventions.

Therapeutic Interventions

Actions/Interventions	Rationales
For the hospitalized or home care patient:	
■ Before mealtime, provide for adequate rest periods.	Fatigue can further contribute to swallowing impairment.
■ Remove or reduce any environmental stimuli (e.g., TV, radio).	With distractions removed, the patient can concentrate on swallowing.
■ Provide oral care before feeding. Clean and insert dentures before each meal.	Oral care stimulates sensory awareness and salivation, which facilitates swallowing.

■ = Independent   ▲ = Interprofessional Collaboration

Actions/Interventions

▲ If a swallowing study was completed, consult with the speech pathologist regarding the level of dysphagia severity and implications for meal planning.

■ Place suction equipment at the bedside, and suction as needed.

■ If decreased salivation is a contributing factor:
  • Before feeding, give the patient a lemon wedge, pickle, or tart-flavored hard candy.
  • Use artificial saliva.

■ Maintain the patient in high-Fowler's position with the head flexed slightly forward during meals.

■ Encourage an intake of food that the patient can swallow; provide frequent small meals and supplements. Use thickening agents as recommended by a speech pathologist.

■ Instruct the patient to (1) hold food in the mouth, (2) close the lips, (3) think about swallowing, and then (4) swallow.

■ Instruct the patient not to talk while eating. Provide verbal cueing as needed.

■ Encourage the patient to chew thoroughly, eat slowly, and swallow frequently, especially if extra saliva is produced. Provide the patient with direction or reinforcement until he or she has swallowed each mouthful.

■ Identify food given to the patient before each spoonful if the patient is being fed.

■ Proceed slowly, giving small amounts; whenever possible, alternate servings of liquids and solids.

■ Encourage a high-calorie diet that includes all food groups, as appropriate. Avoid milk and milk products.

■ If patients pouch food to one side of their mouth, encourage them to turn their head to the unaffected side and manipulate the tongue to the paralyzed side.

■ If the patient has had a stroke, place food in the back of the mouth, on the unaffected side, and gently massage the unaffected side of the throat.

■ Place whole or crushed pills in custard or gelatin. (First ask a pharmacist which pills should not be crushed.) Substitute medication in an elixir form as indicated.

■ Encourage the patient to feed self as soon as possible.

Rationales

Levels on rating scales can range from minimal dysphagia, in which no change in the diet is required, to mild-moderate dysphagia, in which specific swallow techniques and a modified diet may be indicated, to severe dysphagia, in which nothing by mouth is recommended. QSEN: Teamwork and collaboration.

With impaired swallowing reflexes, secretions can rapidly accumulate in the posterior pharynx and upper trachea, increasing the risk for aspiration. QSEN: Safety.

Moistening and use of tart flavors stimulate salivation, lubricate food, and enhance the ability to swallow.

An upright position uses the effect of gravity to facilitate flow of food or fluid through the alimentary tract. Aspiration is less likely to occur with the head tilted slightly forward (this position facilitates elevation of the larynx and posterior movement of the tongue). QSEN: Safety.

Thickened foods with the consistency of pudding, cooked cereal, and semisolid foods are easier for the patient to manage in the mouth and pharynx for controlled swallowing. Thin foods are most difficult; gravy or sauce added to dry foods facilitates swallowing.

Proper instruction and focused concentration on specific steps reduce risks.

Concentration must be focused on swallowing.

Such directions assist in keeping one's focus on the task of swallowing.

Knowledge of the consistency of food to expect can prepare the patient for appropriate chewing and swallowing technique.

This technique helps prevent foods from being left in the mouth.

Dairy products can lead to thickened secretions.

Foods placed in the unaffected side of the mouth facilitate more complete chewing and movement of food to the back of the mouth, where it can be swallowed. These strategies aid in cleaning out residual food.

Massage helps stimulate the act of swallowing.

Mixing some pills with foods helps reduce the risk for aspiration.

With self-feeding, the patient can control the volume of a food bolus and the timing of each bite to facilitate effective swallowing.

Actions/Interventions

▲ If oral intake is not possible or is inadequate, initiate alternative feedings (e.g., nasogastric feedings, gastrostomy feedings, or hyperalimentation).

Follow-up:

▲ Initiate a dietary consultation for calorie count and food preferences.

Rationales

Optimal nutrition is a patient need.

Dietitians have a greater understanding of the nutritional value of foods and may be helpful in guiding treatment. QSEN: Teamwork and collaboration.

Education/Continuity of Care

Actions/Interventions

■ Discuss with and demonstrate the following to the patient or caregiver:
  • Avoidance of certain foods or fluids
  • Upright position during eating
  • Allowance of sufficient time to eat slowly and chew thoroughly
  • Provision of high-calorie meals
  • Use of fluids to help facilitate passage of solid foods
  • Monitoring of the patient for weight loss or dehydration

■ Teach the patient/caregiver exercises to enhance the muscular strength of the face and tongue to enhance swallowing.

■ Facilitate a home care aide or meal provision, if needed.

■ Demonstrate to the patient, caregiver, or family what should be done if the patient aspirates (e.g., chokes, coughs, becomes short of breath). For example, use suction, if available, and the abdominal thrust maneuver if the patient is unable to speak or breathe. If a liquid aspiration occurs, turn the patient three-fourths prone with the head slightly lower than the chest. If the patient has difficulty breathing, call the Emergency Medical System (9-1-1).

■ Encourage family members or the caregiver to seek out cardiopulmonary resuscitation instruction.

Rationales

Both the patient and caregiver may need to be active participants in implementing the treatment plan to optimize safe nutritional intake. QSEN: Safety.

Muscle strengthening can facilitate greater chewing ability and positioning of food in the mouth.

Homebound patients may require additional assistance to maintain adequate nutrition.

Respiratory aspiration requires immediate action by the caregiver to maintain the airway and promote effective breathing and gas exchange. Being prepared for an emergency helps prevent further complications. QSEN: Safety.

Mastery of emergency measures may provide confidence to both the patient and caregiver.

Related Care Plan

Risk for aspiration, Chapter 2

■ = Independent   ▲ = Interprofessional Collaboration

Nursing Diagnosis Care Plans

NDx Impaired Tissue Integrity

Definition: Damage to mucous membrane, cornea, integumentary system, muscular fascia, muscle, tendon, bone, cartilage, joint capsule, and/or ligament

The mucous membranes, cornea, and skin serve as part of a person's first line of defense against threats from the external environment. The tissues of the musculoskeletal system provide structure and function to not only support the person's mobility but also his or her ability to manipulate objects as part of daily living. These tissues can be damaged by physical trauma, including thermal injury (e.g., burns, frostbite); chemical injury such as reactions to drugs, especially chemotherapeutic drugs; radiation; falls; and ischemia. Sometimes damaged tissue is able to regenerate, whereas other times the damaged tissue may be replaced by connective tissue. If untreated, impaired tissue places the person at risk for local or systemic infection and/or necrosis (tissue death). People at risk for impaired tissue integrity include older adults, the homeless, individuals undergoing cancer chemotherapy, and individuals with altered sensation.

Common Related Factors

Extremes of age
Insufficient knowledge about protecting and/or maintaining tissue integrity
Extremes of environmental temperature
Impaired circulation
Chemical injury agent
Pharmaceutical agent
Excessive or insufficient fluid volume
Imbalanced nutritional state (e.g., obesity, malnutrition)
Radiation
Alteration in sensation
Impaired mobility

Defining Characteristics

Damaged tissue
Destroyed tissue

Common Expected Outcome

Patient's tissues return to normal structure and function.

NOC Outcome
Tissue Integrity: Skin and Mucous Membranes
NIC Interventions
Skin Surveillance; Wound Care; Infection Protection

Ongoing Assessment

Actions/Interventions

- Determine the cause of the tissue damage.

- Assess the condition of the tissue.

Rationales

Information about the source of the tissue injury guides specific interventions in the plan of care. QSEN: Patient-centered care.
Redness, swelling, pain, burning, and itching are signs of inflammation and the body's immune system response to localized tissue trauma.

Actions/Interventions

- Assess the characteristics of the wound, including color, size (length, width, depth), drainage, and odor.

- Assess for elevated body temperature.

- Assess the patient's level of discomfort.

- Identify signs of itching and scratching.

Rationales

These data provide information on extent of damage. Pale tissue color is an indication of decreased oxygenation. Odor may arise from infection present in the wound; it may also arise from necrotic tissue. Serous exudate from a wound is a normal part of inflammation and must be differentiated from pus or purulent drainage, which is an indication of infection.

Fever is a systemic manifestation of inflammation and may indicate the presence of infection.

Pain is part of the normal inflammatory response to injury. The extent and depth of a wound may affect pain sensations.

The patient who scratches the skin in attempts to relieve intense itching may open skin lesions and increase risk for infection. QSEN: Patient-centered care.

Therapeutic Interventions

Actions/Interventions

- Remove any embedded material (e.g., glass, metal), as needed.
- Cleanse with normal saline or a nontoxic cleanser, as appropriate.
- ▲ Provide tissue care as needed.

- Maintain sterile dressing technique during wound care.

- ▲ Premedicate for dressing changes as needed.

- Saturate dressings with sterile normal saline solution before removal.
- ▲ Administer antibiotics as ordered.

- Teach the patient to avoid rubbing and scratching the wound area. Provide gloves or clip the nails if necessary.
- Encourage a diet that meets nutritional needs.

Rationales

Removal of foreign material from a wound facilitates healing and decreases the risk for infection. QSEN: Safety.

Cleansing removes debris and pathogens.

Each type of wound is best treated based on its etiology. For example, skin wounds may be covered with wet or dry dressings, topical creams or lubricants, hydrocolloid dressings (e.g., DuoDerm) or vapor-permeable membrane dressings such as Tegaderm. An eye patch or hard, plastic shield may be worn for a corneal injury. The dressing replaces the protective function of the injured tissue during the healing process. QSEN: Evidence-based practice.

This nursing action reduces the risk for wound infection. QSEN: Safety.

Manipulation of deeper wounds or extensive wounds may be painful for the patient.

Saturating dressings will ease dressing removal by loosening adherents and decreasing pain, especially with burns.

Wound infections may be treated more easily with topical agents, although intravenous antibiotics may be indicated.

Rubbing and scratching can cause further injury and delay healing. QSEN: Safety.

A high-protein, high-calorie diet may be needed to promote healing.

■ = Independent   ▲ = Interprofessional Collaboration

Nursing Diagnosis Care Plans

Education/Continuity of Care

Actions/Interventions

■ Teach the patient or caregiver about methods to maintain tissue integrity.

■ Instruct the patient or caregiver in proper care of the wound (i.e., hand washing, wound cleansing, dressing changes, and application of topical medications).

■ Teach the patient or caregiver the signs and symptoms of infection and when to notify the physician or nurse.

Rationales

The patient and caregiver need to learn how to prevent further tissue injury. These measures may include adequate hydration and nutrition, frequent position changes to relieve pressure, appropriate hygiene, safety precautions for specific tissues, and regular inspection of tissues for signs of injury. QSEN: Patient-centered care.

Accurate information increases the patient's ability to manage therapy independently and reduce the risk for infection. QSEN: Patient-centered care.

The patient needs to be aware of potential complications to facilitate prompt intervention in the event of a problem. The patient should report increased wound drainage, increasing pain, local warmth and redness, and fever. QSEN: Safety.

Related Care Plans

Risk for impaired skin integrity, Chapter 2
Burns, Chapter 14
Pressure ulcers (impaired skin integrity), Chapter 14

NANDA-I
NDx Ineffective Peripheral Tissue Perfusion

Definition: Decrease in blood circulation to the periphery that may compromise health

Reduced arterial blood flow causes decreased nutrition and oxygenation at the cellular level. Decreased tissue perfusion can be transient, with few or minimal consequences to the health of the patient, or it can be more acute or protracted, with potentially devastating effects on the patient. Diminished tissue perfusion, which is chronic, invariably results in tissue or organ damage or death.

Management is directed at removing vasoconstricting factors, improving peripheral blood flow, and reducing metabolic demands on the body. In practice, patients often present with a combination of causative factors. Therefore, this care plan will focus on the general assessment and therapeutic interventions common to many causes.

Common Related Factors

Smoking
Hypertension
Diabetes mellitus
Sedentary lifestyle
Insufficient knowledge of disease process
Insufficient knowledge of aggravating factors (e.g., smoking, sedentary lifestyle, trauma, obesity, salt intake, immobility)

Defining Characteristics

Decrease in BP in extremities
Ankle-brachial index < 0.90
Extremity pain
Intermittent claudication
Paresthesia
Alteration in skin characteristics (e.g., color, elasticity, hair, moisture, nails, sensation, temperature)
Color does not return to lowered limb after 1 minute of leg elevation
Skin color pales with limb elevation
Decrease or absence of peripheral pulses
Capillary refill time > 3 seconds
Femoral bruit
Delay in peripheral wound healing

Common Expected Outcomes

Patient maintains optimal peripheral tissue perfusion as evidenced by strong palpable peripheral pulses, reduction in or absence of pain, warm and dry extremities, adequate capillary refill (less than 2 seconds), and prevention of ulceration.

NOC Outcomes
Tissue Perfusion: Peripheral; Knowledge: Disease Process

NIC Interventions
Circulatory Care: Arterial Insufficiency; Teaching: Disease Process

Ongoing Assessment

Actions/Interventions	Rationales
■ Assess for signs of decreased tissue perfusion.	Specific clusters of signs and symptoms as listed in the defining characteristics are general indications of adequacy of tissue perfusion. Evaluation provides a baseline for future comparisons.
■ Assess for possible causative factors of reduced tissue perfusion. Some examples include vasospasm, indwelling arterial catheters, constricting cast, compartment syndrome, embolism or thrombus, and positioning.	Early detection of causes facilitates prompt, effective treatment.
■ Monitor BP for orthostatic changes (drop of 20 mm Hg systolic BP or 10 mm Hg diastolic BP with position changes).	Stable BP is necessary to maintain adequate tissue perfusion. Medication effects such as vasodilation, altered autonomic control, reduced fluid volume, and decompensated heart failure are among many factors that potentially compromise optimal BP.
▲ Use pulse oximetry to monitor oxygen saturation and pulse rate.	Pulse oximetry is a useful tool to detect changes in oxygenation. Appropriate use of safety-enhancing technology reduces the risk of harm to the patient. QSEN: Safety.
▲ Monitor Hgb levels.	Low levels reduce the uptake of oxygen at the alveolar-capillary membrane and reduce oxygen delivery to the tissues.

Therapeutic Interventions

Actions/Interventions	Rationales
▲ Assist with diagnostic testing as indicated.	A variety of tests are available depending on the cause of the impaired tissue perfusion. These include segmental limb pressure measurement such as ankle-brachial index (ABI) for lower extremities, Doppler flow studies, vascular stress testing, and angiograms.
▲ Administer optimal fluid balance. For patients with decreased preload, administer IV fluids as ordered.	Volume therapy may be required to maintain adequate filling pressures and optimize cardiac output needed for tissue perfusion. Oral fluid replacement is indicated for mild fluid deficit. Older patients have a decreased sense of thirst and may need ongoing reminders to drink.
■ Assist with position changes.	Slowly changing from a supine to sitting/standing position can reduce the risk for orthostatic BP changes. Older patients are more susceptible to such drops in pressure with position changes. QSEN: Safety.
▲ Maintain adequate ventilation and perfusion as in the following: • Place the patient in a semi-Fowler's to high-Fowler's position as tolerated. • Administer oxygen therapy as prescribed.	Upright positioning promotes improved alveolar gas exchange. Oxygen saturation needs to be greater than 90%. Increasing arterial oxygen saturation delivers more oxygen to the tissues and relieves oxygen supply and demand imbalances.

■ = Independent ▲ = Interprofessional Collaboration

Actions/Interventions	Rationales
▲ Administer medications as prescribed to treat the underlying problem. Note the response.	These medications facilitate perfusion for most causes of impairment.
• Antiplatelets/anticoagulants (to reduce blood viscosity and coagulation)	
• Peripheral vasodilators (to enhance arterial dilation and improve peripheral blood flow)	
• Antihypertensives (to reduce systemic vascular resistance and optimize cardiac output and perfusion)	
• Inotropes (to improve cardiac output)	
▲ In acute situations, anticipate the need for more invasive therapies as indicated.	Therapies such as percutaneous transluminal angioplasty/stenting, atherectomy, surgical revascularization, embolectomy, and thrombolytic therapy may be indicated. QSEN: Evidence-based practice.
▲ For specific causes, anticipate directed interventions (e.g., fasciotomy for compartment syndrome; bivalving a constricting cast).	Therapies help optimize tissue perfusion.

Education/Continuity of Care

Actions/Interventions	Rationales
■ Provide information on normal tissue perfusion and possible causes for impairment.	Knowledge of causative factors provides a rationale for treatments.
■ Discuss examples of lifestyle factors that can promote improved tissue perfusion (avoiding smoking, reducing risk factors for atherosclerosis [obesity, hypertension, dyslipidemia, inactivity], avoiding crossed legs at the knee when sitting, changing positions at frequent intervals, rising slowly from a supine/sitting to standing position).	Smoking causes vasoconstriction and reduces oxygen supply. Atherosclerosis is a major contributor of reduced blood flow in the peripheral vessels. Attention to position changes can improve circulatory blood flow.
■ Explain all procedures and treatments.	Explaining expected events and sensations can help reduce anxiety associated with the unknown.
■ Instruct the patient to inform the nurse immediately if symptoms of decreased tissue perfusion persist, increase, or return.	Early assessment facilitates prompt treatment.

NANDA-I

NDx Urinary Retention

Definition: Incomplete emptying of the bladder

Urinary retention may occur in conjunction with or independent of urinary incontinence. Urinary retention, the inability to empty the bladder even though urine is present, may occur as a side effect of certain medications, including anesthetic agents, antihypertensives, antihistamines, antispasmodics, and anticholinergics. These drugs interfere with the nerve impulses necessary to cause relaxation of the sphincters, which allow urination. Obstruction of outflow is another cause of urinary retention. Most commonly, this type of obstruction in men is the result of benign prostatic hyperplasia. Women may experience urinary retention if their bladder sags (cystocele) or if it is pulled out of position by a sagging colon (rectocele).

Common Related Factors

Strong sphincter
Anesthesia effects
High urethral pressures (caused by disease, injury, or edema)
Pain, fear of pain
Blockage in urinary tract
Reflex arc inhibition

Defining Characteristics

Small voiding or absent urinary output
Frequent voiding
Sensation of bladder fullness
Bladder distention
Dribbling of urine
Overflow incontinence
Residual urine
Dysuria

Common Expected Outcome

Patient empties bladder completely as evidenced by urine volume greater than or equal to 300 mL with each voiding and residual volume less than 100 mL.

NOC Outcomes
Urinary Continence; Urinary Elimination
NIC Intervention
Urinary Retention Care

Ongoing Assessment

Actions/Interventions	Rationales
■ Evaluate previous patterns of voiding.	There is a wide range of "normal" voiding frequency. Acute urinary retention requires prompt medical intervention. With chronic urinary retention, one is able to urinate but may have trouble starting the stream or emptying the bladder completely. Frequent voiding of small amounts (25-50 mL) of urine or dribbling is associated with urinary retention. The nurse incorporates this information in the planning and evaluation of care and communicates the information to the interprofessional team. QSEN: Patient-centered care.
■ Visually inspect and palpate the lower abdomen for distention. Ask patient regarding feeling of bladder fullness or suprapubic discomfort.	The bladder lies below the umbilicus. The lower abdomen becomes distended as the urine volume increases in the bladder.
■ Evaluate the time intervals between voidings, and record the amount voided each time.	Keeping an hourly log for 48 hours gives a clear picture of the patient's voiding pattern and amounts and can help to establish a toileting schedule.
▲ Use a bladder scan (portable ultrasound instrument) or catheterize the patient to measure residual urine if incomplete emptying is suspected.	These methods determine the amount of residual urine. Retention of urine in the bladder predisposes the patient to urinary tract infection and may indicate the need for an intermittent catheterization program.
■ Assess the amount, frequency, and character (e.g., color, odor, and specific gravity) of urine.	These characteristics allow for assessment of residual urine volumes and risk factors for a urinary tract infection.
■ Determine the balance between intake and output.	An intake greater than output may indicate retention.
■ Determine the probable cause for the problem.	Information guides the design of an optimal treatment plan (e.g., medication side effects versus benign prostatic hyperplasia).
▲ Monitor urinalysis, urine culture, and sensitivity.	Urinary tract infection can cause retention, but it is more likely to cause frequency.
■ If an indwelling catheter is in place, assess for patency and kinking.	An occluded or kinked catheter may lead to urinary retention in the bladder.
▲ Monitor blood urea nitrogen and creatinine.	Elevation in these values will differentiate between urinary retention and renal failure as causes of decreased urine output.

■ = Independent   ▲ = Interprofessional Collaboration

Therapeutic Interventions

Actions/Interventions	Rationales
■ Initiate the following methods to facilitate voiding:	
• Position the patient upright if possible to facilitate successful voiding. Encourage patient to lean forward, supporting upper body with forearms or hands on the thighs.	An upright position on a commode or in bed on a bedpan increases the patient's voiding success through force of gravity; it also decreases embarrassment of soiling self or bed linens.
• Provide privacy.	Privacy helps the patient relax urinary sphincters.
• Encourage the patient to void when the urge is first felt and at least every 4 hours.	Voiding at frequent intervals empties the bladder, reduces bladder overdistention, and reduces risk for urinary retention.
• Encourage the patient to double void by urinating, then resting for 3 to 5 minutes, then attempting to void a second time.	This bladder training technique can more efficiently empty the bladder by allowing the detrusor to contract initially, then relax, and contract again.
• Have the patient listen to the sound of running water, or place the patient's hands in warm water/pour warm water over the perineum.	These actions help stimulate the micturation reflex and promote a sense of relaxation during voiding.
• Offer warm fluids before voiding.	Sufficient urine volume is needed to stimulate the voiding reflex. Warm fluids stimulate the bladder and promote voiding.
• Perform Credé's method over the bladder.	Credé's method (pressing down over the bladder with the hands) increases bladder pressure, which stimulates relaxation of the sphincter to allow voiding.
▲ Insert an indwelling (Foley) catheter as ordered.	With acute urinary retention, treatment begins with the insertion of an indwelling catheter to drain the bladder.
▲ Institute intermittent catheterization.	Because many causes of urinary retention are self-limited, the decision to leave an indwelling catheter in place should be avoided. This may continue for chronic retention problems.
■ Consult with the physician concerning eliminating or adjusting any medication that might contribute to the problem.	Medication side effects may be causing urinary retention. QSEN: Teamwork and collaboration.
▲ Encourage the patient to take bethanechol (Urecholine) as ordered.	Bethanechol stimulates the parasympathetic nervous system to release acetylcholine at nerve endings and to increase the tone and amplitude of contractions of the smooth muscles of the urinary bladder.
■ Encourage fluids unless the patient is on a fluid restriction.	Unless medically contraindicated, fluid intake should be at least 1500 mL/24 hr.
■ Encourage intake of cranberry juice daily.	Cranberry juice keeps urine acidic. This helps prevent infection because cranberry juice metabolizes to hippuric acid, which maintains an acidic urine; acidic urine is less likely to become infected.

Education/Continuity of Care

Actions/Interventions	Rationales
■ Educate the patient or caregiver about the importance of adequate fluid intake (e.g., 8 to 10 glasses of fluids daily) unless the patient is on fluid restriction.	Increased fluid stimulates voiding and decreases the risk for development of urinary tract infections as a result of flushing of bacteria from the genitourinary tract.
■ Instruct the patient or caregiver in measures to stimulate voiding.	Knowledge of a variety of methods to enhance voiding optimizes success.

Actions/Interventions

- Instruct the patient or caregiver in the signs and symptoms of an overdistended bladder (e.g., decreased or absent urine, frequency, hesitancy, urgency, lower abdominal distention, or discomfort).
- Instruct the patient or caregiver in the signs and symptoms of a urinary tract infection (e.g., chills and fever, frequent urination or concentrated urine, and abdominal or back pain).
- Teach the patient or caregiver to perform meatal care twice daily with soap and water and to dry thoroughly.
- Teach the patient to achieve an upright position on the toilet if possible.
- Teach the patient about possible surgical treatment as needed.

Rationales

Knowing the signs and symptoms allows for early recognition of the condition and treatment.

Knowing the signs and symptoms allows the patient or caregiver to recognize them and seek treatment.

Meatal care reduces the risk for infection.

An upright position is the natural position for voiding and uses the force of gravity.

If prostate enlargement is the cause of retention, surgery may be required. Women may need surgery to lift a fallen bladder or rectum. A urethral stent may be required to treat a urethral stricture.

■ = Independent ▲ = Interprofessional Collaboration

CHAPTER

3

Health Promotion and Risk Factor Management Care Plans

This chapter addresses the challenges of working with patients who are seeking to increase their level of well-being. Typical nursing care plans focus on sick care, helping patients manage their medical illnesses. In these disease-focused care plans, nurses assume the more active role, with patients as the recipients of care. Thus this chapter is unique in that it showcases patients who are actively engaged in health-seeking behaviors. The public is beginning to realize that almost half of all premature deaths in the United States are caused by lifestyle-related problems: unhealthy foods, overweight and obesity, tobacco smoking, poorly managed stress, sleep deficit, and sedentary lifestyle, to name a few. Nurses have always done an excellent job educating patients about health and disease; however, research is clear that education, though necessary, is not sufficient for making needed lifestyle changes. Making changes to one's lifestyle

is very complex. Helping a patient adopt new health behaviors requires attention to multifaceted, evidence-based strategies known to facilitate successful behavior change. These strategies include a combination of methods to enhance awareness of risk factors, increase motivation for change, set realistic goals, focus on tailoring the regimen, incorporate self-monitoring, enhance self-efficacy, provide skills in problem-solving, include social support and rewards, and address relapse prevention. Nurses are well positioned to guide patients who are actively seeking to improve their health habits and environment to achieve their optimal level of health and wellness. These care plans demonstrate the important partnership nurses have with patients in assisting them to develop the knowledge and skills needed for making healthy lifestyle decisions and enacting healthy behaviors.

NDx Health-Seeking Behaviors

Health promotion activities include a wide range of topics such as smoking cessation; stress management; weight loss; proper diet for prevention of coronary artery disease, cancer, osteoporosis, and other diseases; exercise promotion; prenatal instruction; safe sex practices to prevent sexually transmitted infections; protective helmets to prevent head trauma; and practices to reduce risks for diabetes, stroke, and other diseases.

Patients of all ages may be involved in improving health habits. Social cognitive theory identifies factors (e.g., behavior, cognition and other personal factors, the environment) that influence how and to what extent people are able to change old behaviors and adopt new ones. Psychosocial factors such as stress and anxiety regarding

perceived risk for disease, along with social support for engaging in the health-promoting behaviors, must be considered. The action plan must be tailored to fit with the patient's values and belief systems. Opportunities for self-monitoring and receiving feedback enhance the behavior change process.

The setting in which health promotion activities occur may range from the privacy of someone's home, group activities (e.g., weight maintenance groups or health clubs), or even the work setting (especially targeted programs for hypertension management and weight reduction). This care plan gives a general overview of health-seeking behaviors.

Common Related Factors

New condition, altered health status
Lack of awareness about environmental hazards affecting personal health
Absence of interpersonal support
Limited availability of health care resources
Unfamiliarity with community wellness resources
Lack of knowledge about health promotion behaviors

Defining Characteristics

Perceives optimum health as a primary life purpose
Expresses desire to seek higher level of wellness
Expresses concern about current health status
Demonstrated or observed lack of knowledge of health promotion behaviors
Actively seeks resources to expand wellness knowledge
Expresses sense of self-confidence and personal efficacy toward health promotion
Verbalizes desire for increased control of health
Anticipates internal and external threats to health status and desires to take preventive action

Common Expected Outcomes

Patient verbalizes accurate information and necessary environmental changes to promote a healthier lifestyle.
Patient engages in desired behaviors to promote a healthier lifestyle.

NOC Outcomes
Health-Promoting Behavior; Health Seeking Behavior; Knowledge: Health Resources
NIC Interventions
Self-Modification Assistance; Health Education; Patient Contracting

Ongoing Assessment

Actions/Interventions	Rationales
■ Assess the patient's individual perceptions of health problems.	According to models such as the Health Belief Model, the patient's perceived susceptibility to and perceived seriousness and threat of disease motivate health-seeking behaviors. In addition, factors such as culture and heritage can affect how people view their health.
■ Question the patient regarding previous experiences and health teaching.	Adults bring many life experiences to learning sessions. Often patients have previously tried unsuccessfully to engage in a specific health practice. Reasons for difficulties need to be explored. QSEN: Patient-centered care.
■ Determine at what stage of change the patient is currently.	The Transtheoretical Model emphasizes that interventions for change should be matched with the stage of change at which patients are situated. For example, if the patient is only "contemplating" starting an exercise program, efforts may be directed toward emphasizing the positive aspects of exercise and reducing barriers; whereas if the patient is in the "preparation" or "action" stages, more specific directions regarding exercise (e.g., places to exercise, equipment, target heart rate, warm-up activities) can be addressed. QSEN: Evidence-based practice; Patient-centered care.
■ Identify the priority of learning needs within the overall care plan.	Patients are more motivated to learn information they feel is most important to them. QSEN: Patient-centered care.
■ Identify any misconceptions regarding material to be taught.	Patients must have accurate information to make appropriate behavior changes.
■ Assess the patient's confidence in his or her ability to perform the desired behavior.	According to the social cognitive theory, positive conviction that one can successfully execute a behavior is correlated with performance and successful outcome. QSEN: Patient-centered care; Evidence-based practice.

■ = Independent ▲ = Interprofessional Collaboration

Actions/Interventions	Rationales
■ Identify the patient's specific strengths and competencies.	Every patient brings unique strengths to the health-planning task (e.g., motivation, knowledge, social support).
■ Identify health goals and areas for improvement.	Systematically reviewing areas for potential change can assist patients in making informed choices.
■ Identify possible barriers to change (e.g., lack of motivation, interpersonal support, skills, knowledge, or resources).	If the patient is aware of possible barriers and has formulated plans for dealing with them, successful behavioral change is more likely to occur. For example, if trying to engage in more exercise, walking in shopping malls can be substituted for outdoor activity during periods of inclement weather.
■ Determine cultural influences on health teaching.	Certain ethnic and religious groups hold unique beliefs and health practices that must be considered when designing educational plans. QSEN: Patient-centered care.

Therapeutic Interventions

Actions/Interventions	Rationales
■ Clearly define the specific behavior to be changed.	The more precisely defined the behavior is, the greater the chance of success.
■ Guide the patient in setting realistic goals.	Goals that are too global, such as "lose 30 pounds," are difficult to achieve and can foster feelings of failure. Shorter-range goals, such as "lose 5 pounds in a month," may be more achievable and therefore offer positive reinforcement. QSEN: Patient-centered care.
■ Promote positive expectations for success.	Patients with stronger self-efficacy to perform a behavior are much more likely to engage in it.
■ Assist the patient in developing a self-contract.	Contracts help clarify the goal and enhance the patient's control over the behavior, creating a sense of independence, competence, and autonomy.
■ Assist in developing a time frame for implementation.	Changes need to be made over time to allow new behaviors to be learned well, integrated into one's lifestyle, and stabilized.
■ Develop a system for the patient to monitor his or her own progress.	Self-management is a key component of a successful change in behavior. QSEN: Patient-centered care.
■ Allow periodic evaluation, feedback, and revision of the health plan as necessary.	This method provides a systematic approach for movement of the patient toward higher levels of health and promotes adherence to the plan. Appropriately timed feedback is critical to successful behavior change. Telephone or Internet feedback can be a convenient source.
■ Reward positive efforts and achievement.	Positive rewards, especially those inherent in the activity (e.g., the enjoyment of outside walking with a partner), should be encouraged because they continue to reinforce the behavior. Other rewards may consist of verbal praise, monetary rewards, special privileges (e.g., earlier office appointment, free parking), or telephone calls from the health care provider.
■ Implement the use of modeling to assist patients.	Observing the behavior of others who have successfully achieved similar goals helps exemplify the exact behaviors that should be developed to reach the goal. The use of videotapes with patients performing the desired behavior has been quite effective.

Actions/Interventions

■ Provide a comprehensive approach to health promotion by giving attention to environmental, social, and cultural constraints.

■ Prepare for lapses and relapses.

Rationales

The various health promotion models emphasize that focusing only on behavior change is doomed to failure without simultaneous efforts to alter the environment and collective behavior.

Relapse prevention needs to be addressed early in the treatment plan. Identifying high-risk situations likely to cause relapse aids problem-solving. The maintenance phase of change is the longest and most challenging to sustain.

Education/Continuity of Care

Actions/Interventions

■ Provide instruction for specific topics or behaviors (e.g., smoking cessation, weight loss).

■ Use a variety of teaching methods to match the patient's preferred learning style.

■ Inform the patient regarding community resources and self-help groups as appropriate.

■ Encourage the participation of family or significant others in proposed changes.

Rationales

Correct information is needed for positive outcomes.

Different people learn in different ways, so using the most effective learning style promotes success. Learning is enhanced when various approaches reinforce the material that is being taught. QSEN: Patient-centered care.

Self-help and support groups provide unique perspectives on "being there" and may be effective in providing alternative treatment modalities. These resources of support often provide the patient with a measure of external accountability to maintain the desired health behaviors.

One's significant others can play an important role in providing support over the long term that may enhance overall adaptation to change.

Readiness for Engaging in a Regular Physical Activity Program

The *2008 Physical Activity Guidelines for Americans* provides an evidence-based prescription for assisting individuals with improving their health through regular physical activity. Based on the Aerobics Center Longitudinal Study, recommendations include both aerobic and muscle-strengthening activities in the following doses: at least 150 minutes per week of moderate aerobic physical activity to obtain general health benefits and muscle-strengthening activities using major muscle groups on 2 or more days per week. Additional health benefits can be achieved in a dose-response fashion, either by increasing the intensity to vigorous activity or by increasing the duration of moderate activity to 300 minutes per week. Health benefits can be achieved in intermittent episodes of even 10 minutes of moderate physical activity. Health benefits are attainable by individuals of all ages, even those with chronic medical problems. Stressful and busy lifestyles, socioeconomic factors, physical constraints, and lack of motivation are all barriers that can contribute to low physical activity. Nursing objectives are to educate patients on the importance of adopting an active lifestyle and to assist patients in finding ways to personalize the recommended exercise prescription.

■ = Independent   ▲ = Interprofessional Collaboration

Defining Characteristics

Expresses willingness to begin a regular physical activity program

Demonstrates attitude toward increasing physical activity congruent with goals

Expresses knowledge of components of a regular physical activity program

Engages in a self-monitoring program

Engages in a prescribed physical activity program

Expresses willingness to use a support group as appropriate

Common Expected Outcomes

Patient verbalizes accurate information about benefits of increasing physical activity and strategies to develop a personal program of increased lifestyle activity.

Patient engages in a tailored aerobic physical activity routine that includes at least 150 minutes of moderate-intensity exercise per week.

Patient performs muscle-strengthening exercise on at least 2 days per week.

NOC Outcomes
Knowledge: Prescribed Activity; Exercise Participation; Physical Fitness; Health Seeking Behavior

NIC Interventions
Exercise Promotion; Exercise Promotion: Strength Training; Teaching: Prescribed Exercise

Ongoing Assessment

Actions/Interventions	Rationales
■ Assess the patient's past experiences with structured physical activity.	Adults bring many life experiences to learning sessions. Many patients have had positive experiences in the past that can serve as a base on which to build. More commonly, patients often have previously tried unsuccessfully to become more active. Reasons for difficulties need to be explored.
■ Determine the patient's level of motivation and confidence for engaging in a regular physical activity program.	It is important that patients have the motivation and commitment not only to begin a program, but to stay with it for the upcoming weeks and months until new lifestyle behaviors are learned. Asking patients to rate their confidence (on a scale of 1 to 10) that they can stick with the program provides important information. QSEN: Patient-centered care.
■ Assess the patient's current level of physical activity, including both lifestyle activity and structured exercise.	This assessment provides a basis for increasing activity. Assessment should be as accurate as possible, and may include such methods as a 1-week activity log or pedometer readings.
■ Assess the patient's level of mobility and physical status before prescribing an activity plan.	Many sedentary patients will have evidence of deconditioning. A baseline assessment of physical status will allow the nurse to safely initiate an exercise regimen specific to patient needs and abilities. Screening tools such as the Physical Activity Readiness Questionnaire (PAR-Q) provide guidance as to when a medical examination may be required before initiating a program. Older adults with chronic conditions may need personalized assessments. QSEN: Safety.

Actions/Interventions

■ Assess possible barriers to increasing physical activity, such as lack of interpersonal support, skills, knowledge, or resources.

■ Monitor the patient's responses to a new exercise routine, such as frequency of participation, length of each session, and any pain or discomfort experienced afterward.

Rationales

If the patient is aware of possible barriers and has formulated plans for dealing with them, successful change is more likely to occur. For example, when trying to engage in a walking program, walking in a shopping mall can be substituted for outdoor activity during periods of inclement weather.

Information on the patient's progress and emotional or physical successes or setbacks provides direction for modifying the exercise routine.

Therapeutic Interventions

Actions/Interventions

■ Provide ongoing education about the benefits of physical activity to both the patient and significant others.

■ Guide the patient in setting realistic short-term and long-term goals for increasing physical activity.

■ Discuss ways to incorporate exercise into daily life, especially by starting a walking program.

■ Introduce an activity calendar, so patients can monitor their physical activity on a daily basis.

Rationales

Patients need information on the many health benefits of exercise and the potential health risks of being sedentary. Physical activity relieves tension and depression that improves general well-being, enhances sleep, reduces risk factors for many chronic conditions, improves physical wellness, and prolongs life. Lack of physical activity can lead to many chronic conditions, including diabetes, heart disease, obesity, and various cancers.

Adults have many options for increasing their current level of activity. Setting realistic achievable goals helps to maintain motivation and eventual success of the exercise regimen. Focus should be on selecting activities that are enjoyable and can be continued all year round. QSEN: Patient-centered care.

Lower-intensity, leisure-time physical activities of a habitual nature are an easy starting point. Walking is the easiest and most effective way to begin an exercise program. Some patients may start with simply walking for 10 minutes a day, whereas others may be ready to commit to 30 minutes. Even brief episodes of activity, as little as 10 minutes each, can add up to the 150 minutes of recommended exercise per week.

Such tracking devices serve as a visual reminder of exercise achievement as well as a self-monitoring technique. Self-monitoring by record-keeping has been shown to be one of the most critical parts of lifestyle change. Self-management is a key component of a successful change in behavior. QSEN: Patient-centered care.

■ = Independent ▲ = Interprofessional Collaboration

Actions/Interventions	Rationales
■ Clarify for the patient the *2008 Physical Activity Guidelines for Americans* (adults and older adults), including aerobic and muscle-strengthening activities, and their associated health benefits:	Adults have many ways to reach their activity goals within their financial means. Beyond simply increasing lifestyle activity, patients can work toward the goal of meeting the national guidelines that include both aerobic (endurance) and muscle-strengthening (resistance) exercises that convey health benefits. Patients need to have accurate information and guidance on how to achieve these goals (if feasible).

- Adults should do 2 hours and 30 minutes (150 minutes) a week of moderate-intensity, or 1 hour and 15 minutes (75 minutes) a week of vigorous-intensity aerobic physical activity, or an equivalent combination of moderate and vigorous physical activity. Greater health benefits are derived from greater amounts of exercise.
- Examples of moderate-intensity exercises include walking briskly at 3 to 4 mph, bicycling slower than 10 mph, doubles tennis, ballroom dancing.
- Examples of vigorous-intensity exercises include jogging, race-walking, running, singles tennis, lap swimming, aerobic dancing, jumping rope.
- Aerobic activities should be completed in increments of at least 10 minutes, spread throughout the week.
- Adults should also engage in muscle-strengthening exercises involving major muscle groups on at least 2 days per week for additional health benefits.
- Examples of muscle-strengthening exercises include resistance training, lifting weights, using resistance bands, doing push-ups, pull-ups, sit-ups, heavy gardening, and carrying heavy loads.

Patients can choose to do aerobic activities for a longer time at a moderate intensity level, for a shorter time at a vigorous level, or a mix of both during the week. Most individuals find that including a variety of exercise activities and routines in their overall activity program prevents boredom.

Actions/Interventions	Rationales
■ Instruct patients in ways to identify prescribed exercise intensity, as appropriate.	Most patients can easily tell the difference between low, moderate, and vigorous levels of exercise intensity. Several approaches can be used to prescribe exercise intensity. Ratings of perceived exertion (RPE) using the Borg scale (range from 6-20) is a common method, with patients encouraged to exercise in a range of 11 to 15 that equates to perceived exertion in the "light" (11) to "somewhat hard" (13) to "hard" (15) range.
■ Instruct patients in monitoring their heart rate (HR) as a measure of intensity of exercise.	The harder one exercises, the more calories are burned and the more one's stamina and endurance is increased. For best effects, patients can be instructed to exercise in their target HR zone, a range usually between 50% and 80% of their maximal HR. Patients can be taught to monitor their HR by palpating their carotid artery. Some patients benefit from wearing an HR monitor to get objective feedback about their level of exercise. These devices are available at many sporting goods stores.
■ Instruct in the importance of warm-up and cool-down period during more strenuous exercise.	Warming up prepares the body for aerobic activity by increasing blood flow to the muscles and raises the body temperature. Jumping into an aerobic workout without preparing the body could lead to such problems as muscle strain or injury. Cooling down after a workout may help gradually reduce the temperature of muscles, especially after a more intense workout. Cooling down may help reduce muscle injury, stiffness, and soreness. QSEN: Safety.

Health Promotion and Risk
Factor Management Care Plans

Actions/Interventions

- Instruct in the importance of wearing comfortable clothing and footwear appropriate for the temperature, humidity, and activity.

- Instruct patients in ways to avoid injury with exercise, especially for older adults (e.g., starting out slowly if previously inactive, selecting the types and amount of exercise appropriate for their fitness and health status, increasing duration before intensity of activity, choosing a safe place to do the activity, reporting any signs of overexertion or health problems to their health care professional).
- Provide education on the use of technology to promote exercise goals, such as Internet and social media sites for monitoring of physical activity or chat rooms to discuss exercise efforts.
- Suggest the patient find an activity or exercise partner.

- Refer patients to community resources such as the YMCA, park districts, or other community activity centers.
- Provide positive reinforcement as indicated. Encourage the patient to plan rewards at appropriate intervals to celebrate successes.

- Assist the patient in preparing for possible lapses and relapses, especially during holidays, when busy at work, during business travel, or during wintry weather.

Rationales

Clothes should allow for appropriate heat loss, especially on hot, humid days. Shoes should fit well to prevent blisters and foot injuries. The feet should be checked regularly for any cuts or breaks in the skin or change in color or temperature, especially in patients with diabetes or peripheral arterial disease.

Initiating a moderate level of physical activity is safe for most people. Actually, people who are physically fit have less of a chance of injury than those less fit. However, for anyone not previously active, activity-induced injuries are possible and the patient should be informed about how best to avoid such problems. Patients with chronic medical conditions should increase their physical activity under the supervision of their health care professional. QSEN: Safety.

Many Internet-based services are available to disseminate information about safe and appropriate activities and to provide a way to correspond with other patients or with the nurse about the patient's progress or setbacks.

Recruiting a support person to share in the activity can increase motivation, fun, and compliance with the regimen.

Patients may not be aware of resources that can be a basis of support and success.

Appropriately timed feedback is critical to successful behavior change. Positive reinforcement encourages a desired behavior. Rewards, both intrinsic and extrinsic, are motivational and can give a sense of satisfaction for a job well done.

A lifetime of physical activity is difficult to maintain. Relapse prevention needs to be addressed early in the treatment plan. Preparing and planning for setbacks will equip patients to positively cope with each challenging situation. Any setbacks should be reframed as learning opportunities and as a normal step in making lifestyle changes.

NDx Readiness for Enhanced Immunization Status

Every year, approximately 50,000 adults in the United States die from diseases that could have been prevented by vaccines. Influenza and pneumonia are the fifth leading cause of death in older adults in the United States. Immunizations are one of the safest, most cost-effective public health measures available to patients to preserve their health. Although many adults do support immunization programs for their children, they are often less informed about the many health benefits of vaccines as adults. The Centers for Disease Control and Prevention (CDC) recommendations clearly identify who is at risk for various diseases and who should be immunized to protect against them.

■ = Independent ▲ = Interprofessional Collaboration

Defining Characteristics

Expresses desire to enhance behavior to prevent infectious disease

Expresses desire to enhance immunization status

Expresses desire to enhance knowledge of immunization standards

Expresses desire to enhance identification of providers of immunizations

Expresses desire to enhance identification of possible problems associated with immunizations

Expresses desire to enhance record-keeping of immunizations

Common Expected Outcomes

Patient acknowledges disease risk without immunization.

Patient obtains adult immunizations recommended by the CDC.

Patient identifies community resources for immunization.

Patient develops and maintains a systematic record-keeping plan for monitoring immunization status.

NOC Outcome
Immunization Behavior
NIC Intervention
Immunization/Vaccination Management

Ongoing Assessment

Actions/Interventions	Rationales
■ Assess the patient's prior history of immunizations as a child and adult.	This information provides a baseline to determine personal protection and adherence to immunization recommendations.
■ Assess the patient's knowledge of the latest CDC recommendations regarding immunization use.	Patients may have basic knowledge about common adult illnesses (e.g., influenza and pneumococcal diseases) but they may have misinformation about vaccinations against less common diseases (e.g., measles, mumps, varicella) that may be needed by adults. QSEN: Patient-centered care.
■ Assess the patient's interest in travel abroad.	Immunizations may be required depending on the country being visited, age and medical status of the patient, and the length of stay.
■ Determine immunization status at every health care visit, especially emergency department visits.	A systematic assessment program can facilitate increased awareness of immunization need by both health care professionals and patients.
■ Identify any contraindications to receiving immunizations.	Vaccines are considered to be quite safe for the general public. However, patients may have had prior anaphylaxis to a vaccine or have a moderate to severe acute illness, putting them at increased risk. Pregnant women need to discuss immunizations with their health care professional. All potential risks need to be weighed against benefits. QSEN: Safety.

Therapeutic Interventions

Actions/Interventions

■ Review information regarding the latest CDC recommendations for the prevention of common diseases. Some of these include the following:

- *Influenza:* The trivalent inactivated influenza vaccine (TIV) is recommended annually for all adults, even healthy adults between the ages of 19 and 49 years without risk factors. Adults age 65 years and older may be given the standard TIV dose or a high dose. Many health care institutions now require every employee to be vaccinated.
- *Pneumonia:* There are two types of pneumococcal vaccine: PCV13 (conjugate) and PPSV23 (polysaccharide). They do not necessarily reduce risk for getting pneumonia, but can reduce associated complications. One or both vaccines may be recommended for all adults, especially those who are 65 years or older, those with a chronic illness, younger adults without a spleen or with a damaged spleen, and people with a compromised immune system.
- *Shingles (herpes zoster):* Zostavax is recommended as a one-time dose for people who are 60 years and older regardless of whether they have had shingles previously.
- *Hepatitis B:* Hepatitis B vaccine is indicated for all people age 18 and older, especially those whose lifestyle (e.g., intravenous [IV] drug users, those with human immunodeficiency virus [HIV], men who have sex with men, people in a nonmonogamous relationship), travel (some international sites), occupation (e.g., health care personnel, public safety personnel, prison staff and inmates), and health conditions (e.g., chronic liver disease, renal disease, dialysis) increase their exposure to hepatitis B.
- *Hepatitis A:* Hepatitis A vaccine is indicated for adults with chronic liver disease, clotting factor disorders, IV drug users, men having sex with men, and people working in or traveling to certain foreign places, except Western Europe, Canada, New Zealand, Australia, and Japan.
- *Tetanus, diphtheria, pertussis:* The combined Td/Tdap vaccine protects against all three diseases and is indicated as a booster for adults younger than 65 years. All adults need tetanus and diphtheria boosters every 10 years throughout life, especially adults in contact with younger infants and health care personnel having direct patient contact.

Rationales

The CDC provides extensive information regarding the many adult vaccines available, for whom the vaccine is recommended, the schedule for the vaccine, and any contraindications and precautions. Health care providers and patients alike need to remain current. QSEN: Evidence-based practice.

■ = Independent   ▲ = Interprofessional Collaboration

Actions/Interventions

- *Varicella (chickenpox):* Varivax is indicated for adults not already immune to the chickenpox virus.
- *Meningitis:* Meningococcal vaccine is recommended for people at risk during an outbreak of the disease, students living in a college dormitory, people with spleen damage, or people traveling to countries in which meningitis is common (sub-Saharan Africa).
- *Measles, mumps, rubella:* Vaccine is recommended for adults born in 1957 or later if there is no evidence of immunity and for high-risk individuals (e.g., health care providers, college students, travelers, women of childbearing age).
- *Human papillomavirus (HPV):* HPV4 or HPV2 is recommended for women starting at age 11 or 12 years through age 26 years to prevent cervical cancer. HPV4 is recommended for men at age 11 or 12 years through age 21 to reduce risk of acquiring genital warts. It may be given to males aged 22 to 26, especially those who have sex with men.

■ Schedule immunizations at appropriate time intervals.

■ Educate the patient using vaccine information statements (VISs).

■ Assist the patient in locating potential sites for obtaining various immunizations.

■ Teach the patient about resources for paying for immunizations (e.g., public health department, insurance coverage).

■ Teach the patient about vaccinations appropriate for international travel to certain countries, referring the patient to a travel clinic, local health department, or the CDC website.

Rationales

Specific guidelines by the CDC are offered to ensure optimal protection, ranging from one-time-only immunizations to 5- to 10-year boosters, to annual flu shots.

The CDC provides VISs available online that explain both the benefits and risks of a vaccine. Federal law requires that a health care professional provide a VIS to a patient before each dose of a certain vaccine. QSEN: Safety.

Providing a listing of sources for vaccinations can facilitate compliance with recommendations. These sources can include family physicians, city or county health departments, local hospitals, pharmacies, or even clinics available in shopping malls, senior centers, and community centers. QSEN: Teamwork and collaboration.

Out-of-pocket expenses for immunizations vary depending on insurance coverage. Patients may need to check into their own health insurance coverage plans regarding their personal benefits. Medicare pays for one influenza immunization each year, one pneumococcal vaccination (along with booster vaccine after 5 years if needed), and hepatitis B vaccination for medium- or high-risk individuals. Medicare Part B will cover other immunizations ONLY if the patient has been exposed to a disease or condition.

Where one travels determines disease risk, though other factors such as age, medical status, length of time in the country, and type of travel (rural areas/backpacking) are also important factors. Exposure to serious disease such as malaria, yellow fever, and hepatitis is higher in developing countries with poor sanitation, such as most parts of Africa and Asia and some parts of South and Central America.

Actions/Interventions

■ Teach the patient about immunizations available for special incidences or outbreaks (e.g., cholera, tuberculosis).

■ Instruct the patient in tools for maintaining personal immunization records.

Rationales

The CDC provides extensive information regarding the many adult vaccines available, for whom the vaccine is recommended, the schedule for the vaccine, and any contraindications and precautions. Health care providers and patients alike need to remain current. QSEN: Evidence-based practice.

Accurate record-keeping helps to ensure that adults are fully protected from vaccine-preventable diseases. Such a mechanism will help prevent gaps in protection, especially when changing health care providers. It also prevents inappropriate revaccination that can occur during a health emergency.

Readiness for Enhanced Nutrition

Definition: A pattern of nutrient intake which can be strengthened

Though people are living longer, living healthy is the more important goal. Eating a nutritious diet is essential for maintaining health, reducing the epidemic of obesity, and reducing the risk of major diseases such as heart disease, diabetes, osteoporosis, and some cancers. However, people who want to adopt a healthy diet pattern find it challenging in today's fast-paced, fast-food, super-sized environment. Readiness to engage in a lifestyle of nutritious eating requires focused time, effort, and practice to learn how to make healthy food choices. National health guidelines such as *The 2015-2020 Dietary Guidelines for Americans* provide people with information about selecting healthy foods. These guidelines focus on the importance of healthy food choices along with physical activity behavior changes. The "healthy diet pattern" described in the guidelines is higher in fruits, vegetables, and whole grains; low-fat or nonfat dairy, seafood, legumes, and nuts; moderate in alcohol; lower in red or processed meat; and lower in sugar-sweetened foods, drinks, and refined grains. The USDA Food Patterns were recently updated to include three diet patterns that meet national recommendations. These patterns provide different approaches to consuming a healthy diet and include the Healthy US-Style Patterns, Healthy Vegetarian Patterns, and the Healthy Mediterranean Patterns. The patterns incorporate variations in calorie levels depending on age, physical activity, and need. Successful nutrition education programs also include information about identifying healthy packaged food products, reading food labels, and selecting healthy foods when eating in restaurants. The guidelines highlight the need to establish a "culture of health" in which healthy lifestyle choices become easy to follow, accessible, affordable, and normative. Ensuring food safety is an additional principle for building healthy eating patterns and includes attention to food preparation, cooking, and storage.

Defining Characteristics

Expresses willingness to enhance nutrition
Attitude toward eating is congruent with health goals
Attitude toward drinking is congruent with health goals
Expresses knowledge of healthy food choices
Expresses knowledge of healthy fluid choices
Consumes adequate food
Consumes adequate fluid
Follows an appropriate standard for intake (*2015-2020 Dietary Guidelines for Americans,* or American Diabetic Association guidelines)
Eats regularly
Safe preparation for foods and fluids
Safe storage for foods and fluids

■ = Independent   ▲ = Interprofessional Collaboration

Health Promotion and Risk Factor Management Care Plans

Common Expected Outcomes

Patient verbalizes the benefits of adopting a healthier eating pattern.

Patient demonstrates appropriate selection of meals or menu planning that incorporates healthy eating recommendations.

Patient engages in desired behaviors to promote healthier nutritional status.

NOC Outcomes

Knowledge: Healthy Diet; Nutritional Status: Food and Fluid Intake; Nutritional Status: Nutrient Intake; Health Seeking Behavior; Adherence Behavior: Healthy Diet

NIC Interventions

Nutrition Management; Nutritional Counseling; Total Parenteral Nutrition (TPN) Administration

Ongoing Assessment

Actions/Interventions

- Assess the patient's motivations for wanting to improve his or her nutritional level.

- Assess the patient's baseline knowledge about healthy food choices.

- Assess the patient's confidence in adopting a healthier eating plan. Suggest patients follow the 80/20 rule.

- Assess the potential barriers for enhancing the patient's nutrition.

Rationales

Individuals may present with a variety of reasons for improving their nutrient health, such as having experienced a negative health event, family illness, or abnormal laboratory values. Understanding motivation helps in designing an individualized plan. QSEN: Patient-centered care.

This information provides the starting point for the educational session. Teaching content the patient already knows wastes valuable time and hinders critical learning.

Research supports the important role that self-efficacy has in promoting successful behavior change. Strategies to enhance self-efficacy need to be part of the plan of care. Motivational interviewing techniques have been successful in enhancing the positive approach to behavior change. The 80/20 rule allows the patient to make healthy choices 80% of the time, which can increase adherence. QSEN: Evidence-based practice.

Knowledge alone does not result in behavior change. Patients need help in reducing potential barriers to success, such as chaotic work or travel schedules, frequently eating out, limited skills in food preparation, access, cost of healthy foods, lack of time for appropriate food preparation, dependence on "comfort" foods, or cultural aspects that affect eating patterns and habits. QSEN: Patient-centered care.

Therapeutic Interventions

Actions/Interventions

- Instruct the patient about the appropriate number of calories that should be consumed daily.

Rationales

Eating the right number of calories to balance one's level of activity is key to maintaining a healthy weight. To curb the obesity epidemic and improve their health, many patients must reduce the number of calories consumed and increase the calories expended through physical activity. The three recommended healthy eating patterns (the Healthy US-Style Patterns, Healthy Vegetarian Patterns, and Healthy Mediterranean Patterns) each incorporate variations in calorie levels depending on age, physical activity, and need.

Actions/Interventions

■ Instruct the patient to eat a variety of nutritious foods from all the food groups. Refer to the National Guidelines for recommended amounts, depending on the specific diet pattern.

• Vegetables and fruits

• Whole-grain foods

• Low-fat milk products

• Seafood

• Lean meats and poultry

■ Instruct the patient to eat fewer foods high in saturated and trans-fats, and to choose mono- and polyunsaturated fats.

Rationales

The 2015-2020 Dietary Guidelines for Americans describes a healthy diet pattern as one that emphasizes nutrient-dense foods and beverages (e.g., vegetables, fruits, whole grains, fat-free or low-fat dairy products, seafood, lean meats and poultry, eggs, beans and peas, nuts and seeds). At all calorie levels, the Healthy Vegetarian Patterns include more legumes, processed soy products, nuts and seeds, and whole grains than the Healthy US-Style Patterns, and contain no meat, poultry, or seafood. The amounts of all other food groups are similar. The Healthy Mediterranean Patterns contain more fruit and seafood selections and fewer dairy items than the Healthy US-Style Patterns. QSEN: Evidence-based practice.

Dietary Guidelines emphasize eating more foods from plants. Vegetables and fruits have high amounts of vitamins, minerals, phytonutrients, antioxidants, and fiber, besides being low in calories and a natural source of energy. These "super foods" are easy to spot because they are very colorful. A rainbow of colors should be part of a healthy diet plan: red tomatoes, orange/yellow squash, and carrots; deep green vegetables such as broccoli and spinach; deep purple/blue eggplant, berries, and plums; and black beans are some examples. People who eat generous amounts of fruits and vegetables are more likely to have reduced risk of chronic diseases. Fruits and vegetables are high in fiber, low in calories, and can fill one up, so they are a great food for both meals and snacks.

Unrefined whole-grain foods contain fiber that helps in managing weight and lowering cholesterol levels. Refined grains such as those found in white bread, white rice, and white pasta should be eaten more sparingly.

Guidelines recommend increasing the intake of fat-free, 1% fat, and low-fat milk products, including yogurt and cheese, or fortified soy beverages.

Fish is a good source of protein and contains many vitamins and minerals. Oily fish provide omega-3 fats, which are known to reduce health risks.

Health guidelines recommend lowering the amounts of red meat consumed, because of its higher levels of saturated fat, and replacing this protein source with poultry, beans, seeds, nuts, and eggs.

Fat is an important component of a balanced diet, but the type of fat eaten is key. Guidelines recommend reducing saturated fat intake to less than 10% of calories per day. Focus is on replacing saturated and trans-fats with healthful monounsaturated and polyunsaturated fats from plant sources and fish. Avocado, seeds, and nuts are great choices for reducing hunger. Mandatory food labeling identifies foods high in trans-fats.

Health Promotion and Risk Factor Management Care Plans

■ = Independent   ▲ = Interprofessional Collaboration

Actions/Interventions

- Instruct the patient to increase the amount of foods with dietary fiber.

- Instruct the patient to limit the intake of added sugar, including sugary drinks, to less than 10% of calories per day.

- Instruct the patient to choose foods that provide more potassium, dietary fiber, calcium, vitamin B$_{12}$, and vitamin D.

- Instruct the patient about how to identify healthy packaged food products.
  - Food industry stamps identify specific high-nutrient foods (e.g., whole grains, high fiber).
  - Reading a food label is informative (e.g., serving size, calories and calories from fat, the nutrients, percent daily value). Consider using an app for a smart phone to be aware of and track what one is eating.

- Instruct the patient about the benefits of drinking water, with caution regarding enhanced water products.

- Instruct the patient about recommended salt intake.

- Instruct the patient about recommended alcohol levels.

- Instruct the patient about portion size.

Rationales

Dietary fiber naturally occurs in plants, helps provide a feeling of fullness, and is important in promoting healthy bowel function. Some of the best sources of dietary fiber are beans and peas, such as navy beans, split peas, lentils, pinto beans, and black beans. Additional sources of dietary fiber include other vegetables, fruits, whole grains, and nuts.

Sugars found naturally in foods are part of the food's total package of nutrients and other healthful components. Foods that contain added sugars often supply calories, but few or no essential nutrients and no dietary fiber. Many desserts are high in calories and low in nutrition.

These nutrients are of concern in American diets. These foods include vegetables, fruits, whole grains, fortified cereals, and milk and milk products.

The food industry has developed stamps to identify nutrient rich foods.

The U.S. Food and Drug Administration (FDA) requires The Nutrition Facts label to provide information on the amount of calories per serving size; beneficial nutrients such as dietary fiber and calcium; and the amount of certain food components that should be limited in the diet, including saturated fat, trans-fat, cholesterol, and sodium. The ingredients list can be used to find out whether a food or beverage contains solid fats, added sugars, whole grains, and refined grains. Restaurant chains now include calorie content of foods on menu boards to assist consumers in making healthy choices.

Water makes up two thirds of the weight of the body and is required for chemical reactions and delivery of nutrients throughout the body. Water is considered the beverage of choice, and recommendations include six to eight glasses a day. However, some energy drinks are high in both sugar and caffeine without any nutritional benefit.

The U.S. Department of Agriculture (USDA) guidelines recommend eating less than 2300 mg of sodium per day Because sodium is found in so many foods, careful choices are needed in all food groups to reduce intake. Strategies to lower intake include using the Nutrition Facts label to compare sodium content of foods and choosing the product with less sodium. The patient needs to be aware that most salt already comes in the food we eat, not from the salt shaker. QSEN: Evidence-based practice.

If someone drinks alcohol, it should be in moderation. Alcohol is also high in calories. Recommendations state one drink per day for women and two drinks per day for men.

There is much "portion distortion" right now, especially with all the super-size choices available. Even eating the right foods in too large an amount can add up in unneeded calories and obesity. Using a smaller plate and starting with smaller portions may be effective. Suggest cutting restaurant portions in half and sharing or bringing home the other half for another meal.

Actions/Interventions

- Instruct the patient about the importance of eating breakfast.

- Assist the patient in selecting healthy foods when eating out in restaurants.

- Assist the patient in making healthier food choices when eating fast food.

- Instruct the patient regarding avoiding raw and undercooked animal food products.

- Instruct the patient about healthy tips for preparing foods.

- Instruct the patient regarding safe food preparation and storage practices, and the need to check expiration dates.

- Assist the patient in enhancing his or her self-efficacy skills toward healthy eating.

Rationales

A healthy breakfast is an important part of a balanced diet and provides some of the vitamins and minerals needed for good health, and a healthy breakfast helps people control their weight. Whole-grain cereal with fruit is an excellent choice.

Foods served fried, crispy, scalloped, pan-fried, sautéed, or stuffed are higher in fat and calories. Better food choices include steamed, broiled, baked, roasted, or grilled entrees, and ones that feature seafood, chicken, and lean meat. The patient needs to recognize that restaurants that offer "all you can eat" choices may be economical but contribute to overeating and weight gain.

Fast food is cheap, convenient, and filling, and often an unhealthy choice. One fast-food meal can include enough calories, salt, and fat for an entire day. Healthy food choices are possible in these settings. Moderation is key. Consider selections such as grilled chicken; veggie burgers; single-patty burgers without cheese, mayonnaise, or special sauces; garden salads with low-fat dressing; yogurt parfaits. Restaurant chains now include calorie content of foods on menu boards to assist consumers in making healthy choices.

Consumption of raw or undercooked animal food products increases the risk for contracting a foodborne illness. Raw or undercooked foods commonly eaten in the United States include eggs (e.g., eggs with runny yolks), ground beef (e.g., undercooked hamburger), milk and milk products (e.g., cheese made from unpasteurized milk), and seafood (e.g., raw oysters). Cooking foods to recommended safe minimum internal temperatures and consuming only pasteurized milk and milk products are the best ways to reduce the risk for foodborne illness from animal products. QSEN: Safety.

Preparing and cooking foods at home provides more control over the nutritional content and overall healthfulness of the foods eaten. Some suggestions include removing the skin from poultry, using egg whites instead of yolks, using low-fat milk or yogurt, using liquid vegetable oil or nonfat cooking sprays, and using little or no salt.

Ensuring food safety is an important principle for building healthy eating patterns. The proportion of foodborne illness outbreaks that can be attributed to unsafe food safety practices in the home is unknown, but is assumed to be substantial. Washing hands, rinsing vegetables and fruits, preventing cross-contamination, cooking foods to safe internal temperatures, and storing foods safely in the home kitchen are the behaviors most likely to prevent food safety problems. The temperature range in which foodborne bacteria can grow is 40°F to 140°F. Foods that remain in this range for more than 2 hours should be discarded. QSEN: Safety.

Employ strategies such as reviewing published guides for tips on eating out, practicing selecting foods off menus from favorite restaurants, suggesting tours at grocery stores to assist in food selection, and personalizing food choices.

Health Promotion and Risk Factor Management Care Plans

■ = Independent   ▲ = Interprofessional Collaboration

Actions/Interventions

■ Encourage the patient to be realistic about his or her approach to healthy eating.

Rationales

Dietitians focus on viewing healthy eating as a lifestyle, not as a diet that one starts and ends. Therefore it is important that some flexibility is provided. One example is the 90-10 rule that states that it is what you eat 90% of the time that matters most, not the 10% of the time. The rule makes lifestyle changes more plausible. An example would be allowing one meal per week that included more restricted foods.

NANDA-I
NDx **Readiness for Enhanced Sleep**

Definition: A pattern of natural, periodic suspension of relative consciousness to provide rest and sustain a desired lifestyle, which can be strengthened

Healthy sleep patterns can be vital to our quality of life. Sleep health is becoming a new field of research, exploring how we sleep and the factors that impact it. The sleep-wake cycle is a dynamic process regulated by complex interactions among neurotransmitters and hormones in the central nervous system. This cycle consists of normal changes in a person's level of consciousness that include rapid eye movement (REM) sleep, non-REM (NREM) sleep, and wakefulness. NREM sleep consists of four stages and accounts for as much as 80% of total sleep time. Body processes decrease during NREM sleep, especially in stages 3 and 4. These changes in body function are related to sleep's function in restoring energy, repairing tissues, and regulating hormone secretion. REM sleep occurs at 90-minute intervals. The length of each REM cycle increases during the night. During REM sleep, brain activity increases to that seen during wakefulness, yet the person is difficult to arouse. Dreams are associated with REM sleep. Research indicates that REM sleep is necessary for learning and memory formation in the brain.

Normal sleep patterns vary based on the person's age. These variations include the total hours of sleep time, the length of each sleep cycle, and the time spent in each stage of the sleep cycle. The majority of healthy adults require 7 to 9 hours of sleep per day. Approximately 20% of sleep time is spent in REM sleep. As the adult ages, the amount of time spent in stage 4 NREM or deep sleep begins to decline. The older adult may have a decline in stage 3 NREM sleep and no stage 4 NREM sleep. As a result of spending more time in the lighter stages of NREM, the older adult may report more frequent night time awakenings. The length of each REM cycle becomes shorter with aging. Older adults sleep less during the night but may take more naps during the day to meet total sleep hour requirements. The quality of sleep for the older adult is affected by the presence of chronic health problems and the use of medications.

Defining Characteristics

Sleep amount is congruent with developmental needs
Expresses a feeling of being rested after sleep
Follows sleep routines that promote sleep habits
Expresses willingness to enhance sleep

Common Expected Outcomes

Patient verbalizes knowledge of a variety of techniques for sleep enhancement.
Patient engages in effective strategies to improve quality of sleep.
Patient achieves age-appropriate total sleep hours.
Patient expresses feeling rested after sleep.

NOC Outcomes
Motivation; Rest; Sleep
NIC Intervention
Sleep Enhancement

Ongoing Assessment

Actions/Interventions	Rationales
■ Determine the patient's usual sleep pattern.	Information about the patient's usual sleep pattern provides a baseline for evaluating measures to improve the patient's sleep quantity and quality. The National Sleep Foundation provides a free Sleep Diary that allows one to track sleep habits and trends. Small portable sleep trackers such as Fitbit wristwatches and sleep-related apps are available for recording hours and patterns of sleep. QSEN: Patient-centered care.
■ Assess the patient's knowledge of age-appropriate recommendations for total sleep time.	This information provides insight into misunderstandings and misconceptions the patient may have about normal sleep patterns. The newest recommendations from the National Sleep Foundation recommend 7 to 9 hours for adults 26 to 64 years of age, and 7 to 8 hours for older adults (65+). Patients can also assess their individual sleep needs by determining if they feel productive and happy on their current hours of sleep, if they feel sleepy while driving, or if they need caffeine products to get through the day.
■ Assess the patient's usual bedtime routines and sleep environment.	Information about the patient's usual sleep habits provides a baseline for identifying measures to promote the quality and quantity of sleep.
■ Determine the patient's motivation for enhancing sleep patterns.	This information provides insight into the patient's expectations for improving sleep. Unrealistic expectations can be addressed as part of patient teaching interventions. The plan of care is based on the patient's willingness to change behavior to achieve goals. QSEN: Patient-centered care.
■ Review medications regularly used by the patient.	Many prescription and over-the-counter medications may interfere with the patient's normal sleep–wake cycle.

Therapeutic Interventions

Actions/Interventions	Rationales
■ Teach the patient about recommended age-appropriate sleep patterns.	Knowledge of the usual sleep pattern for his or her age may help the patient develop realistic expectations about the total number of sleep hours needed for health.
■ Encourage the patient to maintain a consistent time for going to bed and waking up.	A consistent schedule for bedtime and awakening will help the sleep cycle synchronize with the patient's circadian rhythms.
■ Assist the patient in identifying ways to modify the sleep environment:	Creating a more relaxing environment may enhance the patient's sleep pattern.
• Adjust room temperature and ventilation	A room that is too warm or too cold will hinder sleep. Measures to promote air ventilation may include open windows or electric fans.
• Darken room light; consider use of new sleep-enhancing light bulbs	Some patients benefit from using window shades that darken the room from outside light or wearing eye masks for sleep. A darkened room for sleeping is associated with increased production of melatonin. This neurotransmitter facilitates sleep onset. New light bulbs with built-in processors (e.g., Drift Light) can be programmed to gradually fade to dark over a set time (e.g., 30 minutes).

■ = Independent   ▲ = Interprofessional Collaboration

Actions/Interventions	Rationales
• Use low-level background noise or earplugs	The use of low-level noise may promote relaxation and help the patient stay asleep. Machines that generate so-called "white noise" may block the patient's perception of distracting noises. Comfortable earplugs or noise-canceling headphones may facilitate the onset of sleep.
• Change the mattress, pillows, or bed linens or covers	The patient should have a bed with a firmness level that promotes comfort. The patient may try using different pillows and bed covers to find those that promote comfort with sleep.
■ Assist the patient in modifying bedtime habits to promote relaxation and the onset of sleep:	Bedtime activities should promote physical and mental relaxation to facilitate the onset of sleep.
• Light snack high in tryptophan	Tryptophan is an essential amino acid that is part of the chemical structure of serotonin and melatonin. These neurotransmitters play an important role in sleep onset. Proteins from food we eat are the building blocks of tryptophan. A great bedtime snack is one that contains both a carbohydrate and a protein, such as cereal with milk.
• Meditation or prayer	These activities quiet the mind and facilitate relaxation.
• Turning off electronic devices, especially when in bed.	Our bodies need time to shift into a sleep mode, so avoiding stimulating games or work-related activities can facilitate the wind down. For many, the light emanating from the screens of tablets or smart phones can activate the brain. Thus it is important to power-down devices at least 30 minutes before bedtime.
• Enjoyable reading or listening to calming music	These activities may promote physical and mental relaxation. Reading material or music that is stimulating may hinder sleep onset.
• Warm bath	This activity promotes physical relaxation.
• Sexual activity	According to the National Sleep Foundation, sexual activities can reduce cortisol levels, with orgasms releasing prolactin, which helps the body feel relaxed and sleepy.
• Journaling or writing "to-do" lists for the next day	These activities may help the patient put aside worries about the next day and provide an outlet for concerns that interfere with mental relaxation and sleep onset.
• Exercises such as deep breathing and progressive muscle relaxation	Slow, deep breathing for a short period combined with progressive muscle relaxation can enhance the onset of sleep.
■ Teach the patient to limit fluid intake before bedtime.	Reduced fluid intake in the evening will limit awakening during the night to go to the bathroom.
■ Teach the patient to avoid heavy meals close to bedtime.	Full meals close to bedtime may produce gastrointestinal upsets and hinder sleep onset.
■ Teach the patient to limit the intake of caffeine before sleep and to avoid nicotine.	Caffeine, found in food and fluids (coffee, tea, colas, and chocolate), and nicotine stimulate the central nervous system. This stimulation may interfere with the patient's ability to relax and fall asleep.
■ Teach the patient to limit alcohol intake before sleep.	Alcohol produces drowsiness and may facilitate the onset of sleep, but interferes with REM sleep.
■ Assist the patient in modifying medication administration times to minimize the effect on sleep.	Changing the time of day some medications are taken can limit their effect on the patient's sleep. For example, diuretics and corticosteroids taken earlier in the day are less likely to disrupt sleep. The patient can select nondrowsy formulations of over-the-counter medications for cold and allergy symptoms. These medications are less likely to interfere with the patient's normal sleep–wake cycle.

Actions/Interventions

■ Teach the patient to plan strenuous exercise activities no later than 3 hours before bedtime.

■ For the patient who works night shifts, discuss measures to promote relaxation and sleep.
■ For the patient who works variable shifts, discuss the effect that changing work schedules have on sleep.

■ Discuss the use of over-the-counter, herbal, and prescription sleep aids:

• Melatonin

• Valerian, chamomile, lavender, kava

• Antihistamines

• Prescription sedative-hypnotics, antianxiety drugs

▲ Refer to sleep specialist as needed.

Rationales

The onset of sleep is associated with lower body temperature. During exercise, body temperature increases and may take as long as 6 hours to return to preexercise levels. Exercising within 3 hours of bedtime may delay sleep onset and hinder the effectiveness of sleep.

People who are night-active may have more difficulty with effective sleep patterns than day-active people. The patient may benefit from environmental controls that minimize the amount of light and noise. The patient needs to allow time for sufficient relaxation between finishing a work shift and attempting to fall asleep. Those who work variable shifts may have less effective sleep because of disruption of their circadian rhythms. Some research indicates that it may take up to 3 weeks for the body's circadian rhythm to adjust to a change from day-active to night-active sleep–wake cycles.

Short-term use of pharmacological sleep aids may be beneficial when the patient experiences temporary sleep disturbances.

This nutritional supplement acts as a neurotransmitter to promote sleep onset. Older adults seem to tolerate melatonin with minimal side effects.

These herbal preparations are known to have mild sedating effects that promote sleep onset. The patient needs to be careful in selecting herbal products from reputable sources because they are not regulated by the FDA. Some herbal products used for sedation may have significant interactions with other medications taken by the patient.

Many over-the-counter sleep aids contain antihistamines as the active ingredient that promotes sedation. These drugs produce anticholinergic side effects that may be especially troublesome for the older adult. These side effects include dry mouth, constipation, blurred vision, and urinary retention.

These drugs are associated with physical tolerance and dependence with long-term use. Many drugs in this class act through general central nervous system depression and disrupt the normal stages of NREM and REM sleep. With long-term use, side effects include daytime drowsiness, rebound insomnia, and increased dreaming when discontinued.

Not all sleep problems may be easily treated through good sleep hygiene and could signify the presence of a sleep disorder such as sleep apnea, restless leg syndrome, or narcolepsy. QSEN: Teamwork and collaboration.

■ = Independent ▲ = Interprofessional Collaboration

NDx **Readiness for Managing Stress**

Stress is a state of physical and mental readiness. It is not an "event," but rather an approach to an event. Stress is an inevitable part of life and something that cannot be completely eliminated; it should not be, because stress is a natural and important physiological and psychological response to a challenge about which a person is not sure. Living in today's fast-paced, multitasking world, most people accept stress as normal and inevitable. Although stress itself is not harmful, one's response to it can be overwhelming, and even harmful to the body. Prolonged physiological responses to stressors increase stimulation of the sympathetic nervous system and increase the release of cortisol from the adrenal cortex. These neuroendocrine changes may impair cardiovascular and immune function and contribute to the development of chronic disease. The challenge for the individual person is to be able to reduce stress to a manageable and healthy level. Therefore successful stress reduction should be approached as a permanent lifestyle change, not simply a temporary response to a specific life event. Managing stress is about taking charge and not allowing it to control one's life and behavior.

Readiness to engage in a stress management program is a key to success, as it takes focused time, effort, and practice to learn the many stress-reducing techniques. Mastering stress requires establishing a new mindset and habits that become a part of one's everyday life. Different people may benefit from different approaches to stress management, but all successful programs contain the same core components: education, participating in ongoing self-monitoring, cognitive (behavioral) restructuring, incorporating relaxation training into one's daily life, using support people or groups, and paying attention to maintaining lifestyle modifications.

Defining Characteristics

Expresses willingness to enhance ability to manage stress
Demonstrates attitude toward stress management congruent with health goals
Expresses knowledge of stress management techniques
Engages in effective stress management techniques

Common Expected Outcomes

Patient verbalizes the benefits of managing stress in his or her life.
Patient demonstrates knowledge of a variety of techniques available for reducing stress.
Patient engages in effective techniques for managing personal stress.

NOC Outcomes
Knowledge: Stress Management; Stress Level;
  Health Seeking Behavior
NIC Intervention
Relaxation Therapy

Ongoing Assessment

Actions/Interventions

■ Determine the patient's level of motivation for engaging in a stress management program.

Rationales

The assessment of motivation and readiness to start a stress managing program is critical. Stress reduction takes practice and work. Many patients have tried a stress management program many times in the past. Therefore it is important that patients have the motivation and commitment not only to begin a program but to stay with it for the upcoming weeks and months until new lifestyle behaviors are learned. QSEN: Patient-centered care.

Actions/Interventions

- Assess specific stressors.

- Determine how the patient reacts when under stress.

- Assess the patient's baseline knowledge about stress reduction techniques.

- Determine whether any relaxation interventions have been used in the past.

- Assess the patient's confidence in engaging in a stress management program.

Rationales

What is stressful to one person may be viewed as a challenge to another. Thus an accurate appraisal of personal stressors can facilitate development of appropriate coping strategies. QSEN: Patient-centered care.

Individuals have their own pattern for response to stress, especially when experiencing stress for a prolonged period. Responses may include overeating or undereating, overworking, engaging in risky behaviors (e.g., smoking, alcohol), sleeping too much or too little, withdrawing from friends, using drugs to relax, procrastinating, even taking out one's stress on others (angry outbursts). This information provides a basis for future lifestyle changes. QSEN: Patient-centered care.

This information provides the starting point for the educational session. Learning healthier ways to deal with stress is based on two approaches: changing the situation by avoiding or altering the stressor or by changing one's reaction by adapting to or accepting the stressor.

Adults bring many life experiences to learning sessions. Often patients have previously tried a relaxation technique that may have been successful and can be built upon. Any unsuccessful efforts and reasons for difficulties need to be explored.

Research supports the important role that self-efficacy has in promoting successful behavior change. Asking patients to rate their confidence (on a scale of 1 to 10) that they can stick with the program provides important information. Strategies to enhance self-efficacy should be part of the plan of care.

Therapeutic Interventions

Actions/Interventions

- Teach the patient about the body's common responses to stress: physical, mental, emotional, and behavioral symptoms.
- Discuss common sources of stress, focusing on both internal and external sources.

- Assist the patient in setting realistic goals for the stress management program.

Rationales

The patient needs to understand the consequences of maintaining a stressful lifestyle and how it can compromise physical and emotional well-being.

Research has shown that people view events differently. Thus individual differences in perception influence whether one views an event as stressful. Common external sources of stress include commuting in traffic, injury, snowstorms, noise, and the like. Common internal sources of stress relate to one's thoughts and attitudes about a threat or event that contribute to the stress level. Examples include worry, procrastination, taking on too much, catastrophizing, and perfectionism. Physiological sources of stress, such as illness, trauma, or surgery, especially when prolonged or undermanaged, can be detrimental to the patient.

It is important for the patient to realize that life will always have negative events (e.g., death, financial concerns, illness, divorce). A realistic goal is to develop the skills to deal with one's reactions to these events, to master the stress, and not to let it control one's life and behaviors. QSEN: Patient-centered care.

■ = Independent   ▲ = Interprofessional Collaboration

Actions/Interventions

■ Instruct the patient in the importance of keeping a journal or log of stress events and reactions.

■ Provide detailed instruction on the many strategies and techniques available for managing stress:

• Avoid unnecessary stressors

• Challenge stress-producing thoughts

• Use positive self-talk

• Use realistic thinking

Rationales

Self-management is a key component of a successful change in behavior. Self-monitoring by record-keeping has been shown to be one of the most critical parts of lifestyle changes. Self-monitoring of stress might include the date and a record of the average level of stress during the day, then a record of the highest level of stress experienced that day and the place/time/events associated with it. As the patient gains more experience with stress reduction, he or she can add information on thoughts, emotions, and behaviors during the stressful event. This information provides awareness of the triggers associated with higher levels of stress and the patterns for reacting to these events and, over time, provides feedback on progress in controlling one's emotions in similar situations. Record-keeping places the responsibility for change with the patient. QSEN: Evidence-based practice.

A variety of brief interventions can be used toward assisting patients with reducing their levels of stress. Each of them requires practice. Managing stress is about taking charge. The more patients use these stress-management techniques, the better able they will be to master their stress.

A basic approach to stress reduction is to avoid those situations known to cause a stress reaction. This may include avoiding people and relationships that cause stress, avoiding topics that easily escalate into heated discussions (e.g., religion, politics), knowing one's limits and saying no to more than one can handle, taking control of one's environment (e.g., using public transportation to avoid lengthy driving commutes, shopping online to avoid congested stores).

Often patients tend to view a situation or challenge as negative, and these automatic thoughts (not the event itself) produce their stress experience. For example, they always think the worst about something (catastrophize) or they overgeneralize (e.g., "I never do anything right"). By teaching patients to change this thinking pattern, this cycle can be broken.

Negative self-talk with statements (e.g., "I can't do this") increases stress, while positive self-talk (e.g., "I can handle things if I do them one step at a time" or "We all make mistakes") helps to reduce one's stress level.

Realistic thinking works by changing how one interprets potentially stressful situations. It includes examining the evidence for the problem, considering how likely it is to happen, and considering alternative explanations or outcomes, along with an honest appraisal of how bad the consequences would be. Finally, it includes prediction testing to demonstrate how unlikely most feared outcomes really are. A realistic appraisal of "what would really happen if …" can help put life into a more accurate perspective.

Actions/Interventions	Rationales
• Accept things that cannot be changed	Some sources of stress are unavoidable, such as a serious illness. In these situations, practicing acceptance is an important technique. Rather than stressing over what cannot be controlled, acceptance may be easier. Another approach is to look for the upside of a major challenge and view it as an opportunity for personal growth.
• Engage in physical activity	Exercise can improve the body's response to stress by increasing energy levels that make it easier to cope with stressful events, relieving tension and reducing anxiety and depression, and is a good outlet for anger and frustration related to stress.
• Develop some emergency stress stoppers	Being prepared is a great way to handle stressful thoughts. Some stress-relievers can include standing up and stretching, counting to 10 before speaking, going for a walk, laughing, walking away from a stressful situation and planning to handle it later, singing a song, and changing a coffee break to an exercise break.
• Find pleasurable activities	Doing things one enjoys is a great stress reducer. This can be as simple as taking a bubble bath, going for a walk, playing with a pet, watching a favorite movie, or chatting with an old friend.
• Employ better time management	Time pressures are often a big source of personal stress and may be related to taking on too much, not working efficiently, or simply worrying about the level of work rather than completing the task. Several strategies to improve time management include delegating some of the work to others, breaking down big tasks into smaller parts that can be completed, assessing realistic priorities as to what needs to be done today versus this week, sticking to agendas, and learning to say no.
• Get organized	Using tools such as "to do" lists can be a good way to refocus one's efforts and reduce the stress from feeling that too much needs to be done.
• Find opportunities to laugh	Research supports the benefits of laughter in reducing stress and the physiological responses to it. The act of laughing helps the body fight stress in many ways. It can also improve one's perspective on a situation, which can reduce stress.
• Get enough sleep	Attaining quality sleep is important for one's physical and emotional health. Sleep helps the body recover from the day's stressors, and prepares it for the next day. Often people under a lot of stress have difficulty sleeping. Stress management practices can often help one attain better sleep, either by helping to quiet the mind (and putting aside one's worries for the night), or by relaxing the body and encouraging quality sleep.
• Eat a healthy diet	As people get stressed they tend to make poor nutritional choices that can cause increased stress levels and other problems. Eating is often used as a source of comfort for dealing with stress, resulting in weight gain and poor health habits. For others, stress may cause them to not eat, also compromising their nutritional level. Too much stress and a poor diet can sap the body of needed energy. Thus healthy eating is a key component of overall good health. Good health is critical in helping the body manage stress.

Health Promotion and Risk Factor Management Care Plans

■ = Independent   ▲ = Interprofessional Collaboration

Actions/Interventions

- Be spiritual

- Instruct in the variety of methods for muscle relaxation.

- Demonstrate and practice passive relaxation techniques with the patient. Encourage return demonstration.

- Assist in the development of an alternative support system. Encourage participation in self-help groups, if available.

- Provide positive reinforcement as indicated. Encourage the patient to plan rewards at appropriate intervals to celebrate successes.

- Assist the patient in preparing for possible lapses and relapses.

Rationales

Those who are more spiritual tend to view stressful situations as valuable lessons from God. Viewing the situation as a challenge can make the event itself feel less threatening. This can reduce the physical reactions to stress and allow the patient to explore more effective ways to cope, turning a difficult situation into a path to a better life or greater personal growth. Prayer can help people feel more connected with God, leaving them in a calmer state that can act as a buffer against stress. Prayer has been shown to bring benefits similar to the benefits of meditation.

Muscle tension is a consequence of being highly stressed. Managing stress requires breaking the cycle of muscle tension through relaxation efforts. Relaxation can be considered in two forms: active methods (e.g., physical activities, engaging in hobbies) and passive forms (e.g., stretching, deep breathing, imagery, progressive muscle relaxation, yoga, tai chi, meditation).

Correct information for performing each technique is critical for optimal outcomes. Learning is enhanced with repetition from return demonstrations.

When under stress, it is natural to withdraw from the world and focus only on the problem at hand. Although this may be useful, it often is not. Most people have networks of people, either socially or professionally, who can help with problem-solving. These people can provide support and help in a variety of ways: providing resources and information, assisting with problem-solving, or providing needed reassurance. Expressing to someone what one is going through can be very cathartic, even if it doesn't change the situation.

Appropriately timed feedback is critical to successful behavior change. Positive reinforcement encourages a desired behavior. Rewards, both intrinsic and extrinsic, are motivational and can give a sense of satisfaction for a job well done.

Relapse prevention needs to be addressed early in the treatment plan. Identifying high-risk situations likely to cause relapses aids in problem-solving. Any setbacks should be reframed as learning opportunities and as a normal step in making lifestyle changes.

NDx Readiness for Smoking Cessation

Approximately 18% of adults in America are currently smokers. Tobacco use is the leading preventable cause of disease, disability and death in the United States, accounting for approximately 1 in every 5 deaths. The decision to quit smoking is one of the best things people can do to improve their health and add years to their life. Overall, about 70% of smokers say they are "interested" in quitting, but only 10% to 20% plan to quit in the next month. Most smokers try to quit on their own, with a success rate of 2% to 3%. Eventually, half of all smokers are able to quit.

Nicotine is one of the most powerful of all addictions to overcome. Nicotine causes changes in the brain that makes smokers want to use it more. As a result, it is very difficult for the person to stop the smoking habit. Besides the pleasant feeling of smoking, these individuals experience both physiological and psychological withdrawal from nicotine.

Fortunately, there is much evidence available on how to guide smokers in the cessation process. Since 1996 the U.S. Department of Health and Human Services has published clinical practice guidelines for tobacco cessation developed by the Treating Tobacco Use and Dependence Guideline Panel. These guidelines describe five key steps (the 5 A's) to use for patients willing to make a quit attempt. The 5 A's include: (1) Ask—identify if individual uses tobacco; (2) Advise—deliver clear, strong, personal advice about the importance of quitting; (3) Assess—willingness to make a quit attempt; (4) Assist—aid the patient in quitting by setting a quit date and offering pharmacological and behavioral support; and (5) Arrange—for follow-up to prevent relapse.

A wide variety of programs and tools are available to assist the smoker through each stage of the quitting process. Many of these smoking cessation services are available online or through telephone quit lines. Evidence-based studies support that there is a strong dose-response relationship between the intensity of tobacco dependence counseling and its effectiveness. Numerous effective pharmacotherapies are now available. Recent guidelines recommend that all patients expressing an interest in quitting smoking should receive both counseling and pharmacotherapy as appropriate. This care plan is focused on the patient who is motivated to quit smoking.

Defining Characteristics

Expresses willingness to initiate a smoking cessation program
Expresses knowledge of benefits of smoke-free living
Expresses knowledge of components of successful smoking cessation programs
Expresses willingness to set a quit date and sign a no-smoking contract
Engages in a self-monitoring program
Identifies strategies for dealing with personal urges to smoke
Expresses willingness to use a support group as appropriate

Common Expected Outcomes

Patient verbalizes accurate information regarding components of a smoking cessation program.
Patient verbalizes measures necessary to achieve smoking cessation goals.
Patient engages in desired behaviors to quit smoking.

NOC Outcomes
Smoking Cessation Behavior; Health Seeking Behavior
NIC Interventions
Smoking Cessation Assistance; Support System Enhancement

Ongoing Assessment

Actions/Interventions	Rationales
■ Determine the patient's prior history of tobacco use and any previous attempts to quit.	Smoking is considered a chronic disease. Smoking cessation has a high rate of relapse. Reasons for difficulties need to be explored. However, smokers do learn valuable information during each quit attempt.
■ Determine the patient's level of motivation and confidence for beginning a smoking cessation program.	Assessment of the motivation and readiness to quit smoking is critical. Quitting smoking takes work. Most patients have tried many times in the past. Therefore it is important that patients have the motivation and commitment to not only begin a program but also to stay with it for the upcoming weeks and months until new lifestyle behaviors are learned. Asking patients to rate their confidence (on a scale of 1 to 10) that they can stick with the program provides important information. QSEN: Patient-centered care.

■ = Independent ▲ = Interprofessional Collaboration

Actions/Interventions

- Assess the importance and meaning of smoking with the patient.

- Assess for depression.

- Assess the current pattern of smoking by instructing the patient in keeping a diary or log of what, where, when, and why he or she smokes.

- Assess triggers and challenges to be expected in the upcoming quit attempt.

- Determine the degree of addiction to smoking by asking:
  - Do you smoke your first cigarette within 30 minutes of waking up in the morning?
  - Do you smoke 20 cigarettes (a pack) or more each day?
  - At times when you cannot smoke or do not have any cigarettes, do you feel a craving for one?
  - Is it tough to keep from smoking for more than a few hours?
  - When you are sick enough to stay in bed, do you still smoke?

- Assess the patient's knowledge of pharmacotherapy for smoking cessation.

Rationales

Smoking can be a source of pleasure and comfort. Moreover, when smoking is used as a coping mechanism, the emotional needs being met by it will need to be addressed as part of the overall plan for smoking cessation. QSEN: Patient-centered care.

Patients with a history of depression have more difficulty in quitting smoking. This challenge needs to be identified and support provided. They may benefit from the use of antidepressants such as bupropion or nortriptyline, which have been found to be effective pharmacotherapy for smoking cessation.

Self-management is a key component of a successful change in behavior. Much smoking is automatic and occurs with little concentration. Self-monitoring by record-keeping has been shown to be one of the most critical parts of lifestyle changes because it helps patients understand their habit. Self-monitoring includes using daily records of place and time of smoking, thoughts and feelings, and physical and emotional settings in which smoking occurs. This information provides feedback on progress and places the responsibility for change with the patient.

The patient needs to identify the feelings and situations that serve as triggers for smoking, so attention can be directed to breaking these triggers before the quit attempt.

Nicotine is one of the most powerful addictive drugs. These questions from the Fagerstrom Tolerance Test can be used to determine one's level of addiction. If smokers answer "yes" to two or more questions, this is an indication that they have a nicotine addiction. QSEN: Evidence-based practice.

Except in the presence of special circumstances (e.g., adolescents, pregnancy, breastfeeding, light smokers, smokeless tobacco users, and those with special medical contraindications), pharmacotherapy should be used with all patients attempting to quit smoking. It has been found to double the rate of cessation compared to placebo and helps with the symptoms of withdrawal.

Therapeutic Interventions

Actions/Interventions

- Review and reinforce basic information about the benefits of smoking cessation.

Rationales

According to the U.S. Surgeon General and American Heart Association, 12 hours after quitting the carbon monoxide levels in the blood return to normal; after 2 weeks to 3 months the circulation and lung function begin to improve; after 1 year the risk for coronary heart diseases is reduced by 50%; after 5 to 15 years the risk of stroke is that of a nonsmoker; and after 10 years of smoke-free living, the lung cancer death rate is cut by 50%. These benefits and milestones can serve to enhance motivation to continue with smoking cessation efforts. QSEN: Evidence-based practice.

Actions/Interventions

- Choose an approach to quitting most suitable for the specific patient, as in the following:
  - Cold turkey: Abrupt cessation from one's addictive level of smoking
  - Tapering: Smoking fewer cigarettes each day until down to none
  - Postponing: Postponing the time to start smoking each day by a predetermined number of hours, eventually leading to no cigarettes
  - Joining a smoking cessation program
  - Using online quit lines
  - Pharmacotherapy: Nicotine replacement therapy (NRT), bupropion SR, varenicline
  - Acupuncture, hypnosis
- Discuss the evidence regarding use of electronic nicotine delivery systems (ENDS).

- Assist the patient to formally set a date to quit smoking, either verbally or by contract.

- Assist patients in preparing for their "quit day."

- Instruct the patient on the physical symptoms of nicotine withdrawal.

- Discuss with the patient pharmacological agents available for smoking cessation:
  First-line agents:
  - Nicotine replacement therapy (NRT): Patch, gum, inhaler, nasal spray, lozenge
  - Non-nicotine medications (bupropion SR and varenicline)
  Second-line agents:
  - Clonidine
  - Nortriptyline

Rationales

Different approaches appeal to different individuals. Exploration of the most useful treatment options enables the patient to select the approach most acceptable to his or her beliefs, values, and lifestyle. Quit lines, such as 1-800-QUIT-NOW, operated by the National Cancer Institute, help tobacco users quit through a variety of service offerings. Pharmacotherapy should be encouraged based on its effectiveness (except when contraindicated). Acupuncture and hypnosis, if used, should be part of a comprehensive quit-smoking program. QSEN: Evidence-based practice; Patient-centered care.

The U.S. Preventive Services Task Force concluded that the evidence on the use of ENDS for tobacco cessation is insufficient and the balance of benefits and harms cannot be determined from current research. QSEN: Evidence-based practice.

This formality reinforces the intent and behavior being changed. A date should be selected within the first 2 weeks to keep the momentum moving forward. Contracts help clarify the goal and enhance the patient's control over the behavior, creating a sense of independence, competence, and autonomy.

Research supports important activities that enhance the success of quitting. These activities include such things as removing all ash trays and discarding ALL cigarettes at home and work, telling family and friends of their intent to quit, and initiating pharmacotherapy before the start date, as indicated.

The chief physiological obstacle to quitting is the addictive nature of nicotine. Withdrawal from nicotine is characterized by physical symptoms of headache, anxiety, nausea, and craving for tobacco. These symptoms are temporary and can be managed with medications.

Nicotine replacement medications and non-nicotine medications help relieve withdrawal symptoms and cravings for cigarettes and double the smoking cessation rates compared to placebo. Using two types of NRT has been shown to be more effective than using a single type. NRT in combination with bupropion SR may be more effective than bupropion alone, and NRT is safe for patients with a history of cardiovascular disease. If pharmacotherapy is needed for lighter smokers (e.g., 10-15 cigarettes a day), consideration should be given to reducing the dose of the first-line medication. Second-line agents are used for patients who have a contraindication to or lack of success with the first-line agents. QSEN: Evidence-based practice.

■ = Independent ▲ = Interprofessional Collaboration

Actions/Interventions

- Provide practical counseling that includes problem-solving and skills training.

- Assist the patient in finding alternative methods for reducing stress.

- Help the patient plan how to avoid or manage social situations that result in the temptation to smoke (e.g., alcohol use, being with other smokers).

- Promote positive expectations for success.

- Assist the patient in selecting appropriate support people.

- Provide positive reinforcement as indicated. Encourage the patient to plan rewards at appropriate intervals to celebrate successes.

- Discuss concerns about weight gain when no longer smoking.

- Assist the patient in preparing for possible lapses and relapses.

Rationales

Counseling focused on problem-solving and skills training has the greatest outcome. The patient needs to understand the importance of eliminating smoking cues (stimulus control) by changing normal routines. Examples include avoiding situations associated with the pleasurable aspects of smoking, such as having a cocktail before dinner, or taking public transportation to work instead of smoking while driving. Other examples include developing strategies to resist cravings, for example, spending more time with nonsmoking friends; finding new activities that make smoking difficult (e.g., biking or swimming); doing things that require the use of the hands (e.g., gardening, puzzles); and keeping oral substitutes handy (e.g., gum, carrots, apples) that provide oral gratification while reducing the urge to smoke. QSEN: Evidence-based practice.

Physical cravings for cigarettes can cause stress. And for many smokers cigarettes were used as a way to deal with stress. Thus patients need both short-term and long-term solutions for managing stress. Exercise, breathing exercises, and social support are effective methods to relieve tension and overcome the urge to smoke.

The patient needs to learn new strategies to cope with settings that trigger smoking. The use of role-playing or viewing videotapes with people performing the desired behavior can be quite effective.

Patients with a stronger self-efficacy to perform a behavior, such as quitting smoking, are more likely to engage in it.

It is unlikely that one person can meet all types of support that may be required (e.g., listening to challenges and frustrations, discussing shared experiences, helping solve problems). The patient needs to appreciate who can serve as the best supporters at various times.

Appropriately timed feedback is critical to a successful behavior change. Positive reinforcement encourages a desired behavior. Rewards, both intrinsic and extrinsic, are motivational and can give a sense of satisfaction for a job well done.

Acknowledge that weight gain is likely but typically limited to about 6 to 10 pounds. Although this can be challenging, the weight can be lost through healthy eating and exercise. Encourage the patient to focus first on the smoking cessation, then the weight control later. Smoking causes the greatest health risk.

Relapse prevention interventions need to be provided with every smoker who has recently quit. Preventing relapse needs to be addressed early in the treatment plan. Identifying high-risk situations likely to cause relapse aids in problem-solving. Any setbacks should be reframed as learning opportunities and as a normal step in making lifestyle changes. Patients should be encouraged to resume their quit attempt as soon as possible so as not to lose momentum. QSEN: Patient-centered care.

Actions/Interventions

- Inform the patient regarding community resources and self-help groups as appropriate.

- Follow the patient on a long-term basis, if possible, to provide encouragement.

Rationales

Self-help and support groups provide unique perspectives on "being there" and may be effective in providing alternative treatment modalities.

Ongoing follow-up, such as phone calls every few months, to reinforce the importance of maintaining abstinence and acknowledging successes during challenging times promotes long-term outcomes.

NDx   Readiness for Weight Management

Overweight and obesity are common health problems in the United States, and their prevalence is growing globally. Although multiple factors contribute to overweight (genetics, the biology of one's regulatory systems, environment, medications, psychological state), the fact remains that most people gain weight because they consume more calories than they expend. Many overweight people have tried short-term fad diets that resulted in temporary weight loss. However, they soon find that losing weight is much easier than keeping it off.

Successful weight management should be approached as a permanent lifestyle change, not simply a quick fix to lose a few pounds for a special event. Slow and gradual weight loss resulting in about 10% of body weight over a 6-month period is a reasonable expectation and one that has shown health benefits, such as reduced blood pressure and glucose and lipid levels.

Weight loss readiness is a key to success, as it takes focused time and effort to begin a weight loss program.

Making a healthy eating lifestyle change requires establishing a new mindset and habits that become a part of one's everyday life. Different people may benefit from different approaches to weight loss, but all successful weight management programs contain the same core components: paying careful attention to a reduced-calorie, low-fat diet; participating in ongoing self-monitoring; incorporating physical activity into one's daily life; using support people or groups; and paying attention to maintaining lifestyle modifications. Multifactorial programs that include behavioral interventions and counseling are more successful than education alone. This care plan focuses on individuals who are ready to begin a weight management program. Note that basic information about healthy food choices can be found in the care plan *Readiness for Enhanced Nutrition*. Obese individuals with more complex weight issues may benefit from information found in the *Bariatric Surgery* care plan.

Defining Characteristics

Expresses willingness to initiate a weight management program

Demonstrates attitude toward eating congruent with weight goals

Expresses knowledge of components of a healthy eating lifestyle

Expresses knowledge of components of an appropriate physical activity program

Engages in a self-monitoring program

Consumes prescribed meal plan

Engages in a prescribed physical activity program

Expresses willingness to use a support group as appropriate

■ = Independent   ▲ = Interprofessional Collaboration

Common Expected Outcomes

Patient verbalizes accurate information for weight management program.

Patient verbalizes measures necessary to achieve weight-reduction goals.

Patient engages in desired behaviors to promote weight management.

NOC Outcomes

Weight Loss Behavior; Knowledge: Weight Management; Weight Maintenance Behavior; Nutritional Status; Knowledge: Prescribed Diet; Knowledge: Prescribed Activity; Health Seeking Behavior

NIC Interventions

Weight Management; Weight Reduction Assistance; Health Education

Ongoing Assessment

Actions/Interventions	Rationales
■ Determine the patient's level of motivation and confidence for engaging in a weight management program.	Assessment of the motivation and readiness to lose weight is critical. Weight loss takes work. Most patients have tried many times in the past. Therefore it is important that patients have the motivation and commitment to not only begin a program but also to stay with it for the upcoming weeks and months until new lifestyle behaviors are learned. Asking patients to rate their confidence (on a scale of 1 to 10) that they can stick with the program provides important information. QSEN: Patient-centered care.
■ Determine the patient's weight loss goals.	Individuals begin weight loss programs with a variety of expectations as to how much weight they expect to lose in how fast a time. They may be focusing on an unrealistic "ideal weight" rather than the benefits of a "healthier weight." This can be accomplished with a modest 5% to 10% loss in body weight and may translate to 1- to 2-pound weight loss per week (over a 3- to 6-month period). QSEN: Patient-centered care.
■ Determine the baseline weight and body mass index (BMI).	BMI describes relative weight for height and is significantly correlated with total body fat content. BMI is calculated as weight (in kilograms) divided by height squared (in square meters). A BMI between 20 and 24 is associated with healthier outcomes. A BMI greater than 25 is associated with increased morbidity and mortality.
■ Review the patient's weight history.	It is helpful to use milestones to help patients recall the history of their weight gain. Questions such as, "How much did you weigh in high school?" "How much did you weigh when you got married?" and "How much did you weigh after your first child was born?" may help establish when obesity became a problem.
■ Determine any previous attempts at weight loss.	Adults bring many life experiences to learning sessions. Often patients have tried unsuccessfully to engage in weight loss. Reasons for difficulties need to be explored.
■ Perform a nutritional assessment to include: • Daily food intake (type and amount) • Approximate caloric intake • Activity at time of eating • Feelings at time of eating • Location of meals • Meals skipped • Snacking patterns • Social and familial considerations	Assessment of current eating patterns produces a baseline for change. Assessment methods may include a 24-hour recall of foods eaten, food diaries or records, or food frequency recording using typical food groups. QSEN: Patient-centered care.

Actions/Interventions

- Determine behavioral factors that contribute to overeating.

- Identify potential medical causes for being overweight: endocrine or neurological conditions, genetic issues, or medications.
- Explore the importance and meaning of food with the patient, including cultural influences.

- Assess the patient's ability to read food labels.

- Assess the patient's ability to plan a menu and make appropriate food selections.

- Assess the patient's ability to accurately identify appropriate food portions.
- Assess the patient's activity patterns, including a regular exercise program.

Rationales

Overeating may be triggered by environmental cues and behavioral factors unrelated to physiological hunger sensations.

A medical assessment is used to rule out organic causes and assess health risks and the presence of weight-related health problems.

Food is energy and plays a vital role in our daily lives. Without food we cannot survive; however, food is much more than that. It is a source of pleasure and comfort. It is also a symbol of hospitality, social status, and religious or cultural significance. What we select to eat, how we prepare it and serve it, and even how we eat it are all factors profoundly touched by our individual inheritance. Moreover, when food is used as a coping mechanism or as self-reward, the emotional needs being met by the intake of food should be addressed as part of the overall plan for weight reduction. QSEN: Patient-centered care.

Food labels contain information necessary in making appropriate selections, but they can be misleading. Patients need to understand that "low-fat" or "fat-free" does not mean that a food item is calorie-free. In addition, attention should be paid to serving size and the number of servings in the food item.

This information provides the starting point for educational sessions. Teaching content the patient already knows wastes valuable time and hinders critical learning.

Serving sizes must be understood to limit intake according to a planned diet.

This assessment provides a basis for promoting activity. Increasing activity levels may need to begin at a slower pace if the patient has a very sedentary lifestyle.

Therapeutic Interventions

Actions/Interventions

- Assist the patient in setting realistic goals for a weight management program, including food intake and exercise.

- Review and reinforce basic nutrition information.

Rationales

Patients are easily discouraged when they cannot meet unrealistic goals. This sense of failure can lead to overeating. Goals that are too global (e.g., "lose 30 pounds") are difficult to achieve and can foster feelings of failure. Shorter-term goals (e.g., "lose 5 pounds in a month") may be more achievable and therefore reinforcing. Goal-setting needs to be performed by the patient, not the practitioner. QSEN: Patient-centered care.

The key principle of weight management is changing the balance of calories in to calories out, namely to eat fewer calories than are expended so fat stores are used as fuel.

■ = Independent   ▲ = Interprofessional Collaboration

Actions/Interventions	Rationales
■ Instruct the patient in the importance of keeping a diary or food log of what, where, when, and why the patient eats and drinks.	Self-management is a key component of a successful change in behavior. Much eating is automatic and occurs with little concentration. Self-monitoring by record-keeping has been shown to be one of the most critical parts of lifestyle changes. Self-monitoring includes using daily records of place and time of food intake, thoughts and feelings, and physical and emotional settings in which eating occurs. This information provides feedback on progress and places the responsibility for change with the patient. QSEN: Evidence-based practice.
■ Design a meal plan that provides a caloric intake appropriate for achieving weight-loss goals:	An individualized plan is based on knowing how many calories are needed for one's level of activity. As a quick rule of thumb, the average woman needs about 1200 calories and the average man about 1500 calories. One pound of adipose tissue contains 3500 calories. Therefore, to lose 1 pound per week, the patient must have a calorie deficit of 500 calories per day.
• Four food groups or the Food Pyramid/MyPlate	The key principle of weight loss therapy is to eat fewer calories than are expended in order to consume fat stores as fuel. Patients need to learn to eat a variety of foods when changing their eating pattern to ensure lifelong success at weight maintenance.
• Proper serving size	Portion distortion is a growing problem in society; consumers often perceive larger portions as more value for their money, further complicating the problem. Portion size in relation to calories is important in food selection and meal planning. The patient needs to learn strategies to avoid the "portion trap" (e.g., sharing a meal in a restaurant, having the waiter package half the meal before it even gets to the table, not buying super-size bags of anything if too tempting). Using smaller plates and bowls can help the patient reframe the need to fill his or her plate at mealtime and take smaller portions.
• Caloric content of food	Many patients are unaware of the calories present in low-fat foods. Thus it may be valuable to count every calorie and fat gram initially, to increase awareness of amounts eaten.
• Methods of preparation to avoid additional calories	Baking, boiling, broiling, poaching, and grilling are preferable to frying in oil.
■ Teach the patient to read food labels (serving size, calories [and calories from fat], the nutrients, percent daily value).	Food labels can be used to make informed choices. The FDA requires The Nutrition Facts label to provide information on the amount of calories per serving size; beneficial nutrients, such as dietary fiber and calcium; and the amount of certain food components that should be limited in the diet, including saturated fat, trans-fat, cholesterol, and sodium. The ingredients list can be used to find out whether a food or beverage contains solid fats, added sugars, whole grains, and refined grains. Restaurant chains now include calorie content of foods on menu boards to assist consumers in making healthy choices.

Actions/Interventions

■ Encourage water intake.

■ Teach or encourage strategies to modify patient behavior such as keeping problematic foods out of the house or limiting the time and place of eating.

■ Help the patient plan how to avoid or manage social situations that result in overeating.

■ Review complications associated with obesity.

■ Instruct the patient to weigh on a routine schedule—usually once a week.

■ Include the family, caregiver, and food preparer in nutrition counseling.

■ Encourage the patient to be more aware of habits that may contribute to or prevent overeating, such as the following:

  • Realize the time needed for eating.

  • Focus on eating and avoid other diversional activities (e.g., reading, television viewing, telephoning).

  • Observe for cues that lead to eating (e.g., aroma, time, depression, boredom).

  • Eat in a designated place (e.g., at the table rather than in front of the television).
  • Recognize actual hunger versus a desire to eat.

Rationales

Water makes up two thirds of the weight of the body and is required for chemical reactions and delivery of nutrients throughout the body. Weight loss programs typically recommend that people drink eight glasses per day, but this is without scientific evidence. For many, drinking water may assist in curbing the urge to eat. Some research suggests that overweight people may misinterpret physiological sensations of thirst as hunger.

The patient needs to understand the importance of eliminating eating cues (stimulus control) as a successful strategy in weight loss programs. Examples include eating only when sitting down at a designated place, leaving the table as soon as eating is done, not combining eating with other activities, refusing the bread basket at restaurants, and stocking the house with healthier food choices.

The patient needs to learn new strategies to cope with settings that trigger overeating. The use of role-playing or viewing videotapes with people performing the desired behavior can be quite effective.

Patients need to be aware of long-term health problems as a stimulus for change. Medical complications include cardiovascular and respiratory dysfunction, higher incidence of diabetes mellitus, and aggravation of musculoskeletal disorders. Social complications and poor self-esteem may also result from obesity.

The scale should provide feedback on the patient's progress, but not serve as a daily index of whether the program is working. Daily weights are not recommended. Slight variations may unnecessarily encourage or discourage a patient. Adherence to diet and exercise programs will be reflected in gradual and consistent weight loss. Most experts suggest a loss of 0.5 to 1 pound per week.

The patient will be more likely to adhere to changes in food intake when family members are involved in those changes. Research has demonstrated that men whose wives diet with them are more likely to achieve goals than those for whom special food is prepared.

Stimulus control changes involve learning what social or environmental cues encourage undesired eating and then modifying these cues.

Hurried eating may result in overeating because satiety is not realized until 15 to 20 minutes after the ingestion of food.

Doing several activities at once usually results in less attention being devoted to the amount of food eaten and contributes to overeating.

Identifying triggers or situations that prompt eating behaviors is the first step toward developing alternative coping strategies. Awareness and recognition of cues can help the patient substitute other activities for eating.

Controlling environmental stimuli can reduce impulse eating.

Eating when not hungry is a commonly recognized symptom among overeaters.

■ = Independent ▲ = Interprofessional Collaboration

Actions/Interventions

- Plan an exercise program.
  - Pedometer—starting at 4000 steps daily, then gradually increasing to at least 10,000 steps
  - 30 to 60 minutes of moderate-intensity physical activity nearly every day

- Provide positive reinforcement as indicated. Encourage the patient to plan rewards at appropriate intervals to celebrate successes.

- Assist the patient in preparing for possible lapses and relapses.

- Assist the patient in coping with setbacks.

Rationales

Exercise is an integral part of weight reduction programs. The amount of exercise an individual requires for weight loss varies. For most, walking 25 to 30 miles is needed to burn even 1 pound of fat. However, it is not just the calories burned per se that results in weight loss. Research supports that it is increasing physical activity for its enjoyment and overall health benefits that is associated with successful weight loss. And regular physical activity is one of the best predictors of successful weight maintenance. The approach needs to start slow because the patient should view exercise as a lifelong habit. Thus there is no rush in getting started.

Appropriately timed feedback is critical to a successful behavior change. Positive reinforcement encourages a desired behavior. Patients should be taught to use alternative ways to recognize success with weight management besides weight changes on the scale. For example, noticing a better fit in clothing, being able to buy clothes a size smaller, and improved activity tolerance are important signs of success.

Rewards, both intrinsic and extrinsic, are motivational and can give a sense of satisfaction for a job well done. Some people find getting rid of clothes that are now too big can serve as a motivational strategy, for it emphasizes that the patient will work hard to maintain his or her current success. Keeping larger clothes in the closet means that the patient expects to regain weight and thus have the clothes ready for a return to a "fat wardrobe."

Relapse prevention needs to be addressed early in the treatment plan. Identifying high-risk situations likely to cause relapse aids in problem-solving. Any setbacks should be reframed as learning opportunities and as a normal step in making lifestyle changes. Remind patients that missing a day of planned exercise or occasional dietary discretion will inevitably happen and should not be construed failure.

The patient may experience temporary weight plateaus. This can be discouraging to the patient's efforts to continue a weight loss program. Patients need to understand that these changes are expected and that slight modifications in diet or exercise can return the patient to a pattern of continued weight loss. Often patients experience weight cycling, commonly referred to as "yo-yo dieting," that is defined as repeated losses and regains of body weight. The ranges in weight loss can be 5 to 10 pounds in a cycle or for some as large as 50 pounds. Research clearly supports the power of a regular program of moderate- to vigorous-intensity exercise for about 60 minutes each day as the key strategy for successfully maintaining weight loss.

Actions/Interventions

■ Encourage the patient to participate in support groups (e.g., Weight Watchers) for weight loss.

■ Inform the patient about pharmacological agents for weight loss as appropriate.

▲ Consult a dietitian for further assessment and recommendations regarding a weight loss program.

Rationales

Social support is important in successful weight loss and long-term weight management. Regular attendance at sessions enhances weight loss.

Because drugs do nothing to permanently alter eating behaviors, use of drugs for weight management often fails when the patient stops taking the medication. However, drugs may be used as adjunctive therapy in patients with a BMI of 30 or greater or 27 or greater with other obesity-related risk factors or disease. Drugs for weight loss include appetite suppressants (nonadrenergic drugs and serotonin reuptake inhibitors), digestive inhibitors (interfere with digestion and absorption of fat), and fat substitutes as food additives. QSEN: Evidence-based practice.

The dietitian can provide specialized information and ongoing support for weight loss. Some patients require assistance only with meal preparation and choices and can handle other aspects of lifestyle changes. QSEN: Teamwork and collaboration.

■ = Independent   ▲ = Interprofessional Collaboration

Basic Nursing Concepts Care Plans

This chapter has several clinical conditions or situations that may be present in the patient with other medical conditions. These conditions include mood disorders, substance abuse, visual impairment, hearing loss, and death and dying. In addition, this chapter includes several therapeutic interventions that may be used as part of the management of many clinical conditions. These interventions include blood component therapy, central venous access devices, enteral nutrition, and parenteral nutrition. These care plans were in previous editions of the book in the various body systems chapters. The care plan for the patient experiencing surgery focuses on nursing care during the preoperative phase and the postoperative phase of this clinical situation. These care plans have been placed together in this chapter for ease in accessing the information. The care plans follow the same format used for care plans for medical disorders.

Surgical Experience: Preoperative and Postoperative Care

Major; Minor; Elective; Urgent; Emergency; General Surgery; Ambulatory Surgery; Same-Day Surgery; Outpatient Surgery; Minimally Invasive (Fiberoptic) Surgery

Patients undergo surgery for a variety of purposes. These purposes include exploration and diagnosis, excision and removal of diseased body parts, palliation of disease symptoms, restoration or reconstruction of body parts or functions, and cosmetic improvement in physical appearance. Most surgeries are planned and considered elective. Advances in surgical and anesthesia techniques have led to shortened lengths of stay. Many surgical procedures that in the past required several days of inpatient care now are performed in the outpatient or ambulatory setting. The patient is discharged within a few hours after recovery from the effects of anesthesia. Surgical procedures that previously required open incisions are now performed using minimally invasive techniques.

The primary focus of nursing care during the preoperative phase of the surgical experience is teaching the patient and family members. Preoperative teaching includes three types of information: sensory, procedural, and process.

Because the time for patient and family teaching has decreased, a team approach is usually most effective. This interprofessional collaboration to educating the patient and family includes the nurse, the surgeon, the anesthesia care provider, and other members of the team as needed to promote quality outcomes and safety for the patient. Teaching begins in the outpatient setting and is reinforced when the patient arrives at the hospital or surgery center on the day of surgery.

Nursing care during the postoperative phase focuses on pain management, prevention of complications, and preparation for convalescence at home. Patient and family teaching that began preoperatively continues during the postoperative phase and prepares the patient and family to continue care after discharge to home. Because of shorter lengths of stay, patients may be discharged with more complex care requirements.

Preoperative Phase

NDx Deficient Knowledge

Common Related Factors
Insufficient information about proposed surgical experience
Insufficient knowledge from lack of previous surgical experiences
Misinformation presented by others

Defining Characteristics
Insufficient knowledge
Inaccurate follow-through of instruction
Inaccurate performance on a test
Inappropriate behavior

Common Expected Outcomes
Patient and family members verbalize understanding of proposed surgical procedure and realistic expectations for the postoperative course.
Patient and family members verbalize understanding of proposed pain management plan.
Patient demonstrates the ability to cough, deep breathe, use the incentive spirometer, and perform leg exercises.

NOC Outcomes
Knowledge: Treatment Procedure; Information Processing
NIC Interventions
Teaching: Preoperative; Learning Facilitation; Surgical Preparation; Health Literacy Enhancement

Ongoing Assessment

Actions/Interventions

- Assess the patient's knowledge of the proposed surgical procedure and postoperative care.

- Assess the patient's previous experience with surgery.

Rationales

The patient should be aware of the nature of the surgical procedure, as well as risks and benefits of the surgical procedure, the reason it is being done, location of the surgical incision, and expected length of recovery. This information provides a basis for the patient to give informed consent for the surgical procedure. The patient may have received this information from other members of the interprofessional team such as the surgeon and anesthesia care provider.

Patients will base their concept of surgery on their past experiences. Patients who have had surgery in the past may have negative feelings related to the side effects of anesthesia and postoperative pain; they may recall longer hospitalizations than today's typical shorter stays. The patient with no previous surgical experience may have misperceptions of the proposed surgery based on information from family and friends. QSEN: Patient-centered care.

■ = Independent ▲ = Interprofessional Collaboration

Basic Nursing Concepts Care Plans

Actions/Interventions	**Rationales**
■ Assess the patient's level of anxiety.	Surgery is not only a physiological stressor but also a psychological stressor. Preoperative anxiety may be associated with the patient's previous surgical experiences or stories the patient has heard from others. Anxiety will affect the patient's ability to listen and comprehend explanations and teaching. Patients may feel anxious about the surgery and its potential outcomes for their health. The patient may have fear about anesthesia, pain, changes in body appearance and function, or loss of control during surgery. In cases of severe or panic levels of patient anxiety about surgery, the nurse needs to notify the surgical team. The surgery may be postponed until the patient's level of anxiety is reduced. QSEN: Patient-centered care.

Therapeutic Interventions

Actions/Interventions	**Rationales**
■ Explain and reinforce the surgeon's explanations regarding the proposed surgical procedure.	The patient needs to have an accurate understanding of the surgical procedure in order to provide informed consent. The nurse may reinforce explanations provided by the surgeon. The nurse is the patient's advocate in obtaining additional information from the surgical team before the patient signs a consent form or at any time before surgery.
■ Provide procedural information:	These actions reduce the risk for harm to the patient during the surgical experience. The patient uses the information to be a full partner in providing this care during the preoperative phase of surgery. QSEN: Patient-centered care; Safety.
• Fluid and food restrictions (NPO [nothing by mouth] status)	Intake of fluids and food is restricted before surgery to minimize the risk for pulmonary aspiration during surgery. The timing of these restrictions is based on the type of anesthesia and the time of day of the surgery. The patient needs to understand that if these restrictions are not followed, surgery may be delayed or postponed.
• Physical preparation	The patient may be asked to take a shower before surgery to promote general hygiene and reduce the risk for infection. Sometimes the patient will be given an antiseptic solution to use during the shower. Patients having abdominal surgery may need to follow a specific protocol for bowel preparation. This protocol may require the patient to use laxatives or enemas before surgery. Once the patient is in the holding area, the skin on the operative site may be washed again with an antiseptic solution. Excess body hair at the surgical site may be removed. If removed, it will be done by clipping. This method prevents potential sources of infection from microscopic cuts that may occur when shaving is used for hair removal.
• Intravenous (IV) lines	IV lines are inserted before surgery to provide fluid, electrolytes, and emergency IV access. Depending on the type of surgery, the IV lines may be inserted in peripheral veins or central veins.

Actions/Interventions	**Rationales**
• Procedure for anesthesia administration	The nurse needs to reinforce information provided by the anesthesia care provider. This information includes the use of preanesthesia medications, the type of anesthesia used during the procedure, the effects of the anesthesia on the patient's level of consciousness and level of sensation, and the postoperative effects.
• Marking of the surgical site	The Joint Commission has developed patient safety goals for hospital staff to mark the surgical site without ambiguity using indelible markers. This marking should take place while the patient is awake and aware. QSEN: Evidence-based practice.
■ Provide sensory information:	The information helps the patient anticipate sensory experiences during the surgical experience to reduce anxiety. QSEN: Patient-centered care.
• Noise levels and conversations	Preoperative holding areas may be noisy because of the level of activity. The patient may hear conversations among members of the surgical team. The patient needs to know it is appropriate to ask for clarification of questions or comments.
• Cold rooms and skin solutions	Room temperatures in surgical areas tend to be cold. The patient needs to know that it is appropriate to ask for a blanket. The patient may perceive solutions used to prepare the skin before surgery as cold to the touch.
• Bright lights	The lights in holding areas and operating rooms may seem brighter than normal because the patient will be lying on a stretcher or operating table.
• Body positioning for surgery	The nurse needs to explain how the patient may be positioned in the operating room. The patient needs to know that the operating table is narrower than a stretcher or bed. The patient may be anxious about falling off the table. Straps are placed snugly across the patient's thighs to maintain safe positioning on the operating table.
• Unusual odors	Solutions used in the operating room may have unpleasant odors for the patient.
■ Provide process information about the general flow for surgery:	This information helps the patient and family members anticipate activities as part of the preoperative surgical experience. Knowing what to expect can reduce anxiety for both the patient and the family. QSEN: Patient-centered care.
• Holding areas	Patients are brought to the holding area before moving to the specific operating room. Family members may be allowed to stay with the patient in this area. During this time, nurses and other members of the surgical team are reviewing baseline assessments and verifying surgical consent documents with the patient.
• Frequent measurement of vital signs	The patient needs to understand the purpose of frequent measurement of vital signs during the surgical experience. Blood pressure (BP), heart rate (HR), respiratory rate, and body temperature are measured in the preoperative phase to establish baseline data for comparison during surgery and postoperative recovery.

Basic Nursing Concepts Care Plans

■ = Independent   ▲ = Interprofessional Collaboration

Actions/Interventions	Rationales
• Family waiting rooms and methods of obtaining information during surgery	Family members need to know where they may wait while the patient is in the operating room. The nurse needs to inform family members how they will be able to obtain information about the patient's status in surgery and during immediate postoperative recovery. The nurse may need to arrange for appropriate interpreters for family members who do not understand English or have a hearing impairment.
• Transport to operating rooms	The nurse needs to provide the patient and family with information about how the patient will be moved from the holding area to the operating room. The method of transportation depends on the patient's level of consciousness and mobility.
• Postanesthesia recovery area	The patient receiving general anesthesia may be moved from the operating room to a special postanesthesia recovery area after completion of the surgery. Patients who had regional or local anesthesia may be returned to the holding area for additional postoperative monitoring.
• Measures used by the surgical team in the operating room to ensure the correct procedures are performed	Teaching the patient about expectations to promote safety during the procedure may reduce the patient's level of anxiety. The Joint Commission's patient safety goals include performance standards to promote communication among all members of the surgical team at all stages of preparation for the procedure. These standards include a time-out before the start of the procedure to conduct a final assessment that the correct patient, site, and positioning are identified and that all consents, relevant information, and equipment are available. QSEN: Evidence-based practice; Safety.
• Equipment and technology that may be present on awakening from anesthesia	Patients need to know about tubes, drains, dressings, monitors, or other equipment that may have been placed during surgery. This knowledge may help decrease anxiety and sensory distortion of these experiences.
• Personal items and valuables	The nurse needs to provide the patient with information about securing personal items and valuables during surgery. These items may be given to family members or secured according to institution policies.
■ Provide the patient and family with information about preventing postoperative complications:	The information allows the patient to be a full partner in postoperative care to reduce the risk of harm after surgery. QSEN: Patient-centered care; Safety.
• Need for dynamic turning, coughing, deep-breathing exercises, and incentive spirometry; give opportunities for return demonstration	These techniques help prevent pulmonary atelectasis and stasis of secretions, which could lead to pneumonia. Return demonstration allows the patient to receive feedback about his or her effectiveness with these techniques.
• Postoperative leg exercises	Leg exercises help promote venous return and decrease the incidence of deep vein thrombosis.
• Antiembolic stockings or sequential compression devices for patients who remain on bed rest for more than 12 hours	These devices prevent deep vein thrombosis by compressing superficial veins and promoting venous return. At the preference of the surgeon or health care provider, the antiembolic stockings or sequential compression devices (SCDs) may be used during the operation and postanesthesia care even if the patient will not be on extended bed rest.

Actions/Interventions

- Early ambulation

Rationales

This activity helps prevent pulmonary atelectasis, deep vein thrombosis, paralytic ileus, and other complications of immobility. The timing of ambulation depends on the type of surgical procedure and the patient's level of consciousness.

■ Provide the patient and family with information about pain management after surgery.

Adequate pain management allows patients having surgery to participate actively in their care, to ambulate, and to breathe effectively. The patient has a right to be involved in selecting the type of pain management used. The patient needs to know about the importance of reporting the occurrence and intensity of postoperative pain to ensure prompt treatment. The Joint Commission requires implementation of effective pain management strategies for all patients. The nurse develops an individualized plan for pain management that integrates the best clinical evidence, standards of clinical practice, and the patient's values to achieve optimal outcomes for pain management. QSEN: Patient-centered care; Evidence-based practice.

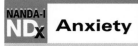
NANDA-I NDx Anxiety

Common Related Factors	**Defining Characteristics**
Change in health status	Apprehensiveness about surgery
Stressors associated with surgery	Fear of errors during surgery
Situational crisis: surgery	Irritability, restlessness, insomnia
	Increased BP, HR, respiratory rate

Common Expected Outcomes

Patient uses effective coping mechanisms.
Patient describes a reduction in the level of anxiety experienced.

NOC Outcomes
Anxiety Level; Anxiety Self-Control; Coping
NIC Interventions
Anxiety Reduction; Coping Enhancement; Presence; Emotional Support; Surgical Preparation

Basic Nursing Concepts Care Plans

Ongoing Assessment

Actions/Interventions

■ Assess the patient's level of anxiety.

Rationales

The level of preoperative anxiety will vary based on the patient's understanding of the surgery, perception of surgical outcomes, previous surgery experience, and personality. Reactions to anxiety may range from mild to severe. The patient may appear calm but express nervousness with mild anxiety. As the level of anxiety increases, the patient may experience increased vital signs and report feeling overwhelmed by the anticipated surgery.

■ = Independent   ▲ = Interprofessional Collaboration

Actions/Interventions

- Determine the patient's concerns about the anticipated surgery.

- Determine how the patient uses defense mechanisms to cope with anxiety.

Rationales

Patients facing surgery may express fear about the wrong procedure being done or other mistakes made by the surgical team. Other concerns may include postoperative pain, body image changes, and changes in role function. QSEN: Patient-centered care.

Assessment of defense mechanisms helps determine the effectiveness of coping strategies used by the patient. Some defense mechanisms may be highly adaptive in managing anxiety. Other defense mechanisms may lead to less adaptive behavior with long-term use.

Therapeutic Interventions

Actions/Interventions

- Acknowledge awareness of the patient's anxiety.

- Assure the patient that he or she is safe. Stay with the patient as necessary during preoperative visits by members of the surgical team.

- Assist the patient in verbalizing anxious feelings and assessing the situation realistically.

- Support the patient's use of coping strategies that the patient has found effective in the past.

- Use simple language and brief statements when teaching the patient about what to expect before surgery.

- ▲ Collaborate with the surgeon to mark the surgical site accurately before the patient is moved to the operating room.

- Review with the patient all surgical consent forms to ensure that the surgical procedure to be done is accurately reported.

- Teach the patient about measures used by the surgical team in the operating room, such as a time-out, to ensure that the correct procedure is done.

Rationales

Acknowledgment of the patient's feelings validates his or her feelings and communicates acceptance of those feelings.

The presence of a trusted person may help the patient feel less threatened in these situations.

Talking about anxiety-producing situations and anxious feelings can help the patient perceive the situation in a less threatening manner.

Using anxiety-reduction strategies enhances the patient's sense of personal mastery and confidence. QSEN: Patient-centered care.

Patients experiencing moderate to severe anxiety may be unable to comprehend anything more than simple, clear, and brief explanations.

Being present with the patient during marking of the surgical site may lessen the patient's concern of the wrong procedure being done. The Joint Commission developed patient safety goals for hospital staff members to mark the surgical site without ambiguity. This marking should take place while the patient is awake and aware. QSEN: Safety; Teamwork and collaboration; Evidence-based practice.

Including the patient in record review allows the patient to have a sense of control for ensuring that the correct procedure is documented on all surgical forms. The patient's anxiety level may be reduced when he or she is a full partner in providing care. Effective use of precautionary measures reduces the risk of errors during the surgical experience. QSEN: Patient-centered care; Safety.

Teaching the patient about expectations to promote safety during the procedure may reduce the person's level of anxiety. The Joint Commission's patient safety goals include performance standards to promote communication among all members of the surgical team at all stages of preparation for the procedure. These standards include a time-out before the start of the procedure to conduct a final assessment that the correct patient, site, and positioning are identified and that all consents, relevant information, and equipment are available. QSEN: Evidence-based practice.

ℯvolve **For additional care plans, go to http://evolve.elsevier.com/Gulanick/.**

Postoperative Phase

Acute Pain

Common Related Factors
Physical injury agent (e.g., operative procedure; presence of drains, tubes)

Defining Characteristics
Self-report of intensity using standardized pain scale
Self-report of pain characteristics using standardized pain instrument
Expressive behavior (e.g., crying, restlessness, vigilance)
Positioning to ease pain
Change in physiological parameter (e.g., BP, HR, respiratory rate, and oxygen saturation)

Common Expected Outcomes
Patient reports satisfactory pain control and a decreased intensity using a standardized pain scale.
Patient uses pharmacological and nonpharmacological pain management strategies.
Patient exhibits increased comfort such as baseline levels for pulse, BP, respirations, and relaxed muscle tone or body posture.

NOC Outcomes
Comfort Status; Pain Control; Pain Level; Medication Response; Surgical Recovery: Immediate Post-Operative

NIC Interventions
Analgesic Administration; Pain Management; Patient-Controlled Analgesia (PCA) Assistance; Sedation Management

Ongoing Assessment

Actions/Interventions

■ Assess the location, quality, onset, frequency, radiation, and duration of pain. Have the patient rate pain intensity using a standardized pain scale (numeric 0 to 10 or FACES).

■ Assess for abdominal distention.

■ Assess the patient's HR, BP, and respiratory rate.

Rationales

Assessment of the pain experience is the first step in providing effective pain management. The patient is the most reliable source of information about his or her pain. Some pain is expected after surgery because of manipulation of tissues during surgery, operative positioning, the presence of drains and tubes, and patient anxiety. The pain should decrease in intensity over time. Persistent intense pain may indicate complications at the surgical site. Appropriate pain management will provide comfort and enable the patient to rest and participate in postoperative care activities such as deep breathing, coughing, and ambulation. QSEN: Patient-centered care.

Distention of the abdomen by accumulation of gas and fluid occurs postoperatively because normal peristalsis does not return until the third or fourth day after surgery; distention stresses suture lines and causes pain.

These assessments provide baseline information. Pain may cause the patient to experience increased HR, BP, and respiratory rate. These changes occur because of increased sympathetic nervous system activity associated with activation of the stress response as part of the pain experience.

Basic Nursing Concepts Care Plans

Therapeutic Interventions

Actions/Interventions	Rationales
■ Assist the patient to a comfortable position.	Repositioning the patient at frequent intervals may promote comfort. A semi-Fowler's position is usually most comfortable for patients with abdominal incisions, because stress on the suture line is relieved.
▲ Administer analgesics, or assist the patient in using patient-controlled anesthesia (PCA) before pain becomes too severe. Evaluate effectiveness and modify doses as needed. (See Acute Pain care plan, Chapter 2.)	It is more difficult to control pain once it becomes severe. Individualizing the pain-relieving regimen recognizes individual differences in pain perception and provides for control that is more effective. Nonsteroidal anti-inflammatory drugs are used alone for mild pain and in combination with opioids for moderate or severe pain. The Joint Commission requires that effective pain management strategies be implemented for all patients experiencing pain. Pain relief is not determined to be effective until the patient indicates that it is acceptable. QSEN: Patient-centered care; Evidence-based practice.
■ Use nonpharmacological treatment measures (e.g., distraction, music, relaxation).	These measures reduce the perception and sensation of pain.
▲ Administer pain medication before painful procedures (e.g., dressing changes, ambulation).	Effective pain management maximizes the patient's ability to tolerate or participate in procedures.

NANDA-I NDx Ineffective Breathing Pattern

Common Related Factors

Neurological impairment
Musculoskeletal impairment
Respiratory muscle fatigue
Body position that inhibits lung expansion
Fatigue
Pain
Anxiety

Defining Characteristics

Dyspnea, tachypnea/bradypnea
Abnormal breathing pattern (e.g., shallow depth)
Use of accessory muscles to breathe
Altered chest excursion

Common Expected Outcome

Patient maintains an effective breathing pattern as evidenced by relaxed breathing at a normal rate and depth and absence of dyspnea.

NOC Outcomes

Respiratory Status: Ventilation; Vital Signs;
  Surgical Recovery: Immediate Post-Operative

NIC Interventions

Airway Management; Respiratory Monitoring;
  Cough Enhancement

Ongoing Assessment

Actions/Interventions	Rationales
■ Assess the rate, rhythm, and depth of respirations.	Respirations may be shallow because the least amount of excursion is less painful, especially when an abdominal incision is present. Shallow breathing increases the risk for developing atelectasis and pneumonia. QSEN: Safety.
■ Auscultate breath sounds.	The bases of the lungs are least likely to be ventilated; therefore breath sounds may be diminished over the bases.

evolve **For additional care plans, go to http://evolve.elsevier.com/Gulanick/.**

Actions/Interventions
- Observe for use of accessory muscles.

- Assess the ability to use an incentive spirometer.

- Assess for pain and abdominal distention.

- Assess the patient's temperature according to postoperative policy.
- Assess the patient's level of consciousness.

- Assess the patient's health history for tobacco use or preexisting pulmonary disease.

Rationales
Work of breathing increases greatly as lung compliance decreases. As moving air in and out of the lungs becomes increasingly more difficult, the breathing pattern alters to include use of accessory muscles to increase chest excursion to facilitate effective breathing. The patient may consciously minimize the depth of each inspiration to reduce the amount of discomfort caused by full expansion of the lungs.

When using an incentive spirometer, the patient inhales and holds a deep breath for a few seconds. Incentive spirometry encourages deep breathing full expansion of alveoli.

Pain and abdominal distention can impair chest excursion and result in an ineffective breathing pattern from shallow breathing.

Elevated temperature in the first 48 hours postoperatively may indicate atelectasis, which can lead to pneumonia.

A decreased level of consciousness, as evidenced by drowsiness and sedation, may be the result of residual effects of anesthesia or analgesic medications. The sedated patient may have a slow respiratory rate and shallow depth of respirations.

Preexisting pulmonary disease or a history of smoking may add to breathing problems associated with anesthesia, analgesic side effects, or pain.

Therapeutic Interventions

Actions/Interventions
- ▲ Manage pain using the prescribed plan for pain management.

- Position the patient with the head of bed elevated 30 degrees.
- Encourage or assist the patient to change positions frequently; position with pillows or positioning devices as needed. Encourage ambulation as tolerated.

- Encourage the patient to do deep-breathing exercises a minimum of 10 times every hour. Encourage the use of an incentive spirometer every 1 to 2 hours.

- Encourage coughing every hour.
- Help the patient splint chest or abdominal incisions by using hands or a pillow.
- ▲ Administer oxygen as prescribed.

Rationales
Effective pain management allows for deeper breathing and coughing. Patients using patient-controlled analgesia may need reinforcement of previous teaching or reminders to push the button during the early postoperative phase until they are fully recovered from anesthesia.

This position enhances diaphragmatic excursion.

Breathing effectiveness and mobilization of secretions are enhanced by position changes and an upright position. Early ambulation enhances breathing and mobilizes secretions.

Deep breathing keeps alveoli from collapsing and promotes a return to full consciousness. Incentive spirometry encourages deep breathing and allows for the full expansion of alveoli. This breathing technique facilitates elimination of anesthetic gases from the body. QSEN: Safety.

Effective coughing clears the bronchial tree of secretions.

Splinting the incision eases the discomfort of coughing and taking deep breaths.

For the patient who received general anesthesia, the administration of oxygen promotes elimination of anesthetic gases.

■ = Independent ▲ = Interprofessional Collaboration

Risk for Deficient Fluid Volume

Common Risk Factors

Active fluid loss (blood loss in surgery; wound or tube drainage; nasogastric suctioning; vomiting)
Inadequate fluid intake (preoperative fluid restriction)

Common Expected Outcome

Patient is normovolemic, as evidenced by systolic BP greater than or equal to 90 mm Hg (or patient's baseline), HR of 60 to 100 beats/min, urine output greater than 30 mL/hr, and normal skin turgor.

NOC Outcomes

Fluid Balance; Hydration; Surgical Recovery: Immediate Post-Operative

NIC Interventions

Fluid Monitoring; Fluid Management; Fluid Resuscitation

Ongoing Assessment

Actions/Interventions	Rationales
■ Monitor and report any postoperative bleeding. Mark the extension of drainage from incisions.	Bleeding from an incision is usually from subcutaneous tissue; this is seen as increased bloody drainage on dressings. Outlining the stain on the surface of the dressing and indicating the time of the assessment allow staff to quantify the amount of drainage and severity of bleeding later.
■ Assess hydration status: • Monitor BP and HR. • Check mucous membranes, skin turgor, and thirst.	Hypotension or tachycardia may indicate fluid volume deficit. Increasing thirst and a coated tongue occur with fluid volume deficit. The patient may report a dry mouth. Tenting of the skin is associated with fluid volume deficit.
• Monitor urine output.	An output of 30 mL/hr or greater indicates adequate hydration.
• Monitor, record, and report output of emesis, nasogastric (NG) tube output, output from surgical drains (check for drainage around drains also), and incisional drainage.	Wound drainage, tube drainage, and emesis can be sources of fluid loss from the body.
▲ Monitor hemoglobin (Hgb), hematocrit (Hct), and coagulation profile.	Decreasing Hgb and Hct levels may indicate internal bleeding. Excessive postoperative bleeding may result from coagulopathy.

Therapeutic Interventions

Actions/Interventions	Rationales
▲ Administer IV fluids as ordered; be prepared to increase fluids if signs of fluid volume deficit appear.	IV fluids are administered to correct fluid volume deficit and maintain fluid balance postoperatively.
▲ Provide oral fluids of the patient's choice, as allowed.	Oral fluids are usually restricted until the patient is fully conscious, peristalsis returns, and the NG tube is removed, because swallowed fluids will be sucked out by the NG tube along with electrolytes; this puts the patient at risk for electrolyte imbalance, especially hypokalemia. However, patients may be allowed ice chips or small sips of clear fluids.
■ Provide oral hygiene every 4 hours.	NPO status and fluid volume deficit will cause a dry, sticky mouth. Oral care stimulates saliva secretion and relieves dry mouth.

Basic Nursing Concepts Care Plans

NDx Risk for Infection

Common Risk Factors

Inadequate primary defenses: altered skin integrity; smoking; stasis of body fluids
Inadequate secondary defenses: immunosuppression; leukopenia; suppressed inflammatory response
Insufficient knowledge to avoid exposure to pathogens
Malnutrition
Invasive procedures
Chronic disease

Common Expected Outcomes

Patient is free of infection, as evidenced by the following:
- Healing incision that is clean, dry, well approximated, and free of redness, swelling, purulent discharge, and pain
- Normal body temperature within 72 hours postoperatively
- IV sites free of redness and purulent drainage
- Clear breath sounds without productive cough

Infection is recognized early to allow for prompt treatment.

NOC Outcomes
Infection Severity; Risk Detection; Wound Healing: Primary Intention; Surgical Recovery: Immediate Post-Operative

NIC Interventions
Infection Control; Infection Protection; Tube Care; Wound Care; Wound Care: Closed Drainage

---

Ongoing Assessment

Actions/Interventions	Rationales
■ Assess the patient's health history for preexisting conditions such as obesity, diabetes mellitus, or smoking. Note the use of any drugs that cause immunosuppression such as corticosteroids.	Preexisting health problems and medication use can impair wound healing and decrease immune system activity necessary for the body's defense against infection. The obese patient is at risk for impaired wound healing and infection because of decreased vascularity of adipose tissue. Diabetes mellitus is known to predispose the patient to delayed wound healing and increased risk for infection. Smoking can contribute to impaired wound healing and risk for infection because of vasoconstriction from nicotine. QSEN: Safety.
■ Monitor temperature.	For the first 48 to 72 hours postoperatively, temperatures of up to 38.5°C (101.3°F) are expected as a normal stress response after major surgery. Beyond 72 hours, temperature should return to the patient's baseline. Temperature spikes, usually occurring in the later afternoon or night, are often indications of infection.
▲ Monitor white blood cell (WBC) counts.	An elevated WBC count is typically an indication of infection; however, in older patients, infection may be present without an increase in WBC count because of normal age-related changes in the immune system.

■ = Independent   ▲ = Interprofessional Collaboration

Basic Nursing Concepts Care Plans

Actions/Interventions	Rationales
■ Assess the incision and wound for redness, drainage, swelling, and increased pain:	Assessment of surgical wounds at regular intervals allows for early detection of changes that indicate infections. QSEN: Safety.
• Closed wounds or incisions	Incisions that have been closed with sutures or staples should be free of redness, swelling, and drainage. Some incisional discomfort is expected. These incisions are usually kept covered by a dry dressing for 24 to 48 hours; beyond 48 hours, there is no need for a dressing if the incision is not draining.
• Open wounds	Wounds left open to heal by secondary intention should appear pink/red and moist, and should have minimal serosanguineous drainage. These wounds are usually packed with sterile gauze moistened with sterile saline. Discomfort is expected on packing.
■ Assess all peripheral and central IV sites for redness, swelling, warmth, purulent drainage, and pain.	IV lines disrupt skin integrity and provide a potential portal of entry for pathogens into the circulatory system. Continual monitoring for signs of inflammation or infection is essential. QSEN: Safety.
■ Assess the color, clarity, and odor of urine.	Cloudy, foul-smelling urine is an indication of urinary tract infection, which can occur as the result of an indwelling catheter.
▲ Obtain specimens of wound drainage, sputum, blood, and urine in sterile containers.	Specimens are sent for analysis to determine if pathogens are present. The identification of pathogens guides clinical decisions about the selection of antimicrobial drugs. QSEN: Evidence-based practice.
■ Assess the quality of breath sounds, cough, and sputum production.	Adventitious breath sounds can indicate a respiratory infection.
■ Assess the stability of tubes and drains.	In-and-out motion of improperly secured tubes and drains allows access by pathogens through stab wounds where tubes and drains are placed.

Therapeutic Interventions

Actions/Interventions	Rationales
■ Wash hands before coming into contact with the postoperative patient.	Handwashing remains the most effective method of infection control. QSEN: Safety.
■ Use aseptic technique during dressing changes, wound care, or handling or manipulation of tubes and drains.	Aseptic technique for dressing changes and wound care limits the introduction of pathogens. QSEN: Safety.
■ Ensure that closed drainage systems (urinary catheter, surgical tubes and drains) are not inadvertently interrupted (opened). Irrigate tubes and drains only by physician prescription; use aseptic technique and a sterile irrigant.	The opening of sterile systems allows access for pathogens and puts the patient at risk for infection. QSEN: Safety.
■ Tape connectors and pin extensions or drainage tubing securely to the patient's gown. Prevent the kinking of drainage tubing.	Stabilizing and securing drainage tubing minimizes tension on tubes and connections. The kinking of tubing prevents the drainage of urine or wound exudate. Stasis contributes to the development of infection.
■ Provide aseptic site care to all peripheral and central venous access devices according to hospital policy.	Aseptic technique prevents transmission of pathogens. QSEN: Safety.
■ Provide care for indwelling urinary catheters according to hospital policy.	Frequent perineal hygiene reduces the number of pathogens around the urinary catheter entrance site.
■ Encourage adequate nutritional intake.	Adequate intake of protein, vitamins, and minerals is essential to promote immune system function and wound healing.

Actions/Interventions

- Educate the patient and family on the signs and symptoms of infection: elevated temperature, redness, swelling of the incisional area, and purulent or foul-smelling wound drainage.
▲ Administer antibiotics and antipyretics as prescribed.

Rationales

Educating the patient and family assists in early recognition of adverse signs and symptoms that may be indictors of infections. QSEN: Safety.

These drugs are used to treat infections and the fever usually associated with infection.

NDx Risk for Impaired Abdominal Wound Healing

Common Risk Factors

Preexisting conditions (e.g., diabetes, obesity, poor nutrition, previous wound dehiscence or evisceration)
Infection
Presence of seroma or hematoma
Increased intra-abdominal pressure
Mechanical force (e.g., stress, tension against wound)

Common Expected Outcome

Patient has an intact wound without complications such as dehiscence, evisceration, or fistula.

NOC Outcomes
Wound Healing: Primary Intention; Tissue Integrity: Skin and Mucous Membranes; Surgical Recovery: Immediate Post-Operative
NIC Interventions
Skin Surveillance; Wound Care; Positioning

Ongoing Assessment

Actions/Interventions

- Assess the wound for hematoma (collection of bloody drainage beneath the skin) or seroma (collection of serous fluid beneath the skin).
- Assess the condition of stitches or staples and retention sutures, if present; report any closures that appear to have loosened or fallen out.

Rationales

The presence of either type of fluid collection predisposes the wound to separation and infection.

Wound edges should remain approximated, without tension, puckering, or open gaps between stitches or staples. An incision is most vulnerable to injury during the first 48 hours, before wound strength begins to develop. Retention sutures (large sutures placed in addition to routine closures) are used when obesity, extreme abdominal distention, intra-abdominal infection, poor nutritional status, or a history of wound evisceration is present. Wound dehiscence (separation of the suture line or wound) occurs with excessive stress on a new incision. Obesity or improper techniques for mobility may add to stress on sutures and contribute to dehiscence. Wounds left open to heal by secondary intention are open only as deep as the subcutaneous tissue is deep; the fascia, muscle, and peritoneum have usually been closed. The deepest portion of the wound will come together, with the presence of tissue beneath being visible.

Basic Nursing Concepts
Care Plans

■ = Independent ▲ = Interprofessional Collaboration

Actions/Interventions	Rationales
■ Assess open wounds for evidence of evisceration (protrusion of abdominal contents).	Evisceration of a surgical wound is a serious complication. The wound should be covered immediately with a sterile dressing moistened with sterile normal saline. The patient is usually returned to the operating room for wound repair.
■ Assess wounds and dressings for suspicious drainage.	The presence of yellow, green, or brown fluid or material with an acrid or fecal odor indicates the presence of a fistula, an opening between some portion of the bowel and the incision or open wound.

Therapeutic Interventions

Actions/Interventions	Rationales
■ Prevent strain on the abdominal incision or wound:	These nursing actions reduce stress on an abdominal incision. Increased incisional stress increases the risk for impaired wound healing. QSEN: Safety.
• Keep the head of bed elevated 30 degrees.	Elevation relaxes abdominal muscles and reduces tension on the incision.
• Encourage the patient to splint the incision with a pillow or the hands before coughing.	Excessive coughing and straining of abdominal muscles and skin can predispose the wound to dehiscence.
• Educate the patient to splint the incision when transferring from the bed to a chair or when getting up to ambulate.	These activities may strain abdominal muscles and increase tension on a suture line. Supporting the area with a pillow or hands when moving reduces the risk for wound separation.
• Ensure proper functioning of the suction machine.	Malfunction of nasogastric suctioning can cause nausea, which may lead to retching and an increased strain on abdominal muscles.
▲ If dehiscence or evisceration occurs or is suspected (i.e., wound edges are separated or abdominal viscera are visible and protruding through the abdominal wound): • Place the patient in Fowler's position.	These nursing actions reduce the risk of harm to the patient. QSEN: Safety. Positioning promotes the relaxation of abdominal muscles and reduces strain on the incision.
• Cover the area with saline solution-soaked sterile gauze.	Keeping viscera moist increases viability.
• Notify the physician of the need for wound evaluation.	This situation usually requires a return to surgery for repair.
▲ If a fistula is suspected, protect the wound edges with petrolatum-based ointment or hydrocolloid.	Intestinal contents can be highly corrosive to skin, denuding it in a matter of hours; this causes pain and may interfere with later attempts to close or pouch the fistula.
▲ Consult with a wound care specialist.	A nurse with advanced education in wound care may provide specialized interventions for the management of incision complications. QSEN: Teamwork and collaboration.

NDx Risk for Deep Vein Thrombosis

Common Risk Factors

Prolonged time in operating room (OR)
Position in OR
Decreased postoperative activity
Dehydration

Common Expected Outcome

Patient remains free of thrombophlebitis and deep vein thrombosis (DVT), as evidenced by bilaterally equal calf circumference and absence of calf pain.

NOC Outcomes
Tissue Perfusion: Peripheral; Surgical Recovery: Immediate Post-Operative

NIC Intervention
Circulatory Care: Venous Insufficiency

Ongoing Assessment

Actions/Interventions	Rationales
■ Assess the legs for swelling.	Except for minor differences, the calves should have the same approximate circumference. Unilateral swelling could indicate thrombophlebitis or DVT.
■ Assess for changes in skin color, temperature, or vein distention in the legs.	Redness, warmth, and edema over a vein are associated with superficial thrombophlebitis. These changes increase the risk for DVT.
■ Assess for pain on compression of the calf or dorsiflexion of the foot (Homans' sign).	Homans' sign may be an indication of DVT. This assessment technique has limited reliability as an indicator of DVT. QSEN: Evidence-based practice.
■ Review the patient's medical record for information about the length of the surgical procedure and the positioning of the patient during surgery.	Prolonged immobility during the surgical procedure contributes to the pooling of blood, slowing of circulation, and thrombus formation. The patient remains in the same position throughout the surgical procedure. Sequential compression devices may be placed on the lower legs during surgery to prevent venous stasis.

Therapeutic Interventions

Actions/Interventions	Rationales
■ Reinforce or encourage leg exercises taught preoperatively; strive for 10 repetitions each hour until fully ambulatory.	Contracting the leg muscles decreases venous stasis and encourages venous return; both decrease the opportunity for thromboembolic developments.
▲ Use antiembolic stockings or sequential compression devices while the patient is in bed.	Both interventions promote venous blood flow and reduce venous stagnation.
■ Discourage gatching of the bed at the knee. Encourage the patient not to cross the legs at the knee or ankle while in bed.	Compression on veins contributes to venous pooling in the legs and decreased venous return. QSEN: Safety.
▲ Encourage ambulation by the patient as soon as possible, according to the physician's prescription.	Being upright is preferable to "dangling" or sitting in a chair because contracted muscles push against the leg vessels and improve venous return most effectively when the patient is upright and the legs are straight.
▲ Administer prophylactic anticoagulant therapy as prescribed.	Low-dose or low-molecular-weight heparin is used to prevent thrombus formation.
▲ Administer IV fluids; encourage oral fluid intake as prescribed.	Adequate hydration reduces hemoconcentration, and reduces the risk for DVT. QSEN: Safety.

Basic Nursing Concepts Care Plans

■ = Independent   ▲ = Interprofessional Collaboration

NANDA-I NDx Deficient Knowledge

Common Related Factors

Insufficient information about postoperative home care
Insufficient knowledge from lack of previous surgical experiences
Misinformation presented by others

Defining Characteristics

Insufficient knowledge
Inaccurate follow-through of instruction
Inaccurate performance on a test
Inappropriate behavior

Common Expected Outcome

Patient verbalizes understanding of and demonstrates ability to provide pain management, wound care, medication administration, advance diet as tolerated, limit activities as appropriate, recognize signs and symptoms of wound infection or other surgical complications, and return for follow-up care.

NOC Outcomes

Knowledge: Prescribed Diet; Knowledge: Treatment Regimen; Knowledge: Prescribed Activity; Surgical Recovery: Immediate Post-Operative

NIC Interventions

Teaching: Disease Process; Teaching: Prescribed Diet; Teaching: Prescribed Exercise; Teaching: Psychomotor Skill; Teaching: Prescribed Medication; Learning Facilitation

---

Ongoing Assessment

Actions/Interventions	Rationales
■ Assess the patient's ability to manage pain, perform wound care, verbalize appropriate activity, advance diet, and administer medications.	A teaching plan will be based on an assessment of the patient's ability to manage postoperative care at home. Shortened hospital stays and early discharges require that patients and families assume more responsibility for self-care during convalescence from surgery. QSEN: Patient-centered care.
■ Assess the patient's understanding of the need for further therapy, if necessary.	Diagnostic surgical procedures may require further therapy, such as chemotherapy, irradiation, immunotherapy, or additional surgery. Some patients may require physical therapy as part of postoperative recovery.
■ Assess the patient's understanding of the need for follow-up care.	Patients who leave the hospital with sutures, staples, or drains in place need to return for their removal or arrange to have a home health caregiver remove them.

Therapeutic Interventions

Actions/Interventions	Rationales
■ Teach the patient to perform appropriate wound care:	The information allows the patient and family members to be full participants in providing care at home after discharge. QSEN: Patient-centered care; Safety.
Closed incision:	
• Staples or sutures and dressings may be removed by the time of discharge, and Band-Aids or Steri-Strips placed on the incision.	Band-Aids or Steri-Strips maintain wound approximation and should be left in place until they fall off. In many situations the Band-Aids may be removed after 3 to 5 days.

Actions/Interventions

Open wounds:

- Wounds require twice-daily wet-to-dry saline solution packings until the wound has granulated enough to close.

■ Teach the patient about resuming activity related to the specific surgical procedure.

■ Teach the patient and family about resuming normal eating patterns.

■ Provide the patient and family with information about follow-up therapy.

■ Provide the patient and family with information about discharge medications.

■ Instruct the patient to seek medical attention for any of the following: unrelieved pain, fever, foul-smelling wound drainage, redness or unusual pain in any incision, and separation of wound edges.

Rationales

The primary purpose of a wet-to-dry dressing is to debride a wound mechanically. The moistened layer of the dressing increases the absorptive ability of the dressing to collect exudates and wound debris. As the dressing dries, it adheres to the wound and debrides the wound of the tissue when the dressing is removed.

The patient and family need specific written guidelines to make appropriate decisions about activities such as lifting, driving, bathing, exercise, and returning to work. Patients and families will need to balance activity and rest to promote effective wound healing and recovery.

Dietary restrictions will vary depending on the type of surgery and the return of peristalsis. A well-balanced diet is desirable for wound healing that continues over a period of weeks after surgery.

Patients and family members may need to schedule appointments for follow-up therapy and need to have specific contact information.

The patient and family need information about the actions of the drugs, possible side effects, and when and how to take them (e.g., analgesics, antibiotics).

For successful recovery, the patient and family must know how to identify problems, and what to do when they occur. QSEN: Safety.

Related Care Plans

Ineffective airway clearance, Chapter 2
Constipation, Chapter 2
Imbalanced nutrition: Less than body requirements,
    Chapter 2

Blood Component Therapy

Whole Blood; Packed Red Blood Cells (RBCs); Random Donor; Platelet Pheresis Packs; Platelets; Fresh Frozen Plasma; Albumin; Coagulation Factors; Autotransfusion

Blood component therapy is used in the management of a variety of clinical disorders. IV administration of blood and blood products is used to restore circulating volume and to replace the cellular components of the blood. Advances in medical technology have significantly improved the safety of blood transfusion therapy. Blood is commonly typed using the ABO system, the Rh system, and human leukocyte antigen found on tissue cells, blood leukocytes, and platelets. Today, specific blood component therapy has essentially replaced the practice of whole blood transfusions. Specific components may consist of packed RBCs, fresh frozen plasma, platelets, specific coagulation factors (e.g., cryoprecipitate, factors VIII and IX), volume expanders such as albumin and plasma protein fraction, and less commonly, granulocytes (WBCs). This use of blood components has expanded the availability of replacement therapy to more patients with reduced risk for side effects. Blood components can be modified in several ways to treat high-risk patients, such as stem cell transplant patients and severely immunocompromised chemotherapy patients.

Several types of transfusion options exist for blood component therapy. Homologous transfusions use blood products collected from random donors. Autologous transfusions use blood products donated by the patient for his or her own use. The blood is collected either by planned preprocedure donations that store blood until needed or by blood salvage, which collects, filters, and then returns the patient's blood that is lost during a surgical procedure or an acute trauma by use of an automatic "cell saver device." Directed transfusions use blood donations by one person that are directed to a specific recipient. Qualified nurses in the hospital, ambulatory care, and home setting can safely administer blood component therapy.

Basic Nursing Concepts Care Plans

NANDA-I NDx **Deficient Knowledge**

Common Related Factors
Unfamiliarity with transfusion process
Misinformation about risks for transfusion

Defining Characteristics
Questioning members of health care team
Verbalized misconceptions
Refusal to permit transfusion

Common Expected Outcomes
Patient or family verbalizes understanding of the need for a transfusion and the screening process performed before the transfusion begins.
Patient or family verbalizes understanding of the surveillance procedures required during the administration of blood components.

NOC Outcomes
Knowledge: Treatment Procedure; Anxiety Self-Control

NIC Interventions
Health Literacy Enhancement; Learning Facilitation; Teaching: Procedure/Treatment

---

Ongoing Assessment

Actions/Interventions	Rationales
■ Assess the patient's knowledge of the transfusion process.	Adults learn best when teaching builds on knowledge or experience.
■ Assess the patient's moral, ethical, and religious background as it relates to the administration of blood.	Informed, competent adult patients have the right to refuse any medical treatment. Some religions prohibit the transfusion of blood products. If a critical need for blood products arises in a patient with such prohibitions, there is a need for sensitive discussion, decision-making, and possible legal action, depending on individual clinical circumstances. Research and clinical trials of oxygen-carrying hemoglobin substitutes may offer alternatives to patients whose religious beliefs prevent the use of donor blood transfusions. Recombinant human erythropoietin injections (e.g., epoetin alfa) may be used before and after some surgeries to reduce the chance that blood transfusion would be needed. Newer surgical techniques can minimize blood loss with surgery. When these techniques are combined with infusion of volume expanders and iron, the patient will have a reduced need for blood component therapy. These approaches are appropriate for patients who refuse blood transfusions. QSEN: Patient-centered care.

Therapeutic Interventions

Actions/Interventions

■ Offer an explanation of precautionary measures used by the blood bank.

■ Explain the specific type of blood product to be transfused and the reason for infusion.

■ Acknowledge concerns. Provide factual information.

■ Explain the procedure for administering blood.

Rationales

Many patients are concerned about the safety of blood transfusions and the risk for disease caused by blood-borne pathogens. However, the blood supply is safer than it has ever been. Blood typing, crossmatching, and testing for various infectious agents are done routinely on all donated blood. All donor blood is quarantined until results of testing are known. This nursing action may reduce the patient's anxiety related to administration of blood products. QSEN: Patient-centered care.

Patients should understand the specific clinical conditions that are being treated and the results or improvements that are anticipated. They should also understand that transfusion administration time frames differ for individual blood components.

Blood transfusion is not without risk. Risks and benefits need to be addressed. Also, patients may have many misconceptions regarding the likelihood of disease transmission, especially that of human immunodeficiency virus (HIV).

Knowledge of routine procedures related to blood component therapy helps ensure that the patient is not concerned when vital signs are taken frequently.

NANDA-I NDx
Risk for Injury: Blood Transfusion Reaction

Common Risk Factors

Blood component transfusion therapy:
• Hemolytic reaction
• Allergic reaction
• Febrile transfusion reaction
• Circulatory overload

Common Expected Outcome

Patient receives blood components without reaction.

NOC Outcomes
Blood Coagulation; Circulation Status; Blood Transfusion Reaction
NIC Interventions
Blood Products Administration; Allergy Management; Shock Management; Emergency Care

---

Ongoing Assessment

Actions/Interventions

■ Assess for previous transfusions or reactions to blood products.

Rationales

The potential for reaction increases in patients who have been previously sensitized to an antigen through transfusion. The patient may require premedication with antihistamines and nonaspirin antipyretics to reduce the risk for an allergic or febrile transfusion reaction. QSEN: Patient-centered care.

■ = Independent ▲ = Interprofessional Collaboration

Actions/Interventions

■ Check for a signed consent form for blood transfusion.

■ Check that the component order is appropriate, that the volume order is within safe range, that the rate of infusion is appropriate, and that no other additives (e.g., medications) will be infused in the same tubing unless the tubing has been flushed clear with normal saline solution.

■ Assess the adequacy and patency of venous access.

■ Follow institutional protocols for confirming the blood product, ABO and Rh compatibility, patient identification, and expiration date.

■ Take vital signs before therapy begins, then 15 minutes later. Follow facility policies and procedures thereafter for frequency. At minimum, assess vital signs every hour until infused. Remain with the patient for the first 15 minutes.

■ Assess for signs and symptoms of a reaction to the blood product:

• Hemolytic reaction: chills, fever, low back pain, rapid thready pulse, tachypnea, hypotension, bleeding (especially hematuria), oppressive feeling, and acute renal failure

• Allergic reaction: flushing, itching, hives, wheezing, laryngeal edema, and anaphylaxis

• Febrile nonhemolytic reaction: sudden chills and fever, headache, flushing, and anxiety

• Circulatory overload: dyspnea, cough, distended neck veins, increased BP, rapid bounding pulse, and crackles heard on pulmonary auscultation

Rationales

A signed consent form ensures that the patient has received information about the benefits and risks associated with blood component therapy. QSEN: Safety.

The patient's cardiopulmonary status must be considered when determining the rate of infusion. This is especially important in older patients, and in those with cardiac and renal impairments to reduce the risk for circulatory overload. QSEN: Patient-centered care; Safety.

An IV cannula no smaller than 19 gauge will accommodate most blood components. Smaller gauges can be used for platelets, albumen, and clotting factors. A larger gauge IV cannula may be required if rapid infusion is indicated.

This nursing action is part of The Joint Commission's National Patient Safety Goals regarding blood transfusion. Discrepancies must be resolved before the product is administered. Mismatches account for the majority of transfusion reactions. Most institutions have written protocols for verifying the compatibility of the blood product for the patient. These protocols include two people verifying the blood product before it leaves the blood bank and again at the bedside before the transfusion is initiated. QSEN: Evidence-based practice; Safety.

This first set of vital signs provides a baseline for comparison during the transfusion. Most reactions occur early during administration and are associated with changes in vital signs. These changes may include hypotension, tachycardia, tachypnea, and fever. Preexisting fever may cause a delay in the transfusion procedure.

Transfusion therapy is not without hazard. Early identification of reactions allows for prompt therapy to be initiated. QSEN: Safety.

Hemolytic reaction is the most serious reaction and is potentially life threatening. It is caused by infusion of incompatible blood products. Some are due to naturally occurring antibodies in the ABO antigen system. Reaction may be immediate or delayed. Delayed reactions usually occur in patients who have been previously sensitized to an antigen through transfusion or pregnancy.

Allergic reactions are caused by sensitivity to plasma protein or a donor antibody that reacts with a recipient antigen. Prompt identification of this type of reaction is necessary to reduce the risk for the reaction progressing to anaphylaxis.

This common transfusion reaction is caused by hypersensitivity to donor WBCs, platelets, or plasma proteins. Use of a leukocyte-reduced product (filtered, washed or frozen) when transfusing blood products to a person with a history of such reactions or who is immunosuppressed may reduce or prevent febrile nonhemolytic reactions.

Circulatory overload occurs when fluid is administered at a rate or volume greater than the circulatory system can manage. This is especially common in older patients or those with cardiac or renal impairment.

Therapeutic Interventions

Actions/Interventions	Rationales
■ Follow institutional policy for obtaining blood products from the blood bank.	Patient safety is a priority. Infusion of the blood product should begin within 30 minutes of receipt of the blood from the blood bank. If there is a delay, the blood must be returned to the blood bank for adequate refrigeration (check institutional policy for any restrictions on returning products). However, blood unrefrigerated for more than 30 minutes cannot be returned. QSEN: Safety.
■ Prime blood tubing with normal saline solution, and connect it to the patient's IV access.	Normal saline is used as a standby for infusion when the blood transfusion is completed or if a reaction occurs. Lactated Ringer's or dextrose solution may induce clotting or hemolysis of RBCs.
▲ Premedicate with prescribed antipyretics, antihistamines, or steroids any patient who has received frequent previous transfusions or who is immunocompromised.	These patients have been sensitized to donor WBC antigens and may experience febrile transfusion reactions if not premedicated. Ensure that an emergency drug kit is available when in the home setting. QSEN: Safety.
▲ Maintain an appropriate infusion rate. Increase the rate as the patient's condition warrants.	Infusion should begin at a slow rate for the first 15 to 20 minutes to monitor for a possible reaction. One unit of packed RBCs can usually be infused over 2 hours, unless the patient is at risk for fluid overload, has cardiopulmonary disease, or is elderly. Blood not infused within 4 hours should be discontinued and returned to the blood bank, as it is at risk of bacterial growth once not refrigerated. QSEN: Safety.
▲ If any type of reaction occurs, stop the transfusion immediately and remove attached tubing. Keep the IV access open with 0.9% sodium chloride (normal saline) solution, and notify the physician and blood bank. Anticipate notifying the Rapid Response Team as needed.	Immediate discontinuation of the transfusion reduces the patient's risk for developing a life-threatening reaction. The Rapid Response Team is a group of health care providers who can be summoned to the bedside to immediately assess and treat the patient with the goal of preventing intensive care unit transfer, cardiac arrest, or death. QSEN: Safety; Teamwork and collaboration.
▲ *For acute hemolytic reaction:*	A hemolytic reaction is usually caused by ABO-incompatible blood or components that are mistakenly given to the patient. It can begin within 15 minutes of infusion. QSEN: Safety.
• Be prepared to treat shock.	Shock is a potentially life-threatening reaction.
• Maintain BP with IV colloids.	Fluid resuscitation is needed to maintain circulatory volume.
• Monitor urine output.	A decreased urine volume indicates hypovolemia and possible shock. Acute renal failure may occur as free hemoglobin obstructs the renal tubules.
• Draw blood samples for serologic testing and collect a urine sample.	Blood sampling permits repeat typing and crossmatch to examine compatibility. Hemolysis of RBCs causes free Hgb to be released into the plasma, which is later filtered by the kidneys and released into the urine. Urine is tested for the presence of RBCs.
• Anticipate a possible transfer to the critical care unit and the initiation of dialysis if renal failure develops.	Specialized care is needed to support the patient's recovery and prevent more serious complications. This type of transfusion reaction may progress to acute renal failure or disseminated intravascular coagulation (DIC).
• Return the blood product and administration tubing to the blood bank.	Testing will be done to reexamine the compatibility of the product and the recipient.

Basic Nursing Concepts Care Plans

■ = Independent ▲ = Interprofessional Collaboration

Nursing Concepts / Care Plans*

Actions/Interventions

▲ *For allergic reaction:*

- Give antihistamines as prescribed.
- Anticipate the need for vasoconstriction medications (e.g., epinephrine) and corticosteroids.
- For severe reactions, anticipate the need for intubation.

▲ *For febrile, nonhemolytic reaction:*

- Give antihistamines as prescribed.

- Give antipyretics as prescribed.
- Send a blood sample, the blood bag, and a urine sample to the laboratory.

▲ *For circulatory overload:*

- Keep the patient in high-Fowler's (upright) position.

- Administer diuretics, oxygen, and morphine, as prescribed.
- Insert a Foley catheter.
- Anticipate a transfer to the critical care unit if pulmonary edema is severe.

Rationales

This reaction is common in patients with a history of allergies and sensitivity to foreign plasma proteins. QSEN: Safety.
These drugs decrease the patient's hypersensitivity response.
Emergency treatment may be needed if severe respiratory distress, hypotension, or shock is present.
Aggressive respiratory measures may be required to maintain an airway.
This reaction occurs because of the recipient's sensitization to the donor's WBCs, platelets, or plasma. QSEN: Safety.
These drugs suppress the inflammatory response in this type of reaction.
These drugs reduce fever and promote patient comfort.
Follow-up testing will be done.

Fluid overload is seen in older patients and in those with cardiac and renal impairment. QSEN: Safety.
This position promotes effective breathing and gas exchange by pooling excess fluid in dependent parts of the body.
These measures promote fluid balance and effective gas exchange.
This measure allows for frequent monitoring of urine output.
Specialized care is required to support the patient's recovery and reduce complications.

Central Venous Access Devices

Implantable Ports; Peripherally Inserted Central Catheter; Tunneled and Nontunneled Catheters

Central venous access devices are indwelling catheters placed in large vessels using a variety of approaches. These catheters or devices are indicated for total parenteral nutrition; blood administration; intermittent or continuous medication administration, especially long-term antibiotics, vesicant agents, or chemotherapy; multiple blood draws; parenteral fluids; and long-term venous access. Central venous access devices are beneficial for patients who receive IV therapies that require the hemodilution from the blood flow in large central veins. Patients with limited peripheral venous access also benefit from placement of a central venous access device for IV therapy and blood draws. These types of access are encountered not only in the hospital, but also in the ambulatory care and home setting. Selection of the appropriate device for venous access depends on the age and size of the patient, the availability of access sites, and the anticipated length of use for the device. Types of devices include the following: nontunneled (or percutaneous) central venous catheter (CVC) suitable for short-term use (typically days or weeks), inserted via the subclavian vein; peripherally inserted central catheters (PICC lines) used for intermediate-length therapy (3 to 12 months) that are inserted via the basilic or cephalic vein into the superior

vena cava; tunneled catheters that can remain in place for several years or more, surgically implanted within a subcutaneous tunnel with an external access on the upper chest; and an implanted infusion port, also used for long-term management (most commonly chemotherapy), that has a catheter attached to a reservoir surgically implanted in a subcutaneous pocket, thereby avoiding an external catheter and its long-term maintenance. Each catheter has specific requirements for flushing, heparinization, and dressing changes.

Mechanical problems (lumen occlusion, migration, dislodgement) and central line–associated bloodstream infections (CLABSI) are serious complications related to the use of these catheters/ports. According to The Joint Commission, central venous catheters are the most frequent cause of health care–associated bloodstream infections. The catheters can be colonized with microorganisms either extraluminally during catheter insertion or intraluminally during ongoing contact and manipulation with the catheter connector or hub, or from contamination of fluid during administration. The Joint Commission and the Institute for Healthcare Improvement provide evidence-based practices and a prevention bundle aimed at reducing these risks.

NANDA-I NDx Risk for Injury: Impaired Catheter Function

Common Risk Factors

Mechanical impairment (e.g., clotting of catheter)
Catheter break, migration, and/or pinch-off syndrome

Common Expected Outcome

Patient's catheter function is maintained, as evidenced by patency with acceptable two-way function (inflow and outflow).

NOC Outcomes
Risk Detection; Risk Control
NIC Interventions
Central Venous Access Device Management; Peripherally Inserted Central Catheter (PICC) Care

---

Ongoing Assessment

Actions/Interventions	Rationales
■ Inspect for catheter integrity:	Early assessment facilitates prompt intervention and reduces complications. QSEN: Safety.
• Verify the type of catheter inserted, its length, and the location of the tip.	This assessment can be done by review of documentation in the patient's medical record, and confirmation by chest x-ray study. Newer catheters may utilize magnet tip locators or electrocardiogram verification.
• Check for patency. Observe gravitational flow (e.g., in transfusion of blood products).	Catheter patency is confirmed by the ability to run an infusion, withdraw blood, or flush the catheter without resistance.
• Observe for kinks; note any leakage.	Kinks will compromise the integrity of the system. Fluid leaking from insertion site can signal catheter rupture.
• Check the patency of the implantable port with a Huber needle.	Implanted ports need to be flushed after each use and at least monthly to maintain patency. Huber noncoring needles are designed with a deflected bevel point to preserve the integrity of the port during access.

Therapeutic Interventions

Actions/Interventions	Rationales
■ Flush the catheter according to established institutional policy and procedure and manufacturer's guidelines. In general the catheter is flushed at the end of every blood-drawing procedure, at the completion of each IV solution and blood product, and before capping the catheter.	Flushing prevents the catheter from clotting. Each catheter has specific requirements for routine flushing. This may include flushing with saline, heparin, or a routine flush with a thrombolytic enzyme such as alteplase. Single-use flushing systems should be used, ideally with a 10-mL syringe.
■ Avoid administering incompatible solutions and medications.	Infusion of incompatible solutions may cause precipitation within the catheter and eventual obstruction. The nurse consults drug and solution compatibility charts before administration. The nurse can consult with the pharmacist, if the charts do not provide sufficiently clear compatibility information. QSEN: Safety; Teamwork and collaboration.
■ Use mechanical IV pumps.	Infusion pumps prevent "dry" IVs and backing up of blood into the catheter. Appropriate use of safety-enhancing technology minimizes the risk of harm to the patient from clotting of the catheter. QSEN: Safety.
■ Avoid BP measurements in the arm with the PICC.	Even short-term compression might compromise blood flow and damage the catheter.

■ = Independent   ▲ = Interprofessional Collaboration

Basic Nursing Concepts Care Plans

Actions/Interventions

- Avoid the use of scissors around the device (especially when changing the dressing); use noncrushing clamps and hemostats when needed.
- ▲ Troubleshoot the catheter and port for common problems (e.g., sluggish inflow, inability to draw blood).

  - Alternate irrigation and aspiration of the catheter using a normal saline solution in a large syringe (at least 10 mL or more). Do not force if resistance is felt.
  - Obtain a prescription for the use of a thrombolytic enzyme such as alteplase or alternative agent for the clearance of an occluded catheter or port if other measures to restore catheter function are unsuccessful.
- Repair external catheter damage according to the manufacturer's recommendations or established procedures.
- Notify the physician of suspected internal catheter damage.

Rationales

Precautions are needed to prevent catheter damage. QSEN: Safety.

These nursing actions maintain function of the catheter and reduce harm to the patient when a nonfunctioning catheter must be replaced. QSEN: Safety.

Gentle irrigation of the catheter with a larger syringe (at least 10 mL) may dislodge small obstructions. Smaller syringes generate too much pressure that can rupture a catheter.

Clots and precipitates in central venous access device are a relatively frequent complication. Alteplase is used to dissolve blood clots, and hydrochloric acid or sodium bicarbonate can be used to remove drug precipitates.

Specially trained nurses familiar with a variety of catheter types should be available to assist as needed (e.g., chemotherapy specialists, nutritional support staff).

Catheter replacement may be indicated.

NANDA-I
NDx Risk for Infection

Common Risk Factors
Indwelling catheter
Manipulation of catheter connecting tubing
Prolonged use of catheter
Neutropenic patient

Common Expected Outcome
Patient is free of infection, as evidenced by normal temperature and no signs of redness, warmth, or drainage at catheter/port site.

NOC Outcomes
Immune Status; Risk Detection; Risk Control

NIC Interventions
Intravenous (IV) Therapy; Central Venous Access Device Management; Peripherally Inserted Central Catheter (PICC) Care

---

Ongoing Assessment

Actions/Interventions

- Check the catheter/port site for signs of infection.

- Assess for fever and chills as needed.

Rationales

Redness, warmth, tenderness, and "streaking" over the subcutaneous tunnel and exudate from the exit or portal pocket or needle insertion site are signs of infection.

An infection within the bloodstream may occur without any indication of a skin infection. Elevated temperature above 38.3°C (101°F) may be related to bacteremia from the central venous catheter.

Basic Nursing Concepts Care Plans

Therapeutic Interventions

Actions/Interventions	Rationales
■ Follow the CLABSI prevention bundle during insertion. Some of the key measures include: • Using an insertion checklist to improve adherence to best practices. • Appropriate hand hygiene • Aseptic technique; chlorhexidine for skin disinfection • Maximal sterile barrier precautions • Sterile gowning, gloving, and masking by person inserting catheter; mask by others in room • Use of preferred insertion sites; avoid use of femoral site in adult patients • Ideally insertion performed under ultrasound guidance to ensure higher rate of success at first-attempt insertions • Use of appropriate catheter securement devices	The interprofessional health care team is responsible for ensuring that the evidence-based guidelines are followed. The Joint Commission emphasizes that the provider's skill during catheter insertion is a key component of patient safety and prevention of CLABSI. QSEN: Safety; Evidence-based practice; Teamwork and collaboration.
■ Follow the CLABSI postinsertion bundle for maintenance care using aseptic technique: • Disinfection of catheter hubs, connectors, and injection ports • Changing IV solutions, tubing, adapters, or caps • Drawing blood; accessing and de-accessing the port • Flushing and heparinizing the catheter • Performing site care using aseptic technique; chlorhexidine preparation with alcohol most commonly used • Changing dressings over the site every 2 days for gauze dressings or every 5 to 7 days for semipermeable dressings; change any dressing that becomes wet or soiled • Ongoing review for necessity of the central line device	Only health care personnel who have attained and maintained competency should access and maintain these catheters/ports. Strict adherence to evidence-based catheter care procedures reduces the possibility of contamination. The antiseptic used for care at the insertion site should be compatible with the catheter material. Each catheter manufacturer provides information about the appropriate antiseptic for their catheter. Transparent dressings such a Tegaderm are used to cover most catheter insertion sites. QSEN: Safety; Evidence-based practice.
▲ If infection is suspected, notify the physician for culturing, treatment, and possible catheter removal.	Aggressive treatment is indicated to prevent the spread of infection. If the catheter is removed, the tip may be sent to the laboratory for testing. QSEN: Safety. If patient is being treated at home, he or she will be admitted to the hospital for IV antibiotic therapy.

Basic Nursing Concepts Care Plans

NANDA-I NDx Deficient Knowledge

Common Related Factors
Insufficient information
Insufficient interest in learning
Misinformation presented by others

Defining Characteristics
Insufficient knowledge
Inaccurate follow-through of instruction

Common Expected Outcomes
Patient verbalizes reasons venous access device has been inserted and common complications associated with it.
In home care setting, caregiver demonstrates correct technique in caring for venous access device.

NOC Outcome
Knowledge: Treatment Procedure
NIC Interventions
Health Literacy Enhancement; Teaching: Procedure/Treatment; Learning Facilitation; Teaching: Psychomotor Skill

■ = Independent   ▲ = Interprofessional Collaboration

Ongoing Assessment

Actions/Interventions

- Assess the patient and caregiver's understanding of:
  - Indications for venous access devices
  - Type of catheter to be used
  - The therapy required
  - Alternatives to the catheter and therapy
  - Hand hygiene and aseptic technique
  - Activity limitations
  - Potential complications to be reported
  - Dressing changes and catheter care
- Assess the patient and caregiver's skill in managing the central venous access device.

- Assess the financial and environmental resources for maintaining equipment and supplies in the home.

Rationales

The Joint Commission includes patient education on these topics as part of the prevention bundle for CLABSI. Assessment provides the starting point for ongoing education. QSEN: Patient-centered care; Evidence-based practice.

Assessment provides the basis for education. This skill can be assessed first in the hospital setting, then again in the home environment by the home health nurse.

Many patients require long-term therapy, which can be costly. Support and resources may be available to reduce stressors.

Therapeutic Interventions

Actions/Interventions

- Instruct the patient and caregiver regarding the importance of and process for maintaining and reordering necessary equipment and supplies (e.g., needles, syringes, tubing, solution bags, pumps) for catheter care and infusion treatment.

- Instruct the patient and caregiver regarding the following:

  - Importance of hand washing and aseptic technique

  - Dressing changes; IV tubing changes

  - Injection cap changes

  - Keeping ports capped and clamped
  - Site care
  - Flushes
- Instruct the patient and caregiver in how to start and discontinue IV therapy as prescribed.
- Instruct the patient regarding the signs of phlebitis and site infection, and to whom to report these signs.
- Inform the patient and caregiver how to notify the home health nurse in case any problems occur.
- Instruct the patient and caregiver to maintain a catheter repair kit at home for use by the home health nurse, as indicated.

Rationales

The patient and caregivers will be responsible for maintaining the correct function of the device and preventing complications associated with long-term IV therapy. QSEN: Patient-centered care.

Attention to these instructions reduces the risk of harm to the patient. QSEN: Safety.

Hand washing is the most effective method of reducing contamination by touch during catheter care.

Frequency and technique will vary depending on the catheter type and whether it is used intermittently or continuously.

These changes are usually performed by the home health nurse in the home and the IV therapy nurse in the hospital.

This procedure prevents air embolus.

Site care prevents infection.

Flushes maintain patency.

A successful treatment plan requires the support and cooperation of the patient and caregiver.

Early assessment facilitates prompt intervention and reduces complications. QSEN: Safety.

Many problems can be handled by telephone triage.

Patient safety is a priority. Prompt repair to a damaged external catheter segment can avoid catheter replacement. QSEN: Safety.

Parenteral Nutrition

Intravenous (IV) Hyperalimentation, Central Vein Parenteral Nutrition; Peripheral Vein
Parenteral Nutrition

Parenteral nutrition (PN) is the administration of nutrients via a central vein or a large peripheral vein. PN therapy is necessary when the gastrointestinal (GI) tract cannot be used or when oral intake is not sufficient to meet the patient's nutritional needs. PN solutions are hypertonic and may contain 20% to 50% glucose and 3.5% to 10% protein (in the form of amino acids), 10% to 30% fat emulsion, electrolytes, vitamins, minerals, and trace elements. These solutions can be modified, depending on the presence of organ system impairment or the specific nutritional needs of the patient. The patient's fluid and electrolyte status requires frequent monitoring while receiving PN. Central vein solutions are usually more hypertonic than peripheral vein solutions. The solution for peripheral vein administration may contain only 10% to 20% glucose. A solution with higher tonicity is more likely to cause phlebitis when infused through a large peripheral vein. PN is often used in hospital, long-term, and subacute care, but it is also used in the home care setting. This care plan addresses nursing care needs that may occur in any of these settings.

NANDA-I NDx Imbalanced Nutrition: Less Than Body Requirements

Common Related Factors
Inability to ingest foods
Inability to digest foods
Inability to absorb nutrients
Biological factors
Psychological disorders
Insufficient dietary intake

Defining Characteristics
Weight loss with adequate food intake
Body weight 20% or more below ideal weight range
Food intake less than recommended dietary allowance (RDA)
Excessive hair loss
Pale mucous membranes
Insufficient interest in food
Sore buccal cavity
Weakness of muscles needed for mastication and/or swallowing

Common Expected Outcome
Patient achieves an adequate nutritional status, as evidenced by weight within 10% of ideal weight range and by improved serum albumin levels.

NOC Outcome
Nutritional Status: Nutrient Intake
NIC Interventions
Nutritional Monitoring; Nutrition Intake; Total Parenteral Nutrition (TPN) Administration

Basic Nursing Concepts
Care Plans

■ = Independent ▲ = Interprofessional Collaboration

Ongoing Assessment

Actions/Interventions	Rationales
■ Obtain an accurate intake and output, and daily weights and calorie counts, including calories provided by PN.	The composition of PN is based on the individual's calculated needs. An interprofessional team will complete a comprehensive baseline assessment before initiating a PN infusion. Team members may include physicians, nurses, dietitians, and pharmacists. Changes in fluid balance, weight, and caloric intake are used to monitor the effectiveness of PN. Daily weights are necessary to determine if nutritional goals are being met. Weight is also used to assess fluid volume status. Weight gain of more than $\frac{1}{2}$ pound per day may indicate fluid retention. QSEN: Patient-centered care; Teamwork and collaboration.
■ Assess wound healing and skin integrity.	Delayed wound healing may indicate a need for PN. Changes in skin integrity and wound healing will be used to monitor PN effectiveness.

Therapeutic Interventions

Actions/Interventions	Rationales
▲ Assist with the insertion and maintenance of central venous or peripherally inserted central catheter (PICC) or an intravenous catheter inserted in a large peripheral vein.	The osmolality of PN solutions requires infusion into a large central or peripheral vein with high-volume blood flow. The tip of a central vein catheter is usually placed in the superior vena cava. X-ray confirmation of accurate catheter placement is necessary before central vein PN administration is initiated. Normal saline or other isotonic solutions may be infused through the central catheter until placement is confirmed.
▲ Administer the prescribed rate of PN solution via an infusion pump.	Giving PN at the prescribed rate is necessary to meet nutritional needs and prevent complications. Electronic infusion pumps are usually used to control the accuracy of the infusion rate. Falling behind on PN administration deprives the patient of needed nutrition; boluses (or too-rapid administration) can precipitate a hyperglycemic crisis because the hormonal response (i.e., insulin) may not be available to allow use of the increased glucose load. QSEN: Safety.
■ Assist with or encourage oral intake, if indicated.	Patients may be fed orally in addition to PN to maximize nutritional support. Patients may benefit psychologically from having oral intake, especially at shared mealtimes with family members.
▲ Collaborate with appropriate members of the interprofessional health care team: nutritional support team, dietitian, pharmacy, home health nurse.	When an experienced nutritional support team supervises administration of parenteral nutrition, nutritional outcomes for the patient are achieved and the risk for most complications is decreased for the hospitalized patient. QSEN: Teamwork and collaboration.

NANDA-I NDx Risk for Deficient Fluid Volume

Common Risk Factors

Hyperglycemia

Inability to respond to thirst mechanisms because of NPO status

Low serum protein level

Common Expected Outcome

Patient is normovolemic as evidenced by systolic BP greater than or equal to 90 mm Hg (or patient's baseline), absence of orthostasis, HR 60 to 100 beats/min, urine output greater than 30 mL/hr, and normal skin turgor.

NOC Outcome
Fluid Balance
NIC Interventions
Fluid Monitoring; Total Parenteral Nutrition (TPN) Administration

Ongoing Assessment

Actions/Interventions	Rationales
■ Assess for the signs and symptoms of fluid volume deficit:	Early identification of changes in fluid balance facilitates prompt interventions. QSEN: Safety.
• Decreased BP	Fluid volume deficit decreases circulatory volume and contributes to a decreased BP.
• Increased HR	A compensatory increase in HR occurs with fluid volume deficit.
• Skin changes	Decreased fluid volume causes dry skin with loss of turgor.
• High urine specific gravity	Urine becomes more concentrated with a decrease in fluid volume.
■ Monitor urine output.	Urine output consistently lower than fluid intake indicates fluid volume deficit and the need for additional fluid to prevent dehydration.
▲ Monitor blood glucose levels at regular intervals according to agency policy.	Hyperglycemia, caused by infusion of a high concentration of glucose in the PN solution, can lead to hyperosmolar, nonketotic coma with subsequent dehydration secondary to osmotic diuresis. A typical schedule for measuring capillary blood glucose is every 6 hours while the patient is receiving PN solution.
▲ Monitor serum protein levels according to agency protocol, usually every 3 to 7 days.	Low serum protein level may lead to a loss of fluids from intravascular spaces, secondary to low colloidal pressures.
■ During the first week of PN administration, weigh the patient daily and record weight; weigh weekly thereafter.	Daily weights are necessary to determine if nutritional goals are being met. Weight is also used to assess fluid volume status. A weight loss of more than ½ pound per day may indicate fluid volume deficit.

Therapeutic Interventions

Actions/Interventions	Rationales
▲ Administer PN at the prescribed, constant rate; if the infusion is interrupted, infuse 10% dextrose in water until the PN infusion is restarted.	This substitute infusion provides needed fluid in addition to protecting the patient from sudden hypoglycemia; hypoglycemia can result when the high glucose concentration to which the patient has metabolically adjusted is suddenly withdrawn.

■ = Independent ▲ = Interprofessional Collaboration

Basic Nursing Concepts Care Plans

Actions/Interventions

- Keep the infusion pump alarms on.

▲ Encourage the oral intake of fluids unless contraindicated. Administer maintenance or bolus fluids as prescribed, in addition to PN.

Rationales

Any interruption in the flow of solution is noted early when alarms sound. QSEN: Safety.

Patients who are NPO and only receiving PN may not be receiving adequate amounts of fluids, especially because PN is initiated in low administration rates; therefore additional fluids may be required.

NANDA-I NDx Risk for Excess Fluid Volume

Common Risk Factors

Overinfusion of PN solution
Inability to tolerate increased vascular load

Common Expected Outcome

Patient is normovolemic as evidenced by urine output greater than or equal to 30 mL/hr, balanced intake and output, stable weight (or loss attributed to fluid loss), absence or reduction of edema, HR 60 to 100 beats/min, and absence of pulmonary crackles.

NOC Outcomes
Fluid Balance; Cardiopulmonary Status

NIC Interventions
Fluid Monitoring; Total Parenteral Nutrition (TPN) Administration

---

Ongoing Assessment

Actions/Interventions

- Assess for the signs and symptoms of fluid volume excess:

  • Edema

  • Shortness of breath and crackles

  • Jugular venous distention

▲ Monitor the patient's serum sodium level.

Rationales

Early identification of changes in fluid balance facilitates prompt interventions. QSEN: Safety.

Edema occurs when fluid accumulates in the extravascular spaces. Edema usually begins in the fingers, facial area, and presacral area. Generalized edema, called *anasarca*, occurs later and involves the entire body. A weight gain of more than $\frac{1}{2}$ pound per day is an indication of fluid volume excess.

These respiratory changes are caused by the accumulation of fluid in the lungs.

Elevated central venous pressure is noticed first as distention of the jugular veins.

Hypernatremia may cause or aggravate edema by holding fluid in the extravascular spaces.

Therapeutic Interventions

Actions/Interventions

- Keep the infusion pump alarms on.

▲ If signs and symptoms of fluid volume excess occur, administer diuretics as prescribed.

- Position the patient in a semi-Fowler's or high-Fowler's position.

- Handle edematous extremities with caution.

Rationales

Any change or interruption in the flow of solution is noted early when alarms sound. QSEN: Safety.

Diuretics aid in the excretion of excess body fluids. Diuretic therapy may include several different types of agents for optimal therapy, depending on the acuteness or chronicity of the patient's problem.

Elevating the head of the bed allows for ease in breathing. This position promotes pooling of fluid in the bases of the lungs and makes more lung tissue available for gas exchange.

Edematous skin is more susceptible to injury and breakdown. QSEN: Safety.

ⓔvolve **For additional care plans, go to http://evolve.elsevier.com/Gulanick/.**

Basic Nursing Concepts Care Plans

NDx Risk for Altered Body Composition

Common Risk Factors

Electrolyte imbalances:
- Hypokalemia (K less than 3.5 mEq/L)
- Hyponatremia (Na less than 115 mEq/L)
- Hypocalcemia (Ca less than 6.8 mg/dL)
- Hypomagnesemia (Mg less than 1.5 mg/dL)
- Hypophosphatemia (PO_4 less than 2.5 mg/dL)

Essential fatty acid deficiency (EFAD)
Hyperglycemia (glucose greater than 200 mg/dL)
Hypoglycemia (glucose less than 60 mg/dL)

Common Expected Outcomes

Patient maintains normal serum electrolyte levels.
Patient maintains normal blood glucose level.

NOC Outcome
Electrolyte and Acid/Base Balance
NIC Intervention
Electrolyte Monitoring

Ongoing Assessment

Actions/Interventions

▲ Assess for the signs and symptoms of electrolyte imbalance:

Hypokalemia
- Alteration in muscle function (e.g., weakness, cramping)
- Electrocardiogram changes (e.g., ventricular dysrhythmias, ST-segment depression, or U wave)
- Changes in level of consciousness (e.g., confusion, lethargy)
- Abdominal distention and loss of bowel sounds

Hyponatremia
- Decreased skin turgor, weakness, tremors or seizures, lethargy, confusion, nausea, vomiting

Hypocalcemia
- Paresthesias, tetany, seizures, positive Chvostek's sign, irregular HR

Hypomagnesemia
- Muscle weakness, cramping, twitching, tetany, seizures, irregular HR

Hypophosphatemia
- Muscle weakness, changes in level of consciousness

■ Assess for signs and symptoms of essential fatty acid deficiency:

- Tendency to bruise and thrombocytopenia

- Dry, scaly skin
- Poor wound healing

Rationales

When patients are receiving PN and no other nutrition, there is a risk, especially early in PN therapy, that all electrolyte needs may not be met. As the physiological condition changes, patients may have altered needs for electrolytes and will require an adjustment of the PN solution. Patients who have had prolonged periods of protein-calorie malnutrition are at risk for developing refeeding syndrome. This syndrome develops as a result of metabolic shifts when the patient begins receiving higher carbohydrate loads with PN. The primary manifestation of refeeding syndrome is hypophosphatemia. The complications associated with refeeding syndrome include rhabdomyolysis, dysrhythmias, seizures, coma, and sudden death. QSEN: Evidence-based practice.

Basic PN solutions contain no fat; fat is a nutritional requirement that allows essential fat-soluble vitamins A, D, E, and K to be absorbed. Patients commonly receive fat emulsions as part of PN solutions, or as a separate infusion.

These findings are caused by coagulopathy secondary to inadequate vitamin K levels.

This change relates to vitamin D and E deficiencies.
This change relates to vitamin A and E deficiencies.

■ = Independent ▲ = Interprofessional Collaboration

Basic Nursing Concepts
Care Plans

Actions/Interventions

▲ Monitor the patient's serum triglyceride level.

■ For patients receiving fat emulsions, monitor for the signs and symptoms of fat embolism (dyspnea, cyanosis, headache, flushing).

▲ Assess for hyperglycemia or hypoglycemia:

Hypoglycemia
- Glucose level less than 60 mg/dL
- Weakness, agitation, clammy skin, tremors

Hyperglycemia
- Glucose level greater than 200 mg/dL
- Glycosuria
- Thirst, polyuria, confusion

Rationales

Patients receiving an IV fat emulsion should have their serum triglyceride monitored any time changes are made in the amount of fat administered.

Fat embolism is a rare but serious complication of fat emulsion infusion.

Signs of hyperglycemia are most likely to be seen on initiation of PN. Signs of hypoglycemia are most likely to be seen when PN infusion rates are decreased or the infusion is stopped.

Therapeutic Interventions

Actions/Interventions

▲ Administer electrolyte replacement therapy as prescribed.

■ When discontinuing PN therapy, taper the rate over 2 to 4 hours.

▲ Use corrective actions if the PN solution stops or must be stopped suddenly:
- For a clotted catheter or if subsequent PN bags are not available, hang 10% dextrose and water at the rate of the PN infusion.
- For hyperglycemia, administer insulin as prescribed.
- For emergency or cardiac arrest situations, stop the PN infusion; administer bolus doses of 50% dextrose.

Rationales

Electrolytes are supplied based on the patient's calculated need. QSEN: Patient-centered care.

This measure prevents a hypoglycemic episode caused by abrupt PN withdrawal. QSEN: Safety.

This solution provides a higher concentration of glucose to prevent sudden hypoglycemia.

This measure facilitates metabolic use of glucose.

These measures prevent hypoglycemia during resuscitation.

Related Care Plans

Risk for unstable blood glucose, Chapter 2
Risk for electrolyte imbalance, Chapter 2
Risk for infection, Chapter 2

Enteral Nutrition

Tube Feeding; Enteral Hyperalimentation; G-Tube; Jejunostomy; Duodenostomy; PEG Tube; Dobhoff Tube

Enteral tube feedings provide nutrition using a nasogastric tube, a gastrostomy tube, or a tube placed in the duodenum or jejunum. Tubes may be inserted through the external nares or may be placed through a small incision into the stomach or small intestine. Enteral tube feedings are indicated for patients who have a functional gastro-intestinal system but are unable to maintain adequate nutritional intake orally. Clinical conditions that may limit the patient's ability to maintain adequate oral intake include cancer, facial fractures, burn injury, and psychiatric problems such as dementia. Research indicates that critically ill patients receiving enteral tube feedings tend to

Basic Nursing Concepts Care Plans

have better outcomes and fewer complications. The problems associated with the administration of enteral tube feedings include pulmonary aspiration of feeding formula, diarrhea, and fluid and electrolyte imbalances. Feedings may be continuous or intermittent (bolus). Enteral tube feedings can be more cost effective than parenteral nutrition (PN). Enteral feeding may occur in the hospital, in long-term care, or in home care. The focus of this care plan is the prevention and management of problems commonly associated with enteral feeding.

NANDA-I NDx Imbalanced Nutrition: Less Than Body Requirements

Common Related Factor

Mechanical problems during feedings, such as clogged tube, inaccurate flow rate, stiffening of tube, delivery pump malfunction

Defining Characteristics

Continued weight loss
Failure to gain weight
Weakness

Common Expected Outcomes

Patient's nutritional status improves, as evidenced by gradual weight gain or stable weight and increased physical strength.
Patient weighs within 10% of ideal weight range.

NOC Outcome
Nutritional Status: Nutrient Intake
NIC Interventions
Nutritional Monitoring; Enteral Tube Feeding; Gastrointestinal Intubation

Ongoing Assessment

Actions/Interventions	Rationales
■ Assess the tubing for patency and free flow of enteral feeding.	A clogged feeding tube decreases the delivery of nutrients.
■ Assess the equipment (pump) used for administration; ensure that the proper flow rate is indicated and that the pump is delivering enteral feeding at the appropriate rate.	A feeding pump regulates formula delivery at a continuous rate. This method of continuous delivery is associated with less diarrhea than occurs with intermittent feedings. QSEN: Safety.
■ Assess the patient's weight every other day or as ordered.	Weight gain is an indicator of improved nutritional status; however, sudden gain of more than 2 pounds in a 24-hour period usually indicates fluid retention. Most commercially available tube-feeding preparations contain 1 kcal/mL. An adult of average size and weight requires 1800 to 2400 kcal/24 hours. QSEN: Patient-centered care.
■ Assess the physical strength of the patient; note any improvement or deterioration.	Improved muscle strength and activity tolerance are indicators of sufficient calories.

Therapeutic Interventions

Actions/Interventions	Rationales
■ Flush the tubing with 20 mL of water after medication administration and any time the flow of solution is interrupted.	Flushing the tube is important to reduce the risk for clogging. Clogging of a feeding tube may require replacement of the tube. Any delay in the administration of the feeding formula decreases the patient's nutrient intake. For intermittent feedings, the tube should be flushed with water before and after each feeding to ensure tube patency. QSEN: Safety.

■ = Independent   ▲ = Interprofessional Collaboration

Actions/Interventions	Rationales
■ Crush medications and dilute them with water.	Whenever possible, liquid forms of medication should be administered through a feeding tube to reduce the risk for clogging. Pills should be crushed to the finest consistency possible and mixed with water before being administered through the feeding tube.
■ Keep the pump alarms on.	Any interruption in the flow of solution is noted early when alarms sound. QSEN: Safety.
■ When a continuous feeding is interrupted for more than 1 hour, recalculate the amount to be given over 8 hours and reset the administration rate.	Rapid administration to "catch up" can precipitate a hyperglycemic crisis because the pancreas may not be able to produce adequate insulin for the increased carbohydrate load. The risk for diarrhea also increases when the rate is suddenly increased.
▲ Consult the dietitian.	The dietitian ensures that ongoing nutritional needs are being met as the patient's condition or situation changes. The dietitian will calculate the patient's caloric and nutritional needs. Using this information, the dietitian provides guidance in selecting the appropriate feeding formulas and any additional nutrient supplements. QSEN: Teamwork and collaboration.

NANDA-I NDx **Risk for Aspiration**

Common Risk Factors

Decrease in level of consciousness
Depressed gag reflex
Incorrect positioning of tube at placement
Migration of the tube after placement
Supine positioning of patient as feeding is administered
Increase in gastric residual volume
Decrease in gastrointestinal motility
Delayed gastric emptying

Common Expected Outcome

Patient maintains a patent airway, as evidenced by normal breath sounds, absence of coughing, no shortness of breath, and no aspiration.

NOC Outcomes

Aspiration Prevention; Respiratory Status: Ventilation

NIC Interventions

Aspiration Precautions; Enteral Tube Feeding; Respiratory Monitoring

Ongoing Assessment

Actions/Interventions	Rationales
▲ Obtain an x-ray study immediately after tube insertion.	Radiological confirmation of the feeding tube position should be obtained after the placement of a nasoenteral tube.
■ Assess the correct position of the tube before the initiation of feeding by aspirating fluid from the tube and checking the color and pH of the fluid.	pH readings of 0 to 5 usually indicate gastric placement of the tube. The color of the gastric fluid varies from off-white to grassy green or brown. Intestinal fluid is golden yellow to brownish green and has a pH of 6 or higher. A pH of 6 or higher in watery yellow fluid may indicate respiratory placement of the tube. This assessment is especially important for gastrostomy tubes because the potential for reflux is increased; duodenostomy and jejunostomy tubes carry somewhat less risk. pH of gastric secretions may be higher than expected if the patient is receiving medications such as histamine-2 antagonists or proton pump inhibitors. Small-bore feeding tubes are more flexible and can easily enter the trachea during insertion or migrate to the trachea at any time after insertion. QSEN: Safety; Evidence-based practice.
■ Assess the level of consciousness (LOC) and gag reflex before the administration of feeding.	A decreased LOC is a prime risk factor for aspiration. High-risk patients are comatose, have a decreased gag reflex, or cannot tolerate the head of bed elevated. Nasoduodenal or gastroduodenal feeding tubes are preferred for high-risk patients because the gastroduodenal sphincter provides additional protection against gastroesophageal reflux. QSEN: Safety.
■ Ask the patient about sensations of gastric fullness, or nausea.	Patients with increased gastric residual volumes may report feeling an uncomfortable fullness for 1 hour or more after a feeding. The patient may report sensations of nausea. These findings may be early indicators of increased gastric residual volumes and an increased risk for aspiration. QSEN: Safety.
■ Assess the pulmonary status for clinical evidence of aspiration. Auscultate breath sounds for the development of crackles or wheezes. Monitor chest x-ray results as ordered.	Aspiration of small amounts of feeding can occur without coughing or a sudden onset of respiratory distress, especially in patients with a decreased LOC. Pulmonary infiltrates on chest x-ray results indicate some level of aspiration has occurred. Coughing and shortness of breath may indicate aspiration.
■ Assess for residual volume before feeding. If the patient is on continuous feedings, check the residual every 4 hours.	Feedings are held if residual volume is greater than 50% of the amount to be delivered in 1 hour. Gastric residuals should be checked frequently when feedings are initiated, and feedings should be held if residual volumes exceed 200 mL
■ Auscultate bowel sounds to evaluate bowel motility, and assess for abdominal distention and firmness.	Decreased gastrointestinal motility increases the risk for aspiration because feeding formula accumulates in the stomach. When combined with a decreased LOC or diminished gag reflex, aspiration is a higher risk. QSEN: Safety.

Therapeutic Interventions

Actions/Interventions	Rationales
■ Elevate the head of the bed to 30 degrees during and for 1 hour after each feeding.	This position facilitates the gravity flow of feeding past the gastroduodenal sphincter and reduces the risk for aspiration. QSEN: Safety.

■ = Independent   ▲ = Interprofessional Collaboration

Basic Nursing Concepts Care Plans

Actions/Interventions

- If the patient has an endotracheal or tracheostomy tube, keep the cuff inflated during feedings and for 1 hour after feedings.
- In case of aspiration:
  - Stop the feeding.
  - Keep the head of the bed elevated.
  - Suction the airway as necessary.
  - Document the time that the feeding was stopped, the patient's appearance, and any change in respiratory status.
  - Document any adventitious breath sounds.

Rationales

This measure protects the patient's airway from inadvertent entry of feedings into the trachea.

Respiratory aspiration requires immediate action by the caregiver to maintain the airway and promote effective breathing and gas exchange. Tracheal suctioning may be necessary to maintain airway patency. QSEN: Safety.

NANDA-I NDx
Risk for Diarrhea

Common Risk Factor
Intolerance to tube feeding formula

Common Expected Outcome
Patient does not experience diarrhea during tube feedings.

NOC Outcomes
Bowel Elimination; Symptom Control
NIC Interventions
Diarrhea Management; Enteral Tube Feeding

Ongoing Assessment

Actions/Interventions

- Assess bowel sounds and for abdominal distention or cramping.

- Assess the number and character of stools.

- Monitor intake and output. Measure the volume of liquid or watery stools.
- Note the osmolarity and fiber content of the feeding.

- Note any history of lactose intolerance.

Rationales

Diarrhea is typically accompanied by hyperactive bowel sounds, distention, and reports of cramping associated with increased peristalsis.

The patient may have an increase in the number of stools per day. The feces may become more watery. Many factors contribute to the development of diarrhea in tube-fed patients. Sorbitol-based elixirs for liquid forms of medications may increase the incidence of diarrhea. *Clostridium difficile* has been found to occur more often in tube-fed hospitalized patients than in non–tube-fed patients. QSEN: Evidence-based practice.

Diarrhea can lead to profound dehydration.

Hyperosmolar or high-fiber feedings draw fluid into the bowel and can cause diarrhea. Isotonic feedings are preferred.

Milk-based feedings contain lactose, which is not tolerated by individuals with lactase deficiency.

Therapeutic Interventions

Actions/Interventions	Rationales
■ Begin feedings slowly; consider a solution concentration that is less than full-strength formula.	Large volumes of hyperosmolar solutions may stimulate osmotic diarrhea. Gradual increase in rate will allow time for the gastrointestinal system to adapt to the increased volume and solutes. The increased osmolality of the full-strength feeding formula pulls fluid from the intravascular and interstitial spaces into the intestinal lumen. The patient may benefit from beginning the feeding with a less than full-strength solution.
■ Instruct the caregiver to increase both the rate and strength to prescribed amounts, but not at the same time.	High-rate feeding combined with high osmolality may precipitate diarrhea.
■ Administer feedings at room temperature.	Administration of a cold feeding formula stimulates peristalsis and increases the risk for diarrhea.
■ Do not allow the formula to hang longer than 4 hours at room temperature.	The risk for bacterial contamination increases the longer a feeding formula remains at room temperature in the feeding delivery system. The American Dietetic Association recommends any feedings that are reconstituted with water or modified in any way should be prepared using aseptic technique and should hang for no more than 4 hours. This includes concentrated liquid and powder formulas, fortified human milk, and any feedings to which other ingredients are added. QSEN: Evidence-based practice.
■ Change the feeding setup daily.	Use of a clean feeding delivery bag and tubing minimizes the risk for bacterial contamination. QSEN: Safety.
■ Keep open containers of feeding formula refrigerated until they are needed.	Open containers of feeding formula will be at risk for bacterial contamination if left at room temperature.

 Deficient Knowledge

Common Related Factors
Alteration in cognitive functioning
Insufficient information
Insufficient interest in learning
Insufficient knowledge of resources
Alteration in memory
Misinformation presented by others

Defining Characteristics
Insufficient knowledge
Inaccurate follow-through of instruction
Inaccurate performance on a test
Inappropriate behavior

Common Expected Outcomes
Patient or caregiver verbalizes reasons for tube feedings and begins to participate in care.
Patient or caregiver demonstrates independence in enteral feeding administration.

NOC Outcome
Knowledge: Treatment Procedure
NIC Interventions
Learning Facilitation; Teaching: Psychomotor Skill; Teaching: Procedure/Treatment; Health Literacy Enhancement

Basic Nursing Concepts Care Plans

■ = Independent   ▲ = Interprofessional Collaboration

Ongoing Assessment

Actions/Interventions	Rationales

■ Assess the patient's or caregiver's knowledge of:
  • Tube feeding purpose, expected length of therapy, and expected benefits
  • Ability to administer feedings
  • Ability to use equipment related to feeding: measuring devices, feeding pump, and tubing
  • Ability to minimize complications related to tube feedings: checking for residual volume, assuming sitting position, and maintaining a bacteria-free feeding system
	Many patients require feedings well beyond hospitalization and can administer feedings to self. Teaching the patient and caregiver is based on their knowledge and ability to manage the equipment and minimize complications. Assessment of their understanding is the foundation for an individualized teaching plan. QSEN: Patient-centered care.

Therapeutic Interventions

Actions/Interventions	Rationales
■ Demonstrate feedings and tube care. Allow for return demonstration.	Supervised practice allows the patient and caregiver to use new information and skills immediately and enhances retention. Repeated practice combined with feedback from the nurse helps the patient and caregiver gain confidence in their ability to manage the enteral feedings. Necessary alteration in the teaching plan can be undertaken. QSEN: Patient-centered care.
■ Arrange for a home care nurse if the patient is unable to feed self.	Community resources provide support for the patient and caregiver as they learn new skills. These agencies may help the patient and family obtain the necessary equipment and feeding formulas in the home setting. QSEN: Teamwork and collaboration.

Related Care Plans

Deficient fluid volume, Chapter 2
Impaired oral mucous membrane, Chapter 2

Hearing Loss

Adults may experience hearing loss as the result of trauma, infection, or exposure to persistently loud occupational and/or environmental noise. Presbycusis is a gradual hearing loss that develops in older adults as part of the normal aging process. Conductive hearing loss is associated with problems affecting the external ear and middle ear. External ear disorders include cerumen impacted against the tympanic membrane and infection. Middle ear disorders include tympanic membrane perforation, or chronic/recurring otitis media. Sensorineural hearing loss occurs with inner ear disorders or impaired function of cranial nerve VIII. Inner ear disorders that contribute to this type of hearing loss include otosclerosis, Ménière's disease, and acoustic neuroma. Persistent noise exposure at levels of higher than 90 dB can result in sensorineural hearing loss. Ototoxicity from some drugs may contribute to this type of hearing loss that is often temporary. When hearing loss is profound and precedes language development, the ability to learn speech and interact with hearing peers can be severely impaired. When hearing is impaired or lost later in life, serious emotional and social consequences can occur, including depression and isolation. Some causes of hearing loss are surgically correctable. Many hearing assistive devices and services are available to help hearing-impaired individuals. Nursing interventions with the hearing impaired are aimed at assisting the individual in effective communication despite the loss of normal hearing.

⊝volve   For additional care plans, go to http://evolve.elsevier.com/Gulanick/.

NANDA-I NDx Impaired Verbal Communication

Common Related Factors

Physiological condition (e.g., conductive or sensorineural hearing loss)

Common Expected Outcome

Patient uses a form of communication to get needs met and to relate effectively with people and his or her environment.

Defining Characteristics

Difficulty comprehending communication
Difficulty in maintaining communication

NOC Outcomes

Hearing Compensation Behavior; Risk Control: Hearing Impairment

NIC Interventions

Communication Enhancement: Hearing Deficit; Ear Care

Ongoing Assessment

Actions/Interventions	Rationales
■ Assess the patient's ability to hear and appropriately respond to normal conversational voice; do this within the patient's sight, then again from out of the patient's sight.	Difficulty responding to normal conversation may be the first indication of impaired hearing. Patients may rely on lip-reading to a greater extent than they are aware. Sensory nerve hearing loss causes an inability to hear high-pitched sounds or comprehend some consonants. QSEN: Patient-centered care.
■ Ask the family or caregivers about their perception of the patient's hearing impairment.	Patients may be unaware of progressive hearing loss; family, friends, and caregivers often first notice requests for verbal repetition, lack of response to verbalizations, and incorrectly answered questions.
■ Review the audiogram, if available.	This diagnostic study indicates the type and amount of hearing loss.
■ Assess the patient's use of adaptive communication techniques to compensate for hearing loss.	Adults with new or progressive hearing loss may have limited use of adaptive techniques that enhance communication. Adults who have had hearing loss since birth or childhood may have acquired the skills, tools, and resources available to cope successfully with hearing impairment. QSEN: Patient-centered care.
■ Review the patient's medical history.	History of head or ear trauma and frequent bouts with ear infections are often associated with hearing loss.
■ Review the patient's exposure to environmental noise as the result of occupation, recreation, or accident.	Repeated or persistent exposure to noise levels exceeding 90 dB puts the individual at risk for sensorineural hearing loss. People who frequent rock concerts or listen to very loud music place themselves at risk for hearing loss. Hearing loss that results from noise may not be reversible.
■ Review any recent use of drugs that are ototoxic.	Aspirin, quinidine, some chemotherapeutic agents, and the aminoglycosides are known ototoxic agents. Withdrawal of these drugs when hearing impairment occurs often allows for full return of hearing.
■ Check the ears for earwax.	Excessive wax may become impacted against the tympanic membrane and prevent sound transmission to the middle ear.

Basic Nursing Concepts Care Plans

■ = Independent   ▲ = Interprofessional Collaboration

Actions/Interventions

- For patients with hearing aids:
  - Note the condition and age of the hearing aid.
  - Note the frequency with which the patient wears a hearing aid.
  - Check the hearing aid for fresh, functional batteries.
  - Check the hearing aid for wax accumulation.
- Assess for drainage from the ear canal.

▲ Culture any drainage from the ear canal.

- Ask the patient whether the ear is painful.

- Assess for dizziness, dysequilibrium.

- Assess the patient's ability to effectively administer ear drops.

Rationales

A hearing aid that is not functioning correctly may be the cause of decreased hearing acuity. The patient may not wear the hearing aid as needed. Wax may clog hearing aids. The patient may have trouble replacing dead batteries or adjusting the volume dial.

Purulent, foul-smelling drainage indicates an infection; serous, mucoid, or bloody drainage may indicate effusion of the middle ear after an upper respiratory tract or sinus infection.

Identification of infectious pathogens guides selection of antibiotic therapy. QSEN: Evidence-based practice.

Pain is a symptom of increased pressure behind the eardrum, usually a result of infection.

Disorders of the ear (e.g., Ménière's disease) may be accompanied by dizziness because of the inner ear's role in maintenance of equilibrium.

Problems with medication administration may limit effectiveness of the drug.

Therapeutic Interventions

Actions/Interventions

- Use touch and eye contact.

- When communicating with the patient, incorporate the following:
  - Reduce or minimize environmental noise.

  - Face the patient in good light, and keep hands away from the mouth.

  - Speak close to the patient's "better" ear and avoid shouting or yelling.

  - Speak slowly and allow time for the patient to respond.

  - Use dry-erase boards, computers, or other writing tools.
  - Provide encouragement to use a hearing aid.

- Explore technology such as amplifiers, modifiers for telephones, and services for the hearing impaired (e.g., closed-captioned TV, telephone hearing-impaired assistance).
- Prepare the patient for ear surgery.

Rationales

Behavioral communication techniques can support effective interactions with the patient. QSEN: Patient-centered care.

The patient with a hearing impairment may have difficulty filtering background noises to hear the speaker.

This nursing action enhances the patient's use of lip-reading, facial expressions, and gesturing to supplement the spoken message.

Loud noise may limit the patient's ability to hear. Drawing attention to the patient's hearing loss may decrease his or her willingness to communicate with others.

The patient may need additional time to process auditory stimuli before responding.

Written media may facilitate communication with profoundly hearing-impaired individuals.

Patients with new hearing aids need time to adjust to the sound produced. Encouragement is often needed, especially among older patients who may decide that the hearing aid is not worth the effort.

These devices may assist the hearing-impaired patient with functioning and participating in meaningful activities.

Tympanoplasty (removal of dead tissue, restoration of bones with prostheses) and mastoidectomy (removal of all or portions of the middle ear structures) are common surgical treatments for hearing loss. Cochlear implants are electronic devices that stimulate auditory nerve fibers. These devices often facilitate hearing for patients who do not benefit from external hearing aids.

Basic Nursing Concepts Care Plans

NANDA-I NDx Deficient Knowledge

Common Related Factors

Insufficient information
Insufficient interest in learning
Insufficient knowledge of resources
Misinformation presented by others

Common Expected Outcomes

Patient verbalizes understanding of importance of hearing protection and of use of adaptive hearing devices.
Patient demonstrates skill in use of hearing protection techniques and of adaptive hearing devices.

Defining Characteristics

Insufficient knowledge
Inaccurate follow-through of instruction
Inaccurate performance on a test
Inappropriate behavior

NOC Outcomes
Knowledge: Hearing Protection; Knowledge: Hearing Aids; Information Processing

NIC Interventions
Learning Facilitation; Teaching: Individual; Ear Care

Ongoing Assessment

Actions/Interventions	Rationales
■ Assess the motivation and willingness of the patient and caregivers to learn about hearing protection and adaptive hearing devices.	Adults must see a need or purpose for learning. Some patients are ready to learn soon after they are diagnosed; others cope better by denying or delaying the need for instruction.
■ Identify any existing misconceptions regarding hearing protection, ear care, or use of adaptive hearing devices.	Assessment provides an important starting point in education. Knowledge serves to correct faulty ideas. Many adults have developed habits for ear care that may contribute to cerumen impaction. Some people are unaware of the risks to hearing with persistent exposure to loud noises.
■ Allow the learner to identify what is most important to him or her.	Allowing the patient to determine the most significant content to be presented first is most effective. Patients may want to focus only on techniques that facilitate improved hearing and are less interested in specifics of the disease process that lead to the hearing impairment. QSEN: Patient-centered care.

Therapeutic Interventions

Actions/Interventions	Rationales
■ Teach the patient or caregiver to administer ear medications.	Drops should be administered at room temperature to avoid pain and dizziness; the tip of the applicator or dropper should not be allowed to come into contact with anything. The head should be positioned to allow the medication to flow into the ear canal; this position should be maintained for 1 to 2 minutes.
■ Instruct the patient or caregiver in safe techniques for cleaning the ears.	Thin washcloths and fingers are best for cleaning ears. Cotton-tipped applicators, bobby pins, toothpicks or other small objects should be avoided to prevent inadvertent injury to the tympanic membrane or pushing cerumen farther into the external ear canal. QSEN: Safety.

Basic Nursing Concepts Care Plans

■ = Independent   ▲ = Interprofessional Collaboration

Actions/Interventions

- Teach the patient or caregiver the use and care of hearing aids and/or other assistive hearing devices.
- Teach the patient about use of hearing protection devices.

- Instruct the patient in the importance of routine examination by an audiologist and reporting symptoms of hearing loss.

Rationales

The patient and caregiver need to be able to care for and maintain the hearing aid in proper working order.

The Occupational Safety and Health Act (OSHA) requires hearing protection in workplaces with noise levels exceeding 90 dB. Hearing protection may include use of noise-canceling headphones, earmuffs, and earplugs. OSHA provides information about noise control strategies for the workplace. QSEN: Safety; Evidence-based practice.

Examinations detect changes in hearing or need for change in hearing aids. Early signs of sensorineural hearing loss may include tinnitus. The patient may report a persistent ringing or buzzing sound.

NANDA-I NDx **Impaired Body Image**

Common Related Factors

Alteration in body function (due to hearing loss)
Alteration in self perception

Defining Characteristics

Preoccupation with change or loss of hearing
Refusal to acknowledge change or use adaptive hearing devices
Change in social involvement

Common Expected Outcome

Patient demonstrates enhanced body image and self-esteem as evidenced by ability to talk about hearing loss, and use adaptive hearing devices and communication techniques.

NOC Outcomes

Body Image; Self-Esteem; Adaptation to Physical Disability

NIC Interventions

Body Image Enhancement; Self-Esteem Enhancement; Grief Work Facilitation; Coping Enhancement

---

Ongoing Assessment

Actions/Interventions

- Assess the patient's perception of change in hearing.

- Assess the social and emotional impact hearing loss may have for the patient.

- Assess the patient's behavior regarding the actual or perceived hearing loss.

Rationales

The extent of the patient's response is related more to the value or importance the patient places on hearing loss than the actual hearing loss. QSEN: Patient-centered care.

Loss of hearing may lead to reclusiveness, isolation, depression, and withdrawal from usual activities. The decision to wear a hearing aid is often resisted because of the social stigma perceived in conjunction with aging and loss of abilities.

There is a broad range of behaviors associated with body image disturbance, ranging from totally ignoring the hearing loss to preoccupation with it. Some patients see a visible hearing aid as a threat to their body image.

Therapeutic Interventions

Actions/Interventions	Rationales
■ Acknowledge the normalcy of the emotional response to the hearing loss and use of adaptive hearing devices.	Experiencing stages of grief over hearing loss is normal and typically involves a period of denial, the length of which varies among individuals. QSEN: Patient-centered care.
■ Demonstrate positive caring in routine activities.	Professional caregivers represent a microcosm of society. The patient will scrutinize the actions and behaviors of members of the interprofessional health team. Positive comments by the nurse may help the patient develop more positive responses to changes in hearing and use of a hearing aid. Patients may stop using a hearing aid if they think it draws attention to the problem and distorts their body image.
■ Provide the patient with information about adaptive hearing devices that are less visible.	Patients may be unaware of miniature models that are now available. Some hearing aids can be molded to fit completely in the external ear canal. Other types of hearing aids are designed to be less visible.

Visual Impairment

Visual impairment occurs with changes in the amount or patterning of stimuli to the optic nerve. This change in visual stimulus results in a diminished, exaggerated, distorted, or impaired perception of the visual image. These changes in vision affect a significant number of people across the life span. Refractive errors are the most common form of visual problem. These correctable visual impairments include myopia, hyperopia, presbyopia, and astigmatism. Correction occurs with glasses, contact lenses, or surgery. Chronic diseases such as diabetes mellitus, glaucoma, and macular degeneration cause visual impairment that may not be correctable and may lead to blindness. Cataracts contribute to visual impairment that may be corrected through surgery and lens replacement. Infections, trauma to the eye, and drug side effects may cause temporary or permanent visual impairment. Diseases or trauma to visual pathways or cranial nerves II, III, IV, and VI secondary to stroke, intracranial aneurysms, brain tumors, myasthenia gravis, or multiple sclerosis may also contribute to visual impairment that is temporary or permanent. Changes in visual acuity may interfere with the person's activities of daily living (ADLs) and productivity at work, school, or home. Loss of vision threatens the safety of the individual and puts the person at risk for falls and other injuries. Visual impairment may affect the person's psychological, emotional, and social well-being as he or she copes with adapting to the loss while attempting to remain independent. Dependence on devices to correct or adapt to visual impairment may affect the person's body image and self-concept.

NANDA-I NDx Deficient Knowledge

Common Related Factors	Defining Characteristics
Insufficient information	Insufficient knowledge
Insufficient interest in learning	Inaccurate follow-through of instruction
Insufficient knowledge of resources	Inaccurate performance on a test
Misinformation presented by others	Inappropriate behavior

■ = Independent   ▲ = Interprofessional Collaboration

Basic Nursing Concepts
Care Plans

Common Expected Outcome

Patient verbalizes understanding of desired content/performs desired skill.

NOC Outcomes
Knowledge: Disease Process; Knowledge: Medication; Information Processing
NIC Interventions
Learning Facilitation; Teaching: Individual

Ongoing Assessment

Actions/Interventions	Rationales
■ Assess the motivation and willingness of the patient and caregivers to learn.	Some patients are ready to learn soon after they develop visual impairment. Others cope better by denying or delaying the need for instruction.
■ Identify the priority of learning needs within the overall teaching plan.	This information provides the starting base for educational sessions. Teaching standardized content that the patient already knows wastes valuable time and hinders critical learning. Adults learn material that is important to them. QSEN: Patient-centered care.
■ Assess the patient's use of aids that improve vision, such as glasses, contact lenses, magnifiers, or bright/natural light.	The teaching plan should include adaptive strategies that the patient has found successful in adjusting to visual impairment. QSEN: Patient-centered care.
■ Evaluate the patient's ability to function within limits of visual impairment.	Personal appearance and condition of clothing and surroundings are good indicators of the patient's adaptation to visual loss. QSEN: Patient-centered care.

Therapeutic Interventions

Actions/Interventions	Rationales
■ Provide information in nonprint formats or large-print formats.	Important teaching information needs to be presented in a format that supports the patient's preferred learning style. Formats that use hearing rather than vision may enhance the patient's learning of new information. Large-print teaching materials combined with visual aids such as magnifiers make it easier for the patient with decreased lens accommodation to use printed material for learning. QSEN: Patient-centered care.
■ Teach the patient about using visual aids when appropriate.	Visual aids such as a magnifying glass or large-type printed books and magazines enhance the patient's engagement in activities such as reading.
■ Reinforce the physician's explanation of medical management and surgical procedures, if any.	Patients and their caregivers may need periodic repetition of information to make informed decisions about treatment and procedures. QSEN: Patient-centered care.
■ Teach general methods of eye care: • Maintain sterility of all eyedroppers, tubes of medications, and other items that come in contact with the tissues of the eye. • Care for contact lenses or eyeglasses as recommended by the manufacturer.	This nursing action reduces the risk for eye infection or injury that may further impair vision. Care and maintenance of corrective lenses enhances the effectiveness of their use to improve vision. QSEN: Safety.
■ Demonstrate the proper administration of eye drops or ointments; allow for return demonstration by the patient and/or caregiver.	Repetition of skills after demonstration promotes the patient's level of confidence in administration of eye medications. QSEN: Patient-centered care.

Actions/Interventions

▲ Consult the occupational therapy staff for assistive devices and educating the patient in their use.

■ Provide the patient and family with information about environmental modifications to reduce to impact of visual glare.

Rationales

Adaptive devices such as magnifiers for reading medication vials or syringes used for injections can increase the patient's self-care independence. QSEN: Teamwork and collaboration.

Vision changes that reduce the ability of the pupil to adjust to light make the patient more sensitive to glare. Using nonglare wall paints and countertop surfaces can minimize glare for the patient. Window treatments such as sheer curtains and adjustable shades will promote visual comfort for the client.

NANDA-I
NDx Risk for Falls

Common Risk Factors

History of falls
Age >65 years
Living alone
Use of assistive devices (e.g., walker, cane, wheelchair)
Visual impairments
Cluttered environment
Insufficient lighting
Unfamiliar setting
Use of throw rugs
Exposure to unsafe environmental conditions (wet floors, ice)

Common Expected Outcomes

Patient will not sustain a fall.
Patient and caregiver will implement strategies to increase safety and prevent falls in the home.

NOC Outcomes

Fall Prevention Behavior; Knowledge: Fall Prevention; Risk Control; Risk Detection

NIC Interventions

Fall Prevention; Environmental Management: Safety; Teaching: Prescribed Exercise; Medication Management

Basic Nursing Concepts Care Plans

Ongoing Assessment

Actions/Interventions

■ Assess central vision, peripheral vision, and acuity with each eye, individually and together.

■ Ask the patient about the ability to read, history of falls, and the ability to ambulate.

Rationales

Changes in the patient's ability to see potential hazards in the environment increases the risk for falls. Vision loss may be unilateral, bilateral, central, and/or peripheral and may not affect both eyes to the same extent. Glaucoma affects peripheral vision; its onset is insidious and has no associated symptoms. Macular degeneration affects central vision and is irreversible.

Visual impairment can contribute to problems in daily activities. The risk for falls increases if the patient has diminished visual acuity. A history of falls increases the patient's risk for falls. QSEN: Safety.

■ = Independent   ▲ = Interprofessional Collaboration

Actions/Interventions

- Assess the patient's use of aids that improve vision, such as glasses, contact lenses, magnifiers, or bright/natural light. Some patients may use a cane when ambulating to identify barriers in their path.

Rationales

The plan of care to reduce fall risk should include adaptive strategies that the patient has found successful in adjusting to visual impairment. QSEN: Patient-centered care.

Therapeutic Interventions

Actions/Interventions

- Provide adequate lighting.

- Guide the patient when ambulating, if appropriate. Describe where you are walking; identify obstacles.

- Instruct the patient to hold both arms of the chair before sitting and to feel for the seat on chairs or sofas without arms.

- Remove environmental barriers to ensure safety. Avoid leaving doors partially open. Do not make unnecessary changes in the environment. Tell the patient of changes that are made.

- Provide the patient and caregivers with information about environmental modifications at home to promote safety and reduce fall risk.

- Encourage the use of touch.

- For the hospitalized patient, place frequently used items (e.g., tissues, water, call light) within the patient's range of vision or reach.

Rationales

Appropriate lighting will allow the patient to see potential barriers in the environment that might contribute to falls. The use of natural or halogen lighting is preferred to improve vision for patients with diminished vision.

This approach helps the patient become oriented to the environment in which he or she will be ambulating. QSEN: Patient-centered care.

These actions reduce the risk for falls when changing positions. QSEN: Safety.

Fully open or closed doors reduce the risk for injury among those with impaired vision. Clutter needs to be removed from the pathway a patient will use in a room. Providing consistency in the patient's environment ensures safety and maintains what the patient has learned. The patient needs time to make new adjustments to any changes in the environment. QSEN: Safety.

Some visual disorders reduce the patient's depth perception. As a result the patient can trip over throw rugs, the edges of steps, and thresholds between rooms. Colored tape at the edge of stair treads makes is easier for the patient to differentiate the edge of one step from the next step. Stairs need to have securely fastened handrails for the full length of the stairs. QSEN: Safety.

Touch provides sensory input to help the patient become familiar with his or her environment. Familiarity with the environment, especially when ambulating, will decrease the risk of falls.

This nursing action promotes the patient's independence and reduces the risk for falls when reaching for objects.

NANDA-I NDx Ineffective Coping

Common Related Factors

High degree of threat
Inaccurate threat appraisal
Ineffective pattern of tension release strategies
Insufficient social support
Inadequate resources
Inadequate opportunity to prepare for visual impairment
Inadequate confidence in ability to deal with visual impairment

Defining Characteristics

Ineffective coping strategies
Inability to make decisions
Inability to ask for help
Insufficient goal-directed behavior
Insufficient problem-solving
Inability to meet role expectations
Alteration in concentration

evolve   **For additional care plans, go to http://evolve.elsevier.com/Gulanick/.**

Common Expected Outcomes

Patient uses available resources and support systems.
Patient describes and initiates effective coping strategies.
Patient describes positive results from new behaviors.

NOC Outcomes
Coping; Stress Level; Decision Making;
  Information Processing
NIC Interventions
Coping Enhancement; Decision-Making Support

Ongoing Assessment

Actions/Interventions	Rationales
■ Determine the nature of the visual symptoms, onset, and degree of visual loss.	Recent visual loss, loss over a long period, and long-standing loss have different implications for the patient's level of adaptation to and coping with the visual impairment. Gradual visual loss may allow the patient time to adjust and begin to develop coping skills.
■ Evaluate the psychological response to visual loss.	Anger, depression, and withdrawal are common responses to visual impairment. Self-esteem is often negatively affected if the patient is becoming less independent with daily activities.
■ Assess the patient's usual coping mechanisms and availability of social support systems.	Coping mechanisms that have been effective for the patient in the past may not be effective in coping with visual impairment. Increasing dependency on others may be a source of anxiety and stress for the patient.
■ Ask the patient about the ability to read, ability to see television, ability to self-medicate, and ability to drive, especially at night.	Visual impairment can contribute to problems in daily activities. Diminished self-care ability may contribute to challenges in coping ability such as increasing dependence on others. The risk for medication errors increases if the patient has diminished visual acuity. Patients with visual impairment such as cataracts may be able to drive on sunny days but not on cloudy days or at night. The loss of the ability to drive may have a significant negative impact on the patient's self-concept and ability to cope with the loss of vision. QSEN: Patient-centered care.

Therapeutic Interventions

Actions/Interventions	Rationales
■ Introduce self to the patient at each encounter and orient the patient to the environment.	This nursing action provides the patient with orientation to an unfamiliar environment and reduced ability to recognize faces. The patient may not be able to recognize people by their voices. Increasing the patient's orientation reduces fear and promotes more effective coping in a new setting. QSEN: Patient-centered care.
■ Use touch when interacting with the patient, as appropriate.	Touch provides sensory input to help the patient become familiar with his or her environment. Familiarity with the environment reduces anxiety and supports effective coping.
■ Encourage the use of radios, audiotapes, and talking books.	Diversional activities that use hearing rather than vision enhance the patient's participation in activities that may support independence, effective coping, and self-concept.

■ = Independent   ▲ = Interprofessional Collaboration

Actions/Interventions

- Explain sounds or other unusual stimuli in the patient's environment.

- Encourage the patient in the use of adaptive devices as appropriate.
- Make appropriate referrals to community resources.

Rationales

This information reduces the patient's anxiety or fear in response of unfamiliar stimuli. Familiarity with the environment supports the patient's coping mechanisms.

Using adaptive devices allows patient to gain independence and supports effective coping.

A variety of community agencies provide resources, information, and support groups for patients and families adapting to visual impairment. Family members may need help to understand the best approaches to support the patient's adaptation and independence. QSEN: Teamwork and collaboration.

Related Care Plans

Anxiety, Chapter 2
Fear, Chapter 2
Disturbed body image, Chapter 2

Substance Use Disorders

The *Diagnostic and Statistical Manual of Mental Disorders,* 5th edition (DSM-V) defines substance use disorders as the recurrent use of alcohol and/or drugs that leads to significant impairment for the individual. This impairment may include development of health problems, disability, and failure to meet major responsibilities at work, school, or home. The most common substance use disorders are alcohol use disorder, tobacco use disorder, cannabis use disorder, stimulant use disorder, hallucinogen use disorder, and opioid use disorder. DSM-V classifies each disorder as mild, moderate, or severe based on the number of diagnostic criteria met by an individual. Each type of substance use disorder has specific pharmacological criteria for diagnosis. In addition, a diagnosis of substance use disorder includes evidence of impaired control, social impairment, and use of the substance in dangerous situations such as driving or operating heavy equipment. The person with impaired control of substance use will exhibit cravings for the substance, develop tolerance to the effects, and may experience withdrawal symptoms. The person with a substance use disorder will spend increased time in activities that support obtaining, using, and recovering from the substance (drug-seeking behavior). Social impairment may be shown as failure to fulfill major role obligations (e.g., at work or within the family), legal problems (e.g., arrest for driving under the influence), and interpersonal problems (e.g., arguments, domestic violence).

The problem of substance use disorders crosses all gender, age, racial, social, and economic boundaries. The pattern of substance use disorder begins with a voluntary choice to use the substance. With continued use of the substance the person loses the ability to choose not to use it. The person's behavior becomes marked by a compulsive need to find and consume the drug or alcohol. This change in behavior is related to prolonged exposure to the substance and its effect on brain function. Substance use disorder is a multidimensional problem. Effective treatment programs address these complex dimensions and their consequences. Substance use disorders may be part of a dual diagnosis in which substance use disorder is the primary or secondary problem with another mental health disorder. Both problems require treatment. A patient may be hospitalized during the initial withdrawal phase of treatment, but treatment must continue on an outpatient basis. Because substance use disorders are often relapsing disorders, remission and recovery require continuous treatments.

NANDA-I NDx Deficient Knowledge

Common Related Factors

Alteration in cognitive functioning
Insufficient information
Insufficient interest in learning
Insufficient knowledge of resources
Alteration in memory
Misinformation presented by others

Common Expected Outcome

Patient verbalizes understanding of substance use disorder and accepts need for treatment.

Defining Characteristics

Insufficient knowledge of substance use disorder
Inaccurate follow-through of instruction for treatment
Inaccurate performance on a test
Inappropriate behavior

NOC Outcomes
Knowledge: Substance Use Control; Information Processing

NIC Interventions
Learning Facilitation; Teaching: Disease Process

Ongoing Assessment

Actions/Interventions

■ Assess the patient's substance use history, including the type of substances used, amount used, routes of administration, and the most recent episode of use.

■ Assess for consequences of substance use such as financial, social, or family problems.

■ Identify the patient's supportive relationships.

Rationales

This information provides the foundation for individualizing a teaching plan based on the patient's use of specific substances. Many patients use and are dependent on more than one substance. The type of substances used by the patient may have changed over time. A variety of assessment tools is available to gather information about a patient's substance use disorder. These tools include Addiction Severity Index, Alcohol Use Disorders Identification Test (AUDIT), CAGE questionnaire, Drug Abuse Screening Test (DAST), Michigan Alcohol Screening Test (MAST), and Substance Abuse Subtle Screening Inventory (SASSI). QSEN: Evidence-based practice.

Substance use disorder presents the patient with problems that pervade virtually every aspect of his or her life. Significant economic resources are needed to support substance use over a prolonged period. The patient may have experienced problems maintaining employment, loss of financial savings, loss of friendships, and loss of stable family relationships. The patient may have a history with the criminal justice system related to substance use disorder. The patient's experience of the consequences of substance use may provide motivation to learn information and follow through with treatment.

The patient may have lost positive supportive relationships as a consequence of substance use. The patient's current relationships may support continued substance use. All relationships are affected by the substance use behavior; significant others who are affected by the substance use disorder also need support and information. The patient's significant others may provide support needed to help the patient acquire new information to manage the substance use disorder.

Basic Nursing Concepts Care Plans

■ = Independent   ▲ = Interprofessional Collaboration

Actions/Interventions

■ Assess the patient's knowledge of behavioral, physical, and psychological effects of substance use disorder.

Rationales

Many patients have accurate information regarding their substance use disorder, yet they continue to use the substance despite this knowledge. QSEN: Patient-centered care.

Therapeutic Interventions

Actions/Interventions

■ Provide accurate information about substance use and treatment:

• Medically assisted detoxification

• Behavioral therapy such as individual or group counseling and 12-step programs

• Medications for opioid and alcohol dependence

Rationales

It is critical that patients have current and accurate information regarding substance use disorders. QSEN: Evidence-based practice; Patient-centered care.

Detoxification and withdrawal are often the first step in the treatment process for a patient with substance use disorders. Patients who use drugs or alcohol may avoid seeking treatment because of fears and misconceptions about withdrawal and detoxification. Medically assisted detoxification provides the patient with medications to reduce the severity of withdrawal symptoms. Drug therapy used during detoxification from alcohol includes benzodiazepines, antiepileptics, and multiple vitamins. An opioid antagonist is administered at the beginning of opioid detoxification. Clonidine is often used in combination with methadone during opioid withdrawal. Benzodiazepines and antipsychotics (e.g., haloperidol) are used during detoxification from other central nervous system depressants and hallucinogens.

Cognitive-behavioral and motivational therapies support the patient's readiness to begin treatment and make behavior changes and help the patient to recognize and cope with situations that stimulate substance use, and to abstain from drugs or alcohol. These treatment approaches may involve individual or group counseling in outpatient or residential treatment settings. The 12-step programs (e.g., Alcoholics Anonymous [AA]) provide guiding principles for the process of recovery from substance use. These 12 principles have been adapted to a variety of recovery programs for other types of substance use and compulsive behavior problems.

Medications are used in the treatment of substance use to reestablish normal brain function, diminish cravings, and help prevent relapse. For patients with opioid use disorder substitution drugs (e.g., methadone, buprenorphine) act on the same brain receptors as the opiates being used by the patient. Drugs for alcohol use disorder include naltrexone, acamprosate, and disulfiram. Naltrexone blocks brain receptors associated with the rewarding effects of drinking, and diminishes the craving for alcohol. Acamprosate is used to support alcohol abstinence following detoxification. The drug acts to maintain a balance between the neurotransmitters glutamate and gamma-aminobutyric acid. Disulfiram blocks metabolism of alcohol and leads to extremely unpleasant symptoms when the patient drinks alcohol. Selective serotonin reuptake inhibitors are used to reduce alcohol cravings.

Actions/Interventions

- Teach the patient and family members about health risks associated with substance abuse:
  - Blood-borne infections
  - Liver disease
  - Cardiovascular and cerebrovascular disease
  - Sexually transmitted infections (STIs)

- Refer family members to support groups and counseling.

- Instruct the patient about symptoms to bring to the attention of the health care provider (e.g., withdrawal symptoms, delirium tremens, paranoid feelings, seeing or hearing things that are not there).

Rationales

Patients and families need to understand the health risks associated with substance use disorders. Patients who use the IV route for substance use and share needles with others are at very high risk for transmission of blood-borne infections such as HIV and hepatitis B. The toxic effects of alcohol are associated with the development of cirrhosis and cancer of the liver. Patients who use drugs or alcohol have a high risk for developing hypertension and stroke. Cocaine use is associated with increased incidence of hemorrhagic stroke in otherwise healthy individuals. The patient may engage in prostitution to obtain money for alcohol or drugs. Unprotected sexual activity may occur under the influence of the abused substance and increase the risk for STI transmission. QSEN: Safety.

Family members may need additional information, support, and counseling to cope with the effects of the patient's substance use disorder. Family members may experience feelings of guilt, despair, and hopelessness. They may have a history of attempts to change the behavior of the patient with little or no success. Many treatment programs offer separate counseling and support sessions for family members. AA offers programs (Al Anon/Alateen) for family members and friends of people with alcohol use disorder. QSEN: Teamwork and collaboration.

Acute symptoms of withdrawal, cravings, or intoxication may signal life-threatening events that require professional care. QSEN: Safety.

Noncompliance With Treatment Program

NANDA-I NDx

Common Related Factors

Values incongruent with plan
Health beliefs incongruent with plan
Cultural incongruence
Spiritual values incongruent with plan
Difficulty in patient-provider relationship
Health care system barriers
Complex treatment regimen
Intensity of regimen
Insufficient knowledge about treatment plan
Financial barriers

Defining Characteristics

Failure to meet outcomes
Nonadherence behavior
Development of complications
Exacerbation of symptoms
"Revolving-door" hospital admissions
Missing appointments

Common Expected Outcomes

Patient follows treatment plan.
Patient's substance screens remain negative.
Patient returns to treatment after relapse.

NOC Outcomes

Adherence Behavior; Compliance Behavior; Participation in Health Care Decisions

NIC Interventions

Self-Responsibility Facilitation; Family Involvement Promotion; Therapy Group; Counseling; Decision-Making Support; Patient Contracting

Basic Nursing Concepts Care Plans

■ = Independent   ▲ = Interprofessional Collaboration

Ongoing Assessment

Actions/Interventions	Rationales
■ Assess the patient's use of denial, rationalization, and blame to sustain his or her substance use habit.	Substance users have an enormous capacity to explain the behaviors they use to support substance use. Rationalization and denial may obstruct a patient's ability to be honest with care providers. QSEN: Patient-centered care.
■ Assess any secondary gains from substance use.	Perceived gains (e.g., friends, income) promote relapse behaviors and continued substance use.
▲ Perform random substance screens.	Support and rewards for compliance are important to recovery.

Therapeutic Interventions

Actions/Interventions	Rationales
■ Support the patient's growing awareness of substance use behaviors.	Positive support may encourage the patient to work toward greater understanding of his or her own behavior. The patient's insight is only the first step toward recovery, and insight without action is meaningless. QSEN: Patient-centered care.
■ Identify the patient's effort to blame or explain and reject change.	Allowing rationalizations to be unchallenged sanctions behavior. Patients must take responsibility for their own behavior. QSEN: Patient-centered care.
■ Promote participation in support groups for recovery.	Professional and self-help programs have been shown to provide immediate help and effective lifelong support for patients recovering from substance use disorders.
■ Plan for small, steady improvements.	It is realistic to expect patients to refrain from alcohol and drugs one day at a time. However, recovery from substance use is marked by relapses.
■ Help the patient learn to identify difficult feelings.	Articulating thoughts and feelings sometimes helps discharge emotions. These emotions may have been triggers for the patient's use of alcohol/drugs.
■ Reward positive actions.	Rewarding positive actions may help sustain them. Success promotes more success.
■ Spend time with the patient, but avoid reinforcing an already low self-esteem.	These patients experience a sense of pervasive worthlessness, helplessness, and hopelessness. It is important to be realistic about the negative, maladaptive behaviors they have used to support their substance use while still being able to affirm their worth as human beings and their individual value to themselves and others.

Related Care Plans

Caregiver role strain, Chapter 2
Ineffective coping, Chapter 2
Imbalanced nutrition: Less than body requirements, Chapter 2
Ineffective health maintenance, Chapter 2
Interrupted family processes, Chapter 2
Powerlessness, Chapter 2
Common mood disorders, ⊜volve
Impaired home maintenance, ⊜volve

⊜volve   **For additional care plans, go to http://evolve.elsevier.com/Gulanick/.**

Death and Dying: End-of-Life Issues

Dying is part of living. It is an active process, but it is rare when we are able to mark the beginning or the middle of an individual's dying. The end, of course, is death. There are individuals who report having come back from death and who have shared their memories of their experiences, but no one has been able to report on the state of actual death. Because death remains an unknown, it is a source of great mystery and endless speculation. Assisting patients and their families with making quality-of-life and end-of-life decisions to achieve a peaceful death is a daunting task for the health care professional in the context of the twenty-first century.

Still, much is known about dying. The process has been observed from time immemorial. Each person dies in his or her own way. This process is influenced by cultural norms, family traditions, and the people and setting among which a person's death takes place. The patient at the end of life may experience both actual and anticipatory losses. Pain, diminished abilities, fear, discomfort, massive dysfunction of organ systems (with or without the application of ever more complicated measures to prolong life),

and the resounding implications his or her death will have on others require the patient to integrate enormous amounts of information and undergo extraordinarily complicated emotions.

Health professionals who understand the inevitability of a patient's death may seek to provide patients with an opportunity for a "good death," or a positive dying experience. Although the characteristics of a good death will vary, most providers agree that patients should be allowed to die with dignity, surrounded by loved ones and free of pain, with everything having been done that could have been done. Caring for patients and their families or significant others at the end of life is the essence of nursing. Nurses experience a rich opportunity to observe the grace and goodness of the human spirit within those final hours. This care plan addresses the emotional aspects of death and dying in accordance with the Hospice and Palliative Nurses Association's Statement on the Scope and Standards of Hospice and Palliative Nursing Practice.

Basic Nursing Concepts Care Plans

NANDA-I NDx Fear

Common Related Factors
Unfamiliar setting
Separation from support system
Learned response
Language barrier
Sensory deficit (e.g., visual, hearing)
Anticipation of pain

Defining Characteristics
Identifies object of fear
Focus narrowed to the source of the fear
Change in physiological response (increased BP, HR, and respiratory rate)
Increase in tension
Apprehensiveness
Impulsiveness
Increase in alertness

Common Expected Outcomes
Patient identifies source of fear related to dying.
Patient uses effective coping strategies to reduce fear response.
Patient verbalizes or manifests a reduction or absence of fear.

NOC Outcomes
Fear Self-Control; Coping

NIC Interventions
Presence; Anxiety Reduction; Security Enhancement; Spiritual Support; Support System Enhancement

■ = Independent   ▲ = Interprofessional Collaboration

Basic Nursing Concepts
Care Plans

Ongoing Assessment

Actions/Interventions	Rationales
■ Assess the nature of the patient's fear by careful, thoughtful questioning and active listening.	Fears are patient-specific. The nurse should not assume that because a patient is dying his or her fears are limited to death. Patients may have fears over leaving dependents behind to fend for themselves or fear of embarrassment. Fear ranges from a paralyzing, overwhelming feeling to mild, nagging concern. QSEN: Patient-centered care.
■ Determine the methods that the patient uses to cope with fear.	This information helps identify the effectiveness of strategies used by the patient to manage the fear. The patient's philosophy about death may influence his or her ability to cope with fear. Some coping strategies may include risk-taking behaviors, denial, or religious rituals. QSEN: Patient-centered care.
■ Assess verbal and behavioral expressions of fear.	The nurse may use behavioral and verbal cues from the patient to determine the patient's fears. Physiological symptoms or complaints will intensify as the level of fear increases. Fear differs from anxiety in that fear is a response to a recognized threat. However, symptoms of fear are similar to those of anxiety. This information provides a basis for planning interventions to support the patient's coping strategies.

Therapeutic Interventions

Actions/Interventions	Rationales
■ Communicate to the patient and family members acceptance of the fears and related feelings experienced by the patient.	In Western culture, there is a great reluctance to discuss death. Some of the social isolation that dying patients feel is the result of trying to protect friends and family members from their need to talk about their impending death and what it means to them. Family members may think that the patient should be protected from the knowledge that his or her condition is terminal. This avoidance limits the patient's ability to talk about and work through these emotions.
■ Confirm that fear is a normal and appropriate response to situations when pain, danger, or loss of control is anticipated or experienced.	This reassurance by the nurse places fear within the scope of normal human experiences.
■ Spend time with the patient.	Patients may fear loneliness and abandonment. Being present and being silent are powerful communication techniques. This presence may involve talking or touching or attending to a physical need. QSEN: Patient-centered care.
■ Encourage reminiscing.	Reminiscing by the patient provides reassurance that one's life has value and eases the fear of meaninglessness. QSEN: Patient-centered care.
■ While interacting with the patient, maintain a calm and accepting manner that expresses care and concern.	Patients who are talking about real feelings need to feel safe in discussing troubling matters.

Actions/Interventions	**Rationales**
■ Provide continuity of care providers.	An ongoing relationship establishes trust and is a basis for communicating fearful feelings. The need for continuity of care providers increases in direct proportion to the intensity of the emotional material on which the patient is working. Patients rarely select a single individual to work on all of their emotional concerns. Rather, patients will share their fears with certain individuals while sharing anger with others. Continuity in care providers creates an environment in which this can best be accomplished. QSEN: Teamwork and collaboration.
■ Educate the patient and family about what to expect as part of the physiologic dying process.	Patients and family members may fear pain associated with the dying process. Knowing about the physical changes that occur as part of dying and measures to manage them may help the patient and family cope more effectively with these changes. For example, the patient approaching death will experience a decreased sensation of pain and touch. The skin becomes cool to touch and pale, mottled, or cyanotic. The patient may appear to stare as the eyelids remain partially open with no blink reflex. The loss of muscle tone may cause the patient's mouth to remain half open. An inability to clear secretions in the posterior pharynx may cause a gurgling sound with respirations. These secretions can be removed with oral suctioning. QSEN: Evidence-based practice.
■ As the patient's fear subsides, encourage him or her to explore specific events preceding the onset of specific fears.	Recognizing factors that precipitate a fear response may help the patient initiate effective coping strategies.
■ Assist the patient in using coping and comfort strategies that were helpful in the past.	Identifying these strategies helps the patient focus on fear as a real and natural part of life that has been and can continue to be dealt with successfully. QSEN: Patient-centered care.
■ Include family members in care activities.	Involvement of family in the care of the dying patient may assist in their sense of worth and decrease their sense of fear and helplessness in the dying process.
■ Adjust the amount of sensory stimulation in the care environment to the preferences of the patient. Remove equipment that is perceived as threatening by the patient.	Fear may escalate with overstimulation or understimulation in the environment. An environment that is too quiet or dark may lead to a patient's fear of being alone. Although staff may be comfortable around high-technology medical equipment, many patients experience more fear with the natural sounds of monitors, infusion pumps, alarms, and other equipment used for patient care and comfort. QSEN: Patient-centered care.
■ Encourage rest and relaxation.	Rest builds inner coping resources. The interprofessional health team will need to pace activities (especially for older adults) to conserve the patient's energy and offset fatigue.
■ Instruct the patient in the performance of self-calming measures:	These measures reduce fear or make it more manageable.
• Breathing exercises	These exercises reduce the physiological response to fear (i.e., increased BP, pulse, respiration).
• Relaxation, meditation, or guided imagery exercises	These exercises promote relaxation and relieve distress.
• Affirmations and calming self-talk exercises	These exercises enhance the patient's self-confidence.

Basic Nursing Concepts Care Plans

■ = Independent   ▲ = Interprofessional Collaboration

NANDA-I NDx Grieving

Common Related Factor

Impending death

Defining Characteristics

Psychological distress
Anger/blaming
Alterations in sleep or dream patterns
Detachment/despair
Disorganization
Suffering
Finding meaning in a loss
Personal growth
Alteration in activity level
Alteration in immune functioning
Alteration in neuroendocrine functioning

Common Expected Outcomes

Patient or family verbalizes feelings regarding impending death.
Patient or family maintains functional support systems.

NOC Outcomes

Grief Resolution; Family Resiliency; Psychosocial Adjustment: Life Change

NIC Interventions

Coping Enhancement; Grief Work Facilitation; Dying Care; Presence; Anticipatory Guidance

---

Ongoing Assessment

Actions/Interventions	Rationales
■ Identify the patient's and family members' grieving process.	Patients and their families will express grief in varied and personal ways. Although the process of grieving has been described as clearly defined phases, grief rarely manifests in a prescribed sequencing of feelings and experiences. Patients and their families revisit the phases of the grief process repeatedly. Grief helps make inevitable loss tolerable. QSEN: Patient-centered care.
■ Assess whether the patient and family members are in different phases of grieving.	Patients and family members may experience turbulent relationships, conflicts, and differences in expectations if they are at different phases of the grief process.
■ Evaluate the effectiveness of support systems available to the patient and family.	Multiple options for support broaden the opportunities for patients and families to personalize their methods of adjusting to the losses associated with dying.
▲ Evaluate the need for referral to hospice, home health, social services, legal consultants, or support groups.	As an increasing number of patients die in their homes, families are assuming more responsibility for end-of-life care. Family members may experience problems associated with the physical, emotional, and economic burden of providing care. Integrating the contributions of pastoral care, home care, social work, counseling, and other interprofessional members of the health care team provides the patient and family with access to a variety of community resources for support and respite care. QSEN: Teamwork and collaboration.

Basic Nursing Concepts Care Plans

Therapeutic Interventions

Actions/Interventions	Rationales
■ Encourage the patient and family members to verbalize feelings.	The patient and family need to complete unfinished business in their relationships through open communication and shared feelings. Exploring issues in a nonthreatening manner will lead to informed decision-making and assist the patient and family in verbalization of the anticipated loss. QSEN: Patient-centered care.
■ Provide a safe and private space for the expression of grief.	The environment needs to support the patient's expressions of grief (e.g., seeing a man cry, mourners making wide gestures with their hands and bodies, loud vocalizations, crying). Expressions of feelings are more likely to occur in a private setting.
■ Assist the patient and family members to understand that verbalizations of anger should not be perceived as personal attacks.	Patients whose emotional responses to life have been fairly predictable in the past may experience turbulent and disrupting grief. Patients and family members may express intense anger as part of the grieving process. The family needs to understand that the dying patient is processing a large amount of highly emotional information and that anger is part of the grieving process of an impending death. QSEN: Evidence-based practice.
■ Provide information about the patient's health status without false reassurances or taking away all hope.	Hope is a basic survival instinct. Because no one knows the future, allow patients and their families to remain hopeful until death is imminent. After being informed of a poor prognosis, many patients and their families experience a defensive retreat from the shock of what they have been told. During this time, patients may engage in denial and wishful thinking. They may become unwilling to participate in self-care or may become indifferent about it. QSEN: Evidence-based practice; Patient-centered care.
■ Encourage family members to talk with a patient who may be unresponsive.	Encouraging family members to talk and visit with the patient, even if the patient is unresponsive, instills hope. It has been shown that the patient is well aware of his or her surroundings (especially audible) beyond the point of responsiveness. QSEN: Evidence-based practice.
■ Facilitate conversations with the patient and significant others on "final arrangements" (e.g., burial, autopsy, organ donation, funeral).	A clear understanding of the patient's and family's belief systems and cultural practices related to death will help in advocating and facilitating open and honest communication regarding these arrangements. QSEN: Patient-centered care.
■ Encourage the patient and family members to share their wishes regarding who should be present at the time of death.	Families and significant others think about this but may feel uncomfortable discussing this issue together. The patient's level of comfort at the time of death may be influenced by who is present.
■ Confirm for family members that not being present at the time of death does not indicate lack of love or caring.	The moment of death cannot be predicted. It is important to remember that individual needs of each of the bereaved are different yet essential to the process of grieving. QSEN: Patient-centered care.
▲ Follow unit policies to identify the patient's critical status (e.g., color-coded door marker).	This identification informs all staff of the patient's status and ensures that staff members do not act or respond inappropriately when encountering the patient or family.
▲ Provide contact with additional support systems (e.g., peer support, groups, clergy) as needed.	Patients and families often become immersed in their grief and forget to access the resources available to them. Others may require expert help in negotiating grief. In either case, the care provider may be able to offer the observation that additional help is available. QSEN: Patient-centered care.

■ = Independent   ▲ = Interprofessional Collaboration

Basic Nursing Concepts
Care Plans

Actions/Interventions

▲ Foster continuity of end-of-life care across settings (e.g., home care, residential care, palliative care, hospice care).

Rationales

When the patient's illness is no longer responsive to treatment, hospice and palliative care provide the patient and family with assistance for decision-making, and disease symptom management, including pain, psychosocial support, spiritual care, and care as death nears. This interprofessional health team approach to end-of-life care includes nurses, physicians, bereavement counselors, social workers, and pastoral care providers. The setting for this care may begin in the hospital and continue in long-term care or the patient's home. QSEN: Teamwork and collaboration.

NANDA-I
NDx **Powerlessness**

Common Related Factors

Dysfunctional institutional environment
Complex treatment regimen
Insufficient interpersonal interactions

Defining Characteristics

Insufficient sense of control
Inadequate participation in care
Alienation
Dependency
Depression
Doubt about role performance
Frustration about inability to perform previous activities

Common Expected Outcomes

Patient participates in care decisions.
Patient makes important end-of-life decisions.

NOC Outcomes

Participation in Health Care Decisions; Health Beliefs: Perceived Ability to Perform; Health Beliefs: Perceived Control

NIC Interventions

Decision-Making Support; Self-Efficacy Enhancement

Ongoing Assessment

Actions/Interventions

■ Assess the patient's need for power and control.

■ Assess for feelings of hopelessness, depression, and apathy.

■ Identify situations or interactions that may increase the patient's feelings of powerlessness.

Rationales

Patients can identify those aspects of self-governance that are most important to them. Actively listen so the patient truly feels heard (e.g., offer your presence). QSEN: Patient-centered care.

These feelings may be components of grief. The patient may experience tremendous guilt associated with any loss of control. Subsequent interventions will be critical to facilitating feelings of well-being and empowerment, especially in older adults.

Many medical routines are superimposed on patients without ever receiving the patient's permission. This can foster a sense of powerlessness in patients. It is important for care providers to recognize the patient's right to refuse procedures. Unresolved loss may trigger feelings of powerlessness and even persist over time. QSEN: Patient-centered care.

Basic Nursing Concepts Care Plans

Actions/Interventions

- Assess the patient's decision-making energy level and ability.

- Assess the patient's wishes for information about end-of-life decisions.

- Determine whether the patient has an advance directive, a durable power of attorney for health care, or a living will:

  • Advance directive

  • Durable power of attorney for health care

  • Living will declaration

Rationales

Powerlessness is not the same as the inability to make a decision. It is the feeling that one has lost the implicit power for self-governance. Energy conservation will help reduce or relieve fatigue so the patient will be better able to use available energy for appropriate decision-making.

This information may help differentiate powerlessness from knowledge deficit. A patient simply experiencing a knowledge deficit may be mobilized to act in his or her own best interest after information is given and options are explored. The act of providing information may heighten a patient's sense of autonomy.

These documents provide the patient with an opportunity to fully participate in end-of-life decisions and designate the person who will act on the patient's behalf to implement those decisions. QSEN: Patient-centered care.

An advance directive is a legal document that expresses the patient's wishes and desires for his or her health care treatment in case he or she becomes terminally ill and unable to articulate wishes and desires. These directives will act in the place of the patient's verbal requests and serve as assurance that the patient's end-of-life decisions will be honored.

This document allows the patient to designate another person to make health care decisions on the patient's behalf. The durable power of attorney for health care becomes effective if the patient becomes unable, either temporarily or permanently, to make his or her own health care decisions. Implicit in this is the fact that the patient has discussed his or her desires with this appointed individual. If the patient becomes able to resume making his or her own decisions, then the durable power of attorney for health care is no longer in effect.

This document contains instructions that a patient be allowed to die if he or she becomes terminally ill and unable to communicate to the extent required by law. It recognizes the patient's desire not to be kept alive artificially and sets parameters on the limits to which health care providers are to go in extending the patient's life.

Therapeutic Interventions

Actions/Interventions

- Support the patient's sense of autonomy by involving the patient in decision-making, by giving and accepting information, and by assisting the patient with controlling the environment as appropriate.
- Assist the patient with developing an advance directive.

- Implement personalized methods of providing hygiene, diet, and sleep. Enhance basic care by offering food, drink, comfort, and security.
- Encourage comfortable furnishings and surroundings.

Rationales

The ultimate decision-making authority lies within the patient. However, the goal of the health care professional is to assist patients in identifying and verbalizing their preferences in making authentic choices. QSEN: Patient-centered care.

An advance directive allows patients to make decisions about their lives even after they are unable to express their own needs and desires.

Allowing or helping the patient decide when and how these things are to be accomplished will increase the patient's sense of autonomy. QSEN: Patient-centered care.

Having comfortable surroundings will enhance the patient's sense of autonomy and acknowledges the patient's right to have dominion over controllable aspects of his or her own life. This gives some normalcy to life during the dying process. QSEN: Patient-centered care.

■ = Independent   ▲ = Interprofessional Collaboration

Actions/Interventions

■ Provide the patient with acceptable opportunities for expressing feelings of anger, anxiety, and powerlessness.

■ Offer continuity of a support network.

Rationales

Verbalizing these feelings may diminish or diffuse the patient's sense of powerlessness. The care provider may need to make a special effort to maintain a careful sense of timing and compassion to alleviate the patient's feelings of loneliness or abandonment.

Encourage personal control by offering continuity in staffing and sustained involvement of significant others.

NANDA-I NDx Spiritual Distress

Common Related Factors

Actively dying
Self-alienation
Social alienation
Increasing dependence on another
Loneliness
Perception of having unfinished business
Sociocultural deprivation

Defining Characteristics

Anxiety
Crying
Fatigue
Questioning identity
Questioning meaning of life
Questioning meaning of suffering
Connections to self
- Anger
- Inadequate acceptance
- Insufficient courage
- Perceived insufficient meaning in life
- Decrease in serenity

Connections with others
- Alienation
- Separation from support system
- Refuses to interact with significant other or spiritual leader

Connections with art, music, literature, and nature
- Decrease in expression of previous pattern of creativity

Connections with power greater than self
- Feeling abandoned
- Hopelessness
- Anger toward a power greater than self
- Inability to experience the transcendent or to be introspective
- Inability to participate in religious activities
- Inability to pray
- Request for a spiritual leader
- Sudden change in spiritual practice

Common Expected Outcomes

Patient expresses hope in and value of his or her own belief system and inner resources.
Patient expresses a sense of well-being through art, music, or writing.
Patient participates in spiritual activities.
Patient expresses connectedness with self, others, or a power greater than self.

NOC Outcomes
Hope; Spiritual Health
NIC Interventions
Spiritual Support; Spiritual Growth Facilitation; Coping Enhancement

Ongoing Assessment

Actions/Interventions

- Assess the patient's history of formal religious affiliation, perceived spiritual needs, and desire to engage in spiritual practices.

- Assess spiritual beliefs and cultural heritage.

- Assess the spiritual meaning of illness and death.
  - "What is the meaning of your illness?"
  - "How does grief affect your relationship with God, your beliefs, or other sources of strength?"
  - "Do your illness and grief interfere with expressing your spiritual beliefs?"
- Assess the patient's need to resolve unfinished business.

Rationales

Eliciting information regarding religious affiliation, spiritual practices, and perceived spiritual needs allows the patient to be a full partner in providing care. QSEN: Patient-centered care.

All people have a spiritual dimension even if they do not express association with a specific religion or faith tradition. The patient's cultural heritage may be a source of important beliefs besides religion that provide strength and inspiration. QSEN: Patient-centered care.

These questions provide a basis for understanding the patient's distress. Some patients may perceive suffering at the end of life as a "punishment from God." The patient's process of introspection will assist him or her in comprehending the loss.

Patients may not find peace or harmony until important affairs are in order such as resolving strained family relationships.

Therapeutic Interventions

Actions/Interventions

- Encourage the verbalization of feelings.

- ▲ When requested by the patient, arrange for clergy, religious rituals, or the display of religious objects.
- If requested, sit with the patient who wishes to pray, and arrange for clergy at the time of death as requested by the patient.

- Do not provide intellectual solutions for spiritual problems.
- Encourage the patient to continue to search for truth by continuing to examine beliefs.

- Offer opportunities to share feelings and experiences in writing, through art, or through taping (audio or video).

Rationales

Patients need the opportunity to express feelings associated with spiritual distress. Support crying by offering caring touch.

Patients may derive comfort and solace from these intimate spiritual experiences.

Being open to cultural and religious differences will allow the patient's traditions and rituals to be a part of their care while providing comfort and compassion to both the patient and family.

Spiritual beliefs are based on faith and are independent of logic.

Reconstitution and reorganization of beliefs often follow times of questioning a philosophical and spiritual construct.

Leaving a historical legacy can help bring meaning to one's life.

Related Care Plans

Acute pain, Chapter 2
Caregiver role strain, Chapter 2
Chronic pain, Chapter 2
Ineffective coping, Chapter 2

Basic Nursing Concepts
Care Plans

■ = Independent   ▲ = Interprofessional Collaboration

CHAPTER
5

Cardiac and Vascular Care Plans

Acute Coronary Syndromes/Myocardial Infarction

Unstable Angina; ST-Segment Elevation Myocardial Infarction; Non–ST-Segment Elevation Myocardial Infarction;

Acute coronary syndromes (ACSs) represent a spectrum of clinical conditions associated with acute myocardial ischemia. Most patients who experience ACS have atherosclerotic changes in the coronary arteries. Chronic inflammatory processes play a key role in the pathogenesis of atherosclerosis. The presence of atherosclerotic plaques narrows the lumen of the arteries, and disruption or rupture of those plaques exposes a thrombogenic surface on which platelets aggregate, contributing to thrombus formation that diminishes blood flow to the myocardium. The resulting imbalance between myocardial oxygen demand and supply is the primary cause of the clinical manifestation in ACS. Other causes of ACS include coronary artery spasm and arterial inflammation related to infection. Noncardiac conditions that increase myocardial oxygen demand can precipitate ACS in patients with preexisting coronary artery disease (CAD). These conditions include fever, tachycardia, and hyperthyroidism. Decreased myocardial oxygen supply can occur in noncardiac conditions such as hypotensive states, hypoxemia, and anemia.

Clinical conditions included in ACS are unstable angina, variant angina, non–ST-segment elevation myocardial infarction (NSTEMI), and ST-segment elevation myocardial infarction (STEMI). Evaluation of chest pain related to these disorders is a major cause of emergency department visits and hospitalizations in the United States. The term *ACS* is used prospectively to diagnose patients with chest pain or other clinical manifestations indicating the need to be triaged for treatment of unstable angina or acute MI. Although their pathogenesis and clinical presentation are similar, they differ primarily by whether ischemia is severe enough to cause sufficient myocardial damage to release

detectable quantities of cardiac biomarkers (e.g., troponin, creatine kinase–myocardial bound [CK-MB], myoglobin) denoting acute MI. Early identification of ACS and intervention to improve myocardial perfusion reduces the risk for sudden cardiac death and acute MI in these patients.

Unstable angina is characterized by (1) angina that occurs when the patient is at rest, (2) angina that significantly limits the patient's activity, or (3) previously diagnosed angina that becomes more frequent, lasts longer, and increasingly limits the patient's activity. Patients typically do not have ST-segment elevation and do not release cardiac biomarkers indicating myocardial necrosis. NSTEMI is distinguished from unstable angina by the presence of cardiac biomarkers, indicating myocardial necrosis. Most patients do not develop new Q waves on the electrocardiogram (ECG). STEMI is characterized by release of cardiac biomarkers and the presence of new Q waves on the ECG.

This care plan focuses on the assessment of and interventions for patients with all of these conditions. The American Heart Association and the American College of Cardiology have developed treatment guidelines for patients with ACSs. Each guideline addresses initial and ongoing drug therapy, indications for fibrinolytic and percutaneous coronary interventions, and discharge considerations. For patients with MI, the therapeutic goals are to establish reperfusion, to minimize the infarct size, to prevent and treat complications, and to provide emotional support and education. This care plan focuses on acute management of ACS. The cardiac rehabilitation care plan presented later in this chapter addresses specific learning needs.

NDx Acute Pain

Common Related Factors

Myocardial ischemia
Myocardial infarction (MI)

Defining Characteristics

Self-reports of chest pain/discomfort using standardized
pain scale
New-onset (<2 months) angina
Changing pattern of previously stable angina
Facial expression of pain
Shortness of breath
Pallor, weakness
Epigastric discomfort/indigestion
Nausea/vomiting
Diaphoresis or cold sweat
Change in physiological parameter (e.g., blood pressure,
heart rate, respiratory rate and oxygen saturation)
Electrocardiogram (ECG) changes: ST-segment depression
or elevation, deep symmetrical T-wave inversion in
multiple leads, or any transient ECG changes occurring
during pain

Common Expected Outcomes

Patient verbalizes satisfactory pain control at a decreased
intensity using a standardized pain scale.
Patient exhibits increased comfort, such as baseline levels
for pulse, BP, respirations, and relaxed muscle tone or
body posture.

NOC Outcomes

Comfort Status; Pain Level; Pain Control;
Medication Response

NIC Interventions

Pain Management; Cardiac Care: Acute

Ongoing Assessment

Actions/Interventions

■ Assess the following pain characteristics:
  • Quality: squeezing, tightening, choking, pressure,
    burning, "viselike," aching
  • Location: substernal area; may radiate to arms, shoul-
    ders, neck, back, jaw
  • Severity: more intense than stable angina pectoris
  • Duration: persists longer than 20 minutes, usually
    several hours
  • Onset: with minimal exertion or during rest or sleep
  • Relieving factors: usually does not respond to sublin-
    gual nitroglycerin (NTG) or rest; may respond to intra-
    venous (IV) NTG; not affected by position change or
    breathing

■ Assess any prior treatments for pain.

Rationales

Patients with presenting symptoms for MI can have a variety
of pain characteristics, making diagnosis difficult. Older
patients, women, patients with diabetes mellitus, and
patients with heart failure often have atypical symptoms.
Sudden shortness of breath and fatigue are more common
than typical substernal chest pain. Associated diaphoresis
may be present. Careful assessment facilitates early or
appropriate treatment when time is critical for saving sal-
vageable myocardium. If patients are phoning the health
care provider about the pain, they should be advised to
seek evaluation in a medical facility. Triage to the appropriate medical setting is a priority task. Patients with significant pain are usually admitted to rule out MI until
serial laboratory data provide definitive diagnosis. QSEN:
Patient-centered care.

The nurse should note treatment that the patient received
before hospital admission. Patients may have tried several
pain relief methods at home, including antacids. Some
patients may have taken sublingual NTG and a single dose
of aspirin before contacting emergency medical services.

Cardiac and Vascular
Care Plans

■ = Independent   ▲ = Interprofessional Collaboration

Actions/Interventions

- Place the patient on the ECG monitor immediately during pain for evidence of myocardial ischemia or injury.

- Note the time since onset of the first episode of chest pain.

▲ Monitor serial cardiac biomarkers.

▲ If cardiac biomarkers are negative, anticipate other diagnostic studies:
  - Exercise stress testing with imaging modality
  - Pharmacological stress testing with dipyridamole, adenosine, or dobutamine, and nuclear imaging

- Monitor heart rate (HR) and blood pressure (BP) during pain episodes and during medication administration.

- Continually reassess the patient's chest pain and response to medication. If no relief is achieved from optimal doses of medication, report to the physician for evaluation for thrombolytic treatment, coronary angiography, percutaneous coronary intervention, or bypass surgery revascularization.

- For patients experiencing an acute ST-segment elevation MI (STEMI), assess for absolute and relative contraindications to thrombolytic agents.

Rationales

MI occurs over several hours. The time course of ST-T wave changes and development of Q waves guides diagnosis and treatment. If the ECG is unchanged from prior tracings, the patient is considered low risk and can be managed on an outpatient basis. QSEN: Safety.

If less than 6 hours since the first pain occurred and patients have evidence of acute ST-segment elevation or new left bundle branch block on ECG, they may be candidates for IV thrombolytic therapy.

Cardiac-specific troponin (troponin I or T) levels should be measured at presentation and 3 to 6 hours after symptom onset in all patients who present with symptoms consistent with acute coronary syndrome (ACS) to identify a rising and/or falling pattern. These can be continued after 6 hours as needed.

According to the American Heart Association guideline, contemporary troponin assay is more sensitive and specific for myocardial injury, in that it remains elevated for 10 to 14 days. Although CK-MB and myoglobin are detectable first, they are not as useful as troponin for the diagnosis of ACS. Cardiac enzymes and proteins do not elevate with unstable angina because there is no cellular death. QSEN: Evidence-based practice.

Exercise and pharmacological stress testing and echocardiography are useful in evaluating ventricular function and myocardial perfusion in patients with acute coronary syndrome (ACS). The choice of test is based on the resting ECG, ability to perform exercise, and technologies available. The results of these tests are used to determine the extent of coronary artery disease (CAD) and the patient's risk for MI. The test results can be used in making decisions about the need for coronary angiography. QSEN: Evidence-based practice.

Pain causes increased sympathetic stimulation, which increases oxygen demands on the heart. Tachycardia and increased BP are seen during pain and anxiety; hypotension is seen with nitrate and morphine administration; bradycardia is seen with morphine and beta-blocker administration. QSEN: Safety.

Ongoing pain can signify prolonged myocardial ischemia that warrants immediate intervention. QSEN: Safety.

Thrombolytic agents do not distinguish a pathological occlusive coronary thrombus from a protective hemostatic clot; therefore patient selection is critical. Guidelines for absolute versus relative contraindications continue to be revised because risk-benefit assessments may change depending on the availability of newer treatment modalities. Guidelines recommend that fibrinolytic agents be given within 30 minutes of hospital admission for STEMI when indicated. QSEN: Evidence-based practice; Safety.

Cardiac and Vascular Care Plans

Therapeutic Interventions

Actions/Interventions	Rationales
■ Instruct the patient to report pain as soon as it starts.	The patient needs to learn the meaning of this chest discomfort/pain as a sign of myocardiac injury, the benefits of obtaining prompt treatment, and the risks of delaying treatment of chest pain.
■ Respond immediately to reports of pain.	Prompt treatment may decrease myocardial ischemia and prevent damage. QSEN: Safety.
■ Obtain a 12-lead ECG during pain episodes.	ST-segment and T-wave changes help provide a definitive diagnosis. Unstable angina and non–ST-segment elevation myocardial infarction (NSTEMI) have similar ECG changes, in contrast to those seen with STEMI.
▲ Administer oxygen as prescribed. Measure oxygen saturation.	When more oxygen is available to the myocardium, ischemia is reduced or reversed. Pulse oximetry is a useful tool to detect changes in oxygenation. Oxygen saturation should be kept at 90% or greater.
▲ Give anti-ischemic therapy as prescribed, evaluating its effectiveness and observing for signs or symptoms of untoward reactions:	Early, effective treatment aids in salvaging at-risk myocardium. Recommendations for anti-ischemic therapy are directed at reducing the risk for harm to the patient. QSEN: Evidence-based practice; Safety.
• Administer non–enteric coated chewable aspirin as ordered.	Aspirin decreases platelet aggregation and significantly improves mortality and morbidity rates when used within 24 hours of onset of chest pain. Use of aspirin is a core performance indicator. Treatment should be started at home or in the emergency department and not delayed until admission. Patients will subsequently be discharged on aspirin therapy
• Administer NTG, either sublingual or spray, at time of admission. Anticipate an NTG drip for unrelieved pain. Titrate the dose until pain is relieved, as long as the systolic BP is greater than 90 mm Hg.	NTG relaxes smooth muscles in the vascular system, causing peripheral arterial and venous vasodilation. This reduction in both preload and afterload results in lower BP, decreased venous return to the ventricle, and decreased myocardial demand.
• Administer morphine sulfate intravenously.	Morphine sulfate is an opioid analgesic that reduces the workload on the heart through venodilation. It reduces anxiety and decreases the patient's perception of pain. Side effects include hypotension, bradycardia, decreased respirations, and nausea.
• Anticipate the administration of anticoagulants or antiplatelet therapy for high-risk patients.	These agents reduce the development or magnitude of MI when administered during the acute phases of ACS. The selection of agents depends on the clinical presentation and whether the patient undergoes early invasive therapies.
• Administer beta-blockers. Anticipate IV administration.	Beta-blockers decrease myocardial oxygen demand, the magnitude of infarction, and the incidence of associated complications. They should be started within the first 24 hours. Research reports reduced mortality rate in acute phase of MI and at 1-year follow-up, as well as chances of reduced reinfarction. Do not give in patients with chronic obstructive pulmonary disease, heart block, bradycardia, decompensated left ventricular failure, hypotension, or cocaine toxicity.
• Administer angiotensin-converting enzyme (ACE) inhibitors or angiotensin receptor blockers (ARBs).	Research supports this therapy in patients with left ventricular ejection fraction less than 40%, and those with hypertension, diabetes mellitus, or chronic kidney disease. They prevent ventricular remodeling and are used indefinitely because the risk for recurrent MI and progression to heart failure and death is reduced.

Cardiac and Vascular Care Plans

■ = Independent ▲ = Interprofessional Collaboration

Actions/Interventions

- Administer calcium channel blockers.

- Provide statin therapy.

- Administer thrombolytic agents according to unit protocol.

■ Anticipate a coronary angiography to diagnose and, depending on the results, anticipate revascularization by percutaneous coronary intervention (e.g., angioplasty) with stenting

Rationales

Calcium channel blockers are indicated for patients with significant hypertension, cocaine toxicity, contraindications to beta-blocker therapy, or refractory ischemia with coronary spasm. They are also used for recurrent ischemia after appropriate use of beta-blockers and nitrates.

High-intensity statin therapy should be initiated or continued to reduce atherosclerotic buildup.

Thrombolytic agents are enzymes that convert plasminogen to plasmin, which has potent fibrinolytic activity. These drugs break down fibrin clots and restore perfusion of myocardial tissue through previously blocked coronary arteries. IV therapy is preferred because it is fastest. Guidelines recommend administration within 30 minutes of hospital arrival ("door to needle goal").

Definitive diagnosis and early revascularization optimize myocardial perfusion and reduce risk for ischemia, infarction, and related complications. If indicated, percutaneous coronary intervention should be done within 90 minutes ("door to balloon inflation goal") of hospital arrival. Patients who initially received thrombolytic therapy still require PCI for more long-term treatment. QSEN: Evidence-based practice.

NANDA-I
NDx Fear

Common Related Factors

Recurrent anginal attacks
Incomplete relief from pain by usual means (NTG and rest)
Threat of MI
Threat of death
Threat of unknown
Unfamiliar environment
Separation from support system

Common Expected Outcomes

Patient verbalizes or manifests a reduction or absence of fear.
Patient uses effective coping mechanisms.

Defining Characteristics

Identifies fearful feelings or object of fear
Restlessness
Increased awareness/tension
Increased questioning
Increased HR, BP, respiratory rate

NOC Outcomes
Fear Self-Control; Coping
NIC Interventions
Anxiety Reduction; Coping Enhancement; Emotional Support; Cardiac Care

---

Ongoing Assessment

Actions/Interventions

■ Assess the level of fear (mild to severe). Note signs and symptoms, especially nonverbal communication.

Rationales

Pain and pending MI can result in a potentially life-threatening situation that will produce high levels of anxiety in the patient and significant other. Fear is associated with the physiological reactions (increased BP and HR) that can increase myocardial oxygen demand.

Actions/Interventions

- Assess the cause of fear.

Rationales

Determining the specific cause guides therapy. The patient may be afraid of the pain experience itself, of interventions associated with emergency care, outcomes such as MI or dying, being separated from loved ones, or being in an unfamiliar environment. QSEN: Patient-centered care.

Therapeutic Interventions

Actions/Interventions

- Acknowledge awareness of the patient's fear.

- Encourage verbalization of fears and feelings.

- Maintain a confident, assured manner.

- Assure the patient and significant others of close, continuous monitoring that will ensure prompt intervention.
- Reduce unnecessary external stimuli.

- Explain all procedures as appropriate, using simple, concrete terms.

- ▲ Administer a mild tranquilizer as needed.

- Establish rest periods between care and procedures.

Rationales

Acknowledgment of the patient's feelings validates the feelings and communicates acceptance of those feelings.

Verbalization provides clarity of the patient's perception and enhances coping.

The staff's anxiety is easily noticed by the patient. The patient's feeling of stability increases in a calm and non-threatening atmosphere.

Continuous monitoring provides a measure of safety and security that can reduce the fear experience for the patient.

Anxiety may escalate with excessive conversation, noise, and equipment around the patient.

Information and open communication help allay anxiety. Patients who are anxious may not be able to comprehend anything more than simple, clear, brief instructions.

Short-term use of antianxiety medications can relieve unpleasant feelings.

Quiet periods assist in relaxation and regaining emotional balance.

NANDA-I
NDx Risk for Decreased Cardiac Output

Common Risk Factors

Prolonged episodes of myocardial ischemia affecting contractility

Acute MI (especially at anterior site) affecting contractility of the heart

Right ventricular infarct (RVI) with reduced right ventricular (RV) contractility

Papillary muscle rupture and mitral insufficiency

Common Expected Outcome

Patient maintains adequate cardiac output, as evidenced by strong peripheral pulses, systolic BP within 20 mm Hg of baseline, HR 60 to 100 beats/min with regular rhythm, urinary output 30 mL/hr or greater, warm and dry skin, clear breath sounds, good capillary refill, and normal level of consciousness.

NOC Outcomes
Cardiac Pump Effectiveness; Vital Signs; Fluid Balance
NIC Interventions
Hemodynamic Regulation; Cardiac Care: Acute; Invasive Hemodynamic Monitoring

Cardiac and Vascular Care Plans

■ = Independent ▲ = Interprofessional Collaboration

Ongoing Assessment

Actions/Interventions	Rationales
■ Monitor the patient's HR and BP.	Sinus tachycardia and an increase in arterial BP are early signs of ventricular dysfunction and occur as compensatory responses.
■ Assess the skin color, temperature, and moisture.	Decreased cardiac output results in a compensatory increase in sympathetic nervous system activity that causes cool, pale, clammy skin.
■ Assess the peripheral pulses, including capillary refill.	Reduced stroke volume and cardiac output cause weak peripheral pulses and slow capillary refill.
■ Assess for any changes in the level of consciousness.	Early signs of cerebral hypoxia are restlessness, anxiety, and difficulty concentrating. Older patients are especially susceptible to reduced perfusion to vital organs. QSEN: Safety.
■ Assess the respiratory rate, rhythm, and breath sounds.	Rapid, shallow respirations and the presence of crackles and wheezes are characteristic of reduced cardiac output. Crackles reflect the accumulation of fluid secondary to impaired ventricular emptying. QSEN: Safety.
■ Assess the patient's urine output.	The renal system compensates for low BP by retaining water. Oliguria is a classic sign of inadequate renal perfusion from reduced cardiac output.
■ Auscultate for the presence of S_3, S_4, or systolic murmur.	S_3 denotes left ventricular (LV) dysfunction; S_4 is a common finding with MI, usually indicating noncompliance of the ischemic ventricle. A loud holosystolic murmur may be caused by papillary muscle rupture.
■ Use pulse oximetry to monitor oxygen saturation; assess arterial blood gases.	Pulse oximetry is a useful tool to detect changes in oxygenation. Oxygen saturation should be kept at 90% or greater. As shock increases, aerobic metabolism ceases and lactic acidosis ensues, raising the level of carbon dioxide and pH. These direct measurements serve as optimal guides for therapy. Appropriate use of safety-enhancing technology reduces the risk of harm by identifying changes in acid-base balance and guiding specific interventions. QSEN: Safety.
■ If the patient had an inferior MI, evaluate the ECG using right precordial leads ($_RV_4$–$_RV_6$) and inferior leads (II, III, aVF). Assess for signs of RVI and RV failure.	These leads may show ECG changes indicative of RVI. RVI is seen in 30% to 50% of patients with symptoms for inferior MI. Signs of RV dysfunction include increased central venous pressure, increased jugular venous distention, absence of crackles, and decreased BP.

Therapeutic Interventions

Actions/Interventions	Rationales
■ Anticipate the insertion of hemodynamic monitoring catheters.	Pulmonary artery diastolic pressure and pulmonary capillary wedge pressure are excellent indicators of filling pressures in the left ventricle; monitoring central venous pressure and right atrial pressure guides management of RVI. Attention to changes in filling pressures and fluid balance reduces the risk of harm to the patient and guides specific interventions. QSEN: Safety.
▲ Administer IV fluids to keep the pulmonary capillary wedge pressure at 16 to 18 mm Hg for optimal filling of the ventricle.	Too little fluid reduces preload or blood volume and BP; too much fluid can overload the heart and lead to pulmonary edema.

Cardiac and Vascular Care Plans

Actions/Interventions	Rationales
▲ If signs of left ventricular failure (LVF) occur: • Administer diuretic and vasodilator medications as prescribed. • Administer IV inotropic medications. • Administer oxygen as needed.	These medications reduce the filling pressures and workload of the infarcted heart and improve fluid balance. These medications improve the contractility of the heart. Oxygen increases arterial saturation. When more oxygen is available to the myocardium, ischemia is reduced or reversed and ventricular pumping may be improved.
▲ If signs of right ventricular failure (RVF) occur: • Anticipate aggressive fluid resuscitation (3 to 6 L/24 hr).	The right ventricle is a low-pressure system that is dependent on a full venous return and strong filling in the ventricle to produce effective cardiac output. The damaged myocardium requires a greater amount of fluid to maintain adequate filling. Aggressive fluid therapy is a key therapy.
• Anticipate inotropic and peripheral vasodilator medications.	These medications improve ventricular contraction and reduce RV and LV afterload, thereby enhancing stroke volume.
▲ Avoid or carefully administer nitrates and morphine sulfate for pain.	These medications reduce preload and filling pressures, which may compromise cardiac output.
■ Anticipate intra-aortic balloon pump (IABP) management if pain and ischemic changes persist despite maximal medical therapy.	IABP increases coronary blood flow during diastole while reducing work by the left ventricle during systolic contraction.

Risk for Decreased Cardiac Output: Dysrhythmias

Common Risk Factor
Electrical instability or dysrhythmias secondary to ischemia or necrosis, sympathetic nervous system stimulation, or electrolyte imbalance (hypokalemia or hypomagnesemia)

Common Expected Outcome
Patient maintains adequate cardiac output as evidenced by strong peripheral pulses, systolic BP within 20 mm Hg of baseline, HR 60 to 100 beats/min with regular rhythm, urinary output greater than or equal to 30 mL/hr, strong peripheral pulses, warm and dry skin, clear breath sounds, good capillary refill, and normal level of consciousness.

NOC Outcomes
Cardiac Pump Effectiveness; Circulation Status
NIC Interventions
Dysrhythmia Management; Hemodynamic Regulation; Cardiac Care: Acute

Ongoing Assessment

Actions/Interventions	Rationales
■ Monitor the patient's HR and heart rhythm continuously. Monitor PR, QRS, and QT intervals and note any changes.	Dysrhythmias produce alterations in both HR and heart rhythm. Changes in electrical properties of myocardial cells occur with prolonged ischemia and infarction. These changes include increased automaticity of ectopic pacemakers and increased refractoriness in normal conduction pathways. Many antidysrhythmic drugs also depress the conduction of normal impulses and can cause further dysrhythmias.

Cardiac and Vascular Care Plans

■ = Independent ▲ = Interprofessional Collaboration

Actions/Interventions

- Observe for or anticipate the following common dysrhythmias:
  - With anterior MI: second-degree heart block, complete heart block, right bundle branch block, left anterior hemiblock, left bundle branch block, or bifascicular block
  - With inferior MI: sinus bradycardia, sinus pause, first- and second-degree heart block (Wenckebach phenomenon), and third-degree heart block
- Monitor with continuous ECG monitoring in the appropriate lead.
  - Monitor in lead II, observing for left anterior hemiblock.

  - If anterior MI with left anterior hemiblock is already present, monitor in a modified chest lead (MCL$_1$) for right bundle branch block.
- Assess for signs of decreased cardiac output that accompany dysrhythmias: hypotension, reduced urine output, weak pulses, cool skin, and a reduced level of consciousness.
- Assess the response to antidysrhythmic treatment.

Rationales

Specific areas of infarction correlate with expected dysrhythmias.

Monitoring facilitates prompt detection of a conduction problem. QSEN: Safety.

Left anterior hemiblock is characterized by normal QRS width and left axis deviation with deep S waves in leads II, III, and aVF. By anticipating these dysrhythmias, early assessment is made and treatment is initiated.

Right bundle branch block is characterized by a QRS complex of greater than 0.12 second and an rSR′ complex in V$_1$ or V$_2$.

The patient's tolerance to the dysrhythmia guides intervention. Hemodynamic status is more important than "treating the dysrhythmia" per se. QSEN: Safety; Patient-centered care.

Follow-up evaluation guides ongoing treatment.

Therapeutic Interventions

Actions/Interventions

- Institute treatments as appropriate and according to protocol:
  - Potassium or magnesium supplements as guided by serum electrolyte levels
  - Amiodarone or procainamide (Pronestyl) for premature ventricular contraction (PVC) and ventricular tachycardia
  - Atropine sulfate for symptomatic bradycardia; external pacemaker on standby
  - Adenosine, beta-blockers, diltiazem, and cardioversion for atrial tachydysrhythmias
  - Temporary pacemaker for Mobitz type II, new complete heart block, new bifascicular bundle branch block, or left bundle branch block with anterior wall MI
  - Implantable cardioverter-defibrillator for recurrent ventricular tachycardia, as indicated
  - Defibrillation for ventricular fibrillation
  - Cardiopulmonary resuscitation as appropriate

Rationales

Current Advanced Cardiac Life Support guidelines provide protocols for the management of dysrhythmias. These medications are based on recommendations from national organizations. QSEN: Evidence-based practice; Safety.

NANDA-I
ND$_x$ **Deficient Knowledge**

Common Related Factors

Insufficient information
Insufficient interest in learning
Misinformation presented by others

Defining Characteristics

Insufficient knowledge
Inaccurate follow-through of instruction
Inappropriate behavior

Cardiac and Vascular Care Plans

Common Expected Outcome

Patient verbalizes understanding of condition, diagnosis or treatment of acute coronary syndrome (ACS), and recovery process.

NOC Outcomes
Cardiac Disease: Self-Management; Knowledge: Anticoagulation Therapy Management; Knowledge: CAD Management

NIC Interventions
Health Literacy Enhancement; Learning Facilitation; Teaching: Disease Process; Teaching: Prescribed Medication

Ongoing Assessment

Action/Intervention	Rationale
■ Assess the patient's knowledge of ACS: causes, treatment, and early recovery process.	Information provides the basis for education. Many patients have been exposed to media information or family and friends experiencing cardiac events. Misconceptions may exist. QSEN: Patient-centered care.

Therapeutic Interventions

Actions/Interventions	Rationales
■ Teach the patient or significant others the following:	Providing information allows the patient to be a full partner in making decisions and assuming responsibility for care at a later time. QSEN: Safety; Patient-centered care.
• Anatomy and physiology of the coronary condition and atherosclerotic process	Information provides rationales for treatment.
• Angina versus unstable angina versus MI	Information aids the patient in assuming responsibility for care at a later time. It is critical that patients are able to recognize when chest pain symptoms require immediate attention.
• Diagnostic procedures (stress test, echocardiogram, or angiogram)	Information can clarify the diagnostic process and reduce anxiety. Follow-up testing is common to assess the response to medical therapy and evaluate functional capacity.
• Medical therapy, as in the following:	Patients are better able to ask questions and seek assistance when they know basic information about prescribed medications. The Clinical Practice Guidelines for Acute Coronary Syndromes require medications known to reduce the consequences of CAD and acute MI. The following nursing actions are based on recommendations from national organizations. QSEN: Evidence-based practice.
• Antiplatelet medicines, especially aspirin and clopidogrel, in setting of MI and percutaneous coronary intervention (PCI)	Antiplatelet medications reduce the risk for thrombosis formation by inhibiting platelet aggregation. Patients who had a PCI require dual antiplatelet therapy.
• Use of NTG if chest pain occurs	NTG causes vasodilation that reduces myocardial demands. Patients need clear directions on self-administration of sublingual or spray NTG.
• Use of ACE inhibitors or ARBs; beta-blockers	These medications decrease myocardial remodeling, mortality, and morbidity rates after MI.
• Use of statins, as indicated	High-intensity statin therapy should be continued. The Joint Commission (TJC) and Clinical Practice Guidelines have this therapy as a core performance measure for patients with dyslipidemia.
• Use of calcium channel blockers	Calcium channel blockers are useful if unstable angina has a spasm component or if beta-blockers are contraindicated.

Cardiac and Vascular Care Plans

■ = Independent   ▲ = Interprofessional Collaboration

Actions/Interventions

- Indicated lifestyle changes (smoking cessation, exercise, diet, hypertension and lipid management)

- Explain that the acute phase of unstable angina is usually over in 4 to 6 weeks and return to prior lifestyle after MI is 2 to 3 months.

- Inform the patient that more extensive teaching sessions will be instituted when the next stage of cardiac rehabilitation is initiated.
- Refer to a cardiac rehabilitation program as indicated.

- Screen for depression.

■ Encourage immunization with the flu vaccine.

Rationales

Modification in risk factors can decrease the risk for CAD events. Smoking cessation counseling is a CMS (Centers for Medicare and Medicaid Services) and TJC quality indictor for acute MI. QSEN: Evidence-based practice.

Recovery from unstable angina is shorter than with an MI because only ischemic, not infarcted, tissue occurs. More than 85% of patients experiencing an MI return to full activity level.

Readiness for learning is key to effective teaching. The complexities of an acute care setting do not provide an optimal environment for learning.

These programs can assist with risk factor reduction and provide education and emotional support.

It is reasonable to screen for depression because the disease process can alter the prognosis and quality of life. Depression is linked to cardiac events.

The flu vaccine is recommended by the National Clinical Practice guidelines because the flu infection has been found to have a direct influence on atherosclerotic plaque, potentially leading to plaque rupture and subsequent cardiac events. QSEN: Evidence-based practice.

Related Care Plans

Activity intolerance, Chapter 2
Ineffective sexuality pattern, Chapter 2
Powerlessness, Chapter 2
Health-seeking behaviors, Chapter 3
Cardiac rehabilitation, Chapter 5
Shock, cardiogenic, Chapter 5
Dysrhythmias, evolve

Angina Pectoris, Stable

Chest Pain

Stable angina pectoris is a clinical syndrome characterized by the abrupt or gradual onset of substernal discomfort (often with radiation to the neck, jaw, shoulder, back, or arm) caused by insufficient coronary blood flow and inadequate oxygen supply to the myocardial muscle. The patient with stable angina will have episodes of chest pain that are usually predictable. Chest pain will occur in response to hypoxia, or is aggravated by physical exertion or emotional stressors. Situations that increase myocardial oxygen demand or decrease oxygen supply include both cardiac and noncardiac causes. Stable angina usually persists for only a few minutes and subsides with cessation of the precipitating factor, rest, or use of nitroglycerin (NTG). Patients may present in ambulatory settings or during hospitalization for other medical problems. Stable angina usually can be controlled with medications on an outpatient basis. Stable angina can significantly affect one's quality of life. A person may limit activities based on fear of precipitating episodes of chest pain.

Cardiac and Vascular Care Plans

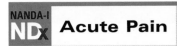

Acute Pain

Common Related Factors

Myocardial ischemia caused by the following:
- Atherosclerosis and/or coronary spasm
- Less common causes: severe aortic stenosis, cardiomyopathy, mitral valve prolapse, hypothyroidism, hypertension, anxiety, tachydysrhythmias, hyperviscosity of blood

Defining Characteristics

Self-report of chest pain or discomfort using a standardized pain scale

Change in physiological parameters (e.g., BP, HR)

No change in the frequency, duration, time of appearance, or precipitating factors of chest pain during the previous 60 days (stable)

Common Expected Outcomes

Patient reports relief of chest discomfort.

Patient exhibits increased comfort, such as baseline levels for pulse, BP, respirations, and relaxed muscle tone or body posture.

NOC Outcomes

Pain Level; Pain Control; Medication Response

NIC Interventions

Pain Management; Cardiac Care

Ongoing Assessment

Actions/Interventions	**Rationales**
■ Assess the following pain characteristics: • Quality: choking, strangling, pressure, burning, tightness, ache, heaviness, griplike, squeezing • Location: substernal area, may radiate to arms and shoulders, neck, back, jaw • Severity: usually low on a scale of 1 to 10 • Duration: typically minutes • Onset and aggravating factors: episodic and usually precipitated by physical exertion, emotional stress, smoking, heavy meal, or exposures to extreme temperature • Relieving factors: rest, use of NTG, or removal of precipitating factor	The discomfort of angina is often difficult for patients to describe, and many patients do not consider it to be "pain." Older patients, patients with diabetes, and women tend to have more fatigue or shortness of breath as anginal symptoms and/or angina equivalents. QSEN: Patient-centered care.
■ Evaluate whether this is a chronic problem (stable angina) or a new presentation.	New-onset angina that is less than 2 months in occurrence, severe, or frequent (more than three times per day) is considered "unstable" angina/ acute coronary syndrome until proved otherwise. It requires immediate assessment (see Acute Coronary Syndromes/Myocardial Infarction, Chapter 5).
■ Assess for the appropriateness of performing an electrocardiogram (ECG) to evaluate ST-segment and T-wave changes.	Differentiating between angina and myocardial infarction (MI) is important in making decisions about implementing appropriate interventions. Anginal changes are transient, occurring during the actual ischemic episode. This measurement is part of the QSEN competency for safety. Differentiating angina from MI can reduce the risk of harm to the patient by guiding specific interventions. QSEN: Safety.
■ Monitor vital signs during chest pain and after nitrate administration.	BP and HR are usually elevated secondary to sympathetic stimulation during pain; however, nitrates cause vasodilation and a resultant drop in BP. Older patients may experience more significant postural hypotension secondary to decreased responsiveness of the baroreceptors. QSEN: Safety.
■ Monitor the effectiveness of interventions.	Chest pain unresponsive to the patient's usual use of rest or NTG requires immediate evaluation. QSEN: Safety.

Cardiac and Vascular Care Plans

■ = Independent   ▲ = Interprofessional Collaboration

Therapeutic Interventions

Actions/Interventions	Rationales
■ At first signs of pain or discomfort, instruct the patient to relax and/or rest.	Decreasing myocardial oxygen demand restores the balance between oxygen supply and demand. When more oxygen is available to the myocardium, ischemia is reversed.
■ Instruct the patient to take sublingual NTG. The patient should sit or lie down when taking NTG and put the pill under the tongue and let it dissolve. If the pain is not relieved in 5 minutes, the patient should take another. If still no relief, the patient should take a third.	The patient needs to learn the meaning of chest pain as a sign of myocardial ischemia and the benefits of prompt therapy. Information allows the patient to be a full partner to initiate effective therapy when needed. A stinging or burning in the mouth should occur if the medication is effective. Many patients find the NTG spray easier to use. QSEN: Patient-centered care.
■ If pain continues after repeating the sublingual NTG dose every 5 minutes for a total of three pills, seek immediate medical attention.	Patients with chronic disease need to be able to recognize important changes in their condition to avert complications. Chest pain unrelieved by NTG may represent unstable angina or MI and should be evaluated immediately. QSEN: Safety.
■ If in a medical setting, administer oxygen as ordered.	Increasing arterial oxygen saturation delivers more oxygen to the myocardium and relieves oxygen supply and demand imbalance.
■ Offer assurance and emotional support by explaining all treatments and procedures and by encouraging questions.	Anxiety can increase cardiac workload and myocardial oxygen demand through stimulation of the sympathetic nervous system.

NANDA-I NDx Deficient Knowledge

Common Related Factors
Insufficient information
Insufficient interest in learning
Misinformation presented by others

Defining Characteristics
Insufficient knowledge
Inaccurate follow-through of instruction
Inappropriate behavior

Common Expected Outcomes
Patient or significant others verbalize understanding of angina pectoris, its causes, and appropriate relief measures for pain.
Patient describes own cardiac risk factors and strategies to reduce them.

NOC Outcomes
Cardiac Disease: Self-Management;
Knowledge: Disease Process; Knowledge:
  Treatment Regimen

NIC Interventions
Health Literacy Enhancement; Learning
  Facilitation; Teaching: Disease Process;
  Teaching: Prescribed Medication; Cardiac
  Care: Rehabilitative

Ongoing Assessment

Actions/Interventions	Rationales
■ Assess the patient's knowledge regarding the causes of angina, diagnostic procedures, treatment plan, and risk factors for CAD.	Information provides a starting base for educational sessions. Teaching standardized content that the patient already knows wastes valuable time and hinders critical learning. QSEN: Patient-centered care.

Actions/Interventions

- Evaluate patient compliance with any previously prescribed lifestyle modifications.

Rationales

Smoking, heavy meals, and obesity can easily precipitate anginal attacks. Behavior change is never easy. This knowledge provides an important starting point in understanding any complexities in implementation of the treatment plan.

Therapeutic Interventions

Actions/Interventions

- Provide information regarding the following:
  - Anatomy and physiology of coronary circulation and the atherosclerotic process.

  - Diagnostic tests for evaluating CAD, such as the following:

    - ECG

    - Exercise stress test and/or stress echocardiogram

    - Pharmacological stress test with nuclear imaging

    - Coronary angiography

  - Differentiating angina from noncardiac pain

  - Differentiating stable versus unstable angina versus MI

  - The need to avoid angina-provoking situations (e.g., heavy meals, physical overexertion, temperature extremes, cigarette smoking, emotional stress, and stimulants such as caffeine or cocaine)
  - The use of sublingual NTG to relieve attacks, as in the following (note that NTG spray may be preferred by some patients):

    - Carry pills at all times.

    - Keep pills in a dark, dry container, away from heat.
    - Replace pills every 3 to 4 months.

Rationales

Patient understanding of the role of normal versus atherosclerotic coronary arteries in supplying oxygen to the myocardial tissue will provide a rationale for treatment.

The appropriate selection of diagnostic testing is based on recommendations from national organizations. QSEN: Evidence-based practice.

Usually ST-segment depression or inverted T wave is present, indicating subendocardial ischemia.

ST-segment changes provide an indirect assessment of coronary artery perfusion. Significant ST-segment depression on stress testing and reversible defects indicate the need for angiography. However, the exercise stress test is not always conclusive for CAD. Exercise echocardiograms are often used to evaluate wall motion abnormality present during myocardial ischemia.

This test is indicated for subgroups of patients who are unable to exercise and who have findings that are highly suggestive of CAD. Scans of the heart identify poorly perfused areas of the myocardium.

Angiography is the definitive test for directly identifying the extent of the CAD.

Chest pain is very challenging to interpret, because pulmonary, gastrointestinal, and musculoskeletal causes can mimic myocardial problems. Patients must have correct information for long-term care.

Patients need to understand the importance of reporting changes in chest pain patterns that may indicate progression of CAD.

Long-term care is the patient's responsibility; enough information is needed for successful intervention.

NTG relaxes smooth muscles in the vascular system, causing peripheral arterial and venous vasodilation, which can lower BP and cause dizziness. Early, effective treatment aids in salvaging at-risk myocardium. The patient needs to understand the importance of obtaining prompt treatment and the risk of delaying treatment. QSEN: Safety.

NTG pills (or spray) must be taken immediately at the first sign of pain.

NTG is volatile and inactivated by heat, moisture, and light.

Once the bottle is opened, NTG begins to lose its strength. Tablets that are effective should sting in the mouth.

■ = Independent ▲ = Interprofessional Collaboration

Actions/Interventions

Rationales

- The use of other medications for long-term management:

  The appropriate selection of medications is based on recommendations from national organizations. QSEN: Evidence-based practice.

  - Long-acting nitrates

    Long-acting nitrites act by producing vasodilation, which increases coronary blood flow and reduces oxygen demands of the heart. They must be used cautiously in older patients, who are more susceptible to postural hypotension secondary to reduced response of baroreceptors.

  - Beta-blockers

    Beta-blockers reduce contractility, HR, and afterload, thereby decreasing myocardial oxygen demand. They must be used cautiously in older patients who have degeneration of the conduction system and who are at risk for bradycardia, conduction heart blocks, and chronic obstructive pulmonary disease (COPD). They are usually prescribed along with a nitrate.

  - Calcium channel blockers

    Calcium channel blockers cause vasodilation, which increases coronary blood flow and reduces oxygen demands of the heart. They are usually prescribed along with a nitrate.

  - Ranolazine

    Ranolazine provides a new approach for treating stable angina. It is one of a new class of drugs called partial fatty acid oxidation inhibitors. It acts by increasing efficiency of oxygen use by the heart by shifting metabolism to a fuel source that requires less oxygen (glucose) to generate the same amount of energy.

  - Antiplatelet aggregation therapy

    Aspirin is strongly recommended as a long-term therapy for those with CAD (angina) who can tolerate it. Aspirin chemically blocks the synthesis of prostaglandins and thromboxane A_2 in platelets. Without prostaglandins, platelets are unable to aggregate and form clots in coronary blood vessels. The effect of aspirin on platelet aggregation is irreversible for the life of the platelet, about 3 to 7 days. Clopidogrel or similar antiplatelet agents can be substituted if aspirin is contraindicated for high-risk patients (determined by testing).

- The need to reduce modifiable risk factors for atherosclerosis:

  The following nursing actions are based on recommendations from national organizations. QSEN: Evidence-based practice.

  - Smoking: Provide counseling, pharmacological therapy, and referral to cessation programs. The American Heart Association, the American Lung Association, and the American Cancer Society provide support groups and interventions.

    Smoking causes vasoconstriction and reduces myocardial oxygen supply. The risk for developing CAD is two to six times greater in cigarette smokers. Risk is proportional to the number of cigarettes smoked.

  - Hypertension: Instruct in the need to maintain healthy weight control, reduce salt intake, initiate an exercise program, and take antihypertensive medications as prescribed. Moderate alcohol intake, a diet high in fruits and vegetables (Dietary Approaches to Stop Hypertension [DASH]), and low-fat dairy products are key.

    The stress of constantly elevated BP can increase the rate of atherosclerosis development. The Joint National Committee (JNC) on Prevention, Detection, Evaluation, and Treatment of High Blood Pressure guidelines provides goals and treatment approaches.

Actions/Interventions

- Elevated serum lipid levels: Emphasize the need to reduce the intake of foods high in saturated fat, cholesterol, or both (e.g., fatty meats, organ meats, lard, butter, egg yolks, dairy products). Arrange for evaluation by a dietitian as needed. Include the spouse or significant others in meal planning. Treatment usually requires antihyperlipidemic medication. Consider adding plant stanols, fiber, and omega-3 fatty acids as appropriate.
- Diabetes: Emphasize its control through lifestyle and medication.

- Obesity: Refer to weight management specialty programs as appropriate.

- Stress: Refer to programs for stress management as appropriate.
- Flu vaccine

- Physical inactivity: Emphasize the benefits of exercise in reducing the risk for heart attack. Refer to a cardiac rehabilitation program as needed. Keep exercise intensity below the angina threshold.

- Therapeutic procedures to relieve angina unresponsive to medications and lifestyle changes:
  - Percutaneous coronary interventions: angioplasty, atherectomy, stent implantation, laser angioplasty
  - Coronary artery bypass graft surgery

  - Enhanced external counterpulsation

- Refer the patient to cardiac rehabilitation services for specialized teaching and assistance with recommended lifestyle changes as appropriate.

Rationales

There is a positive correlation between serum lipids (especially low-density lipoprotein [LDL]) and atherosclerosis. The treatment goal for patients with CAD is an LDL level less than 100 mg/dL (less than 70 mg/dL as a therapeutic option).

Eighty percent of diabetic patients have cardiovascular disease. Diabetes eliminates the lower incidence of cardiovascular disease in women. Diabetes is associated with a high incidence of silent ischemia.

Obesity affects hypertension, diabetes, and lipid levels and contributes to metabolic syndrome, which is highly associated with CAD. The target body mass index (BMI) is 18.5 to 24.9.

Persistent stress causes the release of catecholamines that contribute to elevated BP and CAD.

An annual flu vaccine is recommended for those with cardiovascular disease. The flu has been found to have a direct influence on atherosclerotic plaque, potentially leading to plaque rupture and subsequent cardiac events.

Exercise increases high-density lipoprotein (HDL) levels (good cholesterol), assists with weight loss, lowers hypertension, improves diabetes, and reduces the risk for clot formation (fibrinolytic activity); 150 minutes of moderate activity is recommended per week.

These interventions provide a means to nonsurgically improve coronary blood flow and revascularize the myocardium.

Surgery may be recommended for significant left main CAD, triple vessel disease, and disease unresponsive to other treatments.

Counterpulsation devices use air via cuffs attached to the lower extremities to propel blood back to the heart.

Specialty services may be required to ensure that patients' needs are met and outcomes achieved. QSEN: Teamwork and collaboration.

 NANDA-I NDx **Activity Intolerance**

Common Related Factors	Defining Characteristics
Occurrence or fear of chest pain	Exertional chest pain or dyspnea
Side effects of prescribed medications	Fatigue/weakness
Imbalance between oxygen supply and demand	Abnormal HR or BP response to activity
Sedentary lifestyle	ECG changes reflecting ischemia or dysrhythmias
	Unable to complete desired activities

Cardiac and Vascular Care Plans

Common Expected Outcomes

Patient performs activity within limits of ischemic disease, as evidenced by absence of chest pain or discomfort and no ECG changes reflecting ischemia.

Patient recognizes activity and energy limitations and balances activity and rest.

NOC Outcomes

Activity Tolerance; Knowledge: Prescribed Activity; Energy Conservation

NIC Interventions

Energy Management; Teaching: Prescribed Exercise

Ongoing Assessment

Actions/Interventions	Rationales
■ Assess the patient's level of physical activity before experiencing angina.	Sometimes patients have significantly reduced their activity to avoid anginal symptoms.
■ Assess the patient's BP and HR before, during, and after activity.	Information provides a basis for determining activity intolerance and realistic short- and long-term goals and subsequent therapies. QSEN: Patient-centered care; Safety.
■ Assess the emotional response to limitations in physical abilities.	Depression over the inability to perform desired/required activities can be a source of stress and aggravation.

Therapeutic Interventions

Actions/Interventions	Rationales
■ Assist in reviewing required home, work, or leisure activities and in developing an appropriate plan for accomplishing them (e.g., what to do in morning versus afternoon or how to pace tasks throughout the week).	Devising a plan that facilitates the accomplishment of small, attainable goals can be satisfying. QSEN: Patient-centered care.
■ Evaluate the need for additional support at home (e.g., housekeeper, neighbor to shop, family assistance).	Coordinated efforts are more meaningful and effective in assisting the patient in conserving energy.
■ Encourage adequate rest periods between activities.	Rest between activities provides time for energy conservation and recovery.
■ Remind the patient not to work with the arms above the shoulders for long periods.	Arm activity increases myocardial demands.
■ Remind the patient to continue taking medications (e.g., beta-blockers), despite the side effect of fatigue.	Often the body does adjust to the medications after several weeks.
■ Instruct in the prophylactic use of NTG before physical exertion as needed.	Prophylactic NTG use is an important measure for patients with predictable angina patterns. It is an underutilized therapy.
■ Encourage a program of progressive aerobic exercise. Refer to cardiac rehabilitation as appropriate.	Integrating the contributions of members of the interprofessional team helps the patient and family achieve health goals and allows for shared decision-making to achieve quality patient care. Routine exercise can increase functional capacity, making the heart more efficient. QSEN: Teamwork and collaboration.

Related Care Plans

Ineffective coping, Chapter 2
Health-seeking behaviors, Chapter 3
Cardiac rehabilitation, Chapter 5

Cardiac and Vascular Care Plans

Atrial Fibrillation

Atrial fibrillation is the most common sustained heart rhythm disturbance in the United States, affecting more than 2 million people. It is an abnormal heart rhythm characterized by an irregular or often rapid heartbeat causing reduced cardiac output. In this dysrhythmia, the upper chambers of the heart (atria) fibrillate (quiver) rapidly and erratically, resulting in pooling of blood in the atrium and an irregular ventricular HR and pulse. Although atrial fibrillation itself is not life-threatening, if not adequately treated, it can cause significant side effects resulting in a decreased quality of life and can increase the risk for stroke and heart failure. Because the incidence of atrial fibrillation increases with age, this medical condition is projected to be a huge medical problem as the U.S. and world population ages. Atrial fibrillation is classified by how it terminates: paroxysmal atrial fibrillation refers to occasional occurrences that start and stop on their own; persistent atrial fibrillation is a condition in which the abnormal rhythm continues for more than a week, does not self-terminate, but can be treated to a return to normal rhythm; and permanent atrial fibrillation is a condition in which the abnormal rhythm is chronic and unresponsive to treatment.

The most common causes and risk factors for atrial fibrillation include age older than 60 years, heart disease including valve disease, hypertension, heart failure, prior open heart surgery, thyroid disease, chronic lung disease, exposure to stimulants or excessive alcohol, viral infections, and sleep apnea. Some people develop atrial fibrillation for no apparent reason (termed "lone afib").

Symptoms vary with each person depending on age, cause, and how much the atrial fibrillation affects the contractility of the heart. Symptoms can range from pulse rate that is faster than normal or changing between fast and slow with mild fatigue to shortness of breath, heart palpitations or fluttering, decreased BP, chest tightness or discomfort, dizziness, and lightheadedness. Atrial fibrillation is diagnosed by an electrocardiogram (ECG) while the abnormal rhythm is occurring, but if the rhythm is intermittent, a portable Holter ECG monitor or an event recorder is used to document the dysrhythmia.

Management of atrial fibrillation can vary depending on the type, how long the person has had it, and factors such as age, underlying heart condition, stroke risk, and the severity of associated symptoms. A variety of treatments are available focused on the goals of resetting the rhythm to normal (for first time and more acute episodes) or controlling the ventricular rate (for more persistent and chronic conditions) and preventing blood clots from forming in the fibrillating atria through anticoagulation. Thus treatments may include antiarrhythmic medications, electrical cardioversion, catheter ablation, and a surgical maze procedure. Because atrial fibrillation increases the risk of development of blood clots in the atria, long-term anticoagulation is required for patients at increased risk for stroke. The CHA_2DS_2-VASc Screening Score (see following care plan for description) guides treatment.

NANDA-I NDx Deficient Knowledge

Common Related Factors
Insufficient information
Insufficient interest in learning
Misinformation presented by others

Common Expected Outcome
Patient or significant others verbalize understanding of cause, diagnostic procedures, treatment regimen, possible complications, and long-term management of atrial fibrillation.

Defining Characteristics
Insufficient knowledge
Inaccurate follow-through of instruction
Inappropriate behavior

NOC Outcome
Knowledge: Dysrhythmia Management
NIC Interventions
Health Literacy Facilitation; Learning Facilitation; Teaching: Disease Process; Teaching: Prescribed Medication

Cardiac and Vascular Care Plans

 = Independent ▲ = Interprofessional Collaboration

Ongoing Assessment

Action/Intervention

- Assess the patient's knowledge of atrial fibrillation: type, causative factors, diagnostic procedures, treatment, possible complications, and long-term management.

Rationale

Assessment provides an important starting point in education. Many misconceptions may be present among the lay public. QSEN: Patient-centered care.

Therapeutic Interventions

Actions/Interventions

- Teach the patient about the types of atrial fibrillation: paroxysmal, persistent, and permanent.

- Teach the patient about possible causative factors of atrial fibrillation.

- Teach the patient the physiology of atrial fibrillation.

- Inform the patient of common diagnostic procedures:
  - ECG
  - Ambulatory Holter ECG monitoring
  - Portable event monitor worn for a month
- Teach the patient about the symptoms of atrial fibrillation.

- Teach the patient about the approaches to treating atrial fibrillation: rate control versus rhythm control.

- Instruct the patient regarding treatment versus maintenance medications: dose and method of administration.

Rationales

Knowledge helps the patient become a full partner in decisions about the management of this dysrhythmia. Patients with paroxysmal atrial fibrillation often experience the most symptoms. Those with permanent atrial fibrillation require ongoing medical therapy to reduce the risk for complications.

Understanding the cause of this dysrhythmia is necessary for appropriate follow-through of the treatment plan. Atrial fibrillation is one of the most common dysrhythmias, especially in people older than age 60 and those who have hypertension, coronary artery disease, mitral valve disease, heart failure, recent open heart surgery, viral infections, chronic lung disease, sleep apnea, or thyroid disease. The patient needs to participate in the management of underlying chronic diseases that contribute to atrial fibrillation. QSEN: Patient-centered care.

This information helps the patient understand the complexities of the dysrhythmia and the rationale for therapy, including long-term anticoagulation as needed.

Explanations enhance understanding and reduce anxiety. ECGs can diagnose the dysrhythmia while it is occurring. The ambulatory Holter and event recorders are used for intermittent occurrences of the dysrhythmia.

Patients must understand that each individual may exhibit different symptoms depending on ventricular HR in response to the atrial impulses. These symptoms may vary from none at all when the HR is well-controlled by medications, to fatigue, palpitations, shortness of breath, chest discomfort and/or pain, or dizziness during times of rapid ventricular response.

Treatment for atrial fibrillation must be individualized depending on the acuteness or chronicity of the dysrhythmia, cause, patient age, stroke risk, and the severity of associated symptoms. Treatments available focus on the goals of resetting the rhythm to normal (for first time and more acute episodes) or controlling the ventricular rate (for more persistent and chronic conditions), and preventing blood clots from forming in the fibrillating atria through anticoagulation.

Patients in acute settings may need explanation as to the variety of medications that may be required to successfully treat the problem. Patients with chronic conditions may require long-term self-management.

Cardiac and Vascular Care Plans

Actions/Interventions

- Teach the patient about the side effects of medications.

- Teach the patient about the common complications associated with atrial fibrillation: decreased cardiac output, heart failure, and stroke.

- Provide education concerning risk assessment for stroke (use of CHA$_2$DS$_2$-VASc Screening Scale), antithrombotic drug therapy, and the need for careful monitoring.

- Teach the patient about lifestyle adjustments for managing atrial fibrillation:
  - Diet (if on warfarin)
  - Alcohol and caffeine
  - Smoking cessation
  - Over-the-counter medications
  - Stress reduction

- Instruct the patient and/or family members in the method for checking pulse. State the patient's normal rate and describe the quality of the rhythm that should be reported to the physician.
- Inform the patient of the proper procedure to follow in case dysrhythmia recurs (as evidenced by specific signs and symptoms).

Rationales

Most antidysrhythmics can have significant side effects. If side effects occur, patients need to report them immediately so that appropriate therapy can be initiated.

A rapid ventricular response to the atrial fibrillation impulses can result in reduced ventricular filling time and reduced cardiac output. Atrial fibrillation can also decrease the heart's pumping ability and over time can weaken the heart, leading to heart failure. Heart failure and atrial fibrillation often exist together. Because of the irregular and rapid beating of the atria, blood does not flow through them quickly, causing blood to pool in the chambers where it can develop into a clot. This clot can travel through the heart to the brain, causing a stroke. QSEN: Safety.

Most people who have atrial fibrillation or are undergoing special procedures to treat it are at risk for stroke. The CHA$_2$DS$_2$-VASc score (name derived from first letter of each risk factor) lists these as the major risks for stroke: Congestive heart failure, Hypertension, Age > 75 (more recently updated to >65 to 74), Diabetes, Stroke or transient ischemic attacks, female gender (Sex), and VAScular disease. Points are awarded for each risk factor, generating a "risk" score that guides the need for and level of anticoagulation therapy. QSEN: Evidence-based practice.

Low-risk patients can be treated with aspirin. Higher risk patients require anticoagulation therapy with warfarin or alternative anticoagulation agents such as dabigatran, rivaroxaban, or apixaban. They may be given on a long-term basis to prevent strokes associated with nonvalvular atrial fibrillation. These are powerful medications that can have dangerous side effects if not taken as prescribed. The dose of warfarin requires periodic adjustment based on serum laboratory values of the international normalized ratio (INR). No laboratory testing is required with the newer medications, as they achieve a steady therapeutic state. The downside is that there is no reversal agent available should the patient experience significant bleeding. These recommendations are based on national guidelines. QSEN: Evidence-based practice.

Patients on warfarin need to be aware of foods that are high in vitamin K and can affect clotting factors. Alcohol and caffeine are both known triggers of atrial fibrillation. Nicotine is a cardiac stimulant and can aggravate this dysrhythmia. Some over-the-counter medications (e.g., cold remedies, nasal sprays) contain cardiac stimulants that can aggravate atrial fibrillation. Many patients find that stress can be a trigger for intermittent atrial fibrillation. QSEN: Safety.

Eliciting the patient as a full partner empowers the patient and ensures more appropriate treatment. QSEN: Patient-centered care.

Developing a specific plan of care provides reassurance regarding the ability of the patient to care for self at home. QSEN: Safety.

Cardiac and Vascular Care Plans

■ = Independent   ▲ = Interprofessional Collaboration

NANDA-I
NDx Risk for Ineffective Coping

Common Risk Factors

Misinterpretation of condition or treatment
Situational crisis
Disturbances in self-concept or body image
Disturbances in lifestyle or role
Inadequate coping methods
Prolonged hospitalization
History of ineffective medical treatments
Perceived personal stress resulting from chronic condition
  or treatment
Lack of support system

Common Expected Outcomes

Patient verbalizes acceptance of possible chronic medical
  problem.
Patient describes and maintains effective coping
  strategies.
Patient uses available resources and support systems.

NOC Outcomes
Coping; Social Support
NIC Intervention
Coping Enhancement

Ongoing Assessment

Actions/Interventions	Rationales
■ Evaluate the patient's emotional response to having atrial fibrillation. Assess for coping difficulties.	Palpitations or shortness of breath occurring at home can be especially frightening. For patients in whom dysrhythmias are resistant to therapy, chronic episodes of tachycardia can lead to coping difficulties and even body image disturbances. Behavioral and physiological responses to life-threatening situations provide clues to the level of coping difficulties. QSEN: Patient-centered care.
■ Assess the level of understanding and readiness to learn needed lifestyle changes.	Living with chronic atrial fibrillation requires ongoing medication management and attention to lifestyle adjustments that may be required. Often patients, especially older patients, who are having difficulty coping are unable to hear or assimilate needed information.
■ Evaluate the patient's available resources or support systems.	Patients may have support in one setting, such as during hospitalization, yet be discharged home without sufficient support for effective coping. Resources may include significant others, health care providers such as home health nurse, community resources, and spiritual counseling.

Therapeutic Interventions

Actions/Interventions	Rationales
■ Encourage the patient and family to verbalize feelings about the dysrhythmia, diagnostic procedures and treatment plan, and any lifestyle changes imposed by this medical problem.	Verbalization may help reduce anxiety and open doors for ongoing communication. Eliciting the patient's expressed needs allow the patient to be a full partner in providing care to enhance coping with atrial fibrillation.

Cardiac and Vascular
Care Plans

Actions/Interventions	**Rationales**
■ Provide accurate information about the causes, prognosis, and treatment of the condition in a clear and concise manner to the patient and family.	Many patients have anxiety when diagnosed with a heart problem about which they know little. Information provides rationales for therapy and aids the patient in understanding treatment and assuming responsibility for ongoing care. However, patients who are coping ineffectively have a reduced ability to assimilate information.
■ In an acute setting, maintain an appropriate level of intensity of action when responding to the current dysrhythmia.	Overreaction or excessive response to a patient's dysrhythmia may encourage or increase feelings of anxiety.
■ As necessary, remain with the patient during episodes of the dysrhythmia or during treatments.	The staff's presence is reassuring to the patient.
■ For patients taking anticoagulation medications such as warfarin, explain why frequent and careful monitoring of the INR is required.	People who have atrial fibrillation are at increased risk for stroke. Maintaining INR values within the target range can be challenging for most patients, requiring frequent blood tests to determine how well the medication is working. These measurements serve as optimal guides for therapy. Attention to these INR values reduces the risk of harm to the patient. QSEN: Safety.
■ Provide reassurance that it is possible to lead a normal life with atrial fibrillation.	Professional caregivers represent a microcosm of society, and their actions and behaviors are scrutinized as the patient finds meaning in and adjusts to the new diagnosis. People who have atrial fibrillation—even permanent—can lead normal, active lives.
■ Refer to a support group as indicated.	Participation in a support group may allow the patient to realize that others have the same problem.

Related Care Plans

Activity intolerance, Chapter 2
Decreased cardiac output, Chapter 2
Dysrhythmias, ⊜volve

Cardiac Rehabilitation

Post–Myocardial Infarction; Post–Cardiac Surgery; Post–Percutaneous Transluminal Coronary Angioplasty; Chronic Heart Failure; Stable Angina; Activity Progression; Cardiac Education

Cardiac rehabilitation is the process of actively assisting patients with known heart disease to achieve and maintain optimal physical and emotional health and wellness. It has undergone significant evolution, redesigning itself from a primarily exercise-focused intervention into a comprehensive disease management program. Core components of these programs include baseline and follow-up patient assessments; aggressive strategies for reducing modifiable risk factors for cardiovascular disease (CVD; e.g., dyslipidemia, hypertension, diabetes, obesity); counseling on heart-healthy nutrition, smoking cessation, and stress management; assistance in adhering to prescribed medications; promotion of lifestyle physical activity; exercise training; and psychosocial and vocational counseling. An interprofessional health care team composed of physicians, nurses, health educators, exercise physiologists, dietitians, and behavioral medicine specialists is the most effective approach for providing patients with these integrated services. The nurse commonly serves as the case manager. Cardiac rehabilitation programs typically begin in the hospital setting and progress to supervised (and often electrocardiogram [ECG]-monitored) outpatient programs. However, with shorter hospital stays, little time may be available for adequate instruction regarding lifestyle management and activity progression. Key to providing cost-effective care is an interprofessional team and the provision of interventions based on each patient's unique needs, interests, and skills.

Cardiac and Vascular Care Plans

■ = Independent   ▲ = Interprofessional Collaboration

NANDA-I NDx Activity Intolerance

Common Related Factors

Imposed activity restrictions secondary to medical condition or high-technology therapies or procedures

Pain (ischemic, postsurgery incisional, related to other underlying conditions or health problems)

Generalized weakness or fatigue (sedentary lifestyle before event, lack of sleep)

Reduced cardiac output (secondary to myocardial dysfunction, dysrhythmias, postural hypotension)

Fear or anxiety (of overexerting heart, of experiencing angina or incisional pain)

Defining Characteristics

Abnormal HR or BP in response to activity

Dysrhythmias precipitated by activity

Report of fatigue or weakness

Report of chest pain and/or other pain

Exertional dyspnea

ECG changes reflecting ischemia

Common Expected Outcomes

Patient exhibits activity tolerance as evidenced by HR and BP within prescribed ranges during activity progression, absence of activity-related chest pain or discomfort, absence of dyspnea, no occurrence of or increase in dysrhythmias during activity.

Patient reports readiness to perform activities of daily living (ADLs) and routine home activities.

NOC Outcomes

Activity Tolerance; Physical Fitness; Circulation Status

NIC Interventions

Cardiac Care: Rehabilitative; Teaching: Prescribed Exercise; Exercise Promotion

---

Ongoing Assessment

Actions/Interventions

■ Assess the patient's activity tolerance and exercise habits before the current illness.

■ Assess the patient's HR, BP, cardiac rhythm, and pulse oximetry before initiating an activity or exercise session.

■ Assess the patient's emotional readiness to increase activity.

■ Assess the motivation level and interest regarding initiation of an outpatient exercise program.

Rationales

This information will serve as a basis for formulating short- or long-term goals. Some patients may have participated in regular exercise programs and be quite fit, whereas others may have been incapacitated by stable angina or chronic heart failure or have other health problems that interfere with activity. QSEN: Patient-centered care.

Hospitalized patients with complications need close observation and may require supplemental oxygen and telemetry monitoring. Outpatients may exhibit hemodynamic changes such as orthostatic hypotension secondary to changes in prescribed medications or associated illnesses. QSEN: Safety.

Many patients with myocardial infarction (MI) may still be denying they even had a heart attack and may want to do more than prescribed; some post-MI or surgical patients or older patients with heart failure can be quite fearful of overexerting their hearts or causing discomfort. QSEN: Patient-centered care.

Some patients with no prior history of exercise may benefit from more supervised sessions to facilitate adherence. However, other patients may prefer to exercise independently at home, for example, using a stationary bicycle.

 evolve **For additional care plans, go to http://evolve.elsevier.com/Gulanick/.**

Cardiac and Vascular Care Plans

Actions/Interventions

- Monitor the response to progressive activities. Signs of abnormal responses include:
  - HR outside the target range (depending on the patient's baseline and stage of recovery)
  - Pulse greater than 20 beats/min over baseline or greater than 120 beats/min (while inpatient)
  - Chest pain or discomfort; dyspnea
  - Occurrence of or increase in dysrhythmias (inappropriate bradycardia, symptomatic supraventricular tachycardia)
  - Excessive fatigue and/or weakness
  - Significant decrease of 15 to 20 mm Hg in systolic BP
  - Significant systolic BP of 200 mm Hg or more, or diastolic BP greater than 110 mm Hg
  - ST-segment changes, if ECG is monitored
  - Light-headedness, dizziness
- For inpatients, monitor oxygen saturation.

- Assess the patient's perception of the effort required to perform each activity.

Rationales

Physical activities increase demands on the heart. Close monitoring of the patient's response provides guidelines for optimal activity progression. Attention to these parameters reduces the risk of harm to the patient. QSEN: Safety.

A saturation of greater than 90% is recommended. Lower values require supplemental oxygen during activity and slower activity progression.

The Borg scale uses ratings from 6 to 20 to determine a rating of perceived exertion. A rating of 9 (very light) to 13 (somewhat hard) is an acceptable level for most inpatients, whereas 11 to 15 may be appropriate for outpatients.

Therapeutic Interventions

Actions/Interventions

- Encourage the verbalization of feelings regarding exercise or the need to increase activity.
- Inform the patient about the health benefits and physical effects of activity or exercise.

- ▲ For inpatients, maintain a progression of activities as ordered by the cardiac rehabilitation team or physician and as tolerated by the patient. The following are provided as a guide.

Cardiac rehabilitation activity progression:
- Self-care activities at the bedside
- Selected range-of-motion (ROM) exercises in bed—progressing to a chair
- Sitting up in a chair for 30 to 60 minutes three times a day—progressing "as tolerated"
- Partial bath in a chair progressing to the sink
- Walking 75 to 100 feet in hall two to three times a day—progressing to "ambulate ad lib"
- Calisthenic exercises while standing
- Stair climbing
- Performing a discharge submaximal exercise stress test as prescribed

Rationales

A supportive relationship facilitates problem-solving and successful coping.

Activity prevents complications related to immobilization, improves feelings of well-being, and may reduce the risk of cardiac events (with long-term exercise).

Not everyone progresses at the same rate. Some patients progress slowly because of complicated MI, lack of motivation, inadequate sleep, fear of "overexertion," related medical problems, and previous sedentary lifestyle. In contrast, others who experience small infarcts and who had high fitness and activity levels before hospitalization may progress rapidly. Activities are progressed by increasing either distance or time walked, as the patient tolerates or prefers. QSEN: Safety; Teamwork and collaboration.

Gradual resumption of activities promotes a feeling of independence. ROM exercises reduce the risk for thromboembolism. Early chair sitting reduces postural hypotension and promotes better lung function. Repetition of exercises helps to maintain muscle strength and build confidence. An increase in distance or speed is used to increase the level of activity. Success in stair climbing promotes confidence before discharge. Exercise stress testing is used to risk-stratify patients.

Cardiac and Vascular Care Plans

■ = Independent   ▲ = Interprofessional Collaboration

Actions/Interventions	**Rationales**
▲ For patients with neurological or musculoskeletal problems, refer to physical therapy for the assessment of an ambulatory assistive device.	Assistive aids help reduce energy consumption during physical activity. QSEN: Teamwork and collaboration; Safety.
■ Encourage adequate rest periods before and after activity.	Rest decreases cardiac workload and provides time for energy conservation and recovery.
■ Assist and provide emotional support when increasing activity.	Patients may be fearful of overexertion and potential damage to the heart. Appropriate supervision during early efforts can enhance confidence.
Before discharge:	
■ Provide written guidelines in activity progression for home exercise programs.	Exercise programs must be individualized, because each patient recovers at his or her own rate. Most patients are not enrolled in outpatient rehabilitation until 2 to 3 weeks after hospital discharge (if at all). Thus patients need to initiate some exercise progression on their own. Providing information allows the patient to be a full partner in providing care during recovery. QSEN: Patient-centered care.
■ Include metabolic equivalent task (MET) level guides for determining when to resume various ADLs.	Tables have been developed that indicate the MET level for most ADLs and sports activities. For example, resting in a supine position is 1 MET. Sitting on a bedside commode is about 3 METs, as is walking at 2.5 mph. Walking briskly upstairs is about 7 METs. Shoveling snow is about 8 to 9 METs.
■ Provide instructions for warm-up and cool-down exercises.	Warm-up exercises facilitate the heart and body's transition from rest to physical activity. Cool-down exercises facilitate hemodynamic adjustments and return of HR and BP to near-normal levels. QSEN: Safety.
■ Provide a target HR guide (usually around 20 beats/min above standing resting HR).	Having a target guide aids in monitoring the intensity of exercise. QSEN: Safety.
■ Instruct patients regarding whom (e.g., cardiac rehabilitation nurse, physician) to call if any abnormal response to exercise is noted.	This information enables the patient to take control of the situation.
▲ For older patients or patients with significant medical complications, consider a referral to a home care nurse or physical therapy sessions.	Some patients require more supervision or specialized therapy to regain activity tolerance. QSEN: Teamwork and collaboration.
Outpatient programs:	
■ Assist the patient with setting appropriate short- and long-term goals.	Some patients are only interested in regaining strength after a cardiac event, whereas others are motivated to improve their functional capacities by beginning new lifelong exercise habits. QSEN: Patient-centered care.
■ Determine the patient's projected length of time in a supervised program.	Some insurance carriers reimburse for 36 sessions and others for only 6 sessions. Some patients may prefer home exercise rather than the group environment and may attend only a few sessions to get started.
■ Design an individualized plan, including intensity, duration, frequency, and mode of exercise.	Age and fitness level must be considered in designing the exercise prescription. Although the benefits are the same as for younger patients, older patients need more warm-up and cool-down time. Intensity is usually guided by the target HR, which is about 20 beats/min above standing resting HR. For patients who had symptom-limited exercise stress tests, a more individualized and precise target HR can be calculated. QSEN: Patient-centered care; Safety.
■ Gradually adjust the duration and/or intensity of exercise until the target HR is reached.	For patients less familiar with exercise or with more complications, it may take several sessions to reach the target HR.

Cardiac and Vascular Care Plans

Actions/Interventions

- Provide instruction in appropriate warm-up and cool-down exercises.

- Instruct in the self-monitoring of appropriate and abnormal responses to exercise.

- Teach patients how to self-monitor their pulse rate if appropriate.
- Reinforce positive effects of exercise in improving mortality risk and quality of life.

- Provide positive feedback to patients' efforts.

Rationales

Stretching exercises promote flexibility and prepare the muscles and joints for the upcoming stress from exercise. Cool-down is especially important because it helps to pump blood pooled in the primary muscle groups back to the upper part of the body. It also helps prevent muscle soreness. It is especially important for older patients to perform adequate warm-up and cool-down exercises. QSEN: Safety.

Cardiac patients must be aware of the warning signs that warrant cessation of exercise. Attention to abnormal responses to exercise reduces the risks that overexertion can place on the heart during recovery. QSEN: Safety.

HR is a guide for monitoring intensity or duration of exercise.

Studies of cardiac rehabilitation programs have reported significant reduction in mortality rate in patients with coronary heart disease.

Ongoing feedback facilitates adherence to a sometimes difficult behavior change.

NANDA-I
NDx **Deficient Knowledge**

Common Related Factors

Insufficient information
Insufficient interest in learning
Misinformation presented by others
Insufficient knowledge of resources

Defining Characteristics

Insufficient knowledge
Inaccurate follow-through of instruction
Inappropriate behavior
Inaccurate performance on a test

Common Expected Outcomes

Patient verbalizes understanding of disease state, recovery process, and follow-up care.
Patient identifies available resources for lifestyle changes.

NOC Outcomes

Cardiac Disease: Self-Management; Knowledge: Disease Process

NIC Interventions

Health Literacy Enhancement; Learning Facilitation; Cardiac Care: Rehabilitative; Teaching: Disease Process; Teaching: Prescribed Medications; Teaching: Prescribed Diet; Behavior Modification

---

Ongoing Assessment

Actions/Interventions

- Assess the patient's understanding of the disease process, specific cardiac event, treatments, recovery, and follow-up care.
- Identify specific learning needs and goals before discharge.

Rationales

Teaching standardized content that the patient already knows wastes valuable time and hinders critical learning.

Shortened hospital stays and complex risk factor reduction programs provide challenges to the nurse and patient. Priority needs must be identified and satisfied first. QSEN: Patient-centered care.

Cardiac and Vascular Care Plans

■ = Independent ▲ = Interprofessional Collaboration

Actions/Interventions

For outpatients:

■ Conduct intake interviews regarding prior experiences with risk factor reduction and lifestyle changes that the patient is interested in pursuing.

■ Assess the patient's readiness for and self-efficacy to initiate and maintain recommended behavioral changes.

Rationales

Coronary atherosclerosis is a chronic disease requiring risk factor modification. Patients may have been told to change their lifestyle at an earlier time. Knowledge of prior behaviors serves to guide management plan.

Lifestyle changes can be extremely difficult to make. Many behavior modification techniques based on social learning theory stress the importance of self-efficacy in initiating change.

Therapeutic Interventions

Actions/Interventions

■ Develop a plan for meeting individual goals. Include topics to be covered, format (individual versus group session), frequency (after each exercise session versus monthly), available audiovisual resources (video library, books, Internet, telephone), and specialty personnel (dietitian, exercise physiologist, others).

■ Encourage meetings or conferences with the family or significant others to discuss a home recovery plan.

■ Provide information on the following needed topics:
  • Pathophysiology of the cardiac event (myocardial infarction, heart failure, coronary artery disease, percutaneous transluminal coronary angioplasty, stent, valve disease)
  • Healing process after the cardiac event
  • Incisional pain versus angina versus heart attack
  • Resumption of ADLs (e.g., lifting, household chores, driving a car, climbing stairs, social activities, sexual activity, recreational activity)
  • Return to work

■ Provide information regarding follow-up medications.

■ Provide a referral to comprehensive risk reduction programs as indicated:
  • Lipid management
  • Hypertension management
  • Diabetes management
  • Weight management
  • Counseling on heart-healthy nutrition
  • Smoking cessation
  • Stress management

Rationales

Each patient has his or her own learning style, which must be considered when designing a teaching program. Effective communication with all members of the interprofessional team provides the patient with continuity of cardiac rehabilitation care. QSEN: Patient-centered care; Teamwork and collaboration.

This approach enhances smooth transition to the home and may help guard against "overprotectedness" of the patient by family members and significant others.

Specific instructions, especially in written form, help reduce the patient's postdischarge fears and reduce risks for either overexertion or "cardiac invalidism."

Secondary prevention guidelines recommend that patients should take aspirin (to reduce platelet aggregation), beta-blockers (to reduce mortality risk), lipid-lowering medication (to achieve a low-density lipoprotein level less than 70 to 100 mg/dL), and angiotensin-converting enzyme inhibitors (if ejection fraction is less than 40%). Antihypertensive and glucose-lowering medications are added as needed. QSEN: Evidence-based practice.

Staff is challenged to individualize services. Programs should focus on increasing awareness of personal risk factors and offer clear directions and strategies for risk reduction. QSEN: Teamwork and collaboration.

Cardiac and Vascular Care Plans

Actions/Interventions

■ Stress the importance of the patient's own role in maximizing his or her health status.

■ Provide information on available educational or support resources: American Heart Association, Mended Hearts groups, cardiac rehabilitation programs, stress management programs, smoking-cessation programs, and weight management programs.

Rationales

Patients need to understand that reduction of cardiac risk factors and health maintenance depend on them. Health professionals and family members can only provide information and support.

Lifestyle changes may require the assistance of professionals. Support groups provide contact with other individuals "who have been there" and can be beneficial in reducing anxiety and dealing with the impact of a cardiac event.

NANDA-I NDx **Risk for Ineffective Coping**

Common Risk Factors

Recent changes in health status
Perceived change in future health status
Perceived change in social status and lifestyle
Feeling powerless to control disease progression
Unsatisfactory support systems
Inadequate psychological resources

Common Expected Outcomes

Patient implements an effective coping mechanism.
Patient identifies available resources for psychological and social support.

NOC Outcomes
Coping; Anxiety Self-Control

NIC Interventions
Coping Enhancement; Support System Enhancement; Anxiety Reduction; Teaching: Individual

---

Ongoing Assessment

Actions/Interventions

■ Assess specific stressors.

■ Assess the effectiveness of past and present coping mechanisms.

■ Evaluate the resources or support systems available to the patient in the hospital and at home.

Rationales

Accurate appraisal can facilitate the development of appropriate coping strategies. A patient's concerns may include fear of overexerting the heart with activity, expectation of becoming a cardiac invalid, inability to resume satisfying sexual activity, or inability to maintain recommended lifestyle changes. QSEN: Patient-centered care.

Successful adjustment is influenced by previous coping success. Patients with a history of maladaptive coping may need additional resources.

Patients without family or friends who are willing or able to support them may require additional services.

Therapeutic Interventions

Actions/Interventions

■ Encourage the verbalization of concerns.

Rationales

Acknowledging awareness of the challenges faced by the patient related to recovery from chronic cardiac disease can open doors for ongoing communication.

■ = Independent   ▲ = Interprofessional Collaboration

Cardiac and Vascular Care Plans

Actions/Interventions	Rationales
■ Encourage patients to seek information that will enhance their coping skills.	Patients who are not coping well may need more guidance initially.
■ Provide information that the patient wants or needs. Do not provide more than the patient can handle.	With shortened exposure to cardiac rehabilitation services, patients can easily become overwhelmed by the large number of changes that are expected of them in a short time. Lifestyle changes should be considered over a life-long period. QSEN: Patient-centered care.
■ Provide reliable information about future limitations (if any) in physical activity and role performance.	At least 85% of patients can resume a normal lifestyle. Patients with more complications need guidance in understanding which limitations are temporary during recovery and which may be more permanent.
■ Provide information about the healing process so that misconceptions can be clarified. Refer to famous people (politicians, athletes, movie stars) who had similar cardiac problems or procedures and are now leading productive lives.	Examples of well-known people who have successfully recovered and continued an active life after a cardiac event can provide reassurance and confidence about resuming activities.
■ Explain that patients are often "healthier" after cardiac events.	Patients' blocked arteries may have been opened with revascularization, they are more knowledgeable about their specific risk factors and treatment plan, and they may be taking medication to improve their health.
■ Point out signs of positive progress or change.	Patients who are coping ineffectively may not be able to assess their own progress.
■ Encourage referral to a cardiac rehabilitation program and/or "coronary club."	These programs provide opportunities to discuss fears with specialists and patients experiencing similar concerns. QSEN: Teamwork and collaboration.

Related Care Plans

Disturbed body image, Chapter 2
Ineffective sexuality pattern, Chapter 2
Health-seeking behaviors, Chapter 3

Coronary Bypass/Valve Surgery: Postoperative Care

Coronary Artery Bypass Graft (CABG); Valve Replacement; Minimally Invasive Direct CAB (MIDCAB) Surgery; Off-Pump CABG (OPCAB)

Coronary Bypass Surgery

The surgical approach to myocardial revascularization for coronary artery disease is bypass grafting. An artery from the chest wall (internal mammary) or radial artery, or a vein from the leg (saphenous) is used to supply blood distal to the area of stenosis. Internal mammary arteries have a higher patency rate. Today's coronary artery bypass graft (CABG) patients are older (even octogenarians unresponsive to medical therapy or with failed coronary angioplasties or stents), have poorer left ventricular function, and may have undergone prior sternotomies. Older patients are at higher risk for complications and have a higher mortality rate. Women tend to have CABG surgery performed later in life. They have more complicated recovery courses than men because of the smaller diameter of women's vessels and their associated comorbidity. Women have also been noted to have less favorable outcomes, with more recurrent angina and less return to work. Minimally invasive direct surgical techniques (MIDCAB or "keyhole" surgery) can be used for patients with a lesion confined to the left anterior descending artery. A smaller thoracotomy incision is made, and the left internal mammary artery is dissected and attached to the still beating heart without need for cardiopulmonary bypass. This surgical approach results in smaller incisions and shorter hospital stays, but limits the number of coronary lesions that can be treated.

Newer techniques for revascularization are available, such as transmyocardial revascularization with laser and video-assisted thoracoscopy (robotic surgery or closed-chest heart surgery). These techniques use limited incision and reduce the need for cardiopulmonary bypass and related perioperative complications. Surgical procedures for CABG without cardiopulmonary bypass or cardioplegia (off-pump) hold promise for reductions in postoperative morbidity. This care plan focuses on traditional open heart surgery.

Valve Replacement Surgery

Rheumatic fever, infection, calcification, or degeneration can cause the valve to become stenotic (incomplete opening) or regurgitant (incomplete closure), leading to valvular heart surgery. Whenever possible, the native valve is repaired. (See the nursing care plan under Percutaneous Balloon Valvuloplasty.) If the valve is beyond repair, it is replaced. Replacement valves can be biological (tissue) or prosthetic (mechanical or synthetic). Tissue valves have a short life span; mechanical valves can last a lifetime but require long-term anticoagulation. Patients having a valve replacement undergo an open heart surgery procedure similar to CABG procedure and experience similar complications.

This care plan focuses only on acute care. See *Cardiac Rehabilitation* care plan presented earlier in this chapter for patient education information.

NANDA-I NDx Decreased Cardiac Output

Common Related Factor

Low cardiac output syndrome (occurs to some extent in all patients after extracorporeal circulation [ECC] secondary to reduced ventricular function)

Defining Characteristics

Left ventricular failure (LVF)
- Increased left arterial pressure (LAP), pulmonary capillary wedge pressure, and pulmonary artery diastolic pressure (PADP)
- Tachycardia
- Decreased BP and decreased cardiac output
- Diminished peripheral pulses
- Changes seen on chest x-ray films
- Crackles
- Decreased arterial and venous oxygen
- Acidosis
- Decreasing urine output
- Changes in level of consciousness

Right ventricular failure (RVF)
- Increased right arterial pressure (RAP), central venous pressure (CVP), and HR
- Decreased LAP, pulmonary capillary wedge pressure, and PADP (unless biventricular failure present)
- Jugular venous distention
- Decreased BP, decreased perfusion, decreased cardiac output, change in level of consciousness

Common Expected Outcome

Patient maintains adequate cardiac output, as evidenced by strong peripheral pulses, systolic BP within 20 mm Hg of baseline, HR 60 to 100 beats/min with regular rhythm, urinary output greater than 30 mL/hr, clear breath sounds, good capillary refill, warm and dry skin, and normal level of consciousness.

NOC Outcomes
Cardiac Pump Effectiveness; Cardiopulmonary Status; Circulation Status

NIC Interventions
Hemodynamic Regulation; Invasive Hemodynamic Monitoring

Cardiac and Vascular Care Plans

■ = Independent   ▲ = Interprofessional Collaboration

Ongoing Assessment

Actions/Interventions

- Document the pump time (ECC) during surgery.

- Assess the patient's HR, BP, and pulse pressure. Use direct intra-arterial monitoring as ordered.

- Assess peripheral and central pulses, including capillary refill.
- Assess for changes in the level of consciousness.

- Assess the respiratory rate and rhythm.

- Assess the patient's urine output.

- Use pulse oximetry to monitor oxygen saturation; assess arterial blood gases.

- If hemodynamic monitoring is in place, assess CVP, PADP, pulmonary capillary wedge pressure (PCWP), cardiac output and/or cardiac index, and venous oxygen saturation (Svo_2) levels.

- Auscultate breath sounds.

▲ Monitor serial chest x-ray films.

Rationales

The ECC pump, or the heart-lung machine, is used to divert blood from the heart and lungs, to oxygenate it, and to provide flow to the vital organs while the heart is stopped. For on-pump procedures, the more prolonged the pump run, the more profound the ventricular dysfunction. Newer surgical techniques are performing CABG without extracorporeal bypass (off-pump, or "surgery on the beating heart") to avoid this complication.

Sinus tachycardia and increased arterial BP are seen in the early stages to maintain an adequate cardiac output; BP drops as the condition deteriorates. Older patients have a reduced response to catecholamines; thus their response to a decreased cardiac output may be blunted with less increase in HR. Attention to hemodynamic changes reduces the risk of harm to the patient during the early recovery period. QSEN: Safety.

Pulses are weak with reduced stroke volume and cardiac output. Capillary refill is slow.

Early signs of cerebral hypoxia are restlessness and anxiety, with confusion and loss of consciousness occurring in later stages. Older patients are especially susceptible to reduced perfusion to vital organs. QSEN: Safety.

Rapid shallow respirations are characteristic of decreased cardiac output.

The renal system compensates for low blood pressure by retaining fluid and sodium. Oliguria is a classic sign of inadequate renal perfusion from reduced cardiac output.

Pulse oximetry is a useful tool to detect changes in oxygenation. Oxygen saturation should be kept above 90% or greater. As shock increases, aerobic metabolism ceases and lactic acidosis ensues, raising levels of carbon dioxide and pH. Attention to changes in oxygen levels and acid-base balance reduces the risk of harm to the patient. QSEN: Safety.

CVP provides information on filling pressures of the right side of the heart; PADP and PCWP reflect left-sided fluid volumes. Cardiac output provides information on end-organ perfusion and objective numbers to guide therapy. Svo_2 provides information on tissue oxygenation at the cellular level. Change in oxygen saturation of mixed venous blood is one of the earliest indications of decreased cardiac output. QSEN: Safety.

Crackles are evident in LVF and biventricular failure, but not in RVF.

X-ray studies provide information on an enlarged heart, increased pulmonary vascular markings, and pulmonary edema.

Therapeutic Interventions

Actions/Interventions	Rationales
▲ Maintain hemodynamics within set parameters by the titration of vasoactive drugs, most commonly:	These medications are based on recommendations from national organizations. Appropriate use of these medications reduces the risk of harm to the patient from the effects of vasoactive drugs. QSEN: Evidence-based practice; Safety.
• Nitroglycerin (NTG)	NTG is a vasodilator that acts on the coronary vasculature, decreases spasms of mammary grafts, and dilates venous system.
• Sodium nitroprusside (Nipride)	Sodium nitroprusside is a vasodilator that lowers systemic vascular resistance and decreases BP. Elevated pressure on new grafts may cause bleeding.
• Dopamine	Dopamine is an inotrope and vasopressor that has varying effects at different doses. Low doses increase renal blood flow. Higher doses increase systemic vascular resistance (SVR) and contractility.
• Dobutamine (Dobutrex)	Dobutamine is an inotrope that increases contractility with slight vasodilation.
• Milrinone	Milrinone is a cyclic adenosine monophosohate–specific phosphodiesterase inhibitor that has inotropic and vasodilator effects.
• Norepinephrine (Levophed)	Norepinephrine is a vasopressor that increases SVR and contractility.
• Epinephrine	Epinephrine is an inotrope and vasopressor that increases SVR and contractility.
• Phenylephrine (Neo-Synephrine)	Phenylephrine is a vasopressor that increases SVR.
• Vasopressin	Vasopressin is a vasopressor that increases SVR.
• Nicardipine	Nicardipine is a calcium channel blocker that increases cardiac output and decreases peripheral vascular resistance.
▲ Maintain oxygen therapy as prescribed.	Oxygen saturation needs to be greater than 90%. When more oxygen is available to the myocardial tissues, ventricular function may improve.
■ If the patient is unresponsive to usual treatments, anticipate the use of mechanical assistance.	Mechanical devices such as a ventricular assist device or an intra-aortic balloon pump (IABP) provide temporary circulatory support to improve cardiac output. These devices can be used in cardiac surgery patients who cannot be weaned from cardiopulmonary bypass. The IABP is used to increase coronary artery perfusion and decrease myocardial workload. The nurse needs to follow unit protocols for the management of the patient with a mechanical assist device.

Cardiac and Vascular Care Plans

■ = Independent   ▲ = Interprofessional Collaboration

NANDA-I NDx Deficient Fluid Volume

Common Related Factors

Fluid leaks into extravascular spaces
Diuresis
Blood loss or altered coagulation factors

Defining Characteristics

Decreased filling pressures (CVP, RAP, PADP, pulmonary capillary wedge pressure, LAP)
Hypotension and/or tachycardia
Decreased cardiac output or cardiac index
Decreased urine output with increased specific gravity
If blood loss occurs
• Decreased hemoglobin level or hematocrit
• Increased chest tube drainage

Common Expected Outcome

Patient is normovolemic, as evidenced by normal filling pressures, systolic BP 90 mm Hg or greater, HR 60 to 100 beats/min at regular rate, and urine output at 30 mL/hr or greater.

NOC Outcomes

Circulation Status; Fluid Balance

NIC Interventions

Hemodynamic Regulation; Hypovolemia Management; Invasive Hemodynamic Monitoring

---

Ongoing Assessment

Actions/Interventions	Rationales
▲ Assess the patient's hemodynamic parameters.	Most patients have hypotension and compensatory tachycardia in response to a low fluid volume. Invasive hemodynamic measurements (e.g., CVP, PADP) may be required to determine status and guide therapy. Attention to changes in hemodynamic status reduces the risk of harm to the patient and guides early intervention. QSEN: Safety.
■ Monitor the patient's fluid status: intake, output, and urine specific gravity.	During extracorporeal circulation (ECC), the blood is diluted to prevent sludging in the microcirculation. Total fluid volume may be normal or increased, but because of ECC, changes in membrane integrity cause fluid leaks into extravascular spaces. Concentrated urine denotes fluid deficit.
■ Obtain and assess a report of blood loss from the operating room and the type and amount of fluid replacement.	These data provide key information on the level of fluid balance.
■ Assess the chest tube drainage.	Significant blood loss from chest tubes can contribute to decreased fluid volume.
▲ Monitor the coagulation factors on the complete blood count.	Heparin is used with ECC to prevent clots from forming. Clotting derangements and bleeding are common postoperative problems.
▲ Monitor platelets for thrombocytopenia. If the platelet count drops below 100,000/mm³, or if platelets drop below 50% of the preoperative platelet level, check the heparin-induced platelet antibody (HIPA).	Increasing numbers of patients on heparin develop heparin antibodies that activate platelets, causing new or worsening thrombosis. This heparin-induced thrombocytopenia (HIT) results in a low platelet count. QSEN: Safety.
▲ If the HIPA result is positive, stop all heparin products and obtain a hematology consult.	Patients with HIT are at an increased risk for thrombotic events and should be treated with alternative anticoagulants, such as argatroban, a direct thrombin inhibitor. Each patient must be evaluated individually. QSEN: Teamwork and collaboration.

Cardiac and Vascular Care Plans

Therapeutic Interventions

Actions/Interventions	Rationales
▲ Administer IV fluids as prescribed (e.g., lactated Ringer's solution).	A cell-saver from the ECC is used to replace blood intraoperatively. Further fluid volume replacement is initiated after surgery. These maintain adequate filling pressures.
▲ Ensure that the laboratory has crossmatched blood available.	In case major bleeding occurs, blood replacement must be immediately available.
▲ Administer coagulation drugs as prescribed: vitamin K, protamine.	Specific drugs work for different causes.
▲ Administer blood products (packed red blood cells, fresh frozen plasma, cryoprecipitate).	Transfusion therapy is used to correct deficiencies. Platelet transfusions should be avoided, as they may increase the thrombogenic effect, unless severe bleeding has occurred.

NANDA-I
NDx **Risk for Decreased Cardiac Output: Dysrhythmias**

Common Risk Factors

Dysrhythmias resulting from the following:
- Ectopy (ischemia, electrolyte imbalance, and mechanical irritation)
- Bradydysrhythmias and heart block (edema or sutures in the area of the specialized conduction system)
- Supraventricular tachydysrhythmias (atrial stretching, mechanical irritability secondary to cannulation, or rebound from preoperative beta-blockers)

Common Expected Outcome

Patient maintains optimal cardiac output as evidenced by baseline cardiac rhythm, HR between 60 and 100 beats/min, and adequate BP to meet metabolic needs.

NOC Outcomes
Cardiac Pump Effectiveness; Vital Signs; Electrolyte and Acid/Base Balance
NIC Interventions
Dysrhythmia Management; Electrolyte Monitoring; Electrolyte Management: Potassium, Magnesium, Calcium

---

Ongoing Assessment

Actions/Interventions	Rationales
■ Continuously monitor the patient's cardiac rhythm.	The ability to recognize dysrhythmias is essential to early treatment. Atrial fibrillation, premature ventricular contractions, and heart blocks are the most common postoperative dysrhythmias.
▲ Monitor the 12-lead ECG as prescribed.	Besides providing information on dysrhythmias, the ECG may document intraoperative myocardial ischemia that may also affect cardiac output.
▲ Monitor electrolyte levels, especially potassium, magnesium, and calcium.	Electrolyte imbalances are common causes of dysrhythmias and guide treatment. Potassium and magnesium loss results from diuresis.

■ = Independent   ▲ = Interprofessional Collaboration

Cardiac and Vascular Care Plans

Therapeutic Interventions

Actions/Interventions	Rationales
■ Maintain a temporary pacemaker generator at the bedside.	Dysrhythmias are common after cardiac surgical procedures. Temporary epicardial pacing wires are often placed prophylactically during surgery for use in overdriving tachy-dysrhythmias or for backup pacing bradydysrhythmias. During the first 24 hours the wires may be connected to a pulse generator kept on standby. Appropriate use of safety-enhancing technology minimizes the risk of harm to the patient. QSEN: Safety.
▲ Administer potassium as prescribed to keep the serum level at 4 to 5 mEq/L.	Both hypokalemia and hyperkalemia can initiate cardiac dysrhythmias.
▲ Administer magnesium as prescribed to keep the level greater than 2 mEq/L.	A variety of dysrhythmias can be precipitated by magnesium imbalance.
▲ Administer calcium as prescribed to keep the level at 8 to 10 mg/dL.	Although cardiac dysrhythmias are less common with hypocalcemia, they can be dangerous when present.
▲ Treat dysrhythmias according to unit protocol.	Advanced Cardiac Life Support and other evidence-based clinical guidelines provide direction for treatment. Pacing through epicardial pacing wires is often ordered. These nursing actions are based on recommendations from national organizations. QSEN: Evidence-based practice.
▲ If dysrhythmias are unresponsive to medical treatment, avoid precordial thump. Use countershock instead.	Avoidance of precordial thump reduces the risk for trauma to vascular suture lines.

NANDA-I
NDx Decreased Cardiac Output: Cardiac Tamponade

Common Related Factor	Defining Characteristics
Cardiac tamponade resulting in external compression of cardiovascular structures causing reduced diastolic filling	Decreased BP Narrow pulse pressure Pulsus paradoxus (systolic pressure decreases 10 mm Hg or more during inspiration) Tachycardia Electrical alternans (decreased QRS voltage during inspiration) Equalization of pressures (CVP, RVDP, PADP, pulmonary capillary wedge pressure) Jugular venous distention (JVD) Chest tubes (if present) suddenly stop draining (suspect clot) Distant or muffled heart tones Restlessness, confusion, and anxiety Decrease in hemoglobin and hematocrit Cool, clammy skin Diminished peripheral pulses Decreased urine output Decreased arterial and venous oxygen saturation Acidosis Unwillingness to lie supine

Common Expected Outcome

Patient maintains adequate cardiac output as evidenced by the following: BP within normal limits for patient, strong regular pulses, absence of JVD, absence of pulsus paradoxus, skin warm and dry, and normal level of consciousness.

NOC Outcomes

Cardiac Pump Effectiveness; Fluid Balance; Blood Coagulation

NIC Interventions

Hemodynamic Regulation; Invasive Hemodynamic Monitoring; Fluid Resuscitation; Shock Management: Cardiac; Emergency Care

Ongoing Assessment

Actions/Interventions	Rationales
■ Assess for the classic signs and symptoms associated with acute cardiac tamponade:	The accumulation of blood in the mediastinum or pericardium applies pressure on the heart and causes tamponade with a resulting decrease in cardiac output. Symptoms are related to the degree of tamponade. Cardiac tamponade is a life-threatening condition. Early assessment of reduced cardiac output facilitates early emergency treatment. QSEN: Safety.
• Low arterial BP with narrowed pulse pressure	An initial elevation in BP may occur with compensatory vasoconstriction; however, as venous return is compromised from the cardiac compression, a significant decrease in cardiac output occurs.
• Tachycardia	Tachycardia is related to compensatory catecholamine release.
• Distant or muffled heart sounds	These characteristic sounds are related to fluid accumulation in the pericardial sac.
• Elevated CVP	The CVP may rise to 15 to 20 cm H_2O as a result of impedance to diastolic filling by atrial compression.
• Pulsus paradoxus	Pulsus paradoxus is characterized by a drop of more than 10 mm Hg in systolic BP with inspiration.
• Dyspnea	Dyspnea is related to fluid backup in the pulmonary system.
■ Assess level of consciousness.	Symptoms may range from anxiety to an altered level of consciousness in shock. QSEN: Safety.
■ Monitor the chest tube drainage.	A decrease in chest tube drainage occurring with decreased cardiac output may indicate cardiac tamponade.
▲ Assess the 12-lead ECG.	The ECG may reveal ST-segment elevation, nonspecific ST- and T-wave changes, and/or electrical alternans (caused by pendulum-like movement of the heart within the pericardial effusion).
▲ Assist with the performance of a bedside echocardiogram, if time permits.	Echocardiography evaluation provides the most helpful diagnostic information. Effusions seen with acute tamponade are usually smaller than with chronic tamponade. However, in light of circulatory collapse, treatment may be indicated before the echocardiogram can be performed.
▲ Assess the hemodynamic profile using a pulmonary artery catheter; assess for the equalization of pressures.	The CVP, RVDP, PADP, and pulmonary capillary wedge pressure are all elevated in tamponade and within 2 to 3 mm Hg of each other. These pressures confirm diagnosis. Attention to early changes in hemodynamic status reduces the risk of harm to the patient. QSEN: Safety.
▲ Assess the chest x-ray study.	The x-ray study reveals a widened mediastinum with a normal cardiac silhouette, clear lung fields, and dilation of superior vena cava.

Cardiac and Vascular Care Plans

■ = Independent   ▲ = Interprofessional Collaboration

Therapeutic Interventions

Actions/Interventions	Rationales
■ Implement unit protocols to remove clots from chest and/or mediastinal drainage tubes.	Impaired drainage can cause a buildup of blood in the pericardial sac or mediastinum, resulting in tamponade. QSEN: Safety.
▲ If cardiac tamponade is rapidly developing with cardiovascular decompensation and collapse:	
• Maintain aggressive fluid resuscitation.	Fluids are required to maintain adequate circulating volume as tamponade is evacuated.
• Administer vasopressor agents (dopamine, norepinephrine) as prescribed.	Vasopressor medications maximize systemic perfusion pressure to vital organs.
• Assemble an open chest tray for bedside intervention; prepare the patient for transport to surgery.	Acute tamponade is a life-threatening complication, but immediate prognosis is good with fast, effective treatment.

NDx Risk for Ineffective Myocardial Tissue Perfusion

Common Risk Factors

Spasm of native coronary artery or of bypass grafts
Low flow or thrombosis of vein grafts
Coronary embolus
Perioperative ischemia
Chronic myocardial ischemia

Common Expected Outcome

Risk for perioperative ischemia or infarction is reduced through early assessment and treatment.

NOC Outcomes
Circulation Status; Tissue Perfusion: Cardiac
NIC Interventions
Cardiac Care: Acute; Hemodynamic Regulation

Ongoing Assessment

Actions/Interventions	Rationales
■ Continuously monitor the patient's cardiac rhythm.	Cardiac rhythm changes may occur secondary to myocardial ischemia.
▲ Obtain a 12-lead ECG on admission and as needed. Compare with the preoperative ECG. Note any acute changes: T-wave inversions, ST-segment elevation or depression.	Attention to any changes followed by prompt treatment reduces the risk of harm to the patient. The primary nurse must know which vessels were bypassed and must carefully evaluate the corresponding areas on the 12-lead ECG. Patients commonly have chronic myocardial ischemia that is further compromised during surgery, or they may have spasms in specific coronary arteries:
	• Right coronary artery (RCA): leads II, III, aVF
	• Posterior descending: R waves in leads V_1 and V_2
	• Left anterior descending: leads V_1 to V_4
	• Diagonals: leads V_5 to V_6
	• Circumflex, obtuse marginal: leads I, aVL, and V_5
	QSEN: Safety.

Cardiac and Vascular Care Plans

Actions/Interventions

▲ Monitor cardiac biomarkers (CK-MB and troponin) for signs of perioperative ischemia or infarct per institutional policy.

Rationales

Patients usually do not express characteristic chest pain because of the effects of general anesthesia during surgery. Laboratory data aid in diagnosis. However, many programs no longer measure these postoperatively, because there are no consistent standards to substantiate normal postoperative levels. New wall motion abnormality on echocardiogram can be used to document changes.

Therapeutic Interventions

Actions/Interventions

▲ Maintain an adequate diastolic BP with vasopressors.

▲ Maintain an arterial saturation greater than 95%.
▲ If signs of ischemia are noted, administer medications (IV nitroglycerin and/or calcium channel blocker).
▲ Anticipate the insertion of an intra-aortic balloon.

Rationales

Coronary artery flow occurs during diastole. Adequate pressures of at least 40 mm Hg are needed to drive coronary flow and prevent graft thrombosis.
Adequate oxygenation is required for effective gas exchange.
Nitroglycerin and calcium channel blockers increase coronary perfusion and alleviate possible coronary spasm.
This assist device improves coronary artery blood flow during diastole.

NANDA-I
NDx Risk for Electrolyte Imbalance

Common Risk Factors

Fluid shifts
Diuretics

Common Expected Outcome

Patient maintains normal electrolyte balance, as evidenced by sodium level within 130 to 142 mEq/L; potassium, 4 to 5 mEq/L; chloride, 98 to 115 mEq/L; calcium, 9 to 11 mg/dL; and magnesium, 1.7 to 2.4 mEq/L.

NOC Outcomes
Electrolyte and Acid/Base Balance; Fluid Balance
NIC Intervention
Fluid/Electrolyte Management

Ongoing Assessment

Actions/Interventions

▲ Observe and document serial laboratory data: sodium, potassium, chloride, magnesium, and calcium levels.

■ Monitor the ECG for changes.

Rationales

Serum electrolyte levels may be decreased due to hemodilution from extracorporeal circulation and resultant fluid shifts causing changes in fluid composition.
Widening QRS complex, ST-segment changes, dysrhythmias, and atrioventricular blocks are seen with electrolyte imbalance. Attention to acute changes in the ECG reduces the risk of harm to the patient. QSEN: Safety.

Therapeutic Interventions

Actions/Interventions

▲ Maintain an adequate electrolyte balance by administering desired electrolytes as prescribed.

Rationales

Hypertonic solutions may be used to correct sodium and chloride deficiencies. Potassium, calcium, and magnesium imbalances may be corrected by IV administration of electrolyte solutions.

Cardiac and Vascular Care Plans

■ = Independent ▲ = Interprofessional Collaboration

NANDA-I NDx Risk for Impaired Gas Exchange

Common Risk Factors

Retraction and compression of lungs during surgery
Surgical incision, making coughing difficult
Secretions
Pulmonary vascular congestion

Common Expected Outcome

Patient maintains optimal gas exchange as evidenced by clear breath sounds, normal respiratory pattern, normal arterial blood gases (ABGs), and no further change in level of consciousness.

NOC Outcomes
Respiratory Status: Gas Exchange; Respiratory Status: Ventilation
NIC Interventions
Respiratory Monitoring; Ventilation Assistance; Airway Management; Endotracheal Extubation

---

Ongoing Assessment

Actions/Interventions	Rationales
■ Assess breath sounds, noting any areas of decreased ventilation and presence of adventitious sounds.	Changes in breath sounds may reveal the cause of impaired gas exchange. Diminished breath sounds are associated with poor ventilation.
▲ Monitor serial ABGs and oxygen saturation.	Low Pao_2 and oxygen saturation and increasing $Paco_2$ are characteristic of hypoxemia and respiratory failure. Attention to these parameters reduces the risk of harm to the patient by identifying changes in oxygenation and initiating early intervention. QSEN: Safety.
■ Assess for restlessness or changes in the level of consciousness.	Hypoxemia results in cerebral hypoxia.
▲ Monitor the serial chest x-ray films.	Chest x-ray studies can reveal the cause of the impaired gas exchange. Pleural effusions, pulmonary edema, or infiltrates are contributing factors.
▲ Verify that the ventilator settings are maintained as prescribed: • Tidal volume 10 to 15 mL/kg • Rate 10 to 14/min • Fractional concentration of oxygen inspired gas (Fio_2) to keep Pao_2 greater than 80 mm Hg • Positive end-expiratory pressure (PEEP) starting at 5 cm H_2O	Ongoing titration may be required to maintain ABGs within acceptable limits. Appropriate use of safety-enhancing technology minimizes the risk of harm to the patient. QSEN: Safety.
▲ Monitor rising pulmonary artery pressures and peripheral vascular resistance.	Data provide information on pulmonary hypertension and cor pulmonale.
▲ Anticipate the use of nitric oxide therapy with other ventilation therapy for patients with pulmonary hypertension.	Nitric oxide reduces the pulmonary vascular resistance for patients with persistent pulmonary hypertension.

 For additional care plans, go to http://evolve.elsevier.com/Gulanick/.

Cardiac and Vascular Care Plans

Therapeutic Interventions

Actions/Interventions	Rationales
■ Suction as needed. Hyperventilate and hyperoxygenate the patient during suctioning.	Suctioning removes secretions when the patient is unable to effectively clear the airway while ventilated. However, repeated and prolonged suctioning may lead to desaturation of blood and impaired gas exchange. Hyperoxygenation helps decrease hypoxia related to the suctioning procedure. Hyperventilation helps expand lungs that were deflated during surgery.
▲ Change the ventilator settings as ordered.	Ongoing titration is expected to maintain ABGs within accepted limits. (*NOTE:* Patients with preexisting pulmonary dysfunction will have lower Pao_2 and higher $Paco_2$ values.) PEEP may be increased in increments of 2.5 cm to maintain adequate oxygenation on Fio_2 of 50%. Patients can usually tolerate up to 20 cm H_2O of PEEP if they are not hypovolemic or hypotensive. QSEN: Safety.
■ Initiate calming techniques including sedation if the patient is "fighting" the ventilator.	Patients expend energy and increase oxygen demands when their breathing is asynchronous with the ventilator. This breathing pattern may trigger high-pressure alarms on the ventilator.
■ Instruct the patient or family of the rationale and expected sensations associated with the use of mechanical ventilation.	Adequate educational preparation can reduce anxiety and facilitate adjustment to the mechanical ventilation process.
▲ Administer sedation as needed: • Midazolam (Versed): short-acting central nervous system depressant • Morphine sulfate • Propofol (Diprivan) drip	Sedation with midazolam and/or morphine sulfate helps decrease anxiety, which may reduce myocardial oxygen consumption. Patients are usually kept sedated for at least 4 hours to facilitate hemodynamic stability. Sedation with propofol IV infusion can be used for patients requiring longer mechanical ventilation therapy.
▲ Wean the patient from the ventilator, and extubate as soon as possible.	Initially the cardiac surgical patient requires mechanical ventilation because of the use of general anesthesia. Weaning and extubation occur as soon as the anesthetic agents wear off, after 4 hours in most patients.
■ Encourage coughing and deep breathing. Use a pillow to splint the incision.	Coughing is an effective way to clear secretions. The surgical incision may cause chest discomfort and inhibit deep breathing and coughing. Splinting the chest may enhance coughing efforts.
▲ Use pain medications as needed.	Medications decrease incisional discomfort so the patient will cough and breathe deeply.
▲ Provide supplemental oxygen as indicated.	Oxygen saturation needs to be greater than 90%. Adequate oxygenation is required for effective gas exchange.
■ Instruct in the need to use an incentive spirometer.	Incentive spirometry increases lung volume and reduces alveolar collapse.
■ Encourage dangling of the legs or progressive activity as tolerated.	Progressive activity increases lung volume and ventilation.
■ Consider chest physiotherapy.	Postural drainage and percussion techniques aid in mobilizing respiratory secretions for removal by suctioning or coughing.

Cardiac and Vascular Care Plans

■ = Independent   ▲ = Interprofessional Collaboration

Fear

Common Related Factors

Intensive care unit environment
Unfamiliarity with postoperative care
Altered communication secondary to intubation
Dependence on mechanical equipment
Threat of pain related to major surgery
Threat of death

Defining Characteristics

Feeling of fear and dread
Increased alertness
Jitteriness
Focus narrowed to source of fear
Change in physiological responses (e.g., BP, HR, respiratory rate)

Common Expected Outcomes

Patient appears calm and trusting of medical care.
Patient verbalizes fears and concerns.

NOC Outcomes
Fear Self-Control; Coping
NIC Interventions
Anxiety Reduction; Preparatory Sensory Information; Emotional Support

Ongoing Assessment

Action/Intervention	Rationale
■ Assess the patient's level of fear. Note any signs and symptoms, especially nonverbal communication.	Controlling fear helps reduce physiological reactions that can aggravate the condition and increase oxygen consumption. QSEN: Patient-centered care.

Therapeutic Interventions

Actions/Interventions	Rationales
■ Orient the patient to the intensive care environment.	The noise and continuous lighting in the intensive care unit environment increase the amount of sensory stimuli for the patient and add to the level of anxiety. The patient and family need to be aware of the source of noises such as normal sounds from mechanical ventilators, monitoring equipment, and mechanical ventricular assist devices. Because equipment alarms should not be silenced, nurses need to explain each alarm sound and respond to each alarm as quickly as possible to resolve the problem and restore normal function.
■ Display a calm, confident manner.	This approach increases the patient's feeling of security.
■ Prepare for and explain common postoperative sensations (coldness, fatigue, discomfort, coughing, uncomfortable endotracheal tube). Clarify misconceptions.	Anticipatory preparation can help reduce anxiety associated with the unknown.
▲ Explain the purpose of tubes, monitoring equipment, medication pumps, mechanical ventilators, and other equipment and devices that are part of postoperative care. Explain each procedure before doing it, even if described previously.	Misconceptions about the use of the equipment can add to patients' fear of equipment failure and feelings of dependency on machines. Information can promote trust or confidence in medical management. However, high anxiety levels can reduce attention level and retention of information.

ⓔvolve   **For additional care plans, go to http://evolve.elsevier.com/Gulanick/.**

Cardiac and Vascular Care Plans

Actions/Interventions

- ■ Avoid unnecessary conversations between team members in front of the patient.
- ▲ Provide pain medication at the first sign of discomfort.
- ■ For intubated patients, provide a nonverbal means of communication (slate, paper and pencil, gestures). Be patient with attempts to communicate. Know and anticipate typical patient concerns.
- ■ Ensure the continuity of staff.

- ■ Encourage visiting by family/significant others.

Rationales

This measure can reduce patients' misconceptions and fear or anxiety.

Effective pain management will reduce discomfort and fear.

Patients' inability to talk can add to their anxiety. QSEN: Patient-centered care.

Continuity facilitates communication efforts and provides stability in care.

Visitors can promote a feeling of security; the patient does not feel alone.

Related Care Plans

Surgical experience: Preoperative and postoperative care, Chapter 4
Cardiac rehabilitation, Chapter 5
Mechanical ventilation, Chapter 6
Dysrhythmias, ⊖volve

Heart Failure, Chronic

Congestive Heart Failure; Cardiomyopathy; Left-Sided Failure; Right-Sided Failure; Pump Failure; Systolic Dysfunction; Diastolic Dysfunction

Heart failure is described as a common clinical syndrome resulting in the inability of the heart to meet the hemodynamic and metabolic demands of the body, producing a variety of biochemical and neurohormonal changes and manifesting in a variety of ways. With more than 5 million people in the United States having heart failure, it is a major health problem associated with high mortality rates, major morbidity, and rehospitalization. There is an increased prevalence with age, especially with women, making this a key geriatric concern. Heart failure remains one of the most disabling conditions, carrying a high economic burden related to the frequency of hospital readmissions.

Heart failure is the final syndrome of a wide spectrum of endothelial and myocardial injuries that produce ventricular systolic dysfunction (poor pumping function) and/or diastolic dysfunction (poor relaxation and filling function). Hypertension and coronary artery disease are the most common contributing factors to heart failure, though the list of causative factors is quite extensive. These causes are often described as resulting from myocardial ischemia and chamber enlargement from a variety of causes, volume-related factors, pressure-loading conditions, and restrictive causes. Because of the health consequences of heart failure, attention is being directed to identifying and treating earlier those at risk for heart failure. A lettered classification system has been developed by the American Heart Association and the American College of Cardiology with characteristics defined for stages A, B, C, and D, with A being high risk but without structural problems or heart failure symptoms to D being refractory heart failure requiring specialized interventions. This system somewhat parallels the classic New York Heart Association functional classification system based on severity of symptoms. Class I patients have no symptoms or physical limitations. Class II patients have slight limitations in their physical activity, whereby ordinary physical activities can cause symptoms such as fatigue, palpitations, dyspnea, or angina. Class III patients have marked physical limitations, with less than ordinary level of activities causing symptoms. Class IV patients experience dyspnea even at rest; activity is severely restricted.

The goals of treatment are to prevent progression of heart failure, reduce exacerbations, recognize early signs of decompensation, control symptoms, assist the patient in co-managing the disease, and improve the patient's quality of life. The basis of medical therapy is neurohormonal inhibition. Angiotensin-converting enzyme inhibitors, angiotensin II receptor blockers, beta-blockers, and aldosterone antagonists promote vasodilation, prevent decompensation, and reduce mortality risk. These drugs are used

Cardiac and Vascular Care Plans

in combination with diuretics that reduce fluid overload. Digoxin is sometimes used in appropriate patients but does not reduce mortality rate. Additional therapies such as IV vasodilators and inotropes are indicated as patients deteriorate and experience acute decompensation. Additional device therapies are available for patients with more complicated conditions. These therapies include ultrafiltration to remove excess fluids and sodium, cardiac resynchronization therapy pacemakers to optimize cardiac output, implantable defibrillators to reduce risk for sudden cardiac death, and ventricular assist devices to extend life.

Innovative programs such as cardiac case-managed home care, community-based heart failure case management, telemanagement, and heart failure cardiac rehabilitation programs are being developed to reduce the need for acute care or hospital services for this growing population. Because the goal of therapy is to manage patients outside the hospital, this care plan focuses on treatment in an ambulatory setting for patients with heart failure symptoms (Stage C, Functional Class II-III). *NOTE*: Several national organizations have performance outcome goals related to heart failure: the American Heart Association's Get With the Guidelines—Heart Failure initiative and The Joint Commission's National Patient Safety Goals and National Quality Improvement Goals.

NANDA-I NDx Decreased Cardiac Output

Common Related Factors

Increased or decreased preload
Increased afterload
Impaired contractility
Alteration in HR, heart rhythm, conduction
Cardiac muscle disease
Medication side effects

Defining Characteristics

Low BP
Increased HR/dysrhythmias
Decreased urine output
Decreased peripheral pulses
Cold, clammy skin
Crackles and/or tachypnea
Dyspnea
Orthopnea or paroxysmal nocturnal dyspnea (PND)
Decreased activity tolerance or fatigue
Edema and/or weight gain
Changes in level of consciousness
Abnormal heart sounds (S_3, S_4)

Common Expected Outcome

Patient maintains adequate cardiac output as evidenced by strong peripheral pulses, systolic BP within 20 mm Hg of baseline, HR 60 to 100 beats/min with regular rhythm, urinary output 30 mL/hr or greater, warm and dry skin, normal level of consciousness, and eupnea with absence of pulmonary crackles.

NOC Outcomes

Cardiopulmonary Status; Cardiac Pump Effectiveness

NIC Interventions

Hemodynamic Regulation; Dysrhythmia Management

Ongoing Assessment

Actions/Interventions	Rationales
■ Assess the rate and quality of apical and peripheral pulses, including capillary refill.	Most patients have compensatory tachycardia in response to low cardiac output. Peripheral pulses may be weak, with reduced stroke volume and cardiac output. Capillary refill is slow, sometimes absent.

Actions/Interventions	Rationales
■ Assess the patient's BP, noting any orthostatic changes.	Most patients have significantly reduced BP secondary to a low cardiac output state, as well as the vasodilating effects of prescribed medications. Typically patients can have systolic BPs in the range of 80 to 100 mm Hg and still be adequately perfusing target organs. However, symptomatic hypotension, systolic BP below 80 mm Hg, or a mean arterial pressure less than 60 mm Hg needs to be reported and further evaluated. QSEN: Safety.
■ Assess heart sounds for the presence of S_3 and/or S_4.	S_3 denotes reduced left ventricular ejection and is a classic sign of left ventricular failure (LVF). S_4 occurs with reduced compliance of the left ventricle, which impairs diastolic filling.
■ Assess the respiratory rate, rhythm, and breath sounds. Determine any recent occurrence of PND or orthopnea.	Rapid shallow respirations are characteristic of reduced cardiac output. Crackles reflect accumulation of fluid in pulmonary circulation secondary to impaired left ventricular emptying. They are more evident in the dependent areas of the lung. Orthopnea is difficulty breathing when supine. PND is difficulty breathing during the night. QSEN: Safety.
■ Weigh the patient, and evaluate trends in weight.	Body weight is a more sensitive indicator of fluid or sodium retention than intake and output. A 2- to 3-pound increase in weight usually indicates retention of 1 L of fluid and a need to adjust diuretic drug therapy. Patients need to understand that the focus of daily weighing is on fluid, not changes in body fat.
■ Assess the skin color, temperature, and moisture.	Cool, pale, clammy skin is secondary to compensatory increases in sympathetic nervous system stimulation, low cardiac output, and oxygen desaturation.
■ Assess for reports of fatigue and reduced activity tolerance. Determine at what level of activity fatigue or exertional dyspnea occurs.	Fatigue and exertional dyspnea are common problems with low cardiac output states.
■ Assess urine output. Determine how frequently the patient urinates.	The renal system compensates for low BP by retaining water. Oliguria is a classic sign of decreased renal perfusion. Diuresis is expected with diuretic therapy.
■ Determine any changes in the level of consciousness.	Hypoxia and reduced cerebral perfusion are reflected in restlessness, irritability, and difficulty with concentrating. Older patients are especially susceptible to reduced perfusion. QSEN: Safety.
■ Assess oxygen saturation with pulse oximetry both at rest and after and/or during ambulation.	Changes in oxygen saturation of mixed venous blood is one of the earliest indicators of decreased cardiac output. Hypoxemia is common, especially with activity. QSEN: Safety.
▲ Monitor serum electrolytes, especially sodium and potassium.	Hypokalemia and hypomagnesemia are causative factors for dysrhythmias, which can further reduce cardiac output.
▲ Assess the B-type natriuretic peptide (BNP) as indicated.	BNP is elevated with increased filling pressure and volume in the left ventricle and serves as a critical indicator for heart failure. Changes in this laboratory test aid in differentiating cardiac from noncardiac causes of dyspnea.
▲ Assess the left ventricular (LV) function as ordered.	Several national guidelines recommend that LV function assessment must be completed and documented either before or during the admission or plans made to assess after discharge, because ejection fraction status guides treatment. The integration of these standards of practice into an individualized plan of care help the patient achieve optimal outcomes for the management of heart failure. QSEN: Evidence-based practice.

Cardiac and Vascular Care Plans

■ = Independent   ▲ = Interprofessional Collaboration

Actions/Interventions	Rationales
▲ Monitor the patient for signs and symptoms of digitalis toxicity. Obtain blood specimens to measure the serum digoxin level.	The margin between therapeutic and toxic doses of digoxin therapy is narrow. The margin is further reduced in older patients and in patients with hypokalemia and renal insufficiency. Patients with digitalis toxicity may develop cardiac dysrhythmias such as sinus bradycardia, atrioventricular blocks, and ventricular tachycardia. Serum drug levels greater than 2.5 ng/mL are associated with toxicity. QSEN: Safety.

Therapeutic Interventions

Actions/Interventions	Rationales
■ Administer prescribed medications and evaluate the patient's ability to manage these medications at home::	Heart failure therapy requires the administration of several types of medications. The cornerstone of treatment is angiotensin-converting enzyme (ACE) inhibitors and beta-blockers. Diuretics, aldosterone antagonists, digoxin, and vasodilators are included as appropriate. Polypharmacy is an ongoing challenge for patients with heart failure. These medications are based on recommendations from national organizations. QSEN: Patient-centered care.
• ACE inhibitors or angiotensin II receptor blockers (ARBs)	These medications decrease peripheral vascular resistance and venous tone and suppress aldosterone output, thus reducing BP and demands on heart. This category of drugs has been shown to increase exercise tolerance and is the only one to increase survival in patients with heart failure. It is very important to titrate to symptoms, not BP. National guidelines (American Heart Association, The Heart Failure Society of American, The Joint Commission [TJC]) recommend that the ACE inhibitors or ARBs should be prescribed for patients with ejection fraction less than 40%. In addition, the guidelines require that the reason for contraindication or for any delayed starting needs to be documented. QSEN: Evidence-based practice.
• Beta-blockers	Beta-blockers are used to decrease neurohormonal activity. They have been shown to reduce mortality rate, slow disease progression, and improve quality of life. Careful titration of starting doses is required because some patients exhibit fatigue, mood disturbances, or dizziness when medication is started or titrated up. These drugs should be given with food and separated from other vasodilators to reduce side effects (e.g., carvedilol with breakfast and dinner, ACE inhibitor with lunch) if side effects are troublesome.
• Diuretics (loop, thiazide, K⁺ sparing)	Diuretics reduce circulating volume, enhance sodium and water excretion, and improve symptoms. Loop diuretics are preferred. The correct dose is the dose that works. Often combination therapy is needed.
• Aldosterone antagonists (e.g., spironolactone)	Aldosterone antagonists are not given primarily for their diuretic effect, but rather for the beneficial effects on LV remodeling, reduction in sympathetic activity, and improvement in mortality risk. Patients need to be closely monitored for hyperkalemia.

Cardiac and Vascular Care Plans

Actions/Interventions

- Vasodilators (e.g., nitrates, hydralazine)

- Positive inotropes (e.g., digoxin, dopamine, dobutamine, milrinone)

- Antidysrhythmics (e.g., amiodarone, beta-blockers, potassium and magnesium supplements)

▲ Provide oxygen as indicated by the patient's condition and saturation levels (home oxygen through cannula or partial rebreather).

▲ If increased preload is a problem, restrict fluids and sodium as ordered.

▲ If decreased preload is a problem, increase fluids and monitor closely.

■ If the patient does not respond to therapy, consider referral to an acute care setting or hospital for invasive hemodynamic monitoring, more intensive medical therapy, and mechanical assist devices such as an intra-aortic balloon pump (IABP) and right or left ventricular assist device (VAD).

▲ If chronic life-threatening dysrhythmias are the problem, or if the ejection fraction is less than 35%, anticipate treatment with an ICD.

▲ For patients with intraventricular conduction delay (greater than 0.13 seconds QRS interval), anticipate possible treatment with cardiac resynchronization therapy (CRT) pacemakers.

Rationales

Vasodilators reduce preload, which decreases pulmonary congestion, and reduce afterload, which enhances the pumping ability of the ventricle.

Inotropes improve myocardial contractility. In stable class III to IV patients, intravenous medications may be administered intermittently in the outpatient or home setting.

These medications correct dysrhythmias such as premature ventricular contractions, ventricular tachycardia, and atrial fibrillation. Heart failure is one of the most arrhythmogenic disorders. Unfortunately, management of dysrhythmias in this population is usually unsuccessful or even harmful because some antidysrhythmics have a negative inotropic effect, which may exacerbate heart failure or actually cause additional dysrhythmias. Atrial fibrillation with its resultant loss of atrial kick can cause significant decompensation. Some dysrhythmias require treatment with pacemakers and/or implantable cardioverter-defibrillators (ICDs).

The failing heart may not be able to respond to increased oxygen demand. Oxygen supply may be inadequate when there is fluid accumulation in the lungs. Therefore supplemental oxygen may be indicated.

Fluid restriction decreases extracellular fluid volume and reduces cardiac workload.

Fluids increase extracellular fluid volume to optimize ventricular filling.

Hemodynamic monitoring provides information on filling pressures on the right side (central venous pressure) and left side (pulmonary artery diastolic pressure; pulmonary capillary wedge pressure) of the heart. Mechanical assist devices such as the VAD or the IABP provide temporary circulatory support for the failing ventricle. Newer technologies include portable VADs that allow the patient to ambulate. IABP is used to increase coronary artery perfusion and decrease myocardial workload. QSEN: Evidence-based practice; Safety.

ICDs are typically indicated for documented ventricular tachycardia or ventricular fibrillation that puts patients at risk for sudden death. Newer American Heart Association guidelines recommend ICD therapy for primary prevention of sudden cardiac death in selected patients with dilated cardiomyopathy and ejection fraction of <35% and NYHA class II or III symptoms. QSEN: Evidence-based practice.

Research demonstrates improved LV synchrony and hemodynamics when pacemakers are implanted in both right ventricular (RV) and LV areas. QSEN: Evidence-based practice.

Cardiac and Vascular Care Plans

■ = Independent ▲ = Interprofessional Collaboration

NANDA-I NDx Excess Fluid Volume

Common Related Factors

Decreased cardiac output causing the following:

- Decreased renal perfusion, which stimulates the renin-angiotensin-aldosterone system and causes release of antidiuretic hormone
- Altered renal hemodynamics (diminished medullary blood flow), which results in decreased capacity of nephron to excrete water

Defining Characteristics

Weight gain/edema
Intake greater than output
Decreased urine output
Abnormal breath sounds: crackles
Shortness of breath, orthopnea, and/or dyspnea
Restlessness
Pulmonary congestion on x-ray study
Jugular vein distention (JVD)
Elevated central venous pressure and pulmonary capillary wedge pressure
Ascites and/or hepatojugular reflux
Elevated BP
Tachycardia
Third heart sound (S_3)

Common Expected Outcome

Patient maintains optimal fluid balance, as evidenced by urine output 30 mL/hr or greater, HR less than 100 beats/min, balanced intake and output, stable weight/dry weight (or loss attributed to fluid loss), absence of or reduction in edema, absence of pulmonary congestion.

NOC Outcome
Fluid Balance
NIC Interventions
Fluid Monitoring; Fluid Management

Ongoing Assessment

Actions/Interventions

- Assess for a significant (>2 pounds) weight change in 1 day or a trend over several days. Verify that the patient has weighed consistently (e.g., before breakfast, on the same scale, after voiding, in the same amount of clothing, without shoes).
- Evaluate weight in relation to nutritional status.

- Assess for the presence of edema by palpating the area over the tibia, ankles, feet, and sacrum.

- Assess for crackles in the lungs, a change in respiratory pattern, shortness of breath, or orthopnea.
- Monitor the patient's HR and BP.

Rationales

Body weight is a more sensitive indicator of fluid or sodium retention than intake and output. A 2- to 3-pound increase in weight in a day normally indicates retention of about 1 L of fluid and a need to adjust fluid or diuretic therapy.

In some patients with heart failure, weight may be a poor indicator of fluid volume status. Poor nutrition and decreased appetite over time result in a decrease in weight, which may be accompanied by fluid retention, although the net weight remains unchanged.

Edema occurs when fluid accumulates in the extravascular spaces. Symmetrical dependent edema is characteristic in heart failure; it is graded on a scale of a trace to 4+. Pitting edema is manifested by a depression that remains after the finger is pressed over an edematous area and then removed.

These respiratory changes are signs of fluid accumulation in the lungs.

Sinus tachycardia and elevated BP are seen in early stages. Older patients have a reduced response to catecholamines; thus their response to fluid overload may be blunted with less change in HR. QSEN: Safety.

(side margin) Cardiac and Vascular Care Plans

Actions/Interventions

- Assess for JVD, ascites, nausea, and vomiting.

- If the patient is on fluid restriction, review the daily log for recorded intake.

- Evaluate the urine output in response to diuretics.

- Monitor for an excessive response to diuretics: 2-pound weight loss in 1 day, hypotension, weakness, and a blood urea nitrogen level elevated out of proportion to the serum creatinine level.

▲ Monitor for potential side effects of diuretics: hypokalemia, hyponatremia, hypomagnesemia, an elevated serum creatinine level, and hyperuricemia (gout).

▲ Monitor the chest x-ray reports.

Rationales

Patients with hypertonic overhydration exhibit cellular swelling. Right-sided heart failure causes increased venous pressure and fluid congestion in hepatic and abdominal systems.

All sources of oral fluid need to be recorded. The patient should be reminded to include items that are liquid at room temperature (e.g., gelatin, soup, sherbet, frozen juice bars).

The focus is on monitoring the response to the diuretics, rather than the actual amount voided. It is unrealistic to expect patients to measure each void. Therefore recording two voids versus six voids after a diuretic medication may provide more useful information. (NOTE: Fluid volume excess in the abdomen may interfere with absorption of oral diuretic medications. Medications may need to be given intravenously by a nurse in the home or outpatient setting.)

Significant increased response to diuretic therapy can result in fluid volume deficit and electrolyte imbalances that can cause significant complications. Moreover, excess fluid loss can stimulate compensatory mechanisms to promote activation of renin-angiotensin-aldosterone system. That can begin the vicious cycle of fluid retention.

The electrolyte and other abnormalities related to diuretic therapy can cause significant problems. QSEN: Safety.

As interstitial edema accumulates, the x-ray studies show cloudy white lung fields.

Therapeutic Interventions

Actions/Interventions

- Instruct the patient and/or caregiver regarding fluid restriction as appropriate.

- Provide innovative techniques for monitoring fluid allotment at home. For example, suggest that the patient measure out and pour into a large pitcher the prescribed daily fluid allowance (e.g., 1000 mL). Then, every time the patient drinks some fluid, he or she should remove that same amount from the pitcher.

▲ Administer or instruct the patient to take diuretics as prescribed.

Rationales

Restriction helps reduce extracellular volume. For patients with mild or moderate heart failure, it may not be necessary to restrict fluid intake. In advanced heart failure, fluids may be restricted to 1000 mL/day. Information is key for patients who will be managing their own fluids. QSEN: Patient-centered care.

Strategies such as this provide the patient with a visual guide for how much fluid is still allowed throughout the day, enhancing compliance with the regimen.

Diuretics aid in the excretion of excess body fluids. Therapy may include several different types of diuretic agents for optimal effect, depending on the acuteness or chronicity of the problem. Compliance is often difficult for patients trying to maintain a more normal lifestyle outside the home, who find frequent urination especially troublesome. Some patients prefer taking diuretics later in the day, after their activities. Such creative schedules can increase compliance. QSEN: Patient-centered care.

Cardiac and Vascular
Care Plans

■ = Independent   ▲ = Interprofessional Collaboration

Actions/Interventions

▲ Instruct patients to avoid foods and fluids that are high in sodium. Restrict sodium intake as prescribed.

■ Instruct the patient to discuss with the health care provider "all" the medications he or she is taking.

■ Instruct the patient to notify the health care provider about any significant weight changes, leg swelling, or breathing changes.

■ Teach the patient about measures to relieve dry mouth, such as frequent oral hygiene, sucking on hard candy, or chewing gum.

▲ For significant fluid volume excess, consider admission to an acute care setting for hemofiltration or ultrafiltration.

Rationales

Restriction decreases excess fluid volume. Diets containing 2 to 3 g of sodium are usually prescribed. Patient can begin sodium restriction by eliminating the use of the salt shaker at the table, avoiding obviously salty foods, and not adding salt to food when cooking. The patient needs to learn to read package labels for sources of hidden salt and sodium often used as preservatives and flavoring agents in processed foods. Instruct that soups and many ethnic foods contain high amounts of sodium, especially if eaten in restaurants.

Patients often have many co-morbid conditions requiring treatment with medications that may affect fluid balance or heart function. For example, nonsteroidal anti-inflammatory drugs (NSAIDs) can cause renal insufficiency. Cyclooxygenase (COX)-2 inhibitors (e.g., rofecoxib [Vioxx]) cause fluid retention. Some calcium channel blockers have significant negative inotropic effects.

Early recognition and treatment of symptoms at home can help break the cycle of frequent hospital readmission for heart failure. Patients need to understand their roles in symptom management. Telephone nursing can be initiated to provide for consistent monitoring between office visits. QSEN: Safety.

Patients on fluid restrictions may experience increased thirst and dry mouth. Measures to stimulate saliva secretion will help keep oral mucous membranes moist. The patient with diabetes mellitus may need to use sugar-free gums and candy. The patient should avoid ice chips because they can add to fluid intake. An 8-ounce cup of ice chips equals approximately 4 ounces of water.

These therapies are very effective methods to draw off excess fluid, but patients should be reminded that compliance with medication regimens and sodium restriction will help keep their conditions stable.

NANDA-I NDx ## Activity Intolerance

Common Related Factors
Decreased cardiac output
Deconditioned state
Sedentary lifestyle
Imbalance between oxygen supply and demand
Insufficient sleep or rest periods
Lack of motivation or depression
Side effects of medications

Defining Characteristics
Verbal report of fatigue or weakness
Unable to endure or complete desired activities
Abnormal HR, BP, or respiratory response to activity
Exertional discomfort or dyspnea

Common Expected Outcomes

Patient exhibits activity tolerance, as evidenced by rating of perceived exertion of 3 or less (0 to 10 scale), HR within 20 beats/min of resting HR, systolic BP within 20 mm Hg increase over resting systolic BP, respiratory rate less than 20 breaths/min.

Patient reports ability to perform required ADLs.

Patient verbalizes and uses energy conservation techniques.

NOC Outcomes
Fatigue Level; Activity Tolerance; Energy Conservation; Self-Care: Activities of Daily Living (ADLs)

NIC Interventions
Energy Management; Exercise Promotion

Ongoing Assessment

Actions/Interventions	Rationales
■ Assess the patient's current level of activity. Determine the reasons for limiting activity.	Although newer pharmacological therapies have alleviated many of the disabling symptoms experienced by patients with heart failure, chronic symptoms of activity intolerance and limited exercise capacity often occur. Changes in functional capacity with chronic heart failure have a direct impact on the patient's quality of life. The patient may have restricted activity over time to avoid symptoms. Therefore it is important to ask the patient about tolerance for specific activities, such as walking a specific distance (e.g., 100 feet) or climbing a flight of stairs. QSEN: Patient-centered care.
■ Observe and document the patient's response to activity. Have the patient walk in the hall for several minutes as a nurse evaluates the HR, BP, and oxygen saturation response to exertion. If the patient is able, evaluate the response to stair climbing.	HR increases of more than 20 beats/min, systolic BP drop of more than 20 mm Hg, dyspnea, light-headedness, and fatigue signify abnormal responses to activity. Pulse oximetry provides information on hypoxemia with exertion. QSEN: Safety.
■ Assess the patient's perception of effort to perform each activity.	The Borg scale uses ratings from 6 to 20 to determine ratings of perceived exertion. A rating of 9 (very light) to 13 (somewhat hard) is an acceptable level for most patients with heart failure doing daily work.
■ Evaluate the need for oxygen during increased activity.	Portable pulse oximetry can be used to assess for oxygen desaturation. Supplemental oxygen may help compensate for the increased oxygen demand.

Therapeutic Interventions

Actions/Interventions	Rationales
■ Establish guidelines and goals of activity with the patient and significant others.	Motivation is enhanced if the patient participates in goal setting. Depending on the classification of heart failure, some class I or II patients may be able to successfully work outside the home on a part-time or full-time basis. However, other patients may be class III or IV and be relatively homebound. QSEN: Patient-centered care.
■ Teach a slow progression of activity (e.g., walking in a room, walking short distances around the house, and then progressively increasing distances outside the house, saving energy for the return trip).	Appropriate progression prevents overexerting the heart while attaining short-range goals. Duration and frequency should be increased before intensity. QSEN: Safety.
■ Teach the appropriate use of environmental aids (e.g., bedside commode, chair in bathroom, hall rails).	Appropriate aids enable the patient to achieve optimal independence for self-care.

Cardiac and Vascular Care Plans

■ = Independent   ▲ = Interprofessional Collaboration

Actions/Interventions

- Teach energy conservation techniques, for example:
  - Sitting to do tasks
  - Pushing rather than pulling
  - Sliding rather than lifting
  - Storing frequently used items within easy reach
  - Organizing a work-rest-work schedule
- Recommend the use of light weights (1 to 2 pounds) for upper extremity strengthening.

▲ Consult the cardiac rehabilitation or physical therapy departments for assistance in increasing activity tolerance.

- Instruct the patient to recognize the signs of overexertion.

- Provide emotional support and encouragement while increasing activity levels.

Rationales

These techniques reduce oxygen consumption, allowing for more prolonged activity.

Strength training can enhance endurance and facilitate performance of ADLs; such exercises can be performed while sitting in a chair.

Specialized therapy or cardiac monitoring may be necessary when initially increasing activity. Some exercises may be provided in the home. A structured program of low-intensity exercise can improve functional capacity, increase self-confidence to exert self, improve quality of life, and provide an environment for early triage of symptoms. QSEN: Teamwork and collaboration.

Knowledge promotes awareness of when to reduce activity and provides data for activity progression. Attention to warning signs of overexertion helps reduce the risk of harm to the patient. QSEN: Safety.

Patients may be fearful of overexertion and potential damage to the heart. Appropriate supervision and support during activity progression can enhance confidence.

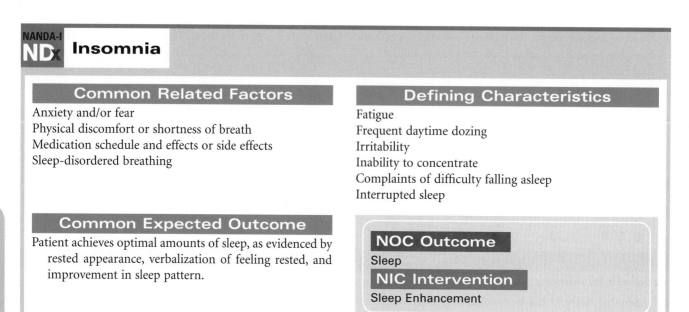

NANDA-I NDx Insomnia

Common Related Factors

Anxiety and/or fear
Physical discomfort or shortness of breath
Medication schedule and effects or side effects
Sleep-disordered breathing

Defining Characteristics

Fatigue
Frequent daytime dozing
Irritability
Inability to concentrate
Complaints of difficulty falling asleep
Interrupted sleep

Common Expected Outcome

Patient achieves optimal amounts of sleep, as evidenced by rested appearance, verbalization of feeling rested, and improvement in sleep pattern.

NOC Outcome
Sleep
NIC Intervention
Sleep Enhancement

Ongoing Assessment

Actions/Interventions

- Assess the patient's current sleep pattern and sleep history.

Rationales

Sleep patterns are unique to each individual. Some patients are unaware of their poor sleep patterns, but their significant others report sleeping problems. QSEN: Patient-centered care.

Actions/Interventions

- Assess for possible deterrents to sleep:
  - Nocturia

  - Volume excess causing dyspnea, orthopnea, and paroxysmal nocturnal dyspnea (PND)
  - Fear of PND

  - Timing of medications

- Assess for a history of signs of sleep-disordered breathing.

Rationales

The supine position during sleep promotes increased venous return and increased renal blood flow. The patient's sleep is interrupted by the need to urinate.

When the patient is supine, the fluid returning to the heart from the extremities may cause pulmonary congestion.

Patients report this as a significant factor in sleeping difficulties.

Patients may be following medication schedules that require awakening in the early morning hours. Diuretics taken in the evening may increase nocturia.

Sleep-disordered breathing is common with heart failure, with reports of occurrence in more than 50% of patients. These patients experience interrupted sleep and periods of desaturation during the nighttime. This disorder is associated with increased dysrhythmias, reduced quality of life, and increased mortality risk.

Therapeutic Interventions

Actions/Interventions

- Instruct the patient to reduce daytime napping and to increase daytime activity.

- Instruct the patient to decrease fluid intake before bedtime.

- Plan a medication schedule so that prescribed medications, especially diuretics, are not given during the late evening or night.
- Encourage the patient to follow as consistent a daily schedule for retiring and arising as possible; avoid caffeine and smoking.
- Encourage the patient to elevate the head with two pillows or put the head of the bed frame on 6-inch blocks.
- Encourage the verbalization of fears.

- Review measures that the patient can take to prevent or treat PND, chest pain, or palpitations.
- Review how the patient can summon help during the night.
- Provide instruction in the use of a continuous positive airway pressure (CPAP) device, if ordered.

Rationales

Napping can disrupt normal sleep patterns. However, older patients do better with frequent naps during the day to counter the shorter nighttime sleep schedule.

Careful scheduling of evening medications and limiting oral fluid intake reduces the need to awaken to void.

Evening fluid restriction facilitates an undisturbed night.

A regular schedule promotes regulation of the circadian rhythm. Stimulation from caffeine and nicotine can disturb sleep.

Elevating the head of the bed can reduce pulmonary congestion and nighttime dyspnea.

Verbalization may help reduce anxiety and open doors for further problem-solving and intervention.

Prevention is key and may require medication adjustments by the physician.

Information enables the patient to take control.

CPAP applied during sleep periods has been shown to improve sleep efforts and reduce episodes of hypopnea and apnea, thereby enhancing oxygen saturation.

NANDA-I
NDx Deficient Knowledge

Common Related Factors

Insufficient information
Insufficient interest in learning
Misinformation presented by others
Insufficient knowledge of resources

Defining Characteristics

Insufficient knowledge
Inaccurate follow-through of instruction
Inappropriate behavior

Cardiac and Vascular Care Plans

■ = Independent   ▲ = Interprofessional Collaboration

Common Expected Outcomes

Patient or significant others verbalize understanding of desired content.
Patient performs desired skills.

NOC Outcomes
Self-Management: Heart Failure; Knowledge: Disease Process
NIC Interventions
Health Literacy Enhancement; Learning Facilitation; Teaching: Disease Process; Teaching: Prescribed Medication; Teaching: Prescribed Diet; Teaching: Prescribed Exercise

Ongoing Assessment

Actions/Interventions	Rationales
■ Assess the patient's knowledge of causes, treatment, and follow-up care related to heart failure.	This information provides a starting base for educational sessions. Teaching standardized content that the patient already knows wastes valuable time and hinders critical learning. QSEN: Patient-centered care.
■ Identify existing misconceptions regarding care.	Understanding any misconceptions the patient may have about the treatment or side effects will guide future interventions.

Therapeutic Interventions

Actions/Interventions	Rationales
■ Educate the patient or significant others about the following:	Patients are better able to ask questions and seek assistance when they know basic information about the disease and treatment. The American Heart Association (AHA), the American Association of Heart Failure Nurses, and The Joint Commission (TJC) provide excellent tools for providing education to meet national guidelines. The following nursing actions are based on recommendations from national organizations. QSEN: Evidence-based practice.
• Normal heart and circulation	Information helps the patient understand the disease process.
• Heart failure disease process	Knowledge of the disease and disease process will promote adherence to suggested medical therapy.
• Overall goals of medical therapy	A discussion of long-range goals will help clarify misconceptions and may promote compliance.
• Importance of adhering to therapy	Heart failure is the most common reason for readmission, especially in the older population. Strict adherence to therapy aids in reducing symptoms and readmission. Therapy must be simplified as much as possible to facilitate adherence. Patients must be encouraged to follow up closely with health care providers and/or heart failure nurses.
• Symptoms (e.g., weight gain, edema, fatigue, dyspnea) and when to report them to health care providers	When patients can identify symptoms that require prompt medical attention, complications can be minimized or possibly prevented. Telemanagement, home care nurses, and heart failure case managers can aid in this education and assessment.
• Dietary modifications to limit sodium ingestion	Understanding the rationale behind dietary restrictions may establish the motivation necessary for making this adjustment in lifestyle. Diet and fluid restriction education is part of national performance guidelines.

Cardiac and Vascular Care Plans

Actions/Interventions

- Activity guidelines

- Medications: instruct in action, use, side effects, and administration

- Psychological aspects of chronic illness

- Smoking cessation

- Community resources
- Provide information on ways to enhance self-management efforts:
  - Recognizing changes in one's condition and their importance
  - Decisions regarding appropriate treatment and evaluation of their effectiveness
- Provide information on medical devices and therapies that may be indicated for optimal cardiac output.

- Encourage questions from the patient or significant others.

Rationales

Providing specific information lessens uncertainty and promotes adjustment to recommended activity levels.

Key medications need to be prescribed and taken to meet national guidelines and reduce morbidity and mortality associated with heart failure. Compliance is improved when patients understand "why" they are expected to take so many medications. Prompt reporting of side effects can prevent drug-related complications.

Living with a chronic illness can be depressing, especially for older patients, who may have limited support systems. Referral to support groups may be indicated.

Anyone who has smoked cigarettes within 12 months, not just current smokers, before admission needs to receive smoking cessation counseling, per national guidelines.

Referral may be helpful for financial and emotional support.

The burden of living with chronic heart failure rests with the patient and caregiver. Patients are at the front line in reacting to changes in symptoms and condition. They need to be able to self-treat for minor changes (e.g., increase diuretics, reduce fluids) before contacting health care providers. QSEN: Patient-centered care.

A select group of patients with heart failure, especially class III and IV, can benefit from adjunct medical therapies, including implantable cardioverter-defibrillator, cardiac resynchronization therapy pacing, ventricular assist device, and heart transplant surgery.

Questions facilitate open communication between the patient and health care provider, and allow the verification of understanding of information given and the opportunity to correct misconceptions.

Related Care Plans

Impaired gas exchange, Chapter 2
Ineffective health management, Chapter 2
Risk for electrolyte imbalance, Chapter 2
Powerlessness, Chapter 2
Death and dying: End of life issues, Chapter 4
Cardiac rehabilitation, Chapter 5
Obstructive sleep apnea, Chapter 6

Hypertension

High Blood Pressure; Isolated Systolic Hypertension

Epidemiological studies report that 1 in 3 U.S. adults have hypertension, with over 70 million people in the United States having BPs 140/90 mm Hg or higher or taking antihypertensive medications. The Eighth Joint National Committee (JNC) on Prevention, Detection and Treatment of High Blood Pressure published revised treatment guidelines in 2104. According to JNC8, in the general population ages 60 years and older, the desired BP is below 150/90 mm Hg. For younger people (<60 years) the desired goal is below 140/90 mm Hg. Patients whose BP values are above these desired goals should be treated with drug therapy.

Age, gender, and ethnic differences are evident. African Americans in the United States develop hypertension earlier, have more significantly elevated BP, and have more

■ = Independent ▲ = Interprofessional Collaboration

target organ disease than Caucasians. Likewise, African-American women have a higher incidence of hypertension than white women.

Although hypertension can be initiated in childhood, it is most evident in middle life. As the population ages, the prevalence of hypertension will increase unless effective prevention measures are implemented. The category of prehypertension identifies a significant segment of the population who are at twice the risk for developing hypertension than people in the normal category. Preventive efforts in this population are aimed at reducing risk factors

through therapeutic lifestyle changes, which are detailed in the JNC guidelines.

BP self-management is key to successful treatment. Ambulatory BP monitoring may be indicated to document changes in BP throughout the day (circadian pattern) and provide information for treating drug-resistant patients and those experiencing hypotension secondary to medication. Several classes of drugs are available for treatment. Usually two or more antihypertensive medications are needed to achieve optimal BP control. This care plan focuses on patients with hypertension in an ambulatory care setting.

NANDA-I NDx Deficient Knowledge

Common Related Factors
Insufficient information
Insufficient interest in learning
Misinformation presented by others
Insufficient knowledge of resources

Defining Characteristics
Insufficient knowledge
Inaccurate follow-through of instruction
Inappropriate behavior

Common Expected Outcomes
Patient verbalizes understanding of the disease and its long-term effects on target organs.
Patient describes strategies for managing hypertension.

NOC Outcomes
Self-management: Hypertension; Knowledge: HTN Management

NIC Interventions
Health Literacy Enhancement; Learning Facilitation; Teaching: Disease Process

---

Ongoing Assessment

Action/Intervention	Rationale
■ Assess the patient's knowledge of the disease and its prescribed management.	Assessment provides an important starting point in education. Patients need to understand that hypertension is a chronic, lifelong disease in which they have a vital role in effective management. QSEN: Patient-centered care.

Therapeutic Interventions

Actions/Interventions	Rationales
■ Encourage questions about hypertension and its prescribed treatments.	Questions facilitate open communication between the patient and health care provider and allow the verification of understanding of given information and the opportunity to correct misconceptions.
■ Involve the family in teaching about hypertension.	Family members play an important role in supporting the patient's efforts to adopt new health behaviors for the management of hypertension. Family members may also need to be screened for hypertension because of its familial tendency. Genetic factors are strong risk factors for hypertension.

evolve For additional care plans, go to http://evolve.elsevier.com/Gulanick/.

Cardiac and Vascular Care Plans

Actions/Interventions

- Instruct the patient that hypertension cannot be diagnosed with only one measurement.

- Instruct the patient to self-measure BP, and suggest home monitoring equipment as appropriate.

- Plan teaching in stages, providing information in the following areas:

  - Definition of hypertension, differentiating between systolic and diastolic pressures; prehypertension

  - Causes of hypertension

  - Risk factors: family history, obesity, diet high in saturated fat and cholesterol, smoking, and stress
  - Nature of the disease and its effect on target organs (e.g., renal damage, visual impairment, heart disease, stroke)
  - Treatment goal: "control" versus "cure"

  - Rationales and strategies for weight reduction (if overweight)

  - Rationales and strategies for adopting the Dietary Approaches to Stop Hypertension (DASH) diet

  - Rationales and strategies for low-sodium diet

  - Common medications: thiazide diuretics, calcium channel blockers, angiotensin-converting enzyme (ACE) inhibitors, and angiotensin II receptor blockers (ARBs)

Rationales

There are wide variations in "normal" blood pressure over the course of a day or week because of biological and diurnal effects. Clinical practice guidelines state that a diagnosis can be established only with the average of two or more BP readings on two or more occasions.

BP self-measurement can be useful in identifying true hypertension versus white-coat hypertension, in documenting response to medication regimen, and in facilitating adherence to treatment. Patients should be guided to only purchase home equipment that meets established criteria for accuracy.

Providing information in short sessions over a longer period of time prevents information overload and promotes comprehension. QSEN: Patient-centered care.

Patients may falsely believe that only elevated diastolic BP requires treatment, when elevated systolic BP is also associated with high risk. Most patients are not aware of the newest classification of prehypertension.

Patients need to realize that 90% of hypertension is not related to a primary cause.

Implementing lifestyle changes is the cornerstone of treatment.

There are few signs and symptoms associated with hypertension until target organ damage occurs.

Hypertension is a chronic, lifelong disease. It is treated with medication and lifestyle changes. Treatment should not be stopped because the patient feels better or has problems with medication side effects.

Of all lifestyle changes, weight reduction has most consistently demonstrated BP-lowering effects. Studies show weight reduction lowers BP at all ages and in both genders. A body mass index (BMI) of 25 or higher is strongly correlated with increased BP. Weight loss of just 10 pounds can lower BP.

The DASH diet is high in fruits, vegetables; high in low-fat dairy products; low in total and saturated fats; and rich in potassium, magnesium, protein, and fiber. The mix of potassium, magnesium, and calcium in the diet serves as a diuretic in helping the body excrete salt. This diet is especially effective in treating African-American patients. QSEN: Evidence-based practice.

Dietary sodium contributes to fluid retention and elevated BP, although not all patients are "salt sensitive" who effectively lower BP with sodium restriction. African-American and older patients seem to be the most salt sensitive.

A wide range of medications is available to help patients reach the desired goal after lifestyle modification. National guidelines provide recommendations for initial therapy, either alone or in combination with other medications for a variety of patient populations: e.g., general nonblack, general black, persons with diabetes or chronic kidney disease, those with resistant hypertension. QSEN: Evidence-based practice.

■ = Independent ▲ = Interprofessional Collaboration

Actions/Interventions

- Establishment of a medication routine considering daily activities and sleep habits
- Possible side effects of medications

- Interaction with over-the-counter drugs such as cough and cold medicines, aspirin compounds, and herbal medications

- Rationales and strategies for the reduction of alcohol intake: no more than two drinks per day for men and one drink per day for women
- Need for potassium-rich foods (e.g., fruit juices, bananas) as appropriate

- Smoking cessation
- Role of physical exercise

- Relaxation techniques to combat stress

- Signs and symptoms to report to the health care provider: chest pain, shortness of breath, edema, weight gain greater than 2 pounds per day or 5 pounds per week, nosebleeds, changes in vision, headaches, and dizziness
- Important safety measures to reduce orthostatic hypotension:
  - Avoid sudden changes in position.
  - Avoid hot tubs and saunas.
  - Avoid prolonged standing; wear support stockings as needed.

■ Provide information about community resources and support groups (e.g., American Heart Association, weight loss programs, smoking cessation programs).

Rationales

A consistent medication schedule will minimize the chance for error and encourage better compliance with therapy.

Side effects are the most common reason for noncompliance with medications. Warning the patient of possible side effects enhances attention on what to do if they occur. Not all people experience side effects. If they do occur and are bothersome (pedal edema, fatigue, hypokalemia, impotence), instruct the patient to discuss them with the health care provider before discontinuing any medications.

Patients should be encouraged to bring in all sources of medications (over-the-counter, complementary, and prescription) to review and rule out iatrogenic causes of hypertension.

Research indicates that increased alcohol intake is associated with high BP.

Some diuretics are potassium wasting; however, most ACE inhibitors and ARBs retain potassium. A potassium-rich diet (DASH) can help reduce elevated BP.

Smoking causes vasoconstriction and an increase in BP.

Research supports a positive effect of aerobic exercise in independently lowering BP, as well as maintaining weight loss.

The physiological response to physical and/or emotional stressors includes neuroendocrine changes associated with increased sympathetic nervous system activity and increased cortisol secretion. These changes produce vasoconstriction and increase sodium and water retention. Unrelieved persistent stress contributes to increased BP. Relaxation techniques can positively influence physiological responses that reduce BP.

Patients need to recognize and report important changes in their condition that could lead to serious outcomes. QSEN: Safety.

Orthostatic hypotension is a common side effect of many drugs used to manage hypertension. Hypotension associated with quickly assuming an upright position is especially evident in older patients with long-standing hypertension that is reduced too rapidly. Hot tubs and saunas cause vasodilation and potential hypotension. Standing can cause venous pooling that lowers systemic BP. Attention to measures to reduce orthostasis minimizes the risk of harm from hypotension. QSEN: Safety.

These resources can assist and support the patient when lifestyle changes are needed.

Cardiac and Vascular Care Plans

Risk for Ineffective Health Management

Common Risk Factors

Complexity of therapeutic regimen
Financial costs
Social support deficits
Conflicting health values
Fears about treatment and possible side effects

Common Expected Outcomes

Patient describes system for taking medications.
Patient describes positive effort to lose weight and restrict
  sodium as appropriate.
Patient verbalizes intention to follow prescribed regimen.
Patient demonstrates ongoing adherence to treatment plan.

NOC Outcomes

Compliance Behavior; Self-Management:
  Hypertension; Participation in Health Care
  Decisions

NIC Interventions

Mutual Goal Setting; Support System
  Enhancement; Teaching: Individual

Ongoing Assessment

Actions/Interventions	Rationales
■ Assess the patient's health values and beliefs.	Health behavior models propose that patients compare factors such as perceived susceptibility to and severity of illness or complications with perceived benefits of treatment in making decisions regarding adherence to therapies. QSEN: Patient-centered care.
■ Assess the previous patterns of adherence.	Past history of noncompliance is a significant risk factor for future adherence problems.
■ Assess for risk factors that may negatively affect adherence to the regimen.	Knowledge of causative factors provides direction for subsequent interventions. Some factors may include contrary beliefs and values, lack of social support, lack of financial resources, and compromised emotional states.

Therapeutic Interventions

Actions/Interventions	Rationales
▲ Simplify the drug regimen.	Many patients require three to four BP-lowering medications to achieve treatment goals. Simplifying the regimen can enhance compliance. Combined medications should be used as available. The more often patients have to take medicines during the day, the greater the risk for noncompliance.
■ Include the patient in planning the treatment regimen.	Patients who become full partners in the management of their hypertension have a greater stake in achieving a positive outcome. Health care providers need to be willing to change unsuccessful regimens and search for those most likely to succeed. QSEN: Patient-centered care.

Cardiac and Vascular
Care Plans

■ = Independent   ▲ = Interprofessional Collaboration

Actions/Interventions	Rationales
■ Instruct in the importance of reordering medications 2 to 3 days before running out. Consider 90-day refills for this chronic condition.	Missing doses of antihypertensive medications while waiting to obtain prescription refills may contribute to rebound hypertension as an adverse reaction. This reaction is most likely to occur with angiotensin-converting enzyme (ACE) inhibitors, alpha-adrenergic blockers, and alpha-2 agonists. Attention to the best time for reordering medications ensures ongoing therapy but is not easy to accomplish because of many insurance rules. The 90-day supplies require refills only 4 times a year versus the typical 12 times.
■ Inform the patient of the benefits of adhering to the prescribed regimen.	Information provides a rationale for therapy and aids the patient in assuming responsibility for care.
■ If negative side effects of prescribed treatment are a problem, explain that many side effects can be controlled or eliminated.	Patients need to be aware that adjustments and substitutions can be made to relieve side effects.
■ Instruct the patient to self-monitor BP.	Self-monitoring provides the patient with immediate feedback and a sense of control.
■ Include significant others in explanations and teaching.	Including significant others encourages support and assistance in reinforcing appropriate behavior and facilitating lifestyle modification.
■ When the patient has inadequate support regarding lifestyle changes, refer him or her to appropriate support groups (e.g., American Heart Association [AHA], weight loss programs, smoking cessation programs, stress management classes, social services).	Groups that come together for mutual support can be beneficial. QSEN: Teamwork and collaboration.

Percutaneous Coronary Intervention

Percutaneous Transluminal Coronary Angioplasty; Atherectomy; Stents; Intracoronary Stenting; Drug-Eluting Stents

Percutaneous coronary intervention (PCI) is a nonsurgical approach for treating obstruction coronary artery disease (CAD) including unstable angina, acute myocardial infarction (MI) and multivessel CAD by improving coronary blood flow and revascularizing the myocardium. Interventional procedures may be performed in combination with the diagnostic coronary angiogram, electively after diagnostic evaluation, or urgently if there is suspicion of coronary artery blockage in the setting of unstable angina or acute MI. PCI uses a balloon-tipped catheter that is positioned at the site of the lesion. Multiple balloon inflations are performed until the artery is satisfactorily dilated to restore blood flow. If the lesion is very calcified, then two additional devices can be employed: a rotating cutter blade that shaves the plaque and collects the tissue in a cone for removal, or a burr-tipped catheter that rotates at high speeds to grind up the hard plaque. These removed pulverized microparticles are released into the distal circulation. In the setting of an acute MI, if a clot is noted on fluoroscopy, a clot retrieval device is engaged to remove the clot and further restore blood flow prior to the balloon inflation.

Stents are expandable metallic coils inserted within the coronary artery after balloon dilation to provide structural support ("internal scaffolding") to the vessel. Both bare metal and drug-eluding stents can be used. Clinical practice guidelines provide direction for antiplatelet therapy prior to, during, and after PCI, depending on the clinical situation. Patients receiving stents are treated with dual antiplatelet therapy (aspirin and a $P2Y_{12}$ receptor inhibitor such as clopidogrel, prasugrel, or ticagrelor) for a minimum of 4 weeks with bare metal stents and a minimum of 12 months for drug-eluding stents. Clinical contraindications for PCI include inability to take or intolerance to long-term antiplatelet therapy.

The cardiac rehabilitation care plan presented earlier in this chapter addresses specific long-term learning needs and risk reduction strategies for patients having these procedures.

NANDA-I NDx Deficient Knowledge

Common Related Factors
Insufficient information
Insufficient interest in learning
Misinformation presented by others

Defining Characteristics
Insufficient knowledge
Inaccurate follow-through of instruction
Inappropriate behavior

Common Expected Outcome
Patient verbalizes understanding of heart anatomy and physiology, coronary artery disease (CAD), anticipated procedure, and follow-up therapies.

NOC Outcomes
Knowledge: CAD Management; Knowledge: Treatment Procedure

NIC Interventions
Health Literacy Enhancement; Learning Facilitation; Teaching: Disease Process; Knowledge: Thrombus Prevention; Teaching: Procedure/Treatment

---

Ongoing Assessment

Action/Intervention

- Assess the patient's knowledge of cardiac anatomy and physiology, CAD, and the anticipated procedure.

Rationale

Patients must have correct information to give informed consent. This may be a first-time procedure for some or a repeat procedure for others because of high restenosis rates and the progressive nature of atherosclerosis. QSEN: Patient-centered care.

Therapeutic Interventions

Actions/Interventions

- Encourage the patient to verbalize questions and concerns.

- Provide information about the following:

  • Heart anatomy and physiology; CAD

  • Indications for interventional procedure

  • Type of procedure

  • Vessels requiring intervention

Rationales

Patients are anxious about the procedure and the possible outcomes and may have difficulty asking questions and interpreting information. Even patients who have undergone prior procedures may be fearful of the possible outcome with this procedure. A lower anxiety level will enable the patient to learn new information and to cooperate better during the procedure.

Providing this information allows the patient to be a full partner in providing care, making decisions as part of informed consent, and achieving optimal learning outcomes. QSEN: Patient-centered care.

This knowledge helps the patient understand the rationale for procedure.

Patients with significant obstruction (70% to 100%) in areas reachable by catheterization are the best candidates.

Some patients want to be involved in decision-making regarding the type of procedure to be performed. However, they may lack knowledge regarding technical aspects and complications that guide such decision-making.

These may be single lesions or vessels or multiple lesions and vessels; the vessels may be calcified or not calcified.

Cardiac and Vascular Care Plans

■ = Independent ▲ = Interprofessional Collaboration

Actions/Interventions	**Rationales**
• Success rate	The success rate is greater than 90% in most cardiac centers. This information may reduce the patient's anxiety about the outcomes of the procedure.
• Procedure room environment: catheterization laboratory	Anxiety can be reduced when the patient knows what to expect.
• Expected length of the procedure	Patients need to understand that the length of the procedure depends on the number of vessels attempted, vessel anatomy, complications, and number of catheters required.
• Sensations that may be experienced during the procedure.	Patients may have less anxiety during the procedure when they know expectations and understand that these sensations are normal. Such sensations may include a warm flushing feeling during dye injection, chest pain, and palpitations.
• The patient will be awake during the procedure.	Maintaining consciousness facilitates any reporting of chest pain and assists in the patient being able to vigorously cough and breathe deeply at designated times to circulate dye, position the catheter, and increase HR and BP.
• Immediate postprocedure care: • Activity restrictions	The patient is instructed to lie flat with affected site straight until the femoral introducer sheath is removed, the vessel has sealed, and hemostasis is achieved. This sheath is usually left in the artery until the activated coagulation time (ACT) is within acceptable range (<180 seconds) or per institution policy.
• Importance of drinking fluids	Patients are allowed nothing by mouth before the procedure and may experience hypovolemia secondary to dye-induced diuresis and the effects of vasodilator medications. Fluids flush the dye from the system, reduce the risk for renal complications, and promote hydration. Older patients may be more susceptible to the hypovolemic effects of the procedure.
• Monitoring for complications	Common complications include bleeding at the site, especially with the use of several simultaneous antiplatelet medications before, during, and after the procedure, and restenosis of the vessel.
• Discharge instructions: • When to notify the physician (e.g., chest pain, bleeding, infection)	Most patients are discharged the same day. Patients need to be aware of the potential complications to facilitate prompt intervention in case of an emergency. QSEN: Safety.
• Medications, especially aspirin and clopidogrel	A variety of medication regimens are used depending on the type of percutaneous coronary intervention performed and whether the procedure was related to an acute coronary syndrome. The primary postprocedure medication focus centers on dual antiplatelet therapy to prevent restenosis. Compliance with prescribed antiplatelets is key to preventing restenosis, especially when drug-eluting stents are used and therapy is required for a minimum of 12 months. QSEN: Evidence-based practice.

Cardiac and Vascular Care Plans

NDx Acute Pain

Common Related Factors

Myocardial ischemia caused by abrupt closure of affected coronary artery, coronary artery spasm, and possible myocardial infarction (MI)

Residual pain from manipulation or dilation of coronary artery

Pain resulting from medical treatment

Defining Characteristics

Self-report of intensity of pain using a standardized pain scale

Self-report of pain characteristics

Restlessness and apprehension

Facial expression of pain

Change in physiological parameter (e.g., blood pressure, heart rate, respiratory rate and oxygen saturation)

ST-segment and/or T-wave changes

Common Expected Outcomes

Patient verbalizes satisfactory pain control at a decreased intensity using a standardized pain scale.

Patient exhibits increased comfort such as baseline levels for BP, pulse, respirations, and relaxed muscle tone or body posture.

NOC Outcomes

Pain Control; Comfort Status; Medication Response

NIC Interventions

Analgesic Administration; Pain Management; Cardiac Care: Acute

---

Ongoing Assessment

Actions/Interventions	Rationales
■ Assess for the chest pain characteristics associated with myocardial ischemia.	Abrupt closure of a coronary artery after the procedure usually has a presenting symptom pattern similar to pain before the interventional procedure.
■ Monitor the electrocardiogram for signs of ST-T wave changes reflective of myocardial ischemia or spasm.	Attention to ECG changes reduces the risk of harm to the patient. ST-segment elevation is commonly seen with abrupt closure of the coronary artery. QSEN: Safety.
■ Assess the patient's HR and BP during episodes of pain.	Attention to hemodynamic signs may help the nurse in evaluating pain; occurrence of pain after the procedure can be very frightening for the patient.
▲ Obtain serial CK-MB measurements (6 to 8 hours and 16 to 24 hours after procedure).	Elevated CK-MB levels five to eight times the upper normal limit is considered to be evidence of an MI and should be treated as such. A downward trend is expected. QSEN: Safety.
■ Monitor the patient's response to the effectiveness of the treatment.	The effects of both oral and IV medications must be monitored. IV medications can be further titrated to relieve pain.

Therapeutic Interventions

Actions/Interventions	Rationales
■ Instruct the patient to report pain immediately.	Abrupt closure results from elastic recoil of the vessel and/or thrombosis. It is important that relief measures be initiated before additional myocardium is jeopardized. It encourages the patient to be a full partner in their care. QSEN: Patient-centered care; Safety.
■ Notify the physician of chest pain immediately.	It is important to differentiate expected residual pain from coronary dilation and manipulation from pain related to vessel closure. The physician needs to make the distinction. QSEN: Safety.

Cardiac and Vascular Care Plans

■ = Independent   ▲ = Interprofessional Collaboration

Actions/Interventions

 Administer medications as ordered:

- Nitroglycerin (NTG)

- Calcium channel blockers
- Morphine sulfate

- Antiplatelet/antithrombotic therapy

■ Anticipate the need for a possible emergency cardiac catheterization and repeat procedure.
■ Stay with the patient during pain.

Rationales

These medications relieve pain through a variety of mechanisms of action that reduce myocardial ischemia. These medications are based on recommendations from national organizations. QSEN: Evidence-based practice.

NTG is useful for arterial spasm that is a common postprocedure complication.

Calcium channel blockers are useful for arterial spasm.

Morphine is useful for analgesic effect and for reducing myocardial ischemia by decreasing preload.

Combinations of medications are available for use, depending on the clinical situation. They include antiplatelets, low-molecular-weight heparin, $P2Y_{12}$ receptor inhibitors (e.g., clopidogrel) to reduce clotting and prevent microembolizzation.

Abrupt closure occurs most often in the catheterization laboratory or during the first 24 hours.

A nursing presence provides emotional support and reassurance.

NANDA-I
NDx Risk for Bleeding

Common Risk Factors

Treatment-related side effects
- Presence of large catheter sheaths usually left in place until clotting times are back to normal
- Medications (heparinization/antiplatelets)
Arterial trauma
Abnormal blood profiles

Common Expected Outcomes

Patient does not experience bleeding.
Patient maintains therapeutic blood level of anticoagulant, as evidenced by partial thromboplastin time (PTT) within desired range.

NOC Outcome
Blood Coagulation
NIC Interventions
Bleeding Precautions; Bleeding Reduction: Wound

Ongoing Assessment

Actions/Interventions

■ Assess the cannulation site for evidence of bleeding. Note the amount of drainage if fresh blood is noted on the dressing. Circle or outline the size of any hematoma.

■ Assess for the signs of retroperitoneal bleeding.

■ After the procedure, monitor vital signs until the patient's condition is stable.

Rationales

Fresh blood on the dressing, oozing, pain, tenderness, swelling, and hematoma are all signs of bleeding. Identifying the size of the hematoma allows for serial comparisons. QSEN: Safety.

Signs of retroperitoneal bleeding may include abdominal, flank, or thigh pain; loss of lower extremity pulses; or drop in hemoglobin. QSEN: Safety.

Increased HR and decreased BP are initial compensatory mechanisms commonly noted with bleeding. QSEN: Safety.

Cardiac and Vascular Care Plans

Actions/Interventions

▲ Monitor the PTT, activated coagulation time (ACT), and platelets as appropriate.

Rationales

These laboratory results provide information on coagulation status. Usually PTT is kept at $1\frac{1}{2}$ to 2 times control time. Sheaths can usually be removed when the ACT is less than 150 to 180 seconds, depending on policy. QSEN: Safety.

Therapeutic Interventions

Actions/Interventions

Before removal of catheter sheaths:

■ Maintain bed rest with the patient in a supine position with the affected extremity straight.

■ Do not elevate the head of the bed more than 30 degrees. Observe appropriate positioning for meals, bowel and bladder elimination, and position changes.

■ Avoid sudden movements of the affected extremity.

■ Instruct the patient to apply light pressure on the dressing when coughing, sneezing, or raising the head off the pillow.
■ Instruct the patient to notify the nurse immediately of signs of bleeding from the cannulation site (e.g., feeling of wetness, warmth, "pop" at catheter sheath site, feeling of faintness).
▲ If significant bleeding occurs:

• Notify the physician immediately.
• Remove the dressing, and apply manual pressure or a mechanical clamp directly above the bleeding site or over the artery.
• Anticipate a fluid challenge.
• Anticipate the removal of catheter sheaths.

After removal of catheter sheaths:
■ Maintain an occlusive pressure dressing on the cannulation site for 20 to 30 minutes.

■ Maintain bed rest in a supine position with the affected extremity straight for the prescribed time.
■ Instruct the patient to avoid sudden movements of the affected extremity.
▲ Resume mobilization and ambulation as prescribed.

Rationales

The length of time for sheath insertion varies according to the type of procedure (stents require longer anticoagulation and longer insertion times), institutional policy, and any procedural complication. QSEN: Safety; Evidence-based practice.
This position facilitates clot formation to preserve hemostasis and minimizes risk for bleeding from the cannulation site. QSEN: Safety.
Significant changes in position cause the catheter to bend or move, which interferes with clot formation and can facilitate bleeding. Comfort issues need to be addressed by nursing staff. QSEN: Safety.
Gradual and controlled position changes prevent displacement of catheter sheaths (may cause bleeding).
These measures facilitate clot formation and prevent dislodgement.

Educating patients on such interventions can prevent complications from a clot being dislodged. QSEN: Safety.

These nursing actions reduce the risk of harm to the patient from bleeding. QSEN: Safety.
Rapid, efficient intervention is required.
Pressure devices provide temporary hemostasis and halt bleeding.

Fluid resuscitation expands blood volume and raises BP.
Sheath removal facilitates more optimal sealing of the insertion site.

Ice packs, sandbags, and mechanical clamps may be used to stop initial bleeding. The selection of an adjunct device depends on physician preference and policy.
This positioning promotes clot formation.

This facilitates clot formation and wound closure at the insertion site. QSEN: Safety.
Protocols may vary according to institutional policy and the type of procedure performed.

Cardiac and Vascular Care Plans

■ = Independent ▲ = Interprofessional Collaboration

NANDA-I NDx **Risk for Ineffective Peripheral Tissue Perfusion**

Common Risk Factors

Mechanical obstruction from arterial and venous sheaths
Arterial vasospasm
Thrombus formation
Embolization
Immobility
Edema
Bleeding or hematoma
Arterial dissection

Common Expected Outcome

Patient maintains optimal peripheral tissue perfusion in affected extremity, as evidenced by strong palpable pulse, reduction in and/or absence of pain, warm and dry extremities, and adequate capillary refill.

NOC Outcomes
Risk Control: Thrombus; Circulation Status; Tissue Perfusion: Peripheral

NIC Interventions
Circulatory Care: Arterial Insufficiency; Bleeding Precautions

Ongoing Assessment

Actions/Interventions

Preprocedure:

■ Assess and document the presence or absence and quality of all distal pulses.

■ Obtain a Doppler ultrasonic reading for faint, nonpalpable pulses. Indicate whether the pulse check is with a Doppler ultrasound. Mark the location of faint pulses with an X.

■ Assess and document the skin color and temperature, the presence or absence of pain, numbness, tingling, movement, and sensation of all extremities.

Postprocedure:

■ Assess the presence and quality of pulses distal to the arterial cannulation site (radial for brachial artery, dorsalis pedis, and/or posterior tibial pulses for femoral artery) until stable.

■ Check the cannulation site for bleeding, swelling, and hematoma.

■ Assess for a pseudoaneurysm (pulsatile mass, systolic bruit, groin pain).

■ Assess for an arteriovenous (AV) fistula (pulsatile mass, groin pain, continuous bruit).

Rationales

The risk for arterial occlusion is high. Distal pulses provide a baseline for serial assessments.

Marking the site of pulse ensures consistency in assessing peripheral pulses.

Knowledge of baseline circulatory status of the extremities will assist in monitoring for postprocedure changes. QSEN: Safety.

Arterial thrombosis at the puncture site may lead to occlusion of the artery or distal thrombosis into the extremity.

A lack of hemostasis at the arterial cannulation site contributes to the development of compartment syndrome by constricting vessels or compressing nerves. Large hematomas can dissect into the retroperitoneum and be life threatening. QSEN: Safety.

A pseudoaneurysm is an extraluminal cavity in communication with the adjacent femoral artery. Its presence is best confirmed by Doppler ultrasound.

An AV fistula is a communication between an artery and vein. Its presence is best assessed by Doppler ultrasound.

Cardiac and Vascular Care Plans

 For additional care plans, go to http://evolve.elsevier.com/Gulanick/.

Actions/Interventions	**Rationales**
■ Assess for a retroperitoneal bleed.	Bleeding behind the retroperitoneal cavity is best confirmed by a stat computed tomography scan of the abdomen. The clinical picture includes abdominal and/or flank pain with an increased pulse and decreased hemoglobin. QSEN: Safety.

Therapeutic Interventions

Actions/Interventions	**Rationales**
Postprocedure:	
■ Ensure safety measures to prevent the displacement of arterial and venous sheaths: 　· Maintain bed rest. 　· Keep the cannulated extremity in a neutral or slightly flexed position. 　· Apply a knee or leg immobilizer or soft restraint. 　· Do not elevate the head of the bed more than 30 degrees. 　· Assist with meals, the use of a bedpan, and position changes appropriate to activity limitations.	Significant changes in position cause the sheath to bend or move, which fosters potential bleeding and dislodgement. QSEN: Safety.
▲ Continue prescribed doses of antiplatelets. Check clotting times periodically after the start of infusions and after changes in dose.	Antiplatelets reduce ischemic complications and systemic clot formation. Patients with a stent implantation require more aggressive anticoagulation until endothelialization occurs around the stent.
■ Do passive range-of-motion (ROM) exercises to the unaffected extremities every 2 to 4 hours as tolerated.	ROM exercises prevent venous stasis and promote effective tissue perfusion.
■ Instruct the patient to report the presence of pain, numbness, tingling, and any decrease or loss of sensation and movement immediately.	The patient needs to understand the meaning these symptoms represent for quick assessment, diagnosis, and treatment of complications. QSEN: Safety.
▲ Immediately report to the physician any decrease or loss of pulse, change in skin color and temperature, presence of pain, numbness, tingling, delayed capillary refill, and decrease or loss of sensation and motion.	Signs of compartment syndrome require immediate intervention to prevent tissue ischemia. QSEN: Safety.
■ If ineffective tissue perfusion is noted, anticipate the removal of the catheter sheath.	The presence of catheter sheaths may obstruct blood flow and cause further complications.
▲ Prepare for a possible embolectomy.	An embolectomy is indicated to remove a blood clot that is obstructing or compromising circulation.

Related Care Plans

Anxiety, Chapter 2
Deficient fluid volume, Chapter 2
Impaired physical mobility, Chapter 2
Cardiac rehabilitation, Chapter 5

Cardiac and Vascular Care Plans

■ = Independent　▲ = Interprofessional Collaboration

Peripheral Arterial Revascularization

Femoral Popliteal Bypass; Percutaneous Transluminal Angioplasty (PTA)

Chronic peripheral arterial occlusive disease (peripheral artery disease, PAD) is most commonly caused by atherosclerosis resulting in reduced arterial blood flow to peripheral tissues. Complications associated with arterial insufficiency include pain in the leg(s), ulcers or wounds that do not heal, and progressive amputation of the affected extremity. Revascularization is indicated when medical management is ineffective. Revascularization procedures are available to treat PAD of the femoral arteries with the goals of improving tissue perfusion, preventing tissue necrosis, reducing pain, and limb salvage. This care plan focuses on preoperative teaching and postprocedure care.

Femoral Popliteal Bypass Surgery: This procedure involves a surgical opening of the upper leg to directly visualize the femoral artery. It is performed to bypass the occluded arterial segment in the femoral artery using another blood vessel such as the saphenous vein or a synthetic material such as Dacron or Gore-Tex that is attached to the popliteal artery either above or below the knee. This allows rerouting the blood flow around the obstruction to optimize peripheral circulation. The distal vessel must be at least 50% patent for the grafts to remain patent. Additional locations along the arterial system can be bypassed. An aortoiliac endarterectomy can also be performed whereby the atheromatous plaque is removed and the vessel is sutured to restore circulation. More recently, minimally invasive surgical techniques are being performed in large medical centers.

Percutaneous transluminal angioplasty (PTA): This minimally invasive endovascular procedure uses balloon-tipped catheters that are positioned at the site of the lesion or blockage. Multiple balloon inflations are performed until the atherosclerotic plaque is compressed and the artery is satisfactorily dilated. A stent (tiny, expandable metal coil) may be inserted into the newly opened area to provide structural support to the vessel. The stent remains in place as the deflated balloon catheter is removed. These stents can reduce restenosis rates. Drug-eluding stents, similar to those used in coronary stenting, are in development.

NANDA-I
NDx **Deficient Knowledge**

Common Related Factors

Insufficient information
Insufficient interest in learning
Misinformation presented by others

Defining Characteristics

Insufficient knowledge
Inaccurate follow-through of instruction
Inappropriate behavior

Common Expected Outcome

Patient verbalizes understanding of anticipated procedure and related care.

NOC Outcomes
Knowledge: Disease Process; Knowledge: Treatment Procedure

NIC Interventions
Health Literacy Enhancement; Learning Facilitation; Teaching: Disease Process; Teaching: Procedure/Treatment

---

Ongoing Assessment

Action/Intervention	Rationale
■ Assess the patient's knowledge regarding the revascularization procedure being planned and the postprocedure management.	A thorough understanding of indications for care related to the revascularization procedure is necessary for the patient to give informed consent. QSEN: Patient-centered care.

Cardiac and Vascular Care Plans

Therapeutic Interventions

Actions/Interventions	Rationales

Actions/Interventions

■ Provide information about the cause and physiology of peripheral arterial disease and the indications for the procedure at this time.

■ Provide information on the revascularization procedure selected for the patient: femoral-popliteal bypass versus percutaneous transluminal angioplasty (PTA) with stenting.

■ Provide information regarding the specifics of the planned procedure:
  • PTAs and/or stents are mostly done as outpatient procedures. The patient is NPO before and immediately after the procedure.
  • Bypass surgery may be performed with general anesthesia (with tracheal intubation) or epidural/spinal induction; PTA is performed with conscious sedation and local anesthesia.
  • For surgical procedures, the incision will be sutured together. For PTA, the insertion site will be held with manual pressure or a closure device may be used.

■ Provide information on postprocedure expectations:

  • Frequent circulatory assessments below the surgical and/or PTA site
  • Activity restrictions: lying flat with the affected and arteriotomy sites straight until hemostasis is achieved
  • Expected discomfort (encourage the patient to notify staff when the anesthetic effect wears off)

  • The need to notify the nurse of any change in sensation in the lower extremities or any bleeding or swelling

■ Instruct in any medications ordered for postprocedure care (e.g., anticoagulants, antiplatelet medication, vasodilators, antibiotics).

■ Instruct in the following signs or symptoms to report after discharge:
  • Increased pain, redness, swelling, or bleeding or other discharge from the leg incision
  • Coolness in the leg or foot
  • Pain, discomfort, tingling, or numbness
  • Fever and/or chills

Rationales

Atherosclerosis is a progressive disease. Once medical management has not improved symptoms and the patient exhibits ischemic pain at rest or significant disability or may be in danger of losing the limb from reduced peripheral circulation, then invasive revascularization measures are indicated.

Some patients want to be involved in decision-making regarding type of procedure to be performed. However, they may lack knowledge regarding the technical aspects and complications that guide such decision-making. Not all disease can be treated with PTA, and not all patients may be candidates for a surgical procedure. The best procedure is based on individual circumstances. QSEN: Patient-centered care.

This information helps patients and families anticipate activities as part of the planned procedure. Knowing what to expect can reduce anxiety for both the patient and family.

Attention to these parameters reduces the risk of harm to the patient. QSEN: Safety.

This information relieves the patient's anxiety about the staff's need for frequent pulse checks.

Crossing the legs may facilitate thrombus formation and graft closure or bleeding from the surgical site.

The site will be tender and sore for several days after the procedure, so early reports of discomfort will facilitate pain management.

This information prevents delays in detecting changes in circulation or any postprocedure complications and allows prompt treatment of any occlusion.

A variety of medication regimens are used depending on the type of revascularization procedure performed. Post-PTA patients require long-term aspirin therapy. Short-term antiplatelet therapy with medications such as clopidogrel is indicated to prevent restenosis.

Information enables the patient to assume control during recovery. Attention to these physical changes can reduce the risk of harm to the patient. QSEN: Safety.

Cardiac and Vascular Care Plans

■ = Independent ▲ = Interprofessional Collaboration

Actions/Interventions

- Instruct in the need for follow-up appointments and vascular testing to ensure vessel patency.
- Clarify that atherosclerosis is a progressive disease and although symptoms have been relieved, the disease has not been cured.
- Explain the importance of lifestyle management (e.g., smoking cessation, hypertension management, exercise, low-fat diet) as appropriate.

Rationales

Duplex ultrasound provides verification of improved blood flow.

Living with a chronic disease is challenging. Atherosclerosis is a systemic disease and may likewise affect other vital organs such as the heart and cerebral circulation.

Information provides rationales for therapy and aids the patient in assuming responsibility for required lifestyle changes.

NANDA-I
NDx **Risk for Ineffective Peripheral Tissue Perfusion**

Common Risk Factors

Graft occlusion
Edema
Hypotension
Hematoma or bleeding
Compartment syndrome
Thrombus formation
Embolization
Arterial vasospasm
Restenosis
Arterial dissection

Common Expected Outcome

Patient maintains optimal peripheral tissue perfusion in affected extremity, as evidenced by adequate arterial pulsation distal to graft and/or percutaneous transluminal angioplasty; no increase in limb pain; resolution of edema/warm skin in affected extremity, and evidence of normal wound healing.

NOC Outcomes
Risk Control: Thrombus; Circulation Status; Tissue Perfusion: Peripheral
NIC Interventions
Circulatory Care: Venous Insufficiency; Lower Extremity Monitoring; Circulatory Status: Venous

---

Ongoing Assessment

Actions/Interventions

- Mark distal pulses (pedal and posterior tibial) with a skin marker, and check every hour. Note the pulse presence and strength. Compare with the side that was not operated on. Use a Doppler ultrasound if needed for nonpalpable pulses.
- Assess the patient's level of pain in the affected limb. Signs of occlusion include the following: pain, pulselessness, poikilothermia (coolness), pallor, paralysis, or paresthesia.

Rationales

The risk for arterial occlusion is high in the immediate postoperative period. Distal pulses indicate arterial patency.

Compartment syndrome can occur from local swelling around the fascial compartment of the leg. Signs include severe pain, decreased sensation, and hard, swollen leg. Saphenous nerve damage may occur as a result of dissection or trauma. Patients with acute arterial occlusion may report pain unrelieved by analgesics. Rapid intervention is critical to preserve circulation to limb. Attention to any changes followed by prompt treatment reduces the risk of harm to the patient. QSEN: Safety.

Actions/Interventions

- Monitor BP.

- During dressing changes, assess for the presence of bleeding, swelling, and/or hematoma. Notify the physician immediately if present.

Rationales

Hypotension can reduce blood flow to the periphery. An increased BP can cause bleeding or hematoma.

These complications may hinder peripheral circulation by constricting vessels or compressing nerves. Large hematomas can dissect into the retroperitoneum and can be life threatening.

Therapeutic Interventions

Actions/Interventions

- Gently reposition the patient every 1 to 2 hours. Instruct in the importance of keeping the affected extremity in a neutral or slightly flexed position.
- Initiate prescribed activities according to institutional policy and the patient's condition.

- ▲ Maintain adequate fluid intake.

- Ensure that the incisional site is easily visualized; instruct the patient or family to notify staff if bleeding is noted.
- Administer anticoagulation therapy as ordered.

- If bleeding is noted, administer IV fluids, colloids, and blood products as prescribed.

Rationales

Ninety-degree flexion of the hip can cause kinking in the graft, which may precipitate clot formation or impair blood flow. QSEN: Safety.

The leg is not usually elevated in bed unless limb edema is evident. When the patient is sitting in a chair, elevate the leg to prevent edema. Progressive ambulation is typically initiated 1 day after the procedure.

Fluids promote effective circulating volume throughout the arterial system.

Vigilant monitoring helps reduce complications.

The risk for graft occlusion by thrombosis and restenosis is high.

Specific deficiencies guide treatment therapy.

NANDA-I
NDx **Acute Pain**

Common Related Factors

Incision
Occlusion
Restenosis
Compartment syndrome

Defining Characteristics

Self-report of intensity of pain using a standardized pain scale
Self-report of pain characteristics
Facial expression of pain
Restlessness and apprehension
Change in physiological parameter (e.g., blood pressure, heart rate, respiratory rate and oxygen saturation)

Common Expected Outcomes

Patient verbalizes satisfactory pain control at a decreased intensity using a standardized pain scale.
Patient exhibits increased comfort such as baseline levels for BP, pulse, respirations, and relaxed muscle tone or body posture.

NOC Outcomes

Pain Control; Comfort Status; Medication Response

NIC Interventions

Pain Management; Cardiac Care: Acute

Ongoing Assessment

Actions/Interventions

- Assess pain characteristics.

Rationales

The description of pain can help differentiate between incisional pain and pain from graft occlusion, restenosis, or compartment syndrome. QSEN: Patient-centered care.

Cardiac and Vascular Care Plans

■ = Independent ▲ = Interprofessional Collaboration

Actions/Interventions	Rationales
■ Monitor the effectiveness of analgesics and/or therapies used to reduce pain.	Pain caused by more than incisional discomfort may not respond to analgesics and may require emergency intervention.

Therapeutic Interventions

Actions/Interventions	Rationales
▲ Anticipate the need for analgesics, and respond immediately to any report of pain.	Patients have a right to effective pain relief. Patient-controlled analgesia devices may facilitate the patient's sense of control and promote increased comfort. QSEN: Patient-centered care.
■ If pain is a result of a bypass graft occlusion, anticipate an immediate evaluation by the physician or surgeon. Prepare the patient for surgical intervention.	Rapid intervention is critical to preserve the limb. Identifying early any changes in circulation guides specific interventions and reduces the risk of harm to the patient. QSEN: Safety.
■ If pain is caused by acute restenosis after percutaneous transluminal angioplasty, anticipate the need for a repeat procedure.	Abrupt closure occurs most often during the first 24 hours after procedure. Repeat balloon inflations have longer-lasting benefit.
■ If pain is caused by compartment syndrome, anticipate the need for a fasciotomy.	Rapid intervention is needed to preserve the limb.

Related Care Plans

Risk for impaired skin integrity, Chapter 2
Risk for infection, Chapter 2
Surgical experience: Preoperative and postoperative care, Chapter 4
Peripheral arterial occlusive disease, chronic, Chapter 5

Peripheral Arterial Occlusive Disease, Chronic

Intermittent Claudication; Arterial Insufficiency; Percutaneous Transluminal Angioplasty (PTA)

Chronic peripheral arterial occlusive disease is most commonly caused by atherosclerosis resulting in reduced arterial blood flow to peripheral tissues, causing decreased nutrition and oxygenation at the cellular level. It can be characterized by four stages: asymptomatic, claudication, rest pain, and necrosis. Management is directed at removing vasoconstricting factors, improving peripheral blood flow, and reducing metabolic demands on the body. Because atherosclerosis is a progressive disease, older patients experience an increased incidence of this disease. Diabetes mellitus and tobacco use are significant risk factors in the development of chronic arterial insufficiency. Complications associated with arterial insufficiency include necrotic skin ulcers and progressive amputation of the affected extremity. Peripheral arterial disease is a major cause of disability, significantly affecting quality of life. It is also a significant predictor of future cardiac and cerebrovascular events and is considered a cardiovascular disease risk equivalent.

Cardiac and Vascular Care Plans

Ineffective Peripheral Tissue Perfusion

Common Related Factors

Atherosclerosis
Vasoconstriction secondary to medications and tobacco
Arterial spasm

Defining Characteristics

Pain, cramping, and ache in extremity
Intermittent claudication (cramping pain or weakness in one or both legs, relieved by rest)
Numbness of toes on walking, relieved by rest
Foot pain at rest
Tenderness, especially at toes
Cool extremities
Pallor of toes or foot when leg is elevated for 30 seconds
Dependent rubor (20 seconds to 2 minutes after leg is lowered)
Capillary refill >3 seconds
Difference in BP in opposite extremity
Decrease in or absent arterial pulses
Shiny skin
Loss of hair
Thickened, discolored nails
Ulcerated areas and gangrene
Bruits

Common Expected Outcome

Patient maintains optimal peripheral tissue perfusion in affected extremity, as evidenced by strong palpable pulse, reduction in/absence of pain, warm and dry extremities, adequate capillary refill, and prevention of ulceration.

NOC Outcomes

Peripheral Artery Disease: Severity; Circulation Status; Tissue Perfusion: Peripheral

NIC Interventions

Circulatory Precautions; Circulatory Care: Arterial Insufficiency

Ongoing Assessment

Actions/Interventions

■ Assess the extremities for pain, pallor, paresthesia, poikilothermia (coolness), pulselessness, and paralysis.

■ Assess the quality of peripheral pulses, noting their presence and strength; assess for bruits in the lower extremities. Note capillary refill. If no pulses are noted, assess arterial blood flow using a Doppler ultrasonic instrumentation.

■ Assess skin color changes upon elevation and dependent positioning.

Rationales

This disease occurs primarily in the legs. The extremities manifest pain, numbness and tingling, coolness and pallor, with shiny hairless skin. Knowledge of baseline circulatory status aids in the selection of appropriate intervention.

Arterial occlusions signify reduced peripheral blood flow and diminished or obliterated peripheral pulses. Routine examination should include palpation of femoral, popliteal, posterior tibial, and dorsalis pedis pulses. The posterior tibial pulse is the most sensitive indicator, in that the dorsalis pedis pulse is absent in approximately 10% of healthy people without disease.

In advanced disease, the lower extremities become pale when the leg is elevated as a result of reduced capillary blood flow, and they become red (rubor) when placed in a dependent position.

Cardiac and Vascular Care Plans

■ = Independent ▲ = Interprofessional Collaboration

Actions/Interventions	Rationales
■ Assess pain, numbness, and tingling for causative factors, time of onset, quality, severity, and relieving factors.	Intermittent claudication is the most common symptom of peripheral vascular disease. It is muscle pain that is precipitated by exercise or activity and is relieved with rest. It commonly occurs in the calf muscles or buttocks. Claudication may not be experienced if patients, especially older patients, have limited their physical activity secondary to cardiac or pulmonary disorders or other contributing problems. Pain that occurs at rest signifies more extensive disease requiring immediate attention. Tingling or numbness represents impaired perfusion to nerve tissue cells. QSEN: Patient-centered care.
■ Assess segmental limb pressure measurements such as ankle-brachial index (ABI).	Normally the BP readings in the lower extremities are higher than in the upper extremities. Normal ratio of ankle systolic pressure divided by brachial systolic pressure is 0.9 or greater. An ABI ratio of less than 0.9 in either leg is diagnostic of peripheral artery disease (PAD). A ratio of 0.4 or greater signifies severe disease.
■ Assess for ulcerated areas on the skin.	Ulcers develop from ischemia and are commonly seen over bony prominences and on the toes and feet. Because of impaired tissue perfusion the ulcers become infected easily. If not treated, they can lead to gangrene.
▲ Monitor the results of diagnostic tests: pulse volume recordings, continuous wave Doppler ultrasound; treadmill exercise testing/6-minute walk; duplex ultrasound; CT or magnetic resonance angiography.	These tests are used to identify the location and severity of disease; angiography is useful for patients requiring surgical intervention. Exercise stress testing helps in reproducing claudication and provides data for evaluating the effectiveness of any treatment.

Therapeutic Interventions

Actions/Interventions	Rationales
■ Maintain the affected extremity in a dependent position.	Gravity can increase peripheral arterial blood flow. However, if edema is present in the lower legs, the feet should be elevated to promote venous return and reduce edema.
■ Keep the extremity warm (socks or blankets).	Warmth promotes vasodilation and comfort. The use of heating pads or hot water bottles for warmth puts the patient at risk for tissue injury.
■ Encourage the need for a progressive activity program, noting claudication.	During exercise, tissues do not receive adequate oxygenation from obstructed arteries and convert to anaerobic metabolism, of which lactic acid is a by-product. Accumulation of lactic acid causes muscle spasm and discomfort. However, gradual progressive exercise helps promote collateral circulation. Patient should be encouraged to walk to the point of claudication, stop and rest, and continue walking.
■ Provide meticulous foot care.	Cleanliness is important to preventing infection. Toenails should be trimmed straight across. Minor trauma can result in skin breakdown.
▲ Administer analgesics as ordered.	The pain caused by chronic PAD is difficult to treat. Analgesics may provide some relief, but antiplatelet and hemorrheological agents, exercise, and percutaneous or surgical procedures may be more effective.

Actions/Interventions

▲ Provide drug therapy as ordered:

- Antiplatelets (aspirin, clopidogrel)

- Cilostazol (Pletal)

- Lipid-lowering agents

■ Explain more invasive therapies as indicated: percutaneous transluminal angioplasty and/or stenting, laser-assisted angioplasty, atherectomy, surgical revascularization.

Rationales

These medications are based on recommendations from national organizations. QSEN: Evidence-based practice.

These medications reduce platelet aggregation and may increase pain-free walking distance and resting limb blood flow.

Cilostazol is indicated to improve symptoms and increase walking distance in those with intermittent claudication. It causes direct arterial dilation, inhibits platelet aggregation, and improves pain-free walking distance. It should not be used in patients with heart failure. Pentoxifylline may be considered as a second-line alternative to cilostazol.

For patients with PAD, the low-density lipoprotein lipid goal is less than 100 mg/dL and lower for patients with additional risk factors for heart attack and stroke.

These therapies are appropriate for symptomatic patients for pain relief, to promote ulcer healing, and for limb salvage.

NANDA-I NDx Deficient Knowledge

Common Related Factors

Insufficient information
Insufficient interest in learning
Misinformation presented by others

Common Expected Outcome

Patient verbalizes understanding of self-care measures required to treat disease and prevent complications.

Defining Characteristics

Insufficient knowledge
Inaccurate follow-through of instruction
Inappropriate behavior

NOC Outcomes

Knowledge: Peripheral Arterial Disease Management; Self-Management: Peripheral Arterial Disease

NIC Interventions

Health Literacy Enhancement; Learning Facilitation; Teaching: Disease Process; Teaching: Prescribed Medication; Teaching: Prescribed Exercise

---

Ongoing Assessment

Action/Intervention

■ Assess the patient's knowledge of the physiology of the disease and its treatment or the preventive techniques prescribed.

Rationale

Peripheral artery disease (PAD) is a lifelong condition. Patients need to understand the self-care strategies for which they are responsible. Attention should be directed toward treating peripheral disease and reducing risk for cardiovascular and cerebrovascular atherosclerosis.

Cardiac and Vascular Care Plans

■ = Independent ▲ = Interprofessional Collaboration

Therapeutic Interventions

Actions/Interventions	Rationales
■ Instruct in the physiology of blood supply to the tissues.	Knowledge of causative factors helps patients understand rationales for therapies.
■ Instruct in prescribed diagnostic tests.	Explaining expected events ahead of time reduces anxiety and facilitates appropriate follow-through.
■ Instruct in how to prevent progression of the disease:	The risk factors for atherosclerosis are smoking, dyslipidemia, hypertension, diabetes mellitus, obesity, sedentary lifestyle, and family history of atherosclerosis. Atherosclerosis is not confined just to the lower extremities; it may occur in the coronary, cerebral, and renal vessels. Risk factor modification early in the disease may slow progression. QSEN: Evidence-based practice; Patient-centered care.
• Smoking cessation	Nicotine is a vasoconstrictor and increases blood viscosity, further decreasing already compromised circulation. Smoking is the single risk factor most commonly implicated in the disease and is said to triple the risk for developing claudication.
• Dietary modification	The National Heart, Lung and Blood Institute's Therapeutic Lifestyle Changes diet is an example of a heart-healthy diet plan to reduce lipids and obesity. Because patients with PAD are considered high risk for systemic atherosclerotic disease, their low-density lipoprotein cholesterol goal is less than 100 mg/dL, with a goal of less than 70 mg/dL for patients with additional risk factors. Lipid-lowering medications may be required.
• Hypertension management	Control of hypertension can improve systemic tissue perfusion.
■ Provide information on a daily exercise program: • Walk on a flat surface to reduce calf pain. • Walk about half a block after intermittent claudication is experienced, unless otherwise ordered by the physician. • Stop and rest until all discomfort subsides. • Repeat the same procedure for a total of 30 minutes two to three times daily.	Exercise is an essential treatment for PAD. When the patient walks to the point of claudication, this ischemic stimulus (buildup of lactic acid) serves to promote enhanced collateral circulation. Once the lactic acid clears from the local blood system with rest, the pain should subside. Repetitive walking sessions serve to increase progress in improving walking ability.
■ Instruct in the prevention of complications:	Teaching content on prevention of complications serves as a nursing action to reduce the risk of harm to the patient. QSEN: Safety.

• Effects of temperature:
  • Keep the extremities warm. Wear stockings to bed.
  • Keep the house or apartment as warm as possible.
  • Never apply hot water bottles or electric heating pads to the feet or legs.
  • Avoid local cold applications and cold temperatures.
	Warmth promotes vasodilation. External heating devices must be used with caution, because burns may occur secondary to impaired nerve function. Cold causes vasoconstriction and reduced blood flow.

• Foot care:
  • Inspect the feet often for signs of ingrown toenails, sores, blisters, and other concerns.
  • Wash the feet daily with warm soap and water. Dry thoroughly by gentle patting. Never rub dry.
  • File or trim toenails carefully and only after soaking in warm water. File or trim straight across. See a podiatrist as needed.
  • Lubricate the skin.
  • Wear clean stockings.
  • Do not walk barefoot.
  • Wear correctly fitting shoes.
	Poor peripheral circulation can result in tissue damage. Early assessment of potential problems reduces complications. Patients with diabetes are at increased risk for injury to the feet. In addition, patients with diabetic neuropathy may have no perception of pain or injury. Ulceration or gangrene of the toe or foot may follow mild trauma.

Cardiac and Vascular Care Plans

Actions/Interventions

- Provide information on more invasive therapies as indicated:
  - Percutaneous transluminal angioplasty (PTA) and stent placements

  - Atherectomy
  - Surgical revascularization

  - Amputation

Rationales

PTA is a nonsurgical procedure using a balloon catheter to dilate an obstructed artery. Stents are used in conjunction with PTA and atherectomy to maintain patency of the blood vessel.

Atherectomy uses a special catheter to "shave" away plaque.

This surgical procedure bypasses atherosclerotic lesions using an autogenous saphenous vein or graft made from synthetic material.

Amputation is required if gangrene is present.

NANDA-I NDx **Impaired Skin Integrity**

Common Related Factors

Pressure over bony prominences
Decreased peripheral tissue perfusion
Trauma to skin

Defining Characteristics

Ulceration over bony prominences, primarily toes and feet
Presence of gangrene
Atrophic skin

Common Expected Outcomes

Patient's skin will be intact without signs of ulcers, redness, or infection.
Patient experiences healing of ulcers.

NOC Outcomes

Tissue Integrity: Skin and Mucous Membranes; Wound Healing: Secondary Intention

NIC Interventions

Skin Care: Topical Treatments; Wound Care

Ongoing Assessment

Action/Intervention

- Assess the skin for signs of redness, open wounds, and vascular ulcers:
  - Location
  - Pain
  - Ulcer characteristics
  - Condition of surrounding tissue

Rationale

Arterial ulcers usually develop over the bony prominences of toes and feet or any point of trauma. The patient may report pain that is burning or sharp. Ulcers have a well-defined border with a pale tissue bed. Eschar may be present. Ulcers may have drainage if infection is present. Surrounding tissue is usually pale on elevation or may have dependent rubor.

Therapeutic Interventions

Actions/Interventions

- Protect the skin from trauma and prolonged pressure.

Rationales

The poor peripheral circulation of peripheral arterial occlusive disease (PAD) combined with decreased sensation places the patient at high risk for injury. Attention to this nursing action minimizes the risk of harm to the patient. QSEN: Safety.

Cardiac and Vascular Care Plans

■ = Independent   ▲ = Interprofessional Collaboration

Actions/Interventions	Rationales
■ Cover noninfected wounds with appropriate dressings.	A variety of dressing materials are available to protect arterial ulcers during the healing process. Hydrocolloid dressings that can be left in place for several days have the benefit of reducing skin trauma and infection associated with frequent dressing changes. The wound healing process is often prolonged.
■ Use sterile technique when caring for broken skin or vascular ulcers.	The patient is at risk for wound infections because of decreased arterial blood flow to the tissue. QSEN: Safety.
▲ Prepare for the debridement of necrotic tissue from the ulcer:	Removal of necrotic tissue from the ulcer is necessary to prevent infection and allow for healing of the wound.
• Surgical debridement	Surgical debridement involves the use of instruments to manually cut away necrotic tissue. The patient usually does not experience pain because tissue is dead. Bleeding will occur when healthy tissue is reached.
• Mechanical debridement	Mechanical debridement is usually accomplished with the application of sterile, wet-to-dry dressings. The wet gauze dressing adheres to the wound surface. Necrotic tissue is pulled away from the wound when the dressing is removed several hours after application.
• Pharmacological debridement	Pharmacological debridement involves the use of enzyme ointments to necrotic tissue in the wound. A sterile dressing is applied.
▲ Administer antibiotics as prescribed.	Antibiotics may be used for infected wounds or to prevent bacteremia. The route of administration may be oral, IV, or topical to the wound itself.
■ Measure the wound with each dressing change. Consult with the wound care management nurse.	The wound should decrease in size as it heals. Regular measurement will aid in evaluating the effectiveness of treatment measures.
	The wound care management nurse has specialized knowledge and skills to evaluate wounds and select the most appropriate wound management interventions. QSEN: Teamwork and collaboration.

Related Care Plans

Peripheral arterial revascularization, Chapter 5
Pressure ulcers (impaired skin integrity), Chapter 14

Pulmonary Edema, Acute

Cardiogenic Pulmonary Edema; Acute Heart Failure

Pulmonary edema is a pathological state in which there is an abnormal and/or excessive diffuse accumulation of fluid in the alveoli and interstitial spaces of the lung. This fluid causes impaired gas exchange by interfering with diffusion between the pulmonary capillaries and the alveoli.

It is commonly caused by left ventricular failure, altered capillary permeability of the lungs, acute respiratory distress syndrome, neoplasms, overhydration, and hypoalbuminemia. Acute pulmonary edema is considered a medical emergency.

Cardiac and Vascular Care Plans

NDx Impaired Gas Exchange

Common Related Factors

Alveolar-capillary membrane changes
Ventilation-perfusion mismatch

Defining Characteristics

Abnormal arterial blood gases (ABGs)
Abnormal breathing pattern (rate, rhythm, depth)
Dyspnea/crackles
Cough
Pink, frothy sputum
Pulmonary capillary wedge pressure greater than 25 to 30 mm Hg (in intensive care unit setting)
Cyanosis or pallor
Restlessness and apprehension
Tachycardia

Common Expected Outcome

Patient maintains optimal gas exchange, as evidenced by ABGs within the patient's usual range, oxygen saturation of 90% or greater, alert responsive mentation or no further reduction in level of consciousness, relaxed breathing, and baseline HR for patient.

NOC Outcomes

Respiratory Status: Gas Exchange; Respiratory Status: Ventilation

NIC Interventions

Respiratory Monitoring; Ventilation Assistance; Medication Administration

---

Ongoing Assessment

Actions/Interventions	Rationales
■ Assess the respiratory rate and depth, presence of shortness of breath, and use of accessory muscles.	Patients will adapt their breathing pattern over time to facilitate gas exchange. In the early stages, there is a mild increase in rate. As it progresses, severe dyspnea, gurgling respirations, use of accessory muscles, and extreme breathlessness, as if "drowning" in one's own secretions, are noted.
■ Assess the character of any secretions.	Frothy, blood-tinged sputum is characteristic of pulmonary edema.
■ Assess breath sounds in all fields, noting aerations and the presence of wheezes and crackles in lung bases.	Bubbling wheezes and crackles are easily heard over the entire chest, reflecting fluid-filled airways. The level of fluid ascends as the pulmonary edema worsens.
■ Assess for headache and any change in the level of consciousness.	These are early nonpulmonary signs of hypoxia and decreased perfusion to the brain. QSEN: Safety.
■ Monitor for changes in the patient's BP, HR, and respiratory rate.	With initial hypoxia and hypercapnia, BP, HR, and respiratory rate all rise. As the hypoxia and/or hypercapnia become severe, BP and HR will drop and dysrhythmias may occur. Respiratory failure may ensue when the patient is unable to maintain the rapid rate of breathing. QSEN: Safety.
▲ Use pulse oximetry to monitor oxygen saturation.	Pulse oximetry is useful to detect changes in oxygenation. Oxygen saturation should be maintained at 90% or greater. QSEN: Safety.

Cardiac and Vascular Care Plans

■ = Independent   ▲ = Interprofessional Collaboration

Actions/Interventions

▲ Monitor serial ABGs and note changes.

■ Assess the skin, nail beds, and mucous membranes for pallor or cyanosis.

▲ Monitor the chest x-ray reports.

Rationales

In early stages, there is a decrease in both Pao_2 and $Paco_2$ secondary to hypoxemia and respiratory alkalosis from tachypnea. In later stages, the Pao_2 continues to drop while the $Paco_2$ may increase, reflecting respiratory acidosis. Attention to changes in acid-base balance reduces the risk of harm to the patient. QSEN: Safety.

Cool, pale skin may be secondary to a compensatory vaso-constrictive response to hypoxemia. As oxygenation and perfusion become impaired, peripheral tissues become cyanotic.

As interstitial edema accumulates, the x-ray films show cloudy, white lung fields.

Therapeutic Interventions

Actions/Interventions

■ Assist the patient to a position of comfort to allow for the most effective breathing pattern.

■ Encourage slow, deep breaths as appropriate.

■ Assist with coughing or suctioning as needed.

▲ Provide oxygen as needed to maintain Pao_2 at an acceptable level.

▲ Anticipate endotracheal intubation and the use of mechanical ventilation.

▲ Administer prescribed medications carefully, as follows:

- Morphine sulfate

- Sodium nitroprusside (Nipride)

- Nitrates
- Diuretics

- Inotropic agents

- Aminophylline

▲ If ABGs are expected to be measured more often than at four 1-hour intervals, suggest the appropriateness of an arterial line.

Rationales

An upright position allows for an increased thoracic capacity and full descent of the diaphragm.

Slow, deep breathing reduces tachypnea and alveolar collapse.

Excessive secretions can interfere with gas exchange in the bronchopulmonary tree. Coughing and suctioning remove secretions to maintain a patent airway, thereby enhancing oxygenation.

Supplemental oxygen may be required to maintain Pao_2 at an acceptable level.

Early intubation and mechanical ventilation are recommended to prevent full decompensation of the patient. Bilateral positive airway pressure (BiPAP) may also be indicated. QSEN: Safety.

These medications are based on recommendations from national organizations. QSEN: Evidence-based practice.

Morphine reduces preload by vasodilation, decreases respiratory rate, and reduces anxiety.

Sodium nitroprusside reduces afterload and is required if systemic vascular resistance is high.

Nitrates reduce preload by dilating venous vessels.

Diuretics reduce intravascular fluid volume and decrease preload.

Inotropic medications such as dobutamine, dopamine, milrinone may be required to support BP and optimize cardiac output.

Aminophylline dilates bronchioles and dilates venous vessels. However, it is also a cardiac stimulant. Patients must be observed for cardiac dysrhythmias.

Arterial cannulation is indicated for the patient's comfort and for ease in obtaining necessary ABG measurements.

NANDA-I NDx Decreased Cardiac Output

Common Related Factors

Increased preload
Increased afterload
Impaired contractility
Altered HR or heart rhythm
Decreased oxygenation

Defining Characteristics

Changes in hemodynamic parameters
Dysrhythmias or electrocardiogram (ECG) changes
Weight gain, edema, and ascites
Abnormal heart sounds (S_3, S_4)
Abnormal breath sounds (crackles)
Anxiety and restlessness
Dizziness, weakness, and fatigue
Decreased peripheral pulses
Pallor, clammy skin
Oliguria
Dyspnea

Common Expected Outcome

Patient maintains adequate cardiac output, as evidenced by strong peripheral pulses, systolic BP within 20 mm Hg of baseline, HR 60 to 100 beats/min with regular rhythm, urinary output 30 mL/hr or greater, warm and dry skin, and normal level of consciousness.

NOC Outcomes

Cardiopulmonary Status; Cardiac Pump Effectiveness

NIC Interventions

Hemodynamic Regulation; Cardiac Care; Invasive Hemodynamic Monitoring

Ongoing Assessment

Actions/Interventions	Rationales
■ Assess skin color, temperature, and moisture.	Cool, pale, clammy skin is secondary to a compensatory increase in sympathetic nervous system stimulation and low cardiac output and desaturation.
▲ Assess the patient's HR, BP, and mean arterial pressure. Use direct intra-arterial monitoring as ordered.	Sinus tachycardia and increased arterial BP are seen in the early stages to maintain an adequate cardiac output. BP drops as the condition deteriorates. Auscultatory BP may be unreliable secondary to vasoconstriction. Mean arterial pressure decreases in shock. Older patients have a reduced response to catecholamines; thus their response to decreased cardiac output may be blunted, with less increase in HR.
■ Assess peripheral pulses, including capillary refill.	Pulses are weak with reduced stroke volume and cardiac output. Capillary refill is slow, sometimes absent.
■ Assess for mental status changes.	Hypoxia and reduced cerebral perfusion are reflected in restlessness, anxiety, and irritability. Older patients are especially susceptible to reduced perfusion to vital organs.
■ Assess the respiratory rate, rhythm, and breath sounds.	Crackles, rhonchi, and wheezes develop as fluid overload worsens. Rapid, shallow respirations are characteristic of reduced cardiac output.
■ Assess fluid balance and weight gain.	Compromised regulatory mechanisms may result in fluid and sodium retention. Body weight is a more sensitive indicator of fluid retention than intake and output.
■ Assess the patient's urine output.	The renal system compensates for low BP by retaining water. Oliguria is a classic sign of inadequate renal perfusion from reduced cardiac output.

Cardiac and Vascular Care Plans

■ = Independent ▲ = Interprofessional Collaboration

Actions/Interventions

■ Assess heart sounds for gallops (S₃, S₄).

■ Assess the cardiac rate and rhythm and the 12-lead ECG.

▲ Use pulse oximetry to monitor oxygen saturation; assess ABGs.

▲ If hemodynamic monitoring is in place, assess the central venous pressure (CVP), pulmonary artery pressure, pulmonary capillary wedge pressure, and cardiac output and/or cardiac index.

Rationales

S_3 denotes a reduced left ventricular ejection and is a classic sign of left ventricular failure. S_4 occurs with reduced compliance of the left ventricle, which impairs diastolic filling.

Cardiac dysrhythmias may occur from low perfusion, acidosis, or hypoxia, as well as from side effects of cardiac medications used to treat this condition. The 12-lead ECG may provide evidence of myocardial ischemia (ST-segment and T-wave changes).

Pulse oximetry is a useful tool to detect changes in oxygenation. Oxygen saturation should be kept at 90% or greater. As the condition worsens, aerobic metabolism ceases and lactic acidosis ensues, raising the level of carbon dioxide and decreasing pH. QSEN: Safety.

CVP provides information on filling pressures of the right side of the heart; pulmonary artery diastolic pressure and pulmonary capillary wedge pressure reflect left-sided fluid volumes. Cardiac output provides an objective number to guide therapy. Attention to changes in cardiac output and fluid balance reduces the risk of harm to the patient. QSEN: Safety.

Therapeutic Interventions

Actions/Interventions

▲ Anticipate the need for hemodynamic monitoring.

■ Position the patient for an optimal reduction of preload (high-Fowler's position, dangling feet at the bedside).
■ Anticipate prescribed medications:

• Positive inotropic agents (e.g., dopamine, dobutamine, milrinone)
• Vasodilators (e.g., nitrates, nitroprusside; angiotensin-converting enzyme inhibitor)
• Diuretics

• Morphine

• Anticoagulants

Rationales

A Swan-Ganz catheter provides pulmonary artery and pulmonary capillary wedge pressure measurements that guide therapy.

This position reduces preload by pooling blood in the lower extremities and decreasing venous return.

These medications are based on recommendations from national organizations. QSEN: Evidence-based practice.

Inotropic medications augment myocardial contractility, increase BP, and increase cardiac output/cardiac index.

Vasodilators reduce preload, reduce afterload, and improve oxygenation.

Diuretics reduce intravascular fluid volume, reduce pulmonary capillary wedge pressure, and enhance sodium excretion.

Morphine reduces pulmonary congestion and relieves dyspnea.

Anticoagulant medications prevent venous thromboembolism.

NANDA-I NDx Anxiety

Common Related Factors	Defining Characteristics
Change in environment (excessive monitoring equipment)	Sympathetic stimulation
Change in health status	Restlessness
Threat of death	Focus on self
	Uncooperative behavior
	Vigilant watch on equipment
	Tachypnea

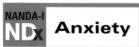 **Evolve** For additional care plans, go to http://evolve.elsevier.com/Gulanick/.

Cardiac and Vascular Care Plans

Common Expected Outcomes

Patient demonstrates reduced anxiety, as evidenced by calm manner and cooperative behavior.

Patient describes a reduction in the level of anxiety experienced.

NOC Outcomes
Anxiety Self-Control; Coping
NIC Interventions
Anxiety Reduction; Calming Technique; Emotional Support

Ongoing Assessment

Actions/Interventions	Rationales
■ Assess the patient's anxiety level (mild, severe). Note any signs and symptoms, especially nonverbal communication.	Acute pulmonary edema is an acute life-threatening situation that will produce high levels of anxiety in the patient as well as in significant others.
■ Assess any prior coping patterns/methods.	Anxiety and ways of decreasing perceived anxiety are highly individualized. Interventions are most effective when they are consistent with the patient's established coping pattern or previously successful coping mechanisms. However, in the acute care setting these techniques may no longer be feasible. QSEN: Patient-centered care.

Therapeutic Interventions

Actions/Interventions	Rationales
■ Acknowledge an awareness of the patient's anxiety.	Acknowledgment validates the patient's feelings and communicates acceptance of those feelings.
■ Maintain a confident, assured manner. Assure the patient and significant others of close, continuous monitoring that will ensure prompt intervention.	The presence of a trusted person helps the patient feel less threatened. The staff's anxiety may be easily perceived by the patient. The patient's feeling of stability increases in a calm, nonthreatening atmosphere.
■ Encourage the verbalization of thoughts and feelings.	Expressing emotions provides clarification of the patient's perceptions and enhances coping.
■ Reduce unnecessary external stimuli by maintaining a quiet environment.	Anxiety may escalate with excessive conversation, noise, and equipment around the patient.
■ Explain all procedures as appropriate, keeping explanations basic.	Information helps allay anxiety. Patients who are anxious may not be able to comprehend anything more than simple, clear, brief instructions.
▲ Administer antianxiety medications as appropriate.	Short-term use of antianxiety medication can enhance patient coping and reduce physiological manifestations of anxiety.

Related Care Plans

Insomnia, Chapter 2
Excess fluid volume, Chapter 2
Ineffective breathing pattern, Chapter 2
Mechanical ventilation, Chapter 6
Dysrhythmias, ⊜volve

Cardiac and Vascular Care Plans

■ = Independent   ▲ = Interprofessional Collaboration

Shock, Cardiogenic

Pump Failure; Acute Pulmonary Edema

Cardiogenic shock is an acute state of sustained decreased tissue perfusion caused by the impaired contractility of the heart. It is usually associated with myocardial infarction (MI), cardiomyopathies, dysrhythmias, valvular stenosis, massive pulmonary embolism, cardiac surgery, or cardiac tamponade. It is a self-perpetuating condition because coronary blood flow to the myocardium is compromised, causing further ischemia and ventricular dysfunction. Patients with massive MIs involving 40% or more of the left ventricular (LV) muscle mass are at highest risk for developing cardiogenic shock. The mortality rate for cardiogenic shock often exceeds 80%. This care plan focuses on the care of an unstable patient in a shock state.

NANDA-I NDx Decreased Cardiac Output

Common Related Factors

Mechanical
- Impaired left ventricular (LV) contractility
- Cardiac muscle disease
- Increased or decreased preload and/or afterload
- Dysrhythmias

Structural
- Valvular dysfunction
- Septal defects

Defining Characteristics

Changes in level of consciousness
Tachycardia
Sustained hypotension with narrowing of pulse pressure
Pale, cool, clammy skin
Cyanosis and mottling of extremities
Oliguria and/or anuria
Pulmonary congestion, dyspnea, and/or crackles
Respiratory alkalosis or metabolic acidosis

Common Expected Outcome

Patient maintains adequate cardiac output as evidenced by strong peripheral pulses, systolic BP within 20 mm Hg of baseline, HR 60 to 100 beats/min with regular rhythm, urinary output 30 mL/hr or greater, warm and dry skin, and normal level of consciousness.

NOC Outcomes

Shock Severity: Cardiogenic; Cardiac Pump Effectiveness; Tissue Perfusion: Cardiac; Tissue Perfusion: Cerebral

NIC Interventions

Cardiac Care: Acute; Invasive Hemodynamic Monitoring; Hemodynamic Regulation; Dysrhythmia Management; Circulatory Care: Mechanical Assist Device; Shock Management: Cardiac

---

Ongoing Assessment

Actions/Interventions

■ Assess skin color, temperature, and moisture.

▲ Assess the patient's HR, BP, and mean arterial pressure. Use direct intra-arterial monitoring as ordered.

Rationales

Cool, pale, clammy skin is secondary to compensatory increase in sympathetic nervous system stimulation and low cardiac output and desaturation.

Sinus tachycardia and increased arterial BP are seen in the early stages to maintain an adequate cardiac output. BP drops as condition deteriorates. Auscultatory BP may be unreliable secondary to vasoconstriction. Reduced mean arterial pressure leads to compensatory responses. Older patients have a reduced response to catecholamines; thus their response to decreased cardiac output may be blunted, with less increase in HR.

evolve   For additional care plans, go to http://evolve.elsevier.com/Gulanick/.

Actions/Interventions

- Assess the peripheral and central pulses, including capillary refill.
- Assess for any changes in the level of consciousness.

- Assess the respiratory rate, rhythm, and breath sounds.

- Assess the patient's urine output.

- Assess fluid balance and weight gain.

- Assess the heart sounds for gallops (S_3, S_4).

- Assess the cardiac rate, rhythm, and electrocardiogram (ECG).

▲ Use pulse oximetry to monitor oxygen saturation; assess arterial blood gases.

▲ If hemodynamic monitoring is in place, assess the central venous pressure (CVP), pulmonary artery diastolic pressure (PADP), pulmonary capillary wedge pressure, and cardiac output/cardiac index.

- Assess serum electrolytes, especially potassium and magnesium.

Rationales

Pulses are weak, with reduced stroke volume and cardiac output. Capillary refill is slow, sometimes absent.

Early signs of cerebral hypoxia are restlessness and anxiety, with confusion and loss of consciousness occurring in later stages. Older patients are especially susceptible to reduced perfusion to vital organs.

Rapid, shallow respirations and the presence of crackles and wheezes are characteristic of shock.

The renal system compensates for low BP by retaining water. Oliguria is a classic sign of inadequate renal perfusion from reduced cardiac output.

Compromised regulatory mechanisms may result in fluid and sodium retention. Body weight is a more sensitive indicator of fluid or sodium retention than intake and urine output.

S_3 denotes reduced left ventricular ejection and is a classic sign of left ventricular failure. S_4 occurs with reduced compliance of the left ventricle, which impairs diastolic filling.

Cardiac dysrhythmias may occur from low perfusion, acidosis, or hypoxia, as well as from side effects of cardiac medications used to treat this condition. The 12-lead ECG may provide evidence of myocardial ischemia (ST-segment and T-wave changes) or pericardial tamponade (decreased voltage of QRS complexes).

Pulse oximetry is a useful tool to detect changes in oxygenation. Oxygen saturation should be kept at 90% or greater. As shock increases, aerobic metabolism ceases and lactic acidosis ensues, raising the level of carbon dioxide and decreasing pH. These direct measurements serve as optimal guides for therapy. Identifying changes in oxygenation and acid-base balance, and initiating early intervention reduce the risk of harm. QSEN: Safety.

CVP provides information on filling pressures of the right side of the heart; PADP and pulmonary capillary wedge pressure reflect left-sided fluid volumes. Cardiac output/cardiac index provides an objective number to guide therapy. Attention to these parameters reduces the risk of harm to the patient from fluid imbalances. QSEN: Safety.

Hypokalemia and hypomagnesemia are causative factors for dysrhythmias, which can further reduce cardiac output.

Therapeutic Interventions

Actions/Interventions

- Place the patient in a position of comfort, usually supine with the head of the bed slightly elevated.
- ▲ Administer oxygen as prescribed.

- ▲ For patients with decreased preload, administer IV fluids.

Rationales

This position promotes venous return and increases cardiac output.

Oxygen may be required to maintain oxygen saturation above 90% or as indicated by order or protocol.

Optimal fluid status ensures effective ventricular filling pressure. Too little fluid reduces circulating blood volume and ventricular filling pressures; too much fluid can cause pulmonary edema in a failing heart. Pulmonary capillary wedge pressure guides therapy.

■ = Independent   ▲ = Interprofessional Collaboration

Actions/Interventions	Rationales
▲ If increased preload is a problem, restrict fluids and sodium as ordered.	Fluid restriction decreases extracellular fluid volume and reduces cardiac workload.
▲ Initiate and titrate drug therapy as ordered:	Therapy is more effective when initiated early. The goal is to maintain systolic BP greater than 90 to 100 mm Hg. These medications are based on recommendations from national organizations. QSEN: Evidence-based practice.
• Inotropic agents: • Dopamine	Dopamine is an inotrope and vasopressor that has varying effects at different doses. Low doses increase renal blood flow. Higher doses increase systemic vascular resistance and contractility.
• Dobutamine	Dobutamine is an inotrope that increases contractility with slight vasodilation.
• Milrinone	Milrinone is a cyclic AMP–specific phosphodiesterase inhibitor that has inotropic and vasodilator effects.
• Vasodilators: • Sodium nitroprusside (Nipride)	Nitroprusside increases cardiac output by decreasing afterload and produces peripheral and systemic vasodilation by direct action to the smooth muscles of blood vessels.
• IV nitroglycerin (NTG)	NTG may be used to reduce excess preload contributing to pump failure and to reduce afterload.
• Diuretics	Diuretics are used when volume overload is contributing to pump failure.
• Antidysrhythmics	Antidysrhythmics are used when cardiac dysrhythmias are further compromising a low-output state.
• Vasopressors (e.g., epinephrine, norepinephrine, phenylephrine)	Vasopressors increase the force of myocardial contraction and constrict arteries and veins. They augment the vasoconstriction that occurs with shock to increase perfusion pressure. They are not routinely used unless aforementioned medications have failed to improve coronary perfusion.
• Morphine	Morphine reduces pulmonary congestion and relieves dyspnea.
▲ Provide electrolyte replacement as ordered.	Electrolyte imbalance may cause dysrhythmias or other pathological states. Laboratory results guide therapy.
▲ If mechanical assistance by counterpulsation is indicated, institute an intra-aortic balloon pump (IABP) or percutaneous ventricular assist device (VAD).	Mechanical assist devices such as VAD or IABP provide temporary circulatory support to improve cardiac output. These devices are used in cardiogenic shock when the patient does not respond to pharmacological interventions. IABP increases myocardial oxygen supply and reduces myocardial workload through increased coronary artery perfusion. The patient's stroke volume increases and thus improves perfusion of vital organs. The nurse needs to follow unit protocols for the management of the patient with a mechanical VAD.
▲ Prepare for surgical intervention as needed.	Acute valvular problems or septal defects may require surgical treatment.

Cardiac and Vascular Care Plans

⊖volve   For additional care plans, go to http://evolve.elsevier.com/Gulanick/.

NANDA-I NDx Impaired Gas Exchange

Common Related Factors

Alveolar capillary membrane changes
Ventilation-perfusion mismatch

Defining Characteristics

Abnormal breathing (rate, rhythm, depth)
Crackles
Hypoxia and/or hypoxemia
Tachycardia
Changes in level of consciousness
Headache
Pallor or cyanosis
Abnormal arterial blood gases (ABGs)

Common Expected Outcome

Patient maintains optimal gas exchange, as evidenced by ABGs within the patient's usual range, oxygen saturation of 90% or greater, alert responsive mentation or no further reduction in level of consciousness, relaxed breathing, and baseline HR for patient.

NOC Outcomes

Shock Severity: Cardiogenic; Respiratory Status: Gas Exchange; Tissue Perfusion

NIC Interventions

Respiratory Monitoring; Airway Insertion and Stabilization; Airway Management; Oxygen Therapy

Ongoing Assessment

Actions/Interventions	Rationales
■ Assess the patient's HR, BP, and rate, rhythm, and depth of respirations.	In the early stages of shock, with initial hypoxia and hypercapnia, the patient's respiratory rate will be rapid. As shock progresses, the respirations become shallow, and the patient will begin to hypoventilate. BP and HR will decrease and dysrhythmias may occur. Respiratory failure develops as the patient experiences respiratory muscle fatigue and decreased lung compliance. QSEN: Safety.
■ Assess the lungs, noting areas of decreased ventilation and the presence of adventitious sounds.	Moist crackles are caused by increased pulmonary capillary permeability and increased intra-alveolar edema.
■ Assess the skin, nail beds, and mucous membranes for pallor or cyanosis.	Cool, pale skin may be secondary to a compensatory vasoconstrictive response to hypoxemia. As oxygenation and perfusion become impaired, peripheral tissues become cyanotic.
■ Assess for restlessness, headache, and changes in the level of consciousness.	These are early nonpulmonary signs of hypoxia. QSEN: Safety.
▲ Use pulse oximetry to monitor oxygen saturation.	Pulse oximetry is useful in detecting changes in oxygenation. Oxygen saturation should be maintained at 90% or greater.
▲ Monitor ABGs, and note any changes.	Increasing $Paco_2$ and decreasing Pao_2 are signs of hypoxemia and respiratory acidosis. As the patient's condition begins to fail, the respiratory rate will decrease and $Paco_2$ will continue to increase. QSEN: Safety.

Therapeutic Interventions

Actions/Interventions	Rationales
■ Place the patient in an optimal position for ventilation.	A slightly elevated head of bed facilitates diaphragmatic movement.
▲ Initiate oxygen therapy as prescribed, attempting to maintain oxygen saturation at 90% or greater.	Supplemental oxygen may be required to maintain the Pao_2 at an acceptable level.

Cardiac and Vascular Care Plans

■ = Independent   ▲ = Interprofessional Collaboration

Actions/Interventions

- Assist with coughing, and suction as needed.

- ▲ Prepare the patient for mechanical ventilation if noninvasive oxygen therapy is ineffective.

Rationales

Suction removes secretions if the patient is unable to effectively clear the airway.

Early intubation and mechanical ventilation are recommended to prevent full decompensation of the patient. Mechanical ventilation provides supportive care to maintain adequate oxygenation and ventilation to the patient. QSEN: Safety.

NANDA-I NDx **Anxiety**

Common Related Factors

Guarded prognosis; mortality rate 80%
Fear of death
Change in health status
Unfamiliar environment

Defining Characteristics

Sympathetic stimulation
Verbalized anxiety
Restlessness and/or agitation
Increased awareness
Increased questioning
Uncooperative behavior
Avoids looking at equipment or keeps vigilant watch over equipment

Common Expected Outcomes

Patient uses effective coping mechanisms.
Patient describes reduction in level of anxiety experienced.

NOC Outcomes
Anxiety Self-Control; Coping
NIC Interventions
Anxiety Reduction; Support System Enhancement; Calming Technique

---

Ongoing Assessment

Actions/Interventions

- Assess the patient's anxiety level (mild, severe). Note any signs and symptoms, especially nonverbal communication.
- Assess the coping techniques commonly used.

Rationales

Shock can result in an acute life-threatening situation that will produce high levels of anxiety in the patient as well as in significant others.

Anxiety and ways of decreasing perceived anxiety are highly individualized. Interventions are most effective when they are consistent with the patient's established coping pattern. However, in the acute care setting these techniques may no longer be feasible. QSEN: Patient-centered care.

Therapeutic Interventions

Actions/Interventions

- Acknowledge an awareness of the patient's anxiety.

- Encourage the verbalization of feelings.

Rationales

Acknowledgment of the patient's feelings validates the patient's feelings and communicates acceptance of those feelings.

Talking about anxiety-producing situations and anxious feelings can help the patient perceive the situation in a less threatening manner.

Actions/Interventions

- Maintain a confident, assured manner while interacting with the patient. Assure the patient and significant others of close, continuous monitoring that will ensure prompt intervention.
- Reduce unnecessary external stimuli by maintaining a quiet environment. If medical equipment is a source of anxiety, consider providing sedation to the patient.
- Explain all procedures as appropriate, keeping explanations basic.

Rationales

The staff's anxiety may be easily perceived by the patient. The patient's feeling of stability increases in a calm and non-threatening atmosphere. The presence of a trusted person may help the patient feel less threatened.

Anxiety may escalate with excessive conversation, noise, and equipment around the patient.

Information helps allay anxiety. Patients who are anxious may not be able to comprehend anything more than simple, clear, brief instructions.

Related Care Plans

Ineffective coping, Chapter 2
Spiritual distress, Chapter 2
Mechanical ventilation, Chapter 6

Shock, Hypovolemic

Hypovolemic shock is an emergency situation that occurs from decreased intravascular fluid volume, resulting from either internal fluid shifts or external fluid loss. This fluid can be whole blood, plasma, or water and electrolytes. Losing about one fifth of total blood volume can produce this condition, resulting in circulatory dysfunction and inadequate tissue perfusion. Common causes include hemorrhage (external or internal), severe burns, vomiting, and diarrhea. Hemorrhagic shock often occurs after trauma, gastrointestinal bleeding, or rupture of organs or aneurysms. Internal fluid losses occur in clinical conditions associated with increased capillary permeability and resulting shifts in fluid from the vascular compartment to interstitial spaces or other closed fluid compartments (e.g., peritoneal cavity). This third-spacing of fluids in the body is seen in patients with extensive burns or with ascites and leads to hypovolemic shock.

Hypovolemic shock can be classified according to the percentage of fluid loss. Mild shock (stage 1) is up to 15% blood volume loss, moderate shock (stage 2) is 15% to 30% blood volume loss, stage 3 is 30% to 40% blood volume loss, and severe shock is a greater than 40% loss. Older patients may exhibit signs of shock with smaller losses of fluid volume because of their compromised ability to compensate for fluid changes. Treatment focuses on prompt fluid and/or blood replacement, identification of causative factors and/or bleeding sites, control of bleeding, and prevention of complications. If aggressive treatment is not prompt during the earlier stages of shock, irreversible multiple organ dysfunction syndrome (MODS) will occur, resulting in eventual cardiac arrest and death.

Cardiac and Vascular Care Plans

■ = Independent   ▲ = Interprofessional Collaboration

NANDA-I NDx Deficient Fluid Volume

Common Related Factors

Inadequate fluid intake and/or severe dehydration
Active fluid volume loss (diuresis, abnormal bleeding or drainage, diarrhea)
Internal fluid shifts
Trauma
Failure of regulatory mechanisms

Defining Characteristics

Tachycardia
Hypotension/orthostasis
Capillary refill greater than 3 seconds
Narrowing pulse pressure
Urine output may be normal (>30 mL/hr) or as low as 20 mL/hr
Cool, clammy skin
Decreased skin turgor
Thirst
Dry mucous membranes
Light-headedness or dizziness
Changes in level of consciousness

Common Expected Outcome

Patient is normovolemic as evidenced by systolic BP greater than or equal to 90 mm Hg (or patient's baseline), absence of orthostasis, HR 60 to 100 beats/min, urinary output greater than 30 mL/hr, and normal skin turgor.

NOC Outcomes

Shock Severity: Hypovolemic; Fluid Balance; Hydration; Vital Signs

NIC Interventions

Fluid Monitoring; Invasive Hemodynamic Monitoring; Fluid Resuscitation; Bleeding Precautions; Bleeding Reduction: Gastrointestinal; Shock Management: Volume; Emergency Care; Hypovolemia Management

Ongoing Assessment

Actions/Interventions	Rationales
■ Assess for the early warning signs of hypovolemia, including changes in the level of consciousness.	Tachycardia, restlessness, headache, and a change in the level of consciousness may be the first signs of impending hypovolemic shock; these may be easily overlooked or attributed to pain, psychological trauma, and fear. QSEN: Safety.
▲ Assess the patient's HR, BP, and mean arterial pressure. Use direct intra-arterial monitoring as ordered.	Sinus tachycardia and increased arterial BP are seen in the early stages to maintain an adequate cardiac output; BP drops as the condition deteriorates. Reduced mean arterial pressure leads to compensatory responses. In young adults, compensatory mechanism responses maintain a normal BP until major blood loss occurs.
■ Monitor BP for orthostatic changes.	Postural hypotension is a common manifestation in fluid loss. Note the significance of the following levels of orthostatic hypotension: • Greater than 10 mm Hg drop—circulating blood volume is decreased by 20% • Greater than 20 to 30 mm Hg drop—circulating blood volume is decreased by 40%
■ Monitor for possible sources of fluid loss.	Specific sources of fluid loss guide therapy. These sources may include diarrhea, vomiting, profuse diaphoresis, polyuria, burns, ruptured organs, trauma, and wound drainage.

Actions/Interventions

- Record and evaluate intake and output.

- Assess skin turgor and mucous membranes.
- If trauma has occurred, evaluate and document the extent of the patient's injuries; use a primary survey (or another consistent survey method) or ABCs: airway with cervical spine control, breathing, circulation.

- Perform a secondary survey after all life-threatening injuries are ruled out or treated.

- If the only visible injury is an obvious head injury, look for other causes of hypovolemia (e.g., long-bone fractures, internal bleeding, external bleeding).
- ▲ If hemodynamic monitoring is in place, assess the central venous pressure (CVP), pulmonary artery diastolic pressure (PADP), pulmonary capillary wedge pressure, and cardiac output/cardiac index.

- If the patient is postsurgical, monitor blood loss (weigh dressings to determine fluid loss, monitor chest tube drainage, mark skin area).
- ▲ Obtain a spun hematocrit, and reevaluate every 30 minutes to 4 hours, depending on the patient's stability.

- ▲ Monitor coagulation studies, including INR, prothrombin time, partial thromboplastin time, fibrinogen, fibrin split products, and platelet counts, as appropriate.

Rationales

Accurate measurement is essential in detecting negative fluid balance and guiding therapy. Concentrated urine denotes a fluid deficit.

Loss of interstitial fluid causes a loss of skin turgor.

A primary survey helps identify imminent or potentially life-threatening injuries. This is a quick initial assessment. QSEN: Safety.

A secondary survey uses a methodical head-to-toe inspection. Anticipate potential causes of the shock state from the ongoing assessment.

Hypovolemic shock following trauma usually results from hemorrhage.

CVP provides information on filling pressures of the right side of the heart; PADP and pulmonary capillary wedge pressure reflect left-sided fluid volumes. Cardiac output/cardiac index provides an objective number to guide therapy. QSEN: Safety.

It is important to note an expanding hematoma or swelling or increased drainage to detect bleeding and/or coagulopathy.

Hematocrit decreases as fluids are administered because of dilution. As a rule of thumb, hematocrit decreases 1% per liter of normal saline solution used. Any other hematocrit decrease must be evaluated as an indication of continued blood loss.

Specific deficiencies guide treatment therapy.

Therapeutic Interventions

Actions/Interventions

- Control the external source of bleeding by applying direct pressure to the bleeding site.

- ▲ Initiate IV therapy. Start two shorter, large-bore peripheral IV lines.

- ▲ Prepare to administer a bolus of 1 to 2 L of IV fluids as ordered. Use crystalloid solutions for adequate fluid and electrolyte balance.

Rationales

External bleeding is controlled with firm, direct pressure on the bleeding site, using a thick dry dressing material. Prompt, effective treatment is needed to preserve vital organ function and life. QSEN: Safety.

Maintaining an adequate circulating blood volume is a priority. The amount of fluid infused is usually more important than the type of fluid (crystalloid, colloid, blood). The volume of fluid that can be infused is inversely related to the length of the IV catheter; it is best to use shorter, large-bore catheters.

The patient's response to treatment depends on the extent of the blood loss. If blood loss is mild (15%), the expected response is a rapid return to normal BP. If IV fluids are slowed, the patient remains normotensive. If the patient has lost 20% to 40% of circulating blood volume or has continued uncontrolled bleeding, a fluid bolus may produce normotension, but if fluids are slowed after the bolus, BP will deteriorate. Extreme caution is indicated in fluid replacement in older patients. Aggressive therapy may precipitate left ventricular dysfunction and pulmonary edema.

Cardiac and Vascular Care Plans

■ = Independent   ▲ = Interprofessional Collaboration

Actions/Interventions

- Encourage oral fluid intake if the patient is able.
- ▲ If hypovolemia is a result of severe burns, calculate the fluid replacement according to the extent of the burn and the patient's body weight.

- ▲ Administer blood products (e.g., packed red blood cells, fresh frozen plasma, platelets) as prescribed. Transfuse the patient with whole blood–packed red blood cells.

- ▲ If hypovolemia is a result of severe diarrhea or vomiting, administer antidiarrheal or antiemetic medications as prescribed, in addition to IV fluids.
- If bleeding is secondary to surgery, anticipate or prepare for a return to surgery.
- ▲ For trauma victims with internal bleeding (e.g., pelvic fracture), military antishock trousers (MAST) or pneumatic antishock garments (PASGs) may be used.

Rationales

The oral route assists in maintaining fluid balance.

Formulas such as the Parkland formula, which follows, guide fluid replacement therapy:

$$\% \text{ BSA (body surface area) burned} \times \text{Weight in kg} \times 4 \text{ mL lactated Ringer's solution} = \text{Total fluid to be infused over 24 hours}$$

Half is given intravenously over 8 hours and half is given over the next 16 hours.

Preparing fully crossmatched blood may take up to 1 hour in some laboratories. Consider using uncrossmatched or type-specific blood until crossmatched blood is available. If type-specific blood is unavailable, type O blood may be used for exsanguinating patients. If available, Rh-negative blood is preferred, especially for women of childbearing age. Autotransfusion may be used when there is massive bleeding in the thoracic cavity.

Treatment is guided by the cause of the problem. (NOTE: Disease must be ruled out first [e.g., *Clostridium difficile*, norovirus].)

Surgery may be the only way to correct the problem.

These devices are useful to tamponade bleeding. Hypovolemia from long-bone fractures (e.g., femur or pelvis) may be controlled by splinting with air splints. Hare traction splints or MASTs and/or PASGs may be used to reduce tissue and vessel damage from the manipulation of unstable fractures.

NANDA-I
NDx Decreased Cardiac Output

Common Related Factors

Fluid volume loss of 30% or more
Late uncompensated hypovolemic shock
Decreased ventricular filling (preload)
Alterations in HR and rhythm

Defining Characteristics

Tachycardia
Hypotension
Capillary refill greater than 3 seconds
Decreased pulse pressure
Decreased peripheral pulses
Cold, clammy skin
Change in level of consciousness
Decreased urinary output (<30 mL/hr)
Abnormal arterial blood gases (ABGs): acidosis and hypoxemia
Cardiac dysrhythmias

Common Expected Outcome

Patient maintains adequate cardiac output, as evidenced by strong peripheral pulses, systolic BP within 20 mm Hg of baseline, HR 60 to 100 beats/min with regular rhythm, urinary output 30 mL/hr or greater, warm and dry skin, and normal level of consciousness.

NOC Outcomes

Shock Severity: Hypovolemic; Cardiac Pump Effectiveness; Tissue Perfusion

NIC Interventions

Invasive Hemodynamic Monitoring; Hemodynamic Regulation; Emergency Care; Shock Management: Volume

Cardiac and Vascular Care Plans

Ongoing Assessment

Actions/Interventions

- Assess skin color, temperature, and moisture.

- ▲ Assess the patient's HR, BP, and mean arterial pressure. Use direct intra-arterial monitoring as ordered.

- Assess the peripheral and central pulses, including capillary refill.
- Assess for any changes in the level of consciousness.

- Assess the patient's urine output.

- Assess the respiratory rate, rhythm, and breath sounds.

- Assess the cardiac rhythm for dysrhythmias.

- ▲ Use pulse oximetry to monitor oxygen saturation; assess ABGs.

- ▲ If hemodynamic monitoring is in place, assess the central venous pressure (CVP), pulmonary artery diastolic pressure (PADP), pulmonary capillary wedge pressure, and cardiac output/cardiac index.

Rationales

Cool, pale, clammy skin is secondary to a compensatory increase in sympathetic nervous system stimulation and low cardiac output and desaturation.

Sinus tachycardia and increased arterial BP are seen in the early stages to maintain an adequate cardiac output. BP drops as the condition deteriorates. Auscultatory BP may be unreliable secondary to vasoconstriction. Reduced mean arterial pressure leads to compensatory responses. Older patients have a reduced response to catecholamines; thus their response to decreased cardiac output may be blunted, with less increase in HR.

Pulses are weak with reduced stroke volume and cardiac output. Capillary refill is slow, sometimes absent.

Early signs of cerebral hypoxia are restlessness and anxiety, with confusion and loss of consciousness occurring in later stages. Older patients are especially susceptible to reduced perfusion to vital organs.

The renal system compensates for low BP by retaining water. Oliguria is a classic sign of inadequate renal perfusion from reduced cardiac output.

Rapid, shallow respirations and the presence of crackles and wheezes are characteristic of shock.

Cardiac dysrhythmias may occur from low perfusion, acidosis, or hypoxia, as well as from side effects of cardiac medications used to treat this condition.

Pulse oximetry is a useful tool to detect changes in oxygenation. Oxygen saturation should be kept at 90% or greater. As shock increases, aerobic metabolism ceases and lactic acidosis ensues, raising the level of carbon dioxide and decreasing pH. The ability of the patient to attain high oxygen delivery parameters correlates with improved chance of survival. QSEN: Safety.

CVP provides information on filling pressures of the right side of the heart; PADP and pulmonary capillary wedge pressure reflect left-sided fluid volumes. Cardiac output provides an objective number to guide therapy. These direct measurements serve as optimal guides for therapy. Attention to these fluid parameters reduces the risk of harm to the patient. QSEN: Safety.

Therapeutic Interventions

Actions/Interventions

- ▲ Administer fluid and blood replacement therapy as described in the prior nursing care plan, *Deficient Fluid Volume.*

- ▲ If possible, use a fluid warmer or rapid fluid infuser.

- ▲ Provide electrolyte replacement as ordered.

Rationales

Maintaining an adequate circulating blood volume is a priority.

Fluid warmers keep core temperatures warm. Infusion of cold blood is associated with myocardial dysrhythmias and paradoxical hypotension. Macropore filtering IV devices should also be used to remove small clots and debris.

Electrolyte imbalance may cause dysrhythmias and other pathological states.

Cardiac and Vascular Care Plans

■ = Independent   ▲ = Interprofessional Collaboration

Actions/Interventions

▲ If the patient's condition progressively deteriorates, initiate cardiopulmonary resuscitation or other lifesaving measures according to Advanced Cardiac Life Support guidelines, as indicated.

Rationales

Shock unresponsive to fluid replacement can deteriorate to cardiogenic shock. Depending on etiological factors, inotropic agents, antidysrhythmics, vasopressors, or other medications can be used. These medications are based on recommendations from national organizations. QSEN: Evidence-based practice.

NANDA-I
NDx **Anxiety**

Common Related Factors
Health status change
Unfamiliar environment
Threat of death

Defining Characteristics
Verbalized anxiety
Restlessness and agitation
Apprehensive
Sympathetic stimulation
Increased awareness
Difficulty concentrating

Common Expected Outcomes
Patient uses effective coping mechanisms.
Patient describes a reduction in level of anxiety experienced.

NOC Outcomes
Anxiety Self-Control; Coping
NIC Interventions
Anxiety Reduction; Calming Technique

Ongoing Assessment

Actions/Interventions

■ Assess the patient's anxiety level (mild, severe). Note the signs and symptoms, especially nonverbal communication.
■ Assess the coping techniques commonly used.

Rationales

Shock can result in an acute life-threatening situation that will produce high levels of anxiety in the patient as well as in significant others.

Anxiety and ways of decreasing perceived anxiety are highly individualized. Interventions are most effective when they are consistent with the patient's established coping pattern. However, in the acute care setting these techniques may no longer be feasible. QSEN: Patient-centered care.

Therapeutic Interventions

Actions/Interventions

■ Acknowledge an awareness of the patient's anxiety.

■ Encourage the verbalization of feelings.

■ Maintain a confident, assured manner. Assure the patient and significant others of close, continuous monitoring that will ensure prompt intervention.

Rationales

Acknowledgment of the patient's feelings validates the patient's feelings and communicates acceptance of those feelings.

Talking about anxiety-producing situations and anxious feelings can help the patient perceive the situation in a less-threatening manner.

The staff's anxiety may be easily perceived by the patient. The patient's feeling of stability increases in a calm and nonthreatening atmosphere. The presence of a trusted person may help the patient feel less threatened.

Actions/Interventions

- Reduce unnecessary external stimuli by maintaining a quiet environment.
- Explain all procedures as appropriate, keeping explanations basic.

Rationales

Anxiety may escalate with excessive conversation, noise, and equipment around the patient.

Information helps allay anxiety. Patients who are anxious may not be able to comprehend anything more than simple, clear, brief instructions.

Related Care Plans

Impaired gas exchange, Chapter 2
Shock, cardiogenic, Chapter 5
Acute respiratory distress syndrome (ARDS), Chapter 6
Gastrointestinal bleeding, Chapter 8
Burns, Chapter 14

Shock, Septic

Distributive Shock; Sepsis; Bacteremia; Endotoxic Shock; Disseminated Intravascular Coagulation (DIC); Multiple Organ Failure

Septic shock is associated with severe infection and occurs after bacteremia of gram-negative bacilli (most common) or gram-positive cocci. Septic shock is mediated by a complex interaction of hormonal and chemical substances through an immune system response to bacterial endotoxins. In the early stages of sepsis, the body responds to infection by the normal inflammatory response. As the infection progresses, sepsis becomes more severe and leads to decreased tissue perfusion and oxygen delivery and multiple organ dysfunction syndrome (MODS). Septic shock occurs as an exaggerated inflammatory response that leads to hypotension even with adequate fluid resuscitation. The primary effects of septic shock are massive vasodilation, maldistribution of blood volume, and myocardial depression. The maldistribution of circulatory volume results in some tissues receiving more than adequate blood flow and other tissues receiving less than adequate blood flow. As shock progresses, disseminated intravascular coagulation may occur, resulting in a serious imbalance between clotting and bleeding.

Older patients are at increased risk for septic shock because of factors such as impaired immune response, impaired organ function, chronic debilitating illnesses, impaired mobility that can lead to pneumonia, decubitus ulcers, and loss of bladder control requiring indwelling catheters. Patients with central lines that provide a direct access point for microorganisms are at risk for central line–associated bloodstream infections (CLABSIs). The mortality rate from septic shock is very high, especially in older patients. Immunocompromised patients and those with chronic diseases are also at increased risk. Patients are usually treated in an intensive care unit. Treatment is focused on providing fluid volume resuscitation and antibiotic therapy based on causative bacteria and/or cocci and supporting major organ dysfunction. The Surviving Sepsis Campaign Bundles are the core of the sepsis improvement efforts. Each hospital's sepsis protocol may be customized, but it must meet the standards created by the Bundle.

Cardiac and Vascular Care Plans

■ = Independent   ▲ = Interprofessional Collaboration

NDx Infection

Common Related Factors

An infectious process of either gram-negative or gram-positive bacteria

The most common causative organisms are as follows:

- *Escherichia coli*
- *Klebsiella pneumoniae*
- *Proteus*
- *Pseudomonas aeruginosa*
- *Staphylococcus aureus*
- *Streptococcus*
- *Candida albicans*

Common Expected Outcome

The patient is free of infection, as evidenced by normal body temperature, normal white blood cell count, negative cultures, absence of chills, and normal level of consciousness.

Defining Characteristics

Changes in level of consciousness
Fever or chills
Ruddy appearance with warm, dry skin (early stage)
Cool clammy skin (later stage)
Leukocytosis
Positive blood cultures

NOC Outcomes

Shock Severity: Septic Shock; Infection Severity; Thermoregulation

NIC Interventions

Vital Signs Monitoring; Medication Administration; Temperature Regulation

---

Ongoing Assessment

Actions/Interventions	Rationales
■ Monitor the patient's HR and BP.	Septic shock can present in two phases. During the early, more treatable phase (high-output shock), there is an increase in cardiac output reflected by tachycardia and normal or elevated BP. However, as shock continues and the septic phase ensues, blood vessels dilate, causing hypovolemia and hypotension. Refractory hypotension despite optimal fluid therapy is a criterion for diagnosing septic shock.
■ Assess for the presence of chills and a febrile state.	Chills often precede temperature spikes. Temperature provides information about the patient's response to invading organisms. Temperature may be higher than 38°C or lower than 36°C.
■ Assess the skin turgor, color, temperature, and peripheral pulses.	In early septic shock, warm, dry, flushed skin and bounding pulses are evident as a result of initial vasodilation (warm shock). As the shock state continues, skin becomes cool, clammy, and cyanotic with reduced peripheral pulses.
■ Assess the level of consciousness.	Altered cerebral tissue perfusion may be the first sign of compensatory response to the septic state. The patient may experience fatigue, malaise, anxiety, or confusion. Mild disorientation is common in older adults.
▲ Use pulse oximetry to monitor oxygen saturation.	Pulse oximetry is a useful tool to detect changes in oxygenation. Oxygen saturation should be kept at 90% or greater.
▲ Assess arterial blood gases (ABGs).	Initially, respiratory alkalosis from hyperventilation may be evident. As shock increases, aerobic metabolism ceases and lactic acidosis ensues, raising the level of carbon dioxide and decreasing pH.

Cardiac and Vascular Care Plans

Actions/Interventions

- Assess the related factors of infection thoroughly:
  - *Lungs:* Assess lung sounds and the presence of sputum, including color, odor, and amount. Note the presence of crackles and decreased breath sounds.
  - *Genitourinary:* Monitor urinalysis reports, assess the color and opacity of urine, and assess for the presence of drainage or pus around the Foley catheter.
  - *Gastrointestinal:* Check for abdominal distention, and assess for bowel sounds and abdominal tenderness.
  - *Central lines/IV catheters:* Assess all insertion sites for redness, swelling, and drainage.
  - *Surgical wounds:* Assess all wounds for signs of infection, including redness, swelling, and drainage.
  - *Pain:* Obtain the patient's subjective statement of the location and description of pain or discomfort. This may help localize a site.

- ▲ Initiate the bundle for resuscitation and management of severe sepsis:

  - Monitor serum lactate levels.

  - Obtain culture and sensitivity (C&S) samples as ordered before administering antibiotics.

- ▲ Draw peak and trough antibiotic titers as needed.

- ▲ Monitor white blood cell counts.

- ▲ Monitor for toxicity from antibiotic therapy, especially in patients with hepatic and/or renal insufficiency or failure and in older patients.

Rationales

The cause of shock guides the treatment plan. Initial antibiotics are selected depending on the most likely site of infection. As culture reports are obtained, the most effective antibiotics will be selected. QSEN: Evidence-based practice.

The Surviving Sepsis Campaign Bundle provides key assessments that should be performed within 3 hours of time of presentation with severe sepsis as they guide further treatment. QSEN: Evidence-based practice.

Lactate levels will rise as oxygenation and tissue perfusion are compromised.

Evidence of infection through a positive blood culture is a criterion for diagnosis. C&S reports show which antibiotic will be effective against the invading organism.

Serum drug levels help ensure an appropriate and safe level of antibiotic for the patient.

A white blood cell count provides data on the progression of sepsis and the response to treatment.

Aminoglycosides should be followed with urinalysis and serum creatinine levels at least three times per week. Chloramphenicol should be restricted in patients with liver disease.

Therapeutic Interventions

Actions/Interventions

- ▲ Initiate the early administration of broad-spectrum antibiotics as prescribed.

- Manage indwelling catheters (e.g. central lines, urinary catheter, IV catheter) to minimize the risk of infection. Change catheters as needed should an infection result.

Rationales

The Surviving Sepsis Campaign Bundle for resuscitation and management of septic shock recommends that antibiotic therapy begins with broad-spectrum antibiotics (after the C&S is obtained but before the actual C&S report is received). The Joint Commission's National Patient Safety Goals recommend that gram-negative IV antibiotics be given before causative organisms are identified. After the C&S report is received, the physician should be notified if the organism is not sensitive to the present antibiotic coverage. The antibiotic may then be changed or supplemented. QSEN: Evidence-based practice.

Infection prevention begins with removing possible sites for bacterial entry into the body. Invasive catheters disrupt skin and mucous membranes and interfere with the body's first line of defense against infection. QSEN: Safety.

Cardiac and Vascular Care Plans

■ = Independent   ▲ = Interprofessional Collaboration

Actions/Interventions

▲ Maintain a temperature in the optimal range:
- Administer antipyretics as prescribed.
- Apply a cooling mattress.
- Administer tepid sponge baths.
- Limit the number of blankets/linens used to cover patients.

▲ Initiate appropriate isolation measures.

▲ Assist with the incision and drainage of wounds, irrigation, and sterile application of saline-soaked 4 × 4s as indicated.

▲ Manage the cause of infection, and anticipate a surgical consult as necessary.

▲ If signs of disseminated intravascular coagulation (DIC) occur, refer to the nursing care plan for Disseminated Intravascular Coagulation, Chapter 10.

Rationales

Normothermia prevents stress on the cardiovascular system and promotes comfort.

Isolation prevents the spread of infection. QSEN: Safety. Early treatment promotes recovery.

Surgical treatment may be indicated to drain pus or abscess, resolve obstruction, or repair a perforated organ.

Disseminated intravascular coagulation is a coagulation disorder that prompts overstimulation of the normal clotting cascade and results in simultaneous thrombosis and hemorrhage. Specific interventions guide therapy to treat the underlying cause and manage complications from this life-threatening complication.

NANDA-I
NDx **Deficient Fluid Volume**

Common Related Factors

Early septic shock
Decrease in systemic vascular resistance
Increased capillary permeability
Increased metabolic rate (fever, infection)
Failure of regulatory mechanisms

Defining Characteristics

Hypotension
Tachycardia and/or weak pulse
Decreased urine output (<30 mL/hr)
Concentrated urine
Decreased skin turgor
Dry mucous membranes
Weakness

Common Expected Outcome

Patient experiences adequate fluid volume as evidenced by urine output greater than 30 mL/hr, HR less than 100 beats/min, systolic BP greater than or equal to 90 mm Hg (or patient's baseline), and normal skin turgor.

NOC Outcomes
Shock Severity: Septic Shock; Fluid Balance
NIC Interventions
Fluid Monitoring; Fluid Resuscitation; Invasive Hemodynamic Monitoring; Hemodynamic Regulation; Shock Management: Vasogenic

---

Ongoing Assessment

Actions/Interventions

■ Assess the patient's HR, BP and mean arterial pressure (MAP).

■ Assess the patient's urine output.

Rationales

During the early phase of shock, tachycardia and normal BP are evident, but as shock progresses with subsequent vasodilation, hypotension ensues.

The renal system compensates for low BP by retaining water. Oliguria is a classic sign of inadequate renal perfusion from reduced cardiac output. As shock continues and the kidneys fail, urine output may stop, resulting in buildup of metabolic waste products.

Cardiac and Vascular Care Plans

Actions/Interventions

■ Assess fluid balance, noting skin turgor and mucous membranes.

▲ If hemodynamic monitoring is in place, assess the central venous pressure (CVP), pulmonary artery diastolic pressure (PADP), pulmonary capillary wedge pressure, and cardiac output/cardiac index.

▲ When initiating fluid challenges, closely monitor the patient.

Rationales

Compromised regulatory mechanisms may result in fluid and sodium retention. Loss of interstitial fluid causes loss of skin turgor. As sepsis continues, toxins cause leakage of fluid into tissues and cause swelling.

CVP provides information on filling pressures of the right side of the heart; PADP and pulmonary capillary wedge pressure reflect left-sided fluid volumes. Cardiac output/cardiac index provides an objective number to guide therapy during fluid resuscitation and vasopressor administration. Identifying early changes in fluid balance guides specific interventions. QSEN: Safety.

Close monitoring prevents iatrogenic volume overload. However, patients with sepsis usually have refractory hypotension despite aggressive fluid therapy.

Therapeutic Interventions

Actions/Interventions

▲ Perform fluid resuscitation aggressively as ordered, using crystalloids for hypotension or elevated lactate levels. Use caution with fluid replacement in older patients.

▲ If there is a poor or no response to fluid resuscitation, administer vasoactive substances, such as phenylephrine hydrochloride (Neo-Synephrine), norepinephrine bitartrate (Levophed), or dopamine, as prescribed to maintain MAP at 65 mm Hg or more.

Rationales

Fluid administration is necessary to support tissue perfusion. Infusion rates will vary depending on clinical status. The 6-hour Surviving Sepsis Campaign Bundle directs administration of vasopressors for hypotension persistent despite volume resuscitation. The fluid needs in septic patients may exceed 8 to 20 L in the first 24 hours. Older patients may be more prone to congestive heart failure. In these patients, monitor closely for signs of iatrogenic fluid volume overload. QSEN: Evidence-based practice.

In early septic shock the cardiac output is high or normal. At this point, the vasoactive agents are administered for their alpha-adrenergic effect to raise BP.

Decreased Cardiac Output

Common Related Factors

Late septic shock: a decrease in tissue perfusion leads to increased lactic acid production and systemic acidosis, which causes a decrease in myocardial contractility

Gram-negative infections may cause a direct myocardial toxic effect

Hypovolemia

Defining Characteristics

Decreased peripheral pulses

Cold, clammy skin

Hypotension

Tachycardia

Change in level of consciousness

Decreased urinary output less than 30 mL/hr

Elevated lactate levels

Abnormal arterial blood gas levels: acidosis and hypoxemia

Cardiac and Vascular Care Plans

■ = Independent   ▲ = Interprofessional Collaboration

Common Expected Outcome

Patient maintains adequate cardiac output, as evidenced by strong peripheral pulses; systolic BP within 20 mm Hg of baseline, HR 60 to 100 beats/min with regular rhythm; urine output greater than 30 mL/hr; warm and dry skin, and normal level of consciousness.

NOC Outcomes
Shock Severity: Septic Shock; Cardiac Pump Effectiveness

NIC Interventions
Invasive Hemodynamic Monitoring; Hemodynamic Regulation; Acid-Base Management: Metabolic Acidosis; Shock Management: Vasogenic

---

Ongoing Assessment

Actions/Interventions	Rationales
■ Assess the skin's warmth and the quality of the peripheral pulses.	Compensatory peripheral vasoconstriction in the late stages of septic shock causes cool, pale, diaphoretic skin. Pulses are weak with reduced stroke volume and cardiac output.
■ Assess for any changes in the level of consciousness.	Early signs of cerebral hypoxia are restlessness and anxiety, with confusion and lethargy occurring in later stages.
▲ Assess the patient's HR, BP, and MAP. Use direct intra-arterial monitoring as ordered.	Sinus tachycardia and increased arterial BP are seen in the early stages to maintain an adequate cardiac output. However, as sepsis progresses, toxins are produced by the bacterial cells in the body, resulting in release of cytokines that cause extensive vasodilation and dangerously low BPs. The lowered BP compromises perfusion to vital organs. Auscultatory BP may be unreliable secondary to vasoconstriction.
■ Assess the patient's urine output.	The renal system compensates for low BP by retaining water. Oliguria is a classic sign of inadequate renal perfusion from reduced cardiac output. As shock continues and the kidneys fail, urine output may stop, resulting in buildup of metabolic waste products. QSEN: Safety.
■ Assess the cardiac rhythm for dysrhythmias.	Cardiac dysrhythmias may occur from the low perfusion state, acidosis, or hypoxia, as well as from side effects of cardiac medications used to treat this condition.
▲ If hemodynamic monitoring is in place, assess the central venous pressure (CVP), pulmonary artery diastolic pressure (PADP), pulmonary capillary wedge pressure, and cardiac output.	CVP provides information on filling pressures of the right side of the heart; PADP and pulmonary capillary wedge pressure reflect left-sided fluid volumes. QSEN: Safety.

Therapeutic Interventions

Actions/Interventions	Rationales
▲ Place the patient in the physiological position for shock: head of the bed elevated 10 degrees while hypotensive and the lower extremities elevated 20 to 30 degrees with the knees straight.	This position promotes venous return and increases cardiac output.
▲ Administer inotropic and vasopressor agents: dobutamine hydrochloride, dopamine, digoxin, or milrinone. Continuously monitor their effectiveness. Administer sodium bicarbonate to treat acidosis.	These medications improve myocardial contractility and cardiac output. Sodium bicarbonate buffers the excess lactic acid released by anoxic tissues. These medications are based on recommendations from the Surviving Sepsis Campaign Bundle. QSEN: Evidence-based practice.

Risk for Ineffective Breathing Pattern

Common Risk Factors
Progressive shock state
Lactic acidosis

Common Expected Outcome
Patient will maintain an effective breathing pattern, as evidenced by relaxed breathing at normal rate.

NOC Outcome
Respiratory Status: Ventilation
NIC Interventions
Respiratory Monitoring; Ventilation Assistance

Ongoing Assessment

Actions/Interventions	Rationales
■ Assess the respiratory rate, rhythm, and depth.	Rapid, shallow respirations may occur from hypoxia or from acidosis with sepsis. As shock continues, lung function deteriorates, causing fluid to accumulate in the lungs. Development of hypoventilation indicates that immediate ventilator support is needed. QSEN: Safety.
■ Assess for any increase in the work of breathing: shortness of breath and the use of accessory muscles.	As septic shock progresses, patients may experience acute respiratory distress syndrome. QSEN: Safety.
■ Assess the lungs, noting areas of decreased ventilation and the presence of adventitious sounds.	Moist crackles are caused by increased pulmonary capillary permeability and increased intra-alveolar edema. Older patients, who most commonly experience septic shock, may have difficulty clearing their airways, resulting in atelectasis and pneumonia.
▲ Use pulse oximetry to monitor oxygen saturation; assess arterial blood gases.	Oxygen saturation should be kept at 90% or greater. As shock increases, aerobic metabolism ceases and lactic acidosis ensues, raising the level of carbon dioxide and decreasing pH. Identifying changes in oxygenation and acid-base balance, and initiating early intervention reduces the risk for harm. QSEN: Safety.

Therapeutic Interventions

Actions/Interventions	Rationales
■ Position the patient with proper body alignment for an optimal breathing pattern.	If not contraindicated, a sitting position allows for adequate diaphragmatic and lung excursion.
■ Assist with coughing, and suction as needed.	Productive coughing is the most effective way to remove moist secretions. If the patient is unable to perform coughing, suctioning may be needed to promote airway patency.
■ Provide reassurance and allay anxiety by staying with the patient during episodes of respiratory distress.	Respiratory distress can produce an extremely anxious state that can result in rapid, shallow respirations and increase noneffective breathing efforts.
▲ Administer oxygen as prescribed.	Oxygen may be required to maintain oxygen saturation at 90% or greater. Desaturation leads to tissue hypoxia, acidosis, dysrhythmias, and a decreased level of consciousness.

Cardiac and Vascular Care Plans

■ = Independent ▲ = Interprofessional Collaboration

Actions/Interventions

■ Anticipate the need for intubation and mechanical ventilation if the patient is unable to maintain adequate gas exchange.

Rationales

Rapid, efficient intervention is critical to preserve vital organ function and life. Appropriate use of safety-enhancing technology minimizes the risk of harm to the patient. QSEN: Safety.

NANDA-I NDx Deficient Knowledge

Common Related Factors

Insufficient information
Insufficient interest in learning
Misinformation presented by others

Common Expected Outcome

Patient or significant others verbalize understanding of disease process and treatments used.

Defining Characteristics

Insufficient knowledge
Inaccurate follow-through of instruction
Inappropriate behavior

NOC Outcomes

Knowledge: Disease Process; Knowledge: Infection Management

NIC Interventions

Health Literacy Enhancement; Learning Facilitation; Teaching: Disease Process; Infection Protection

---

Ongoing Assessment

Action/Intervention

■ Evaluate the patient's understanding of septic shock and the patient's overall condition.

Rationale

Information guides the starting point for educational intervention. QSEN: Patient-centered care.

Therapeutic Interventions

Actions/Interventions

■ Keep the patient or significant others informed of the disease process and present status of the patient.
■ Explain the common factors that placed the patient at risk for septic shock:
  • Advanced age with a declining immune system
  • Malnourishment and/or poor hydration
  • Debilitating chronic illnesses
  • Insertion of an indwelling catheter
  • Surgical and diagnostic procedure
  • Decubitus ulcer or wounds
  • Cross-contamination or exposure to resistant organisms
■ Instruct regarding general hygiene measures to reduce the risk for infection.

Rationales

Patients are better able to ask questions when they have basic information about what to expect.
Patients may be unaware of situations or procedures that can place them at risk.

Practices such as good personal hygiene, hand washing, adequate rest, balanced diet, exercise, and oral care all promote reduced infection risks. QSEN: Safety.

Cardiac and Vascular Care Plans

Related Care Plans

Fear, Chapter 2
Imbalanced nutrition: Less than body requirements,
    Chapter 2
Ineffective peripheral tissue perfusion, Chapter 2
Central venous access devices, Chapter 4
Shock, hypovolemic, Chapter 5
Acute respiratory distress syndrome (ARDS),
    Chapter 6
Disseminated intravascular coagulation, Chapter 10
Acute kidney injury, Chapter 11

Thrombosis, Deep Vein

Venous Thromboembolic Disease; Phlebitis; Phlebothrombosis

Thrombophlebitis is the inflammation of the wall of a vein, usually resulting in the formation of a blood clot (thrombosis) that may partially or completely block the flow of blood through the vessel. Venous thrombophlebitis usually occurs in the lower extremities. It may occur in superficial veins, which, although painful, is not life threatening and does not require hospitalization, or it may occur in a deep vein, which can be life threatening because clots may break free (embolize) and cause a pulmonary embolism. Three factors contribute to the development of deep vein thrombosis (DVT): venous stasis, hypercoagulability, and endothelial damage to the vein. Prolonged immobility is the primary cause of venous stasis. Hypercoagulability is seen in patients with deficient

fluid volume, oral contraceptive use, smoking, and certain malignancies. Venous wall damage may occur secondary to IV infusions, certain medications, fractures, and contrast x-ray studies. DVT most commonly occurs in lower extremities, where it is often asymptomatic and resolves in a few days. In the inpatient setting, all patients are required to be assessed for venous thromboembolism (VTE). The Joint Commission has a VTE bundle to guide prophylaxis and treatment for this high-risk condition. More proximal DVTs are associated with more severe symptoms and carry a higher risk for dislodgement and migration. Treatment is supportive, usually with anticoagulant therapy. Goals are to reduce risk for complications and prevent recurrence.

NANDA-I NDx Ineffective Peripheral Tissue Perfusion

Common Related Factors

Venous stasis
Injury to vessel wall
Hypercoagulability of blood

Defining Characteristics

Usually involves changes in femoral, popliteal, or small calf
    veins:
• Pain
• Edema (unilateral)
• Tenderness
• Increased warmth in leg
• Pain during palpation of calf muscle
• May be asymptomatic

Common Expected Outcomes

Patient maintains optimal peripheral tissue perfusion in affected extremity, as evidenced by strong palpable pulses, reduction in or absence of pain, warm and dry extremities, and adequate capillary refill.
Patient does not experience pulmonary embolism, as evidenced by normal breathing, normal heart rate, and absence of dyspnea and chest pain.

NOC Outcomes

Thrombus Prevention; Risk Control: Thrombus;
    Tissue Perfusion: Peripheral

NIC Interventions

Embolus Care: Peripheral; Teaching: Disease
    Process

Cardiac and Vascular Care Plans

■ = Independent   ▲ = Interprofessional Collaboration

Ongoing Assessment

Actions/Interventions

- Assess for the signs and symptoms of deep vein thrombosis (DVT). (See Defining Characteristics.)
- Assess for contributing factors: immobility, leg trauma, intraoperative positioning (especially in older patients), dehydration, smoking, varicose veins, venous stasis, pregnancy, obesity, surgery, malignancy, and the use of oral contraceptives.
- Measure the circumference of the affected leg with a tape measure.

▲ Monitor the results of diagnostic tests:

- Duplex ultrasound

- D-dimer assay

- Impedance plethysmography
- Contrast venography

▲ Monitor the coagulation profile (prothrombin time [PT]/ international normalized ratio [INR]/partial thromboplastin time [PTT]).

Rationales

DVT can be challenging to diagnose, especially if it involves a distal vein.

Many patients are asymptomatic. Knowledge of high-risk situations aids in early detection. QSEN: Patient-centered care; Safety.

Measurement will document progression or resolution of swelling. The affected leg will be larger. In some patients, unequal leg circumference may be the only sign of DVT.

These tests are used to document the location of a clot and the status of the affected vein.

Ultrasound uses a Doppler probe to document reduced flow, especially in popliteal and iliofemoral veins.

D-dimer is a global marker for clot lysis. It does not provide any information about the site of the problem.

This test uses BP cuffs to record changes in venous flow.

In this test radiopaque contrast medium is injected through a foot vein to localize thrombi in the deep venous system.

The results of coagulation studies are used to measure the effectiveness of anticoagulant therapy. The PTT is used for patients receiving IV heparin. The PT/INR is used for patients receiving warfarin. Baseline values are obtained before the first dose of anticoagulant is administered. Repeated tests are done at prescribed intervals to adjust drug dosages to achieve desired changes in coagulation. *Note:* Newer anticoagulants (e.g., rivaroxaban) do not require laboratory monitoring because they achieve a steady therapeutic state. QSEN: Safety.

Therapeutic Interventions

Actions/Interventions

- Encourage and maintain bed rest with the affected leg elevated (depending on size and location of clot) as indicated.

▲ Administer/instruct in the use of anticoagulant therapy as ordered:
- Unfractionated heparin
- Low-molecular-weight heparin (enoxaparin, dalteparin, apixaban)
- Bivalirudin/Lepirudin
- Warfarin (Coumadin)

Rationales

Bed rest, the cornerstone of past treatments, may not be required for clots in the lower leg, because these are less likely to embolize. It may be required for upper extremity clots. Elevation of the leg will reduce venous pooling and edema.

Anticoagulation therapy will prevent further clot formation by decreasing normal activity of the clotting mechanism. A variety of direct thrombin inhibitors is available, the choice depending on the patient's clinical situation. Unfractionated heparin was the cornerstone of treatment. However, it can also reduce platelet aggregation, resulting in heparin-induced thrombocytopenia. Today, low-molecular-weight heparin and newer derivatives are more commonly used. Oral anticoagulant therapy (warfarin) will be initiated while the patient is still receiving heparin because the onset of action for warfarin can be up to 72 hours. Heparin will be discontinued once the warfarin reaches therapeutic levels. These medications are based on recommendations from national organizations. QSEN: Evidence-based practice.

Actions/Interventions

▲ Administer analgesics as indicated.
■ Maintain adequate hydration.

■ Provide warm, moist heat to the affected site.
▲ Apply below-knee compression stockings as prescribed. Ensure that the stockings are the correct size and are applied correctly.
▲ With a massive DVT severely compromising tissue perfusion, anticipate thrombolytic therapy.

▲ If the patient shows no response to conventional therapy or if the patient is not a candidate for anticoagulation, anticipate surgical treatment:
  • Thrombectomy

  • Placement of a vena cava filter

Rationales

Analgesics relieve pain and promote comfort.
Hydration prevents an increased viscosity of blood, which contributes to venous stasis and clotting.
Heat relieves pain and inflammation.
These stockings promote venous blood flow and decrease venous stagnation. Inaccurately applied stockings can serve as a tourniquet and can facilitate clot formation.
Thrombolytic therapy is reserved for severe cases. Clot lysis carries a higher risk for bleeding than anticoagulation because it dissolves both undesired and therapeutic clots. Therefore its use is restricted to patients with a severe embolism that significantly compromises blood flow to the tissues. Therapy must be initiated soon after the onset of symptoms (within 5 days).

Thrombectomy is a procedure to excise the clot if a major vein is occluded.
This filter traps any migrating clots and prevents pulmonary embolism. It is recommended for patients who cannot take anticoagulants or those with recurrent DVT despite anticoagulant therapy.

NANDA-I
NDx **Risk for Bleeding**

Common Risk Factors

Anticoagulation therapy for deep vein thrombosis (DVT)
Abnormal blood profiles

Common Expected Outcomes

Patient maintains therapeutic blood level of anticoagulant, as evidenced by prothombin time (PT), international normalized ratio (INR), and partial throboplastin time (PTT) within desired range.
Patient does not experience bleeding.

NOC Outcomes
Risk Control; Blood Coagulation
NIC Interventions
Bleeding Precautions; Bleeding Reduction

Ongoing Assessment

Actions/Interventions

▲ Monitor platelet counts and coagulation test results (INR, PT, PTT).

Rationales

The effects of anticoagulation therapy must be closely monitored to reduce the risk for bleeding. The type of test depends on the anticoagulation medication administered. Newer anticoagulants are easier to use than warfarin because there is less bleeding risk without the monitoring required for warfarin. They achieve a therapeutic steady state. QSEN: Safety.

Cardiac and Vascular Care Plans

■ = Independent   ▲ = Interprofessional Collaboration

Actions/Interventions

- Assess for the signs and symptoms of bleeding.
- ▲ Monitor platelets and the heparin-induced platelet aggregation (HIPA) status.

Rationales

Early assessment facilitates prompt treatment. QSEN: Safety.

Severe platelet reduction can occur with heparin use, especially unfractionated heparin therapy, and is known as heparin-induced thrombocytopenia (HIT). HIT is less commonly seen with the use of low-molecular-weight heparin.

Therapeutic Interventions

Actions/Interventions

- ▲ Administer anticoagulant therapy as prescribed (continuous IV heparin/subcutaneous low-molecular-weight heparin; oral anticoagulants).

- ▲ If bleeding occurs while on IV heparin:
  - Stop the infusion.
  - Recheck the PTT level stat.
  - Reevaluate the dose of heparin on the basis of the PTT result.
- ▲ Convert from IV anticoagulation to oral anticoagulation after the appropriate length of therapy. Monitor INR, PT, and PTT levels.
- ▲ If HIPA is positive, stop all heparin products and anticipate a hematology consult.

Rationales

Anticoagulants are given to prevent further clot formation. The type of medication varies per protocol and severity of the clot. These medications are based on recommendations from national organizations. QSEN: Safety; Evidence-based practice.

Laboratory data guide further treatment. The guide for the PTT level is 1.5 to 2 times normal. QSEN: Safety.

PT or INR levels should be in an adequate range for anticoagulation before discontinuing heparin.

Continuation of heparin products further complicates the situation. Specialty expertise is needed. QSEN: Teamwork and collaboration.

NANDA-I
NDx Deficient Knowledge

Common Related Factors

Insufficient information
Insufficient interest in learning
Misinformation presented by others

Defining Characteristics

Insufficient knowledge
Inaccurate follow-through of instruction
Inappropriate behavior

Common Expected Outcome

Patient and/or significant others verbalize understanding of DVT process, management, and prevention.

NOC Outcomes
Knowledge: Thrombus Prevention; Knowledge: Disease Process; Knowledge: Treatment Regimen

NIC Interventions
Health Literacy Enhancement; Learning Facilitation; Teaching: Disease Process; Teaching: Prescribed Medication

Cardiac and Vascular Care Plans

 evolve For additional care plans, go to http://evolve.elsevier.com/Gulanick/.

Ongoing Assessment

Action/Intervention	Rationale
■ Assess the patient's understanding of the causes, treatment, and prevention plan for deep vein thrombosis (DVT).	This information provides an important starting point in education. DVT requires preventive action to reduce the risk for recurrence. QSEN: Patient-centered care.

Therapeutic Interventions

Actions/Interventions	Rationales
■ Explain the contributing factors that place people at risk for blood clots.	Knowledge of causative factors provides direction for subsequent treatment. Preventing thrombus formation is an ongoing concern.
■ Explain the rationale for the treatment of DVT.	DVT may range from mild to life threatening and may require additional treatment with anticoagulation.
■ Explain the need for activity restriction and elevation of the leg.	Activity restriction and elevation of the leg prevent embolization seen with more significant DVT.
■ Instruct the patient in the correct application of compression stockings.	Stockings applied incorrectly can act as a tourniquet and facilitate clot formation.
■ Instruct the patient to avoid rubbing or massaging the calf.	Avoidance will prevent breaking off the clot, which may circulate as an embolus.
■ Instruct the patient to take medications as prescribed, explaining their actions, dosages, and side effects.	Accurate knowledge reduces future complications. Analgesics and anti-inflammatory medications may be needed for short-term symptom relief. Patients may require anticoagulation for weeks or long term, depending on the risks.
■ Discuss and give the patient a list of signs and symptoms of excessive anticoagulation.	Patients need to self-manage their condition. Early assessment facilitates prompt treatment. QSEN: Safety.
■ Inform the patient of the need for routine laboratory testing while on warfarin.	Continued regular assessment of warfarin is necessary to prevent both recurrence of clots and active bleeding. Newer anticoagulants are easier to use than warfarin because there is less bleeding risk without the monitoring required for warfarin.
■ Discuss the following measures to prevent recurrence:	Information enables the patient to assume control during recovery. Attention to these parameters reduces the risk of harm to the patient. QSEN: Safety.
• Avoiding staying in one position for long periods; when traveling, move the feet/legs often	Avoidance will prevent venous stasis (at home, on a train or plane, or at a desk).
• Not sitting with the legs crossed	The patient should avoid any position that compresses the veins and limits venous return.
• Maintaining a healthy body weight	Obesity contributes to venous insufficiency and venous hypertension through the compression of the main veins in the pelvic region.
• Maintaining an adequate fluid status	Adequate hydration prevents hypercoagulability.
• Wearing properly sized, correctly applied compression stockings as prescribed	Patients with DVT are at high risk for redevelopment and may need to wear stockings over the long term.
• Avoiding constricting garters or socks with tight bands	Wearing constricting clothing reduces optimal blood flow and promotes clotting.
• Quitting smoking	Nicotine is a vasoconstrictor that promotes clotting.
• Participating in an exercise program	Walking, swimming, and cycling help promote venous return through the contraction of the calf and thigh muscles. These muscles act as a pump to compress veins and support the column of blood returning to the heart.

Cardiac and Vascular Care Plans

■ = Independent   ▲ = Interprofessional Collaboration

Actions/Interventions	Rationales
■ For patients with DVT, instruct in the following signs of pulmonary embolus: • Sudden chest pain • Tachypnea • Tachycardia • Shortness of breath • Restlessness	These symptoms may be the result of a clot that breaks off from the original clot in the leg and travels to the lung. QSEN: Safety.
■ Discuss the safety or precautionary measures to use while on anticoagulant therapy: the need to inform the dentist or other caregivers before treatment, the use of an electric razor, the use of a soft toothbrush.	These measures help reduce the risk for bleeding. QSEN: Safety.

Related Care Plan

Pulmonary embolism, Chapter 6

Venous Insufficiency, Chronic

Postphlebitic Syndrome; Peripheral Venous Hypertension; Venous Stasis Ulcer

Chronic venous insufficiency occurs from a disruption in the venous system that results in the pressure from the venous blood column no longer being supported toward the heart. This pressure is directed as backflow to the ankle area. The most common causes are congenital venous valve insufficiency, acquired valve incompetence from venous valve prolapse (often from history of deep vein thrombosis [DVT] or varicose veins), venous obstruction from tumor or fibrosis, or calf muscle pump malfunction from sedentary lifestyle or muscle wasting disease. The increased backflow and pressure cause dilation of the venules of the skin, primarily in the ankle area, with resulting movement of fluid from the vascular bed to the tissue bed. Because the endothelium of the venules is subjected to higher than normal pressures, red blood cells move across the vessel wall into the interstitial spaces. When these red blood cells break down, they deposit hemosiderin in the tissues. The presence of hemosiderin in the tissues produces the characteristic skin color changes in venous insufficiency. The clinical manifestations of chronic venous insufficiency include dull aching, tenderness, pain in leg; leg pain getting worse when standing or when legs are raised; edema; skin color changes; dermatitis; and venous stasis ulcers. Once skin ulceration occurs, it is difficult to heal. Ulcers may recur with minimal skin trauma.

NANDA-I NDx Risk for Ineffective Peripheral Tissue Perfusion

Common Risk Factors

Increased venous pressure
Dependent edema

Common Expected Outcomes

Patient maintains optimal peripheral tissue perfusion in affected extremity, as evidenced by strong palpable pulse, reduction in and/or absence of pain, warm and dry extremities, and adequate capillary refill.
Patient demonstrates measures to increase venous return and decrease leg edema.

NOC Outcomes
Tissue Perfusion: Peripheral; Circulation Status
NIC Interventions
Circulatory Care: Venous Insufficiency; Lower Extremity Monitoring

Cardiac and Vascular Care Plans

Ongoing Assessment

Actions/Interventions	Rationales
■ Assess the lower extremities for the following:	
• Edema (by measuring the leg circumference)	Edema of chronic venous insufficiency may not be relieved with elevation of the extremity. Assessment provides data on the response to therapy.
• Skin color	Skin may have a dark brown discoloration caused by deposition of hemosiderin in the tissues. This condition is sometimes referred to as brawny edema or stasis dermatitis.
• Pain	The patient may report a dull aching or heaviness in the legs.
• Skin changes	The patient may have areas of induration as a result of liposclerosis. Areas of the skin may be thinned or scarred from previous stasis ulcers.
▲ Monitor the results of Doppler flow studies.	This diagnostic test assesses venous flow and any obstruction.

Therapeutic Interventions

Actions/Interventions	Rationales
■ Encourage the patient to keep the legs elevated when not ambulating. The patient may benefit from the placement of the foot of the bed on 6-inch blocks to enhance venous return while sleeping.	The goal of treatment is to reduce venous hypertension and reduce tissue edema. Elevation uses the effects of gravity to promote venous return.
▲ Apply appropriate venous compression devices such as support hose or pneumatic compression.	Prescription support hose are worn below the knee to support venous return. Hosiery should apply about 40 mm Hg of compression. Above-the-knee hosiery is not needed because the thigh muscle pump is usually adequate. Also, patients are less compliant with thigh-high compression because of difficulty with application and discomfort. Full-leg pneumatic compression devices may be used for short-term management of severe edema.
■ Encourage the patient to avoid standing for prolonged periods.	Standing in one position for a long time without walking will increase venous pressure and edema.
■ Teach the patient to change positions at frequent intervals.	Remaining in one position for more than a couple of hours causes vein compression and venous stasis.
■ Teach the patient to avoid crossing the legs at the knee when sitting.	The patient should avoid any position that compresses the veins and limits venous return.
■ Encourage weight reduction for overweight patients.	Obesity contributes to venous insufficiency and venous hypertension through compression of the main veins in the pelvic region.
■ Encourage the patient to begin an exercise program.	Walking, swimming, and cycling help promote venous return through contraction of the calf and thigh muscles. These muscles act as a pump to compress veins and support the column of blood returning to the heart.
▲ Administer prescribed diuretics.	Diuretic therapy may be used as an adjunct treatment to help mobilize fluid and reduce tissue edema.

Cardiac and Vascular Care Plans

■ = Independent   ▲ = Interprofessional Collaboration

NANDA-I NDx Impaired Skin Integrity

Common Related Factors
Venous stasis ulcers
Stasis dermatitis

Defining Characteristics
Loss of epidermis and dermis in areas of chronic edema around medial malleolus or tibial area
Irregular-bordered ulcer with granulation tissue at base or soft yellow necrosis

Common Expected Outcome
Patient will have intact skin without signs of infection.

NOC Outcomes
Circulation Status; Wound Healing: Secondary Intention; Knowledge: Treatment Regimen

NIC Interventions
Circulatory Care: Venous Insufficiency; Wound Care; Skin Care: Topical Treatments; Teaching: Procedure/Treatment; Teaching: Prescribed Exercise

Ongoing Assessment

Actions/Interventions	Rationales
■ Assess ulcer characteristics:	
• Location	Venous stasis ulcers are usually located around the medial malleolus or in the pretibial and laterotibial areas of the ankle.
• Size	Initially a venous stasis ulcer will be small, but it increases in size over time. The borders of venous ulcers tend to be irregular.
• Tissue bed	New ulcers will have a beefy red color consistent with the presence of granulating tissue. Older ulcers may have soft tissue necrosis at the base of the ulcer. This tissue may be yellowish green and have a stringy consistency.
• Surrounding tissue	Tissue surrounding the ulcer will be edematous. Skin may have a dark brown color and may be dry and flaky (chronic stasis dermatitis). The patient may report severe itching.
■ Measure the surface of the ulcer area at regular intervals; use pictures as appropriate.	Assessment provides data on the response to therapy.
■ Monitor for signs of infection.	Many ulcers are already colonized. Aggressive wound care is indicated at first sign of infection or breakdown. QSEN: Safety.
▲ Obtain specimens for culture of any wound drainage.	If the ulcer is infected, cultures need to be obtained before appropriate antimicrobial therapy can be started.

Therapeutic Interventions

Actions/Interventions	Rationales
■ Elevate the legs as needed.	Reducing venous hypertension and edema is important for healing.
■ Cleanse the wound using saline or noncytotoxic cleanser before any dressing change.	Preparation of the wound bed is necessary to promote healing; necrotic tissue may require removal before treatment is started.

 For additional care plans, go to http://evolve.elsevier.com/Gulanick/.

Cardiac and Vascular Care Plans

Actions/Interventions	Rationales
▲ Apply appropriate dressings to protect the ulcer during healing:	These ulcers heal through secondary intention. The use of long-term dressings with compression allows the patient to be ambulatory.
• Unna boot	The Unna boot is the mainstay of treatment of venous ulcers. This traditional dressing covers the ulcer and provides compression. It is made of gauze dressing impregnated with zinc oxide, calamine lotion, and glycerin. Once applied, it forms a soft cast from the toes to just below the knee. The boot is covered with an elastic wrap. It can remain in place for 7 days or longer. Disadvantages include discomfort, limitations on bathing, and odor if drainage leaks through the dressing.
• Hydrocolloid (DuoDERM) or vapor-permeable dressing (OpSite, Tegaderm)	These dressings promote wound debridement and healing. Do not use with heavy exudate–producing wounds.
• Hydrogels (Aqua Skin, Carrasyn V)	These dressings are used for shallow ulcers without exudates. They promote wound debridement and healing.
• Alginates (Kalginate, Kaltostat, Sorbsan)	These dressings are for ulcers with exudates or moderate drainage; avoid with dry or heavily bleeding ulcers.
• Gauze with sodium chloride solution	These dressings maintain a moist environment but require multiple dressing changes.
▲ Consult with a wound care management nurse.	The wound care management nurse has specialized knowledge and skills to evaluate a venous ulcer and select the most appropriate wound management interventions. QSEN: Teamwork and collaboration.
▲ If the ulcer is not healing, anticipate surgical intervention.	Nonhealing ulcers may require debridement and skin grafting. For patients with repeated stasis ulcers, the removal of veins with incompetent valves may be indicated. In some cases, valve transplantation may be used.
▲ Administer prescribed antibiotics.	Antibiotics are indicated if cellulitis is present in the affected area.
■ Once the ulcer is healed, teach the patient about measures to prevent new ulcer development:	Once skin integrity has been compromised in venous insufficiency, it is less resistant to trauma. With the slightest trauma, the skin will break. An ulcer forms as a way to relieve pressure in the chronically edematous tissue. QSEN: Safety.
• Continue wearing external compression hosiery as prescribed.	Maintaining compression to reduce venous hypertension is important in preventing new ulcers. Stockings should be applied when first getting up in the morning and removed at bedtime.
• Replace compression hosiery every 3 to 6 months.	Even without signs of wear, the compression effectiveness is lost with long-term use.
• Inspect the skin around the ankles daily.	Venous stasis ulcers usually develop around the perforator veins in the pretibial and medial malleolar areas of the ankles. The first sign may be a small reddened area that is tender to the touch.
• Keep the skin clean and well lubricated.	The patient should avoid moisturizers that contain alcohol because of the drying effect on the skin.
• Exercise care when ambulating.	Even minor trauma to the skin can result in ulcer formation.

Cardiac and Vascular Care Plans

■ = Independent   ▲ = Interprofessional Collaboration

CHAPTER

6

Pulmonary Care Plans

Acute Respiratory Distress Syndrome (ARDS)

Acute Lung Injury; Noncardiogenic Pulmonary Edema; Stiff Lung; Wet Lung

Acute respiratory distress syndrome (ARDS) is a form of respiratory failure characterized by noncardiogenic pulmonary edema and a refractory hypoxemia. It is also known as acute lung injury. The pathology results from damage to the alveolar-capillary membrane. This damage is caused by cytokines released by primed neutrophils during a massive immune response (systemic inflammatory response syndrome). These cytokines increase vascular permeability to such an extent that a massive noncardiac pulmonary edema develops. This edema not only interferes with gas exchange but also damages the pulmonary cells that secrete surfactant. Loss of surfactant allows alveoli to collapse and results in very stiff, noncompliant lungs. Fibrin and cell debris build up, forming a membrane (hyaline) and further decreasing gas exchange. The combined edema, loss of surfactant, alveoli collapse, and hyaline membrane formation lead to a progressive refractory hypoxemia and eventually death.

Anyone with a recent history of severe cell damage or sepsis is at risk for developing ARDS. Examples include individuals who have aspirated or who have suffered trauma, burns, multiple fractures, severe head injury, pulmonary contusions, drowning (salt water aspiration seems to be slightly higher risk than fresh water aspiration), smoke inhalation, carbon monoxide exposure, drug overdose, oxygen toxicity, shock, and so on.

No specific therapy exists for ARDS. The mortality rate for ARDS is 40% to 60%, and even those who survive may have permanent lung damage. With such a high mortality rate, it is clear that early detection and prevention are critical, as is treatment of any causal factors. Thus careful assessment of all at-risk individuals for early warning signs of developing respiratory distress is a nursing responsibility. Unfortunately, the only early warning sign may be labored breathing and tachypnea. Once ARDS develops, nursing care focuses on maintenance of pulmonary functions. Despite evidence that ARDS is the result of an inflammatory response, anti-inflammatory therapy is not effective, and with time, acute lung injury with severe respiratory distress usually results. The Joint Commission's (TJC's) National Patient Safety Goals require the following of meticulous infection control guidelines to prevent ARDS. This care plan focuses on acute care in the critical care setting where the patient's condition is typically managed with intubation and mechanical ventilation.

NANDA-I NDx Ineffective Breathing Pattern

Common Related Factors

Decreased lung compliance
- Low amounts of surfactant
- Fluid transudation

Fatigue and decreased energy
- Increased work of breathing
- Primary medical problem
- Buildup of fibrin and cellular debris (hyaline membrane development)

Defining Characteristics

Dyspnea
Abnormal breathing pattern
Restlessness and/or change in level of consciousness
Tachypnea
Cough
Use of accessory muscles to breathe
Respiratory depth changes
Cyanosis
Arterial pH less than 7.35
Decreased Pao_2 level (<50 to 60 mm Hg)
Increased $Paco_2$ level (50 to 60 mm Hg or higher)

Common Expected Outcomes

Patient maintains an effective breathing pattern, as evidenced by relaxed breathing at normal rate and depth, absence of dyspnea, and blood gas results within patient's normal parameters.

Patient verbalizes ability to breathe comfortably without sensation of dyspnea.

NOC Outcomes

Respiratory Status: Gas Exchange; Respiratory Status: Airway Patency; Respiratory Status: Ventilation

NIC Interventions

Respiratory Monitoring; Airway Management; Mechanical Ventilation Management: Invasive; Oxygen Therapy

Ongoing Assessment

Actions/Interventions	Rationales
■ Assess the respiratory rate, rhythm, and depth.	Respiratory rate and rhythm changes are early warning signs of impending respiratory difficulties. With a stiff, noncompliant, wet (pulmonary edema) lung, gas exchange is decreased, leading to hypoxemia, which leads to an increase in the depth and rate of ventilations.
■ Assess for the use of accessory muscles.	The work of breathing increases greatly as lung compliance decreases. Moving air in and out of the lungs becomes increasingly more difficult, and passive ventilation is no longer adequate to meet oxygenation needs. The breathing pattern alters to include use of the accessory muscles to increase chest excursion to facilitate effective breathing.
■ Assess the lungs for normal or adventitious breath sounds.	As pulmonary edema increases and fluid moves into the alveoli, adventitious breath sounds (crackles) are heard throughout the lung fields.
■ Assess for the sensation of dyspnea.	The sensation of dyspnea is associated with hypoxia and may cause anxiety, which leads to increased oxygen demand and may further affect breathing patterns.
■ Assess for cyanosis of the tongue, oral mucosa, and skin.	Cyanosis of the tongue, oral mucosa, and skin indicates an increased concentration of deoxygenated blood and that the breathing pattern is no longer effective to maintain adequate oxygenation of tissues.

■ = Independent   ▲ = Interprofessional Collaboration

Actions/Interventions	**Rationales**
▲ Use pulse oximetry to monitor oxygen saturation; assess arterial blood gases (ABGs).	Pulse oximetry and ABG measurements provide an objective indication of oxygenation status (and therefore effectiveness of breathing pattern). With acute respiratory distress syndrome (ARDS), oxygen saturation decreases. It should be kept at 90% or greater. The ABGs will indicate developing respiratory acidosis and hypoxemia. QSEN: Safety.
■ Assess for cough.	Increased pulmonary edema and fibrin buildup stimulate the cough reflex.
■ Assess the patient's energy level.	As compliance decreases and breathing patterns alter to include the use of accessory muscles, the work of breathing increases dramatically, leading to patient fatigue. Energy expenditure increases oxygen demand. Eventually the patient may be incapable of adequately maintaining oxygenation needs. QSEN: Patient-centered care.
■ Assess for changes in the level of consciousness.	Increased restlessness, confusion, and/or irritability are early indicators of insufficient oxygenation of the brain and require further intervention.

Therapeutic Interventions

Actions/Interventions	**Rationales**
■ Provide reassurance and allay anxiety by staying with the patient during acute episode of respiratory distress.	The presence of a trusted person may help the patient feel less threatened and can reduce anxiety, thereby reducing oxygen requirements. QSEN: Patient-centered care.
■ Position the patient to optimize ventilation, including the prone position. Observe for changes in oxygen saturation levels with position changes. If saturation drops or fails to return promptly to baseline, reposition the patient for optimal oxygenation.	Prone positioning is a technique used to improve oxygenation in patients with ARDS who are receiving mechanical ventilation. The exact mechanism leading to the improvement of oxygenation in this position is unknown. Proposed mechanisms include recruitment of collapsed alveoli, redistribution of ventilation from the ventral (collapsed in the prone position) to dorsal regions (recruited in the prone position), and mobilization of secretions. This nursing action reduces harm by identifying changes in oxygenation and initiating early intervention. QSEN: Safety.
■ Arrange daily activities to provide periods of rest between activities.	Fatigue is common with the increased work of breathing. Activity increases metabolic rate and oxygen requirements. Rest helps mobilize energy for more effective breathing and coughing efforts.
▲ Maintain oxygen saturation at or above 90%.	Oxygen saturation below 90% leads to tissue hypoxia, anaerobic cellular metabolism, acidosis, electrolyte shifts, dysrhythmias, decreased level of consciousness, increasing hypoxia, and ultimately death. Use caution with FIO_2 greater than 40% because of the increased risk for oxygen toxicity.
▲ Administer medications as indicated (e.g., steroids, antibiotics, bronchodilators, antianxiety medications).	No specific pharmacologic therapy exists for ARDS. Steroids may help reduce inflammation. Antibiotics may be necessary to treat the underlying cause of the inflammatory response. Bronchodilators may be useful to decrease the work of breathing and provide airway clearance. Antianxiety drugs relieve anxiety and may increase cooperation with ventilatory efforts and procedures. QSEN: Evidence-based practice.

Actions/Interventions

■ Provide suctioning as needed.

■ Keep all team members informed of the patient's respiratory status.

▲ Anticipate the need for intubation and mechanical ventilation.

Rationales

Suctioning cleans secretions from pulmonary congestion and reduces the work of breathing. Its use should be guided by objective data, not preset time intervals.

To be successfully treated, ARDS requires aggressive intervention by multiple team members. The nurse is often the first team member to recognize changes in effective breathing patterns that may require other team members to intervene. QSEN: Teamwork and collaboration.

Early intubation and mechanical ventilation using a low tidal volume strategy are recommended to prevent full decompensation of the patient. Mechanical ventilation provides supportive care to maintain adequate oxygenation and ventilation. This nursing assessment reduces harm by identifying changes in oxygenation and initiating early intervention. QSEN: Safety.

NANDA-I
NDx   Impaired Gas Exchange

Common Related Factors

Diffusion defect
- Abnormal A-a gradient (greater difficulty for oxygen and carbon dioxide to cross alveolar-capillary membrane)
- Increased shunting leading to an abnormal $\dot{V}/\dot{Q}$ ratio
- Increased dead space (areas with decreased pulmonary circulation)

Defining Characteristics

Hypoxia and/or hypoxemia
Hypercapnea
Restlessness, irritability
Confusion
Abnormal arterial blood gases
Abnormal breathing pattern (rate, rhythm, depth)
Tachycardia
Abnormal skin color (pale, dusky)
Dyspnea

Common Expected Outcome

Patient maintains optimal gas exchange as evidenced by arterial blood gas (ABG) levels within patient's usual range; alert, responsive mentation or no further reduction in level of consciousness; relaxed breathing; and baseline heart rate (HR) for patient.

NOC Outcomes

Respiratory Status: Gas Exchange; Respiratory Status: Ventilation

NIC Interventions

Respiratory Monitoring; Oxygen Therapy; Mechanical Ventilation Management: Invasive

---

Ongoing Assessment

Actions/Interventions

■ Assess the respiratory rate, rhythm, and depth.

■ Assess for changes in the level of consciousness.

Rationales

Respiratory rate and rhythm changes are early warning signs of impending respiratory difficulties. Rapid, shallow breathing patterns affect gas exchange. Hypoxia is associated with increased breathing effort.

Restlessness and irritability are early indicators of development of further hypoxia and decreased perfusion to the brain.

■ = Independent   ▲ = Interprofessional Collaboration

Actions/Interventions	Rationales
■ Assess the lungs for areas of decreased ventilation and the presence of adventitious breath sounds.	As pulmonary edema increases and fluid moves into the alveoli, adventitious breath sounds (crackles) are heard throughout the lung fields, indicating increased hypoxia; decreased breath sounds are indicative of collapsed alveoli.
▲ Use pulse oximetry to monitor oxygen saturation.	Pulse oximetry is a useful tool in the clinical setting to detect changes in oxygenation. Oxygen saturation should be maintained at 90% or greater.
▲ Closely monitor ABGs, and note changes.	This nursing assessment reduces harm by identifying changes in oxygenation and acid-base balances, and initiating early intervention. QSEN: Safety.
	In ARDS, a progressive hypoxemia is apparent on serial ABG measurements despite increased concentrations of inspired oxygen. Initially, hypocapnia (a decrease in $Paco_2$) may be present as a result of hyperventilation. However, respiratory acidosis with an increase in $Paco_2$ occurs in later stages as a result of an increase in dead space and a decrease in lung compliance and alveolar ventilation.
▲ Assess the cardiac rhythm for dysrhythmias.	Electrolyte shifts, hypoxia, and mechanical ventilation, especially with positive end-expiratory pressure (PEEP), place the patient at risk for cardiac dysrhythmias and decreased cardiac output.
▲ Monitor chest x-ray reports, noting improvement or worsening.	Chest x-ray studies will show bilateral diffuse infiltrates with a normal cardiac silhouette to a complete whiteout of both lung fields; x-ray studies of lung edema lag behind clinical presentation.
▲ Assess the pulmonary artery pressure and pulmonary capillary wedge pressure, if present.	These direct measurements serve as optimal guides for therapy. Attention to fluid balance reduces the risk of harm to the patient. Initially pulmonary artery pressure will be normal, but with PEEP and continuing deterioration, pulmonary artery pressure may increase, leading to further pulmonary edema. QSEN: Safety.
▲ Assess pulmonary function tests.	Decreased vital capacity, minute volume, and functional residual capacity; decreased pulmonary compliance of greater than 50 mL/cm H_2O; and increased shunt fraction greater than 15% to 20% (normal 3% to 4%) are indicative of worsening lung status.
▲ Assess lactic acid levels.	Increasing lactic acid levels are indicative of anaerobic cellular metabolism.
▲ Assess fluid balance through daily weights, intake and output, and appropriate laboratory values as available.	Overhydration or dehydration places the patient at further risk. Tight fluid control is essential to maintaining hydration without increasing edema.

Therapeutic Interventions

Actions/Interventions	Rationales
▲ Use a team approach in planning care with the physician, respiratory therapist, patient, family, and other team members.	Timely and accurate communication of assessments is required to keep pace with needed change in Fio_2, PEEP, and activity levels. QSEN: Teamwork and collaboration.
■ Plan activity and rest to maximize the patient's energy. Temporarily discontinue activity if saturation drops, and make any necessary Fio_2, PEEP, or sedation changes to improve saturation.	Activity increases metabolic rate and oxygen requirements. Rest helps mobilize energy for more effective breathing and coughing efforts. QSEN: Patient-centered care.

Actions/Interventions

■ Elevate the head of bed; change the patient's position every 1 to 2 hours.

■ Institute prone positioning as indicated.

■ Provide suctioning as needed.

▲ Administer medication as indicated (e.g., steroids, sedation, antibiotics, bronchodilators).

▲ Anticipate the need for intubation and mechanical ventilation.

■ If the patient is intubated, anticipate (assess for) the need for PEEP or continuous positive airway pressure (CPAP).

Rationales

Increasing the head of bed to more than 30 degrees prevents aspiration and ventilator-associated pneumonia. Repositioning facilitates movement and drainage of secretions, increases patient comfort, and maintains skin integrity.

Prone positioning is a technique used to improve oxygenation in patients with ARDS who are receiving mechanical ventilation. The exact mechanism leading to the improvement of oxygenation in this position is unknown. Proposed mechanisms include recruitment of collapsed alveoli, redistribution of ventilation from the ventral (collapsed in the prone position) to dorsal regions (recruited in the prone position), and mobilization of secretions. QSEN: Evidence-based practice.

Suctioning clears secretions and increases airway patency to improve gas exchange. Its use should be guided by objective data, not preset time intervals.

No specific pharmacologic therapy exists for ARDS. Steroids may help reduce inflammation. Sedation may be ordered to decrease the patient's energy expenditure during mechanical ventilation and to allow for adequate synchrony of the ventilator so that the patient can be adequately ventilated. Antibiotics may be necessary to treat the underlying cause of the inflammatory response. Bronchodilators may be useful to decrease the work of breathing and provide airway clearance. QSEN: Evidence-based practice.

Early intubation and mechanical ventilation using a low tidal volume strategy are recommended to prevent full decompensation of the patient. Mechanical ventilation provides supportive care to maintain adequate oxygenation and ventilation to the patient. This nursing assessment reduces harm by identifying changes in oxygenation and initiating early intervention. QSEN: Safety.

Hypoxemia leads to tissue damage, causing an increased release of inflammatory mediators, which leads to further lung damage. Artificial positive pressure (PEEP or CPAP) assists in keeping alveoli open. Treatment with low tidal volumes and increased respiratory rates has been shown to be effective in counteracting decreased lung compliance seen in ARDS. Airway pressure-release ventilation and high-frequency oscillatory ventilation are alternative modes of mechanical ventilation that can improve gas exchange in more severe cases.

NANDA-I
NDx **Risk for Decreased Cardiac Output**

Common Risk Factors

Mechanical ventilation
Positive-pressure ventilation

■ = Independent   ▲ = Interprofessional Collaboration

Common Expected Outcome

Patient maintains adequate cardiac output, as evidenced by strong peripheral pulses, systolic blood pressure (BP) within 20 mm Hg of baseline, HR 60 to 100 beats/min with regular rhythm, urine output greater than 30 mL/hr, warm and dry skin, and normal level of consciousness.

NOC Outcomes

Cardiac Pump Effectiveness; Tissue Perfusion: Peripheral; Tissue Perfusion: Abdominal Organs; Circulation Status

NIC Interventions

Hemodynamic Regulation; Mechanical Ventilation Management: Invasive

---

Ongoing Assessment

Actions/Interventions	Rationales
▲ Obtain a cardiac output measurement after positive-pressure ventilation changes.	Attention to changes in cardiac output reduces the risk of harm to the patient. Artificial positive pressure (positive end-expiratory pressure [PEEP] or continuous positive airway pressure [CPAP]) assists in keeping alveoli open; however, the positive pressure compresses the great vessels returning to the heart, which, in turn, decreases the cardiac output. QSEN: Safety.
▲ Assess vital signs and the level of consciousness every hour and with changes in positive-pressure ventilation and inotrope administration.	Mechanical ventilation can cause decreased venous return to the heart, resulting in decreased BP, compensatory increases in HR, and decreased cardiac output. This may occur abruptly with ventilation changes (rate, tidal volume, or positive-pressure ventilation). The level of consciousness will decrease if cardiac output is severely compromised. Therefore close monitoring during ventilation changes is imperative. QSEN: Safety.
■ Assess peripheral pulses, capillary refill, and skin temperature.	Cold, clammy skin is secondary to compensatory increase in sympathetic nervous system stimulation and low cardiac output and oxygen desaturation. Peripheral pulses are weak with reduced stroke volume and cardiac output. Capillary refill is slow with reduced cardiac output.
■ Monitor fluid intake, urine output, and daily weight.	Optimal hydration status is needed to maintain effective circulating blood volume and counteract the ventilator's effect on cardiac output. With positive-pressure ventilation, pressure from the diaphragm decreases blood flow to the kidneys and could result in a drop in urine output. The brain is very sensitive to a decrease in blood flow and may respond by releasing antidiuretic hormone (to increase water and sodium retention), further reducing urinary output. Daily weight is an excellent indicator of fluid status.

Therapeutic Interventions

Actions/Interventions	Rationales
▲ Administer medications as prescribed, noting the response and observing for side effects.	Inotropic medications may be used to increase cardiac output. Sedatives and analgesics are used to relieve pain and agitation. Neuromuscular blocking agents are given to promote synchronous breathing with mechanical ventilation.

ⓔvolve   For additional care plans, go to http://evolve.elsevier.com/Gulanick/.

Actions/Interventions

▲ Administer IV fluids, as prescribed.

■ Anticipate the need to decrease the level of PEEP to a range that facilitates improved cardiac output, if fluid administration and inotropes are not successful.

Rationales

Conservative fluid therapy may be required to maintain optimal fluid balance and increase cardiac output without causing edema.

An "optimal PEEP" level is one that achieves maximal oxygenation benefits without causing a decrease in cardiac output.

 NANDA-I NDx **Risk for Ineffective Protection**

Common Risk Factors

Decreased pulmonary compliance
Dependency on ventilator
Improper ventilator settings
Improper alarm settings
Positive-pressure ventilation
Increased secretions

Common Expected Outcomes

Patient remains free of injury, as evidenced by appropriate ventilator settings and arterial blood gas (ABG) values within normal limits for patient.

Potential for injury from ventilator-associated pneumonia (VAP) and barotrauma is reduced by ongoing assessment and early intervention.

NOC Outcomes
Respiratory Status: Ventilation; Risk Detection
NIC Interventions
Mechanical Ventilation Management:
  Pneumonia Prevention; Mechanical
  Ventilation Management: Invasive

Ongoing Assessment

Actions/Interventions

▲ Closely monitor ventilator settings. Ensure that ventilator alarms are on. Notify the respiratory therapist of any discrepancy in ventilator settings immediately.

▲ Use pulse oximetry to monitor oxygen saturation; assess ABGs, as appropriate.

■ Assess the rate and rhythm of the patient's respiratory pattern, including the work of breathing.
▲ Assess for signs of pulmonary infection.

Rationales

Patient safety is a priority. Assessment ensures that the patient is receiving the correct mode, rate, tidal volume, FIO_2, positive end-expiratory pressure (PEEP), and pressure support. Immediate attention to details can prevent problems. TJC's National Patient Safety Goals requires that alarm systems are activated and functional at all times. QSEN: Safety; Evidence-based practice.

Pulse oximetry is a useful tool to detect changes in oxygenation; oxygen saturation should be at 90% or greater. ABG measurement provides additional information about developing respiratory acidosis and hypoxemia. QSEN: Safety.

It is important to maintain the patient in synchrony with the ventilator and not permit "fighting" it.

VAP is a major contributor to the morbidity and mortality in the ICU. Most ventilator-associated infections are caused by bacterial pathogens, with gram-negative bacilli being common.

■ = Independent   ▲ = Interprofessional Collaboration

Actions/Interventions

■ Assess for signs of barotrauma: crepitus, subcutaneous emphysema, altered chest excursion, asymmetrical chest, change in ABGs, shift in trachea, restlessness, evidence of pneumothorax on chest x-ray film. Notify the physician of these signs immediately.

▲ Monitor chest x-ray film reports daily, and anticipate the ordering of a stat portable chest x-ray film if barotrauma is suspected.

▲ Monitor plateau pressures with the respiratory therapist.

Rationales

Barotrauma is damage to the lungs from positive pressure, as seen in ARDS when high pressures are needed to ventilate the stiff lungs or when PEEP is used. Frequent assessments are needed because barotrauma can occur at any time and the patient will not show signs of dyspnea, shortness of breath, or tachypnea if heavily sedated to maintain ventilation. Being prepared for an emergency helps prevent further complications. QSEN: Safety.

Vigilant monitoring helps reduce complications.

Monitoring for barotrauma can involve measuring plateau pressure, which is the pressure after delivery of the tidal volume but before the patient is allowed to exhale. The ventilator is programmed so that after delivery of the tidal volume the patient is not allowed to exhale for half a second. Therefore pressure must be maintained to prevent exhalation. Elevation of plateau pressures increases both the risk and incidence of barotrauma when a patient is on mechanical ventilation. QSEN: Safety; Teamwork and collaboration.

Therapeutic Interventions

Actions/Interventions

▲ Institute measures to reduce VAP:

• Wash hands before and after suctioning, touching ventilator equipment, and/or coming into contact with respiratory secretions.

• Use a continuous subglottic suction endotracheal tube for intubation that is expected to be longer than 24 hours.

• Keep the head of the bed elevated to 30 to 45 degrees or perform subglottic suctioning unless medically contraindicated.

• Brush teeth two or three times per day with a soft toothbrush. Chlorhexidine-based rinses may also be incorporated into oral care protocols.

• Use sterile suctioning procedures.

■ Listen for alarms. Know the range in which the ventilator will set off the alarm.

▲ If signs of barotrauma are noted, anticipate the need for chest tube placement, and prepare as needed.

Rationales

Nosocomial infections such as VAP are a leading cause of hospital deaths. Prevention of VAP is a national initiative to promote quality and safety. Research continues to identify the most effective "ventilation bundle" order sets to prevent VAP. QSEN: Safety; Evidence-based practice.

An artificial airway bypasses the normal protective mechanisms of the upper airways. Handwashing reduces the transmission of microorganisms.

This intervention prevents the accumulation of secretions that can be aspirated.

Elevation promotes better lung expansion. It also reduces gastric reflux and aspiration.

Oral care reduces colonization of oropharynx with respiratory pathogens that can be aspirated into the lungs.

This technique decreases the introduction of microorganisms into the airway.

The ventilator is a lifesaving treatment that requires a prompt response to alarms. TJC's National Patient Safety Goals require that alarm systems be activated and functional at all times. Appropriate use of safety-enhancing technology minimizes the risk of harm to the patient. QSEN: Safety.

If barotrauma is suspected, intervention must follow immediately to prevent tension pneumothorax while the patient is on the ventilator.

NANDA-I NDx   Anxiety

Common Related Factors
Inability to breathe adequately without support
Inability to maintain adequate gas exchange
Unknown outcome
Inability to speak if intubated
Change in environment
Change in health status

Defining Characteristics
Restlessness/apprenhensiveness
Fear of sleeping at night/insomnia
Uncooperative behavior
Worried
Tachypnea
Vigilant watch on equipment/Scanning behavior
Facial tension
Self-focused

Common Expected Outcomes
Patient demonstrates reduced anxiety, as evidenced by calm manner and cooperative behavior.
Patient uses effective coping mechanisms.
Patient describes a reduction in level of anxiety experienced.

NOC Outcomes
Anxiety Self-Control; Coping
NIC Interventions
Anxiety Reduction; Presence; Emotional Support

Ongoing Assessment

Actions/Interventions	Rationales
■ Assess for signs of anxiety.	Acute respiratory distress syndrome (ARDS) is an acute, life-threatening condition that will produce high levels of anxiety in the patient and significant others. Anxiety can affect the respiratory rate and pattern, resulting in rapid, shallow breathing and leading to arterial blood gas abnormalities and the patient "fighting" the ventilator.
■ Assess the patient's understanding of ARDS and treatment.	ARDS is an acute problem with which most patients have not had prior experience. Fear of the unknown can increase anxiety. QSEN: Patient-centered care.

Therapeutic Interventions

Actions/Interventions	Rationales
■ Display a confident, calm manner and an understanding attitude. Keep the patient or significant others informed of the patient's current status.	The presence of a trusted person may be helpful during periods of anxiety. ARDS is a serious syndrome with a high mortality rate. Significant others must be informed of changes. These patients are typically managed with intubation and mechanical ventilation and require critical care nursing in an acute care setting. Many causal factors are related to ARDS, and the patient or significant others should be informed of the need to treat the underlying cause. QSEN: Patient-centered care.
■ Orient the patient and significant others to intensive care unit surroundings, routines, equipment alarms, and noises. Explain all procedures to the patient before performing them.	The intensive care unit is a busy environment that can be very upsetting and scary to the patient or significant others. Information helps decrease the patient's anxiety. An informed patient who understands the treatment plan will be more cooperative and relaxed.
■ Reduce distracting stimuli. Explain that alarms may periodically sound, which may be normal, and that the staff will be in close proximity.	Reducing stimuli provides a quiet environment that enhances rest. Anxiety may escalate with excessive noise, conversations, and equipment around the patient.

■ = Independent   ▲ = Interprofessional Collaboration

Actions/Interventions	Rationales
■ Explain the need for frequent assessments (i.e., vital signs, auscultation of lung sounds, ventilator checks).	This explanation helps reduce anxiety by providing a basis for actions.
■ Explain the need for suctioning as needed.	Information can help reduce the anxiety associated with the procedure.
■ Encourage visiting by family and friends, as appropriate.	The presence of significant others reinforces feelings of security for the patient. However, family and/or friends can sometimes be a source of anxiety in certain situations.
■ Encourage sedentary diversional activities (e.g., television, reading, being read to, writing, occupational therapy).	These activities enhance the patient's quality of life and help pass time.
■ Provide relaxation techniques (e.g., tapes, imagery, progressive muscle relaxation).	Using anxiety-reduction techniques enhances the patient's sense of personal mastery and confidence.
■ If impaired communication is the problem, provide the patient with word-and-phrase cards, a writing pad and pencil, or a picture board.	These tools broaden the opportunity for communicating, which may reduce frustration.
▲ Refer to a psychiatric liaison clinical nurse specialist, psychiatrist, or hospital chaplain, as appropriate.	Specialty expertise may provide a wider range of treatment options and may be needed to achieve successful outcomes. QSEN: Teamwork and collaboration.

Related Care Plans

Decreased cardiac output, Chapter 2
Imbalanced nutrition: Less than body requirements, Chapter 2
Impaired physical mobility, Chapter 2
Impaired verbal communication, Chapter 2
Mechanical ventilation, Chapter 6
Respiratory failure, acute, Chapter 6
Tracheostomy, ⊖volve

Asthma

Bronchial Asthma; Status Asthmaticus

Asthma is a chronic inflammatory disorder that is characterized by airflow obstruction. This inflammatory response causes bronchoconstriction, increased mucus production, and hyperresponsiveness of the airways to a variety of stimuli. Although the stimuli for this exaggerated bronchoconstrictive response are individually defined, respiratory infection, cold weather, physical exertion, some medications, and allergens are common triggers. When a hypersensitive individual is exposed to a trigger, a rapid inflammatory response with subsequent bronchospasm occurs. Proinflammatory cells, primarily mast cells, signaled by immunoglobulin E (IgE), release inflammatory mediators that produce swelling and spasm of the bronchial tubes. This causes adventitious sounds (wheezing), coughing, increased mucus production, and feelings of "not being able to breathe" (dyspnea). Eosinophils and neutrophils rush to the area, and additional cytokines are released, some of which are long acting and result in epithelial damage, late-phase airway edema, continued mucus hypersecretion, and additional hyperresponsiveness of the bronchial smooth muscle. Reversal of the airflow obstruction usually occurs spontaneously or with treatment. Status asthmaticus occurs when the asthma attack is refractory to the usual treatment, with clinical manifestations that are more severe, prolonged, and life threatening. With repeated attacks, remodeling of the airway occurs through hypertrophy and hyperplasia of normal tissues.

Although this care plan focuses on acute care in the hospital setting, current thinking is to prevent the hypersensitivity reaction and thus keep airway remodeling at a minimum. For this reason, the emphasis of treatment is on an asthma plan individualized for each patient and for optimal outpatient management.

NDx Ineffective Breathing Pattern

Common Related Factor

Swelling and spasm of the bronchial tubes in response to allergies, drugs, stress, infection, inhaled irritants

Defining Characteristics

Dyspnea and/or orthopnea
Respiratory depth changes
Abnormal breathing pattern (rate, rhythm, depth)
Prolonged expiratory phase
Nasal flaring
Use of accessory muscles to breathe

Common Expected Outcome

Patient maintains optimal breathing pattern, as evidenced by relaxed breathing, normal respiratory rate or pattern, and absence of dyspnea.

NOC Outcomes

Respiratory Status: Ventilation; Vital Signs

NIC Interventions

Respiratory Monitoring; Vital Signs Monitoring; Medication Administration

Ongoing Assessment

Actions/Interventions	Rationales
■ Assess the respiratory rate, rhythm, and depth.	Respiratory rate and rhythm changes can be early warning signs of impending respiratory difficulties.
■ Assess the relationship of inspiration to expiration.	Reactive airways allow air to move into the lungs more easily than out of the lungs. If the patient is gasping and frantically trying to "get air," an intervention to assist the patient in developing a more effective breathing pattern may be necessary.
■ Assess for conversational dyspnea.	Shortness of breath during normal conversation indicates respiratory distress.
■ Assess for dyspnea, retractions, flaring of nostrils, and the use of accessory muscles.	These signs signify an increase in respiratory effort. As moving air into and out of the lungs becomes more difficult, the breathing pattern alters to include the use of accessory muscles. This nursing assessment reduces harm by identifying changes in breathing pattern and initiating early intervention. QSEN: Safety.
■ Assess breath sounds, and note wheezes or other adventitious sounds.	Adventitious breath sounds may indicate a worsening condition or an additional developing pathology such as pneumonia. Wheezing occurs as a result of bronchospasm. Diminishing wheezing and inaudible breath sounds are ominous findings and indicate impending respiratory failure.
▲ Use pulse oximetry to monitor oxygen saturation.	Pulse oximetry is a useful, noninvasive tool to detect early changes in oxygenation. Oxygen saturation should be at 90% or higher, with oxygen applied as ordered by the physician. QSEN: Safety.

■ = Independent   ▲ = Interprofessional Collaboration

Actions/Interventions

▲ Monitor arterial blood gases.

▲ Monitor peak expiratory flow rates and forced expiratory volumes as obtained by the respiratory therapist.

■ Assess the patient's level of anxiety.

■ Assess for fatigue and the patient's perception of how tired he or she feels.

■ Assess the patient's vital signs as needed while in distress.

■ Assess for the presence of pulsus paradoxus of 12 mm Hg or greater.

Rationales

During a mild to moderate asthma attack, patients may develop a respiratory alkalosis. Hypoxemia leads to increased respiratory rate and depth, and carbon dioxide is blown off. An ominous finding is respiratory acidosis, which usually indicates that respiratory failure is pending and that mechanical ventilation may be necessary. QSEN: Safety.

The severity of the exacerbation can be measured objectively by monitoring these values. The peak expiratory flow rate is the maximum flow rate that can be generated during a forced expiratory maneuver with fully inflated lungs. It is measured in liters per second and requires maximal effort. When done with good effort, it correlates well with forced expiratory volume in 1 second (FEV_1) measured by spirometry and provides a simple reproducible measure of airway obstruction. QSEN: Teamwork and collaboration.

Hypoxia and the sensation of being "not able to breathe" can be frightening and may cause anxiety.

Fatigue may indicate increasing distress, leading to respiratory failure. QSEN: Patient-centered care.

With initial hypoxia and hypercapnia, BP, HR, and respiratory rate increase. As the hypoxia and/or hypercapnia become severe, BP and HR drop and respiratory failure may ensue.

Pulsus paradoxus is an accentuation of the normal drop in systolic arterial BP with inspiration. Normally the difference in systolic BP at expiration and inspiration is less than 10 mm Hg. A pulsus paradoxus of 12 mm Hg or greater with asthma is a predictor of severe airflow obstruction.

Therapeutic Interventions

Actions/Interventions

■ Keep the head of bed elevated.

■ Encourage slow deep breathing. Instruct the patient to use pursed-lip breathing for exhalation. Instruct the patient to time breathing so that exhalation takes two to three times as long as inspiration.
■ Plan for periods of rest between activities.

▲ Use beta-2 agonist drugs by a metered-dose inhaler or nebulizer (per respiratory therapist) as prescribed.

Rationales

This position allows for adequate diaphragm excursion and lung expansion.

Pursed-lip breathing during exhalation produces a positive distending pressure within the bronchioles, which facilitates expiratory airflow by helping to keep the bronchioles open. Prolonged expiration prevents air trapping.

Fatigue is common with the increased work of breathing from the ineffective breathing pattern. Activity increases metabolic rate and oxygen requirements.

Short-acting beta-2–adrenergic agonist (SABA) drugs relax airway smooth muscle and are the treatment of choice for acute exacerbations of asthma. These short-acting inhaled bronchodilators work quickly to open the air passages, making it easier to breathe and decrease bronchoconstriction.

Actions/Interventions

▲ Administer other medications as ordered or instruct the patient in methods.

Rationales

Pharmacologic management of asthma is based on a step category for severity and treatment. Corticosteroids are the most effective anti-inflammatory drugs for the treatment of reversible airflow obstruction. They may be given parenterally, orally, or inhaled, depending on the severity of the attack. Inhaled steroids should be administered after beta-adrenergic agonists. During severe attacks, anticholinergics (e.g., ipratropium bromide [Atrovent]) may be effective when used in combination with beta-adrenergic agonists. They produce bronchodilation by reducing intrinsic vagal tone to the airway and have been found to be synergistic in their effect with beta-adrenergic agonists. QSEN: Evidence-based practice.

NANDA-I
NDx **Ineffective Airway Clearance**

Common Related Factors

Bronchospasm
Excessive mucus
Ineffective cough and fatigue

Defining Characteristics

Adventitious breath sounds (rhonchi, wheezes)
Alteration in respiratory pattern
Dyspnea
Verbalized chest tightness
Absence of cough
Abnormal arterial blood gas (ABG) levels

Common Expected Outcome

Patient will maintain clear open airways, as evidenced by normal or improved breath sounds, normal rate and depth of respirations, ability to effectively cough up secretions, and normal ABGs or oxygen saturation of 90% or greater on pulse oximeter.

NOC Outcomes

Respiratory Status: Airway Patency; Symptom Control

NIC Interventions

Airway Management; Cough Enhancement; Ventilation Assistance; Calming Technique; Airway Suctioning

---

Ongoing Assessment

Actions/Interventions

■ Auscultate the lungs for adventitious breath sounds (rhonchi and wheezes).

■ Assess any secretions, noting the color, viscosity, odor, and amount.

■ Assess the respiratory rate, rhythm, and depth.

Rationales

Assessment allows for early detection and correction of abnormalities. Rhonchi suggest secretions in the lower airways. Wheezing may indicate partial obstruction or resistance.

Thick, tenacious secretions increase airway resistance and the work of breathing and may be indicative of dehydration. Colored or odorous secretions may indicate bleeding (brown, red) or infections (green, yellow, salmon-colored).

Respiratory rate and rhythm changes are warning signs of impending respiratory difficulties. An increase in respiratory rate may be compensation for airway obstruction.

■ = Independent   ▲ = Interprofessional Collaboration

Actions/Interventions	Rationales
■ Assess cough for effectiveness and productivity.	Coughing is the most helpful way to remove most secretions. Possible causes of an ineffective cough are respiratory muscle fatigue; severe bronchospasm; and thick, tenacious secretions.
■ Assess for color changes in the lips, buccal mucosa, and nail beds.	Cyanosis indicates increased concentration of deoxygenated blood, and that breathing is no longer effective to maintain adequate oxygenation of tissues.
■ Use pulse oximetry to monitor oxygen saturation.	Pulse oximetry is a useful tool to detect changes in oxygenation. Oxygen saturation should be maintained at 90% or greater.
▲ Monitor laboratory work as ordered:	These direct measurements serve as optimal guides for therapy. Attention to changes from baseline reduces the risk of harm to the patient. QSEN: Safety.
• Theophylline level (if on theophylline)	Theophylline increases anxiety and causes tachycardia. It has a narrow window of therapeutic effectiveness, placing the patient at risk for subtherapeutic levels or toxicity.
• ABGs	Carbon dioxide retention occurs as the patient becomes fatigued from the increased work of breathing caused by the bronchoconstriction. Once the patient is intubated and mechanically ventilated, permissive hypercapnia may be used to maintain plateau pressure less than 30 to 35 cm H_2O.
• Complete blood count with special attention to white blood cell (WBC) count	An increased WBC count is associated with infection.
• Serum potassium level	Beta-adrenergic agonists cause potassium to shift intracellularly and can result in decline in serum potassium levels.
▲ Monitor chest x-ray reports.	The chest x-ray report provides information about lung hyperinflation, presence of infiltrates, or presence of barotrauma.

Therapeutic Interventions

Actions/Interventions	Rationales
■ Keep the patient as calm as possible.	Anxiety during an asthma attack can further potentiate the exacerbation. QSEN: Patient-centered care.
■ Pace activities.	Fatigue can increase the work of breathing and decrease cough effectiveness.
▲ Ensure that respiratory treatments are given as prescribed; notify the respiratory therapist as the need arises. Obtain peak expiratory flow rate (PEFR) or forced expiratory volume in 1 second (FEV_1) before and after treatments.	PEFR is the fastest airflow rate reached at any time during exhalation. It should improve with effective therapy. FEV_1 is the volume of air expired in 1 second. QSEN: Teamwork and collaboration.
■ Encourage the patient to cough, especially after treatments. Teach effective coughing techniques.	Controlled coughing techniques help mobilize secretions from smaller airways to larger airways because the coughing is done more effectively.
▲ Maintain oxygen as prescribed.	Oxygen therapy decreases the risk for hypoxia. Oxygen saturation should be maintained at 90% or greater.
▲ Administer medications and intravenous (IV) fluids as prescribed.	In severe exacerbations, IV access is needed for the administration of IV corticosteroids and for emergency medication administration. Although aggressive hydration is no longer recommended, fluid administrations may be necessary for those who present with dehydration.

Actions/Interventions

- Anticipate the need for intubation and mechanical ventilation if ABGs begin to deteriorate ($Paco_2$ 55 mm Hg or greater), the work of breathing continues to increase, PEFR is less than 40% of baseline with failure of PEFR to improve after treatment, and the patient has subjective feelings of doom and/or decreasing alertness.
- Encourage an increased fluid intake (up to 3000 mL/day) if there are no contraindications, such as cardiac or renal disease.

Rationales

Being prepared for an emergency helps prevent further complications. Intubation may be needed to facilitate the removal of tenacious secretions and provide sources for augmenting oxygenation. QSEN: Safety.

Fluids are lost from mouth-breathing and oxygen therapy. Mucous membranes dry out. Maintaining hydration increases ciliary action to remove secretions and decreases viscosity of secretions.

NANDA-I NDx Anxiety

Common Related Factors
Respiratory distress
Hypoxia
Change in health status
Change in environment

Defining Characteristics
Reports of inability to breathe
Alteration in respiratory pattern
Increase in heart rate
Facial tension
Restlessness
Apprehensiveness
Frequent requests for someone to be in room

Common Expected Outcomes
Patient demonstrates reduced anxiety as evidenced by calm manner and cooperative behavior.
Patient uses effective coping mechanisms.
Patient describes a reduction in level of anxiety experienced.

NOC Outcome
Anxiety Self-Control
NIC Interventions
Anxiety Reduction; Calming Technique

Ongoing Assessment

Actions/Interventions

- Assess for signs of anxiety (e.g., tachycardia, alterations in breathing pattern/rate, restlessness, apprehension).

- ▲ Use pulse oximetry to monitor oxygen saturation.

- ▲ Assess theophylline levels if the patient is on theophylline.

Rationales

Anxiety increases as breathing becomes more difficult. Also, anxiety can affect the respiratory rate and rhythm, causing rapid, shallow breathing.

Anxiety increases with increasing hypoxia and may be an early warning sign that the patient's oxygen levels are decreasing.

Theophylline increases anxiety and causes tachycardia. Therapeutic serum levels range from 10 to 20 mcg/mL. This narrow window of therapeutic effectiveness places the patient at risk for subtherapeutic or toxic levels. Short-acting beta-agonists may also cause anxiety. QSEN: Safety.

Therapeutic Interventions

Actions/Interventions

- Stay with the patient, and encourage slow, deep breathing. Assure the patient and significant others of close, continuous monitoring that will ensure prompt intervention.

Rationales

The presence of a trusted person may help the patient feel less threatened. QSEN: Patient-centered care.

■ = Independent   ▲ = Interprofessional Collaboration

Actions/Interventions

- Explain all procedures to the patient before starting; be simple and concise.

- Explain the importance of remaining as calm as possible.

- Keep significant others informed of the patient's progress. Avoid excessive reassurance.

- Encourage the expression of feelings.

- Teach relaxation techniques such as progressive muscle relaxation if the patient's condition permits.

Rationales

Providing information allows the patient to be a full partner in making decisions and assuming responsibility for care at a later time. QSEN: Patient-centered care.

An informed patient who understands the treatment plan will be more cooperative and less anxious.

Maintaining calmness will decrease oxygen consumption and the work of breathing.

Anxiety may be readily transferred to the patient from family members. Information can help relieve apprehension. Excessive reassurance may actually increase anxiety for many people.

Talking about anxiety-producing situations and anxious feelings can help the patient perceive the situation in a less-threatening manner. Expressing emotions can enhance the patient's coping strategies. QSEN: Patient-centered care.

Although anxiety as the result of hypoxia requires correcting the hypoxic condition, some patients will experience anxiety as a learned response to the asthma attack. If this is the case, relaxation techniques may be effective in decreasing the anxiety.

NANDA-I NDx Deficient Knowledge

Common Related Factors

Insufficient information
Insufficient interest in learning
Misinformation presented by others

Defining Characteristics

Insufficient knowledge
Inaccurate follow-through of instruction
Inappropriate behavior
Inaccurate performance on a test

Common Expected Outcome

Patient or significant others verbalize knowledge of disease and its management and community resources available to assist the patient in coping with chronic disease.

NOC Outcomes

Knowledge: Health Behavior; Knowledge: Medication; Knowledge: Asthma Management

NIC Interventions

Health Literacy Enhancement; Learning Facilitation; Teaching: Disease Process; Teaching: Prescribed Medication

---

Ongoing Assessment

Actions/Interventions

- Assess the patient's knowledge of asthma triggers and asthma medications:
  - Ability to distinguish between rescue (reliever) medications and controllers
  - Correct use of metered-dose inhaler (MDI) and spacers
  - Use of spacers with an MDI
  - Sequence to use medications
  - Treatment for status asthmaticus

Rationales

Asthma is a chronic disease that requires important patient self-management. The patient will need to learn to manage exposure to asthma triggers. The correct use of medications is important to control and reduce the frequency of acute attacks. Improper use of an MDI will result in the medications not getting deep enough to influence the tracheobronchial tree. QSEN: Patient-centered care.

---

evolve **For additional care plans, go to http://evolve.elsevier.com/Gulanick/.**

Actions/Interventions

- Assess past and present therapies, as well as the patient's response to them.

- Evaluate self-care activities: preventive care and home management of an acute attack.
- Assess the patient's knowledge of care for status asthmaticus, as appropriate.
- Assess the patient's tobacco use.

Rationales

Knowledge of what has been successful and unsuccessful in the past guides the selection of interventions. The nurse incorporates this information in the planning and evaluation of care and communicates the information to the interprofessional team. QSEN: Patient-centered care.

The patient is living with a chronic disease and will be required to self-manage the disease.

Adequate preparation on how to handle this potential emergency can be lifesaving. QSEN: Safety.

Although assessment of tobacco use is critical for all patients, it is especially important for patients suffering from lung disease. If the patient is a tobacco user, smoking cessation interventions need to be offered.

Therapeutic Interventions

Actions/Interventions

- Explain the disease to the patient and significant others.

- Instruct the patient how to avoid asthma triggers (e.g., cigarette smoke, aspirin, nonsteroidal anti-inflammatory drugs [NSAIDs], air pollution, allergens, seasonal variations).
- Instruct in the use of peak flow meters and develop an individualized plan on how to adjust medications and when to seek medical advice. Establish the patient's "personal best" peak expiratory flow rate (PEFR).

- Reinforce the need for taking controller medications as prescribed.

Rationales

Asthma self-management education reduces the use of health care resources (hospitalizations, urgent care visits) and morbidity. A common misconception held by patients and families is that asthma attacks can be averted without medication through self-control and discipline.

Information enables the patient to take control. Environmental trigger control can reduce the frequency of attacks and improve the patient's quality of life. QSEN: Safety.

Peak flow meters are the standard against which future measurements are evaluated. Use the zone system, individualized to the patient. Personal best is established by having the patient obtain and document peak flow each morning before medication use and in the late afternoon for 2 weeks. Personal best is the highest peak flow reading regularly blown, which is then used to calculate the patient's zone. Monitoring peak flow is particularly important for those who cannot accurately perceive worsening airflow obstruction ("poor perceivers") and more severe levels of asthma.

- *Green zone:* 80% to 100% of personal best.
- *Yellow zone:* 50% to 80% of personal best; this signals caution, and an acute exacerbation may be present. A temporary increase in medication may be indicated.
- *Red zone:* Below 50% of personal best; this signals a medical alert. A beta-2–adrenergic agonist should be taken, and if there is no improvement in PEFR to yellow or green zones, the physician should be notified. QSEN: Evidence-based practice.

Asthma is a chronic condition that is present even when attacks are not occurring. Medications, including anti-inflammatory agents, chromones and leukotriene modifiers, and bronchodilators, reduce the incidence of attacks.

■ = Independent   ▲ = Interprofessional Collaboration

Actions/Interventions	Rationales
■ Review all medications with the patient including a discussion of short- versus long-acting medications, a review of zones, and the dosage of each medication in each zone.	Short-acting beta-agonists are the rescue medication of choice. Long-acting beta-2–adrenergic agonists take too long to act in an emergency. Anti-inflammatory medications, such as mast cell stabilizers or leukotriene modifiers are designed to prevent the release of inflammatory mediators. Once an attack is present, the inflammatory mediators are already at work, and blocking release is not immediately effective. Beta-2–adrenergic agonists should be used before inhaled steroids because they open the airways and allow the anti-inflammatory medication to reach deeper into the lung fields. Rinsing the mouth after using an inhaled steroid prevents a yeast infection. Increase each medication's effectiveness by correct use of spacers; slow, deep inhalation; and breath-holding after inhalation. QSEN: Patient-centered care.
■ Teach how to administer nebulizer treatments, MDIs, spacers, dry powder capsules, or Diskus inhalers with the correct technique. Instruct patients to rinse the mouth with water after using inhalants containing a steroid component to avoid an oral yeast infection.	Return demonstrations on techniques are necessary to ensure appropriate delivery of the medication.
■ Teach the warning signs and symptoms of an asthma attack and the importance of early treatment of an impending attack. Provide a written copy of daily and exacerbation management.	Patients need to have their own written treatment plans to reinforce information that is taught. Early treatment within 6 hours of onset may reduce hospitalizations. QSEN: Safety.

■ Reinforce what to do in an asthma attack:
  • Home management
  • When to go to the emergency department
  • Prevention
	Information enables the patient to take control and reduce life-threatening situations. Medical help should be sought for severe exacerbations, ineffective response to treatment, and deteriorations in condition. QSEN: Safety.

■ Instruct the patient to keep emergency phone numbers readily available.	Advance planning avoids delay in securing assistance.
■ Address long-term management issues.	Environmental controls, control of allergens, avoidance of precipitators, controlling air pollutants (avoidance of smoke, perfumes, aerosol sprays, powder, or talc), and good health habits help avoid attacks.
■ Discuss the need for the patient to obtain vaccines for pneumococcal pneumonia and a yearly vaccine for influenza.	Regular immunizations decrease the occurrence and severity of these diseases.
■ Discuss use of a medical alert bracelet or other identification.	These forms of identification alert others to an asthma history to facilitate the delivery of safe, effective medical care. QSEN: Safety.
▲ Refer to support groups, as appropriate.	Community resources can provide support for patients as they learn disease management and appropriate health behavior changes such as smoking cessation.

Chest Trauma

Pneumothorax; Tension Pneumothorax; Flail Chest; Fractured Ribs; Pulmonary Contusion; Hemothorax; Myocardial Contusion; Cardiac Tamponade

Chest trauma is a blunt or penetrating injury of the thoracic cavity that can result in a potentially life-threatening situation secondary to hemothorax, pneumothorax, tension pneumothorax, flail chest, pulmonary contusion, myocardial contusion, and/or cardiac tamponade. This care plan focuses on acute care in the hospital setting.

NANDA-I NDx Ineffective Breathing Pattern

Common Related Factors

Pain
Simple pneumothorax
Tension pneumothorax
Flail chest
Simple hemothorax (<400 mL blood)
Massive hemothorax (1500 mL blood)
Pulmonary contusion

Defining Characteristics

Shortness of breath and/or dyspnea
Tachypnea and/or shallow respirations
Decreased breath sounds on affected side
Asymmetrical chest expansion
Tracheal deviation
Paradoxical chest movements (flail chest)
Tachycardia
Chest pain
Use of accessory muscles to breathe
Abnormal arterial blood gas (ABG) levels
Oxygen saturation less than 90%
Confusion/restlessness

Common Expected Outcome

Patient maintains effective breathing pattern, as evidenced by relaxed breathing at normal respiratory rate and pattern, absence of dyspnea, and normal blood gas values within patient parameters.

NOC Outcome
Respiratory Status: Ventilation
NIC Interventions
Respiratory Monitoring; Airway Management; Ventilation Assistance

Ongoing Assessment

Actions/Interventions	Rationales
■ Assess the respiratory rate, rhythm, and depth.	Respiratory rate and rhythm changes are early warning signs of impending respiratory difficulties.
■ Assess the lungs for adventitious and decreased breath sounds; percuss the lungs to note changes.	Decreased breath sounds may be evident on affected side. Hyperresonance to percussion on the affected side is present with pneumothorax. Dullness is present with hemothorax.
■ Assess for the use of accessory muscles.	As moving air in and out of lungs becomes more difficult, the patient uses accessory muscles to increase chest excursion and facilitate effective breathing.
■ Assess for changes in the level of consciousness.	Restlessness, confusion, and/or irritability are early indicators of hypoxia to brain tissue. This nursing assessment reduces harm by identifying changes in oxygenation and initiating early intervention. QSEN: Safety.
■ Assess skin color and temperature.	Cool, pale skin may be secondary to a compensatory vasoconstrictive response to hypoxia.
■ Assess chest excursion.	Paradoxical movement is a sign of flail chest. Decreased chest expansion on the affected side is a sign of pneumothorax and/or hemothorax.
■ Assess for pain quality, location, and severity and whether it increases with inspiration.	Pain that increases with inspiration can be a sign of rib fracture.
■ Assess the position of the trachea.	Tracheal deviation from the midline to the unaffected side is a sign of tension pneumothorax.

■ = Independent ▲ = Interprofessional Collaboration

Actions/Interventions

- Use pulse oximetry to monitor oxygen saturation; assess ABGs.

- Assess and inspect the chest wall for obvious injuries that allow air to enter the pleural cavity. Assess for the presence of contusions, abrasions, and bruising on the chest.

- ▲ Monitor chest x-ray films.

- Palpate the chest for subcutaneous emphysema or crepitus.
- Assess for a tension pneumothorax: respiratory distress, tachycardia, cyanosis, tachypnea, hypotension, mediastinal shift (toward unaffected side), changes in breath sounds, distant heart sounds, subcutaneous emphysema.

- Assess the history of the traumatic event: what happened, when, pain, and so forth.

Rationales

Pulse oximetry is a useful tool to monitor oxygen saturation and detect early changes in oxygenation. Increasing $Paco_2$ and decreasing Pao_2 are signs of respiratory failure. QSEN: Safety.

Air entering the pleural cavity would cause pneumothorax. Wound size and location may be the cause of the ineffective breathing pattern. Further injuries may have occurred beneath these integumentary manifestations of trauma (e.g., fractured ribs, pulmonary contusion, myocardial contusion). QSEN: Safety.

The chest x-ray film is used to determine pneumothorax or hemothorax size, confirm the suspected diagnosis, confirm the correct placement of chest tubes, indicate signs of improvement of pneumothorax or hemothorax, and indicate the presence of rib fractures.

Emphysema is a sign of air escaping into the subcutaneous tissues.

Tension pneumothorax is a medical emergency. As pressure within the thorax increases, the great vessels and the lung become compressed, resulting in severe cardiovascular and pulmonary compromise that can quickly become fatal. Immediate identification of the problem is essential. QSEN: Safety.

A history of the traumatic event will assist in alerting the health care team to injury not immediately visible that may be causing the ineffective breathing pattern.

Therapeutic Interventions

Actions/Interventions

- Place the patient in a sitting position, if not contraindicated.
- ▲ Provide pain relief.

- ▲ Provide oxygen therapy.

- Encourage the patient to clear his or her own secretions with effective coughing, helping to splint the chest as needed. If not effective, suction as needed.

- If flail chest is present, tape the flail segment or place manual pressure over the flail segment.

- If an open pneumothorax is present, cover the chest wall defect with 4 × 4 dressing. Tape on three sides with waterproof tape.

Rationales

A sitting position allows for adequate diaphragmatic and lung excursion and chest expansion.

Pain interferes with deep breathing and effective ventilation. Pain relief enhances the ability to deep breathe and cough.

Supplemental oxygen may be needed to maintain an oxygen saturation of 90% or greater for adequate oxygenation.

Productive coughing is the most effective way to remove secretions. Splinting will provide the patient's injured chest wall with support and stability to reduce pain with coughing. If the patient is unable to perform independently and/or effectively, suctioning may be needed.

Patients with increasing respiratory distress may require external pressure to stabilize the chest until a more definitive treatment (intubation, surgical stabilization) is initiated. This nursing action will prevent the outward motion of flail chest. The flail segment will still move inward with respirations, but stopping the outward motion will help decrease the pendulum-like motion to the mediastinum and great vessels.

An untaped side allows air to escape from the pleural cavity (flutter-valve effect) so that tension does not continue to increase.

Actions/Interventions

▲ If a tension pneumothorax is suspected, prepare for a needle thoracostomy.

▲ If severe respiratory distress or respiratory status is steadily deteriorating, prepare for chest tube placement. Connect the chest tube to water seal drainage.

▲ Prepare for intubation if the patient's condition warrants.

Rationales

A needle thoracostomy reduces a tension pneumothorax to a pneumothorax. QSEN: Safety.

Chest tubes are inserted to assist in reinflating the lung. Patients with small pneumothoraces, hemothoraces, and minimal symptoms may not require a chest tube. However, if the patient's condition deteriorates with the need to be intubated or mechanically ventilated, a chest tube will be required, even with small pneumothoraces, because of the high risk for developing a tension pneumothorax in that circumstance. Larger chest tubes are inserted for hemothorax than for pneumothorax to help alleviate chest tube clotting. QSEN: Safety.

Appropriate use of safety-enhancing technology minimizes the risk of harm to the patient. Patients with flail chest may be stable initially because of compensatory mechanisms (e.g., splinting of flail segment and shallow respirations). As these compensatory mechanisms fail, increasing respiratory distress develops. Intubation and positive-pressure ventilation are a means of stabilizing the flail segment by preventing the patient from breathing independently, resulting in inward movement of the flail segment. QSEN: Safety.

NANDA-I
NDx Deficient Fluid Volume

Common Related Factors

Trauma
Active fluid loss (hemothorax)
Chest tube drainage

Defining Characteristics

Decreased urine output
Alteration in skin turgor
Thirst
Dry mucous membranes
Tachycardia
Hypotension and/or orthostasis
Cool, clammy skin
Alteration in mental status
Weakness
Increase in urine concentration

Common Expected Outcome

Patient is normovolemic, as evidenced by urine output greater than 30 mL/hr, systolic BP greater than or equal to 90 mm Hg (or patient's baseline), HR less than 100 beats/min, normal skin turgor, and moist mucous membranes.

NOC Outcomes

Fluid Balance; Blood Loss Severity; Vital Signs; Tissue Integrity: Skin and Mucous Membranes

NIC Interventions

Fluid Monitoring; Fluid Management; Fluid Resuscitation; Bleeding Reduction; Blood Products Administration; Shock Management: Volume

---

■ = Independent ▲ = Interprofessional Collaboration

Ongoing Assessment

Actions/Interventions	Rationales
■ Assess the patient's BP and HR.	Tachycardia is an early indication of fluid volume deficit and a compensatory mechanism to maintain cardiac output. BP is not a good indicator of early shock.
▲ Assess the central venous pressure (CVP).	Changes in CVP will distinguish hypotension caused by hypovolemia (low CVP reading of <6 cm H_2O) versus hypotension caused by pericardial tamponade/tension pneumothorax (high CVP reading of >10 cm H_2O). Attention to any changes followed by prompt treatment reduces the risk of harm to the patient. QSEN: Safety.
■ Assess for jugular venous distention (JVD).	JVD may occur with cardiac tamponade as a result of the increased heart pressures, or with tension pneumothorax from the shifting of the mediastinum toward the unaffected side.
■ Assess the patient's restlessness and anxiety level.	Mild to moderate anxiety may be the first early warning sign before vital sign changes. Anxiety may also indicate pain and/or psychological traumas.
■ Monitor and document fluid intake and urine output.	Urine output of less than 30 mL/hr may indicate early acute tubular necrosis and acute kidney injury secondary to hypovolemia.
▲ Monitor laboratory test results for complete blood count, electrolytes, blood urea nitrogen (BUN), creatinine levels, blood type and crossmatch, and urine specific gravity.	Serum sodium, BUN and/or creatinine ratio, and hematocrit are elevated with decreased fluid volume because they are measures of concentration. Increasing urine specific gravity reflects increased urine concentration.
■ If a chest tube is in place: • Assess, measure, and document the amount of blood in the chest tube collection chamber. • Monitor the chest tube drainage every 10 to 15 minutes until blood loss slows to less than 25 mL/hr. • Maintain and check the tube patency; avoid dependent loops. • Maintain the prescribed fluid level within the collection system.	Excessive chest tube drainage may indicate hemorrhage. The obstruction of drainage from chest tubes interferes with lung expansion. Accumulated drainage in dependent loops obstructs tube drainage and increases pressure within the lungs. Maintaining the prescribed water seal and suction levels helps prevent complications. Newer systems are available that offer waterless options. QSEN: Safety.
■ Assess for orthostatic hypotension and weakness.	Orthostatic hypotension is an early sign of hypovolemia. Note the significance of the following levels of orthostatic hypotension: • Greater than 10 mm Hg drop: circulating blood volume is decreased by 20%. • Greater than 20 to 30 mm Hg drop: circulating blood volume is decreased by 40%. QSEN: Safety.

Therapeutic Interventions

Actions/Interventions	Rationales
▲ Provide oral fluids as ordered and tolerated.	Oral fluid replacement is indicated for a mild fluid deficit or as a supplement to IV fluids.
■ Assist the patient in sitting or standing if orthostatic hypotension is present.	Hypotension may produce lightheadedness and dizziness. This nursing action reduces the patient's risk for falls. Orthostasis is especially evident in older patients. QSEN: Safety.

Actions/Interventions

- Attempt to control the bleeding source by using direct pressure with a sterile 4 × 4 dressing.
- ▲ Insert one to two large-bore peripheral IV lines. Administer crystalloid or colloid fluids as prescribed.

- ▲ Prepare the patient for transfusions, if prescribed, with typed and crossmatched blood if it is available and time permits.

- ▲ Prepare the patient for autotransfusion.

- Prepare the patient for possible surgery as the condition warrants.

Rationales

Significant pressure may be required to halt bleeding.

Parenteral fluid replacement is indicated to prevent or treat hypovolemic complications. The rule for fluid replacement: infuse 3 mL IV fluid for every 1 mL blood volume lost.

Blood transfusion may be required to correct fluid loss. Type-specific blood may be used if unable to obtain a type and crossmatch. Type O-negative blood may be used as a last resort.

Autotransfusion is used in cases of blunt or penetrating injuries isolated to the chest area.

An open thoracotomy may be required to correct the source of bleeding.

NANDA-I
NDx Decreased Cardiac Output

Related Factors

Acute pericardial tamponade
Tension pneumothorax
Severe fluid volume loss
Decreased ventricular filling (preload)

Defining Characteristics

Hypotension
Narrow pulse pressure
Decreased peripheral pulses
Pulsus paradoxus (systolic BP falls >15 mm Hg during inspiration)
Tachycardia
Capillary refill greater than 3 seconds
Electrical alternans (decreased QRS voltage during inspiration)
Equalization of pressures (central venous pressure [CVP], pulmonary artery pressure, and pulmonary capillary wedge pressure)
Jugular venous distention (JVD)
Distant or muffled heart tones
Restlessness
Cool, clammy skin
Decreased urine output
Decreased arterial or venous oxygen saturation

Common Expected Outcome

Patient maintains adequate cardiac output as evidenced by BP within normal limits for patient, HR 60 to 100 beats/min with regular rhythm, urine output 30 mL/hr or greater, strong peripheral pulses, absence of JVD, absence of pulsus paradoxus, warm and dry skin, and normal level of consciousness.

NOC Outcomes

Cardiac Pump Effectiveness; Circulation Status; Vital Signs

NIC Interventions

Vital Signs Monitoring; Invasive Hemodynamic Monitoring; Hemodynamic Regulation

---

■ = Independent   ▲ = Interprofessional Collaboration

Ongoing Assessment

Actions/Interventions	Rationales
■ Assess for the classic signs associated with acute pericardial tamponade:	Pericardial tamponade can decrease cardiac output as the pericardial sac fills with blood to the point that it compresses the myocardium, causing a decreased ability of the heart to pump blood out and take blood in. QSEN: Safety.
• Low arterial BP with narrowing pulse pressure	An initial elevation in BP may occur with compensatory vasoconstriction. However, as venous return is compromised from the cardiac compensation, a significant drop in cardiac output occurs.
• Pulsus paradoxus	Pulsus paradoxus is an accentuation of normal drop in systolic arterial BP with inspiration. Normally the difference in systolic BP at expiration and inspiration is less than 10 mm Hg.
• Distant or muffled heart sounds	Muffled heart sounds are caused by distention in pericardial sac, creating a cushion between stethoscope and heart sounds.
• Sinus tachycardia	Sinus tachycardia is related to compensatory catecholamine release.
• Distended neck veins	The jugular neck veins become distended as a result of impaired venous return to the heart.
■ Assess for changes in the level of consciousness.	Restlessness, irritability, and anxiety are early indicators of hypoxia and reduced cerebral perfusion.
■ Assess the peripheral pulses, capillary refill, and skin temperature.	Cool, pale, clammy skin is secondary to a compensatory increase in the sympathetic nervous system and low cardiac output. Peripheral pulses are weak with reduced stroke volume and cardiac output. Capillary refill is slow.
▲ Assess ECG changes.	A slowly developing tamponade may present like heart failure with nonspecific ECG changes. Low voltage of ECG complexes is also a common finding.
■ Monitor the chest tube drainage for an increase or decrease in drainage.	A sudden cessation of chest tube drainage suggests a clot.
▲ Assist with the performance of an echocardiogram if time permits.	An echocardiogram provides the most helpful diagnostic information. Effusions seen with acute tamponade are usually smaller than with chronic tamponade. However, to prevent circulatory collapse, treatment may be indicated before the echocardiogram can be performed.
▲ If the patient is in the intensive care unit, assess the hemodynamic profile using a pulmonary artery catheter; assess for the equalization of pressure.	Attention to changes in cardiac output reduces the risk of harm to the patient. The right atrial pressure, right ventricular diastolic pressure, pulmonary artery diastolic pressure, and pulmonary capillary wedge pressure are all elevated in tamponade and are within 2 to 3 mm Hg of each other. These pressures confirm the diagnosis. QSEN: Safety.
▲ Monitor serial chest x-ray films.	The chest x-ray film is used to evaluate for a widened mediastinum or increased heart size.
■ Assess for a midline shift of the trachea.	Tension pneumothorax will cause a midline shift of the trachea and mediastinum to the opposite side with compression of the great vessels, causing a decrease in cardiac output.

Therapeutic Interventions

Actions/Interventions	Rationales
▲ Keep the patient and significant others informed.	With a tamponade, the patient may be feeling well and suddenly develop restlessness and feelings of doom. This can be confusing and frightening for patients and their loved ones. QSEN: Patient-centered care.
■ Place the patient in an optimal position to increase venous return.	Positioning is guided by the extent of the chest trauma injuries.
▲ Initiate oxygen therapy.	Supplemental oxygen will maximize oxygen saturation at 90% or greater.
▲ Establish a large-bore IV access. Maintain aggressive fluid resuscitation as ordered.	Fluids may be required to raise venous pressure above pericardial pressure and optimize cardiac output. IV access provides for rapid fluid resuscitation and blood administration.
▲ Anticipate blood product replacement.	Blood replacement therapy corrects existing hematological or coagulation factor alterations.
■ Have emergency resuscitative equipment and medications readily available.	Pericardiocentesis is the emergency treatment of choice for cardiac tamponade. Vasopressor medications maximize systemic perfusion pressure to vital organs. QSEN: Safety.
▲ Assemble a pericardiocentesis tray or open chest tray for bedside intervention of pericardial tamponade, or prepare the patient for transport to surgery.	Acute tamponade is a life-threatening complication, but immediate prognosis is good with fast, effective treatment. Tamponade must be relieved to improve cardiac output. It is indicated when systolic BP is reduced more than 30 mm Hg from baseline. Bedside pericardiocentesis can be a high-risk lifesaving procedure. If the patient's condition can be stabilized, the drainage of fluid should be delayed until surgical or open resection and drainage can be performed. Pericardiocentesis should be performed under sterile conditions.
▲ If repeated pericardiocentesis fails to prevent the recurrence of acute tamponade, anticipate a surgical correction.	Surgical pericardiotomy (pericardial window) or resection of a portion of the pericardium may be indicated.
▲ Assemble a thoracentesis tray or chest tube drainage system for the treatment of tension pneumothorax.	If tension pneumothorax is suspected, interventions must be rapid to lessen the compression of the mediastinum and great vessels, which results in decreased cardiac output and shock.
▲ Administer vasopressor agents (dopamine, norepinephrine bitartrate [Levophed]), as ordered.	These medications maximize systemic perfusion pressure to vital organs.

NANDA-I NDx Acute Pain

Common Related Factors	Defining Characteristics
Rib fractures	Self-report of intensity using a standardized pain scale
Chest tube incision	Self-report of pain characteristics using a standardized pain instrument
Contusions or abrasions	Facial expression of pain
Penetrating wounds	Change in physiological parameter (e.g., blood pressure, heart rate, diaphoresis)
Pleural irritation	Shallow respirations to minimize pain
	Agitation and/or restlessness

■ = Independent   ▲ = Interprofessional Collaboration

Common Expected Outcomes

Patient reports satisfactory pain control at a decreasing intensity using a standardized pain scale.

Patient exhibits increased comfort such as baseline levels for HR, BP, and respirations, and relaxed muscle tone or body position.

NOC Outcomes
Comfort Status; Pain Control; Medication Response

NIC Interventions
Pain Management; Analgesic Administration; Distraction

Ongoing Assessment

Actions/Interventions

■ Assess the patient's pain level and its characteristics.

■ Evaluate the effectiveness of all pain management, including medications and nonpharmacological interventions.

■ Assess how the patient has successfully dealt with pain in the past.
■ Assess the patient's cultural beliefs about reporting pain.

Rationales

Assessment is important to determine the type of pain the patient is experiencing to aid in the diagnosis and appropriate treatment.

All patients with chest trauma will need some type of pain medication. Unlike other body fractures, rib fractures cannot be casted to reduce pain. The rib cage is in continuous motion; therefore the pain is more difficult to manage. Pain management is easiest if the pain is not allowed to peak but is consistently controlled. If one medication or complementary technique is not effective, other interventions will need to be implemented. QSEN: Patient-centered care.

Patient responses to pain are highly varied and must be explored with each patient.

Many factors influence a patient's willingness to report pain. Some are afraid of addiction to pain medications and will need reassurance that addiction is not a problem in treatment of acute pain. Others believe "toughing it out" is the way to handle pain. This knowledge deficit would need to be addressed. Finding out how the patient has dealt with pain in the past gives insight as to how best to effectively relieve current pain. QSEN: Patient-centered care.

Therapeutic Interventions

Actions/Interventions

▲ Anticipate the need for analgesics, and respond immediately to reports of pain.

■ Assist the patient in splinting the chest with a pillow.

▲ Give the patient as much control over pain management as the condition allows.

▲ Assist with the insertion or maintenance of an epidural catheter or intercostal nerve block, as appropriate.
■ Plan care activities for times when the patient is most pain-free, if possible.
■ Use distraction techniques.

Rationales

In the midst of painful experiences, a patient's perception of time may become distorted. Prompt responses to reports of pain may result in decreased anxiety in the patient.

Splinting minimizes discomfort and assists with effective coughing and deep breathing.

The ability to actively participate and control pain management may decrease the patient's fear of pain. QSEN: Patient-centered care.

A variety of measures may be used to effectively manage pain and improve ventilation.

This facilitates more active participation by the patient.

Distraction techniques heighten one's concentration on nonpainful stimuli to decrease awareness and experience of pain.

Actions/Interventions

- Teach additional nonpharmacological interventions such as massage therapy, music therapy, heat or cold therapy, imagery, controlled breathing, and so on when pain is relatively controlled.
- Eliminate additional stressors or sources of discomfort whenever possible.

Rationales

Chest trauma results in significant pain. Offering a variety of alternative therapies, such as cutaneous stimulation or cognitive-behavioral strategies, may be useful.

Patients may experience an exaggeration in pain or a decreased ability to tolerate painful stimuli when environmental, intrapersonal, or intrapsychic stressors are present.

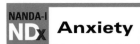

NANDA-I NDx   Anxiety

Common Related Factors

Acute injury
Unfamiliar environment
Hypoxia
Threat of death

Defining Characteristics

Apprehensiveness
Restlessness
Alteration in concentration
Increased BP
Increase in HR

Common Expected Outcomes

Patient uses effective coping mechanisms.
Patient describes a reduction in level of anxiety experienced.

NOC Outcomes
Anxiety Self-Control; Coping
NIC Interventions
Anxiety Reduction; Emotional Support; Presence

Ongoing Assessment

Actions/Interventions

- Assess the patient's anxiety level (mild, severe). Note any signs and symptoms, especially nonverbal communication.
- Assess coping factors.

Rationales

Chest trauma can result in an acute life-threatening injury that will produce high levels of anxiety in the patient as well as in significant others. QSEN: Patient-centered care.

Anxiety and ways of decreasing perceived anxiety are highly individualized. Interventions are most effective when they are consistent with the patient's established coping patterns. QSEN: Patient-centered care.

Therapeutic Interventions

Actions/Interventions

- Acknowledge an awareness of the patient's anxiety; encourage the patient to express fears.
- Maintain a confident, assured manner. Assure the patient and significant others of close, continuous monitoring that will ensure prompt interventions.

- Reduce unnecessary external stimuli (e.g., clear unnecessary personnel from the room; decrease the volume of the cardiac monitor).
- Reduce the patient's or significant others' anxiety by explaining all procedures and treatment. Keep explanations basic.

Rationales

Acknowledgment validates the patient's feelings and communicates acceptance of those feelings.

The presence of a trusted person may help the patient feel less threatened. The staff's anxiety may be easily perceived by the patient. The patient's feeling of stability increases in a calm, nonthreatening atmosphere.

Anxiety may escalate with excessive conversation, noise, and equipment around the patient.

Information helps allay anxiety. Patients who are anxious may not be able to comprehend anything more than simple, clear, brief instructions.

■ = Independent   ▲ = Interprofessional Collaboration

Actions/Interventions

■ Support the patient's use of coping strategies that have been effective in past.

▲ Refer to other support systems (e.g., clergy, social workers, other family and friends) as appropriate.

Rationales

Using anxiety-reduction strategies enhances the patient's sense of personal mastery and confidence. This approach allows the patient to be a full partner in providing care that meets the patient's expressed needs for effective coping. QSEN: Patient-centered care.

Specialty expertise may be needed to achieve successful outcomes. QSEN: Teamwork and collaboration.

Related Care Plans

Impaired gas exchange, Chapter 2
Risk for infection, Chapter 2
Blood component therapy, Chapter 4
Respiratory failure, acute, Chapter 6
Thoracotomy, ⊜volve

Chronic Obstructive Pulmonary Disease

Chronic Bronchitis; Emphysema

Chronic obstructive pulmonary disease (COPD) is the fourth leading cause of death in the world. It refers to a group of diseases, including chronic bronchitis and emphysema, that cause a reduction in expiratory outflow. It is usually a slow, progressive, debilitating disease, affecting those with a history of heavy tobacco abuse and prolonged exposure to respiratory system irritants such as air pollution, noxious gases, and repeated upper respiratory tract infections. It is also regarded as the most common cause of alveolar hypoventilation with associated hypoxemia, chronic hypercapnia, and compensated acidosis. According to GOLD (Global Initiative for Chronic Obstructive Lung Disease), assessment of COPD is based on the patient's level of symptoms, future risk of exacerbations, the severity of the spirometric abnormality, and the presence of comorbid conditions. Spirometry is required to make a diagnosis of COPD. The spirometric classification of airflow limitation is divided into four grades: GOLD 1 = mild; GOLD 2 = moderate; GOLD 3 = severe; and GOLD 4 = very severe, using the fixed ratio of post-bronchodilator forced expiratory volume in 1 second (FEV_1) to forced vital capacity (FVC) of <0.70 to define airflow limitation.

This care plan focuses on exacerbation of COPD in the acute care setting and chronic care in the ambulatory setting or chronic care facility. It does not include surgical treatments such as lung volume reduction surgery or lung transplant.

NANDA-I NDx Ineffective Airway Clearance

Common Related Factors

Hyperplasia and hypertrophy of mucus-secreting glands
Increased mucus production in bronchial tubes
Thick secretions
Decreased ciliary function
Alveolar wall destruction
Decreased energy and fatigue
Impaired exhalation
Bronchospasm
Smoking

Defining Characteristics

Coarse lung sounds and/or wheezing
Alteration in respiratory pattern
Persistent cough for months
"Smoker's cough"
Ineffective cough
Retained secretions
Loud, prolonged expiratory phase
Dyspnea
Altered arterial blood gas (ABG) levels (compensated hypercapnia)

 For additional care plans, go to http://evolve.elsevier.com/Gulanick/.

Common Expected Outcomes

Patient will maintain clear open airway, as evidenced by normal breath sounds, normal rate and depth of respirations, and ability to cough up secretions.

Patient demonstrates effective coughing techniques.

NOC Outcome
Respiratory Status: Airway Patency
NIC Interventions
Cough Enhancement; Airway Management

Ongoing Assessment

Actions/Interventions	Rationales
■ Auscultate the lungs after coughing as needed to note and document any significant change in breath sounds:	Patients with chronic obstructive pulmonary disease (COPD) have hypertrophy and hyperplasia of goblet cells with increased mucus production. Impaired ciliary movement contributes to retained secretions and less effective coughing. These patients have decreased breath sounds in varying degrees depending on their stage of illness.
• Decreased or absent breath sounds	Decreased or absent breath sounds may indicate the presence of a mucus plug or other major airway obstruction.
• Coarse sounds	Coarse sounds indicate the presence of fluid along larger airways.
• Presence of fine crackles	Fine crackles may indicate cardiac involvement or secretion trapping.
■ Assess for changes in the respiratory rate, depth, and use of accessory muscles or tripod positioning.	Respiratory rate and rhythm changes are early signs of respiratory compromise. As compromise becomes greater, the use of accessory muscles becomes evident and the patient assumes a tripod posture with the forearms resting on the thighs to facilitate breathing. QSEN: Safety.
■ Assess the characteristics of or changes in secretions: consistency, quantity, color, odor.	A sign of infection is discolored sputum; an odor may be present. Thick, tenacious secretions increase hypoxemia and may be indicative of dehydration.
■ Note any color changes in the lips, buccal mucosa, or nail beds.	Cyanosis is more common in patients with chronic bronchitis. The patient with emphysema develops cyanosis in the later stages of this disease.
■ Assess the patient's hydration status: skin turgor, mucous membranes, and tongue.	Airway clearance is impaired with inadequate hydration and subsequent secretion thickening.
▲ Use pulse oximetry to monitor oxygen saturation; assess ABGs.	Hypoxia can result from increased pulmonary secretions and respiratory fatigue. Oxygen saturation should be maintained at 90% or greater. ABGs may demonstrate compensated hypercapnia. QSEN: Safety.
■ Assess the patient's physical capabilities with activities of daily living (ADLs), including the ability to expectorate sputum. Note if the patient has conversational dyspnea.	Fatigue can limit cough effectiveness. Hypoxemia can limit activity tolerance. Shortness of breath during normal activities indicates respiratory distress. QSEN: Patient-centered care.
▲ Assess lung function spirometry results as available.	Lung function parameters define the disease severity, prognosis, and response to therapy.

■ = Independent   ▲ = Interprofessional Collaboration

Therapeutic Interventions

Actions/Interventions	Rationales
▲ Administer beta-2–adrenergic agonists (e.g., albuterol, levalbuterol) by a metered-dose inhaler (MDI) or nebulizer, as prescribed.	These short-acting inhaled bronchodilators work quickly to open the air passages, making it easier to breathe and decreasing bronchoconstriction.
▲ Administer anticholinergics such as ipratropium bromide (Atrovent) by an MDI or nebulizer or tiotropium (Spiriva) dry powder inhalation only in conjunction with beta-2–adrenergic agonist.	These medications have been shown to work synergistically with beta-2–adrenergic agonists to relieve bronchoconstriction.
▲ Anticipate the administration of IV corticosteroids (followed by oral steroids) during the acute exacerbation. Anticipate the addition of xanthines and chromones as indicated.	These medications are based on recommendations from national organizations. Treatment guidelines recommend a stepped approach for selecting medications depending on the severity of the problem and the patient's response to prior treatments. QSEN: Evidence-based practice.
■ Encourage the patient to cough out secretions.	Coughing is the most helpful way to remove most secretions.
■ Assist with effective coughing techniques: • Splint the chest. • Have the patient use abdominal muscles. • Use cough techniques as appropriate (e.g., quad, huff).	Controlled cough techniques help mobilize secretions from smaller airways to larger airways because coughing is done more effectively. Forced expiratory coughing through an open airway (while saying "huh") may be effective to move the trapped mucus into the larger airways for the patient to cough up.
▲ Assist in mobilizing secretions to facilitate airway clearance: • Increase room humidification. • Administer mucolytic agents as prescribed. • Perform chest physiotherapy: postural drainage, percussion, and vibration. • Encourage 2 to 3 liters of fluid intake unless contraindicated. • Encourage activity and position changes every 2 hours.	Increasing the humidity of inspired air will decrease the viscosity of secretions and facilitate their removal. These agents help liquefy secretions. Chest physiotherapy helps to loosen and mobilize secretions in smaller airways that cannot be removed by coughing. Fluids prevent dehydration from increased insensible loss and keep secretions thin. Activity helps mobilize secretions and prevents pooling in the lungs.
■ Perform nasotracheal suctioning as indicated if the patient is unable to effectively clear secretions. Use a well-lubricated soft catheter.	Suctioning is indicated when patients are unable to remove secretions from the airways by coughing because of weakness, thick mucus plugs, or excessive secretions. It can also stimulate a cough. Suctioning with a lubricated catheter minimizes irritations.
▲ Anticipate intubation and mechanical ventilation, if needed, with transfer to the acute care setting.	Early intubation and mechanical ventilation may be needed to prevent full decompensation and a potentially life-threatening situation. Appropriate use of safety-enhancing technology minimizes the risk of harm to the patient from airway obstruction. QSEN: Safety.

Impaired Gas Exchange

Common Related Factors

Increase in dead space caused by the following:
- Loss of lung tissue elasticity
- Atelectasis
- Increased residual volume

Increased upper and lower airway resistance caused by the following:
- Overproduction of secretions along bronchial tubes
- Bronchoconstriction

Defining Characteristics

Altered inspiratory and/or expiratory (I/E) ratio (prolonged expiratory phase)

Active expiratory phase: use of accessory muscles of breathing

Increase in rate and depth of respiration

Hypoxemia and/or hypercapnia

$Paco_2$ greater than 55 mm Hg

Pao_2 less than 55 mm Hg

Tachycardia

Restlessness and/or irritability

Confusion and/or somnolence

Pale, dusky skin color and/or cyanosis

Common Expected Outcome

Patient maintains optimal gas exchange, as evidenced by arterial blood gases (ABGs) within the patient's usual range, oxygen saturation of 90% or greater, alert response mentation or no further reduction in level of consciousness, relaxed breathing, and baseline HR for patient.

NOC Outcomes
Respiratory Status: Gas Exchange; Vital Signs; Knowledge: Treatment Regimen

NIC Interventions
Respiratory Monitoring; Oxygen Therapy; Teaching: Psychomotor Skill

Ongoing Assessment

Actions/Interventions	Rationales
■ Assess for altered breathing patterns: • Increased work of breathing • Abnormal rate, rhythm, and depth of respiration • Use of accessory muscles • Abnormal chest excursions	The patient with chronic obstructive pulmonary disease (COPD) has hyperinflation of the alveoli. This change leads to an increased anteroposterior chest diameter (barrel chest) and flattening of the diaphragm. As a result the patient may have decreased chest excursion and increased accessory muscle use. Patients will adapt their breathing patterns over time to facilitate gas exchange. Both rapid, shallow breathing patterns and hypoventilation affect gas exchange. Hypoxia is associated with increased breathing efforts.
■ Assess the patient's generalized appearance and favored position for breathing.	Patients usually appear thin with reduced muscle mass. Posture, upright positioning, and mental alertness cue the nurse to the severity of the COPD exacerbation. The patient with COPD may adopt a tripod sitting position, with the forearms resting on the thighs. This position decreases the work of breathing. QSEN: Patient-centered care.
■ Assess for restlessness and changes in the level of consciousness.	Restlessness is an early sign of hypoxia. Lethargy and somnolence are late signs.
■ Monitor vital signs.	Hypoxia or hypercarbia may cause initial hypertension, tachycardia, and increased respiratory rate.
■ Assess the patient's level of anxiety.	Dyspnea often increases anxiety, and anxiety increases oxygen use by tissues. Anxiety may be an indication of worsening hypoxemia.

■ = Independent   ▲ = Interprofessional Collaboration

Actions/Interventions

▲ Use pulse oximetry to monitor oxygen saturation; assess ABGs.

■ If the patient is on theophylline, monitor for therapeutic levels and side effects.

Rationales

Increasing $Paco_2$ and decreasing Pao_2 are signs of respiratory failure. As the patient's condition begins to fail, the respiratory rate will decrease and $Paco_2$ will begin to rise. The patient with COPD has a significant decrease in pulmonary reserves, and any physiological stress may result in acute respiratory failure. The noninvasive measurement of oxygen saturation by pulse oximetry provides for early recognition of impaired oxygenation status. QSEN: Safety.

Theophylline increases anxiety and causes tachycardia. Therapeutic serum levels range from 10 to 20 mcg/mL. This narrow window of therapeutic effectiveness places the patient at risk for subtherapeutic or toxic levels.

Therapeutic Interventions

Actions/Interventions

▲ Promote a more effective breathing pattern for better gas exchange:
  - Instruct in positioning for optimal breathing.

  - Teach the patient pursed-lip breathing.

  - Teach the patient to use abdominal and other accessory muscles.

  - Teach the patient to take bronchodilators and anticholinergics as prescribed.

▲ Administer low-flow oxygen therapy as indicated (e.g., 2 L/min by nasal cannula). If insufficient, switch to high-flow oxygen apparatus (e.g., Venturi mask) for more accurate oxygen delivery.

▲ If the Pao_2 level is significantly lower or if the $Paco_2$ level is higher than the patient's usual baseline (varies from patient to patient), anticipate the following:
  - Vigorous pulmonary toilet and suctioning
  - Increase in Fio_2 with the use of a controlled high-flow system
  - Possible need for intubation and mechanical ventilation with placement in the acute care setting

▲ Use caution in the administration of respiratory depressants such as opioids and tranquilizers.

Rationales

Attention to these strategies reduces the risk of harm to the patient. QSEN: Safety.

Upright and high-Fowler's positions favor better lung expansion; the diaphragm is pushed downward. If the patient is bedridden, turning from side to side at least every 2 hours promotes better aeration of all lung lobes, thus minimizing atelectasis.

Pursed-lip breathing promotes positive airway pressure during exhalation. This breathing technique decreases carbon dioxide retention, allows for increased tidal volume, decreases breath rates, allows for a longer period of time for oxygen and/or carbon dioxide diffusion, and increases alveolar ventilation. It is especially useful during activity or exertion.

The use of abdominal muscles facilitates movement of the diaphragm, and the use of accessory muscles increases chest excursion.

These drugs decrease the work of breathing by decreasing airway resistance.

COPD patients who chronically retain carbon dioxide depend on "hypoxic drive" as their stimulus to breathe. When applying oxygen, close monitoring is imperative to prevent unsafe increases in the patient's Pao_2, which could result in apnea. QSEN: Safety.

Signs of respiratory failure include increasing $Paco_2$ and decreasing Pao_2, paradoxical breathing, fatigue, somnolence, and increased respiratory rate. Treatment focuses on airway management, oxygen therapy, and more aggressive therapy using mechanical ventilation as needed to correct acidosis and hypoxemia. QSEN: Safety.

These medications reduce respiratory drive, thereby promoting hypoxemia. This nursing action is part of the QSEN competency for safety to reduce harm to the patient and to achieve outcomes for effective gas exchange.

ⓔvolve **For additional care plans, go to http://evolve.elsevier.com/Gulanick/.**

Actions/Interventions

▲ Plan activity with interspersed rest periods and after bronchodilator treatments. Work with the respiratory therapist for the best time sequence of pulmonary treatment.

▲ Administer bronchodilators, expectorants, anti-inflammatory agents (steroids), and antibiotics, as ordered.

▲ Work with the rehabilitation team and patient to establish discharge planning.

Rationales

Activities will increase oxygen consumption and should be planned so that the patient does not become hypoxic. Pacing activities will help the patient conserve energy. QSEN: Teamwork and collaboration.

These medications reduce airway resistance, treat infection, and facilitate secretion removal.

COPD is a chronic debilitating disease that requires an interprofessional team approach to assist the patient in maximizing quality of life. QSEN: Teamwork and collaboration.

NANDA-I NDx Imbalanced Nutrition: Less Than Body Requirements

Common Related Factors

Increased metabolic need caused by increased work of breathing
Poor appetite resulting from fever, dyspnea, and fatigue
Indifference to food

Defining Characteristics

Body weight 20% or more below ideal weight range
Food intake less than recommended daily allowance for metabolic demands of disease state
Insufficient muscle tone

Common Expected Outcome

Patient's optimal nutritional status is maintained as evidenced by body weight within ideal weight range and adequate caloric intake.

NOC Outcomes

Nutritional Status: Food and Fluid Intake; Knowledge: Prescribed Diet

NIC Intervention

Nutrition Management

Ongoing Assessment

Actions/Interventions

▲ Compile a nutritional history, including preferred foods and dietary habits. Consult with the dietitian.

■ Assess the patient's physical ability to eat (energy level).

■ Assess the oral cavity.

▲ Monitor laboratory values that indicate nutritional status: serum albumin, total protein, ferritin, transferrin.

■ Assess the patient's weight weekly.

Rationales

The dyspnea of chronic obstructive pulmonary disease (COPD) may make it hard for patients to eat sufficient calories. Eating meals may increase dyspnea. Excessive mucus and coughing may decrease the appetite and alter the taste of foods. The dietitian can estimate the patient's daily caloric requirements. QSEN: Patient-centered care; Teamwork and collaboration.

The work of breathing may allow little energy for other activity, including eating.

Dry mucous membranes and poor dentition may contribute to a decreased appetite and nutritional status.

Serum prealbumin and albumin levels reflect protein status; ferritin and transferrin reflect iron status. Decreased values may be indicative of poor nutritional status or other pathology.

Patients may be unaware of their actual weight. Objective data guide the treatment plan. During aggressive nutritional support, the patient can gain up to $\frac{1}{2}$ pound per day.

■ = Independent   ▲ = Interprofessional Collaboration

Therapeutic Interventions

Actions/Interventions	Rationales
■ Encourage small feedings of nutritionally dense, soft food or liquids. Add nutritional supplements as appropriate.	Small feedings are easier to digest and require less chewing.
■ Instruct the patient to avoid very spicy foods, gas-producing foods, and carbonated beverages.	Avoidance prevents possible abdominal distention. Cold foods may give less sense of fullness than hot foods.
■ Instruct the patient to eat high-calorie foods first and have favorite foods available.	When anorexia is a problem, these strategies can be useful to maintain nutrition. In addition, adding butter, mayonnaise, margarine, sauces, or gravies to food can add calories.
■ Avoid fluid intake with meals, and instead encourage fluids between meals.	Fluid intake gives a sense of fullness with meals, thereby reducing the desire for solid foods.
■ Instruct the patient to plan activities and rest periods during the day.	Planning activities allows rest before eating.
■ Instruct the patient to eat slowly, use pursed-lip breathing between bites, and use bronchodilators before meals.	These techniques decrease dyspnea with eating.
■ Reinforce the need to substitute nasal prongs for an oxygen mask during mealtime.	This change in oxygen delivery equipment will maintain the patient's oxygenation.
■ Stress the importance of frequent oral care.	Oral care promotes mouth comfort and can enhance one's appetite.
■ Provide companionship at mealtime.	Attention to the social aspects of eating is important in both the hospital and home settings.
■ Assist with meals as needed, and cut up food if patients take longer than 1 hour to complete a meal.	These measures facilitate optimal intake.
■ Encourage the patient to sit up during meals.	This position reduces hypoxia and the danger of aspiration.

NANDA-I
NDx Risk for Infection

Common Risk Factors
Retained secretions (good medium for bacterial growth)
Poor nutrition
Impaired pulmonary defense system secondary to chronic obstructive pulmonary disease (COPD)
Use of respiratory equipment
Chronic disease

Common Expected Outcome
The patient remains free of infection as evidenced by normal temperature, negative sputum cultures, normal white blood cell count, and breath sounds clear to auscultation.

NOC Outcomes
Risk Control; Knowledge: Infection Management
NIC Intervention
Infection Protection

Ongoing Assessment

Actions/Interventions	Rationales
■ Auscultate the lungs to monitor for significant changes in breath sounds.	Bronchial breath sounds and crackles may indicate pneumonia.

Actions/Interventions

- Assess for any of the following significant changes in sputum:
  - Sudden increase in production
  - Change in color (rusty, yellow, greenish)
  - Change in consistency (thick)
- Assess for other signs and symptoms of infection: fever, chills, increase in cough, elevated white blood cell (WBC) count, shortness of breath, nausea, vomiting, diarrhea, anorexia.
- Assess the patient's understanding of techniques to prevent infection, such as careful handwashing, adequate rest and nutrition, and avoidance of crowds.
- Assess the patient's vaccination status (flu and pneumococcal vaccines).

Rationales

These signs may indicate the presence of infection. QSEN: Safety.

Prompt assessment of infection facilitates early intervention.

This knowledge helps the patient understand the rationale for interventions to reduce infection risk. QSEN: Safety.

These vaccines prevent some types of infection and are recommended by such organizations as the American Lung Association and the American Thoracic Society. QSEN: Evidence-based practice.

Therapeutic Interventions

Actions/Interventions

- Encourage an increase in fluid intake, unless contraindicated.

- Ensure that the oxygen humidifier is properly maintained. Reinforce not to add new water to old water.
- Minimize retained secretions by encouraging the patient to cough and expectorate secretions frequently. If the patient is unable to cough and expectorate, instruct the patient or caregiver in nasotracheal and oropharyngeal suctioning.
- Follow standard precautions, including proper handwashing techniques, to minimize microorganism transmission.

Rationales

Fluid intake maintains good hydration. Insensible loss is markedly increased during infection because of fever and an increase in respiratory rate.
Stagnant old water is a medium for bacterial growth.

Retained secretions provide bacterial growth medium.

Friction and running water effectively remove microorganisms from the hands. QSEN: Safety.

NANDA-I NDx **Deficient Knowledge**

Common Related Factors
Insufficient information
Insufficient interest in learning
Misinformation presented by others
Insufficient knowledge of resources

Defining Characteristics
Insufficient knowledge
Inaccurate follow-through of instruction
Inappropriate behavior

Common Expected Outcome
Patient verbalizes understanding of COPD and its treatment.

NOC Outcomes
Knowledge: Disease Process; Knowledge: COPD Management; Self-Management: COPD
NIC Interventions
Health Literacy Enhancement; Learning Facilitation; Teaching: Disease Process; Teaching: Prescribed Medication; Teaching: Prescribed Exercise; Teaching: Psychomotor Skill

■ = Independent   ▲ = Interprofessional Collaboration

Ongoing Assessment

Actions/Interventions	Rationales
■ Assess the patient's knowledge base of chronic obstructive pulmonary disease (COPD).	Patients need to understand that COPD is a progressive disease that requires self-management to reduce episodes of dyspnea, hypoxia, and acidosis. QSEN: Patient-centered care.
■ Assess the patient's cognitive function and emotional readiness to learn.	Cognitive impairments need to be assessed so an appropriate teaching plan can be designed. Patients with chronic hypoxia may have learning challenges.

Therapeutic Interventions

Actions/Interventions	Rationales
■ Allow the patient to identify what is most important to him or her.	This information clarifies learner expectations and helps the nurse match the information to be presented to the patient's needs. Adult learning is problem oriented. Providing information allows the patient to be a full partner in making decisions and assuming responsibility for care at a later time. QSEN: Patient-centered care.
■ Instruct the patient in basic anatomy and physiology of the respiratory system, with attention to its structure and airflow.	Information helps patients understand the complexities of their airway problems.
■ Discuss the relation of the disease process to the signs and symptoms that the patient experiences.	The recognition of key signs prevents delays in seeking help and facilitates appropriate self-management.
■ Discuss the purpose and method of administration for each medication.	Information enables the patient to self-manage the disease. Return demonstrations on metered-dose inhaler (MDI) spacers, dry powder capsules, or Diskus inhaler techniques are necessary to ensure appropriate delivery of the medications. If a steroid component is used, teach the patient to rinse the mouth after use to avoid fungal mouth infections.
■ Instruct the patient to avoid central nervous system depressants.	Depressants can depress respiratory drive.
■ Discuss appropriate nutritional habits, including supplements, as appropriate.	Patients with COPD have increased nutritional needs because of the work of breathing.
■ Discuss the concept of energy conservation.	Patients need to learn self-management skills to reduce dyspnea from fatigue. A variety of measures are appropriate to conserve energy, such as pacing activities, avoiding working with the arms raised, or reorganizing home items so that most frequently used ones are within easy reach.
■ Discuss the signs and symptoms of infection and when to contact the health care provider.	Respiratory infections can increase the work of breathing and precipitate respiratory failure. Teaching content on prevention of complications serves as a nursing action to reduce the risk of harm to the patient. QSEN: Safety.
■ Discuss the common factors that lead to exacerbations of lung problems: smoking, environmental temperature, and humidity.	Chemical irritants and allergens can increase mucus production and bronchospasm.
■ Refer the patient or significant others to smoking cessation support groups as appropriate.	Smoking or chronic exposure to tobacco smoke is the leading cause of COPD. Supportive groups provide emotional support and information.

⊖volve   **For additional care plans, go to http://evolve.elsevier.com/Gulanick/.**

Actions/Interventions	Rationales

■ Instruct in indoor and outdoor air quality:
  • Avoid smoke-filled rooms, sudden changes in temperature, aerosol sprays.
  • Use air conditioning in hot weather.
  • Stay indoors when pollen counts are high or when outdoor air quality is poor or during ozone alerts.
  • Use scarves or masks over the face in cold weather.
	Patients need to learn how to control air quality to promote effective breathing. Smoke and other factors resulting in poor air quality can cause bronchospasm. Similarly, cold air can induce bronchospasm.

■ Discuss the importance of specific therapeutic measures:
  • Breathing exercises
    • Exercise 1—TECHNIQUE:
      1. Lie supine with one hand on the chest and one hand on the abdomen.
      2. Inhale slowly through the mouth, raising the abdomen against the hand.
      3. Exhale slowly through pursed lips while contracting abdominal muscles and moving the abdomen inward.
	This exercise strengthens muscles of respiration.

• Exercise 2—TECHNIQUE:
      1. Walk; stop to take a deep breath.
      2. Exhale slowly while walking.
	This exercise develops slowed, controlled breathing.

• Exercise 3—TECHNIQUE:
      1. For pursed-lip breathing, inhale slowly through the nose.
      2. Exhale twice as slowly as usual through pursed lips.
	This exercise decreases air trapping and airway collapse.

• Cough: Lean forward; take several deep breaths with the pursed-lip method. Take a last deep breath, cough with an open mouth during expiration, and simultaneously contract abdominal muscles.	Controlled cough techniques help mobilize secretions.
• Forced expiratory technique: Instruct to take a deep breath, exhale forcefully without coughing through an open mouth while saying "huh." Repeat as many times as needed.	This technique moves the trapped mucus into the larger airways for the patient to cough up.
• Chest physiotherapy or pulmonary postural drainage: Demonstrate correct methods for positioning (including postural drainage), percussion, and vibration.	Chest physiotherapy, including postural drainage, facilitates the expectoration of secretions and prevents the waste of energy.
• Hydration: Discuss the importance of maintaining good fluid intake. Recommend 1.5 to 2 L/day.	Hydration decreases the viscosity of secretions.
• Humidity: Discuss various forms of humidification.	Humidity prevents the drying of secretions.
■ Discuss home oxygen therapy: • Type and use of equipment (compressed oxygen in tanks; liquid oxygen; oxygen concentrator).	Medicare guidelines for the reimbursement of home oxygen require a Pao_2 less than 55 mm Hg and/or oxygen saturation of 88% or less on room air. Patients or others who are primarily responsible for oxygen therapy at home should be able to demonstrate how to start oxygen flow and regulate the flowmeter; the flow rate of oxygen at rest, at night, and with activity; and the use of a portable oxygen system for ambulating.
• Safety precautions using oxygen.	Oxygen is not combustible itself but can feed a fire if one occurs. Providing the patient and the caregiver with this information reduces harm from oxygen therapy in the home setting. QSEN: Safety.

■ = Independent   ▲ = Interprofessional Collaboration

Actions/Interventions	Rationales
■ Discuss the available resources for securing equipment or managing the disease.	Home care agencies and patient support groups provide patients with resources to maintain compliance with a treatment program.
▲ Discuss or arrange for the patient to participate in a pulmonary rehabilitation program.	Pulmonary rehabilitation improves on baseline physical conditioning, increases optimal capabilities, and teaches the patient techniques to control breathing and energy conservation. QSEN: Teamwork and collaboration.
■ Discuss the need for the patient to obtain vaccines for pneumococcal pneumonia and a yearly vaccine for influenza.	Vaccines decrease the occurrence or severity of these diseases.
■ Discuss the use of a medical alert bracelet or other identification.	These forms of identification alert others to the patient's COPD history.

Related Care Plans

Activity intolerance, Chapter 2
Insomnia, Chapter 2
Ineffective health management, Chapter 2
Self-care deficit, Chapter 2

Head and Neck Cancer: Surgical Approaches

Radical Neck Surgery; Laryngectomy

Head and neck cancer includes cancer of the mouth, nose, sinuses, salivary glands, throat, and lymph nodes in the neck. Ninety percent of head and neck cancers are squamous cell carcinomas, with the remaining 10% divided among lymphomas and minor salivary gland tumors. Tobacco use, heavy alcohol use, and infection with the Epstein-Barr virus and the human papillomavirus (HPV) increase risk of many of the types of head and neck cancer. This cancer is three times more common in men, and its incidence increases with age, especially after age 50. Patients with HPV-associated head and neck cancer tend to be younger. If caught early, this cancer is curable. However, most cancers are diagnosed at later stages when a patient presents with a mass in the neck, hoarseness, or respiratory distress. A computed tomography (CT) scan of the head and neck, along with a fine-needle biopsy, are the most common diagnostic tools. Treatment for early-stage disease with surgery and possibly another adjunct therapy results in a cure for the majority of patients. For more locally advanced disease, treatment consists of combined modalities, such as surgery, radiation, and/or chemotherapy, in hopes of achieving the best outcome possible. The focus of this care plan is the surgical management of patients with head and neck cancer.

NANDA-I NDx Ineffective Airway Clearance

Common Related Factors	Defining Characteristics
Presence of artificial airway: tracheostomy tube and/or laryngectomy tube	Adventitious breath sounds (rhonchi, wheezes, crackles)
Thick, copious secretions	Ineffective cough
Pain	Dyspnea
Edema	Alteration in respiratory pattern (rate or depth)
Decreased energy and fatigue	Orthopnea
Inability and/or refusal to cough	Excessive sputum

◉volve   For additional care plans, go to http://evolve.elsevier.com/Gulanick/.

Common Expected Outcome

Patient maintains clear, open airways, as evidenced by normal breath sounds, normal rate and depth of respirations, and ability to effectively cough up secretions after treatment and deep breaths.

NOC Outcome

Respiratory Status: Airway Patency

NIC Interventions

Airway Management; Cough Enhancement; Airway Suctioning

Ongoing Assessment

Actions/Interventions	Rationales
■ Assess the respiratory rate, rhythm, and effort.	Respiratory rate and rhythm changes may be a compensatory response for airway obstruction and are early warning signs of impending respiratory difficulties.
■ Assess the effectiveness of cough.	An effective mucus-clearing cough is essential for adequate airway clearance. Pain may interfere with coughing. Thick, tenacious secretions may be difficult to expectorate.
■ Assess the color, consistency, and quantity of secretions.	Abnormalities may be the result of infection, smoking history, or other abnormalities. Discolored sputum, thick tenacious secretions, and a sudden increase in sputum production are signs of infection.
■ Auscultate the lungs after coughing for normal and abnormal sounds, as in the following: decreased or absent breath sounds, wheezing, coarse crackles.	Diminished breath sounds or the presence of adventitious sounds may indicate an obstructed airway.
▲ Use pulse oximetry to monitor oxygen saturation; assess arterial blood gases.	This nursing assessment reduces harm by identifying changes in oxygenation and acid-base balances, and initiating early intervention. Increasing $Paco_2$ and decreasing Pao_2 and pulse oximetry readings can result from increased pulmonary secretions and respiratory fatigue. QSEN: Safety.
■ Assess the color of skin, nail beds, and mucous membranes.	Color changes such as cyanosis indicate an increased concentration of deoxygenated blood and that inadequate oxygenation of tissues is occurring.
■ Assess changes in the level of consciousness.	Increasing confusion, restlessness, and/or irritability are early signs of cerebral hypoxia.
■ Assess for pain.	Postoperative pain can result in shallow breathing and an ineffective cough.

Therapeutic Interventions

Actions/Interventions	Rationales
■ Maintain humidified oxygen through the tracheostomy collar.	Humidification thins secretions for easier expectoration with coughing. With radical neck surgery, a total laryngectomy may be done, in which the entire larynx and pre-epiglottic region are removed and a permanent stoma is created. In other surgical procedures a tracheostomy may be performed to avoid potential airway complications in the immediate postoperative period.
■ Encourage the patient to deep breathe every 2 hours while awake and to cough. Encourage effective coughing after taking deep breaths.	Deep breathing prevents atelectasis and enhances gas exchange. Coughing is the most helpful way to remove most secretions, especially when combined with deep breathing.

■ = Independent　▲ = Interprofessional Collaboration

Pulmonary Care Plans

Actions/Interventions

- Suction the tracheostomy or stoma with sterile technique if the patient is unable to clear his or her own secretions.

- Position the patient with the head of the bed elevated.

- Encourage and assist the patient in changing positions every 2 hours, and increase activity as tolerated.
- Keep the same size sterile tracheostomy tube at the bedside.

Rationales

A patent airway is a priority. Suctioning is indicated when patients are unable to remove secretions by coughing. Sterile technique is important because patients with impaired immune systems as a result of cancer and surgery are at risk for infection. QSEN: Safety.

This position decreases surgical edema and increases lung expansion.

Frequent position changes facilitate the mobilization of secretions.

This standby tube is for insertion if dislodgement should occur.

NANDA-I NDx Impaired Verbal Communication

Common Related Factors

Laryngectomy (results in permanent loss of voice)
Tracheostomy (may temporarily cause inability to create sound)

Defining Characteristics

Inability to speak
Difficulty vocalizing words
Difficulty maintaining usual communication pattern

Common Expected Outcome

Patient uses a form of communication to get needs met and to relate effectively with persons and his or her environment.

NOC Outcome
Communication: Expressive
NIC Intervention
Communication Enhancement: Speech Deficit

Ongoing Assessment

Actions/Interventions

- Assess the patient's communication ability.

- Assess for additional obstacles to communication (e.g., the patient is hard of hearing, has low literacy, or has arthritis of the hands).
- Frequently assess the patient's need to communicate.

- Assess the effectiveness of nonverbal communication methods.

Rationales

With total laryngectomy, the vocal cords are removed, so sound is not produced. An assessment of the best nonverbal method for communication guides subsequent efforts. With a tracheostomy the majority of air bypasses the vocal cords. In some patients, no sound is made. In others, sound is "breathy" or weak. The speech therapy staff should evaluate the patient to determine if the use of a speaking valve is appropriate. QSEN: Teamwork and collaboration; Patient-centered care.

An accurate assessment of the full scope of limitations guides the selection of appropriate communication aids. QSEN: Patient-centered care.

Early recognition of and prompt response to the patient's need to communicate decreases anxiety and helps establish trust. QSEN: Patient-centered care.

The patient may use hand signals, facial expressions, and changes in body posture to communicate with others. However, others may have difficulty in interpreting these nonverbal techniques. Each new method needs to be assessed for effectiveness and altered as necessary. QSEN: Patient-centered care.

Therapeutic Interventions

Actions/Interventions	Rationales
■ Ensure that unit personnel are aware of the patient's inability to speak.	This knowledge may reduce the patient's sense of frustration when attempting to communicate with unit staff. QSEN: Teamwork and collaboration.
■ Keep the call light within reach at all times. Answer the call light promptly.	Prompt response decreases the patient's anxiety and feelings of helplessness.
■ Allow the patient time to communicate his or her needs.	The nurse should set aside enough time to attend to all of the details of patient care. Care measures may take longer to complete in the presence of a communication deficit.
■ Provide emotional support to the patient and significant others.	Difficulties communicating are a source of frustration to all involved.
■ Instruct the patient and significant others in alternative methods of communication: hand gestures, writing tablet with pen, picture board, word board, electronic communication system, electronic voice box.	Providing a variety of communication aids allows the patient more channels through which information can be communicated and broadens the group of people with whom the patient can communicate.
▲ Consult the speech therapy staff regarding alternative forms of speech. The following may be used for the patient:	Integrating the contributions of members of the interprofessional team helps the patient and family achieve health goals and allows for shared decision-making to achieve quality patient care. QSEN: Teamwork and collaboration.
• For tracheostomy only: speaking valve	The speaking valve is "one-way," allowing air to enter through the tracheostomy, then forcing exhalation via the upper airway. As air flows over the vocal cords, the vibrations create sound. The patient's oxygen saturation must be monitored at 30 minutes following initial placement. Always remove it for sleeping.
• Voice prosthesis (tracheoesophageal prosthesis [TEP])	The voice prosthesis is inserted into a fistula made between the esophagus and trachea. The prosthesis prevents aspiration but allows air from the lungs to enter the esophagus and out of the mouth with speech being produced by movement of the tongue and lips.
• Electrolarynx	The electrolarynx is a battery-operated, handheld device that uses sound waves to create speech while being held against the neck. The pitch is low, and the sound is electronic.
• Esophageal speech	Esophageal speech is a method of swallowing air and "belching" it to create sound.
■ Encourage the patient to obtain an audiotape for home use that can be played when emergency service is called.	The patient will feel more secure in the home environment with a means for rapid communication in an emergency. QSEN: Safety.
■ Encourage the patient to wear a medical alert bracelet to inform emergency personnel; "neck breather" is generally used.	This form of communication may be helpful in times of stress and emergency.

NANDA-I NDx   Risk for Ineffective Tissue Perfusion

Common Risk Factors

Tissue edema
Malfunction of wound drainage tubes
Preoperative radiation to surgical area
Extensive surgical dissection of blood vessels
Infection of surgical area

■ = Independent   ▲ = Interprofessional Collaboration

Pulmonary Care Plans

Common Expected Outcome

Patient maintains adequate tissue perfusion, as evidenced by normal incisional healing, gradual decrease in edema, gradual decrease in wound drainage, and no signs and symptoms of infection.

NOC Outcomes
Tissue Perfusion: Peripheral; Wound Healing: Primary Intention
NIC Interventions
Wound Care; Wound Care: Closed Drainage

Ongoing Assessment

Actions/Interventions	Rationales
■ Assess the surgical wound drainage system for the amount and color of drainage.	An abrupt cessation of drainage can indicate a clogged tube. Excessive drainage can indicate a leaking vessel in the area. Purulent drainage can indicate infection. White or "milky" drainage may indicate a chyle leak. Any of these *may* constitute a medical emergency. QSEN: Safety.
■ Assess for edema at the surgical wound.	Excessive edema can impede blood flow to or from the area and result in necrosis or infection.
■ Assess the color of the wound and its surrounding skin for signs of decreased circulation: pale, blue, or dark in color.	Changes in perfusion can compromise skin flap integrity.
■ Assess the wound edges for approximation.	Wound edges should be proximate (next to each other). Wound dehiscence can occur with excessive edema, necrosis, and infection.
■ Assess for hematoma formation: oozing from the skin edges, swelling, an increase in bruising, airway compromise.	Bleeding into the subcutaneous tissue may indicate a vessel leak and can result in a surgical emergency. QSEN: Safety.
■ Monitor the patient's body temperature.	Fever is a sign of infection.

Therapeutic Interventions

Actions/Interventions	Rationales
▲ Gently compress the drainage tubes as needed. Maintain suction as prescribed (e.g., Jackson-Pratt drain).	These procedures maintain patency and prevent the buildup of fluid at the surgical site, which would cause excessive edema and possible infection or necrosis.
■ Keep the head of the bed elevated.	This position decreases surgical edema.
■ Perform tracheostomy tube and site cleaning as needed.	This keeps respiratory secretions away from the surgical wound and reduces the risk for infection.
■ Promptly change tracheostomy or wound dressings when wet.	Attention to tube and dressing changes prevents maceration of the skin.

NANDA-I
NDx Imbalanced Nutrition: Less Than Body Requirements

Common Related Factors
Inability to ingest food (e.g., nothing by mouth (NPO) status)
Insufficient dietary intake (due to decreased appetite, difficulty swallowing)
Biological factors (due to side effects from radiation therapy and/or chemotherapy)

Defining Characteristics
Body weight 20% or more below ideal weight range
Food intake less than recommended dietary allowance (RDA)
Weakness of muscles needed for mastication and/or swallowing
Sore buccal cavity

 For additional care plans, go to http://evolve.elsevier.com/Gulanick/.

Common Expected Outcomes

Patient or caregiver demonstrates and verbalizes selection of foods or meals that will achieve a cessation of weight loss and intake of RDA.

Patient weighs within 10% of ideal weight range.

NOC Outcomes

Nutritional Status: Food and Fluid Intake; Nutritional Status

NIC Intervention

Nutrition Management

Ongoing Assessment

Actions/Interventions	Rationales
■ Monitor the patient's weight at regular intervals.	These data provide encouragement when eating habits are impaired and identify ineffective interventions.
▲ Monitor laboratory test results: serum albumin, protein, electrolytes, glucose.	These test results provide data on the extent of the nutritional deficiency.
■ Assess the types of foods that the patient enjoys.	A selection of favorite foods may enhance interest in eating and improve caloric intake. Eliciting the patient's food preferences allows the patient to be a full partner in providing care and achieving outcomes for improved nutrition. QSEN: Patient-centered care.
■ Observe the patient during the initial oral feeding.	In tracheostomy patients, signs of aspiration of food or fluid from the tracheostomy, such as choking, may occur when oral feeding is started. After laryngectomy, patients may have difficulty swallowing because of edema or surgical reconstruction. There is no longer any common pathway for food and air following a laryngectomy, so aspiration is a risk only for patients undergoing partial laryngectomies or other surgeries in which a tracheostomy is performed. QSEN: Safety.

Therapeutic Interventions

Actions/Interventions	Rationales
■ Instruct the patient in the importance of adequate caloric intake.	The patient may not understand the importance of caloric intake to promote incisional healing as well as to enhance overall nutritional status. QSEN: Patient-centered care.
▲ Consult with a dietitian.	The dietitian will determine caloric requirements specific to the patient, assess the caloric intake, and suggest enteral feedings, as appropriate. QSEN: Teamwork and collaboration.
■ Instruct in the need for enteral feedings if prescribed. Instruct in the procedure for the administration of home enteral feedings if prescribed.	Enteral feedings are initially used postoperatively until suture lines have healed. The feeding tube is put in place during surgery.
■ Assist the patient in performing oral hygiene.	Oral hygiene keeps the mouth fresh and promotes an interest in eating.
▲ Consult speech therapy staff for swallowing evaluation as needed.	If a total laryngectomy is performed, swallowing should not be a problem because there is no connection between the esophagus and trachea. If a supraglottic laryngectomy is done, swallowing is more difficult because the epiglottis has been removed. QSEN: Teamwork and collaboration.
■ Encourage the oral intake of soft foods when allowed.	Soft foods and thicker liquids are easier to swallow than thin liquids. If aspiration is suspected, instruct the patient in aspiration precautions and consult the speech therapy staff or occupational therapy staff for a swallowing evaluation.
■ Maintain a suction setup at the bedside for safety. Stay with the patient during initial oral feedings.	Suction may be needed during or after feedings to keep the airway patent. QSEN: Safety.

■ = Independent ▲ = Interprofessional Collaboration

NANDA-I NDx Disturbed Body Image

Common Related Factors

Alteration in body function (due to visible incision, facial and neck edema, tracheostomy or laryngectomy stoma, alteration in verbal communication, dysphagia, diagnosis of cancer, etc.)

Alteration in self-perception

Common Expected Outcome

Patient demonstrates enhanced body image and self-esteem as evidenced by ability to look at and talk about body changes, planning for discharge, showing interest in learning, and using alternative communication methods.

Defining Characteristics

Verbalization of negative feelings about body
Preoccupation with change
Refusal to look at face and neck
Withdrawal
Change in social behavior
Decreased motivation for self-care

NOC Outcome

Body Image

NIC Interventions

Body Image Enhancement; Support System Enhancement

Ongoing Assessment

Actions/Interventions

■ Assess the patient's mood and behavior for signs of difficulty in coping with changes in body appearance or function.

■ Assess the patient's perception of life changes precipitated by cancer treatments (occupational, interpersonal).

Rationales

There is a broad range of behaviors associated with body image disturbance, ranging from totally ignoring the altered structure to preoccupation with it. QSEN: Patient-centered care.

This assessment may give some perspective on any perceived misconceptions by the patient that could affect recovery.

Therapeutic Interventions

Actions/Interventions

■ Encourage the patient to view the tracheostomy or stoma site.

■ Suggest the use of a loose scarf or shirt over the stoma to camouflage it.

■ Encourage the patient and significant others to communicate fears or concerns regarding the diagnosis of cancer treatment.

■ Encourage visits, both in the hospital and at home, from significant others.

■ Refer to support services (e.g., Lost Cords, American Cancer Society, and International Association of Laryngectomees).

■ Arrange for a visit from a person who has had a laryngectomy.

Rationales

Looking at the site is often the first indication that the patient is ready to deal with the change in appearance.

Decreasing the visibility of the tracheostomy or stoma site may promote enhanced self-esteem.

Misconceptions may need to be clarified.

Visitors help the patient feel accepted and promote communication and support.

Rehabilitation after radical neck surgery is a long process, and support services can have a positive impact on the patient's recovery.

Laypersons in similar situations offer a different type of support that is perceived as helpful.

NANDA-I NDx   Deficient Knowledge: Preoperative and Postoperative

Common Related Factors

Insufficient information
Insufficient interest in learning
Misinformation presented by others
Insufficient knowledge of resources

Defining Characteristics

Insufficient knowledge
Inaccurate follow-through of instruction
Inappropriate behavior

Common Expected Outcome

Patient demonstrates an understanding of diagnostic process; treatment plan options; surgical procedures; tracheostomy and stoma care and/or suctioning techniques; and individualized course of postoperative treatment (e.g., radiation therapy).

NOC Outcomes
Knowledge: Disease Process; Knowledge: Treatment Regimen

NIC Interventions
Health Literacy Enhancement; Learning Facilitation; Teaching: Disease Process; Teaching: Psychomotor Skill

---

Ongoing Assessment

Actions/Interventions	Rationales
Preoperative:	
■ Assess the patient's knowledge of the diagnosis and treatment options.	This information provides the starting point for the educational session. This type of cancer is less publicized in the media and is one with which many patients have no experience.
Postoperative:	
■ Assess the patient's knowledge of postoperative care and follow-up cancer treatment.	A lack of knowledge of postoperative care can compromise the patient's ability to care for self at home, especially with a tracheostomy or laryngectomy stoma. The follow-up treatment plan depends on several factors, including the exact location of the tumor, the cancer stage, and other comorbid conditions. QSEN: Patient-centered care.
■ Assess the patient's support systems.	Living with a serious disease is challenging and carries an emotional burden. Assessment helps determine home care needs.

Therapeutic Interventions

Actions/Interventions	Rationales
■ Encourage questions and provide information on the nature of the cancer and the usual methods for diagnosis.	Questioning facilitates open communication between the patient and health care provider, and allows a verification of understanding of given information. Besides the usual physical examination and routine laboratory tests, the examination of tissue by biopsy is needed to confirm the diagnosis.
■ Provide information about the selected treatment plan and its implications.	Treatment is individualized but usually consists of a combination of surgery, radiation, and/or chemotherapy. Head and neck surgery usually affects the patient's ability to chew, swallow, or talk. Radiation causes side effects such as redness to the face, dry mouth and thick saliva, changes in taste, and difficulty swallowing. The side effects of chemotherapy depend on the agents being used.

■ = Independent   ▲ = Interprofessional Collaboration

Pulmonary Care Plans

Actions/Interventions	Rationales
■ Provide information about pain control.	Pain is a frequent and distressing in head and neck cancer. It can occur from radiation burns, and especially from damaged oral mucosa. The pain makes it difficult to talk and swallow. It can occur for a few weeks to a month or more after radiation/chemotherapy is completed. It is usually controlled with a fentanyl patch or liquid vicodin or morphine, along with mucositis cocktails with lidocaine that the patient swishes and spits out.
■ Provide information on postoperative procedures and treatments (e.g., regarding drainage tubes, dressings, feeding tube).	An understanding of the importance of caring for these devices may increase patient cooperation.
■ Teach the patient and caregiver as appropriate:	Providing information allows the patient to be a full partner in making decisions and assuming responsibility for care at a later time. QSEN: Patient-centered care; Safety.
	Early assessment facilitates prompt treatment.
• Signs and symptoms of infection and when to notify the health care provider	
• Indications for suctioning	A patent airway is a priority. Retained secretions can lead to a mucus plug.
• Procedure for tracheal suction. Use a mirror for teaching; include return demonstration.	Patients may need visual reinforcement to be successful with this procedure.
• Procedure for cleaning the inner cannula	This information decreases the incidence of a clogged tracheostomy tube.
• Procedure for changing and securing tracheal ties	This information decreases the incidence of a tracheostomy dislodgement.
▲ Once healing has occurred, consult with the speech therapy staff for the appropriate intraluminal device for individual patients.	Speech therapists can work with patients to develop the best plan for the patient's lifestyle. QSEN: Teamwork and collaboration.
■ Instruct the patient to cover the stoma when coughing to expectorate. The stoma should also be covered to prevent the inhalation of foreign materials (e.g., when shaving or applying makeup). Swimming is contraindicated to prevent the aspiration of water through the stoma.	Covering the stoma when coughing helps reduce the transmission of pathogens. Covering the stoma at other times helps prevent the inhalation of foreign materials and reduces aspiration risk. QSEN: Safety.
▲ Arrange for home health nurse care or visit as needed.	Continuity of care is facilitated through support services.
■ Discuss plans for radiation therapy, including what to expect, the probable time schedule for the series, and possible side effects.	Postoperative radiation therapy may be used to control the patient's metastasis.
■ Teach the importance of adequate calorie intake.	Caloric intake facilitates an optimal nutritional balance.
■ Teach exercises after radical neck surgery for strengthening the shoulder and neck muscles.	Restricted movement affects the ability to perform many ADLs.
■ Discuss the use of a medical alert bracelet or other identification to alert others to the disease process or stoma.	These forms of identification alert others to facilitate the delivery of safe, effective medical care. QSEN: Safety.

Related Care Plans

Grieving, Chapter 2
Disturbed body image, Chapter 2
Impaired verbal communication, Chapter 2
Ineffective coping, Chapter 2
Risk for impaired skin integrity, Chapter 2
Risk for aspiration, Chapter 2
Surgical experience: Preoperative and postoperative care, Chapter 4

Lung Cancer

Squamous Cell Carcinoma; Small Cell Carcinoma; Non–Small Cell Carcinoma; Adenocarcinoma; Large Cell Tumors

Lung cancer is the second most commonly occurring cancer among men and women, and despite all available therapies, lung cancer remains the leading cancer-related cause of death for men and women. Because of the late stage at which it is usually diagnosed, the 5-year survival rate for lung cancer patients is only 17%. But it is one of the most preventable cancers. The American Cancer Society estimates that more than 85% of all lung cancers are related to cigarette smoking. The U.S. Preventive Services Task Force (USPSTF) recommends that individuals at high risk for lung cancer (i.e., between ages of 55 and 80 years who have a 30 pack-year history of smoking and are current smokers or have quit within last 15 years) undergo annual low-dose CT screening as a means to improve lung cancer survival rates by finding the disease at an earlier and more treatable stage.

Lung cancer is divided into two major cell types: non–small cell lung cancer (NSCLC) and small cell lung cancer (SCLC). NSCLC accounts for more than 80% of cases, with adenocarcinomas being most common (approximately 40%), then squamous cell carcinoma, large cell carcinoma, and mixed cell tumors. SCLC is biologically and clinically distinct from the other histological types and accounts for approximately 15% of cases. The diagnosis and stage of lung cancer subtype are critical to the determination of appropriate treatment. NSCLC can be surgically resected in the early stages and treated with chemotherapy and/or radiation therapy based on stage. SCLC cannot be surgically resected and is always treated with chemotherapy and radiation therapy.

Prevention is essential. Providing smoke-free environments, testing for radon, and providing educational programs remain the most powerful interventions. Smoking cessation interventions are a part of all care plans for patients who smoke. Although there are currently no effective screening tests or tumor markers used for the general population, promising research focuses on making the immune system and chemical messengers more effective in responding to early cellular changes of lung cancer. Work continues in the development of chemical messengers that control and stop abnormal cell growth (antioncogene therapy), the use of monoclonal antibodies that recognize and destroy only abnormal lung cells, and stimulation of the immune system by learning to control cytokines such as interleukin 2 and the interferons. In the future, systemic treatment (chemotherapy and targeted therapy) may be selected based on patients' cellular mutation status. This care plan focuses on the educational aspects of lung cancer.

NANDA-I NDx Deficient Knowledge

Common Related Factors

Insufficient information
Insufficient interest in learning
Misinformation presented by others
Insufficient knowledge of resources

Common Expected Outcomes

Patient describes probable cause of his or her cancer.
Patient describes the diagnostic evaluation for lung cancer.
Patient explains the treatment regimen for own type of lung cancer.
Patient verbalizes resources available for additional information and support.

Defining Characteristics

Insufficient knowledge
Inaccurate follow-through of instruction
Inappropriate behavior

NOC Outcomes

Knowledge: Disease Process; Knowledge: Treatment Procedure

NIC Interventions

Health Literacy Enhancement; Learning Facilitation; Teaching: Disease Process; Teaching: Procedure/Treatment; Smoking Cessation Assistance

■ = Independent   ▲ = Interprofessional Collaboration

Ongoing Assessment

Actions/Interventions	Rationales
■ Assess the patient's understanding of the causes, diagnostic evaluation, and treatment interventions for lung cancer.	Educational programs are individualized to meet the patient's level of previous knowledge. Many patients are exposed to someone with lung cancer, yet many misconceptions continue to exist.
■ Assess the patient's readiness to learn.	Some patients are ready to learn soon after they are diagnosed; others cope better by denying or delaying the need for instruction. Learning also requires energy, which patients may not be ready to use. Physical and emotional pain, grieving, denial, anxiety, and anger are barriers to learning, and information presented may not be learned. QSEN: Patient-centered care.
■ Assess the family's and significant other's willingness to participate in the teaching and learning process.	Often during the acute stages, the family or significant others may require the most teaching. This can assist them in providing support to the patient. Individuals do have a right to refuse educational services.

Therapeutic Interventions

Actions/Interventions	Rationales
■ Involve the patient and significant others in developing the teaching plan.	Allowing the patient to actively participate in the teaching plan increases motivation and helps ensure that the information most significant to the patient is presented first and in a comfortable format. Significant others are important in the educational process because chronic illness and potentially fatal illnesses involve not only the patient but also the patient's loved ones. QSEN: Patient-centered care.
■ Provide information on community resources, websites, and additional sources of support.	The American Lung Association (www.lung.org), the American Cancer Society (www.cancer.org), the National Cancer Institute (www.cancer.gov/about-cancer), the National Comprehensive Cancer Network (NCCN) (www.nccn.org), and many other sources have numerous teaching aids available to support and reinforce learning. Support groups can assist in the learning process by reinforcing learning and increasing motivation to learn. Warn the patient about resources that do not provide correct information (e.g., "Dr. Rob's Lung Cancer Cure Website").
■ Explain the possible causes of lung cancer.	The patient may benefit from understanding the broad range of causes of lung cancer, including passive exposure to smoke, radon, asbestos; air pollution containing benzopyrenes and hydrocarbons; and exposure to occupational agents such as petroleum, chromates, and arsenic. The role of genetic factors is an ongoing area of study.
■ If the patient is a smoker: • Discuss tobacco-dependence treatment for smoking cessation, such as the use of pharmacological cessation aids, nicotine-replacement therapies, behavior modification, and smoking-cessation support groups.	Smoking cessation following the diagnosis of lung cancer will improve clinical outcomes. However, the perceived pressure to stop smoking is an added stressor to the patient with newly diagnosed lung cancer.
• Communicate information on the risk to children and nonsmokers caused by environmental second-hand tobacco smoke.	Second-hand passive smoke is a known carcinogen in individuals with long-term exposure. Children exposed to smoke also have an increased incidence of respiratory complications or disease.

Actions/Interventions	Rationales
■ Discuss the evaluation of the home for the detection of radon and its inexpensive removal, if necessary.	By its own action and by its interaction with cigarette smoking, radon is considered the second leading cause of lung cancer in the United States.
■ Discuss the diagnostic evaluation:	The appropriate selection of diagnostic testing is based on recommendations from national organizations. QSEN: Evidence-based practice.
• Chest x-ray film	Chest x-ray films are repeated at frequent intervals and may be the initial test performed when new symptoms are reported.
• Imaging tests	Imaging tests use x-rays, magnetic fields, sound waves, or radioactive substances to find cancer. Monoclonal antibodies tagged with technetium concentrate in areas of tumor cells and are detected by single-photon emission computed tomography (SPECT).
• Collection of sputum for cytological evaluation	Sputum cytological examination may help identify tumors that involve the bronchial wall.
• Bronchoscopy	Brush biopsies and multiple bronchial washings are performed to obtain a tissue diagnosis. Bronchoscopy is mandatory for small cell cancer.
• Percutaneous transthoracic needle aspiration (TTNA) or biopsy under fluoroscopy, and/or computed tomography (CT)	This procedure is indicated for non–small cell cancer. It is done if bronchoscopy has not yielded an adequate tissue diagnosis or if the lesion is not central and accessible by bronchoscopy.
• Mediastinoscopy	Mediastinoscopy is performed if the previous two procedures have not yielded a tissue diagnosis. It is used to sample lymph nodes and is mandatory for staging non–small cell cancer if surgery is being contemplated.
• Pulmonary function tests	These tests predict whether lung function is sufficient to tolerate a surgical resection. Most patients with lung cancer are long-term smokers with poor lung function.
• Positron emission tomography (PET) scan	PET scan is done to identify mediastinal and distant metastases. It is recommended for staging all non–small cell lung cancer (NSCLC).
• Open surgical biopsy	Surgical biopsies are required when a larger piece of tissue is needed, especially for molecular testing.
• Blood tests	Serum blood tests are done to determine whether there is liver or bone metastasis.
■ Describe the following tests for patients with small cell cancer:	The appropriate selection of diagnostic testing is based on recommendations from national organizations. QSEN: Evidence-based practice.
• Brain or head CT and magnetic resonance imaging (MRI) scans	These scans determine the presence of brain metastases.
• Liver and abdominal CT scans	These scans evaluate the liver and adrenal glands for signs of metastasis.
• Bone scan	These scans are done if the patient has bone pain (optional if PET scan obtained).
■ Discuss staging classifications for the following: *For small cell cancer:*	Staging by TNM (described below) is not used with small cell cancer because of the aggressiveness of the tumor at diagnosis.
• Limited stage	*Limited* usually means one lung and lymph nodes on the same side of the chest that can be encompassed in a single radiation therapy port. Port refers to the anatomical location designated to receive radiation therapy.

■ = Independent   ▲ = Interprofessional Collaboration

Actions/Interventions

- Extensive stage

For non–small cell cancer:
- Tumor, node, metastasis (TNM) staging classification

■ Explain "Performance Status Assessment."
- Fully ambulatory patients tolerate therapy better and live longer.
- Patients with restricted activities and out of bed more than 50% of the day survive longer than more restricted patients.
- Totally bedridden patients tolerate all forms of therapy poorly and have short survival.

■ Explain the treatments for non–small cell cancer:

- Chemotherapy: systemic treatment with platinum-based combination therapy
- Radiation therapy for a regional inoperable tumor

- Molecular targeted therapy

- Surgery for resectable disease (stages I to IIIA)

- Pneumonectomy

- Lobectomy

- Wedge resection

■ Explain treatments for small cell cancer:

- Chemotherapy

Rationales

The *extensive* stage includes all other disease and means that cancer has spread to the other lung, to lymph nodes on the other side, or to distant organs.

The clinical diagnostic stage is based on pretreatment scans, radiographs, biopsies, and mediastinoscopy and is used to determine extent of disease and resectability. The postsurgical pathological stage is based on the analysis of tissue obtained at thoracotomy and is used to determine prognosis and the need for additional treatment. Tumor size, spread to the lymph nodes, and metastasis to distant organs are staged from 0 to IV. The lower the number, the less the cancer has spread. Tumor staging classification is helpful to determine the optimal treatment plan.

This assessment probably is the most important prognostic factor for nonresectable cases. QSEN: Patient-centered care.

The following nursing actions are based on recommendations from national organizations. The 5-year survival rate for patients with early stages I to III disease range from 30% to 50%. QSEN: Evidence-based practice.

Chemotherapy offers palliation of symptoms.

Radiation relieves symptoms in a significant percentage of patients, especially those with superior vena cava syndrome, dyspnea, cough, hemoptysis, and pneumonia secondary to obstruction.

These agents (gefitinib, erlotinib) stop tumor growth by blocking molecules essential to the growth and progression of tumors.

Surgical resection offers the best chance for long-term survival. Selection of the type of operation is determined by the tumor location and size.

Removal of the affected lung is reserved for extensive disease that is technically resectable.

Lobectomy is performed when the tumor is contained within a lobe and adequate margins can be obtained or when lymph node extension is limited to lobar nodes totally encompassed in the en bloc dissection.

Wedge resection is performed for small (<2 cm) peripheral nodules without lymph node or other extensive involvement.

The following nursing actions are based on recommendations from national organizations. QSEN: Evidence-based practice.

Because small cell cancer more often spreads from the primary site and because of its increased sensitivity to chemotherapy, combination chemotherapy is the major treatment and has improved survival fivefold.

Actions/Interventions

- Prophylactic cranial irradiation (PCI)

■ Explain any treatment options or potential clinical trials the physician may feel would be beneficial to the patient, and how the patient can get additional information about these other therapies.

Rationales

PCI can improve both disease-free and overall survival in patients in complete remission. PCI should be considered after chemotherapy in patients with stage I disease who have had a complete resection.

Gene therapy, the use of cytokines, and enhanced immune system therapy are topics in the national news. Patients may have questions about the appropriateness of these therapies for their cancer.

Pulmonary Care Plans

NDx Cancer-Related Fatigue

Common Related Factors

Tumor and metastatic disease
Chemotherapy and/or targeted therapy
Radiation
Pain
Distress (spiritual or emotional)
Anxiety and/or fear
Malnutrition
Anemia

Defining Characteristics

A sense of physical or emotional tiredness that is not proportional to recent activity or treatment and interferes with the individual's daily functioning.
Inability to restore energy, even after sleep
Verbalization of an overwhelming lack of energy

Common Expected Outcomes

Patient reports reduction in fatigue, as evidenced by reports of increased energy and ability to perform desired activities.
Patient reports use of energy-conservation principles.

NOC Outcomes

Activity Tolerance; Endurance; Energy Conservation; Self-Care: Activities of Daily Living (ADL)

NIC Interventions

Energy Management; Nutrition Management; Sleep Enhancement; Exercise Promotion

Ongoing Assessment

Actions/Interventions

■ Assess for fatigue regularly using a numeric rating scale of 0 to 10 and defining characteristics.

■ Refer to Fatigue (Chapter 2).

Rationales

Fatigue has become the most common and distressing complaint for patients with cancer, especially during treatment. Regular assessment allows the nurse to evaluate the fatigue and response to interventions and to develop and alter the plan accordingly. QSEN: Patient-centered care.

■ = Independent ▲ = Interprofessional Collaboration

Therapeutic Interventions

Actions/Interventions	Rationales
In addition to the Fatigue care plan in Chapter 2, consider the following:	
■ Educate the patient regarding these treatments:	Providing information allows the patient to be a full partner in making decisions and assuming responsibility for self-management at a later time. QSEN: Patient-centered care.
• Energy-conservation strategies	Conserving energy will allow the patient to achieve the most desired goals and feel a sense of accomplishment. Energy conservation may include setting priorities, delegating tasks, frequent rest periods, work simplification, and the use of assistive devices.
• Limiting naps to 20 to 30 minutes	Limiting the amount of sleep during naps will help the patient sleep at night.
• Use of psychostimulants after ruling out other causes	These medications have been used cautiously and demonstrate improved symptoms of fatigue in some patients.
• Treatment for anemia as indicated	Anemia in patients with cancer results from the disease itself and treatment. Correcting the anemia may improve the patient's energy level.
• Cognitive-behavioral therapy (CBT)	Fear and anxiety associated with the patient's response to cancer and its treatment requires expenditure of energy. CBT facilitates psychological adjustment by helping certain patients recognize and change their maladaptive thoughts.
• Nutrition consultation	Protein caloric malnutrition may contribute to weakness and fatigue. A dietitian can counsel the patient and family on how to maximize the patient's intake during treatment for optimal nutritional needs. QSEN: Teamwork and collaboration.

NANDA-I NDx Risk for Ineffective Protection

Common Risk Factors

Cancer
Chemotherapy and/or targeted therapies
Radiation
Myelosuppression

Common Expected Outcome

Risk for ineffective protection is reduced by early assessment of complications and appropriate treatment.

NOC Outcomes

Immune Status; Blood Loss Severity; Neurologic Status: Consciousness

NIC Interventions

Surveillance; Bleeding Precautions; Neurologic Monitoring; Electrolyte Monitoring; Respiratory Monitoring

Ongoing Assessment

Actions/Interventions

- Assess for common oncological emergencies:
  - Superior vena cava syndrome (SVCS)
  - Cardiac tamponade
  - Spinal cord compression

- Assess for common paraneoplastic syndromes:
  - Endocrine disorders: seen with small cell lung cancer: syndrome of inappropriate antidiuretic hormone (SIADH)
  - Hypercalcemia
  - Hematologic disorders, such as disseminated intravascular coagulation (DIC)

Rationales

An oncological emergency is an acute, life-threatening event either directly or indirectly related to the patient's cancer and its treatment. If untreated it can lead to permanent damage or death. Common examples include SVCS caused by partial or complete obstruction of blood flow through the superior vena cava by tumor or thrombosis; cardiac tamponade caused by accumulation of fluid-containing tumor cells in the pericardial sac and by encasement of the heart by the tumor; and spinal cord compression caused by tumor in the epidural space of the spinal cord. QSEN: Safety.

Paraneoplastic syndromes are a set of signs and symptoms that are the consequence of cancer in the body, caused by hormones secreted by tumor cells. These symptoms may precede the diagnosis of lung cancer. Because of their complexity and variety, the clinical presentation of these syndromes may vary greatly.

Therapeutic Interventions

Actions/Interventions

- ▲ Anticipate the treatment for oncological emergencies.
  - For SVCS: radiation therapy to site of obstruction, chemotherapy, surgery
  - For cardiac tamponade:
    - Decompression of the heart either surgically or by pericardiocentesis
    - To prevent reaccumulation of fluid of effusions:
      - Catheter drainage with instillation of a sclerosing agent
      - Radiation therapy
      - Surgical intervention with the creation of a pericardial window
  - For spinal cord compression, treat with radiation therapy, corticosteroids, surgical decompressive laminectomy.
- ▲ Anticipate the appropriate treatment for each type of paraneoplastic syndrome.
  - For SIADH: correct sodium–water imbalance, including free water restriction and adequate sodium intake.
  - For hypercalcemia: hydration therapy and infusion of bisphosphonates
  - For DIC: heparin, cryoprecipitates, platelets, and packed red blood cells

Rationales

These life-threatening problems require immediate treatment. Being prepared for an emergency helps prevent further complications. QSEN: Safety.

A variety of systemic effects called paraneoplastic syndromes occur with lung cancer. The optimal approach is to treat the underlying tumor. Specific manifestations guide treatment. QSEN: Evidence-based practice.

■ = Independent ▲ = Interprofessional Collaboration

NANDA-I NDx Acute Pain

Common Related Factors

Original tumor and metastatic disease
Chemotherapy and/or targeted therapy
Radiation

Defining Characteristics

Self-report of intensity using a standardized pain scale
Self-report of pain characteristics using a standardized pain instrument
Facial expression of pain
Change in physiological parameter (e.g., blood pressure, heart rate, respiratory rate and oxygen saturation)

Common Expected Outcomes

Patient reports satisfactory pain control at a decreased intensity using a standardized pain scale.
Patient exhibits increased comfort such as baseline levels for BP, HR, and respirations, and relaxed muscle tone or body posture.

NOC Outcomes

Pain Control; Medication Response; Comfort Status

NIC Interventions

Pain Management; Analgesic Administration

Ongoing Assessment

Actions/Interventions	Rationales
■ Assess for pain characteristics.	Assessment of the pain experience is the first step in planning pain management strategies. Each patient may exhibit a slightly different pain presentation.
■ Assess the patient's expectations for pain relief.	Some patients may be content to have pain decreased; others may expect complete elimination of pain. Their expectation affects their perception of the effectiveness of the treatment modality and their willingness to participate in additional treatment. QSEN: Patient-centered care.
■ Monitor the effectiveness of pain-relief therapies.	Patients have a right to effective pain relief. The use of visual analogue scales may provide objective data. Evidence of relaxed appearance and baseline HR, BP, and respiration support the achievement of comfort goals. QSEN: Patient-centered care.
■ Assess the concerns and fears related to pain medication.	There remain many myths about pain. Some patients fear addiction to medication or incomplete pain relief. These concerns may enhance the perception of pain or decrease the patient's use of safe, effective, pain-relieving medications.
■ Assess the side effects of pain therapies, including constipation.	Analgesics produce side effects. These side effects should be monitored and appropriate interventions taken. Constipation is preventable and should be anticipated and appropriate interventions planned.

Therapeutic Interventions

Actions/Interventions	Rationales
▲ Administer prescribed medications as follows (based on World Health Organization [WHO] analgesic ladder and National Comprehensive Cancer Network [NCCN] guidelines for cancer pain):	These medications are based on recommendations from national organizations. Various medications may be given by a variety of routes, including patient-controlled analgesia, in which the patient can control the amount of medication delivered. QSEN: Evidence-based practice.
• Nonsteroidal anti-inflammatory drugs (NSAIDs)	NSAIDs are used to treat muscle spasms associated with progressive tumor spread.
• Short- and long-acting opioid analgesics	These opioid medications are used for acute and chronic cancer pain, including bone metastases. It is essential to work for pain relief and patient comfort and not fear escalating doses as opioid tolerance develops or patients manifest symptoms of disease progression.
• Transdermal opioids	Transdermal administration may be indicated for patients unable to take oral medications.
■ Teach nonpharmacological interventions for pain relief.	Massage, distraction, music therapy, and support groups are examples of techniques and/or resources that may enhance pharmacological interventions.
■ Consult a pain specialist as needed.	Specialty expertise may be required to manage severe chronic or intractable pain. QSEN: Teamwork and collaboration.

Related Care Plans

Acute pain, Chapter 2
Chronic pain, Chapter 2
Fatigue, Chapter 2
Imbalanced nutrition: Less than body requirements, Chapter 2
Death and dying: End-of-life issues, Chapter 4
Surgical experience: Preoperative and postoperative care, Chapter 4
Cancer chemotherapy, Chapter 10
Cancer radiation therapy, Chapter 10
Thoracotomy, ⊜volve

Mechanical Ventilation

Ventilator; Endotracheal Tube; Intubation; Ventilator-Associated Pneumonia

Mechanical ventilation can be a temporary or chronic lifesaving therapy. Its purpose is to maintain adequate ventilation by delivering preset concentrations of oxygen at an adequate tidal volume while reducing the work of breathing. The patient who requires mechanical ventilation must have an artificial airway (endotracheal tube) or tracheostomy. It is used most often in patients with hypoxemia and alveolar hypoventilation. Although the mechanical ventilator will facilitate movement of gases into and out of the pulmonary system (ventilation), it cannot ensure gas exchange at the pulmonary and tissues levels (respiration). It provides either partial or total ventilatory support for patients with respiratory failure. Mechanical ventilation may be used short-term in the acute care setting (e.g., after surgery; during general anesthesia) or long term in the subacute, rehabilitation, or home care setting. Ventilator-associated pneumonia (VAP) is a significant nosocomial infection that is associated with endotracheal intubation and mechanical ventilation. Prevention of VAP is a primary focus of the 100,000 Lives Campaign to promote quality care and patient safety. Many VAP bundles have been developed and are available to guide prevention of this complication. This care plan focuses on patient care in a hospital setting.

Pulmonary Care Plans

■ = Independent ▲ = Interprofessional Collaboration

Pulmonary Care Plans

NANDA-I NDx Impaired Spontaneous Ventilation

Common Related Factors

Metabolic factors
Respiratory muscle fatigue
Acute respiratory failure

Defining Characteristics

Arterial pH less than 7.35
Decreased Pao_2 level (<50 to 60 mm Hg)
Increased $Paco_2$ level (50 to 60 mm Hg or higher)
Decreased oxygen saturation (Sao_2 < 90%)
Apprehension
Restlessness
Increased or decreased respiratory rate
Dyspnea
Apnea
Decreased tidal volume
Forced vital capacity less than 10 mL/kg
Inability to maintain airway (depressed gag reflex, depressed cough, emesis)
Adventitious breath sounds
Diminished lung sounds

Common Expected Outcomes

Patient maintains spontaneous gas exchange resulting in normal arterial blood gases (ABGs) within patient parameters, return to normal pulse oximetry, and decreased dyspnea.
Patient demonstrates no complications from the mechanical ventilation.

NOC Outcomes

Respiratory Status: Ventilation; Respiratory Status: Gas Exchange

NIC Interventions

Respiratory Monitoring; Ventilation Assistance; Airway Insertion and Stabilization; Artificial Airway Management; Mechanical Ventilation Management: Invasive; Oxygen Therapy

Ongoing Assessment

Actions/Interventions	Rationales
Before intubation:	
■ Assess the patient's BP and HR.	Hypotension and tachycardia may result from hypoxia and/or hypercarbia.
■ Assess the respiratory rate, pattern, and depth, including the use of accessory muscles.	Respiratory rate and rhythm changes are early signs of impending respiratory difficulties. As moving air in and out of the lungs becomes more difficult, the breathing pattern alters to include the use of accessory muscles to increase chest excursion. QSEN: Safety.
▲ Use pulse oximetry, as available, to monitor oxygen saturation.	Pulse oximetry is useful in detecting early changes in oxygenation. Oxygen should be at 90% or greater.
■ Assess ABGs as appropriate.	Increasing $Paco_2$ and decreasing Pao_2 are signs of respiratory failure. If the patient's condition begins to fail, the respiratory rate and depth decrease and $Paco_2$ begins to rise. QSEN: Safety.
	Identifying changes in oxygenation and acid-base balances facilitates the initiation of early intervention. QSEN: Safety.

 evolve For additional care plans, go to http://evolve.elsevier.com/Gulanick/.

Actions/Interventions

- Assess for changes in the level of consciousness.

- Assess the skin color, checking nail beds and lips for cyanosis.

- Assess the lungs for normal or adventitious breath sounds.

After intubation:
- Assess for correct endotracheal (ET) tube placement:
  - Auscultation of bilateral breath sounds
  - Observation of a symmetrical rise of both sides of the chest
  - X-ray confirmation (after the ET tube is taped)
- Assess the ventilator settings and alarm system every hour.

- Assess for patient comfort and the ability to cooperate with therapy.

Rationales

Restlessness, confusion, and irritability can be early signs of hypoxia. Lethargy and somnolence are later signs. QSEN: Safety.

Cyanosis indicates an increased concentration of deoxygenated blood and that the breathing pattern is no longer effective to maintain adequate oxygenation of tissues.

Changes in lung sounds are important in making an accurate diagnosis of impaired ventilation. Assessment allows for early detection of deterioration or improvement.

Correct ET tube placement is necessary for effective mechanical ventilation. QSEN: Safety.

Assessment ensures that settings are accurate and alarms are functional. Appropriate use of safety-enhancing technology minimizes the risk of harm to the patient. QSEN: Safety.

Patient discomfort may be related to incorrect ventilator settings that result in insufficient oxygenation. Once intubated and breathing on the mechanical ventilator, the patient should be breathing easily and not "fighting" the ventilator. QSEN: Patient-centered care.

Therapeutic Interventions

Actions/Interventions

Before intubation:
- Maintain the patient's airway. Use the oral or nasal airway as needed.
- Encourage the patient to breathe deeply and cough.

- If coughing and deep breathing are not effective, use nasotracheal suction as needed.

- Place the patient in high-Fowler's position, if tolerated. Check the position often.

Prepare for endotracheal intubation:
- ▲ Notify the respiratory therapist to bring a mechanical ventilator.

- If possible, before intubation, explain to the patient the need for intubation, the steps involved, and the temporary inability to speak because of the ET tube passing through the vocal cords.
- Prepare the equipment:
  - ET tubes of various sizes, noting the size used

  - Syringe, benzoin, and waterproof tape or other securing methods

Rationales

A patent airway is a priority. An artificial airway is used to prevent the tongue from occluding the oropharynx.

Deep breathing facilitates oxygenation. Coughing is the most helpful way to remove most secretions.

Suctioning is indicated when patients are unable to remove secretions from the airway by coughing. It can also stimulate cough.

This position promotes lung expansion and improved air exchange. Do not let the patient slide down; this causes the abdomen to compress the diaphragm, which would cause respiratory change.

A variety of ventilator types are available, depending on the extent and type of the patient's problem. Positive-pressure ventilators are used most frequently.

Preparatory information can reduce anxiety and promote cooperation with intubation.

Adult sizes range from 7 to 9 mm. Selection is based on the size of the patient.

A syringe is used to inflate the balloon (cuff) after the ET tube is in position. Tape and benzoin are used to secure the ET tube.

■ = Independent   ▲ = Interprofessional Collaboration

Actions/Interventions

- Local anesthetic agent (e.g., benzocaine [Cetacaine] spray, cocaine, lidocaine [Xylocaine] spray or jelly, and cotton-tipped applicators)
- Stylet, laryngoscope, and blades

▲ Administer sedation as prescribed.

Assist with intubation:

■ Place the patient in a supine position, hyperextending the neck (if not contraindicated) and aligning the patient's oropharynx, posterior nasopharynx, and trachea.

▲ Oxygenate and ventilate the patient with an Ambu bag and mask as needed before and after each intubation attempt. If intubation is difficult, the physician will stop periodically so that oxygenation is maintained with artificial ventilation by the Ambu bag and mask.

▲ Apply cricoid pressure as directed by the physician.

After intubation:

▲ Assist with the verification of correct ET tube placement as described under "Assessment" earlier in this care plan. Use a carbon dioxide detector as indicated.

■ Continue with manual Ambu bag ventilation until the ET tube is stabilized. Assist in securing the ET tube once tube placement is confirmed.

■ Document the ET tube position, noting the centimeter reference marking on the ET tube.

▲ Institute mechanical ventilation with prescribed settings.

■ Insert an oral airway and/or bite block for the orally intubated patient.

■ Institute aseptic suctioning of the airway.

■ Apply bilateral soft wrist restraints as needed, explaining the reason for their use.

Rationales

These anesthetic agents suppress the gag reflex and promote general comfort.

A stylet makes the ET tube firmer and gives additional support to direction during intubation. The scope and blades facilitate opening of the upper airway and visualization of the vocal cords for placement of oral ET tubes.

Sedation facilitates comfort and ease of intubation.

This position is necessary to promote visualization of landmarks for accurate tube insertion.

This provides assisted ventilation with 100% oxygen before intubation. Increasing oxygen tension in the alveoli may result in more oxygen diffusion into the capillaries.

Pressure is used to occlude the esophagus and allow easier intubation of the trachea. It may also prevent vomiting and aspiration.

Correct placement is needed for effective mechanical ventilation and to prevent complications associated with malpositioning (e.g., gastric distention, vomiting, lung trauma, hypoxia). The carbon dioxide detector is attached to the ET tube immediately after intubation to verify tracheal intubation. Other capnography devices that provide numerical measurements of end-tidal carbon dioxide (normal value is 35 to 45 mm Hg) and capnograms may also be used. Appropriate use of safety-enhancing technology minimizes the risk of harm to the patient. QSEN: Safety.

Stabilization is necessary before initiating mechanical ventilation.

Documentation provides a reference for determining possible tube displacement, usually 23 cm at the lips for men and 21 cm for women.

Modes for ventilating (assist/control, synchronized intermittent mandatory ventilation), tidal volume, rate per minute, fraction of oxygen in inspired gas (FIO_2), pressure support, positive end-expiratory pressure, and the like must be preset and carefully evaluated for response. Appropriate attention to prescribed settings minimizes the risk of harm to the patient. QSEN: Safety.

An oral airway and/or bite block prevents the patient from biting down on the ET tube.

Suction maintains a clear airway. A Yankauer suction device should be available. Suctioning procedures should be based on need rather than preset time intervals to reduce the risk for infection and airway trauma. QSEN: Safety.

These restraints may prevent self-extubation of the ET tube. Although not all patients require restraints to prevent extubation, many do.

Actions/Interventions

▲ Administer muscle-paralyzing agents, sedatives, and opioid analgesics as indicated.

■ Anticipate the need for nasogastric and/or oral gastric suction.

■ Respond to alarms, noting that high-pressure alarms may be from patient resistance or the patient's need for suctioning. A low-pressure alarm may be a ventilator disconnection. If the source of the alarm cannot be located, ventilate the patient with an Ambu bag until assistance arrives.

■ Check the cuff volume by assessing whether the patient can talk or make sounds around the tube or whether exhaled volumes are significantly less than volumes delivered. To correct, slowly reinflate the cuff with air until no leak is detected. Notify the respiratory therapist to check cuff pressure.

Rationales

These medications decrease the patient's work of breathing, decrease myocardial work, and may facilitate effective gas exchange.

Abdominal distention may indicate gastric intubation and can also occur after cardiopulmonary resuscitation when air is inadvertently blown or bagged into the esophagus, as well as the trachea. Suction prevents abdominal distention. Oral gastric suctioning may also reduce the risk for sinusitis.

The key is that the patient receives oxygenation support at all times until mechanical ventilation is no longer required. TJC's National Patient Safety Goals requires that alarm systems be activated and functional at all times. Appropriate use of safety-enhancing technology minimizes the risk of harm to the patient. QSEN: Safety; Evidence-based practice.

Cuff pressure should be maintained at 20 to 30 mm Hg. Maintenance of low-pressure cuffs prevents many tracheal complications formerly associated with ET tubes. Notify the physician if the leak persists. The ET tube cuff may be defective, requiring the physician to change the tube. QSEN: Safety; Teamwork and collaboration.

NANDA-I
NDx **Risk for Ineffective Protection**

Common Risk Factors

Dependency on ventilator
Improper ventilator settings
Improper alarm settings
Disconnection of ventilator
Positive-pressure ventilation
Decreased pulmonary compliance
Increased secretions

Common Expected Outcomes

Patient remains free of injury as evidenced by appropriate ventilator settings and arterial blood gases (ABGs) within normal limits for patient.

Potential for injury from ventilator-associated pneumonia (VAP) and barotrauma is reduced by ongoing assessment and early intervention.

NOC Outcomes

Respiratory Status: Ventilation; Risk Detection

NIC Interventions

Mechanical Ventilation Management: Invasive; Mechanical Ventilation Management: Pneumonia Prevention

---

■ = Independent   ▲ = Interprofessional Collaboration

Ongoing Assessment

Actions/Interventions	Rationales
▲ Check the ventilator settings every hour. Notify the respiratory therapist of any discrepancy in the ventilator settings immediately.	Assessment ensures that the patient is receiving correct mode, rate, tidal volume, F_{IO_2}, positive end-expiratory pressure (PEEP), and pressure support. Immediate attention to details can prevent problems. Appropriate use of safety-enhancing technology minimizes the risk of harm to the patient. QSEN: Safety.
• Mode: • Synchronized intermittent mandatory ventilation (SIMV)	SIMV ensures a preset rate in synchronization with the patient's own spontaneous breathing.
• Controlled mandatory ventilation (CMV)	CMV ensures a preset rate with no sensitivity to the patient's respiratory effort. The patient cannot initiate breaths or alter the pattern.
• Assist control (AC)	AC ensures that the preset rate is sensitive to the patient's inspiratory effort. It delivers a preset tidal volume for each patient-initiated breath.
• Rate of mechanical breaths	Although patient dependent, the usual rate is between 10 and 14 breaths/min.
• Tidal volume (TV)	Typical ranges for TV are 6 to 8 mL/kg of ideal body weight. Research supports lower standard TVs to reduce barotrauma.
• F_{IO_2}	The amount of oxygen prescribed depends on the patient's condition and ABG results.
• PEEP	PEEP serves to improve gas exchange and prevent atelectasis.
• Pressure support (PS)	PS provides positive airway pressure during the inspiratory cycle of a spontaneous inspiratory effort.
■ Ensure that the ventilator alarms are on.	Alarms alert the caregiver to ventilation problems. A prompt response to alarms ensures the correction of problems and maintenance of adequate ventilation. TJC's National Patient Safety Goals requires that alarm systems be activated and functional at all times. Appropriate use of safety-enhancing technology minimizes the risk of harm to the patient. QSEN: Safety; Evidence-based practice.
▲ Use pulse oximetry to monitor oxygen saturation; assess ABGs as appropriate.	Objective data guide the ventilator settings and appropriate interventions. QSEN: Safety.
■ Assess the rate or rhythm of the respiratory pattern, including the work of breathing.	It is important to maintain the patient in synchrony with the ventilator and not permit "fighting" it.
▲ Assess for the signs of pulmonary infection: fever, purulent secretions, elevated white blood cell count, positive bacterial cultures, and evidence of pulmonary infection on chest x-ray studies.	VAP is a major contributor to morbidity and mortality in the intensive care unit. Most ventilator-associated infections are caused by bacterial pathogens, with gram-negative bacilli being common. QSEN: Safety.
▲ Assess for the signs of barotrauma: the patient with crepitus, subcutaneous emphysema, altered chest excursion, asymmetrical chest, abnormal ABG values, shift in trachea, restlessness, evidence of pneumothorax on chest x-ray studies.	Barotrauma is damage to the lungs from positive pressure as seen in patients with acute respiratory disease when high pressures are needed to ventilate stiff lungs or when PEEP is used. Frequent assessments are needed because barotrauma can occur at any time and the patient will not show signs of dyspnea, shortness of breath, or tachypnea if heavily sedated to maintain ventilation. QSEN: Safety.
▲ Monitor chest x-ray reports daily and obtain a stat portable chest x-ray film if barotrauma is suspected.	Vigilant monitoring helps reduce complications.

Actions/Interventions

▲ Monitor plateau pressures with the respiratory therapist.

Rationales

Monitoring for barotrauma can involve measuring plateau pressure, which is the pressure after delivery of the tidal volume but before the patient is allowed to exhale. The ventilator is programmed so that after delivery of the tidal volume the patient is not allowed to exhale for a half second. Therefore pressure must be maintained to prevent exhalation. Elevation of plateau pressures increases both the risk and incidence of barotrauma when the patient is on mechanical ventilation. There has been less occurrence of barotrauma since guidelines have recommended lower standard tidal volumes. QSEN: Teamwork and collaboration.

Therapeutic Interventions

Actions/Interventions

■ Institute measures to reduce VAP.

- Wash hands before and after suctioning, touching ventilator equipment, and/or coming into contact with respiratory secretions.
- Use a continuous subglottic suction endotracheal (ET) tube for intubation that is expected to be longer than 24 hours.
- Keep the head of the bed elevated to 30 to 45 degrees or perform subglottic suctioning unless it is medically contraindicated.
- Brush teeth two or three times per day with a soft toothbrush. Chlorhexidine-based rinses may also be incorporated into oral care protocols.
- Use sterile suctioning procedures.

▲ Listen for alarms. Know the range in which the ventilator will set off the alarm and how to troubleshoot:

- High peak pressure alarm

- Low-pressure alarm

- Low exhale volume

- Apnea alarm

▲ Notify the physician of signs of barotrauma immediately; anticipate the need for chest tube placement, and prepare the patient as needed.

Rationales

Nosocomial infections are a leading cause of hospital deaths. Prevention of VAP is a national initiative to promote quality and safety. Research is ongoing to identify the most effective ventilator bundle order sets to prevent VAP. QSEN: Safety; Teamwork and collaboration.

An artificial airway bypasses the normal protective mechanisms of the upper airways. Handwashing reduces germ transmission. QSEN: Safety.

This intervention prevents the accumulation of secretions that can be aspirated.

Elevation promotes better lung expansion. It also reduces gastric reflux and aspiration.

Oral care reduces colonization of the oropharynx with respiratory pathogens that can be aspirated into the lungs.

This technique decreases the introduction of microorganisms into the airway.

The ventilator is a life-sustaining treatment that requires prompt response to alarms. TJC's National Patient Safety Goals requires that alarm systems be activated and functional at all times. Appropriate use of safety-enhancing technology minimizes the risk of harm to the patient. QSEN: Safety; Teamwork and collaboration.

The high peak pressure alarm indicates bronchospasm, retained secretions, obstruction of ET tube, atelectasis, acute respiratory distress syndrome (ARDS), or pneumothorax, among others.

The low-pressure alarm indicates a possible disconnection or mechanical ventilator malfunction.

The low exhale alarm indicates that the patient is not returning delivered TV (through leak or disconnection).

The apnea alarm is indicative of a disconnection or absence of spontaneous respirations.

If barotrauma is suspected, intervention must follow immediately to prevent tension pneumothorax.

■ = Independent   ▲ = Interprofessional Collaboration

NANDA-I NDx Ineffective Airway Clearance

Common Related Factors
Endotracheal intubation
Copious secretions
Decreased energy and fatigue

Defining Characteristics
Excessive secretions
Ineffective cough
Abnormal breath sounds
Dyspnea
Anxiety
Restlessness
Increased peak airway pressure

Common Expected Outcome
Patient will maintain clear, open airways, as evidenced by normal breath sounds after suctioning.

NOC Outcome
Respiratory Status: Airway Patency
NIC Interventions
Airway Management; Airway Suctioning

Ongoing Assessment

Actions/Interventions	Rationales
■ Assess the lungs for the presence of normal or adventitious breath sounds.	Diminished lung sounds or the presence of adventitious sounds may indicate an obstructed airway and the need for suctioning.
■ Observe the quantity, color, consistency, and odor of sputum.	Thick, tenacious secretions increase airway resistance and the work of breathing. A sign of infection is discolored sputum, often with an odor.
▲ Assess arterial blood gases (ABGs).	This nursing assessment reduces harm by identifying changes in oxygenation and acid-base balances, and initiating early intervention. Signs of respiratory compromise include decreasing Pao_2 and increasing $Paco_2$. QSEN: Safety.
▲ Monitor for peak airway pressures and airway resistance.	Increases in these parameters signal the accumulation of secretions or fluid and the potential for ineffective ventilation. QSEN: Safety.
■ Assess oxygen saturation before and after the suctioning procedure.	This assessment provides an evaluation of the effectiveness of therapy.

Therapeutic Interventions

Actions/Interventions	Rationales
■ Explain the suctioning procedure to the patient; give reassurance throughout the procedure.	Suctioning can be frightening to the patient. Reinforce the need to maintain a patent airway. Provide sedation and pain relief as needed.
■ Institute suctioning of the airway "as needed" based on the presence of adventitious breath sounds and/or increased ventilatory pressure.	The frequency of suctioning should be based on the patient's clinical status, not on a preset routine such as every 2 hours. Oversuctioning can cause hypoxia and injury to bronchial and lung tissue. QSEN: Patient-centered care.
■ Avoid saline instillation before suctioning.	Saline instillation before suctioning has an adverse effect on oxygen saturation.
■ Use closed in-line suction.	This technique decreases the infection rate, may reduce hypoxia, and is often less expensive. Sterile technique is a priority.

ⓔvolve   For additional care plans, go to http://evolve.elsevier.com/Gulanick/.

Pulmonary Care Plans

Actions/Interventions

▲ Hyperoxygenate as ordered.

▲ Administer pain medications, as appropriate, before suctioning.

■ Silence any ventilator alarms during suctioning. Reset the alarms after suctioning.

▲ Administer an adequate fluid intake (IV and nasogastric, as appropriate).

■ Turn the patient every 2 hours.

▲ Consult a respiratory therapist for chest physiotherapy as indicated.

Rationales

Hyperoxygenation before, during, and after endotracheal suctioning decreases hypoxia and cardiac dysrhythmias related to the suctioning procedure.

These medications decrease peak periods of pain and assist with effective cough needed to clear secretions.

Silencing alarms decreases the frequency of false alarms during suctioning and reduces stressful noise to the patient. Alarms need to be turned on again after suctioning to ensure safety. QSEN: Safety.

Maintaining hydration increases ciliary action to remove secretions and reduces viscosity of secretions. It is easier to mobilize thinner secretions with coughing and suctioning.

Turning mobilizes secretions and helps prevent ventilator-associated pneumonia.

Chest physiotherapy includes the techniques of postural drainage and chest percussion to loosen and mobilize secretions. QSEN: Teamwork and collaboration.

NANDA-I
NDx **Risk for Decreased Cardiac Output**

Common Risk Factors

Mechanical ventilation
Positive-pressure ventilation

Common Expected Outcome

Patient maintains adequate cardiac output, as evidenced by strong peripheral pulses; systolic BP within 20 mm Hg of baseline; HR 60 to 100 beats/min with regular rhythm; urine output greater 30 mL/hr, warm and dry skin; and normal level of consciousness.

NOC Outcomes
Cardiac Pump Effectiveness; Circulation Status; Respiratory Status: Ventilation
NIC Interventions
Hemodynamic Regulation; Mechanical Ventilation Management: Invasive

---

Ongoing Assessment

Actions/Interventions

▲ Assess the patient's vital signs, level of consciousness, and hemodynamic parameters if in place (central venous pressure, pulmonary artery diastolic pressures [PADP] and/or pulmonary capillary wedge pressure, cardiac output).

■ Assess the peripheral pulses, capillary refill, and skin temperature.

Rationales

Mechanical ventilation can cause decreased venous return to the heart, resulting in decreased BP, compensatory increased HR, and decreased cardiac output. This may occur abruptly with ventilator changes: rate, tidal volume, or positive-pressure ventilation. The level of consciousness will decrease if cardiac output is severely compromised. Therefore close monitoring during ventilator changes is imperative. These direct measurements serve as optimal guides for therapy. QSEN: Safety.

Pulses are weak with reduced stroke volume and cardiac output. Capillary refill is slow with reduced cardiac output. Cold, pale, clammy skin is secondary to compensatory sympathetic nervous system stimulation and associated with low cardiac output and oxygen desaturation.

■ = Independent ▲ = Interprofessional Collaboration

Actions/Interventions

■ Monitor fluid balance and urine output.

■ Monitor for dysrhythmias.

▲ Notify the physician immediately of signs of a decrease in cardiac output, and anticipate possible ventilator setting changes.

Rationales

Optimal hydration status is needed to maintain effective circulating blood volume and counteract the ventilatory effects on cardiac output. With positive-pressure ventilation, pressure from the diaphragm decreases blood flow to the kidneys and could result in a drop in urine output. The brain is very sensitive to a decrease in blood flow and may respond by releasing antidiuretic hormone (ADH) (to increase water and sodium retention), further reducing urinary output. After the initial decrease in venous return to the heart, volume receptors in the right atrium signal a decrease in volume, which triggers an increase in the release of ADH from the posterior pituitary and retention of water by the kidneys.

Cardiac dysrhythmias may result from the low perfusion state, acidosis, or hypoxia.

Vigilant monitoring reduces the risk for complications. Hypotension and decreased cardiac output may be related to positive-pressure ventilator itself or use of positive end-expiratory pressure (PEEP) mode. QSEN: Safety.

Therapeutic Interventions

Actions/Interventions

▲ Maintain an optimal fluid balance.

▲ Administer medications (diuretics, inotropic agents) as ordered.

Rationales

Volume therapy may be required to maintain adequate filling pressures and optimize cardiac output. However, if PADP and/or pulmonary capillary wedge pressure rises and cardiac output remains low, fluid restriction may be necessary.

Diuretics may be useful to help maintain fluid balance if fluid retention is a problem. Inotropic agents may be useful to increase cardiac output.

 Anxiety

Common Related Factors

Inability to breathe adequately without support
Inability to maintain adequate gas exchange
Inability to communicate verbally
Unknown outcome
Change in environment
Change in health status

Defining Characteristics

Restlessness
Uncooperative behavior
Withdrawal
Tachypnea
Vigilant watch on equipment
Facial tension
Self-focused

Common Expected Outcomes

Patient uses effective coping mechanisms.
Patient describes a reduction in level of anxiety experienced.
Patient demonstrates reduced anxiety as evidenced by calm manner and cooperative behavior.

NOC Outcomes
Anxiety Self-Control; Coping

NIC Interventions
Anxiety Reduction; Presence; Emotional Support

Ongoing Assessment

Actions/Interventions

- Assess the patient for signs of anxiety.

- Assess the patient's understanding of the need for mechanical ventilation.

Rationales

Being on a mechanical ventilator can be a drastic change that will produce high levels of anxiety. Anxiety can affect the respiratory rate and pattern, resulting in rapid, shallow breathing and leading to arterial blood gas abnormalities and the patient "fighting" the ventilator.

This approach allows the patient to be a full partner in providing care that meets the patient's expressed needs for improved ventilation and reducing anxiety. Accurate appraisal can facilitate the development of appropriate treatment strategies. QSEN: Patient-centered care.

Therapeutic Interventions

Actions/Interventions

- Display a confident, calm manner and understanding attitude. Be available to the patient for support, as well as for explanations of the patient's care and progress.

- Reduce distracting stimuli. Inform the patient of alarms on the ventilatory system, and reassure the patient about the close proximity of health care personnel to respond to alarms.
- Encourage visiting by family and friends.

- Encourage sedentary diversional activities (e.g., television, reading, being read to, writing, occupational therapy).
- Provide relaxation techniques (e.g., tapes, imagery, progressive muscle relaxation).
- If impaired communication is the problem, provide the patient with word-and-phrase cards, a writing pad and pencil, or a picture board.
- ▲ Refer to members of the interprofessional teams, such as the psychiatric liaison clinical nurse specialist, psychiatrist, or hospital chaplain, as appropriate.

Rationales

The presence of a trusted person may be helpful during periods of anxiety. An ongoing relationship establishes a basis for comfort in communicating anxious feelings. QSEN: Patient-centered care.

Reducing stimuli provides a quiet environment that enhances rest. Anxiety may escalate with excessive noise, conversation, and equipment around the patient. An informed patient who understands the treatment plan will be more cooperative.

The presence of significant others reinforces feelings of security for the patient.

These activities enhance the patient's quality of life and help pass time.

Using anxiety-reduction techniques enhances the patient's sense of personal mastery and confidence.

These tools broaden the opportunity for communicating, which may reduce frustration.

Specialty expertise may provide a wider range of treatment options and may be needed to achieve successful outcomes. Integrating the contributions of members of the interprofessional team helps the patient and family achieve health goals and allows for shared decision-making to achieve quality patient care. QSEN: Teamwork and collaboration.

NANDA-I
NDx Deficient Knowledge

Common Related Factors

Insufficient information
Insufficient interest in learning
Misinformation presented by others

Defining Characteristics

Insufficient knowledge
Inaccurate follow-through of instruction
Inappropriate behavior

Common Expected Outcome

Patient or significant others demonstrate knowledge of mechanical ventilation and care involved.

NOC Outcome
Knowledge: Treatment Procedure
NIC Interventions
Health Literacy Enhancement; Learning Facilitation; Teaching: Individual

---

■ = Independent   ▲ = Interprofessional Collaboration

Ongoing Assessment

Actions/Interventions	Rationales
■ Assess the patient's perception and understanding of mechanical ventilation. ■ Assess the patient's readiness and ability to learn.	This information provides an important starting point in education. Educational interventions must be designed to meet the learning limitations, motivation, and needs of the patient. Patients in acute care may not be able to take in much information because of fatigue, pain, sensory overload, hypoxemia, and the like. QSEN: Patient-centered care.

Therapeutic Interventions

Actions/Interventions	Rationales
■ Encourage the patient or significant others to express feelings and ask questions.	Questions facilitate open communication between the patient and health care professionals and allow the verification of understanding and the opportunity to correct misconceptions.
■ Explain that the patient will not be able to eat or drink while intubated but assure him or her that alternative measures (IV fluids, gastric feedings, or hyperalimentation) will be taken to provide nourishment.	The risk for aspiration is high if the patient eats or drinks while intubated. In long-term care settings, patients may be allowed to eat and drink after a swallow evaluation.
■ Explain to the patient the reason for the inability to talk while intubated. Explain alternative efforts for communicating.	The endotracheal tube passes through the vocal cords, and attempts to talk can cause more trauma to the cords. However, patients must understand how to use supplementary methods for communication (paper, pen, pictures).
■ Explain that alarms may periodically sound off, which may be normal, and that the staff will be in close proximity.	Explaining expected events can help reduce anxiety.
■ Explain the need for frequent assessments (vital signs, auscultation of breath sounds, ventilator checks).	This information also helps reduce anxiety by providing a basis for actions.
■ Explain the need for suctioning as needed.	This information can help reduce the anxiety associated with the procedure.
■ Explain the weaning process, and explain that extubation demonstrates adequate respiratory function and a decrease in pulmonary secretions.	This information aids the patient in maintaining some control.
■ If long-term ventilation is anticipated, discuss or plan for long-term ventilator care management and use appropriate referrals: long-term ventilator care facilities versus home care management.	Continuity of care is facilitated through the use of specialty resources.

Related Care Plans

Impaired verbal communication, Chapter 2
Imbalanced nutrition: Less than body requirements, Chapter 2
Impaired gas exchange, Chapter 2
Impaired physical mobility, Chapter 2
Dysfunctional ventilatory weaning response, ⊝volve
Tracheostomy, ⊝volve

⊝volve   **For additional care plans, go to http://evolve.elsevier.com/Gulanick/.**

Obstructive Sleep Apnea

Sleep-Disordered Breathing

Sleep-disordered breathing (SDB) affects at least 20 million people in the United States and is defined as a cessation of breathing during sleep that is caused by repetitive partial or complete obstruction of the airway and pharyngeal structures. There are two types: (1) the most common form, obstructive sleep apnea (OSA), and (2) central sleep apnea. The manifestations of OSA include episodes of loud snoring, decreased oxygen saturation, brief periods of apnea, and arousal from sleep. These episodes may occur several times during sleep. OSA is strongly linked to cardiovascular diseases—especially hypertension and coronary artery disease, which eventually leads to heart failure—so the prevalence in patients with heart failure rises to approximately 50%. Consequences of OSA include altered alertness, daytime somnolence, cognitive impairment, and increased risk of morbidity and mortality. Common screening methods include pulse oximetry, blood gas analysis, and/or ambulatory airflow measurements, but the diagnosis of OSA is confirmed by overnight sleep laboratory studies.

Treatment for mild OSA includes conservative measures such as weight loss, abstaining from the use of alcohol and sedatives, avoiding the supine position during sleep, and sometimes oropharyngeal appliances or surgery. However, continuous positive airway pressure (CPAP) is the most consistently effective treatment for clinically significant OSA and appears to substantially improve the condition. Unfortunately, some patients complain that the CPAP mask is uncomfortable, so compliance with the treatment is often low. As technology advances, the treatment of OSA will become more comfortable and less cumbersome. Patients must be encouraged to try different equipment to adapt to their own facial structure because patients who use CPAP report less fatigue, better BP control, and improved quality of life.

NANDA-I NDx Ineffective Breathing Pattern

Common Related Factors

Enlarged tonsils and adenoids
Narrowing of respiratory passages
Decreased airway muscle tone during sleep

Common Expected Outcomes

Patient maintains effective breathing pattern, as evidenced by relaxed breathing at normal rate and depth and decreased snoring and apneic episodes.
Patient adheres to continuous positive airway pressure (CPAP) device regimen as prescribed.

Defining Characteristics

Bradypnea and/or periods of apnea
Snoring
Decreased oxygen saturation

NOC Outcomes

Respiratory Status: Airway Patency; Respiratory Status: Ventilation

NIC Interventions

Airway Management; Respiratory Monitoring

Ongoing Assessment

Actions/Interventions	Rationales
■ Assess the current sleep pattern and sleep history. Assess quality of sleep using a tool such as the Epworth Sleepiness Scale. This tool requires the patient to score his likelihood of falling asleep during eight common activities of daily living.	Periodic changes in the sleep pattern need to be differentiated from true obstructive sleep disorder and/or apnea. QSEN: Patient-centered care.
■ Ask the patient's partner or significant other whether the patient snores or has apneic episodes during the night.	Most patients are unaware of their own snoring and apnea. The partner may have complained about loud snoring followed by stopping breathing and a loud gasp or snort when the patient is aroused by the apnea.

■ = Independent   ▲ = Interprofessional Collaboration

Actions/Interventions

- Assess for characteristics of sleep-disordered breathing (SDB): loud snoring, apneic episodes (5 to 10 per hour), jerky or restless leg movements during sleep, daytime somnolence and fatigue.

- Assess for contributing factors to obstructive sleep apnea (OSA): obesity (body mass index [BMI] > 30), large neck circumference, having a large uvula, having a narrowed airway (enlarged tonsils or adenoids), having chronic nasal congestion, small recessive jaw, oropharyngeal edema, being a certain age (around 18-60 years), being black or male, smoking and using alcohol.

- Assess the physiological effects resulting from comorbid conditions affected by OSA.

Rationales

Although a variety of manifestations may occur, patients may only be aware of the daytime fatigue and sleepiness.

Research has shown that body type affects diagnosis. Excess body weight can result in the accumulation of fat on the sides of the upper airway, causing it to become narrow. Increasing neck size has been correlated with the severity of apnea. Aging causes the loss of muscle mass replaced by fat, again leaving the airway narrow and soft. Anatomical abnormalities affect the upper airway musculature. Alcohol use results in the excessive relaxation of muscles in the upper airway during sleep.

During sleep apneic periods, there is a fall in Pao_2 levels with a buildup of $Paco_2$. The immediate "arousal" to breathe causes surges in sympathetic activity that affect many organ systems, especially the cardiovascular system. The sympathetic stimulation can lead to cardiac dysrhythmias, systemic vascular resistance, and reduced cardiac output in patients with compromised heart failure. Research has demonstrated a high prevalence of OSA in patients with heart failure, hypertension, coronary artery disease, and stroke, although the exact relationship is unclear. OSA can aggravate conditions such as heart failure because of the increased physiological demands put on the heart during sleep.

Therapeutic Interventions

Actions/Interventions

- ▲ Suggest a referral for a nighttime sleep study if not already performed.

- In diagnosed patients, explain the mechanisms by which sleep apnea occurs:
  - Relaxation of the muscles of the soft palate during sleep results in a reduced airway size and partial or complete closure.
  - This closure causes the cessation of breathing (apnea).
  - During the apneic period, the body struggles to breathe and is aroused to awaken, which reopens the airway.
  - The obstructive periods are associated with reduced oxygen saturation.
  - This sleep apnea–arousal–awaken cycle repeats on an ongoing basis, preventing the patient from reaching the deep stages of rapid eye movement sleep.

Rationales

The most definitive test is the overnight sleep study—polysomnography. Using electrodes, it records the type and depth of sleep, eye movement observations, respiratory effort and movement, oxygen saturation, and muscle movement. Patients can use simpler "screening" techniques such as home sleep monitoring (although it is difficult to maintain equipment during sleep) or overnight pulse oximetry to document drops in oxygen saturation during the apneic periods. QSEN: Teamwork and collaboration.

The more the patient understands the condition, the better he or she is able to participate in the treatment plan. QSEN: Patient-centered care.

Actions/Interventions	Rationales
■ Teach the patient about nonsurgical therapies to treat OSA:	
• Weight loss—indicated for mild sleep apnea	Weight loss has been shown to improve this condition, although the amount of weight loss required varies among patients.
• Nonsupine positioning—indicated for mild sleep apnea	Supine sleeping causes the most significant relaxation of upper airway muscles, causing the tongue to more easily fall back and occlude the airway or airway muscles and tissues such as the tonsils to relax and block the airway. Turning on one's side can reduce episodes of apnea. Suggested techniques include sewing or attaching a sock filled with tennis balls lengthwise down the back of a pajama top. This reminds the patient to stay positioned on the side.
• Oral appliances resembling mouth guards (tongue-retaining or mandibular advance devices)—indicated for mild sleep apnea	Repositioning the muscles may prevent the apneic episode. These devices should be fitted by a specialty dentist. The devices are more appropriate for milder forms of OSA.
• Continuous positive airway pressure (CPAP)—indicated for mild to severe apnea	CPAP is a treatment that delivers positive pressurized air during the breathing cycle to "stabilize" the airway and maintain patency. CPAP uses a nasal or facial mask held in place with secure straps. Appropriate mask fitting is key to success. The mask is usually worn for at least 4 hours during the night's sleep. It should be used daily, although patients with milder levels may need the device only a few days a week. Newer CPAP models are available which slightly reduce pressure on exhalation to increase patient comfort and compliance.
• Bilateral positive airway pressure (BiPAP)—a variation of CPAP	Variable positive airway pressure (known as bilevel or BiPAP) delivers a higher pressure during inhalation and a lower amount during exhalation. Patients often find the BiPAP device more tolerable than CPAP.
• Nasal trumpets—indicated to bypass any nasal, soft palate, or sometimes tongue obstructions and commonly used in postanesthesia settings	These devices may reduce mucosal trauma, but they are not readily tolerated by patients on a long-term basis.
• Supplementary oxygen	Supplementary oxygen raises oxygen saturation.
■ Emphasize compliance issues, especially related to CPAP.	Patients frequently have difficulty getting masks or nasal devices to fit properly, or they may feel claustrophobic while wearing the devices. The CPAP device is effective only while in use, making compliance a key issue. Many patients find the nasal device easier to tolerate than the mask. Patients can use more portable units. Patients need to take the device with them when they anticipate sleeping away from home (e.g., on vacations, for work travel, or on long plane flights, especially if they already have heart failure).
■ Instruct patients to bring their CPAP/BiPAP devices to the hospital for personal use while hospitalized. Notify the hospital team, especially the anesthesiologist, of OSA problems so that ventilation needs can be correctly assessed.	It is more effective for patients to use their own face mask and devices that have been properly fitted. Use of the positive pressure aids ventilation, maintains tissue oxygen saturation, and reduces the workload of the heart. QSEN: Teamwork and collaboration.
■ Instruct the patient to reduce or avoid drinking alcohol.	Alcohol causes relaxation of the muscles of the upper airway and can aggravate the condition.

■ = Independent ▲ = Interprofessional Collaboration

Actions/Interventions	Rationales
■ Instruct the patient regarding possible surgical technique (uvulopalatopharyngoplasty; implants), as indicated.	A minimally invasive procedure (Pillar Procedure) is available that consists of placing three tiny rods in the soft palate to stiffen and support the tissue to reduce upper airway collapse. The uvulopalatopharyngoplasty procedure involves removal of part of the soft palate, uvula, and redundant peripharyngeal tissues to eliminate snoring. It does not always prevent the apneic periods. The procedure can be done surgically or with laser assistance. It is indicated for individuals who cannot tolerate CPAP.
■ Instruct the patient regarding medication for patients experiencing excessive daytime sleepiness.	Modafinal is a medication that assists in promoting daytime wakefulness.
▲ Refer to a sleep specialist as needed.	Specialists may provide additional treatment strategies. QSEN: Teamwork and collaboration.

NANDA-I NDx Sleep Deprivation

Common Related Factors

Sleep apnea
Sleep stage shifts
Cycle of sleep apnea–arousal–sleep that interferes with rapid eye movement (REM) sleep

Defining Characteristics

Daytime drowsiness
Decrease in ability to function
Fatigue
Irritability
Change in reaction time
Alteration in concentration
Confusion

Common Expected Outcome

Patient achieves optimal amounts of sleep, as evidenced by rested appearance, verbalization of feeling rested, and improvement in sleep pattern.

NOC Outcomes
Sleep; Rest
NIC Intervention
Sleep Enhancement

Ongoing Assessment

Actions/Interventions	Rationales
■ Assess for reports of waking up feeling tired or fatigued and experiencing daytime somnolence.	The cycle of interrupted sleep results in reduced REM sleep, which the body requires for rest and to replenish itself. Interrupted sleep is associated with feelings of tiredness and often reports of feeling worse on awakening than when retiring for sleep. Patients are often embarrassed by episodes of falling asleep such as in movie theaters, during work meetings, or while watching television.
■ Assess for safety issues at work and at home.	Memory and cognitive changes can significantly affect the ability to perform ADLs and occupational activities. Decreased alertness and impaired concentration during the day places the patient at risk for accidents. QSEN: Safety.
■ Assess any history of automobile accidents.	The "drowsy driver syndrome," which has been linked to frequent automobile accidents, may be caused by OSA and lack of alertness and slowed reflexes while driving.

Actions/Interventions	**Rationales**
■ Assess for other factors that contribute to fatigue such as alcohol and medications.	It is critical that patients with OSA do not aggravate their condition through the use of sedatives, analgesics, opioids, tranquilizers, other prescribed medications, or alcohol that also contribute to reduced alertness and fatigue.
■ Assess whether interpersonal relationships and quality of life have been affected by chronic fatigue, irritability, or mood changes.	Lack of sleep can contribute to irritability and depression, making it difficult to maintain healthy personal relationships. Impotence is also related to OSA and may affect feelings of intimacy. The patient's sleep partner may experience disrupted sleep because of the patient's loud snoring. Many sleep partners and other family members report remaining awake waiting for the patient to breathe again after a period of apnea. QSEN: Patient-centered care.

Therapeutic Interventions

Actions/Interventions	**Rationales**
■ Explain the relationship of REM sleep and of feeling refreshed when awakening.	REM sleep is characterized by rapid eye movements and is essential to waking up feeling refreshed. It is the deepest level of relaxation. This level is not reached when patients are continually being aroused from sleep and restarting their sleep cycles.
■ Reinforce the importance of adhering to the prescribed treatment.	Most treatments need to be initiated on a daily basis (weight management, positioning, use of continuous positive airway pressure [CPAP]). Knowledge of the physiological basis for restful sleep may provide the rationale for compliance with treatments.
■ Instruct the patient to consider alternative transportation (carpool, public transportation) until achieving a more restful sleep.	Daytime somnolence, reduced alertness, impaired concentration, and delayed reaction time place the patient at greater risk for injuring self and others. Using alternative modes of travel reduces this risk. QSEN: Safety.
▲ Refer to a social worker as needed for assistance with personal relationships.	Specialized expertise may be needed to help the patient gain insight into problems. QSEN: Teamwork and collaboration.

Related Care Plans

Ineffective health management, Chapter 2
Imbalanced nutrition: More than body requirements, Chapter 2
Fatigue, Chapter 2
Readiness for enhanced sleep, Chapter 3

■ = Independent   ▲ = Interprofessional Collaboration

Pneumonia

Pneumonitis; Community-Acquired Pneumonia (CAP); Hospital-Acquired Pneumonia (HAP); Aspiration Pneumonia

Pneumonia is caused by a bacterial, viral, or fungal infection that results in an inflammatory process in the lungs. It is an infectious process that is spread by droplets or by contact and is one of the most common causes of death in older adults. Risk factors include upper respiratory tract infection, excessive alcohol ingestion, central nervous system depression, cardiac failure, any debilitating illness, chronic obstructive pulmonary disease (COPD), endotracheal (ET) intubation, and postoperative effects of general anesthesia. Pneumonia is a particular concern in persons older than 65 years or anyone who is bedridden, is immunosuppressed, has chronic illness, is malnourished, or is hospitalized, and patients exposed to methicillin-resistant *Staphylococcus aureus* (MRSA), as well as the very young and very old.

The most common causes of viral pneumonia are influenza viruses and respiratory syncytial virus (RSV), and a common cause of bacterial pneumonia is *Streptococcus pneumoniae*. Pneumonia that develops in the community is called community-acquired pneumonia (CAP). Pneumonia that developed during or following a stay in a health care facility is termed health care–associated pneumonia and includes hospital-acquired pneumonia (HAP) and ventilator-associated pneumonia (VAP). Treatment is determined by the specific cause, setting, and severity of the pneumonia. Although antibiotics can be used to treat bacterial pneumonia, the most common cause, they do not work for viral pneumonia. Specific antiviral drugs can be used to treat specific viral infections.

In healthy people with responsive immune systems, treatment can be administered in the outpatient setting. This care plan focuses on acute care treatment of pneumonia. See also discussion of VAP in the Mechanical Ventilation care plan.

NDx Infection

Common Related Factor

Invading bacterial, viral, or fungal organisms

Defining Characteristics

Fever
Chills
Elevated white blood cell (WBC) count
Positive sputum culture report
Tachypnea
Dyspnea
Cough with purulent sputum
Tachycardia

Common Expected Outcomes

Patient experiences improvement in infection as evidenced by normal body temperature, normal WBC count, and negative sputum culture report.
Patient demonstrates hygiene measures such as handwashing and control of infectious sputum.

NOC Outcomes

Medication Response; Thermoregulation; Infection Severity; Risk Control: Infectious Process.

NIC Interventions

Infection Protection; Medication Administration

Pulmonary Care Plans

Ongoing Assessment

Actions/Interventions	Rationales
■ Assess the patient's description of the current illness.	Classic signs of pneumonia include chills, fever, pleuritic chest pain, cough, dyspnea, sputum changes.
■ Assess for predisposing risk factors: recent exposure to illness; alcohol, tobacco, or drug abuse; chronic illness; immunosuppressive therapy; malnutrition; prolonged immobility; tube feedings.	Patients are at risk from a variety of sources. Both cause and causative organisms relate to the setting. For example, an intubated immobilized patient will have a different pathogenic risk and treatment than a patient with community-acquired pneumonia (CAP).
■ Assess the patient's immunization status.	Immunizations with pneumococcal vaccine and seasonal influenza vaccine are recommended by the Centers for Disease Control and Prevention (CDC) for high-risk groups, especially older adults, to reduce the risk for developing pneumonia. QSEN: Evidence-based practice.
■ Assess the patient's temperature, closely monitoring for fluctuations.	Fever suggests infection. Other causes of continued fever may be a drug allergy, drug-resistant bacteria, superinfection, or inadequate lung drainage.
■ Monitor breath sounds.	Bronchial breath sounds are evident in areas of lung consolidation. Egophony (often called *E to A changes*) is a simple technique to identify areas of consolidation in the lungs. Wheezing is evident if inflammation or narrowing of the airways occurs. Crackles are evident if fluid is present in interstitial or alveolar lung areas.
▲ Obtain fresh sputum for a Gram stain and for a culture and sensitivity, as prescribed. Assess for drug resistance.	This testing determines the correct antibiotic coverage for the patient. A blood culture obtained before the initial antibiotic is given is an indicator or benchmark used to measure the quality of care in hospitals. In the outpatient setting, patients will often be treated empirically. QSEN: Evidence-based practice.
▲ Monitor WBC counts and blood cultures.	A rising WBC count indicates the body's efforts to fight pathogens. Patients admitted to the emergency department or intensive care unit should have a blood test for the presence of bacteria in their blood within 24 hours of hospital arrival (National Patient Safety Goal). QSEN: Evidence-based practice.
■ Assess the patient's hydration status.	Water loss is increased with fever and can result in dehydration if not adequately treated.
▲ Use pulse oximetry to monitor oxygen saturation; assess arterial blood gases (ABGs) as indicated.	Pulse oximetry and ABGs provide an objective indication of oxygenation status. It should be 90% or greater. ABGs will indicate developing respiratory acidosis and hypoxemia. Oxygenation assessment is a National Patient Safety Goal. QSEN: Evidence-based practice; Safety.
▲ Monitor serial chest x-ray reports.	Pneumonia causes increased areas of density on the chest x-ray film, occurring in an isolated segment or lobe, either unilaterally or bilaterally. Serial changes guide the subsequent treatment.

■ = Independent   ▲ = Interprofessional Collaboration

Pulmonary Care Plans

Therapeutic Interventions

Actions/Interventions	Rationales
▲ Administer prescribed antimicrobial agents within 4 hours of hospital arrival (e.g., cephalosporins, penicillins, vancomycin).	This timeline is an indicator or benchmark used to measure the quality of care in hospitals—the focus is on giving an antibiotic early. As culture results become available, patients with CAP should be receiving appropriate antibiotics within 24 hours of hospital arrival. Parenteral IV antibiotics are usually given for the first few days of acute cases and then changed to oral antibiotics, which may be adequate for milder cases from the first day. To prevent a relapse of pneumonia, the patient needs to complete the course of antibiotics as prescribed. Antiviral drugs (e.g., amantadine, rimantadine) are available for parenteral administration for viral respiratory infections. Antibiotics are not effective against viral pneumonia but may be used when concurrent viral and bacterial pneumonias are present. In CAP, patients are frequently started on oral antibiotics. QSEN: Evidence-based practice.
▲ Use the appropriate therapy for elevated temperatures: antipyretics, cold therapy.	These treatments maintain normothermia and reduce metabolic needs.
■ Provide tissues and waste bags for the disposal of sputum.	Careful disposal of contaminated tissues reduces the transmission of microorganisms.
■ Wash hands frequently and instruct the patient and/or family to do the same.	Handwashing is the most effective method for preventing the spread of infection.
■ Keep the patient away from other patients who are at high risk for developing pneumonia by careful room assignment when patients are in semiprivate rooms.	Immunocompromised patients are at high risk for developing nosocomial pneumonia.
■ Isolate patients as necessary after reviewing culture and sensitivity results.	Isolation prevents the potential spread of the disease. If the patient is positive for methicillin-resistant *Staphylococcus aureus* (MRSA), a private room with isolation is required. Appropriate use of isolation procedures minimizes the risk of harm to the patient and others from transmission of microorganisms. QSEN: Safety.

NANDA-I
NDx Ineffective Airway Clearance

Common Related Factors	Defining Characteristics
Increased sputum production in response to respiratory infection Decreased energy and increased fatigue Aspiration	Abnormal breath sounds (e.g., rhonchi, bronchial lung sounds, egophony) Decreased breath sounds over affected lung areas Ineffective cough Purulent sputum Dyspnea, tachypnea Change in respiratory status Infiltrates seen on chest x-ray film Hypoxemia

Common Expected Outcome

Patient will maintain clear, open airways, as evidenced by normal breath sounds, normal rate and depth of respirations, and ability to effectively cough up secretions after treatments and deep breathing.

NOC Outcome

Respiratory Status: Airway Patency

NIC Interventions

Airway Management; Cough Enhancement; Airway Suctioning

Ongoing Assessment

Actions/Interventions	Rationales
■ Assess respirations, noting the rate, rhythm, depth, and use of accessory muscles.	An increase in the respiratory rate and depth may be a compensatory response to airway obstruction. The breathing pattern may alter to include the use of accessory muscles to increase chest excursion to facilitate effective breathing. QSEN: Safety.
■ Assess cough for effectiveness and productivity.	Coughing is the most effective way to remove secretions. Patients may have an ineffective cough because of fatigue or thick tenacious secretions.
■ Observe the characteristics of sputum: color, viscosity, and odor; report any significant changes.	A sign of infection is discolored sputum (no longer clear or white). An odor may be present. Thick, tenacious secretions increase airway resistance and the work of breathing.
■ Assess the patient's hydration status.	Airway clearance is impaired with inadequate hydration and the thickening of secretions. Thick, tenacious secretions increase hypoxemia.
■ Auscultate the lungs, noting areas of decreased ventilation and the presence of adventitious sounds.	Bronchial lung sounds are commonly heard over areas of lung density or consolidation. Crackles are heard when fluid is present.
▲ Use pulse oximetry to monitor oxygen saturation; assess arterial blood gases (ABGs).	Oxygen saturation should be maintained at 90% or greater. Increasing $Paco_2$ and decreasing Pao_2 and pulse oximeter readings can result from increased pulmonary secretions and respiratory fatigue. QSEN: Safety.

Therapeutic Interventions

Actions/Interventions	Rationales
■ Assist the patient with coughing, deep breathing, and splinting, as necessary.	Coughing is the most helpful way to remove most secretions. Deep breathing improves the productivity of cough. Frequent nonproductive coughing can result in hypoxemia. Splinting the abdomen promotes more effective coughing by increasing abdominal pressure and upward diaphragmatic movement. If coughing is painful, medicate for pain.
■ Assist with suctioning if necessary.	If coughing is ineffective, nasotracheal suctioning may be required to remove secretions. However, suctioning can cause increased hypoxemia, especially without hyperoxygenation before, during, and after suctioning.
■ Encourage ambulation.	Ambulation mobilizes secretions and reduces atelectasis.
■ Maintain adequate hydration.	Fluids are lost by diaphoresis, fever, and tachypnea. Maintaining hydration increases ciliary action to remove secretions and reduce the viscosity of secretions. It is easier for the patient to mobilize thinner secretions with coughing.

■ = Independent   ▲ = Interprofessional Collaboration

Actions/Interventions	Rationales
■ Use humidity (humidified oxygen or humidifier at bedside).	Increasing the humidity of inspired air will decrease the viscosity of secretions and facilitate their removal. Clean the humidifier according to its instructions to inhibit a reservoir for bacterial growth.
■ Assist the patient with the use of an incentive spirometer.	Incentive spirometry serves to improve deep breathing and prevent atelectasis.
■ For patients with reduced energy, pace activities.	Effective coughing is hard work and may exhaust an already compromised patient. Fatigue is a contributing factor to ineffective coughing.
▲ Consult the respiratory therapist for chest physiotherapy and nebulizer treatments, as appropriate and as ordered.	Chest physiotherapy includes the techniques of postural drainage and chest percussion to loosen and mobilize secretions in smaller airways that cannot be removed by coughing or suctioning. A nebulizer may be used to humidify the airway to thin secretions to facilitate their removal; it can also be used to deliver bronchodilators and mucolytic agents. QSEN: Teamwork and collaboration.
▲ Administer medications such as antibiotics and expectorants for productive coughs and cough suppressants for hacking nonproductive coughs as prescribed, noting their effectiveness; administer inhaled bronchodilators and inhaled steroids, as prescribed, to open the airway and decrease inflammation.	A variety of medications are available to treat specific problems. Most promote the clearance of airway secretions and may reduce airway resistance. If treating the patient in the outpatient setting, review medication administration, timing, and adverse effects with the patient. QSEN: Evidence-based practice.
▲ Assist with bronchoscopy and thoracentesis, as appropriate.	Bronchoscopy is done to obtain lavage samples for culture and sensitivity and to remove mucus plugs; thoracentesis is done to drain associated pleural effusions.
▲ Anticipate the possible need for supplemental oxygen or intubation if the patient's condition deteriorates.	Oxygen may be needed to correct associated hypoxemia. Intubation may be needed to facilitate deep suctioning efforts and to provide a source for augmenting oxygenation. QSEN: Safety.

NANDA-I NDx Impaired Gas Exchange

Common Related Factors
Collection of mucus in airways
Inflammation of airways and alveoli
Fluid-filled alveoli
Ventilation-perfusion mismatch (especially with bacterial pneumonia)
Lung consolidation with decreased surface area available for gas exchange

Defining Characteristics
Dyspnea
Hypoxemia and/or hypercapnia
Pale, dusky, cyanotic skin color
Tachypnea
Tachycardia
Hypotension
Restlessness/irritability
Disorientation or confusion
In older patients, functional decline with or without fever

Common Expected Outcome
Patient maintains optimal gas exchange as evidenced by arterial blood gases (ABGs) within the patient's usual range, oxygen saturation of 90% or greater, alert response mentation or no further reduction in level of consciousness, relaxed breathing, and baseline HR for patient.

NOC Outcome
Respiratory Status: Gas Exchange
NIC Interventions
Respiratory Monitoring; Oxygen Therapy

Ongoing Assessment

Actions/Interventions	Rationales
■ Assess respirations: note the quality, rate, rhythm, depth of respiration; dyspnea on exertion; use of accessory muscles; and the position assumed for easy breathing.	Patients will adapt their breathing patterns over time to facilitate gas exchange. Both rapid, shallow breathing patterns and hypoventilation affect gas exchange. Hypoxia is associated with signs of increased breathing effort. Conversational dyspnea and tripod posturing are evidence of significant dyspnea. Respiratory failure may ensue with the patient unable to maintain the rapid respiratory rate. QSEN: Safety.
■ Monitor for changes in HR and BP.	With initial hypoxia and hypercapnia, BP and HR rise. As the hypoxia and/or hypercapnia become more severe, BP may drop; HR tends to continue to be rapid with dysrhythmias.
■ Assess the skin, nail beds, and mucous membranes for pallor or cyanosis.	Cool, pale skin may be secondary to a compensatory vasoconstrictive response to hypoxemia. As oxygenation and perfusion become impaired, peripheral tissues become cyanotic.
■ Assess for restlessness and changes in the level of consciousness.	Increased restlessness, confusion, and/or irritability are early indicators of insufficient oxygenation of the brain and require further intervention. Always check the pulse oximetry results with any mental status changes in older adults. QSEN: Safety.
▲ Use pulse oximetry to monitor oxygen saturation; assess ABGs.	Pulse oximetry is a useful tool to detect changes in oxygenation. Oxygen saturation should be at 90% or greater. The ABGs provide information about developing hypoxemia and respiratory acidosis. Increasing $Paco_2$ and decreasing Pao_2 are signs of respiratory failure. QSEN: Safety.

Therapeutic Interventions

Actions/Interventions	Rationales
▲ Maintain an oxygen administration device as ordered. Avoid high concentrations of oxygen in patients with chronic obstructive pulmonary disease (COPD).	Supplemental oxygen therapy maintains an oxygen saturation of 90% or greater to provide for adequate oxygenation. Patients with COPD who chronically retain carbon dioxide depend on a "hypoxic" drive as their stimulus to breathe. When applying oxygen, close monitoring is imperative to prevent unsafe increases in the oxygen level.
■ Plan activity and rest periods to minimize the patient's energy.	Activities increase metabolic rate and oxygen consumption and should be planned so the patient does not become hypoxic. Rest helps conserve the energy needed for more effective breathing and coughing efforts.
■ Anticipate the need for intubation and possibly mechanical ventilation if the condition worsens.	Early intubation and mechanical ventilation are recommended to prevent full decompensation of the patient and a potentially life-threatening situation. QSEN: Safety.

■ = Independent   ▲ = Interprofessional Collaboration

Pulmonary Care Plans

NANDA-I NDx Acute Pain

Common Related Factors
Pain resulting from disease
Coughing

Defining Characteristics
Self-report of intensity using a standardized pain scale
Self-report of pain characteristics using a standardized pain instrument
Facial expression of pain
Change in physiological parameter (e.g., blood pressure, heart rate, respiratory rate and oxygen saturation)

Common Expected Outcomes
Patient reports satisfactory pain control at a decreasing level using a standardized pain scale.
Patient verbalizes understanding of nonpharmacological interventions for pain relief.
Patient exhibits increased comfort such as baseline levels for HR, BP, and respirations, and relaxed muscle tone or body posture.

NOC Outcomes
Pain Control; Medication Response
NIC Interventions
Pain Management; Analgesic Administration

Ongoing Assessment

Actions/Interventions

■ Assess reports of pain with breathing or coughing.

■ Determine how the patient has effectively dealt with pain in the past.

Rationales

The assessment of pain/discomfort is the first step in planning pain management strategies. Pain can result in shallow breathing and poor cough effort.
This evaluation provides an opportunity to consider the patient's reactions to and expectations for pain relief. QSEN: Patient-centered care.

Therapeutic Interventions

Actions/Interventions

▲ Administer appropriate medications to treat the cough:

  • Do not suppress a productive cough; use moderate amounts of analgesics to relieve pleuritic pain.

  • Use cough suppressants and humidity for a dry, hacking cough.
▲ Administer analgesics as prescribed and as needed. Encourage the patient to take analgesics before discomfort becomes severe. Evaluate the medication's effectiveness.
■ Use additional measures, including positioning and relaxation techniques.

Rationales

Persistent coughing can be painful and require suppression. Careful balancing of the dosage is needed to prevent reduction in respirations seen with some analgesics.
Coughing is necessary to mobilize secretions. Cough suppression will cause retained secretions and delay the resolution of infection.
An unproductive hacking cough irritates airways and should be suppressed.
Medications allow for pain relief and the ability to deep breathe and cough. Analgesics prevent peak periods of pain.
These measures facilitate effective respiratory excursion.

NANDA-I NDx Deficient Knowledge

Common Related Factors

Insufficient information
Insufficient interest in learning
Misinformation presented by others
Insufficient knowledge of resources

Defining Characteristics

Insufficient knowledge
Inaccurate follow-through of instruction
Inappropriate behavior

Common Expected Outcome

Patient and caregiver demonstrate understanding of disease process and compliance with treatment regimen and isolation procedures.

NOC Outcomes

Knowledge: Disease Process; Knowledge: Pneumonia Management; Self-Management: Pneumonia

NIC Interventions

Health Literacy Enhancement; Learning Facilitation; Teaching: Disease Process; Teaching: Prescribed Medication; Immunization/Vaccination Management

Ongoing Assessment

Actions/Interventions	Rationales
■ Determine the patient's understanding of pneumonia complications and their treatment.	This information provides an important starting point in education. Providing information allows the patient to be a full partner in making decisions and assuming responsibility for care at a later time. QSEN: Patient-centered care.
■ Assess potential home care needs.	Therapy will continue after hospital discharge. Home care needs will depend on the availability of supportive people and the patient's energy level and cognitive level.

Therapeutic Interventions

Actions/Interventions	Rationales
■ Teach the patient deep breathing exercises and techniques to cough effectively.	These techniques facilitate clearance of secretions and prevent atelectasis.
■ Discuss with the patient or caregiver the need to complete the full course of antibiotics, as prescribed, and for adequate rest for recuperation.	A full antibiotic course is needed to prevent a relapse or the development of a resistant organism. A prolonged period of convalescence may be needed for older patients.
■ Provide information about the need to do the following: • Maintain a natural resistance to infection through adequate nutrition, rest, and exercise. • Avoid contact with people with upper respiratory infections. • Obtain a chest x-ray examination after the completion of therapy. • Obtain immunizations against influenza if older and with chronic health problems.	These preventive measures reduce the recurrence of disease and promote a healthy immune system. A chest x-ray examination after therapy completion confirms the resolution of the pneumonia and verifies the absence of other lung pathology obliterated by the pneumonia. Pneumococcal vaccination is recommended by the CDC for adults who are 65 or older, and those adults with certain medical conditions. QSEN: Safety; Evidence-based practice.
■ Provide smoking-cessation advice as indicated.	One of the National Patient Safety Goals is to provide advice about stopping smoking to patients while hospitalized. QSEN: Evidence-based practice.

■ = Independent   ▲ = Interprofessional Collaboration

Related Care Plans

Activity intolerance, Chapter 2
Impaired gas exchange, Chapter 2
Imbalanced nutrition: Less than body requirements,
    Chapter 2
Mechanical ventilation, Chapter 6

Pulmonary Embolism

Thromboembolism (VTE); Deep Vein Thrombosis (DVT)

Pulmonary embolism (PE) occurs when a thrombus (blood clot) originating in the venous system or the right side of the heart obstructs blood flow in the pulmonary artery or one of its branches. The clinical picture varies according to the size and location of the embolus, making diagnosis challenging. Careful analysis of risk factors aids in diagnosis; these factors include prolonged immobility, use of central venous catheters, deep vein thrombosis, recent surgery, pregnancy, trauma to vessel walls, hypercoagulable states, obesity, smoking, and certain disease states such as heart failure and trauma. Treatment approaches vary depending on the degree of cardiopulmonary compromise associated with the PE. They can range from thrombolytic therapy in acute situations to anticoagulant therapy and general care measures to optimize respiratory and vascular status (e.g., oxygen, compression stockings). PE is a frequent hospital-acquired condition and is one of the most common causes of death in hospitalized patients. Prevention of thrombus formation is a critical nursing role. In the inpatient setting, all patients need to be assessed for VTE. TJC has a VTE bundle to guide prophylaxis and treatment for this high-risk condition. This care plan focuses on acute care treatment for PE.

NANDA-I NDx **Ineffective Breathing Pattern**

Common Related Factors
Hypoxia
Chest pain
Anxiety

Defining Characteristics
Dyspnea
Tachypnea
Use of accessory muscles to breathe
Tachycardia
Hypoxemia
Restlessness
Abnormal values for arterial blood gases (ABGs)

Common Expected Outcome
Patient maintains effective breathing pattern, as evidenced by relaxed breathing at normal rate and depth, and absence of dyspnea.

NOC Outcome
Respiratory Status: Ventilation
NIC Interventions
Airway Management; Respiratory Monitoring

Ongoing Assessment

Actions/Interventions	Rationales
■ Assess the respiratory rate, rhythm, and depth. Assess for any increase in the work of breathing: shortness of breath, and the use of accessory muscles.	Respiratory rate and rhythm changes are early warning signs of impending respiratory difficulties. Tachypnea is a typical finding of pulmonary embolism (PE). The rapid, shallow respirations result from hypoxia. The development of hypoventilation (a slowing of respiratory rate) without improvement in the patient's condition indicates respiratory failure. QSEN: Safety.
▲ Monitor ABGs, and note any changes.	ABG tests of these patients typically exhibit hypoxemia and respiratory alkalosis from a blowing off of carbon dioxide. The development of respiratory acidosis in this patient indicates respiratory failure, and immediate ventilator support is indicated. QSEN: Safety.
▲ Use pulse oximetry to monitor oxygen saturation.	Pulse oximetry is a useful tool to detect early changes in oxygenation. The goal is oxygen saturation levels greater than 90% on room air.
■ Assess the characteristics of pain, especially in association with the respiratory cycle.	Pain is usually sharp or stabbing and gets worse with deep breathing and coughing. It can result in shallow respirations, further impairing effective gas exchange.
■ Assess the patient's level of anxiety.	PE is a sudden, acute condition that can produce anxiety. Anxiety can result in rapid, shallow respirations and increase dyspnea. It can be a sign of decreasing hypoxemia. QSEN: Safety.

Therapeutic Interventions

Actions/Interventions	Rationales
■ Position the patient in a sitting position, and change the position every 2 hours.	If not contraindicated, a sitting position allows good lung excursion and chest expansion. Repositioning facilitates movement and the drainage of secretions.
▲ Administer oxygen as prescribed.	Supplemental oxygen maintains adequate oxygenation, decreases the work of breathing, relieves dypsnea, and promotes comfort. The appropriate amount of oxygen needs to be continuously delivered so the patient does not become desaturated.
■ Provide reassurance and allay anxiety by staying with the patient during acute episodes of respiratory distress.	The presence of a trusted person may be helpful during periods of anxiety.
■ Prepare the patient for diagnostic tests (e.g., chest x-ray examination, ABG measurement, D-dimer assay, computed tomography [CT] scan, ventilation-perfusion scan, and pulmonary arteriogram).	Common tests such as a chest x-ray examination and D-dimer assay (marker for clot lysis) are readily available in acute care settings, especially to rule out PE. If there is a high suspicion for PE, then a CT scan and other scans are added to make a diagnosis. A pulmonary arteriogram is the definitive test.
■ Assist the patient with coughing and deep breathing. Suction as needed.	Coughing is the most productive way to remove secretions. The patient may be unable to perform independently. Suctioning is indicated when patients are unable to remove secretions from the airways by coughing. These maneuvers help keep airways open by clearing secretions.
■ Anticipate the need for intubation and mechanical ventilation.	Intubation and positive-pressure ventilation are a means to stabilize breathing and ventilation and prevent decompensation of the patient. QSEN: Safety.

■ = Independent   ▲ = Interprofessional Collaboration

Pulmonary Care Plans

Impaired Gas Exchange

Common Related Factors

Decreased perfusion to lung tissues caused by obstruction in pulmonary vascular bed by embolus

Increased alveolar dead space

Increased physiological shunting caused by collapse of alveoli resulting from loss of surfactant

Defining Characteristics

Confusion and/or somnolence

Restlessness and/or irritability

Hypoxemia

Hypercapnia

Tachycardia

Dyspnea

Headache

Abnormal skin color

Oxygen saturation less than 90%

Abnormal values for arterial blood gases (ABGs)

Common Expected Outcome

Patient maintains optimal gas exchange, as evidenced by ABGs within the patient's usual range, oxygen saturation of 90% or greater, alert response mentation or no further reduction of level of consciousness, relaxed breathing, and baseline HR for patient.

NOC Outcomes

Respiratory Status: Gas Exchange; Tissue Perfusion: Pulmonary

NIC Interventions

Respiratory Monitoring; Oxygen Therapy; Acid-Base Management

Ongoing Assessment

Actions/Interventions	Rationales
■ Monitor vital signs, noting any changes.	In initial hypoxia and hypercapnia, the BP, HR, and respiratory rate all rise. As the hypoxia and/or hypercapnia becomes more severe, BP may drop, HR tends to continue to be rapid and includes dysrhythmias, and respiratory failure may ensue, with the patient unable to maintain the rapid respiratory rate. QSEN: Safety.
■ Auscultate lung sounds, noting areas of decreased ventilation and the presence of adventitious sounds.	Common clinical findings with pulmonary embolism (PE) include crackles.
■ Assess the skin, nail beds, and mucous membranes for color changes.	Cool, pale skin may be secondary to a compensatory response to hypoxemia. As oxygen and perfusion become impaired, peripheral tissues become cyanotic.
■ Assess for the signs and symptoms of hypoxia.	Hypoxia results from increased dead space (ventilation without perfusion) that reduces effective gas exchange. Signs include tachycardia, restlessness, diaphoresis, headache, lethargy or confusion, and skin color changes. QSEN: Safety.
■ Assess for the presence of signs and symptoms of pulmonary infarction.	A large pulmonary embolus or multiple small clots in a specific area of the lung can cause an ischemic necrosis and/or infarction of the lung area. Signs include cough, hemoptysis, pleuritic pain, consolidation, pleural effusion, bronchial breathing, pleural friction rub, fever.
▲ Monitor ABGs, and note any changes.	ABG analysis can be normal or show hypoxemia and hypocapnia because of tachypnea. Later signs of respiratory failure include low Pao_2 and elevated $Paco_2$. Metabolic acidosis results from a lactic acid buildup from tissue hypoxia. QSEN: Safety.

 evolve **For additional care plans, go to http://evolve.elsevier.com/Gulanick/.**

Actions/Interventions

▲ Use pulse oximetry, as available, to continuously monitor oxygen saturation.

■ Assess for calf tenderness, swelling, redness, and/or hardened areas.

Rationales

Pulse oximetry is a useful tool in the clinical setting to detect changes in oxygenation. Oxygen saturation should be at 90% or greater.

PE often arises from a deep vein thrombosis and may have been previously overlooked.

Therapeutic Interventions

Actions/Interventions

▲ Administer oxygen as needed.

■ Position the patient properly to facilitate ventilation-perfusion matching.

▲ Anticipate the need to start anticoagulant therapy and, if there is a massive thromboembolism, the use of thrombolytic therapy.

Rationales

Supplemental oxygen maintains adequate oxygenation, decreases the work of breathing, relieves dyspnea, and promotes comfort. The appropriate amount of oxygen needs to be continuously delivered so the patient does not become desaturated.

Upright and sitting positions optimize diaphragmatic excursions and lung perfusion. When the patient is positioned on one side, the affected area should not be dependent.

Unfractionated heparin was the cornerstone of treatment. However, it can decrease platelet aggregation resulting in heparin-induced thrombocytopenia. Today low-molecular-weight heparin is more commonly used to prevent the recurrence of emboli. These medications do not dissolve clots that already exist. A variety of direct thrombin inhibitors are available, depending on the clinical situation. If a massive thrombus is present or the patient is hemodynamically unstable, thrombolytic therapy (e.g., alteplase [Activase] or reteplase [Retavase]) is used to directly lyse or dissolve the clot. These medications are based on recommendations from national organizations. QSEN: Evidence-based practice.

NANDA-I
NDx **Risk for Bleeding**

Common Risk Factors

Anticoagulant or thrombolytic therapy
Abnormal blood profiles

Common Expected Outcomes

Patient does not experience bleeding.
Patient maintains prothrombin time (PT), partial thromboplastin time (PTT), and international normalized ratio (INR) within desired range.

NOC Outcomes
Blood Coagulation; Risk Control
NIC Interventions
Bleeding Precautions; Bleeding Reduction

■ = Independent ▲ = Interprofessional Collaboration

Ongoing Assessment

Actions/Interventions	Rationales
■ Assess for the history of a high-risk bleeding condition: liver disease, kidney disease, severe hypertension, cavitary tuberculosis, bacterial endocarditis, and heparin-induced thrombocytopenia.	Because anticoagulation therapy is the hallmark treatment for PE, prior patient experiences with bleeding or antico-agulants must be assessed before treatment. Risks versus benefits of treatment must be assessed. QSEN: Patient-centered care; Safety.
▲ Monitor the IV dosage and delivery system (tubing or pump).	IV anticoagulation is administered using an electronic infusion pump. This device reduces the risk for overcoagulation or undercoagulation. This nursing action reduces the risk of harm to the patient from over or under-dosing of medications. QSEN: Safety.
▲ Monitor platelet counts, coagulation test results (INR, PT, activated partial thromboplastin time [aPTT]), and hemoglobin and hematocrit. Notify the physician immediately if a higher or lower than designated range occurs.	The effects of anticoagulation therapy must be closely monitored to reduce the risk for bleeding. The type of test depends on the anticoagulation medication administered.
▲ Monitor platelets and the heparin-induced platelet aggregation (HIPA) status.	Severe platelet reductions can occur with heparin use, especially unfractionated heparin therapy, and are known as heparin-induced thrombocytopenia (HIT). HIT is less commonly seen with the use of low-molecular-weight heparin.
■ Assess for the signs and symptoms of bleeding: petechiae, purpura, hematoma; bleeding from catheter insertion sites; gastrointestinal or genitourinary bleeding; bleeding from the respiratory tract; bleeding from mucous membranes; decreased hemoglobin and hematocrit.	Early assessment facilitates the prompt administration of the appropriate antidote. QSEN: Safety.

Therapeutic Interventions

Actions/Interventions	Rationales
▲ Administer anticoagulant therapy as prescribed (bolus, continuous IV heparin and/or subcutaneous low-molecular-weight heparin), oral anticoagulants or direct thrombin inhibitors).	Anticoagulants are given to prevent further thrombus formation. The type of medication varies per protocol. New nonheparin agents are also available for patients who cannot tolerate heparin. These medications are based on recommendations from national organizations. QSEN: Evidence-based practice.
▲ If the patient is HIPA positive, stop all heparin products and consult a hematologist.	Continuation of heparin products is contraindicated in the patient who is HIPA positive. Integrating the contributions of members of the interprofessional team helps the patient and family achieve health goals. QSEN: Teamwork and collaboration.
▲ If bleeding occurs while on heparin, anticipate the following: • Stop the infusion. • Recheck the aPTT level stat. • Take vital signs often. • Reevaluate the dose of heparin on the basis of the aPTT result. • Notify the blood bank to ensure blood availability if needed.	Laboratory data guide further treatments; the aPTT guide is 1.5 to 2 times normal. QSEN: Safety.

Actions/Interventions	**Rationales**
▲ Convert from IV anticoagulation to oral anticoagulation after the appropriate length of therapy. Monitor the INR, PT, and aPTT levels.	The onset of anticoagulation with warfarin is 2 to 3 days. There needs to be an overlap of these medications to ensure adequate PT levels or INR levels for anticoagulation before discontinuing heparin. Newer medications do not require laboratory testing as they achieve a steady therapeutic state. The downside is that no reversal agent is available should the patient experience significant bleeding.
▲ Administer thrombolytic therapy as prescribed.	Lytic agents are indicated for patients with a massive PE that results in hemodynamic compromise. Be aware of the following contraindications for thrombolytic therapy to minimize complications: recent surgery, recent organ biopsy, pregnancy, recent stroke, or recent or active internal bleeding.
▲ Institute precautionary measures for thrombolytic therapy per protocol.	Preventive care is given per institutional policy. Such measures to reduce the risk for bleeding include using only compressible vessels for IV sites; compressing IV sites for at least 10 minutes and arterial sites for 30 minutes; limiting physical manipulation of patients; providing gentle oral care; avoiding intramuscular (IM) injections; drawing all laboratory specimens through an existing arterial line or venous heparin-lock line; and sending the specimen for type and crossmatch. QSEN: Safety; Evidence-based practice.
■ Anticipate treatment for excessive bleeding.	Protamine sulfate is an antidote for heparin. Vitamin K is an antidote for warfarin. Clotting factors, Amicar (aminocaproic acid), and fresh frozen plasma are antidotes for fibinolytic therapy. QSEN: Safety; Evidence-based practice.

NANDA-I
NDx **Deficient Knowledge**

Common Related Factors

Insufficient information
Insufficient interest in learning
Misinformation presented by others

Defining Characteristics

Insufficient knowledge
Inaccurate follow-through of instruction
Inappropriate behavior

Common Expected Outcome

Patient verbalizes understanding of desired content: importance of medications, signs of excessive anticoagulation, and means to reduce risk for bleeding and recurrence of emboli.

NOC Outcomes

Knowledge: Disease Process; Knowledge: Medication

NIC Interventions

Health Literacy Enhancement; Learning Facilitation; Teaching: Disease Process; Teaching: Prescribed Medication

---

■ = Independent ▲ = Interprofessional Collaboration

Ongoing Assessment

Action/Intervention

- Assess the patient's knowledge of pulmonary embolus: its severity, prognosis, risk factors, and therapy.

Rationale

Pulmonary embolism (PE) can be a sudden acute condition for which the patient has no prior experience. Assessment provides an important starting point in education.

Therapeutic Interventions

Actions/Interventions

- Provide information on the cause of the problem, common risk factors, and effects of PE on body functioning.

- Instruct the patient about medications, their actions, dosages, and side effects.

- Inform the patient of the need for routine laboratory testing while on oral anticoagulation.

- Discuss with and provide the patient with a list of what to avoid when taking certain anticoagulants:
  - Do not use a blade razor (electric razors preferred).
  - Do not take new medications without consulting the physician, pharmacist, or nurses.
  - Do not change a diet of foods high in vitamin K (e.g., dark-green vegetables, cauliflower, cabbage, bananas, tomatoes).
  - Discuss drug, herb, alcohol, and food interactions with the medication. Emphasize that significant diet changes and all over-the-counter medications and complementary therapies need to be discussed with the physician or nurse practitioner before initiation.

- Discuss with and give the patient a list of measures to minimize the recurrence of emboli:
  - Perform leg exercises as advised, especially during long automobile and airplane trips.
  - Do not cross the legs at the knees.
  - Use elastic stockings as prescribed.
  - Maintain adequate hydration.

- Discuss and give the patient a list of signs and symptoms of excessive anticoagulation: easy bruising, severe nosebleed, black stools, blood in urine or stools, joint swelling and pain, coughing up of blood, severe headache.

- Discuss the use of a medical alert bracelet or other identification.

- If the patient is heparin-induced platelet aggregation (HIPA) positive, instruct about the importance of avoiding heparin.

Rationales

Preventing thrombus formation is an ongoing concern. An informed patient is more likely to avoid common risk factors.

Teaching content on risk factors and the prevention of complications reduces the risk of harm to the patient. QSEN: Safety.

Patients may require anticoagulation for weeks, months, or more, depending on their risks. Accurate knowledge reduces future complications.

Continued regular assessment of anticoagulation is necessary to prevent both recurrence of clots and active bleeding. Newer direct thrombin inhibitors such as Xarelto achieve a steady therapeutic state and do not require laboratory testing.

These safety measures reduce the risk for bleeding. Many medications and foods interact with warfarin, altering the anticoagulation effect. QSEN: Safety.

These measures reduce the potential for thrombus formation.

Patients need to self-manage their condition. Early assessment facilitates prompt treatment.

These forms of identification alert others of the patient's anticoagulation history to facilitate safe, effective medical care.

Heparin use can result in formation of antiheparin antibodies, which puts the patient at risk.

Actions/Interventions

- Explain the need for a vena cava filter device if clotting is a chronic problem.

Rationales

In high-risk patients this filter and/or interruption device can trap a thrombus migrating from a deep vein thrombosis (DVT) in the leg.

Related Care Plans

Decreased cardiac output, Chapter 2
Anxiety, Chapter 2

Respiratory Failure, Acute

Ventilatory Failure; Oxygenation Failure

Acute respiratory failure is a life-threatening inability to maintain adequate pulmonary gas exchange. Persons with acute respiratory failure cannot carry out the two major functions of gas exchange: delivery of adequate amounts of oxygen into the arterial blood (oxygenation failure), removal of a corresponding amount of carbon dioxide from the mixed venous blood (ventilatory failure), or both. Diagnostic criteria in patients without chronic lung disease include Pao_2 less than 60 mm Hg on room air, or $Paco_2$ above 45 mm Hg with acidosis, *and* arterial oxygen saturation below 90%. Respiratory failure can result from obstructive disease (e.g., emphysema, chronic bronchitis, asthma), restrictive disease (e.g., atelectasis, acute respiratory distress syndrome [ARDS], pneumonia, multiple rib fractures, postoperative abdominal or thoracic surgery, central nervous system depression), or ventilation-perfusion abnormalities (e.g., pulmonary embolism). This care plan focuses on acute care management of respiratory failure.

NANDA-I
NDx Impaired Spontaneous Ventilation

Common Related Factors

Respiratory muscle fatigue
Metabolic factors
Central nervous system depression
Drug overdose

Defining Characteristics

Shortness of breath and/or dyspnea
Increased $Paco_2$ level ($\geq$50 to 60 mm Hg)
Decreased Pao_2 level (<50 to 60 mm Hg)
Arterial pH less than 7.35
Decreased in arterial oxygen saturation (Sao_2 < 90%)
Decreased tidal volume
Increase in HR
Restlessness

Common Expected Outcome

Patient maintains spontaneous gas exchange resulting in normal arterial blood gases (ABGs) within parameters for patient, return to normal pulse oximetry, and decreased dyspnea.

NOC Outcomes

Respiratory Status: Gas Exchange; Respiratory Status: Ventilation; Vital Signs

NIC Interventions

Respiratory Monitoring; Ventilation Assistance; Mechanical Ventilation Management: Invasive; Oxygen Therapy

---

■ = Independent   ▲ = Interprofessional Collaboration

Ongoing Assessment

Actions/Interventions	Rationales
■ Assess the respiratory rate, pattern, and depth. Assess for dyspnea and note the position assumed for breathing.	Respiratory rate and rhythm changes are early warning signs of impending respiratory difficulties. Dyspnea is a classic sign of respiratory failure. A tripod position or orthopnea is associated with breathing difficulty. QSEN: Safety.
■ Assess for the use of accessory muscles.	The work of breathing increases greatly as lung compliance decreases. As moving air into and out of lungs becomes more difficult, the breathing pattern alters to include the use of accessory muscles to increase chest excursion to facilitate breathing.
■ Assess the patient's HR and BP.	Hypotension and tachycardia may result from hypoxia and/or hypercarbia.
■ Assess for changes in the level of consciousness.	Increased restlessness, confusion, and/or irritability are early indicators of insufficient oxygenation of the brain and require further intervention. QSEN: Safety.
■ Assess for the presence of cough and, if effective, the amount expectorated, frequency, and color.	These may be indicative of a cause for the alteration in breathing pattern.
■ Auscultate the lungs for normal and adventitious sounds: wheezing, crackles, or rhonchi.	Changes in lung sounds may reveal specific problems that guide treatment.
■ Monitor for dysrhythmias.	Cardiac dysrhythmias may result from hypoxia, catecholamine release in response to low oxygen levels, and acidosis.
■ Use pulse oximetry to monitor oxygen saturation.	Pulse oximetry provides an objective indication of oxygen saturation. It should be kept at 90% or greater.
▲ Closely monitor ABGs carefully, and note any changes.	This nursing assessment reduces harm by identifying changes in oxygenation and acid-base balances, and initiating early intervention. Increasing $Paco_2$ and/or decreasing Pao_2 are signs of respiratory failure. QSEN: Safety.

Therapeutic Interventions

Actions/Interventions	Rationales
■ Position the patient to optimize ventilation.	If not contraindicated, a sitting position allows for adequate diaphragmatic and lung excursion and chest expansion.
■ Plan activity and rest periods to maximize the patient's energy.	Fatigue is common with the increased work of breathing. Activity increases the metabolic rate and oxygen requirements. Rest helps mobilize energy for more effective breathing and coughing efforts.
▲ Administer oxygen as needed. For patients with severe chronic obstructive pulmonary disease (COPD), give oxygen cautiously, preferably with a Venturi device.	Oxygen is needed to correct associated hypoxemia. Patients with COPD who chronically retain carbon dioxide depend on "hypoxic drive" as their stimulus to breathe. When applying oxygen, close monitoring is imperative to prevent unsafe increases in the patient's Pao_2, which could result in apnea. The Venturi device is a high-flow oxygen delivery system with a stable Fio_2 that is unaffected by the patient's respiratory rate or tidal volume.
■ Assist with ventilatory support measures as appropriate:	Appropriate use of safety-enhancing technology minimizes the risk of harm to the patient. QSEN: Safety.
• Bilevel positive airway pressure (BiPAP)	BiPAP is a noninvasive form of positive-pressure ventilation.
• When necessary, prepare for intubation and mechanical ventilation.	Early intubation and mechanical ventilation may be needed to maintain adequate oxygenation and ventilation and to prevent full decompensation of the patient and a potentially life-threatening situation.

NANDA-I NDx Risk for Ineffective Airway Clearance

Common Risk Factors

Copious and tenacious tracheobronchial secretions
Inability to cough
Tracheobronchial infection
Presence of artificial airway (endotracheal tube)
Fatigue/decreased energy
Impaired respiratory function

Common Expected Outcome

Patient will maintain clear, open airways, as evidenced by normal breath sounds, normal rate and depth of respiration, and ability to cough up secretions.

NOC Outcome
Respiratory Status: Airway Patency
NIC Interventions
Airway Suctioning; Airway Management

Ongoing Assessment

Actions/Interventions	Rationales
■ Assess the lungs for adventitious breath sounds (e.g., rhonchi, wheezes).	Airway obstruction from fluid accumulation produces crackles and rhonchi. Wheezes are caused by bronchospasm.
■ Assess the respiratory rate, rhythm, and depth.	An increase in respiratory rate and rhythm may be a compensatory response for airway obstruction. Hypoxia is associated with an increased breathing effort. QSEN: Safety.
■ Assess the characteristics of sputum: color, consistency, amount, odor.	Abnormalities may be a result of infection, bronchitis, chronic smoking, or other conditions. A sign of infection is discolored sputum (no longer clear or white); an odor may be present. Thick, tenacious secretions increase hypoxemia and may be indicative of dehydration.
■ Assess cough for effectiveness and productivity.	Patients may have an ineffective cough because of respiratory muscle fatigue, severe bronchospasm, or thick, tenacious secretions.

Therapeutic Interventions

Actions/Interventions	Rationales
■ Use an upright position (if tolerated, the head of the bed at 45 degrees). Instruct the patient or assist in changing the position every 2 hours.	An upright position provides for better lung expansion and improved air exchange. Position changes mobilize secretions.
▲ Maintain humidified oxygen as prescribed.	Increasing the humidity of inspired air will reduce the viscosity of secretions and facilitate removal.
■ Instruct the patient to deep breathe adequately, to cough effectively, and to use incentive spirometry, as ordered.	These measures improve lung capacity and gas exchange. Coughing is the most effective way to remove most secretions.
▲ If cough is ineffective, use nasotracheal suction as ordered.	Suctioning is indicated when patients are unable to remove secretions from the airway by coughing because of weakness, thick mucus plugs, or excessive or tenacious mucus production. It can also stimulate a cough.

■ = Independent   ▲ = Interprofessional Collaboration

Actions/Interventions

After intubation:
▲ Institute suctioning of the airway as needed (not routinely).

Rationales

The frequency of suctioning should be based on the presence of adventitious sounds and/or increased ventilatory pressure, not time intervals. Oversuctioning can cause hypoxia and injury to bronchial and lung tissues.

NANDA-I
NDx   Risk for Infection

Common Risk Factors

Increased secretions
Suctioning of airway
Endotracheal (ET) intubation

Common Expected Outcome

Patient remains free of infection, as evidenced by normal body temperature, normal white blood cell (WBC) count, negative cultures, normal vital signs, and absence of purulent drainage from tubes.

NOC Outcomes
Immune Status; Risk Control: Infectious Process
NIC Intervention
Infection Protection

Ongoing Assessment

Actions/Interventions

■ Assess the patient for fever.

▲ Monitor the WBC count.

■ Observe the patient's secretions for color, consistency, quantity, and odor.
▲ Monitor sputum cultures and sensitivities.

Rationales

Fever may be a manifestation of an infection or an inflammatory process. If the patient is receiving steroid therapy, detecting infections may be more difficult.
A rising WBC count indicates the body's efforts to combat pathogens.
Increased amounts of sputum and colored or odorous secretions may indicate infection. QSEN: Safety.
Identification of the infecting microorganism is important to determine antibiotic coverage.

Therapeutic Interventions

Actions/Interventions

■ Practice conscientious bronchial hygiene, good handwashing techniques, and sterile suctioning.

■ Administer mouth care (e.g., mouthwash, mouth swabs, mouth spray) every 2 hours and as needed; brush the patient's teeth at least every 12 hours.
■ Institute airway suctioning as needed.

■ If the patient was placed on a mechanical ventilator, keep the head of the bed elevated greater than 30 degrees.

Rationales

TJC's National Patient Safety Goals provide meticulous infection control guidelines. Many infections are transmitted by hospital personnel. QSEN: Evidence-based practice; Safety.
Mouth care helps limit oral bacterial growth and promotes patient comfort.

Accumulation of secretions provides a medium for bacterial growth.
Upright positioning helps prevent ventilator-associated pneumonia (VAP). VAP carries a high mortality rate. Most infections are caused by bacterial pathogens, with gram-negative bacilli being common.

Actions/Interventions

■ Institute measures to reduce VAP.

  · Wash hands before and after suctioning, touching ventilator equipment, and/or coming into contact with respiratory secretions.
  · Use a continuous subglottic suction ET tube for intubation expected to be longer than 24 hours.
  · Keep the head of the bed elevated to 30 to 45 degrees or perform subglottic suctioning unless medically contraindicated.
  · Brush teeth two or three times per day with a soft toothbrush. Chlorhexidine-based rinses may also be incorporated into oral care products.
  · Use sterile suctioning procedures.

Rationales

Nosocomial infections such as VAP are a leading cause of hospital deaths. Prevention of VAP is a national initiative to promote quality and safety. Research continues to identify the most effective ventilator bundle order sets to prevent VAP. QSEN: Evidence-based practice.

An artificial airway bypasses the normal protective mechanisms of the upper airways. Handwashing reduces the transmission of microorganisms.

This intervention prevents the accumulation of secretions that can be aspirated.

Elevation promotes better lung expansion. It also reduces gastric reflux and aspiration.

Oral care reduces colonization of the oropharynx with respiratory pathogens that can be aspirated into the lungs.

This technique decreases the introduction of microorganisms into the airway.

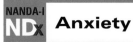

NANDA-I
NDx **Anxiety**

Common Related Factors	Defining Characteristics
Unknown outcome	Restlessness
Change in health status	Uncooperative behavior
Change in environment	Withdrawal
Inability to speak if intubated	Vigilant watch on equipment
Inability to maintain adequate gas exchange	Tachypnea
	Facial tension

Common Expected Outcomes

Patient demonstrates reduced anxiety, as evidenced by calm manner and cooperative behavior.
Patient uses effective coping mechanisms.
Patient describes a reduction in level of anxiety experienced.

NOC Outcomes
Anxiety Self-Control; Coping
NIC Interventions
Anxiety Reduction; Presence; Emotional Support

Ongoing Assessment

Action/Intervention

■ Assess the patient for signs of anxiety.

Rationale

Respiratory failure is an acute life-threatening condition that will produce high levels of anxiety in the patient as well as significant others. Anxiety can affect the respiratory rate and pattern, resulting in rapid, shallow breathing and leading to arterial blood gas abnormalities. QSEN: Patient-centered care.

■ = Independent   ▲ = Interprofessional Collaboration

Therapeutic Interventions

Actions/Interventions	Rationales
■ Display a confident, calm manner and understanding attitude. Assure the patient and significant others of close, continuous monitoring that will ensure prompt interventions. Reassure the patient of the staff's presence.	The presence of a trusted person may be helpful during periods of anxiety. The staff's anxiety may be easily perceived by the patient. The patient's feeling of stability is increased in a calm, nonthreatening atmosphere. QSEN: Patient-centered care.
■ Encourage visiting by family or significant others.	The presence of significant others may reinforce feelings of security for the patient.
■ Anticipate questions. Provide explanations of mechanical ventilation and the alarm systems on monitors and ventilators.	The intensive care unit is a busy environment that can be scary and upsetting to the patient and significant others. Information helps reduce anxiety. An informed patient who understands the treatment plan will be more cooperative and relaxed.
■ If impaired communication is the problem, provide the patient with word-and-phrase cards, a writing pad and pencil, or a picture board.	These tools provide a channel through which information can be communicated.
▲ Use other supportive measures (e.g., medications, psychiatric liaison, clergy, social services) as indicated.	Medication and supportive resources may be used if the patient's anxiety continues to escalate. Specialty expertise may provide a wider range of treatment options. QSEN: Teamwork and collaboration.

NANDA-I NDx Deficient Knowledge

Common Related Factors
Insufficient information
Insufficient interest in learning
Misinformation presented by others
Insufficient knowledge of resources

Defining Characteristics
Insufficient knowledge
Inaccurate follow-through of instruction
Inappropriate behavior

Common Expected Outcome
Patient verbalizes understanding of disease process, procedures, and treatment.

NOC Outcomes
Knowledge: Disease Process; Knowledge: Treatment Regimen

NIC Interventions
Heath Literacy Enhancement; Learning Facilitation; Teaching: Disease Process; Teaching: Individual

Ongoing Assessment

Action/Intervention	Rationale
■ Assess the patient's perception and understanding of the disease process that led to respiratory failure and of oxygen therapy and deep breathing and coughing techniques.	This provides an important starting point in education. Teaching interventions must be designed individually to meet specific patient needs. Patients in acute care may not be able to take in much information because they may need to focus efforts on effective breathing rather than on the educational session. QSEN: Patient-centered care.

Therapeutic Interventions

Actions/Interventions	Rationales
■ Explain the disease process to the patient or significant others, and correct misconceptions. Include the family and significant others in the plan of care.	During the acute phase, the family or significant others may require the most teaching. This will reduce their feelings of helplessness and assist them in supporting the patient. Acute respiratory failure is a serious condition.
■ Explain all tests and procedures before they occur.	An informed patient is more cooperative.
■ Explain the necessity of oxygen therapy, including its limitations.	Oxygen is used to support arterial saturation.
■ Instruct the patient to deep breathe and cough effectively.	These techniques facilitate the clearance of secretions.
■ Instruct the patient in preventive measures as appropriate (e.g., avoidance of exposure to smoke and fumes, cold air, and allergens such as pollens, dust, and dander).	Attention to these parameters reduces the risk of harm to the patient. These efforts serve to prevent further respiratory difficulties. QSEN: Safety.
■ Provide guidelines for activities and the advancement of activities, the need for home oxygen, and timing for follow-up visits with health care providers.	Information aids in the transition from hospital to home.
■ Discuss with the patient and significant others the reversibility of the condition, advance directives, and medical power of attorney.	Patients must make very clear what they want regarding life-sustaining treatments. Providing this information allows the patient to be a full partner in providing care, making decisions as part of informed consent, and achieving optimal learning outcomes. QSEN: Patient-centered care.

Related Care Plans

Acute respiratory distress syndrome (ARDS), Chapter 6
Chest trauma, Chapter 6
Chronic obstructive pulmonary disease, Chapter 6
Mechanical ventilation, Chapter 6
Pneumonia, Chapter 6

■ = Independent   ▲ = Interprofessional Collaboration

CHAPTER

7

Neurological Care Plans

Alzheimer's Disease/Dementia

Multi-Infarct Dementia (MID); Dementia of the Alzheimer Type (DAT)

Dementia is characterized by a progressive impairment of cognitive function, personality, and behavior. The person with dementia experiences loss of memory, disorientation, impaired language skills, decreased concentration, and impaired judgment. In advanced stages, the person experiences behavior and personality changes such as aggressiveness, mood swings, wandering, and confusion. These changes interfere with the person's ability to carry out role responsibilities and activities of daily living. The causes of dementia are numerous and include degenerative disorders of the nervous system, vascular disorders, autoimmune disorders, and traumatic brain injury such as concussions. Multi-infarct dementia develops in people who have sustained brain injury from multiple strokes. This type of irreversible dementia occurs more often in men than women. People in the later stages of acquired immunodeficiency syndrome (AIDS) may develop dementia. Alcoholism and Parkinson's disease are known to contribute to dementia.

Alzheimer's disease (AD) is an irreversible disease of the central nervous system that manifests as a cognitive disorder. Onset is usually between 50 and 60 years and is characterized by progressive deterioration of memory and cognitive function. Disease progression begins with memory impairment, speech and motor difficulties, disorientation of time and place, impaired judgment, memory loss, forgetfulness, and inappropriate affect, followed by loss of independence, complete disorientation, wandering, hoarding, communication difficulties, complete memory loss, and the final stage with blank expression, irritability, seizures, emaciation, and absolute dependence until death.

Although the cause is unknown, research has found specific genetic loci associated with the development of AD. Chronic inflammation, stroke, and cellular damage from free radicals have been identified as risk factors for AD. Drug therapy for AD includes cholinesterase inhibitors and N-methyl-D-aspartate (NMDA) antagonists. These drugs have been shown to delay the progression of cognitive impairment. Some patients may experience improved memory function with these drugs.

This care plan addresses needs for patients with a wide variety of dementia, of which AD is a type. Focus is on the home care setting. Family members and caregivers of the patient with AD may be the focus for nursing action as part of this care plan.

 NANDA-I NDx **Risk for Violence: Self-Directed or Other-Directed**

Common Risk Factors

Alteration in cognitive functioning
Impulsiveness
Pattern of other-directed violence (e.g., hitting/kicking/ spitting on others)
Pattern of threatening violence (e.g., cursing, verbal threats against people)
Insufficient personal resources (e.g., achievement, affect poorly controlled)
Social isolation

Common Expected Outcomes

Patient avoids self-directed harm.
Patient does not harm others.

NOC Outcomes

Aggression Self-Restraint; Cognition; Dementia
    Level; Mood Equilibrium; Risk Control

NIC Interventions

Anger Control Assistance; Behavior
    Management: Self-Harm; Impulse Control
    Training; Mood Management; Environmental
    Management: Violence Prevention

Ongoing Assessment

Actions/Interventions

- Assess cognitive factors that may contribute to the development of violent behaviors, including the following:
  - Decreased ability to solve problems
  - Alteration in sensory and perceptual capacities
  - Impairment in judgment
  - Psychotic or delusional thought patterns
  - Impaired concentration or decreased response to redirection
- Assess for physical factors that may foster violence: physical discomfort, such as being wet or cold, and sensory overload (overstimulation), such as noise.

- Assess the emotional factors that can lead to violence: the inability to cope with frustrating situations, expressions of low self-esteem, noncompliance with the treatment plan, and a history of aggressive behaviors as a means of coping with stress.

- Evaluate the impact of the medication regimen on behaviors in terms of its contribution to agitation.

Rationales

A decline in cognitive ability contributes to the patient's over-responsiveness to environmental stimuli, leading to agitation and combativeness. The agitation may be manifested as physical aggression or verbal aggression. The patient may have poor impulse behavior control. A decreased attention span and memory loss can contribute to the patient's inability to respond to environmental stimuli. QSEN: Patient-centered care.

Many physical factors will increase stimulation and lead to increased confusion. Patients with Alzheimer's disease (AD) may experience increased confusion, restlessness, and agitation in the late afternoon and early evening. These changes are called sundowner's syndrome. The increased confusion may be related to anxiety that occurs in response to an accumulation of sensory stimuli during the day, fatigue, or an inability to see in the dark. QSEN: Patient-centered care.

A thorough assessment of precipitating factors is needed so that preventive measures can be instituted. Changes in the patient's environment and daily routines may increase his or her level of anxiety and cause outbursts of aggressive behavior. The person may perceive these changes as threats to his or her safety. QSEN: Safety.

Neuroleptics and antipsychotics may cause extrapyramidal side effects, manifested as restlessness.

Therapeutic Interventions

Actions/Interventions

- Involve the patient on a cognitive level as much as possible. Instruct the caregiver in the following techniques. Begin with the least restrictive measures, and progress to the most restrictive measures as the patient's behavior becomes more aggressive.

Rationales

This approach allows the patient some measure of control over the environment. Feeling a sense of control may increase the patient's cooperation with caregivers. Providing the caregiver with information about techniques to manage the patient's behavior reduces the risk of harm to the patient and to the caregiver. QSEN: Patient-centered care; Safety; Evidence-based practice.

Neurological Care Plans

■ = Independent   ▲ = Interprofessional Collaboration

Actions/Interventions	Rationales

Level I

Nonaggressive behaviors: may include wandering or pacing, restlessness or increased motor activity, climbing out of bed, changing clothes or disrobing, hand wringing or handwashing.

- Give verbal feedback, and institute interpersonal approaches.

At this level of dementia, the patient may still have insight about the losses he or she is experiencing.

- Initiate measures such as reorientation, reduced stimuli, and consistent schedules.

Sensory stimulation needs to be reduced. Frequent reorientation to the person's environment increases the ability to trust others. Consistency in schedules and the physical environment promotes orientation and reduces anxiety.

- Speak in slow, clear, soothing tones. Make comments brief and to the point. Repeat as needed.

Attention to technique helps avoid communication conflicts. The patient may have declines in short-term memory that require frequent repetition of new information.

- Use distraction.

Impaired short-term memory may allow the introduction of new stimuli to calm agitated behavior.

- If the patient wanders or paces, consider the need to provide visual supervision, especially if the patient expresses the need to leave.

Providing for safety is a priority. Doors to the outside may need to be locked or have alarms installed to prevent the patient from leaving. Alarms will notify caregivers if the patient attempts to open a door to the outside.

Level II

Verbally aggressive behaviors: may include cursing, yelling, screaming, unintelligible or repetitious speech, and threats or accusations.

- Attempt verbal control; attempt feedback about behavior (for less cognitively impaired), distraction (for cognitively impaired), or limit setting (although this may increase agitation at times).

These techniques can decrease sensory stimuli. Providing the patient with feedback about his or her verbal aggression allows him/her to stop the behavior.

- If feasible, allow the patient more personal space.

If the patient's memory span is short, leaving the room briefly may decrease his or her agitation.

- Acknowledge the patient's fear of loss of control; evaluate the use of touch and hand-holding.

Touch may be calming to some and aggravating to others.

- Provide diversional activities (e.g., folding towels, handling worry beads, walking with the patient).

These activities may assist in increasing the patient's feelings of self-worth and meet his or her need for activity. Repetitive activities can reduce agitation and provide a release of energy.

Level III

Physically aggressive behaviors: may include hitting, kicking, spitting or biting, throwing objects, pushing or pulling others, and fighting.

- Permit the verbalization of feelings associated with agitation.

Verbalization of feelings may diffuse aggressive behavior.

- Offer acceptable alternatives to unacceptable behaviors, such as undressing in public, by allowing the patient to select his or her own clothing.

Providing the patient some measure of control over the environment may diffuse perceptions of threats in the environment.

- If the patient poses a potential threat of injury to self or others, consider the use of soft physical restraints, such as cloth wrist-, hand-, leg-, belt-, or vest-type restraints.

As initial measures become ineffective, more extreme measures may be indicated to ensure the safety of the patient or caregiver.

- Initiate safety measures such as drawer and cabinet locks in the bathroom and kitchen.

This action reduces the patient's access to hazardous items.

Neurological Care Plans

Actions/Interventions

▲ Use pharmaceutical restraints, such as antidepressants or antipsychotics, only if agitation has reached a point where soft restraints are inadequate to protect the patient from injury.

Rationales

Medication may be indicated to decrease the potential risk for injury. The use of the atypical antipsychotics in patients with dementia remains controversial. The use of these drugs may increase the risk of adverse effects such as stroke. The positive benefits have been identified as reduced agitation and increased participation in activities of daily living. Some research studies identify reduced caregiver depression when the patient is taking one of these medications. QSEN: Evidence-based practice; Safety.

NANDA-I NDx

Self-Care Deficit: Bathing, Dressing, Feeding

Common Related Factors

Alteration in cognitive functioning
Anxiety
Decrease in motivation
Perceptual impairment
Weakness

Defining Characteristics

Impaired ability to wash body
Impaired ability to put on or remove various items of clothing
Impaired ability to prepare food
Impaired ability to self-feed in an acceptable manner

Common Expected Outcome

Patient participates in self-care activities, as evidenced by appropriately dressing, bathing, and feeding self.

NOC Outcomes

Self-Care: Bathing; Self-Care: Dressing; Self-Care: Eating

NIC Interventions

Self-Care Assistance: Bathing/Hygiene; Self-Care Assistance: Dressing/Grooming; Self-Care Assistance: Feeding

Neurological Care Plans

Ongoing Assessment

Actions/Interventions

■ Assess for cognitive deficits or behaviors that would create difficulty in bathing self, performing oral hygiene, selecting and putting on appropriate clothing, choosing food menu items, and feeding self.

■ Assess the patient's level of independence in completing self-care.

Rationales

In the early stages of the disease, the patient may have problems with forgetfulness, information processing, and the retrieval of information necessary to make decisions about self-care activities.

The patient with impaired thought processes is unable to self-monitor personal grooming, hygiene, and nutrition needs adequately. The nurse needs to reassess the patient's self-care ability at regular intervals to provide assistance for the patient and caregivers. QSEN: Patient-centered care.

■ = Independent   ▲ = Interprofessional Collaboration

Therapeutic Interventions

Actions/Interventions	Rationales
Instruct the caregiver in strategies to facilitate self-care activities, as in the following:	Providing the caregiver with information about strategies to support the patient with self-care activities allows the patient a measure of control with self-care and allows the caregiver to be a full partner in providing care and achieving optimal outcomes for self-care. QSEN: Patient-centered care; Safety.
▪ Stay with the patient during self-care activities if his or her judgment is impaired.	This approach promotes safety and provides necessary redirection. The caregiver may need to provide verbal cues to help the patient initiate each step of a self-care activity.
▪ Allow enough time in a quiet environment; limit distractions.	Rushing the patient with self-care activities promotes frustration and failure. Distractions interrupt the patient's concentration when performing an activity.
▪ Follow established routines for self-care, if possible, or develop a routine that is consistently followed.	An established routine becomes easier for the patient to follow and requires less decision-making.
▪ Provide a simple, easy-to-read, large-print list of self-care activities to complete each day (e.g., brush teeth, comb hair).	Reminders for the patient may enhance functional abilities.
▪ Assist, as needed, with perineal care each morning and evening (or after each episode of incontinence).	Poor hygiene after elimination increases the risk for skin breakdown.
▪ Assist, as needed, in selecting clothing. Allow the patient to choose if possible (e.g., put out one or two sets of clothing and allow a choice).	Giving the patient some control over the choices about clothing reduces anxiety.
▪ Encourage the patient to dress as independently as possible. Provide easy-to-wear clothes (elastic waistbands, snaps, large buttons, loop-and-pile closures).	It is important for the patient to maintain functional ability for as long as possible.
▪ Assist in selecting nutritious, high-bulk foods. Allow the patient to choose foods he or she prefers, if possible.	These measures promote adequate intake.
▪ Assist in the setup of the meal as needed (e.g., open containers, cut food).	Easy access promotes better nutritional intake.
▪ If judgment is impaired, cool down hot liquids to palatable temperatures before serving.	This measure is necessary to avoid injury.
▪ Limit the number of choices of food on the plate or tray.	It is important to reduce the number of decisions that the patient is required to make. Too many choices may add to the patient's confusion and agitation.
▪ Provide easy-to-eat finger foods if motor coordination is impaired. Provide nutritious between-meal snacks if nutritional intake is inadequate.	This approach promotes meeting the patient's nutritional needs.
▪ If the patient has difficulty with complex tasks: break the task into smaller steps; use a calm, unhurried voice to offer praise and encouragement.	Disorientation and impaired memory can limit the patient's ability to process information and respond appropriately to directions and environmental stimuli. These techniques make it easier for the patient to participate in self-care activities.

NANDA-I
NDx Impaired Social Interaction

Common Related Factors	Defining Characteristics
Disturbance in self-concept	Dysfunctional interactions with others
Disturbance in thought processes	Family reports of changes in interaction
Impaired mobility	Discomfort in social situations
	Impaired social functioning

Common Expected Outcome

Patient engages in social interactions, as evidenced by positive contacts with caregiver or significant others.

NOC Outcomes
Social Involvement; Social Interaction Skills
NIC Interventions
Socialization Enhancement; Behavior Modification: Social Skills

Ongoing Assessment

Actions/Interventions	Rationales
■ Assess for cognitive deficits or behaviors that interfere with forming relationships with others.	As the disease progresses, the ability to maintain attention and memory deteriorates. Behavior may be socially unacceptable.
■ Assess for previous patterns of interaction.	Knowledge of the patient's past patterns of interaction will help the caregiver understand the patient's current pattern of interaction. The ability and/or willingness to interact may vary with the patient's mood, perceptions, and reality orientation. QSEN: Patient-centered care.
■ Assess the patient's potential to interact in a community day care situation.	Confusion, disorientation, and loss of social inhibitions may result in socially inappropriate and/or harmful behavior to self or others. Community-based programs vary in capacity for handling patients in the later stages of dementia and Alzheimer's disease (AD). QSEN: Safety.

Therapeutic Interventions

Actions/Interventions	Rationales
■ Within the context of the nurse-patient relationship, provide regular opportunities for frequent, brief contacts.	Being present demonstrates caring and provides the patient with an opportunity for social interaction.
■ Assist the caregiver in doing the following:	These actions reduce the risk of harm for the patient with social interactions and allow the caregiver to be a full partner in providing care and achieving outcomes for the patient's social interactions. QSEN: Patient-centered care; Safety.
• Support the patient's participation in social activities appropriate to the patient's level of cognitive functioning, such as small family parties.	Large gatherings become more problematic as symptoms intensify. The patient may not be able to tolerate excessive stimuli in large gatherings.
• Redirect the patient when behaviors become socially embarrassing or inappropriate	The patient's short-term memory loss allows the nurse or the caregiver to redirect the patient's behavior and thinking and promote reality orientation.
• Discuss subjects in which the patient is interested but that do not require short-term recall.	Interactions that require short-term recall become difficult and frustrating for the patient.
• When discussing past experiences, assist the patient in connecting them with here-and-now.	Past coping strategies may assist with current situations. Reminiscence promotes long-term memory skills and can relieve depression.
• Do not correct the patient's ideas or confront them as delusional.	Challenges to the patient's thinking can be perceived as threatening. The confused patient may become anxious and agitated.
• Consider the impact of environment on social interaction. Avoid an overstimulating environment (noise, lights, activity).	Sensory overload aggravates impaired cognitive thinking and increases the patient's agitation in social settings. The patient may not be able to cope with changes in environmental routines. New social settings and strangers may increase the patient's anxiety and agitation.

Neurological Care Plans

■ = Independent ▲ = Interprofessional Collaboration

Actions/Interventions

- Involve the patient in developing a daily schedule that includes time for social activity, as well as quiet time.

- Provide information on community day care programs that will help the patient maintain social interaction.

Rationales

The patient is more likely to participate in activities that match his or her talents, interests, and abilities. A schedule that includes activities interspersed with rest periods allows the patient to have energy for social interaction.

Involvement with group activities is determined by various factors, including group size, activity level, and the patient's tolerance level. Fluctuations in mood and affect may influence the ability to respond appropriately to others. Adult day care also provides needed respite for the caregiver.

NANDA-I
NDx **Impaired Home Maintenance**

Common Related Factors

Alteration in cognitive functioning
Insufficient family organization/planning
Insufficient knowledge of home maintenance
Insufficient knowledge of neighborhood resources
Insufficient role model
Insufficient support system

Defining Characteristics

Difficulty maintaining a comfortable home environment
Insufficient equipment/supplies for maintaining home
Poor fiscal management
Request for assistance
Unsanitary environment
Pattern of disease or infection caused by unhygienic conditions (e.g., disease, illness, injury)

Common Expected Outcomes

Caregiver or family provides safe home environment.
Caregiver or family describes nursing or community resources available for home care.

NOC Outcomes

Family Functioning; Safe Home Environment; Self-Care: Instrumental Activities of Daily Living (IADLs)

NIC Interventions

Family Support; Self-Care Assistance; Home Maintenance Assistance

---

Ongoing Assessment

Actions/Interventions

- Determine the adequacy of the home environment.

- Assess the patient's ability to recognize danger (smoke, fire).
- Assess the frequency of disorientation, wandering, and becoming lost in familiar surroundings.

- Assess the family or caregiver's understanding of the patient's needs or deficits, resources to provide adequate supervision and behavior management, the family's ability to cope, and internal or external support systems.

Rationales

The patient's home needs to provide a physically safe living environment (e.g., hand rails on stairs, door locks, smoke alarms). Correcting safety hazards increases the potential for the patient to remain in the home. QSEN: Safety.

Cognitive impairment limits the patient's ability to perceive potential threats in the environment. QSEN: Safety.

These behaviors are the most frequent reason given by family members for placing the patient in a closely supervised care setting.

A thorough assessment is needed to determine potential problems and complications. Families may not have sufficient money to pay for basic home maintenance or repair. Grants or special funds can sometimes be used to modify the home to suit the needs of a cognitively challenged patient. Other supports and services are available to reduce financial stress. QSEN: Patient-centered care.

---

evolve **For additional care plans, go to http://evolve.elsevier.com/Gulanick/.**

Neurological Care Plans

Therapeutic Interventions

Actions/Interventions	Rationales
■ Involve the patient, family, or caregiver in all home planning.	In the initial stages, the patient will be able to contribute to care decisions and should not be excluded from home planning. QSEN: Patient-centered care.
■ Discuss the need to wear an identification bracelet at all times.	This approach allows patients to be identified quickly if they become lost. QSEN: Safety.
■ Suggest a daily program of supervised exercise or walking.	Structured activity may decrease wandering behavior and meet the patient's need for exercise.
■ Provide information about home security devices, such as keyed door locks and audible alarms.	Attention to security measures may decrease wandering behavior and notify the caregiver if the patient attempts to open a door to the outside. QSEN: Safety.
■ Recommend procedures for getting help (e.g., calling police, notifying neighbors) in case the patient becomes lost.	Caregivers need to have up-to-date photographs and physical description information readily available for people who will search for the lost patient.
■ Help the family to identify and mobilize available support networks such as home health services, support groups, church groups, and senior citizens organizations.	A network of family members, friends, and community resources can facilitate home patient care. Using these services promotes independence and reduces caregiver burden. Support groups often have the best practical tips and suggestions to help the patient remain in the home environment.
■ Provide literature and references related to caring for cognitively impaired people in the home.	The Alzheimer's Association has a broad range of resources to help families and caregivers.

NANDA-I NDx **Caregiver Role Strain**

Common Related Factors

Complexity of care activities
Knowledge deficit regarding management of care
Around-the-clock responsibilities
Change in nature of care activities
Unpredictability of care situation
Caregiver has competing role commitments
Caregiver has no respite from caregiver demands
Insufficient resources
Insufficient social support

Defining Characteristics

Difficulty in performing/completing required tasks
Apprehensiveness about future ability to provide care
Apprehensiveness about well-being of care receiver if unable to provide care
Preoccupation with care routine
Insufficient time to meet personal needs
Insufficient coping strategies
Difficulty watching care receiver with illness
Caregiver expresses negative feeling about patient or relationship
Caregiver neglects patient care
Caregiver expresses change in own health status (e.g., fatigue, gastrointestinal upset, headache, weight changes, disturbed sleep, frustration, stress)

Common Expected Outcomes

Caregiver expresses satisfaction with caregiver role.
Caregiver demonstrates competence and confidence in performing the caregiver role by meeting care recipient's physical and psychosocial needs.
Caregiver reports that formal and informal support systems are adequate and helpful.
Caregiver demonstrates flexibility in dealing with problem behavior of care recipient.

NOC Outcomes

Caregiver Well-Being; Caregiver Role Endurance; Caregiver-Patient Relationship

NIC Intervention

Caregiver Support

Neurological Care Plans

■ = Independent ▲ = Interprofessional Collaboration

Ongoing Assessment

Actions/Interventions	Rationales
■ Assess the caregiver–care recipient relationship.	A healthy family or caregiver relationship based on familiarity and compassion provides a strong foundation for the evolving dynamics of caregiving. Mutually rewarding relationships foster a therapeutic caregiving experience. Dysfunctional relationships can result in ineffective, fragmented care or even lead to neglect or abuse.
■ Assess the caregiver's appraisal of the caregiving situation, level of understanding, and willingness to assume caregiver role.	Caregivers need to have a realistic perspective of the situation and the scope of responsibility. The demands of caring for the patient with dementia may be long-term, in which both the caregiver and recipient need to accept a new normal in their lives. Individual responses to caregiving situations are mediated by an appraisal of the personal meaning of the situation. For some, caregiving is viewed as "a duty"; for others, it may be an act of love. QSEN: Patient-centered care.
■ Assess family communication patterns.	Open communication among all family members creates a positive environment, whereas families with communication issues or who conceal feelings creates problems for the caregiver and care recipient.
■ Assess family resources and support systems.	Family and social support is related positively to coping effectiveness. Some cultures are more accepting of this responsibility. However, factors such as blended family units, aging parents, geographical distances between family members, and limited financial resources may hamper the caregiver's coping effectiveness.
■ Determine the caregiver's knowledge and ability to provide patient care, including bathing, skin care, safety, nutrition, medications, and ambulation.	Lack of knowledge and a limited ability to provide care may cause caregiver anxiety. Caregiver frustration can lead to anger directed toward the patient. These emotions may result in verbal or physical abuse or neglect of the patient. QSEN: Safety.

Therapeutic Interventions

Actions/Interventions	Rationales
■ Provide information on the disease process and management strategies.	Accurate information increases understanding of the care recipient's condition and behavior, including the knowledge that regardless of the quality of care, the disease will progress and care requirements will continually increase. Families need to understand the importance of consistency when caring for the patient with dementia. QSEN: Patient-centered care.
■ Encourage the caregiver to identify available family and friends who can assist with caregiving.	As the patient's cognitive function declines, he or she requires more hours of direct supervision. Nighttime wandering may keep family members from getting adequate sleep. Caring for a family member can be a mutually rewarding and satisfying family experience. Successful caregiving should not be the sole responsibility of one person. It often "takes a village" or network of people to care for the patient The contributions of family and friends can be special skills, time, money, or knowledge of additional resources. In some situations there may be no readily available resources; however, often family members hesitate to notify other family members or significant others because of unresolved conflicts in the past.

Actions/Interventions

- Suggest that the caregiver use available community resources such as respite care, home health care, adult day care, and the Alzheimer's Association.

- ▲ Consult a social worker for referral for community resources and/or financial aid, if needed.

- Encourage the caregiver to set aside time for self.

- Acknowledge to the caregiver his or her role and its value.

Rationales

Resources provide the opportunity for multiple competent providers and services on a temporary basis or for a more extended period. Using these resources may allow family members to continue job responsibilities and other family activities.

The social worker can provide the family with guidance in planning for long-term care, estate planning, powers of attorney, and living wills for the patient. QSEN: Teamwork and collaboration.

The caregiver may need reminders to attend to his or her own physical and emotional needs. Having "respite" time helps conserve physical and emotional energy. Simple activities such as a relaxing bath, time to read a book, or going out with friends help to maintain the caregiver's physical and mental well-being. QSEN: Patient-centered care.

Caregivers have identified how important it is to feel appreciated for their efforts. The patient may not be able to express this himself or herself. QSEN: Patient-centered care.

Related Care Plans

Chronic confusion, Chapter 2
Impaired memory, Chapter 2
Ineffective coping, Chapter 2

Headache: Migraine, Cluster, Tension

Headache is defined as pain in the head or face, classified as either "primary" or "secondary" in origin. Migraine, cluster, and tension headaches are classified as primary because the pain occurs without a known pathological cause. Secondary headaches are a result of a known pathologic condition, such as cranial tumor or aneurysm. Migraine headache, a recurring unilateral or bilateral headache, is the most common type of vascular headache. Multiple theories have been proposed to explain the cause of migraine headache. Evidence suggests that increased muscle tension, changes in cerebrovascular tone, and biochemical factors are involved in producing the pain of a migraine headache. Women are affected three times more often than men. Migraines may begin in early childhood and adolescence, and 65% of patients with migraine headaches have a family history of migraine headache. Migraines may occur with or without an aura. The aura is a collection of neurological symptoms that precede the onset of pain by 10 to 30 minutes. These symptoms include changes in level of consciousness, vision,

behavior, and motor or sensory function. Many patients develop a migraine headache without a precipitating event. For other patients a variety of precipitating events trigger migraine headaches, including stress, foods high in tyramine, hunger, sleep disturbances, and for women, alterations in reproductive hormone levels. Manifestations are associated with autonomic nervous system dysfunction.

Tension headaches are the most common form of headache, occurring in women more often than men. The usual age of onset is 20 to 25 years old. The pain is usually mild to moderate and described as a tightening or sensation of pressure around the head. This type of headache is thought to be the result of muscle tension in the jaw and neck with hypersensitivity of pain fibers in the trigeminal nerve. The exact mechanisms for the pain are unknown. Many patients may experience both migraine and tension headaches.

Cluster headaches are defined as pain episodes that occur for several days or weeks at a time followed by long periods

■ = Independent ▲ = Interprofessional Collaboration

of remission. The person may experience several short headaches in one day. Men are affected more often than women, with the age of occurrence between 20 and 50 years old. The pain is described as severe, with tearing, burning, and reddening of the eye on one side of the face. The mechanisms of cluster headaches are thought to be similar to those causing migraine headaches. The exact mechanisms remain unknown but may include vascular and neurogenic alterations of the hypothalamus associated with changes in serotonin transmission.

This care plan focuses on the classic migraine, which is believed to be a dysfunction of the hypothalamic and upper brainstem areas. Diagnosis, treatment, and follow-up care are usually accomplished in an outpatient setting.

NANDA-I NDx Deficient Knowledge

Common Related Factors

Insufficient information
Insufficient interest in learning
Insufficient knowledge of resources
Misinformation presented by others

Defining Characteristics

Insufficient knowledge
Inaccurate follow-through of instruction
Inappropriate behavior

Common Expected Outcomes

Patient identifies perceived learning needs about headaches and headache management.
Patient verbalizes understanding of migraine headache etiological factors and treatment.
Patient verbalizes understanding of prevention protocol for recurrent headaches and successful prevention of recurrent headaches.

NOC Outcomes
Knowledge: Disease Process; Knowledge: Medication

NIC Interventions
Health Literacy Enhancement; Learning Facilitation; Teaching: Disease Process; Teaching: Prescribed Medication

---

Ongoing Assessment

Actions/Interventions	Rationales
■ Assess the patient's current understanding of the cause of headache, prevention, and treatment.	An individualized teaching plan is based on the patient's level of understanding, current knowledge, and need for new information. The patient needs to be open to learning ways to manage the headaches. The strategies may require lifestyle changes and new behaviors for managing headache triggers. QSEN: Patient-centered care.
■ Question the patient regarding previous experience and health teaching about headaches and headache management.	Adults bring many life experiences to each learning session. Adults learn best when teaching builds on previous knowledge or experience. This experience is the foundation for an individualized teaching plan.
■ Determine the patient's self-efficacy to learn and apply new knowledge.	A first step in teaching may be to foster increased self-efficacy in the learner's ability to learn the desired information about headaches or skills for prevention and management of recurrent headaches. QSEN: Patient-centered care.

Neurological Care Plans

Therapeutic Interventions

Actions/Interventions	Rationales
■ Explain the etiological factors of migraine headache: • Changes in the neurotransmitter levels of serotonin, dopamine, and norepinephrine cause cerebral vasodilation and headache. • Serotonergic cells are hyperactive during migraine (can be seen on positron emission tomography [PET]), and serotonin levels are more easily manipulated than other neurotransmitters.	Providing knowledge may reduce the patient's anxiety and clear up common misconceptions about the cause and treatment of migraine headache. Many approaches to prevention and treatment of migraine headache are directed at modifying activity at serotonin receptors, prostaglandins, and trigeminal nerve pathways.
▲ Explain and facilitate diagnostic testing (may include a computed tomography [CT] scan, PET scan, magnetic resonance imaging [MRI] scan, and/or electroencephalogram).	These tests are done to rule out other possible causes of headache such as aneurysms or tumors. For the patient with migraine headache the results should be negative.
■ Discuss the avoidance of foods known to precipitate migraine, such as caffeinated drinks, chocolate, most alcohol (especially red wine), citrus fruits or drinks, pickled or cured foods, some cheeses, and monosodium glutamate (MSG).	Foods high in the amino acid tyramine are known to trigger migraine headache. Tyramine stimulates the release of epinephrine and norepinephrine.
■ Help the patient recognize and prevent situations that seem to cause headache, such as exhaustion, fatigue, stress, fever, or bright lights.	Prevention of migraine headache is a primary focus of treatment. Changing lifestyle and behavior is usually the most difficult aspect of the treatment plan for migraine sufferers. QSEN: Patient-centered care.
■ Ensure a thorough understanding of the prescribed medication therapy for the prophylaxis of migraine headache. Prescriptive choices include the following:	Preventive medications are shown to have increasing importance in the management of migraine headache. Accurate knowledge helps the patient make decisions for achieving the maximum benefit from drug therapy. QSEN: Evidence-based practice; Patient-centered care.
• Tricyclic antidepressants	Tricyclic antidepressants block the uptake of serotonin and catecholamines. Amitriptyline is the primary drug in this class use for prevention of migraine.
• Calcium channel blockers	Calcium channel blockers are thought to prevent migraines by altering cerebral vessel constriction.
• Beta-adrenergic blockers	Beta-blockers are a commonly used drug for migraine prophylaxis. This group of drugs inhibits serotonin uptake and prevents vasodilation.
• Ergotamine preparations	The drugs in this group are used for pain management of migraines. The drugs are antagonists of specific serotonin (5-hydroxytryptamine [5HT]) receptors. These drugs may be administered by a variety of routes including oral, rectal suppository, sublingual, and nasal spray.
• Divalproex sodium (Depakote)	This antiepilepsy drug has been approved by the Food and Drug Administration (FDA) for migraine prophylaxis. Women of childbearing age need complete information about the risks and benefits of the drug because of its adverse effects on the fetus.
■ Provide support group information: • National Headache Foundation • American Council for Headache Education	These resources provide the patient with additional information and best practices about coping with headaches.

Neurological Care Plans

■ = Independent ▲ = Interprofessional Collaboration

Neurological Care Plans

NANDA-I
NDx Acute Pain

Common Related Factor
Biological injury agent (cerebral artery vasoconstriction causing increased serotonin levels, followed by vasodilation)

Defining Characteristics
Self-report of intensity using standardized pain scale
Self-report of pain characteristics using standardized pain instrument

Common Expected Outcomes
Patient reports satisfactory pain control and a decreased intensity using a standardized pain scale.
Patient uses pharmacological and nonpharmacological pain management strategies.
Patient exhibits increased comfort such as baseline levels for HR, BP, and respirations, and relaxed muscle tone or body posture.

NOC Outcomes
Comfort Status; Pain Control; Pain Level; Medication Response
NIC Interventions
Analgesic Administration; Pain Management

Ongoing Assessment

Actions/Interventions	Rationales
■ Obtain a detailed headache history, including the following:	The patient is the most reliable source of information about his or her pain. Detailed information is necessary to differentiate from other serious neurological problems and to determine the etiological factors and type of headache before a specific treatment protocol can be designed. QSEN: Patient-centered care.
• Family history	Many patients will report a history of other family members experiencing migraine headache.
• Age of onset, frequency, and duration	Many patients experience their first migraine headache in early adolescence. Migraine headache pain may reach peak intensity an hour after onset. The pain may continue for several hours or even days.
• Typical location	About 60% of patients with migraine will report pain that begins on one side of the head and spreads to include both sides.
• Type of pain	Patients may describe the pain as deep, steady, throbbing, or stabbing.
• Precipitating factors	Identifying headache triggers is important in developing a plan for prevention. These triggers may include foods, stress, weather changes, fatigue, or hormonal changes during the menstrual cycle.
• Aggravating factors	Bright lights and noise may intensify headache pain. Some patients will report an increase in the throbbing characteristic of the pain with activity.
• Associated symptoms (aura)	Associated symptoms may occur before, during, or after the headache. The symptoms may include nausea, vomiting, numbness, visual disturbances, sensitivity to light (photophobia), vertigo, scalp tenderness, neck muscle contraction, and sensitivity to odors. Approximately 10% of patients with migraine will experience an aura.

Actions/Interventions

- Relief measures

- Effect on activities of daily living

■ Assess the patient's willingness or ability to explore a range of techniques aimed at controlling pain.

■ Assess for depression and suicide risk.

Rationales

Patients may have tried a variety of treatments to cope with headache pain. Those measures that have been successful should be included in the individualized care plan.

For some patients, migraine headaches are incapacitating. The patient may report a feeling of exhaustion with headache. Headache episodes can disrupt the patient's ability to work and participate in family or social activities.

Some patients may be unaware of the effectiveness of nonpharmacological methods and may be willing to try them, either with or instead of traditional analgesic medications. Often a combination of therapies (e.g., mild analgesics with distraction or heat) may be more effective. Some patients will feel uncomfortable exploring alternative methods of pain relief. However, patients need to be informed that there are multiple ways to manage pain. QSEN: Patient-centered care.

Many patients experience anxiety and depression with recurrent and disabling headaches. The treatment plan needs to include a holistic approach to support effective coping strategies.

Therapeutic Interventions

Actions/Interventions

■ Encourage the patient to lie down in a quiet, dark room.

■ Provide a gentle head massage if tolerated.

■ Apply cold packs.

■ Support the head and neck with pillows.

▲ Administer attack-aborting medications, as prescribed.

▲ Administer analgesics for mild to moderate pain.

Rationales

Darkness diminishes photophobia, and quiet decreases neural stimulation. If implemented at the onset of pain, these measures may reduce the intensity and duration of the headache.

Massage may promote the relaxation of scalp muscles and reduce pain intensity.

The application of cold therapy to the forehead, temples, or back of the neck may decrease headache intensity.

Position changes reduce muscle tension, which aggravates pain.

These medications are taken at the earliest onset of a migraine headache to reduce the severity and duration of the headache. Selective serotonin receptor agonists (e.g., sumatriptan) and nonselective serotonin agonists (ergot alkaloids) act by constricting cerebral arteries. Opioid analgesics may be used in patients with hypertension when the use of a vasoconstricting drug might be contraindicated. A variety of routes of administration are available to facilitate patient management of this approach to headache relief. The routes include oral, intranasal spray, and subcutaneous injection. QSEN: Evidence-based practice.

Acetaminophen and nonsteroidal anti-inflammatory drugs (e.g., aspirin, ibuprofen, naproxen) may be useful to relieve mild to moderate migraine pain. These drugs act on peripheral pain receptors and relieve inflammation. Many over-the-counter drugs marketed specifically for migraine headache contain these active ingredients. Opioid analgesics may be prescribed for relief of more severe headache pain. QSEN: Evidence-based practice.

Neurological Care Plans

■ = Independent ▲ = Interprofessional Collaboration

Actions/Interventions

- Provide information on additional pain- or stress-relieving measures, including relaxation techniques, physical therapy, exercise, and biofeedback.

Rationales

Patients can decrease the frequency of migraine headaches by avoiding precipitating events that trigger pain episodes. Regular sleep patterns, exercise, and stress management activities can reduce headache frequency.

Related Care Plan

Ineffective coping, Chapter 2

Intervertebral Disk Disease

Low Back Pain, Herniated Disk; Slipped Disk; Ruptured Disk; Sciatica; Laminectomy

Deterioration and herniation of lumbar intervertebral disks are common causes of low back pain in the adult. Age of onset is typically between 30 and 50 years of age, with men affected more often than women. Etiological factors include trauma, degenerative diseases (e.g., osteoarthritis and ankylosing spondylitis), and congenital defects (e.g., scoliosis). Weak back and abdominal muscles combined with strenuous activity and heavy lifting form a common scenario for disk herniation in the lumbar spine. In many cases the disk is spontaneously reduced or reabsorbed without treatment, but more often the problem becomes chronic with pain and disability depending on the location

and severity of the herniation. The amount of disk (nucleus pulposus) herniated into the spinal canal affects the narrowing of the space and the degree of compression on the lumbar or sacral spinal roots. A variety of surgical procedures may be done to reduce nerve compression and relieve lower back pain. Conservative management (rest, heat or ice, and nonsteroidal anti-inflammatory drugs [NSAIDs]) is usually accomplished in the ambulatory setting and is the focus of this care plan. Duration of treatment depends on location of herniation and symptoms. Hospitalization is necessary only if pain and sensorimotor deficits are incapacitating.

NANDA-I NDx **Acute Pain**

Common Related Factor

Physical injury agent (trauma, muscle spasm, nerve root compression)

Defining Characteristics

Self-report of intensity using standardized pain scale
Self-report of pain characteristics using standardized pain instrument
Protective behavior
Positioning to ease pain
Guarding behavior

Common Expected Outcomes

Patient reports satisfactory pain control and a decreased intensity using a standardized pain scale.
Patient uses pharmacological and nonpharmacological pain management strategies.
Patient exhibits increased comfort such as baseline levels for pulse, BP, and respirations, and relaxed muscle tone or body posture.

NOC Outcomes

Comfort Status; Pain Level; Pain Control; Medication Response

NIC Interventions

Pain Management; Positioning; Medication Management

Ongoing Assessment

Actions/Interventions

- Obtain a detailed pain history, including the following:
  - Location and onset of pain
  - Presence of radiating pain
  - Recurrent (duration and frequency) or continuous pain
  - Precipitating factors
  - Relief factors (preference for standing or lying down)
  - Aggravating factors (sitting, jarring movements)

- Assess for changes in sensorimotor function, including:
  - Absent lumbar lordosis
  - Lumbar scoliosis
  - Limited movement or flexion
  - Slight motor weakness
  - Decreased knee and ankle reflexes
  - Paresthesia or numbness
  - Changes in bowel or bladder function
- ▲ Facilitate diagnostic testing, if needed: spinal x-ray films, computed tomography (CT), magnetic resonance imaging (MRI), lumbar puncture for cerebrospinal fluid (protein will be high with normal cell count), myelogram, and/or nerve conduction studies.
- Evaluate the effectiveness of previous treatments.

- Assess the patient's willingness or ability to explore a range of techniques aimed at controlling pain.

Rationales

Assessment of the pain experience is the first step in planning pain management strategies. The patient is the most reliable source of information about his or her pain. Remission and exacerbation of pain in the patient with a lumbar herniation often occur because of decreased edema and root compression, as well as spontaneous reduction of the disk into its normal position and reabsorption of disk exudate. Lumbar disk disease may cause pain that radiates along the path of the sciatic nerve into the leg and groin area. Muscle weakness may occur with the pain. QSEN: Patient-centered care.

A decrease in motor function is often a guarding behavior, a protective action or inaction to control pain. The cervical and lumbar spines are affected most often because they are the most flexible segments of the spine. A herniated disk can press against adjacent nerves, causing pain and paresthesias. The specific level of injury will determine the symptoms experienced by the patient. Alterations in gait and posture may represent nerve injury or adaptation to chronic pain.

Serial testing may be done to determine the progression of the herniation.

Patients may have tried multiple home remedies for relief of low back pain before seeking professional care. Measures that have been successful should be included in the plan of care.

Some patients may be unaware of the effectiveness of nonpharmacological methods and may be willing to try them, either with or instead of traditional analgesic medications. Often a combination of therapies (e.g., mild analgesics with distraction or heat) may be more effective. Some patients will feel uncomfortable exploring alternative methods of pain relief. However, patients need to be informed that there are multiple ways to manage pain. QSEN: Patient-centered care.

Therapeutic Interventions

Actions/Interventions

- Teach the patient to do the following:
  - Begin bed rest on a firm mattress.
  - Use a pillow under the knees (lumbar).

Rationales

Rest reduces pressure on nerve roots, relieves muscle spasms, and promotes comfort during the healing process. A firm mattress provides back support. A board can be placed underneath a soft mattress for support. Most patients find positioning in a semi-Fowler's position with the knees flexed reduces pressure on nerve roots and promotes muscle relaxation. A supine position may aggravate pain. The use of appropriate sleep aids for body positioning will promote comfort and decrease stress on nerve roots.

Neurological Care Plans

■ = Independent   ▲ = Interprofessional Collaboration

Actions/Interventions

▲ Initiate drug therapy, possibly including analgesics, muscle relaxants, anti-inflammatory drugs, and/or sedatives as ordered.

▲ Refer the patient for a physical therapy consult.

■ Instruct the patient in the use of back braces, corsets, or traction therapy (pelvic belt).

■ Assist the patient in using nonpharmacological pain management modalities, such as heat and cold applications, relaxation therapy, imagery, and anxiety reduction.

Rationales

These drugs reduce inflammation and muscle spasm. Medications and dosage depend on the patient's symptoms and the amount of relief.

The physical therapist can provide a variety of treatments for muscle relaxation and pain relief, including ultrasound and thermal treatments. The physical therapist can help the patient learn exercises to strengthen back muscles and prevent further injury. QSEN: Teamwork and collaboration.

These devices limit spinal movement and relieve pressure on nerve roots. Traction does not seem to have a direct effect on disk placement but does provide relief from muscle spasms and decreases pressure on nerve roots, thereby providing pain relief.

Nonpharmacological pain interventions will contribute to effective pain management. These strategies may reduce the development of problems associated with the overuse of opioid analgesics. Cold packs or heat may be effective when used early in the acute pain episode by reducing inflammation and relieving muscle spasms.

NANDA-I NDx **Deficient Knowledge**

Common Related Factors

Insufficient information
Insufficient interest in learning
Insufficient knowledge of resources
Misinformation presented by others

Defining Characteristics

Insufficient knowledge
Inaccurate follow-through of instruction
Inappropriate behavior

Common Expected Outcome

Patient verbalizes understanding of treatment program and demonstrates skills necessary for protecting vertebrae.

NOC Outcomes

Knowledge: Disease Process; Knowledge: Treatment Regimen

NIC Interventions

Health Literacy Enhancement; Learning Facilitation; Teaching: Disease Process; Teaching: Prescribed Exercise

---

Ongoing Assessment

Actions/Interventions

■ Assess the patient's understanding of the diagnosis and treatment plan.

■ Assess the motivation and willingness of the patient and caregivers to learn.

Rationales

Patients often have misunderstandings about the cause of back pain and measures for effective management. The effectiveness of the treatment plans requires the patient's cooperation and willingness to make necessary changes in lifestyle behaviors. QSEN: Patient-centered care.

Some patients are ready to learn soon after they are diagnosed; others cope better by denying or delaying the need for instruction. Learning also requires energy, which patients may not be ready to use.

Neurological Care Plans

Actions/Interventions

■ Identify the priority of learning needs within the overall care plan.

Rationales

This information provides the starting base for educational sessions. Teaching standardized content that the patient already knows wastes valuable time and hinders critical learning. Adults learn material that is important to them. QSEN: Patient-centered care.

Therapeutic Interventions

Actions/Interventions

■ Reinforce the information provided by other members of the interprofessional health team about treatment options.

■ Teach the patient about the components of a conservative treatment plan:
- Exercise program: muscle strengthening exercise is prescribed

- Proper body mechanics: for safe lifting and the avoidance of repetitive motion and body movements

- Medications: analgesics, NSAIDs, muscle relaxants

- Application and use of support garments and traction equipment
- Weight control

- Remission and exacerbation

■ Reinforce information about the surgical intervention:
- Type of surgery:
  - Minimally invasive techniques—intradiscal electrothermoplasty; radiofrequency discal nucleoplasty; interspinous process decompression
  - Disk replacement with artificial disk
  - Diskectomy—partial removal of the lamina
  - Laminectomy—excision of the posterior arch of the vertebra (lamina)
  - Spinal fusion—fusion of the vertebrae with bone grafts, rods, plates, or screws
- Pain: immediately postoperative (spasms, incisional)

Rationales

The patient needs information about treatment options to guide decision-making. The long-term effectiveness of nonsurgical and surgical approaches to treatment is similar for patients with mild to moderate disease. Surgical therapy is associated with better outcomes for patients with moderate to severe disease. QSEN: Patient-centered care.

This nursing action reduces the risk of injury with activity. QSEN: Safety.

Exercise helps support the spinal column. These exercises focus on strengthening abdominal and paravertebral muscles. The patient may need to continue specific back exercises for a lifetime.

Improper body mechanics can aggravate weakened disks. Extremes of spinal flexion and rotation are discouraged. The patient may need to learn ways to modify the home and work environment to protect the back during activities.

The appropriate use of medications for pain relief will help the patient maintain desired activity levels.

The use of supportive back braces and corsets minimizes injury and relieves nerve root compression.

Obesity and increased abdominal adipose tissue adds to the strain on the lumbar spine and paravertebral muscles. Weight reduction, as part of the treatment plan, decreases the risk of exacerbations.

Patients experience periods of improvement and exacerbation of symptoms because of changes in the amount of inflammation at the level of herniation until the area is healed.

Surgery may be required for patients who suffer severe herniation resulting in cord compression, loss of function, and unrelenting pain. A variety of minimally invasive procedures may be done to relieve pain, decompress the disk, and reduce spinal stenosis. More traditional surgical procedures such as laminectomy may be done after poor response to conservative treatment or minimally invasive techniques. QSEN: Evidence-based practice.

Patients need to understand that incisional pain is part of the normal postoperative experience. This pain is managed with analgesics. Patients who have experienced long-term radiating pain and paresthesias may continue to have these symptoms for several postoperative weeks. This pain will diminish over time. QSEN: Patient-centered care.

Neurological Care Plans

■ = Independent ▲ = Interprofessional Collaboration

Actions/Interventions	Rationales
• Postoperative expectations: initial immobility, relearning how to move	Physical therapy will be required in the home and as an outpatient to strengthen muscles, to learn to move, and to protect the spine. QSEN: Teamwork and collaboration.
• Recurrent herniation: may occur near the site of the original herniation or at another location	Degenerative or other changes may predispose the patient to repeat herniation and repeat laminectomy, despite following the prescribed treatment plan.

Related Care Plans

Chronic pain, Chapter 2
Impaired physical mobility, Chapter 2
Ineffective coping, Chapter 2

Multiple Sclerosis

Disseminated Sclerosis; Demyelinating Disease

Multiple sclerosis (MS) is a chronic progressive and degenerative nervous system disease characterized by scattered patches of demyelination and glial tissue overgrowth in the white matter of the brain and spinal cord. These structural changes in nerve tissue lead to decreased nerve conduction. As the inflammation or edema diminishes, some remyelination may occur and nerve conduction returns. Over time the growth of glial tissue in the areas of repeated inflammation and demyelination leads to scarring (plaque) of the white matter and loss of nerve conduction. Among the clinical symptoms associated with MS are extremity weakness, visual disturbances, ataxia, tremor, incoordination, sphincter impairment, and impaired position sense. The clinical manifestations occur randomly with no predictable pattern of progression. Remissions and exacerbations are associated with the disease. Although the specific cause is unknown, etiological hypotheses include environmental, viral, and genetic factors. Infection with the Epstein-Barr virus in genetically susceptible individuals is thought to trigger an immune response that begins the inflammatory process causing demyelination. Loss of myelin disrupts nerve conduction. MS lesions are found in the cerebral white matter, optic nerves, brainstem, cerebellum, and cervical spinal cord. MS is considered the disease of young adults. The McDonald Criteria, from the International Panel on Diagnosis of MS, allow for earlier diagnosis of MS based on MRI results and clinical presentation. The criteria have application in the diagnosis of MS across cultures. The onset of MS is typically between 15 and 50 years of age. Women are affected more often than men. This care plan focuses on maintenance care in the ambulatory care setting.

NANDA-I
NDx Deficient Knowledge

Common Related Factors

Alteration in cognitive functioning
Insufficient information
Insufficient interest in learning
Insufficient knowledge of resources
Alteration in memory
Misinformation presented by others

Defining Characteristics

Insufficient knowledge
Inaccurate follow-through of instruction
Inaccurate performance on a test
Inappropriate behavior

 evolve For additional care plans, go to http://evolve.elsevier.com/Gulanick/.

Neurological Care Plans

Common Expected Outcome

Patient or significant others verbalize understanding of disease process of MS, medications used, adverse effects, and follow-up care.

NOC Outcomes
Knowledge: Disease Process; Knowledge: Treatment Regimen

NIC Interventions
Health Literacy Enhancement; Learning Facilitation; Teaching: Disease Process; Teaching: Procedure/Treatment; Teaching: Prescribed Medication

Ongoing Assessment

Actions/Interventions	Rationales
■ Assess the patient's knowledge of the disease, exacerbations, remissions, medical regimen, and resources.	Lack of knowledge about MS and its progressive nature can compromise the patient's ability to care for self and cope effectively. QSEN: Patient-centered care.
■ Assess the motivation and willingness of the patient and caregivers to learn.	Adults must see a need or purpose for learning. Some patients are ready to learn soon after they are diagnosed; others cope better by denying or delaying the need for instruction. Learning also requires energy, which patients may not be ready to use.
■ Assess the ability to learn, remember, or perform desired health-related care.	Cognitive impairments need to be identified so an appropriate teaching plan can be designed. For example, the Mini-Mental State Examination (MMSE) can be used to identify memory problems that would interfere with learning. Physical limitations (e.g., impaired vision, poor hand coordination) can likewise compromise learning and must be considered when designing the educational approach. QSEN: Patient-centered care.

Therapeutic Interventions

Actions/Interventions	Rationales
■ Discuss the disease process in a simple, straightforward manner, as follows: • MS is a chronic, slowly progressive nervous system disease that affects nerve conduction.	Accurate information about MS reduces anxiety and allows the patient to comprehend the disease process. The patient and family members need to understand the disease process to make informed decisions concerning financial resources, long-term care, power of attorney, and living wills. QSEN: Patient-centered care.
• Diagnostic tests are used in conjunction with a careful history and physical examination, such as magnetic resonance imaging (MRI), visual-evoked potentials (VEP), and cerebrospinal fluid (CSF) analysis.	The diagnosis of MS is based on criteria from the Revised International Panel on MS Diagnosis (Revised McDonald Criteria). The patient needs to provide a detailed history to assist in an accurate diagnosis of MS. Patients may experience symptoms for many months before a diagnosis is made. MRI is used to detect the presence of MS plaques. VEP tests are useful in confirming a diagnosis of MS. The demyelination that occurs with MS results in a slowing of response time. An analysis of CSF is done to detect increased immune cells indicative of MS. QSEN: Evidence-based practice.

■ = Independent ▲ = Interprofessional Collaboration

Actions/Interventions	Rationales
• There is no specific cure.	Drug therapy is initiated to reduce disease activity and disease progression. Others aspects of the treatment plan such as nutrition and exercise are designed to help the patient maintain functional independence as long as possible.
• MS can result in weakness, visual disturbances, walking unsteadiness, and sometimes urine or bowel problems.	The patient and family need to plan strategies for the management of exacerbations of MS. The patient and family should be able to identify signs of the exacerbation of MS and implement strategies for its management.
■ Instruct the patient or significant others when to contact the health care team (e.g., urinary symptoms; motor, sensory, visual disturbances; exacerbations).	Prompt treatment of exacerbations can be initiated when the patient and family know what to report.
■ Instruct the patient and family about drugs that modify or suppress the immune system.	These drugs include beta-interferon (Betaseron), glatiramer acetate, and mitoxantrone. The drugs work by modifying or suppressing immune system activity. The risk for infection increases with the use of these immunosuppressant drugs. Many of the drugs are administered as subcutaneous injections by the patient. The cost of treatment is expensive and may be covered by the patient's health insurance or assistance programs through pharmaceutical companies. QSEN: Evidence-based practice; Safety.
■ Instruct the patient or significant others about steroid therapy: • Side effects (e.g., sodium retention, fluid retention, pedal edema, hypertension, gastric irritation)	Steroid therapy decreases edema and the acute inflammatory response within evolving plaques. Prednisone and adrenocorticotropic hormone are used most often for acute exacerbations.
• Measures to control side effects (e.g., low-sodium diet, daily weighing, leg elevation, support hose, BP monitoring, antacids, adequate rest, and avoiding contact with people with infectious disease)	These measures reduce fluid retention and the risk for infection and gastric ulcers. QSEN: Safety.
■ Teach about the drugs used to manage muscle spasticity.	Muscle spasticity can be managed with muscle relaxants. The FDA approved Botox for the management of muscle spasticity. Drugs may be used for short-term or long-term therapy. QSEN: Evidence-based practice.
■ Instruct in the following: • Importance of maintaining the most normal activity level possible	When the patient can have a normal activity pattern, it helps maintain functional ability and improve body image.
• Avoiding hot baths	Heat increases metabolic demands and may increase weakness.
• Sleeping in a prone position	Good positioning during sleep decreases flexion spasms.
• Need to inspect areas of impaired sensation for serious injuries	Careful attention to these areas decreases the risk for injury. Patients may have decreased temperature sensation that increases the risk for burns. A patient with decreased pressure sensation is at risk for skin breakdown.
• Need to use energy conservation techniques	The fatigue in MS is from nerve demyelination, not muscle fatigue. A balance of daily rest and exercise is indicated. Drugs such as amantadine or pemoline are helpful in treating fatigue.
■ Instruct the patient to avoid potentially exacerbating activities: emotional stress, physical stress or fatigue, infection, pregnancy, physically "run down" condition.	Young female patients may choose to become pregnant. Symptoms of MS often diminish during pregnancy, but exacerbation is common and sometimes severe during the postpartum period. Stress is the most common cause of exacerbations.

Actions/Interventions

- Refer the patient and family to the Multiple Sclerosis Society, support groups, and/or counseling, as desired.

Rationales

The MS Society may provide the patient and family with information about best practices for managing the disease. Support groups can assist with issues such as family relationships, work, parenting, and sexuality. Professional counselors, as members of the interprofessional health team, have the specialized knowledge and skills to provide appropriate therapy. Developmentally, this age group is typically in its most productive years, therefore MS has the potential for causing major life cycle alterations. Depression and cognitive impairment are common problems for the patient with MS. QSEN: Teamwork and collaboration.

NANDA-I NDx

Impaired Physical Mobility

Common Related Factors

Physical deconditioning
Alteration in cognitive function
Neuromuscular impairment
Insufficient muscle strength
Insufficient knowledge of mobility strategies

Defining Characteristics

Impaired ability to reposition self in bed
Impaired ability to turn from side to side
Impaired ability to move between sitting and supine positions
Impaired ability to move between long sitting and supine positions
Impaired ability to move between prone and supine positions

Common Expected Outcomes

Patient performs physical activity independently or within limits of disease.
Patient demonstrates use of adaptive techniques that promote ambulation and transferring.
Patient is free of complications of immobility, as evidenced by intact skin, absence of thrombophlebitis, normal bowel pattern, and clear breath sounds.

NOC Outcomes

Ambulation; Mobility; Transfer Performance

NIC Interventions

Environmental Management; Teaching: Prescribed Exercise; Exercise Therapy: Muscle Control

Neurological Care Plans

Ongoing Assessment

Actions/Interventions

- Assess the patient's gait, muscle strength, weakness, coordination, and balance.
- Assess the patient's endurance level and stamina (e.g., number of stairs the patient can climb, distance the patient can walk, ability to work, ability to perform activities of daily living [ADLs] independently).

Rationales

Changes in these findings are a gauge to assess the progression and remission of MS.

Motor dysfunction contributes to weakness with MS. Cerebellar dysfunction causes tremors, poor coordination, and ataxia. These symptoms can interfere with ADLs and mobility. Restricted movement affects the ability to perform most ADLs. A variety of assessment tools are available, depending on the clinical setting. Such tools provide objective data for baselines. For example, the Functional Independence Measure (FIM) scale assesses 18 self-care items related to eating, bathing, grooming, dressing, toileting, bladder and bowel management, transfer, ambulation, and stair climbing. Fatigue and reduced functional ability may be more pronounced in the evening. QSEN: Evidence-based practice.

■ = Independent   ▲ = Interprofessional Collaboration

Actions/Interventions

- Determine the patient's ability to use assistive devices (cane, walker) and adaptive techniques (using larger muscle groups).

Rationales

The proper use of assistive devices can promote mobility and reduce the risk for falls. QSEN: Safety.

Therapeutic Interventions

Actions/Interventions

- Encourage self-care as tolerated and seeking assistance when necessary; arrange for home care when needed.

- Suggest placing frequently needed items (cooking material, personal care items, cleaning supplies) within easy reach.

- Encourage stretching exercises and ROM daily. Suggest scheduled rest periods.

- Instruct the patient in the use of adaptive techniques and equipment. These may include wrist weights, adaptive equipment such as stabilized plates and nonspilling cups, stabilization of the extremity, and training the patient to use the trunk and head.

- ▲ Consult members of the interprofessional health team about the use of assistive or ambulatory devices and ADLs evaluation.

Rationales

The patient and family need to have a plan for providing care when exacerbations become more frequent and longer in duration as the disease progresses. QSEN: Patient-centered care.

Home modifications can help the patient maintain a desired level of functional independence with mobility and reduce fatigue with activity. QSEN: Patient-centered care.

These activities promote venous return, prevent flexion contractures, and maintain muscle strength and endurance. Exercises and early ambulation require much energy. Rest periods help reduce the level of fatigue.

Aids can compensate for impaired function and increase the level of activity. The goal for using adaptive devices is to promote safety, increase mobility, prevent falls, and conserve energy. QSEN: Safety.

A physical therapist and an occupational therapist can provide guidance for the patient and caregivers about appropriate assistive devices to promote mobility. These professionals can evaluate the home environment for modifications as needed to support patient mobility. QSEN: Teamwork and collaboration.

NDx Risk for Impaired Vision

Common Risk Factor

Optic nerve demyelination

Common Expected Outcome

Patient achieves optimal functioning within limits of visual impairment, as evidenced by ability to care for self, to navigate environment safely, and to engage in meaningful activities.

NOC Outcomes

Risk Control: Visual Impairment; Vision Compensation Behavior

NIC Intervention

Communication Enhancement: Visual Deficit

Ongoing Assessment

Actions/Interventions

- Assess for visual impairment.

Rationales

Common symptoms in MS include diplopia, blurred vision, nystagmus, visual loss, scotomas (blind spots), and impaired color perception.

---

evolve **For additional care plans, go to http://evolve.elsevier.com/Gulanick/.**

Neurological Care Plans

Actions/Interventions

- Ask the patient about specifics such as the ability to read or see television, a history of falls, or the ability to self-medicate.
- Assess for factors or aids that improve vision, such as glasses, contact lenses, or bright and/or natural light.

- Evaluate the patient's ability to function within the limits of visual impairment.

- Evaluate the psychological response to visual loss.

Rationales

Visual impairment can contribute to problems in daily activities. The risk for falls and medication errors increases if the patient has diminished visual acuity. QSEN: Safety.

Nursing interventions should include strategies that enhance the patient's adaptive abilities. QSEN: Patient-centered care.

Personal appearance and the condition of clothing and surroundings are good indicators of the patient's adaptation to visual loss.

Anger, depression, and withdrawal are common responses to vision changes. Self-esteem is often negatively affected.

Therapeutic Interventions

Actions/Interventions

- Encourage the patient to ask for orientation to new environments, such as the location of bathrooms, stairs, and other features in unfamiliar homes, restaurants, and businesses.
- Encourage the patient and family to place objects within reach. Do not change familiar home environments without informing the patient.
- Provide an eye patch for diplopia; encourage alternating the patch from eye to eye.

- Instruct the patient to rest the eyes when fatigued.
- Advise the patient of the availability of large-type reading materials and talking books.
- Teach the patient to turn the head from side to side when entering an unfamiliar environment.

Rationales

The patient may be embarrassed or hesitant to ask for assistance.

The consistent placement of belongings enhances independence. QSEN: Patient-centered care.

Alternating the patch from one eye to another alleviates diplopia. Using adaptive techniques can help the patient cope with visual changes. Corrective lenses may be beneficial for changes in visual acuity.

Fatigue can aggravate visual problems.

These resources allow the patient to retain desired activities for work and leisure.

Visual scanning will help the patient who has decreased peripheral vision. QSEN: Safety.

NDx Risk for Urinary Retention/Incontinence

Common Risk Factor

Neurogenic bladder

Common Expected Outcomes

The patient maintains residual urine of less than 100 mL.
The patient does not experience urinary tract infection (UTI).
The patient remains dry between voluntary voiding.

NOC Outcomes
Urinary Continence; Urinary Elimination
NIC Interventions
Urinary Retention Care; Urinary Incontinence Care

Ongoing Assessment

Actions/Interventions

- Inquire about the symptoms of urinary retention, frequency, urgency, pain, and abdominal distention.

Rationales

Patients may experience either a spastic bladder, characterized by frequency and dribbling, or a flaccid bladder, in which an absence of the sensation to void results in urine retention.

■ = Independent   ▲ = Interprofessional Collaboration

Neurological Care Plans

Actions/Interventions

- Assess for the signs of UTI.

- Assess the pattern of fluid intake.

Rationales

This assessment approach reduces harm by identifying early signs of UTI and guiding specific interventions. Retention predisposes to infection. Infection can trigger an exacerbation of MS. QSEN: Safety.

Fluid intake is related to bladder filling and voiding. Patients may reduce fluid intake to control incontinence. Decreased intake increases the risk for UTI.

Therapeutic Interventions

Actions/Interventions

- Initiate an individualized bladder training program. Instruct the patient about the Credé method and intermittent catheterization for residual urine if signs of retention are present.

- Encourage the patient to drink 2 to 3 L of fluid daily.

- Instruct the patient about the signs and symptoms of UTI.

- Explain the prescribed medications.

- Recommend vitamin C and a liberal intake of cranberry juice.

Rationales

These methods of managing urinary retention allow the patient to maintain independence with urinary elimination. Residual urine greater than 100 mL predisposes the patient to UTIs. Bladder Credé methods stimulate complete emptying of the bladder. QSEN: Patient-centered care.

Increased fluid intake increases urine output and reduces the risk for infection. QSEN: Safety.

Patients need to be able to recognize the symptoms of UTI so that treatment can be started as soon as possible. QSEN: Patient-centered care.

Cholinergic drugs are indicated for flaccid bladder, and anticholinergic drugs are indicated for spastic bladder.

These nutrients acidify urine and reduce bacterial growth.

NANDA-I NDx **Risk for Falls**

Common Risk Factors

Use of assistive devices (e.g., walker, cane, wheelchair)
Visual impairments
Urinary or bowel incontinence
Alteration in cognitive functioning
Difficulty with gait
Impaired balance
Neuropathy
Decreased lower extremity strength

Common Expected Outcomes

Patient will not sustain a fall.
Patient and caregiver will implement strategies to increase safety and prevent falls in the home.

NOC Outcomes

Fall Prevention Behavior; Knowledge: Fall Prevention; Risk Control; Risk Detection

NIC Interventions

Fall Prevention; Environmental Management: Safety; Teaching: Prescribed Exercise; Medication Management

Neurological Care Plans

Ongoing Assessment

Action/Intervention	Rationales
■ Assess for factors known to increase the level of fall risk for a patient with MS on admission to a care facility, after any change in the patient's physical or cognitive status, whenever a fall occurs, periodically during a hospital stay, or at defined times in home or long-term care settings:	The level of risk and subsequent fall precautions can be determined using standard risk assessment tools that incorporate these intrinsic and extrinsic factors. Examples of commonly used tools include Morse Fall Scale, and the Hendrich II Fall Risk Model. QSEN: Evidence-based practice; Safety.
• History of falls	Evidence indicates that falls are a common problem for the patient with MS. A person who has sustained one or more falls in the past 6 months is more likely to fall again.
• Mental status changes	The patient with MS may experience cognitive changes such as memory loss and impaired judgment. These changes increase the patient's risk for falls.
• Visual deficits	Impaired vision associated with MS limits the patient's ability to recognize hazards in the environment.
• Use of mobility assistive devices	Evidence suggests that the patient with MS who uses a mobility aid has an increased risk for falls. Factors that require the use of mobility aids (e.g., muscle weakness and impaired balance) may be more significant fall risks than the mobility devices. Improper use and maintenance of mobility aids such as canes, walkers, and wheelchairs increase the patient's risk for falls.
• Disease-related symptoms	Increased incidence of falls has been demonstrated in people with MS symptoms such as urinary incontinence, muscle spasticity, muscle weakness, fatigue, and confusion.

Therapeutic Interventions

Actions/Interventions	Rationales
■ Encourage the patient to wear shoes or slippers with nonskid soles when ambulating.	Nonskid footwear provides sure footing for the patient with diminished foot and toe lift when walking.
■ Provide the patient with a chair that has a firm seat and arms on both sides. Consider locked wheels as appropriate.	This chair style is easier to get out of, especially when the patient experiences weakness and impaired balance when transferring from bed to chair.
■ Teach the patient and all caregivers about the use of mobility and transfer aids.	The use of gait belts by all health care providers can promote safety when assisting patients with transfers from bed to chair. Canes, walkers, and wheelchairs can provide the patient with improved stability and balance when ambulating. Raised toilet seats can facilitate safe transfer on and off the toilet. QSEN: Safety.
■ Instruct the patient to notice foot placement when ambulating.	This technique compensates for a decreased position sense and balance that may contribute to the patient's fall risk.
▲ Collaborate with physical therapy and occupational therapy.	These professional members of the health care team can assist with teaching the patient about gait techniques and provide the patient with assistive devices for transfer and ambulation. They can evaluate the patient's home for modifications as needed to promote safety. QSEN: Teamwork and collaboration.

Related Care Plans

Grieving, Chapter 2
Disturbed body image, Chapter 2
Ineffective sexuality pattern, Chapter 2
Self-care deficit, Chapter 2
Powerlessness, Chapter 2

Neurological Care Plans

■ = Independent   ▲ = Interprofessional Collaboration

Parkinson's Disease
Parkinsonism

Parkinson's disease (PD) is a movement disorder associated with dopamine deficiency in the brain. As a result, the patient develops a neurotransmitter imbalance between dopamine and acetylcholine. This imbalance affects the extrapyramidal system of the brain responsible for control and regulation of movement. There is no specific diagnostic test. A diagnosis of PD is based on thorough evaluation of presenting clinical manifestations. The four characteristic signs are tremor at rest, rigidity, postural instability, and slowness of movement. Other clinical manifestations include shuffling gait, masklike facial expressions, and muscle weakness affecting writing, speaking, eating, chewing, and swallowing. Onset is usually around 60 years of age; however, a significant number of young adults have PD. Etiological hypotheses include exposure to environmental toxins and age-related degeneration of brain neurons. Some theories suggest gene mutation may play a role in the development of PD. Free radical formation has also been considered as a contributing factor. Secondary parkinsonism is associated with traumatic brain injury and side effects of the phenothiazine drug group. There is no cure for PD. Treatment is focused on slowing disease progression and symptom management. Drug therapy is the primary treatment for PD. As the disease progresses and tremors become more severe, surgical therapy may be used. Patient care is usually managed in the outpatient setting.

NANDA-I NDx Impaired Physical Mobility

Common Related Factors
Neuromuscular impairment
Insufficient muscle strength
Insufficient knowledge of mobility strategies

Common Expected Outcomes
Patient performs physical activity independently or within limits of muscle rigidity and tremors.
Patient demonstrates use of adaptive techniques that promote ambulation and transferring.
Patient is free of complications of immobility, as evidenced by intact skin, absence of thrombophlebitis, normal bowel pattern, and clear breath sounds.

Defining Characteristics
Impaired ability to move between sitting and supine positions
Impaired ability to move between long sitting and supine positions

NOC Outcomes
Ambulation; Mobility
NIC Interventions
Exercise Therapy; Teaching: Prescribed Exercise; Environmental Management

---

Ongoing Assessment

Actions/Interventions

- Assess the patient's ability to perform activities of daily living (ADLs) effectively and safely on a daily basis using an appropriate assessment tool, such as the Functional Independence Measures (FIM).

Rationales

Restricted movement affects the ability to perform most ADLs. A variety of assessment tools are available, depending on the clinical setting. Such tools provide objective data for baselines. For example, the FIM measures 18 self-care items related to eating, bathing, grooming, dressing, toileting, bladder and bowel management, transfer, ambulation, and stair climbing. QSEN: Patient-centered care; Evidence-based practice.

evolve   For additional care plans, go to http://evolve.elsevier.com/Gulanick/.

Actions/Interventions

- Assess for rigidity:

  - Cogwheel

  - Plastic
  - Lead pipe
- Assess the extent of tremors.

- Assess the patient's posture, coordination, and ambulation.

- Assess for bradykinesia.

- Evaluate the need for ambulatory aids (e.g., single point cane, quad cane, walker)

- Evaluate the safety of the immediate environment.

- Evaluate the need for home assistance (e.g., physical therapy, home care nurse).

Rationales

Rigidity is a common sign of PD. It may be unilateral or bilateral. Rigidity impairs muscle movement and mobility.

Cogwheel rigidity is an interrupted but rhythmic muscle movement.

Plastic rigidity represents more resistance to movement.

This type of rigidity is a complete resistance to movement.

Tremors are a common sign of PD. Typically tremors are more prominent at rest and are aggravated by emotional stress. Hand tremors may present as a "pill-rolling" movement at rest. Tremors occur as a result of unopposed acetylcholine activity from the dopamine deficiency.

Clinical manifestations may range from only a slight limp to the typical shuffling, propulsive gait with rigidity. These changes are more common in advanced PD.

The patient with PD will have difficulty initiating movement or changing the direction of movement. This results from poor coordination of opposing muscle groups. The patient's movements will be slow and hesitant.

Proper use of canes, walkers, and other ambulatory aids can promote activity and reduce dangers of falls. The specific aid required depends on the amount of weight bearing that is tolerated, and the ability of the patient to balance safely. QSEN: Safety.

Obstacles such as throw rugs and children's toys, wet floors, uneven surfaces can impede one's ability to ambulate safely. Moveable chairs need to be locked. QSEN: Safety.

Obtaining appropriate assistance for the patient can ensure safe and proper progression of activity. QSEN: Teamwork and collaboration.

Therapeutic Interventions

Actions/Interventions

- Encourage the patient to perform range of motion (ROM) to all joints daily.
- Encourage the patient to use a sturdy, high-seated chair with arms.

- Reinforce the need for regular activity and ambulation.

- Encourage the family to supervise and assist with ambulation as needed.
- Teach the patient and the family caregivers about the appropriate use of assistive devices for mobility. Encourage family members about use of a gait belt for safety when assisting the patient with ambulation.

Rationales

Exercise reduces muscle rigidity, maintains joint mobility, and prevents muscle atrophy.

This type of chair provides more support and is easier for the patient to get up from a sitting position. Using the arms of the chair when getting up reduces the risk for falls with changes in position. QSEN: Safety.

Activity is important to reduce the hazards of immobility. Some patients have shown improvement in rigidity and tremors with rhythmic exercise programs such as yoga or tai chi. QSEN: Evidence-based practice.

The use of mobility aids such as canes and walkers promotes stability and reduces the risk for falls. QSEN: Safety.

Canes or walkers may assist the patient with mobility. These aids can compensate for impaired function and increase level of activity. The patient should wear a gait belt for safety so the nurse or family member can guide the patient to reduce the risk for falling. However, some patients may refuse to use assistive devices because they attract attention to a perceived disability. QSEN: Patient-centered care; Safety.

■ = Independent   ▲ = Interprofessional Collaboration

Actions/Interventions

- Encourage the patient to lift the feet and take large steps while walking.

- Discuss the need for removing environmental barriers in the home.
- Instruct the family to allow sufficient time for ADLs.

- Encourage the patient to rest between activities that are tiring. Teach energy-saving techniques.

- ▲ Consult physical and occupational therapists about aids to facilitate ADLs and safe ambulation and to promote muscle strengthening.

Rationales

Rigidity and weakness may make it difficult for the patient's foot to clear the floor when taking a step. The patient needs to be intentional in lifting the foot off the floor while walking. A broad-based gait helps improve balance and reduces shuffling.

Bradykinesia may make it difficult for the patient to change direction to avoid environmental barriers. QSEN: Safety.

The family often wants to perform the task rather than enabling the patient to do it. The goal is to help the patient maintain functional independence as long as possible.

Rest periods are necessary to conserve energy. The patient must learn to respect the limitations of his or her restrictions.

Ambulatory aids can increase mobility and allow the patient some control over the environment. QSEN: Teamwork and collaboration.

NANDA-I NDx Imbalanced Nutrition: Less Than Body Requirements

Common Related Factors

Inability to ingest foods
Insufficient dietary intake

Defining Characteristics

Body weight 20% or more below ideal weight range
Food intake less than recommended dietary allowance (RDA)
Weakness of muscles needed for mastication and/or swallowing

Common Expected Outcomes

Patient verbalizes and demonstrates selection of foods to prevent weight loss and maintain nutrient intake.
Patient weighs within 10% of ideal weight range.

NOC Outcomes
Nutritional Status: Nutrient Intake; Respiratory Status: Airway Patency
NIC Interventions
Nutrition Management; Aspiration Precautions

Ongoing Assessment

Actions/Interventions

- Assess the degree of swallowing difficulty with fluids, solids, and/or medications.

- Inquire about episodes of choking, drooling, and nasal regurgitations.

- Assess the patient's ability to feed self.

- Monitor the patient's weight at each visit. Encourage the patient or family to keep a weight and/or diet log.

Rationales

Swallowing difficulty accompanied by fatigue and fine motor impairment causes a diminished appetite and poor nutritional intake. Swallowing problems are associated with the later stages of the disease.

Poor muscle coordination and weakness in the mouth and throat increase the risk for aspiration. Drooling indicates an inability to swallow saliva because of muscle weakness. QSEN: Safety.

Bradykinesia, tremors, and rigidity may interfere with feeding self-care, chewing, and swallowing. QSEN: Patient-centered care.

Weight loss is usually the result of decreased intake.

Therapeutic Interventions

Actions/Interventions	Rationales
■ Reinforce the need for a high-Fowler's position for eating and drinking.	This position reduces the risk for aspiration. QSEN: Safety.
■ Elicit family supervision during meals. Avoid distractions.	The patient needs to focus on chewing and swallowing to avoid aspiration.
■ Stress the importance of allowing adequate time for meals; avoid rushing the patient.	It may be difficult for patients to swallow under pressure. Bradykinesia may require more time for feeding self-care. QSEN: Patient-centered care.
■ Suggest high-calorie, low-volume supplements between meals.	Additional caloric intake may be required for optimal nutrition.
■ Suggest that the patient take small bites of food. Encourage the patient to swallow two to three times after taking a bite of food.	Smaller bites may require less effort for chewing and may be easier to swallow. The patient may require multiple swallows to move a bolus of food from the mouth through the esophagus.
■ Suggest fluids that are thickened rather than watery fluids.	Thin liquids are more difficult to control when swallowing. A variety of thickening agents are available. Foods thickened to the consistency of honey are often easier for the patient to control when swallowing. QSEN: Patient-centered care.
■ Suggest four to five small meals per day and at least 2000 mL of fluids (if fluids are not restricted for another health reason).	Small meals may be tolerated with greater success than three meals daily. This meal plan is associated with improved nutritional intake.
■ Encourage oral hygiene after meals.	Toothbrushing and rinsing the mouth are useful in removing residual and pocketed food that can be aspirated later. QSEN: Safety.
▲ Consult members of the interprofessional health team.	A dietitian can recommend alterations in food selections to promote adequate calorie and nutrient intake. A speech therapist may be needed to design plans to improve the patient's ability to swallow. An occupational therapist can provide the patient with adaptive equipment to promote feeding self-care. Hand and wrist braces may help control tremors. Plates with rim guards and adaptive utensils may improve the patient's ability to feed self. QSEN: Teamwork and collaboration.

NANDA-I NDx Impaired Verbal Communication

Common Related Factor

Physiological condition (e.g. weakened musculoskeletal system)

Defining Characteristics

Difficulty forming words (e.g., slow, slurred speech, dysarthria, stammering)
Difficulty in use of body expressions or facial expressions

Common Expected Outcome

Patient uses a form of communication to get needs met and to relate effectively with people and his or her environment.

NOC Outcome

Communication: Expressive

NIC Intervention

Communication Enhancement: Speech Deficit

Neurological Care Plans

■ = Independent ▲ = Interprofessional Collaboration

Ongoing Assessment

Actions/Interventions	Rationales
■ Determine the patient's primary and preferred means of communication (e.g., verbal, written, gestures).	Patients may have skill with many forms of communication, yet they will prefer one method for important communication. QSEN: Patient-centered care.
■ Evaluate the patient's ability to speak, as well as to understand spoken words, written words, and pictures.	As the disease progresses, cognitive abilities diminish. The patient with PD may have slurred speech as a result of dysarthria.
■ Assess the patient's voice quality.	As PD progresses, the patient's voice may become lower-pitched and softer.

Therapeutic Interventions

Actions/Interventions	Rationales
■ Maintain eye contact when speaking.	This approach promotes patient focus and attention.
■ Allow the patient time to articulate.	The patient may be discouraged and give up if rushed. The patient needs time to organize thoughts before speaking. QSEN: Patient-centered care.
■ Encourage face and tongue exercises.	Regular exercise can reduce rigidity and facilitate the muscle relaxation needed to form words.
■ Encourage the patient to practice reading aloud or singing.	Activities that involve the affected muscles help the patient practice muscle control.
■ Avoid speaking loudly unless the patient is hard of hearing.	Loud talking does not improve the patient's ability to understand.
▲ Consult a speech therapist if indicated.	The speech therapist can evaluate the patient's need for adaptive devices such as voice synthesizers or computers. QSEN: Teamwork and collaboration.
■ Provide alternative communication aids as needed, such as picture or word boards.	These aids reduce the patient's frustration with verbal communication.

NANDA-I NDx **Chronic Low Self-Esteem**

Common Related Factors

Alteration in body image, especially drooling, tremors, gait, slurred speech
Alteration in social role
Functional impairment

Defining Characteristics

Situational challenge to self-worth
Self-negating verbalizations
Indecisive, nonassertive behavior
Underestimates ability to deal with situation
Helplessness

Common Expected Outcomes

Patient verbalizes positive self-acceptance.
Patient describes successes in current situations.

NOC Outcomes

Body Image; Self-Esteem; Personal Resiliency

NIC Interventions

Body Image Enhancement; Self-Esteem Enhancement; Coping Enhancement

Ongoing Assessment

Actions/Interventions	Rationales
■ Review with the patient past and current accomplishments: emotional, social, interpersonal, intellectual, vocational, and physical.	Patients experiencing situational stress from progression of PD often lose sight of their past successes in managing similar situations. QSEN: Patient-centered care.
■ Listen to statements the patient makes about himself or herself.	Low self-esteem is often expressed as feeling unloved, unworthy, or incompetent. The patient may be self-critical especially about his or her ability to manage the symptoms of PD. Patients may attempt to hide tremors. Over time, they may withdraw from social interactions because they are embarrassed by their symptoms
■ Assess the degree to which the patient feels loved and respected by others.	The manner in which others respond to the patient influences self-esteem. Feeling loved and respected despite disabilities implies that one is valued by others and supports self-esteem.
■ Evaluate the patient's support system.	A positive social network can promote effective coping with the changes of PD.

Therapeutic Interventions

Actions/Interventions	Rationales
■ Encourage the patient to verbalize fears and concerns. Listen attentively.	The verbalization of actual or perceived threats can help reduce anxiety. Patients may express concern about increasing dependency on others for mobility and ADLs. QSEN: Patient-centered care.
■ Discuss the patient's feelings about the symptoms: tremors, drooling of saliva, slurred speech.	Patients may be ashamed about changes in their appearance and their inability to control symptoms.
■ Discuss the impact of alteration in health status on the patient's self-esteem.	Disturbances in self-esteem are natural responses to significant changes. Reconstruction of the individual's self-esteem occurs after grieving has taken place and acceptance has followed.
■ Instruct the family to avoid overprotection of the individual; promote social interaction as appropriate.	Patients should not be forced into uncomfortable situations. Overprotection by family members may reinforce the patient's feelings of unworthiness and dependence on others.
■ Encourage the patient to attend to grooming, hygiene, and dressing daily.	These actions may increase the patient's self-esteem. The patient may need to learn to use adaptive equipment to facilitate independence with these activities.
■ Instruct the family to provide privacy, if desired, especially when performing ADLs and eating.	The patient may be embarrassed about eating in public places because of swallowing difficulties; family meals should be encouraged.
■ Explore strengths and resources with the patient.	Attention to the patient's strengths will reinforce a more positive self-esteem.
■ Encourage family members to support the patient's efforts at self-care.	Success with self-care activities promotes a more positive self-esteem. QSEN: Patient-centered care.
■ Advise of the realistic need for additional support in coping with this lifelong illness. Refer to support groups.	As this disease progresses, self-care and home care issues become more evident, especially for older people who may live alone or with an equally elderly or a frail spouse. The use of lay support groups or individuals may help the patient recognize positive aspects even in the face of disease.
■ Refer to the American Parkinson's Disease Association.	Local chapters of the organization provide information and resources such as support groups.

Neurological Care Plans

■ = Independent　▲ = Interprofessional Collaboration

NANDA-I NDx Deficient Knowledge

Common Related Factors

Alteration in cognitive functioning
Insufficient information
Insufficient interest in learning
Insufficient knowledge of resources
Misinformation presented by others

Defining Characteristics

Insufficient knowledge
Inaccurate follow-through of instruction
Inaccurate performance on a test
Inappropriate behavior

Common Expected Outcome

Patient or caregiver verbalizes understanding of disease process and special needs related to activity, exercises, ambulation, medication, diet, and elimination.

NOC Outcomes

Knowledge: Disease Process; Knowledge: Treatment Regimen

NIC Interventions

Health Literacy Enhancement; Learning Facilitation; Teaching: Disease Process; Teaching: Prescribed Medication; Teaching: Prescribed Exercise

Ongoing Assessment

Actions/Interventions	Rationales
■ Assess the motivation and willingness of the patient and caregivers to learn.	Adults must see a need or purpose for learning. Some patients are ready to learn soon after they are diagnosed; others cope better by denying or delaying the need for instruction. Learning also requires energy, which patients may not be ready to use.
■ Evaluate the patient's and the caregiver's understanding of the disease process, diagnostic tests, treatments, and outcomes.	This information provides the starting base for educational sessions. An individualized teaching plan is based on the patient's previous knowledge and desire for additional information. Teaching standardized content that the patient already knows wastes valuable time and hinders critical learning. QSEN: Patient-centered care.

Therapeutic Interventions

Actions/Interventions	Rationales
■ Reinforce the explanation of the disease and its treatment: • Disease has a gradual onset and progression; there is no known cure. • Treatment is aimed at relieving symptoms and preventing complications.	This information helps the patient and family become full partners in making decisions about long-term care, financial resources, living arrangements, power of attorney, and living wills. Knowledge of the disease process and treatment may assist the patient with developing coping skills to be used as PD progresses to later stages. QSEN: Patient-centered care.
■ Encourage independence and avoid overprotection by encouraging the patient to do things for self: feeding, dressing, ambulation.	In the early stages and with medication therapy, most ADLs can be continued (driving, working), but as the disease progresses, assistance will be required.

Actions/Interventions	Rationales
■ Discuss with the patient, family, and caregiver the use and the potential side effects of the following:	Patients may find it challenging to find the right medications for PD to manage symptoms effectively with minimal side effects. The patient and family will be a source of important information to allow the adjustment of medication dosages. Providing information allows the patient to be a full partner in making decisions and assuming responsibility for medication management at a later time. QSEN: Patient-centered care; Evidence-based practice; Safety.
• Anticholinergics: benztropine mesylate (Cogentin), procyclidine (Kemadrin), cycrimine (Pagitane), trihexyphenidyl (Artane)	These drugs decrease tremors by blocking acetylcholine activity. Side effects include constipation, dry mouth, confusion, blurred vision.
• Dopamine precursors: levodopa, carbidopa/levodopa (Sinemet)	These drugs cross the blood-brain barrier, and they are converted to dopamine in the brain. The addition of carbidopa decreases peripheral conversion of levodopa and makes more of the drug available to the brain. Side effects include nausea, hypotension, confusion, and dyskinesia. The patient may develop a tolerance to these drugs, producing an "on-off" phenomenon. The management for this phenomenon is to reduce the dosage or give the patient a drug holiday.
• Dopamine agonists: bromocriptine (Parlodel), ropinirole (Requip), pergolide (Permax)	This class of drugs mimics the activity of dopamine on postsynaptic receptors. These drugs are used in combination with carbidopa/levodopa. Side effects are increased sleepiness, confusion, and hypotension.
• Monoamine oxidase B inhibitor: selegiline (L-deprenyl)	This drug potentiates the effect of carbidopa/levodopa. Patients may experience sleep problems as a side effect. Adverse interactions with meperidine have been reported.
• Indirect agonist: amantadine (Symmetrel)	This antiviral medication has both anticholinergic and dopaminergic effects in patients with PD. It also reduces the development of dyskinesia from other PD drugs. Side effects may include dry mouth, ankle swelling, and a reddish blue mottling of the skin (livedo reticularis).
• Catechol-*O*-methyltransferase inhibitor (COMT): tolcapone (Tasmar), entacapone (Comtan)	These drugs block peripheral conversion of levodopa, making more of the drug available to cross the blood-brain barrier. They decrease the development of tolerance to levodopa. Liver toxicity is associated with the use of these drugs.
■ Discuss the potential surgical interventions for patients who develop severe tremors:	
• Stereotactic pallidotomy	Stereotactic pallidotomy involves the use of electrical stimulation of selected neuron centers to diminish rigidity or tremors by creating permanent lesions.
• Stereotactic thalamotomy to relieve tremors and rigidity	Stereotactic thalamotomy uses thermal coagulation of neuron centers to reduce tremors.
• Neurotransplantation of dopamine-producing cells and stem cell research	Transplantation of dopamine-producing cells from fetal tissue is considered an experimental procedure. Sources of fetal tissue are either human or porcine. The procedure is considered high risk, but many patients demonstrate symptomatic improvement.
• Deep brain stimulation	Deep brain stimulation using an implanted pulse generator, similar to a cardiac pacemaker, provides control of tremors in patients whose drug therapy has been unsuccessful.

Neurological Care Plans

■ = Independent ▲ = Interprofessional Collaboration

Related Care Plans

Activity intolerance, Chapter 2
Caregiver role strain, Chapter 2
Risk for aspiration, Chapter 2
Self-care deficit, Chapter 2

Seizure Activity

Epilepsy; Seizure Disorder; Convulsion

A seizure is an unpredictable, excessive disorderly discharge of neuronal activity from the cerebral cortex causing behavioral and physical disturbances. Epilepsy is a disease that is diagnosed when a patient experiences at least two seizures occurring more than 24 hours apart. Seizures may be classified as generalized or focal. Generalized seizures involve activity in both hemispheres of the brain. This type of seizure activity is associated with changes in consciousness and convulsive motor activity. Focal seizures arise in one area of the brain without changes in consciousness. Convulsive motor activity is not associated with focal seizures unless the seizure spreads to the other hemisphere of the brain. The onset of seizure activity can occur across the life span. The most common onset is usually before 20 years of age. However, new onset of seizures has been noted in older adults with no previous history of seizure activity. Genetics may play a role in the development of seizures. Patients with new onset of seizure activity after age 20 may have a history of structural or metabolic disorders such as traumatic brain injury, brain tumor, degenerative neurologic disorders, or stroke. Fever, low blood glucose level, drug and alcohol abuse, acid-base imbalances, electrolyte imbalances, and medication side effects may also contribute to the onset of seizures. Seizure activity has three distinct phases. The preictal phase is that time before the actual seizure. This phase of seizure activity is most characteristic of focal seizures rather than generalized seizures. During the preictal phase the patient may experience symptoms that warn of an impending seizure. This unusual sensation is called an aura. During the ictal phase, the patient experiences a progression of neuromuscular changes as a result of the disorganized neuron activity. These neuromuscular changes include an increase in muscle tone (tonic phase) with stiffening of the extremities and a rhythmic contraction/relaxation of muscles (clonic phase). This clonic phase presents as a jerking activity of the extremities. The postictal phase is the period immediately following seizure activity. This phase represents brain recovery and return to baseline status. During the postictal phase the patient may experience confusion, headache, fatigue, and memory loss for the event. Some patients may sleep for several minutes to an hour during this period of brain recovery. The long-term consequences of seizures include many psychosocial challenges for the patient. These challenges include employment opportunities, driving restrictions, and the social stigma of seizures. A patient with new onset of seizures may require hospitalization for diagnosis and initiation of treatment. Follow-up care is in the outpatient setting. This care plan focuses on self-care in the ambulatory setting.

NANDA-I
NDx Deficient Knowledge

Common Related Factors

Alteration in cognitive functioning
Insufficient information
Insufficient interest in learning insufficient knowledge of resources
Misinformation presented by others

Defining Characteristics

Insufficient knowledge
Inaccurate follow-through of instruction
Inappropriate behavior

Common Expected Outcome

Patient and family caregivers verbalize understanding of the disease process, treatment, and safety measures.

NOC Outcomes

Knowledge: Disease Process; Knowledge: Treatment Regimen; Seizure Self-Control

NIC Interventions

Health Literacy Enhancement; Learning Facilitation; Seizure Precautions; Seizure Management; Teaching: Disease Process; Teaching: Procedure/Treatment

---

Ongoing Assessment

Actions/Interventions	Rationales
■ Assess the primary concerns of the patient about the diagnosis of seizures.	The patient may have experienced challenges for employment, education, and social interactions because of his or her seizure diagnosis. The nurse should address these concerns as an important part of the individualized teaching plan. QSEN: Patient-centered care.
■ Assess the patient's knowledge concerning seizures and seizure management.	This information provides a baseline on which to design an individualized teaching plan. The patient and family members may have misconceptions about the causes and treatment of seizures. Teaching standardized content that the patient already knows wastes valuable time and hinders critical learning. Adults learn material that is important to them.
■ Assess the frequency, duration, and type of seizure activity. Ask the patient and family about a seizure history, and if precipitating factors are involved, such as odors, visual stimulation, fatigue, stress, fever, menstruation, or alcohol consumption. Inquire about warnings before the seizure (aura, prodromal signs).	Each individual may present with his or her own pattern of seizure activity. Understanding the pattern is necessary for planning appropriate treatments and creating an individualized teaching plan. QSEN: Patient-centered care.
■ Determine the physical effects of prior seizures, such as a change in the level of consciousness preceding seizure activity, the body part in which the seizure started, automatism, length of the seizure, head and eye turning, pupillary reaction, associated falls, oral secretions, urinary or fecal incontinence, cyanosis, and postictal state.	Knowledge of changes that occur with each phase of seizure activity may help the patient and family plan appropriate care to prevent seizures and prevent injury during a seizure. QSEN: Safety.

Therapeutic Interventions

Actions/Interventions	Rationales
■ Provide information about the patient's specific type of seizure.	Generalized seizures affect the entire brain and are bilateral and symmetrical. There is usually no aura, but there is a loss of consciousness. Generalized seizures range from staring spells to the stiffening (tonic) and jerking (clonic) of extremities. Partial seizures, or focal onset seizures, affect a specific region of the cerebral cortex with physical effects depending on where the seizure originated. Partial (simple) seizures are typically just motor or sensory and do not cause a loss of consciousness. Partial (complex) seizures are psychomotor-like partial simple seizures but also involve changes in consciousness such as confusion and memory loss. This seizure can spread through the cerebrum and culminate in a generalized seizure.

■ = Independent ▲ = Interprofessional Collaboration

Neurological Care Plans

Actions/Interventions	Rationales
■ Discuss the disease process, including aura and prodrome.	Knowledge of these warnings allows the patient to use safety measures that can be implemented, such as sitting or lying down or pulling over if driving. QSEN: Safety.
■ Teach the patient and family about specific antiepilepsy drugs (AEDs):	Drug therapy is the primary approach to the management of seizure activity. Patients may need to take a combination of medications to achieve effective seizure control. Providing information allows the patient to be a full partner in making decisions and assuming responsibility for safe and effective medication management at a later time. QSEN: Patient-centered care; Evidence-based practice; Safety.
• Hydantoins: phenytoin (Dilantin), fosphenytoin (Cerebyx)	This class of drugs is a mainstay of drug therapy for seizures. Patients need to implement routine dental care to decrease the development of gingival hyperplasia. This side effect occurs with long-term use of these drugs.
• Iminostilbenes: carbamazepine (Tegretol), oxcarbazepine (Trileptal)	These drugs are used for partial complex and generalized seizures. The side effects of these drugs include nausea, diplopia, hepatic toxicity, and leukopenia. The patient may need periodic blood work done to monitor for drug side effects. Some patients taking these drugs may experience Stevens-Johnson syndrome, a skin disorder with life-threatening consequences.
• Phenobarbital	This drug is a long-acting barbiturate. It is used in combination with hydantoins in the management of partial complex and generalized seizures. The drug is a class IV controlled substance. Dependency can develop with long-term use.
• Valproates: valproic acid (Depakene), divalproex sodium (Depakote)	These drugs are used in the management of partial, partial complex, and generalized seizures. With long-term use the patient may develop weight gain, alopecia, hepatic toxicity, and thrombocytopenia. Periodic blood work needs to be done to monitor for side effects. The patient needs to implement safety precautions to prevent bleeding.
■ Discuss the danger of seizure activity with the abrupt withdrawal of medications.	Patients sometimes believe they no longer need medication because they have not experienced a seizure in some time. Patients may be able to discontinue drug therapy if they are seizure-free for 2 to 5 years. The patient should only discontinue medications with close supervision by a health care provider. Abrupt discontinuation of anticonvulsants may trigger seizure activity. QSEN: Safety.
■ Discuss the need for periodic follow-up checks on anticonvulsant blood levels and a possible complete blood count check.	Anemia and other blood dyscrasias occur with anticonvulsant therapy. QSEN: Safety.
■ Provide information for patients undergoing continuous video electroencephalogram monitoring.	This assessment technique is used for patients who have new-onset seizures or seizures that do not respond to drug therapy. Documentation of the brain location of seizure activity and type of seizure will guide decisions about drug therapy and other treatment. The patient may be hospitalized for several days until a seizure is documented.
■ Reinforce the information about surgical therapy for seizure management.	Patients who do not respond to drug therapy may be candidates for surgical intervention. Procedures range from destruction of a single seizure focus to disconnection of nerve pathways between brain hemispheres. Surgery may be curative or palliative to reduce the number and frequency of seizures.

Actions/Interventions

- Reinforce the information about nerve and brain stimulation therapies for seizure management.

- Explain to the patient, caregiver, or significant others what to do during a seizure:
  - If the patient is on the floor, remove furniture or other potentially harmful objects from the area.
  - Do not restrain the patient during a seizure. Loosen clothing.
  - Turn the patient to the side. Do not place a tongue blade or other objects in the patient's mouth.

- If seizures persist longer than 5 minutes or are incessantly repetitive, instruct the caregiver to call 9-1-1.

- Educate the patient about safety measures:

  - Driving

  - Home safety: The patient should have someone else present when cooking and bathing to reduce the risk for injury
  - Work safety: Avoid construction work, ladder climbing, heavy equipment operation
  - Personal safety: Dive or swim with a companion; wear medical alert identification; be aware of the effect of alcohol and drugs

- ▲ Refer the patient to a dietitian if a ketogenic diet is prescribed.

- Refer to the Epilepsy Foundation of America.

- Provide information, as appropriate, about specially trained animals for epileptics.

Rationales

Neurostimulation therapies include vagus nerve stimulation (VNS) and responsive neurostimulation (RNS). VNS therapy reduces the frequency and duration of seizures through changes in neurotransmitter levels. RNS therapy involves placement of a microcomputer in the skull with electrodes placed on the brain surface. This device can detect a seizure and deliver an electrical stimulus to disrupt the seizure.

Injury prevention is a priority during seizure activity. QSEN: Safety.

Physical restraint applied during seizure activity can cause musculoskeletal or soft tissue injury.

This position is important to promote gravity drainage of secretions and maintain airway patency. Inserting objects into the mouth often causes more harm, such as dislodging teeth, causing lacerations, and obstructing the airway by pushing the tongue farther into the pharynx.

The patient may require administration of rescue antiepileptic drugs to stop status epilepticus. These drugs may include IV phenytoin, IV lorazepam, or IV or rectal diazepam.

This information helps the patient reduce the risk for injury. QSEN: Safety.

Laws about driving after the onset of a seizure disorder vary from state to state. In most states, the patient must be seizure-free for 6 months to 2 years before resuming driving a motor vehicle.

The patient and family need to have a plan to provide appropriate supervision of the patient in the home setting.

Most states have laws prohibiting workplace discrimination against people with epilepsy.

There is an increased risk for seizures produced by the interaction of alcohol with anticonvulsant drugs. A "buddy system" for athletic or recreational activities promotes safety and prompt intervention if the patient experiences a seizure.

Diet therapy is usually attempted only for severe, unrelenting seizures that do not respond to drug therapy. The diet is a high-fat, low-carbohydrate, low-protein diet, divided into several small meals per day. The diet is complex and requires education about the careful selection of foods. The patient needs to eat 4 g of fat for each gram of carbohydrates and protein. QSEN: Teamwork and collaboration.

This organization provides information and resources to support effective coping and seizure management.

Some dogs can be trained to detect a seizure prodrome and warn the patient so safety measures can be implemented before the seizure begins.

Neurological Care Plans

■ = Independent ▲ = Interprofessional Collaboration

Risk for Chronic Low Self-Esteem

Common Risk Factors

Alteration in social role
Functional impairment with seizure activity
Inadequate recognition
History of rejection and discrimination

Common Expected Outcome

Patient verbalizes positive statements about self in relation to living with a seizure disorder.

NOC Outcome
Self-Esteem

NIC Intervention
Self-Esteem Enhancement

Ongoing Assessment

Actions/Interventions	Rationales
■ Review with the patient past and current accomplishments: emotional, social, interpersonal, intellectual, vocational, and physical.	Patients experiencing situational stress often lose sight of their past successes in managing similar situations. QSEN: Patient-centered care.
■ Assess the patient's feelings about self, the seizure diagnosis, and long-term therapy.	Patients may express frustration, anxiety, and unrealistic expectations because of the unpredictability of their seizures and dependence on medications. Many patients begin to identify themselves as chronically ill and express feelings of loss of independence.
■ Assess the patient's perceived implications of the disorder and its effect on socialization.	Patients may have a fear of or have experienced actual discrimination in jobs and schooling, as well as a fear of loss of control and embarrassment in public if a seizure occurs. QSEN: Patient-centered care.

Therapeutic Interventions

Actions/Interventions	Rationales
■ Encourage the patient's ventilation of feelings through active listening and open-ended questions.	Talking about feelings can support effective coping and improved insight. These communication techniques allow the patient to express concerns, fears, and ideas without interruption. This approach to the patient will convey a sense of respect for the patient's abilities and strengths in addition to recognizing problems and concerns. QSEN: Patient-centered care.
■ Incorporate the family and significant others in the care plan.	A strong social support system may promote more effective coping and positive self-esteem for the patient.
■ Dispel common myths and fears about convulsive disorders.	Historically, epilepsy has been seen as a mental disorder with negative connotations and social stigma; but with good health habits and maintenance of a medication schedule, most seizure disorders are controllable and have no relationship to mental capabilities or intellect.
■ Refer to a support group if possible.	These groups provide practical assistance in dealing with social and personal issues.

Neurological Care Plans

ⓔvolve **For additional care plans, go to http://evolve.elsevier.com/Gulanick/.**

Actions/Interventions

▲ Consult with members of the interprofessional health team to address specific patient concerns and challenges.

Rationales

A social worker can assist the patient and family with financial and vocational issues. A mental health professional can help the patient if anxiety, depression, and lifestyle changes become troublesome. The patient may benefit from talk therapy to promote effective coping and support positive self-esteem. Human rights organizations and/or labor relations departments may need to be contacted if job security or discrimination is evident. QSEN: Teamwork and collaboration.

Related Care Plans

Impaired home maintenance, Chapter 2
Risk for aspiration, Chapter 2

Spinal Cord Injury

Tetraplegia; Quadriplegia; Paraplegia; Neurogenic Shock; Spinal Shock

Spinal cord injury (SCI) is damage to the spinal cord at any level from C1 to L1 or L2, where the spinal cord ends. Primary causes of SCI are motor vehicle accidents, followed by sporting accidents, falls, and penetrating injuries (gunshot or knife wounds). Motor vehicle accidents are the leading cause among people younger than age 65. Among people older than 65 years, a fall is the leading cause of SCI. Approximately 50% of people who sustain SCI are men between 15 and 29 years of age. Injury may result in a complete cord lesion with no preservation of motor and sensory function below the level of injury. An incomplete lesion results in residual and mixed motor and sensory function below level of injury and some potential for improvement in function. Complete cord injury above C7 results in tetraplegia (also called quadriplegia); injury from C7 to L1 causes paraplegia.

Neurogenic (or spinal) shock often follows cervical and high thoracic SCI. Spinal shock can last from 7 to 10 days to weeks or months after injury. It temporarily results in (1) total loss of all motor and sensory function below the injury; (2) sympathetic disruption, resulting in loss of vasoconstriction and leaving parasympathetics unopposed, leading to bradycardia and hypotension; (3) loss of all reflexes below the injury; (4) inability to control body temperature, secondary to the inability to sweat, shiver, or vasoconstrict below the level of injury; (5) ileus; and (6) urinary retention. When neurogenic shock resolves, it is followed by a stage of spasticity.

The long-term consequences of SCI affect all aspects of the patient's life and become part of the rehabilitation process. Physically, the patient needs to learn about strategies to maintain mobility, skin integrity, urinary elimination, and bowel elimination. The patient needs access to knowledge, skills, and resources to support adjustment in the areas of psychological, social, and spiritual well-being, independence with ADLs, sexuality, education, and employment. This care plan focuses on the acute care of a patient with SCI.

NANDA-I
NDx **Risk for Ineffective Breathing Pattern**

Common Risk Factors

Neuromuscular impairment from high cervical cord injury
Respiratory muscle weakness and fatigue

Neurological Care Plans

 = Independent   ▲ = Interprofessional Collaboration

Common Expected Outcome

The patient maintains an effective breathing pattern, as evidenced by relaxed breathing at normal rate and depth and absence of dyspnea.

NOC Outcomes
Respiratory Status: Airway Patency; Respiratory Status: Ventilation

NIC Interventions
Respiratory Monitoring; Airway Management

Ongoing Assessment

Actions/Interventions	Rationales
■ Monitor the patient's respiratory rate, depth, and effort.	An injury at C4 or above causes paralysis of the diaphragm, necessitating intubation. All patients with tetraplegia will have some degree of respiratory insufficiency as a result of intercostal muscle weakness or paralysis. If the patient has a C5 to T6 cord injury, abdominal and intercostal muscle innervation will be absent or diminished and the patient may be unable to take deep breaths and cough. This situation increases the patient's risk for atelectasis and respiratory infection. QSEN: Safety.
■ Auscultate the patient's breath sounds.	Hypoventilation occurs with diaphragmatic respirations as a result of decreased vital capacity and tidal volume. Lung sounds will be diminished.
▲ Use pulse oximetry to monitor oxygen saturation; assess arterial blood gases as ordered.	Oxygen saturation should be at 90% or greater. Spinal cord edema (even with an incomplete lesion at or below C4) and hemorrhage can affect phrenic nerve function and cause respiratory insufficiency. The patient may have a chronically low Pao_2 level and elevated $Paco_2$ level. QSEN: Safety.
▲ Monitor the patient's vital capacity.	Monitoring detects changes early, so ventilatory support may be initiated before full decompensation occurs.

Therapeutic Interventions

Actions/Interventions	Rationales
▲ Administer oxygen as needed.	Initially, supplemental oxygen is necessary to maintain a high Pao_2 level and oxygen saturation at 90% or higher.
■ Provide reassurance and allay anxiety by staying with the patient during acute episodes of respiratory distress.	The presence of a trusted person may help the patient feel less threatened and can reduce anxiety, thereby reducing oxygen requirements. Anxiety increases dyspnea, respiratory rate, and the work of breathing. QSEN: Patient-centered care.
▲ Assist with intubation and ventilatory support, if indicated.	Patients with a high cervical cord injury (above C4 or C5) are at the greatest risk for apnea and respiratory arrest. Blind nasotracheal intubation or fiberoptic endotracheal intubation without neck involvement will be performed. The duration of intubation depends on the extent of the spinal cord damage. Long-term airway management may require a tracheostomy. Mechanical ventilation may be needed for the tetraplegic patient who cannot maintain spontaneous respirations. QSEN: Safety.
■ Suction the patient as needed. When stabilized, implement postural drainage and chest percussion.	These measures mobilize secretions to prevent pneumonia or atelectasis.

Actions/Interventions

- Teach an assisted cough technique.

- Encourage the use of an incentive spirometer.
- ▲ Apply an abdominal binder.

- Plan activity and rest to maximize the patient's energy.

- ▲ Consult with members of the interprofessional health team.

Rationales

The low tetraplegic and the paraplegic patient can use a coughing technique that employs manual abdominal pressure to support air movement with coughing.

This device promotes deep breathing.

A binder supports weak abdominal muscles used to promote diaphragmatic breathing.

Fatigue is common with the increased work of breathing. Activity increases metabolic rate and oxygen requirements. Rest helps mobilize energy for more effective breathing and coughing efforts.

The respiratory therapist can provide ongoing monitoring of respiratory function and guide decisions about the best strategies to support effective breathing patterns for the patient. QSEN: Teamwork and collaboration.

NANDA-I NDx Risk for Decreased Cardiac Output

Common Risk Factors

Neurogenic shock (traumatic sympathectomy) as a result of spinal cord injury (SCI) at T5 or above
Hypotension
Bradycardia

Common Expected Outcome

Patient has adequate cardiac output as evidenced by systolic BP within 20 mm Hg of baseline, HR 60 to 100 beats/min with regular rhythm, urine output 30 mg/hr or greater, strong peripheral pulses, warm and dry skin, eupnea with absence of pulmonary crackles, and orientation to person, time, and place.

NOC Outcomes
Cardiopulmonary Status; Circulation Status; Vital Signs

NIC Interventions
Hemodynamic Regulation; Invasive Hemodynamic Monitoring

Neurological Care Plans

Ongoing Assessment

Actions/Interventions

- Assess the patient's HR and BP closely.

- Assess the patient's level of consciousness.

- Assess the peripheral pulses and capillary refill.

- Assess respiratory rate and rhythm and breath sounds.

Rationales

The loss of sympathetic innervation results in bradycardia and the vasodilation of vessels below the injury resulting from an unopposed parasympathetic nervous system. The patient will be hypotensive.

Restlessness is an early sign of hypoxia and decreased cerebral perfusion from decreased cardiac output.

Peripheral vasodilation decreases venous return, further decreasing cardiac output and blood pressure.

Rapid, shallow respirations are characteristic of reduced cardiac output. Crackles reflect accumulation of fluid secondary to impaired left ventricular emptying. They are more evident in the dependent areas of the lung. QSEN: Safety.

■ = Independent   ▲ = Interprofessional Collaboration

Therapeutic Interventions

Actions/Interventions	Rationales
▲ Administer IV fluids as ordered to maintain BP.	Patients with neurogenic shock secondary to SCI have a relative hypovolemia. Circulatory blood volume is unchanged but the space in the circulatory system is increased with decreased systemic vascular resistance. IV fluids need to be infused carefully to prevent fluid volume excess. Because of abnormal autonomic hemodynamics, overhydration may lead to pulmonary edema. QSEN: Safety.
■ Avoid elevating the head of the bed.	Because of sympathetic disruption and the resultant loss of vasoconstrictor tone below the injury, head elevation will result in a further drop of BP. The supine position promotes venous return to the heart and supports cardiac output.
▲ Administer vasopressors if needed.	These drugs are titrated to maintain a mean arterial pressure of 80 mm Hg or higher. Atropine may be given to correct bradycardia.
▲ Apply a military antishock trouser (MAST) suit or sequential compression boots (SCBs).	These devices help compensate for lost muscle tone and decrease venous pooling. Improving venous return to the heart will support cardiac output.

Neurological Care Plans

NANDA-I NDx Impaired Physical Mobility

Common Related Factors

Neuromuscular impairment
Insufficient muscle strength (paraplegia or tetraplegia)
Insufficient knowledge of mobility strategies

Defining Characteristics

Impaired ability to reposition self in bed
Impaired ability to turn from side to side
Impaired ability to move between sitting and supine positions
Impaired ability to move between long sitting and supine positions
Impaired ability to move between prone and supine positions

Common Expected Outcomes

Patient performs physical activity independently or within limits of activity restrictions.
Patient demonstrates use of adaptive techniques that promote ambulation and transferring.
Patient is free of complications of immobility, as evidenced by intact skin, absence of thrombophlebitis, normal bowel pattern, and clear breath sounds.

NOC Outcomes

Mobility; Transfer Performance; Ambulation: Wheelchair; Immobility Consequences: Physiological

NIC Interventions

Positioning; Neurologic Monitoring; Exercise Therapy: Joint Mobility

Ongoing Assessment

Actions/Interventions

- Perform a neurological assessment to estimate the level of injury.

  - Evaluate the movement of major muscle groups in the upper and lower extremities: at the toes, ankles, knees, hips, fingers, elbows, and shoulders.
  - Assess the patient's motor strength, checking for the level of progression, symmetry and asymmetry, ascending and descending paralysis, and paresthesia.

  - Evaluate sensations to pinpricks (spinothalamic tract). Start at the toes and ascend gradually up to the face. If sensations change, mark the skin.
  - Assess sensations to light touch (anterior spinothalamic track). Start at the toes and ascend as described.
  - Check for proprioception (joint position sense that reflects posterior columns). Ask the patient to close the eyes. Move the toes and fingers up and down slowly to determine whether the patient can perceive motion.

  - Evaluate the deep tendon reflexes: biceps, triceps, knee, and ankle.
- Serially monitor the patient for any deviation from the initial baseline examination, noting any signs of complete or incomplete injury.

- Assess the patient's ability to perform ADLs effectively and safely on a daily basis using an appropriate assessment tool, such as the Functional Independence Measures (FIM).

Rationales

The information will help determine the degree of immobility and the need for adaptive equipment. QSEN: Patient-centered care; Safety.
The patient's functional ability for mobility will depend on the level of injury.

Injury to the corticospinal tracts results in the loss of motor strength and limits the patient's mobility. The patient's motor strength will determine the type of adaptive equipment needed to promote mobility independence.
The spinothalamic tracts transmit sensations of deep pressure, pain, and temperature. Loss of this sensation puts the patient at risk for complications of immobility.
The anterior spinothalamic tract transmits sensations of light touch.
Changes in proprioception are the result of injury to the dorsal column spinal tract. Loss of proprioception increases the patient's risk for injury.

Changes in reflexes will be related to the level of injury.

If the patient has a worsening deficit or higher evolving sensory deficit, additional studies such as magnetic resonance imaging (MRI) or myelography are indicated. A change from flaccid to spastic paralysis indicates the resolution of spinal shock.
Restricted movement affects the ability to perform most ADLs. A variety of assessment tools are available, depending on the clinical setting. Such tools provide objective data for baselines. For example, the FIM measures 18 self-care items related to eating, bathing, grooming, dressing, toileting, bladder and bowel management, transfer, ambulation, and stair climbing. QSEN: Patient-centered care; Evidence-based practice; Safety.

Therapeutic Interventions

Actions/Interventions

- Apply a low-air-loss mattress to the bed before the patient is placed in the bed. Immobilize the patient. Maintain the patient in a collar and on a backboard. Once all studies are completed and the patient is stabilized, remove the backboard.

▲ Insert a nasogastric tube if appropriate.

- If the spine is stable, logroll and reposition the patient at least every 2 hours.
- Perform ROM exercises.

Rationales

Immobilization is necessary to prevent additional injury from active or passive movements of the spine. Early removal of the backboard reduces the potential for pressure ulcer formation. Special mattresses promote an even distribution of pressure to reduce the risk for skin breakdown. QSEN: Safety.
The immobilization of the head and neck prevents the patient from protecting the airway if vomiting occurs. QSEN: Safety.
Frequent turning relieves pressure and reduces the risk for skin breakdown.
These exercises reduce the potential for contractures, which may occur once neurogenic shock advances to the next stage of spasticity.

Neurological Care Plans

■ = Independent   ▲ = Interprofessional Collaboration

Actions/Interventions	Rationales
■ Provide support to the feet.	A high-top sneaker or special device may be helpful to prevent footdrop from unopposed plantar flexion.
▲ Administer methylprednisolone as prescribed.	Methylprednisolone decreases spinal cord ischemia, improves impulse conduction, represses the release of free fatty acids from the spinal cord, and restores extracellular calcium. Clinical practice guidelines recommend high-dose methylprednisolone be administered within 8 hours of injury to reduce the extent of permanent paralysis. QSEN: Evidence-based practice.
▲ Administer anticoagulants as prescribed.	Subcutaneous administration of low-dose or low-molecular-weight heparin may be indicated to reduce the risk for deep vein thrombosis.
▲ Collaborate with members of the interprofessional health team (physical and occupational therapists).	An interprofessional health team approach needs to be initiated early in the patient's care to promote effective mobility in the rehabilitation phase of care. Splints and braces may be used to maintain joints and extremities in a position of anatomical function. The selection of a wheelchair is important to provide stability of the trunk, to maximize the use of remaining function to propel the chair, and to prevent pressure ulcers. The physical therapist will help the patient learn safe transfer techniques. The occupational therapist will provide the patient with adaptive devices to promote independence with ADLs. QSEN: Teamwork and collaboration.
■ Prepare the patient and family for possible surgical intervention.	Spinal decompression, realignment, and/or stabilization can be accomplished with traction or surgery depending on the site and extent of the spinal cord damage. Early surgery to remove bone fragments, relieve cord compression, and repair open wounds improves the chances for good recovery and achieve outcomes for maximum mobility.

NANDA-I
NDx Risk for Impaired Skin Integrity

Common Risk Factors
Immobility
Impaired sensation

Common Expected Outcome
Patient maintains intact skin, as evidenced by no redness over bony prominences and capillary refill less than 6 seconds over areas of redness.

NOC Outcomes
Tissue Integrity: Skin and Mucous Membranes; Risk Control; Risk Detection
NIC Interventions
Pressure Ulcer Prevention; Skin Surveillance

Ongoing Assessment

Actions/Interventions	Rationales
■ Assess the general condition of the patient's skin, noting the color, moisture, texture, and temperature, especially at pressure points.	Pressure ulcers are a common complication of SCI. Healthy skin varies among individuals but should have good turgor (an indication of moisture), feel warm and dry to the touch, be free of impairment (scratches, bruises, excoriation, rashes), and have quick capillary refill (less than 6 seconds). Areas where skin is stretched tautly over bony prominences are at higher risk for breakdown because the possibility of ischemia to skin is high as a result of compression of skin capillaries between a hard surface (e.g., mattress, chair) and the bone. Pressure areas initially appear as persistent reddened areas in light pigmented skin. In darker skin tones, the area may appear as red, blue, or purple hue spots. Early identification of stage I pressure ulcers allows for the prompt initiation of pressure relief interventions. QSEN: Patient-centered care; Safety.
■ Assess the patient's awareness of the sensation of pressure.	The patient with a SCI is not aware of pressure because of impaired sensation. As a result, the patient does not change position to relieve the pressure. Normally, individuals shift their weight off pressure areas every few minutes; this occurs more or less automatically, even during sleep. Patients with decreased sensation are unaware of unpleasant stimuli (pressure) and do not shift weight. This results in prolonged pressure on skin capillaries and ultimately in skin ischemia. QSEN: Patient-centered care.
■ Use an objective tool for pressure ulcer risk assessment. • Braden Scale • Norton Scale	These are validated tools for risk assessment. The Braden Scale is the most widely used. It consists of six subscales: sensory, perception, moisture, activity and mobility, nutrition, and fraction/sheer. Assessment should be carried out on admission and every 24 to 48 hours or sooner if the patient's condition changes. QSEN: Evidence-based practice.

Therapeutic Interventions

Actions/Interventions	Rationales
■ Keep the skin clean and dry.	Moisture accumulation leads to skin maceration and skin breakdown over pressure points. Increased skin moisture, especially in skin folds, adds to the risk for development of fungal skin infection.
■ Apply a thin dressing of DuoDerm or similar product to bony prominences.	Various dressings are available to protect and maintain intact skin.
■ Turn the patient every 2 hours. Use lift sheets when repositioning the patient.	Because of sensory disturbance, the patient will be unable to detect painful pressure. Lift sheets reduce shear forces, which further contribute to skin breakdown.
■ Provide an appropriate prophylactic use of pressure-relieving devices.	These devices should be used on the patient's bed and wheelchair. QSEN: Safety.
■ Instruct the patient in a wheelchair to shift positions every 20 to 30 minutes.	Frequent position changes prevent pressure areas from developing. The patient needs to use his or her arms to lift the upper body and trunk off the surface of the chair.
■ Provide adequate nutritional intake.	A high-protein, high-carbohydrate, and high-calorie diet is needed to counteract the catabolic effects of injury and maintain healthy, intact skin. Enteral feedings may be necessary.

Neurological Care Plans

■ = Independent   ▲ = Interprofessional Collaboration

Actions/Interventions

■ Teach the patient and caregivers to inspect the skin daily. Provide a long-handled, angled mirror.

Rationales

Skin breakdown is an ongoing, lifetime concern for the patient with SCI. The use of a mirror allows the patient independence in performing skin inspection. QSEN: Patient-centered care.

NANDA-I NDx Disturbed Body Image

Common Related Factors

Alteration in body function (due to paralysis from SCI)
Alteration in self perception

Defining Characteristics

Preoccupation with change or loss
Avoids looking at or touching one's body
Focusing behavior on changed body part/function
Alteration in body structure or body function
Change in social involvement

Common Expected Outcome

Patient demonstrates enhanced body image and self-esteem, as evidenced by ability to look at, touch, talk about, and care for parts of body with reduced function.

NOC Outcomes

Body Image; Self-Esteem; Adaptation to Physical Disability

NIC Interventions

Coping Enhancement; Body Image Enhancement; Self-Esteem Enhancement

Ongoing Assessment

Actions/Interventions

■ Assess the patient's perception of dysfunction.

■ Assess the perceived impact on ADLs, personal relationships, and occupational activity.

■ Assess the impact of body image disturbance in relation to the patient's developmental stage.

■ Inquire about coping skills used before the injury.

■ Assess the patient's social support system.

Rationales

The patient may perceive changes that are not present or real. The effects of neurogenic shock will seem permanent to the patient, even if the injury is an incomplete lesion. QSEN: Patient-centered care.

The patient needs to understand that decisions about relationships and occupation need not be made immediately because prior knowledge and beliefs about disability may change during the rehabilitative stage of care.

Adolescents and young adults may be particularly affected by changes a SCI has for their bodies. This is a time when developmental changes are normally rapid and at a time when developing social and intimate relationships is particularly important.

Previous coping skills may not be sufficient or appropriate to help the patient adjust to the dramatic life changes from SCI. QSEN: Patient-centered care.

The patient will have a new level of dependency. A strong social support network can help the patient achieve an appropriate level of functional independence that promotes self-esteem.

Neurological Care Plans

⊖volve **For additional care plans, go to http://evolve.elsevier.com/Gulanick/.**

Therapeutic Interventions

Actions/Interventions

Rationales

■ Acknowledge the normalcy of the emotional response to the change in body function. Allow the patient to grieve.

Stages of grief over a loss of body function are normal (e.g., losing the function of one's legs is like a "death" of the body part as well as the "death" of future plans). The grieving process may take years.

■ Help the patient verbalize feelings regarding impairment.

The expression of feelings supports coping and the development of insights about the impact of the injury. QSEN: Patient-centered care.

■ Help the patient identify helpful coping mechanisms such as interacting with family and friends, spiritual rituals, perseverance, or distraction.

As a result of the overwhelming nature of SCI, prior coping skills may not be effective. Family and friends will provide feedback as the patient integrates the impact of injury into a new perception of self.

▲ Consult with members of the interprofessional health team as needed.

Both the patient and caregivers may benefit from professional counselors in developing effective coping and adjustment strategies. QSEN: Teamwork and collaboration.

NANDA-I
NDx ## Deficient Knowledge

Common Related Factors

Insufficient information
Insufficient interest in learning
Insufficient knowledge of resources
Misinformation presented by others

Defining Characteristics

Insufficient knowledge
Inaccurate follow-through of instruction
Inaccurate performance on a test
Inappropriate behavior

Common Expected Outcome

Patient and caregivers verbalize understanding of the SCI, prognosis, ongoing care measures, and rehabilitation expectations.

NOC Outcomes
Knowledge: Disease Process; Knowledge: Treatment Regimen

NIC Interventions
Health Literacy Enhancement; Learning Facilitation; Teaching: Disease Process; Teaching: Procedure/Treatment; Discharge Planning

Neurological Care Plans

Ongoing Assessment

Actions/Interventions

Rationales

■ Assess the patient's knowledge of the injury and its prognosis.

An understanding of the prognosis is necessary to progress to rehabilitation. This information provides the starting base for educational sessions. Teaching standardized content that the patient already knows wastes valuable time and hinders critical learning. During the acute stages of recovery from SCI, the family or significant others may require the most teaching. QSEN: Patient-centered care.

■ Assess the patient's understanding of the treatment and rehabilitation process.

An effective teaching plan will build on the previous knowledge of treatment. A rehabilitation program may take several weeks or months to achieve effective results for the patient.

■ = Independent ▲ = Interprofessional Collaboration

Neurological Care Plans

Actions/Interventions

■ Assess the motivation and willingness of the patient and caregivers to learn.

Rationales

Adults must see a need or purpose for learning. Some patients are ready to learn soon after they are diagnosed; others cope better by denying or delaying the need for instruction. Learning also requires energy, which patients may not be ready to use. QSEN: Patient-centered care.

Therapeutic Interventions

Actions/Interventions

■ Explain what is happening as care and tests (ventilatory support, x-ray films, laboratory tests) are performed.

■ Explain spinal cord function and the effects of injury on body functions (respiration, mobility, bowel and bladder function). Expect to see a grieving process. Wait until the patient is ready for more information.

■ Encourage the patient and caregiver to participate in care while the patient is hospitalized. Explain about positioning, skin care, pressure ulcer prevention, bowel and bladder management, nutrition, and medications.

■ Initiate a discussion concerning the caregiver's ability to provide long-term home care, especially if the patient requires mechanical ventilation, and if special equipment or transportation is required.

▲ Collaborate with members of the interprofessional health team for social service referrals.

■ Encourage participation in support groups.

Rationales

Knowledge is power. This information will assist the patient with eventual coping once the situation has stabilized. Many patients are young and may have no previous experience with illness or hospitalization. QSEN: Patient-centered care.

The patient and family need to develop realistic expectations about the patient's long-term needs for assistance with self-care activities and ADLs.

Patients and caregivers need time to develop new skills for meeting ADLs and other dimensions of SCI care. Providing information allows the patient and the caregiver to be full partners in making decisions and assuming responsibility for care at a later time that prevents complications of SCI. QSEN: Patient-centered care; Safety.

Family members need to learn to balance their desire to help the patient and the patient's need to achieve functional independence. Family members may perceive the demands of supportive care as an overwhelming burden.

Although care at home is less costly, many third-party payers may not cover special equipment, supplies, home alterations, or utility costs. The patient and family may need help with financial resources to support long-term care. QSEN: Teamwork and collaboration.

Support groups assist the patient in coping with the long-term effects of SCI.

Related Care Plans

Anxiety, Chapter 2
Bowel incontinence, Chapter 2
Caregiver role strain, Chapter 2
Constipation, Chapter 2
Hopelessness, Chapter 2
Ineffective coping, Chapter 2
Ineffective sexuality pattern, Chapter 2
Risk for infection, Chapter 2
Risk for impaired skin integrity, Chapter 2
Self-care deficit, Chapter 2
Urinary retention, Chapter 2

⊝volve **For additional care plans, go to http://evolve.elsevier.com/Gulanick/.**

Stroke

Brain Attack; Cerebrovascular Accident (CVA); Ischemic Stroke; Thrombotic Stroke; Embolic Stroke; Hemorrhagic Stroke

Stroke is a disease that affects the arteries leading to and within the brain. Strokes are classified as either ischemic (as a result of a cerebral thrombus or an embolus) or hemorrhagic (as a result of a rupture of a cerebral blood vessel). Stroke is the leading cause of serious, long-term disability in the United States and Canada. It is the third leading cause of death in the United States. A significant majority of those affected by strokes are older than 65 years of age. African Americans have a higher incidence of stroke than Caucasians or Hispanics. Risk factors for stroke include poorly controlled hypertension, diabetes mellitus, high cholesterol levels, smoking, cocaine use, alcohol abuse, obesity, high-dose estrogen drug therapy, and cerebral aneurysm. Acute ischemic stroke is a medical emergency requiring prompt treatment with thrombolytic therapy within 3 to 4.5 hours after symptom recognition ("time is brain"). Evidence suggests that up to one third of all ischemic strokes can be classified as cryptogenic strokes, meaning the exact cause of the stroke cannot be determined. This type of ischemic stroke may be related to undiagnosed cardiac emboli associated with atrial fibrillation. These patients benefit from transthoracic or transesophageal echocardiography to detect cardiac emboli. Hemorrhagic stroke needs to be ruled out before treatment with thrombolytics. Stroke severity is determined using the National Institutes of Health Stroke Scale (NIHSS). Much attention is directed to providing safe, efficient and quality care to patients with stroke. National guidelines by the American Stroke Association and the Brain Attack Coalition provide direction for stroke care provided by hospitals. The Get With the Guidelines—Stroke continuous quality improvement program provides a mechanism for physicians and hospital staff to monitor their performance. The Joint Commission provides certification for Primary Stroke Centers.

The clinical manifestations of stroke and outcomes for the patient vary, depending on the area of the brain affected. The area of the brain supplied by the middle cerebral artery is the most common site for stroke. A stroke in the nondominant hemisphere often causes spatial-perceptual deficits, changes in judgment and behavior, and unilateral neglect. A stroke in the dominant right hemisphere typically causes dysphasia, dysarthria, left-sided sensory loss and homonymous hemianopia, a decreased awareness of the left side of the body, left-sided paralysis and/or paresis, apraxia, impaired judgment, increased emotional lability, and deficits in handling new spatial information. A stroke in the dominant left hemisphere can cause repetitive or expressive dysphasia, dysarthria, right-sided sensory loss and homonymous hemianopia, right-sided paralysis and/or paresis, increased emotional lability, and a deficit in handling new language information. In this type of stroke there is typically intact judgment, infrequent apraxia, and usually a normal awareness of both sides of the body. This care plan focuses on acute care management of ischemic stroke in the hospital.

NDx Impaired Cerebral Tissue Perfusion

Common Related Factors

Intracranial hemorrhage
Ischemia (embolism or thrombosis)

Defining Characteristics

Altered mental status
Changes in motor response
Changes in papillary reactions
Behavioral changes
Speech abnormalities
Dysphagia
Headache

■ = Independent ▲ = Interprofessional Collaboration

Neurological Care Plans

Common Expected Outcome

Patient maintains optimal cerebral tissue perfusion, as evidenced by National Institutes of Health Stroke Scale (NIHSS) score less than 4, Glasgow Coma Scale (GCS) score greater than 13, absence of new neurological deficits, and stable BP.

NOC Outcomes

Tissue Perfusion: Cerebral; Neurological Status; Blood Coagulation; Medication Response

NIC Interventions

Cerebral Edema Management; Cerebral Perfusion Promotion; Neurological Monitoring; Medication Management

Ongoing Assessment

Actions/Interventions

- Assess the patient's neurological status (serially) using the NIHSS or GCS.

- Assess for a past history of cardiac dysrhythmias, hypertension, smoking, and transient ischemic attacks.

- Monitor the patient's vital signs as needed.

- ▲ Monitor the baseline electrocardiogram, and observe for changes.
- Monitor the fluid intake and urine output.

- ▲ Use pulse oximetry to monitor oxygen saturation; assess arterial blood gases as ordered.

Rationales

This information is used to determine the effects of stroke and identify life-threatening complications such as increased intracranial pressure (ICP). The NIHSS is a standardized assessment of consciousness, vision, sensory and motor responses, speech, and language function. Scores may range from 0 (no stroke) to 42 (severe stroke). Current practice guidelines recommend that patients with an initial score greater than 4 may benefit from thrombolytics. The GCS measures changes in the level of consciousness based on verbal, motor, and pupillary responses. Scores range from 0 to 15. A score less than 13 is associated with a decreased level of consciousness. QSEN: Evidence-based practice.

A cardiac workup is warranted if the stroke is embolic; atrial fibrillation is a major cause of embolic stroke. Some patients may have undiagnosed paroxysmal atrial fibrillation. These patients require transthoracic or transesophageal echocardiography to detect emboli in the left atrium or left ventricle of the heart. Hypertension seems to be related to hemorrhagic stroke. Atherosclerosis and transient ischemic attacks are associated with thrombotic stroke.

The frequent assessment of BP is essential. A normotensive state is desired to promote effective cerebral perfusion pressure. QSEN: Evidence-based practice.

Stroke can produce cardiac electrical changes and dysrhythmias.

A decrease in urine output may indicate decreased renal perfusion and an associated decrease in cerebral perfusion. Because of cerebral edema, fluid balance must be regulated. Fluids may be restricted if the patient has a significant increase in ICP, or volume expanders may be used if the patient is hypotensive with decreased cerebral perfusion.

Oxygen saturation should be 90% or greater for adequate cerebral perfusion. $Paco_2$ greater than 45 mm Hg induces cerebral vasodilation and increases ICP. QSEN: Safety.

Neurological Care Plans

Therapeutic Interventions

Actions/Interventions	Rationales
▲ Administer the following medications, as ordered:	Administration of medications is guided by clinical practice guidelines from many national organizations for stroke care. QSEN: Evidence-based practice.
• Thrombolytics	Thrombolytics are given to dissolve clots in cerebral vessels. These drugs work best when administered within 3 to 4.5 hours of an ischemic stroke. Tissue plasminogen activator (tPA) is the first drug of choice. Alteplase (Activase) is the only thrombolytic approved by the FDA for use in ischemic strokes. Early administration of tPA is associated with reduced neurological damage and stroke severity.
• Anticoagulants and antiplatelet drugs	Anticoagulants and antiplatelet drugs are given to reduce clot formation and prevent the extension of existing clots.
• Antihypertensives	Antihypertensives are given to control severe hypertension and maintain cerebral perfusion.
• Osmotic diuretics	Osmotic diuretics are given to decrease ICP by reducing cerebral edema.
■ Raise the head of the bed no higher than 30 degrees.	Current evidence suggests that elevating the head of the bed reduces ICP by increasing cerebral venous outflow. This position may also reduce cerebral perfusion and contribute to an increased risk for cerebral infarction. QSEN: Evidence-based practice.
■ Keep the patient's head and neck in a neutral position.	This position promotes venous drainage from the brain and decreases ICP.
■ Avoid unnecessary care activities.	Frequent stimulation of the patient can serve as a noxious stimulus and increases brain activity and ICP. Clustering care activities in a short period also increases ICP. QSEN: Safety.
▲ Maintain normothermia with antipyretics, antibiotics, and a cooling blanket.	Controlling fever reduces the metabolic demands of the brain and reduces ICP.
▲ Maintain the patient's volume status by replacing or restricting fluids, as prescribed.	Fluid balance will be adjusted to reduce cerebral edema and prevent a hypercoagulable state.

Neurological Care Plans

NANDA-I NDx Risk for Ineffective Airway Clearance

Common Risk Factors

Neuromuscular impairment
Retained secretions
Airway obstruction

Common Expected Outcome

Patient maintains clear, open airways, as evidenced by normal breath sounds, normal rate and depth of respirations, and ability to cough up secretions after treatments and deep breaths.

NOC Outcome
Respiratory Status: Airway Patency
NIC Interventions
Cough Enhancement; Airway Management; Airway Suctioning

■ = Independent ▲ = Interprofessional Collaboration

Ongoing Assessment	
Actions/Interventions	**Rationales**
■ Monitor the patient's respiratory rate and rhythm, breath sounds, and ability to handle secretions.	Airway obstruction may occur with stroke as a result of impaired cranial nerve function leading to diminished airway protective reflexes and impaired chewing and swallowing. Weakness of the hypoglossal nerve may allow the tongue to fall back in the pharynx and obstruct the airway. Diminished cough and gag reflexes increase the risk for aspiration of oral secretions and food. QSEN: Safety.
■ Check for the presence of a gag reflex and dysphagia.	Brainstem strokes may diminish cranial nerve function and cause impaired function of airway protective reflexes. An impaired gag reflex increases the risk for aspiration and airway obstruction. Impaired swallowing may occur with stroke. The use of a formal dysphagia screening protocol significantly decreases the risk for aspiration pneumonia. The Joint Commission quality indicators for Stroke Center Certification include screening all patients with stroke for dysphagia before oral intake. This is a safety issue to prevent aspiration pneumonia. QSEN: Evidence-based practice; Safety.

Therapeutic Interventions	
Actions/Interventions	**Rationales**
■ Position the patient upright.	This position reduces the work of breathing and promotes more effective coughing to promote airway patency.
■ If the patient is comatose, use an oropharyngeal airway.	An artificial airway keeps the tongue from obstructing the airway. Cranial nerve involvement (hypoglossal nerve) may cause unilateral weakness and tongue deviation.
■ Encourage deep breathing and coughing.	Coughing is the most helpful way to remove most secretions. The patient may be unable to perform coughing independently. The sitting position and splinting the abdomen promote more effective coughing by increasing abdominal pressure and upward diaphragmatic movement.
■ Suction the mouth and airways to remove secretions.	Impaired cranial nerve function may result in decreased cough effectiveness. Impaired swallowing may lead to the aspiration of oral secretions and airway obstruction. Suctioning helps the patient more effectively manage airway secretions. QSEN: Patient-centered care.
▲ Provide respiratory support:	These nursing actions reduce the risk of harm from airway obstruction. QSEN: Safety.
• Administer supplemental oxygen.	This measure reduces hypoxemia, which can cause cerebral vasodilation and increased intracranial pressure.
• Anticipate endotracheal or tracheal intubation.	The patient with a persistent decreased level of consciousness may require intubation to optimize airway clearance.

Neurological Care Plans

NDx **Impaired Physical Mobility**

Common Related Factors

Alteration in cognitive function
Musculoskeletal impairment
Neuromuscular impairment
Insufficient muscle strength
Imposed restrictions of movement, including mechanical and medical protocol
Insufficient knowledge of mobility strategies

Defining Characteristics

Impaired ability to reposition self in bed
Impaired ability to turn from side to side
Impaired ability to move between sitting and supine positions
Impaired ability to move between long sitting and supine positions
Impaired ability to move between prone and supine positions

Common Expected Outcomes

Patient performs physical activity independently or within limits of impaired muscle function.
Patient demonstrates use of adaptive techniques that promote ambulation and transferring.
Patient is free of complications of immobility, as evidenced by intact skin, absence of thrombophlebitis, normal bowel pattern, and clear breath sounds.

NOC Outcomes

Ambulation; Mobility; Body Positioning: Self-Initiated; Transfer Performance; Ambulation

NIC Interventions

Exercise Therapy: Muscle Control; Exercise Therapy: Balance; Fall Prevention; Self-Care Assistance: Transfer

Ongoing Assessment

Actions/Interventions

■ Assess the patient's ability to move and change position, to transfer and walk, to perform ROM to all joints, for fine muscle movement, and for gross muscle movements.

■ Observe for activities or situations that increase or decrease muscle tone.

■ Monitor the patient's skin integrity for areas of blanching or redness.

■ Evaluate the patient for safe patient handling and movement, using standardized tool if available.
  • Ability of patient to provide assistance (independent; partial assist; dependent)
  • Weight-bearing capability (full, partial, none)
  • Upper-extremity strength (yes/no)
  • Ability of patient to cooperate and follow instructions (cooperative; unpredictable)
  • Height/weight/BMI (body mass index)
  • Special circumstances likely to affect transfer or repositioning tasks (e.g., amputation, abdominal wound, history of falls, fractures, tube insertion)
  • Specific physician orders or physical therapy recommendations that relate to transferring or repositioning patients (e.g., hip abduction during transfer)

Rationales

The patient may have differing degrees of involvement on the affected side. Paralysis, paresis, and sensory loss are contralateral to the side of the brain affected by the stroke. In the early phase of stroke recovery the patient may be completely immobile. As brain recovery progresses, paresis or paralysis may be limited to one side of the body or just one extremity. QSEN: Patient-centered care.

Initially muscles demonstrate hyporeflexia, which later progresses to hyperreflexia. Activities that cause the patient to have a spastic response can be postponed until later in recovery.

Impaired mobility increases the risk for skin breakdown. Early identification of stage 1 pressure ulcers allows for the prompt initiation of measures to relieve pressure and promote skin integrity. QSEN: Safety.

Patient handling and movement activities are a basic part of nursing care. Use of a patient assessment tool can provide a standardized way to assess patients and make appropriate decisions about how to safely perform high-risk tasks, which promote mobility and prevent injury to the patient and care providers. QSEN: Evidence-based practice; Safety.

Neurological Care Plans

■ = Independent   ▲ = Interprofessional Collaboration

Actions/Interventions

- Refer to a safe patient handling and movement algorithm if available, for example:
  - Transfer to and from bed to chair, toilet
  - Lateral transfer to and from bed to stretcher
  - Reposition in bed: side to side, up in bed
  - Reposition in chair
  - Transfer a patient up from floor
  - Bariatric (BMI > 50) handling of above examples

- ▲ Collaborate with members of the interprofessional health team to evaluate the need for ambulatory aids (e.g., single point cane, quad cane, crutches, walker).

- ▲ Collaborate with members of the interprofessional health team to evaluate the need for home assistance.

Rationales

Best practices algorithms or decision tools help nurses assess patient needs to determine the technique, equipment, and number of staff required for performing high-risk patient handling tasks. The Veterans Health Administration provides algorithms for selecting the right combination of equipment and personnel needed to handle or move patients safely. A sample algorithm is available at www.visn8.med.va.gov/visn8/patientsafetycenter/safePt Handling/default.asp. QSEN: Evidence-based practice.

A physical therapist can evaluate the patient's need for ambulation assistive devices. Proper use of canes, walkers, and other assistance can promote activity and reduce the danger of falls. The specific aid required depends on the amount of weight bearing that is tolerated, and the ability of the patient to balance safely. QSEN: Teamwork and collaboration.

Obtaining appropriate assistance for the patient can ensure safe and proper progression of activity through the rehabilitation phase of care and discharge planning to an appropriate setting (home vs. long-term care). Social workers, physical therapists, occupational therapists, and home care nurses can evaluate the patient's needs and the home environment. QSEN: Teamwork and collaboration.

Therapeutic Interventions

Actions/Interventions

- Change the position of the patient at least every 2 hours, keeping track of the position changes with a turning schedule.

- Perform active and passive ROM exercises in all extremities several times daily. Increase functional activities as strength improves and the patient is medically stable.

- Perform activities in a quiet environment with few distractions.

- Teach the patient and family exercises and transfer techniques.

Rationales

Position changes optimize circulation to all tissues and relieve pressure. Patients may not feel increases in pressure or have the ability to adjust positions. A loss of motor control can contribute to abnormal posturing. QSEN: Safety.

ROM activities preserve muscle strength and prevent contractures, especially in spastic extremities. Early mobilization and ROM exercises should begin as soon as the patient is stable and no longer requires intensive care. QSEN: Patient-centered care.

Impaired cognitive function that occurs with stroke may decrease the patient's attention span and concentration during mobility activities. The patient may be easily distracted, resulting in an increased risk for falls. QSEN: Safety.

Once medically stable, the patient may have long-term deficits such as altered spatial perception and motor strength. Exercise will increase strength and endurance, promote the patient's use of the affected side, and promote transfer safety. On discharge, the patient and family will need to continue an exercise program to maintain the patient's mobility. QSEN: Patient-centered care.

Actions/Interventions

- Encourage the appropriate use of assistive devices. Use gait belts for safety as indicated.

- Use pressure-relieving devices on the bed and chair.
- Initiate rehabilitation techniques in the hospital setting as soon as medically possible.

For balance and coordination problems:
- Assist the patient in performing movements or tasks. Begin with tasks that require a small range of movements and encourage control (e.g., sitting upright and maintaining balance).

- Encourage focusing on proximal muscle control initially and then distal muscle control, such as beginning with limb positioning and progressing to self-feeding and writing.
- Ensure that the center of gravity is over the pelvis or equally distributed over a stance for sitting and standing activities; provide a safe environment for these activities.
- Teach the patient and family exercises and techniques to improve balance and coordination.
- Reinforce safety precautions with the patient and family.

For increased muscle tone (spasticity):
- Instruct the family in the concepts of spasticity and ways to reduce tone.

- Perform muscle-stretching activities in gentle, rhythmical motions.
- ▲ Apply splinting devices to spastic extremities as prescribed, with ongoing assessment for increasing tone.

Rationales

Crutches, canes, or walkers may be provided to assist the patient with mobility. These aids can compensate for impaired function and increase level of activity. The patient should wear a gait belt for safety so a member of the interprofessional health team or family member can guide the patient during transfer and ambulation to reduce the risk for falling. The goal for using assistive devices is to promote safety, increase mobility, prevent falls, and conserve energy. However, some patients may refuse to use assistive devices because they attract attention to a disability. Additional home evaluation may be needed to promote a safe environment. QSEN: Safety.

These devices decrease the risk for pressure ulcer development.

Early rehabilitation in the medically stable patient prevents further systemic deterioration and facilitates the transition to long-term rehabilitation.

Mobility interventions follow a pattern of progressive activity for the patient with a stroke. Activities to encourage balance are the first step and begin with the patient sitting on the side of the bed. As muscle tone improves and the patient gains some voluntary muscle control, the focus shifts to activities that support transfer from the bed to a chair and finally ambulation. QSEN: Patient-centered care.

Larger muscle groups are easier to focus on and control.

Patients may have impaired righting reflexes and a wide-base stance. Spatial deficits make it difficult for patients to determine their position in space. QSEN: Safety.

Support from significant others will encourage compliance and success.

Spatial deficits, impaired judgment, and a loss of motor function increase the patient's risk for falls, perceptual accidents (bumping into things), wandering, and impulsive behavior. QSEN: Safety.

Spasticity is a sign of improvement. Muscles that remain flaccid are not likely to recover. Spasticity will gradually diminish as the control of muscles is regained. As spasticity decreases, a phenomenon known as synergy often occurs. Synergy is the involuntary movement of part of an extremity after an initial voluntary movement of the whole extremity.

This approach reduces the stimuli that contribute to muscle spasticity.

Devices are used to prevent muscle shortening that occurs with chronic flexion. This approach helps prevent contractures. QSEN: Safety.

Neurological Care Plans

■ = Independent ▲ = Interprofessional Collaboration

NANDA-I NDx Risk for Impaired Verbal Communication

Common Risk Factors

Physiological condition (e.g., left brain hemisphere stroke, weakened orofacial musculoskeletal system)
Insufficient stimuli

Common Expected Outcome

Patient uses a form of communication to get needs met and to relate effectively with people and his or her environment.

NOC Outcomes
Communication: Expressive; Communication: Receptive; Information Processing
NIC Interventions
Active Listening; Communication Enhancement: Hearing Deficit; Communication Enhancement: Speech Deficit

---

Ongoing Assessment

Actions/Interventions	Rationales
■ Assess the patient's verbal communication ability.	The patient with expressive forms of dysphasia will have difficulty finding words. Speech will be nonfluent, with use of single words or short phrases to communicate ideas. Writing will be difficult. The patient with receptive forms of dysphasia will have fluent speech but produce meaningless language. Rhythm, cadence, and articulation are normal. The patient is unable to correct errors in speech, such as words that sound alike or have similar meaning. QSEN: Patient-centered care.
■ Assess the patient's ability to comprehend language.	Verbal comprehension is usually intact with expressive dysphasia. Some patients with expressive dysphasia may experience changes in reading comprehension. The patient with receptive dysphasia has impaired verbal and reading comprehension.
■ Assess the function of facial and hypoglossal cranial nerves.	Weakness of the tongue and facial muscles necessary for speech contribute to dysarthria. The patient will have difficulty forming clear sounds and have slurred speech.
■ Assess the patient's energy level.	Fatigue and shortness of breath can make communication more difficult for the patient.

Therapeutic Interventions

Actions/Interventions	Rationales
■ Acknowledge the patient's frustration with impaired communication.	The inability to express needs or feelings is most distressing to patients. The staff needs to be sensitive to the dignity of the patient. QSEN: Patient-centered care.
■ Minimize the stimuli in the environment.	Communication can be facilitated and distractions minimized by turning off the television or radio, or by closing the door.
■ Provide clear, simple directions.	The patient with dysphasia requires directions to be repeated frequently. Tasks need to be explained in very simple steps and presented one at a time.

---

 evolve For additional care plans, go to http://evolve.elsevier.com/Gulanick/.

Actions/Interventions

- Incorporate multimodality input, such as music, song, and visual demonstration.
- Use written materials (if appropriate).

- Use prompting cues, such as gestures or holding an object that is being discussed.
- Allow adequate time for the patient's response.

- Provide opportunities for spontaneous conversation.

- Anticipate the patient's needs until an alternative means of communication can be established.

- Provide reality orientation and focus attention, but avoid constantly correcting errors.
- ▲ Collaborate with a speech therapist.

- Encourage the family to communicate with the patient; explain the type of dysphasia and methods of communication that can be tried.

- Provide the patient with feedback about any progress made with verbal communication.

Rationales

These different inputs enhance the function of the intact speech-language areas of the brain.

These materials (e.g., communication board with pictures, numbers, words, and/or alphabet) supplement auditory input. If the patient has homonymous hemianopia, place material in the unaffected field of vision. Homonymous hemianopia affects the field of vision in both eyes, opposite the side of the brain affected by the stroke.

Visual cueing can enhance the patient's understanding of verbal messages.

If the patient feels rushed, communication problems are worsened. The patient needs more time to cognitively process information and formulate a verbal response.

The patient needs frequent opportunities to talk without the expectation of a desired outcome. This method decreases the patient's anxiety about communication abilities.

The nurse should plan enough time to attend to all the details of patient care. Care measures may take longer to complete in the presence of a communication deficit.

Constant correction of communication errors increases the patient's frustration, anxiety, and anger.

A comprehensive interprofessional plan of care may be required to improve the patient's communication ability. QSEN: Teamwork and collaboration.

Consistency in the approach by professional caregivers and family members promotes more effective communication for the patient. Family members may need reminders to let the patient respond rather than talking for the patient.

Positive feedback increases confidence and facilitates the patient's ongoing efforts to communicate verbally.

NDx Risk for Disturbed Sensory Perception (Tactile)

Common Risk Factor
Stroke within the sensory transmission and/or integration pathways of the brain

Common Expected Outcome
Patient's skin remains free of injuries, including pressure ulcers.

NOC Outcomes
Risk Detection; Risk Control
NIC Intervention
Peripheral Sensation Management

Ongoing Assessment

Actions/Interventions
- Assess the patient's ability to sense light touch, pinpricks, and temperature. Touch the skin lightly with a pin, cotton ball, or hot or cold object, and ask the patient to describe the sensation and point to where the touch occurred.

Rationales
Early assessment determines the level of alteration and identifies specific areas of risk. Tactile deficits increase the risk for injury related to the patient's inability to sense deep pressure, pain, or temperature. QSEN: Safety.

■ = Independent ▲ = Interprofessional Collaboration

Neurological Care Plans

Actions/Interventions

■ Using the patient's toes or fingers, assess his or her position sense (ability to sense whether the joint is moved in an upward or downward position).

Rationales

The loss of position sense occurs in patients with strokes affecting the anterior cerebral artery, basilar artery, and posterior cerebral artery. Spatial-perceptual deficits increase the patient's risk for injury.

Therapeutic Interventions

Actions/Interventions

■ Perform regular skin inspections, and instruct the patient and family members in techniques to do the same. Explain the consequences of prolonged pressure on the skin.

■ Provide tactile stimulation to the affected limbs using rough a cloth or hand, and instruct the patient or family in the methods used.

■ Explain how a stimulus might feel (e.g., cool water, soft flannel).

■ Teach the patient to check the temperature of water with the unaffected side before using the water (thermal screening).

■ Instruct the patient to regularly move the affected limbs.

■ Teach the patient and family strategies to modify the home environment.

▲ Collaborate with members of the interprofessional health team to help the patient and family learn adaptive skills for sensory deficits.

Rationales

Pressure on the affected side should last no longer than 30 minutes. The inability to sense pressure increases the risk for skin breakdown. QSEN: Safety.

The frequent application of stimuli helps patients learn to recognize sensations.

Verbal descriptions improve the patient's understanding of the stimulus.

Diminished temperature sensation, especially for heat, increases the risk for accidental burn injury. QSEN: Safety.

Movement promotes circulation. An impaired sensitivity to pain or numbness increases the likelihood of prolonged stationary positioning.

Optimal safety can be achieved by modification in the environment. Some modifications include lowering the temperature setting on the hot water heater, moving sharp-edged furniture out of areas and pathways frequently used by the patient, and lighting hallways. QSEN: Safety.

Patients and caregivers need to learn adaptive skills to reduce the risk for injury. A physical therapist or occupational therapist can provide knowledge and teach adaptive skills for use in the home environment. QSEN: Teamwork and collaboration.

NANDA-I
NDx Risk for Unilateral Neglect

Common Risk Factor

Stroke in the nondominant hemisphere or the dominant right side

Common Expected Outcomes

Patient incurs no injuries as a result of deficit.
Patient can cross midline with eyes and unaffected arm.
Patient observes and touches affected side during ADLs.
Patient begins to wash, dress, and eat with attention to both sides.
Patient and family verbalize cognitive awareness of deficit.

NOC Outcomes
Body Positioning: Self-Initiated; Self-Care:
  Activities of Daily Living (ADLs); Personal
  Safety Behavior
NIC Intervention
Unilateral Neglect Management

Ongoing Assessment

Actions/Interventions	Rationales
■ Assess the patient's response to touch, pain, and temperature.	Assessment data determine the actual level of sensation for comparison with how the patient uses the affected side. Use may be different from actual ability. QSEN: Patient-centered care.
■ Perform a visual fields confrontation test.	The patient may not be able to see on the affected side (hemianopia). Injury to the parietal lobe in the nondominant hemisphere makes it difficult for the patient to recognize the contralateral side of the body, even if visual fields are intact.
■ Observe the patient's performance of ADLs.	This information determines the patient's recognition of the affected side. The patient may not, for example, bathe the affected side, forgetting that it is there.
■ Assess for distorted spatial relationships.	Impaired spatial awareness and proprioception interferes with the patient's awareness of the affected side of the body.

Therapeutic Interventions

Actions/Interventions	Rationales
■ Approach the patient from the unaffected side when the patient initially regains consciousness.	Approaching the patient from the unaffected side increases awareness of the presence of people in the environment and facilitates the ability to interact with others. QSEN: Patient-centered care.
■ As the patient becomes more alert, approach from the affected side while calling the patient's name.	This approach will enhance the patient's awareness of the affected side of the body. QSEN: Patient-centered care.
■ Ensure a safe environment by placing a call light on the patient's unaffected side.	Hemianopia limits the patient's ability to see objects in the affected visual field. If the patient cannot find the call light, he or she may attempt to get up without assistance. This behavior increases the risk for falls. QSEN: Safety.
■ Provide tactile stimulation to the affected side.	Frequent stimulus application increases short-term memory of sensation.
■ Place all food in small quantities, arranged simply on a plate.	This approach diminishes spatial and visual deficits. Small quantities make it easier to delineate foods because of the space between food items.
■ Attach a watch or bright bracelet to the affected arm.	This technique draws the patient's attention to the affected side.
■ Encourage the patient to wash the affected side of the body and to dress the affected side of the body first.	This approach to ADLs increases the patient's awareness of the affected side of the body. Increased tactile and visual awareness of the affected side promotes the neural perception and integration of external stimuli.
■ Practice drawing and copying figures with the patient.	These activities help develop fine motor skills and relearn spatial relationships.
■ Draw a bright mark on the sides of a newspaper or book when the patient is reading.	This technique cues the end of a line and the return for the next line.
■ Teach compensatory strategies such as visual scanning (turning the head to visualize the entire area).	The patient needs to learn strategies to reduce the chance of injury and increase visual awareness of the entire field of vision. QSEN: Safety.
▲ Collaborate with members of the interprofessional health team.	Physical and occupational therapists can help the patient learn adaptive skills to promote increased self-care and decrease the risk for injury. QSEN: Teamwork and collaboration.

Neurological Care Plans

■ = Independent ▲ = Interprofessional Collaboration

NDx Deficient Knowledge

Common Related Factors

Alteration in cognitive functioning
Insufficient information
Insufficient interest in learning
Insufficient knowledge of resources
Alteration in memory
Misinformation presented by others

Defining Characteristics

Insufficient knowledge
Inaccurate follow-through of instruction
Inaccurate performance on a test
Inappropriate behavior

Common Expected Outcome

Patient and/or caregivers verbalize understanding of stroke process, treatment, rehabilitation, and potential outcomes.

NOC Outcomes
Knowledge: Disease Process; Knowledge: Treatment Regimen; Knowledge: Medication; Knowledge: Personal Safety
NIC Interventions
Health Literacy Enhancement; Learning Facilitation; Teaching: Disease Process; Teaching: Prescribed Exercise

Ongoing Assessment

Actions/Interventions	Rationales
▪ Determine the stroke-related deficits that may affect learning.	The teaching plan will be individualized based on the patient's ability to comprehend and remember new information. Cognitive impairments and communication deficits may limit the patient's attention span, concentration, and understanding of new information.
▪ Assess the patient's and family's perception of the diagnosis and care needs.	Patients are more receptive to learning if their own identified needs and goals are being met. Teaching standardized content that the patient already knows wastes valuable time and hinders critical learning. Adults learn material that is important to them. During the acute stages, the family or significant others may require the most teaching. QSEN: Patient-centered care.

Therapeutic Interventions

Actions/Interventions	Rationales
▪ Discuss the type of stroke, progress, treatments, rehabilitation, and preventive measures.	Explaining physical and mental changes that occur with stroke helps reduce anxiety and limit the onset of depression. Knowing what to expect during stroke recovery promotes effective coping and the motivation to participate in the rehabilitation process. QSEN: Patient-centered care.
▪ Prepare the patient and family for possible changes in patient behavior and judgment.	Patients may experience mood changes and depression within 6 months of the initial stroke injury. Emotional lability may continue for several months.
▪ Include the caregiver in the rehabilitation process to learn and assist with care, as well as to provide emotional support for the patient's efforts.	Almost all stroke victims will have some degree of disability and will require assistance and emotional support. Family members need to understand how a stroke may influence their social and personal roles and activities.

Actions/Interventions

- Teach measures to manage or reduce the risk factors for repeated stroke.

- Provide education concerning long-term medication use for stroke prevention.

- Encourage the use of community resources and support groups.

▲ Refer the patient and family to members of the interprofessional health team for counseling and social services.

Rationales

Knowing the risk factors is the first step in controlling them and decreasing the chance of further stroke. Risk factors include hypertension, heart disease, smoking, polycythemia, alcohol use, obesity, hypercholesterolemia, diabetes mellitus, and sedentary lifestyle. QSEN: Safety.

Clinical practice guidelines from the American Heart Association and American Stroke Association recommend daily use of antiplatelet medications for recurrent stroke prevention. These medications may include low-dose aspirin combined with extended release dipyridamole, and clopidogrel. Oral anticoagulants may be indicated for patients with embolic strokes from atrial thrombi. The addition of cholesterol-lowering statin drugs may benefit patients with thrombotic strokes from cerebral atherosclerosis. QSEN: Evidence-based practice.

The family needs information about how community resources can promote effective coping and decrease feelings of caregiving as a burden. Stroke victims are often older people whose disabilities may be overwhelming to an equally elderly or frail spouse. The responsibility of caregiving can increase fear and stress for the family member.

Some patients may experience depression that interferes with learning. Professional counseling may be necessary to facilitate more effective learning by the patient and family. The involvement of social services will facilitate planning for rehabilitation and the return home. QSEN: Teamwork and collaboration.

Related Care Plans

Anxiety, Chapter 2
Constipation, Chapter 2
Decreased intracranial adaptive capacity, Chapter 2
Imbalanced nutrition: Less than body requirements, Chapter 2
Ineffective coping, Chapter 2
Ineffective sexuality pattern, Chapter 2
Risk for aspiration, Chapter 2
Risk for falls, Chapter 2
Risk for impaired skin integrity, Chapter 2
Self-care deficit, Chapter 2
Situational low self-esteem, Chapter 2

Neurological Care Plans

■ = Independent   ▲ = Interprofessional Collaboration

Traumatic Brain Injury

Head Trauma; Closed Head Trauma; Skull Fracture; Subdural Hematoma; Concussion

Traumatic brain injury (TBI) is a leading cause of death in the United States for people 1 year to 42 years of age. An estimated 3 million people suffer TBIs every year. About half of all severe TBIs result from accidents involving automobiles, motorcycles, bicycles, and pedestrians. People who do not use appropriate safety equipment (e.g., seat belts, helmets) have a significant increase in TBI with accidents. Approximately 20% of TBIs are associated with violence, such as blunt force trauma and firearms. Recent evidence identifies TBI from concussions sustained by athletes playing contact sports and military personnel during combat. The severity of TBI is defined by the traumatic coma data bank on the basis of the Glasgow Coma Scale (GCS): Severe brain injury = GCS score of 8 or less; moderate brain injury = GCS score of 9 to 12. Most brain injuries are blunt (closed) trauma to the brain. Secondary injuries associated with TBI include scalp lacerations, skull fractures, increased intracranial pressure, extracerebral bleeding, and intracerebral bleeding. Patients with moderate to severe TBI are usually observed in a critical care unit where immediate intervention can be achieved. Most deaths occur in the first few hours after brain trauma as a result of internal bleeding or worsening cerebral edema. Patients with minor TBI (concussion) are most often treated in the Emergency Department and discharged with instructions for observation at home. Symptoms of mild TBI usually resolve within 48 to 72 hours. Postconcussion syndrome occurs when symptoms persist longer than 72 hours. Older adults are most often affected with postconcussion syndrome, characterized by decreased neurological function 2 weeks to 2 months after the initial injury and often caused by slow subdural bleeding. This care plan focuses on moderate to severe TBI in the acute care setting.

Neurological Care Plans

NANDA-I NDx Decreased Intracranial Adaptive Capacity

Common Related Factors
Brain injury (e.g., cerebrovascular impairment, trauma)
Decreased cerebral perfusion

Defining Characteristics
Repeated increase in intracranial pressure (ICP)
≥ 10 mm Hg for ≥ 5 minutes following external stimuli
Baseline ICP ≥ 10 mm Hg
Wide amplitude ICP waveform

Common Expected Outcome
Patient maintains optimal cerebral tissue perfusion, as evidenced by stable neurological status, ICP less than 10 mm Hg, and cerebral perfusion pressure (CPP) from 60 to 90 mm Hg.

NOC Outcomes
Neurological Status: Consciousness; Neurological Status: Autonomic; Tissue Perfusion: Cerebral; Fluid Balance

NIC Interventions
ICP Monitoring; Neurologic Monitoring; Cerebral Edema Management; Cerebral Perfusion Promotion

Ongoing Assessment

Actions/Interventions	Rationales
■ Assess the patient's neurological status including the level of consciousness (LOC) pupil size, symmetry, and reaction to light; extraocular movement; gaze preference; motor function; abnormal Babinski reflex; and postural rigidity.	Early detection of changes is necessary to prevent permanent neurological dysfunction. Deteriorating neurological signs indicate increased cerebral ischemia. A decreased LOC is the first sign of increased ICP. This change in LOC usually presents as increasing restlessness, irritability, or agitation. The patient may become disoriented and confused. Changes in pupil size, symmetry, and reactivity to light will occur with increased ICP. When the patient's head is turned there will be lack of conjugate gaze and absence of the oculocephalic reflex response (doll's eyes). The patient may exhibit postural rigidity as ICP rises. These postural changes may be flexion (decorticate) or extension (decerebrate). As ICP increases the patient will exhibit fanning of the toes with dorsiflexion of the great toe when testing the Babinski reflex. QSEN: Safety.
■ Assess for rhinorrhea (cerebrospinal fluid [CSF] drainage from nose), otorrhea (CSF drainage from ear), Battle's sign (ecchymosis over the mastoid process), and raccoon eyes (periorbital ecchymosis).	These signs may indicate frontal, orbital, or basal skull fractures.
■ Evaluate the presence or absence of protective reflexes (e.g., swallowing, gagging, blinking, and coughing).	A loss of protective reflexes occurs with increasing ICP and puts the patient at risk for injuries such as aspiration or corneal abrasions. QSEN: Safety.
■ Monitor the patient's vital signs.	This assessment reduces harm by identifying early changes in intracranial pressure and guiding specific interventions. Continually increasing ICP results in life-threatening hemodynamic changes; early recognition is essential to survival. As compensatory mechanisms fail to regulate ICP, the patient may exhibit a full, bounding pulse with a gradually slowing rate. The BP begins to show a widening pulse pressure. The respiratory rate begins to slow, and the patient may develop breathing pattern changes such as Cheyne-Stokes breathing. Core body temperature may be unstable as increasing ICP exerts pressure on the hypothalamus. QSEN: Safety.
▲ Monitor ICP with an appropriate measurement device. Report ICP greater than 10 mm Hg for 5 minutes. Serially monitor ICP pressure and waveforms.	Insertion of a ventriculostomy catheter is the traditional method for monitoring ICP. Newer methods use fiberoptic catheters that measure not only ICP but also cerebral oxygenation. These direct measurements serve as optimal guides for therapy. QSEN: Safety.
■ Analyze changes in ICP waveforms.	Waveform analysis provides information to identify patients experiencing changes in brain compliance and decreased intracranial adaptive capacity. Changes in the pulse component (P1, P2, P3) of the ICP waveform are associated with alterations in arterial pulsations in the large cerebral vessels. Increased ICP and decreased intracranial compliance produce elevations in the amplitude of the pulse component waveforms. QSEN: Evidence-based practice.
■ Calculate the CPP (CPP = Mean systemic arterial pressure − ICP).	CPP should be 90 to 100 mm Hg. There is little or no perfusion if CPP is less than 50 mm Hg.

Neurological Care Plans

■ = Independent ▲ = Interprofessional Collaboration

Actions/Interventions

- ▲ Monitor arterial blood gases and/or pulse oximetry (recommended parameters: Pao₂ greater than 80 mm Hg and Paco₂ less than 35 mm Hg with normal ICP). If the patient's lungs are being hyperventilated to decrease ICP, Paco₂ should be between 25 and 30 mm Hg.
- ■ Assess for pain, fever, and shivering.

Rationales

A $Paco_2$ less than 20 mm Hg may decrease cerebral blood flow (CBF) because of profound vasoconstriction that produces hypoxia. $Paco_2$ greater than 45 mm Hg induces vasodilation with increase in CBF, which may trigger increase in ICP. QSEN: Safety.

These symptoms increase CBF and ICP.

Therapeutic Interventions

Actions/Interventions

- ■ Report a deteriorating neurological status immediately to members of the health care team.

- ▲ Elevate the head of the bed 30 degrees, and keep the head in a neutral alignment.

- ▲ Limit nursing and medical procedures to those that are absolutely necessary.
- ■ Reorient the patient to the environment, and provide familiar objects and pictures.
- ▲ Administer mannitol, as ordered.

- ■ Avoid Valsalva maneuvers.

- ■ Hyperventilate and hyperoxygenate before suctioning the endotracheal (ET) tube or trachea.

Rationales

Immediate surgical intervention may be necessary to preserve cerebral function. QSEN: Safety; Teamwork and collaboration.

Elevation promotes venous outflow and contributes to a decrease in cerebral blood volume and ICP. Exceptions to this positioning may include shock and cervical spine injuries associated with head trauma. A neutral head position prevents venous obstruction.

Both prescribed and unnecessary procedures can serve as a noxious stimulus that can further increase ICP.

These measures decrease anxiety and help maintain stable ICP levels.

Mannitol is a hyperosmotic agent that should be used carefully because it can induce cerebral ischemia. It is contraindicated with hypovolemic symptoms. A diuretic response can be anticipated within 30 to 60 minutes. A Foley catheter should be in place. An IV filter should be used when mannitol is infused. Electrolytes, osmolality, and serum glucose must be monitored during mannitol infusion.

Valsalva maneuver, as occurs with straining, increases intrathoracic pressure and CBF, thereby increasing ICP.

This measure avoids hypoxemia, hypercapnia, and hypotension, which contribute to increased ICP. QSEN: Safety.

NANDA-I
NDx **Risk for Deficient Fluid Volume**

Common Risk Factors

Active fluid loss (diuresis secondary to use of hyperosmotic agents)

Compromised regulatory mechanisms (diabetes insipidus [DI])

Inadequate fluid intake

Common Expected Outcome

Patient is normovolemic as evidenced by systolic BP greater than or equal to 90 mm Hg (or patient's baseline), absence of orthostasis, HR 60 to 100 beats/min, urine output greater than 30 mL/hr, normal skin turgor, and urine specific gravity between 1.005 and 1.025.

NOC Outcomes
Fluid Balance; Hydration

NIC Interventions
Fluid Monitoring; Fluid Management; Fluid Resuscitation

Neurological Care Plans

Ongoing Assessment

Actions/Interventions	Rationales
■ Monitor the patient's fluid intake and urine output. Report a urine output greater than 200 mL/hr for 2 consecutive hours.	DI occurs when the renal tubules are unable to conserve water because of decreased antidiuretic hormone (ADH). Disruption of the neurohypophyseal system may occur with traumatic brain injury and decrease the production and release of ADH. QSEN: Safety.
■ Assess the urine specific gravity.	A decrease in urine specific gravity to less than 1.005 occurs with DI.
▲ Monitor serum and urine electrolytes and osmolarity.	DI causes hypernatremia, increased serum osmolality, and decreased urine osmolality and urine sodium concentration. These direct measurements serve as optimal guides for therapy. QSEN: Evidence-based practice.
■ Monitor for the signs of dehydration (decreased skin turgor, increased HR, decreased BP).	Increased urine volume with DI causes decreased circulatory blood volume and BP. The HR will increase as a compensatory response to the reduced circulatory blood volume.
■ Monitor daily weights.	Polyuria causes weight loss in the patient with DI.

Therapeutic Interventions

Actions/Interventions	Rationales
▲ Replace fluid output as directed.	The patient with DI has intense thirst. Oral intake in response to thirst may correct the problem. IV fluid administration may be needed if the patient is unable to maintain oral fluid intake in response to thirst.
▲ Administer vasopressin as ordered.	Vasopressin is a synthetic ADH that will reduce serum concentration and decrease urine output. Careful monitoring of the urine output and serum sodium and osmolarity is mandatory when vasopressin is administered.

NANDA-I
NDx **Risk for Excess Fluid Volume**

Common Risk Factor

Compromised regulatory mechanism (syndrome of inappropriate antidiuretic hormone [SIADH])

Common Expected Outcome

Patient is normovolemic as evidenced by urine output greater than or equal to 30 mL/hr, balanced intake and output, stable weight (or loss attributed to fluid loss), absence or reduction of edema, HR 60 to 100 beats/min, absence of pulmonary crackles, and urine specific gravity between 1.005 and 1.025.

NOC Outcomes
Fluid Balance; Cardiopulmonary Status
NIC Interventions
Fluid Monitoring; Fluid Management

Neurological Care Plans

■ = Independent ▲ = Interprofessional Collaboration

Neurological Care Plans

Ongoing Assessment

Actions/Interventions	Rationales
■ Assess the patient's fluid intake and urine output, and monitor weight.	SIADH occurs from persistently high levels of circulating antidiuretic hormone (ADH). Urine output will be significantly less than fluid intake. Urine volume may be less than 30 to 40 mL/hr. Weight gain occurs in SIADH without the signs of peripheral edema. This assessment approach reduces harm by identifying early changes in urine output and guiding specific interventions. QSEN: Safety.
▲ Assess serum and urine electrolytes and osmolality.	These tests provide information on fluid volume excess (usually determined by hyponatremia and lowering of serum osmolarity). The secretion of ADH is no longer regulated by changes in plasma osmolarity. These direct measurements serve as optimal guides for therapy. QSEN: Evidence-based practice.
■ Assess for the signs of hyponatremia (confusion, headache, fatigue, vomiting, muscle twitching, or seizures).	These clinical manifestations are associated with hyponatremia. SIADH may cause cerebral edema and increased intracranial pressure (ICP).

Therapeutic Interventions

Actions/Interventions	Rationales
▲ Restrict oral or IV fluids as ordered. In a patient with a nasogastric tube and feedings, normal saline solution can be used for flushing after feedings.	Fluid restriction of 1 to 1.2 L/day usually corrects hyponatremia associated with SIADH. IV D_5W is inappropriate because of excess free water and should not be used for piggyback medications.
▲ If fluid restriction fails to correct hyponatremia, anticipate an order for 3% saline solution infusion given with furosemide (Lasix) and potassium.	Administration of a hypertonic solution may cause cardiac problems from further fluid overload. Furosemide promotes diuresis. Potassium supplementation corrects diuretic-induced potassium excretion.

NANDA-I
NDx Risk for Seizures

Common Risk Factors

Cortical laceration
Intracranial bleeding
Hyponatremia
Hypoxia
Multiple contusions
Penetrating injuries to brain

Common Expected Outcomes

Patient does not sustain injury with seizure activity.
Patient does not experience seizure activity.

NOC Outcomes
Seizure Self-Control; Risk Detection; Risk Control; Medication Response

NIC Interventions
Seizure Precautions; Seizure Management

Ongoing Assessment

Actions/Interventions

- Observe the patient for seizure activity. Record and report the following observations:
  - Time of onset
  - Body part involved; order of involvement and character of movement
  - Tonic-clonic stages
  - Incontinence
  - Duration of seizure
  - Postictal state (e.g., confusion, drowsiness, sleep)

- Monitor for signs of airway obstruction.

Rationales

Any cerebral irritation puts the patient at risk for seizure activity. Seizures occur in about 5% of patients with nonpenetrating traumatic brain injury; the risk is greater with penetrating injuries. Seizures increase cerebral metabolism and oxygen demand. Ischemic injury from the primary trauma can be aggravated by seizure-induced hypoxia. Careful documentation of seizure activity helps in diagnosing the specific type of seizure. Generalized tonic-clonic seizures are more likely to occur with increased intracranial pressure (ICP). QSEN: Evidence-based practice.

Loss of motor control during a seizure can compromise the airway if the tongue falls back into the upper airway. QSEN: Safety.

Therapeutic Interventions

Actions/Interventions

- Implement seizure precautions: side rails up and padded, bed in the low position, head protection if needed.
- ▲ Administer anticonvulsants as directed.

- If a seizure occurs, remain with the patient, do not attempt to put anything in the patient's mouth, and maintain the airway.
- Turn the patient's head to the side, suction, and administer oxygen if needed.

Rationales

These measures reduce the risk for injury during seizure activity. QSEN: Safety.

Phenytoin (Dilantin) can only be mixed in normal saline. Precipitation will be noted when mixed with D_5W. Infuse no faster than 50 mg/min to prevent hypotension.

Inserting objects will often cause more harm, such as broken teeth, soft tissue injury, and airway obstruction. QSEN: Safety.

This position is used to maintain airway patency during the postictal state.

NANDA-I NDx

Risk for Imbalanced Nutrition: Less Than Body Requirements

Common Risk Factors

Inability to ingest foods (facial trauma, decreased level of consciousness)
Insufficient dietary intake

Common Expected Outcome

Patient weighs within 10% of ideal weight range.

NOC Outcomes
Nutritional Status: Food and Fluid Intake;
Nutritional Status: Nutrient Intake

NIC Interventions
Nutritional Monitoring; Nutrition Therapy;
Nutrition Management

Ongoing Assessment

Actions/Interventions

- ▲ Monitor the patient's albumin, protein, glucose, and electrolytes.

Rationales

These laboratory tests are indicative of the patient's general nutritional state and provide a guide for an individualized nutrition plan. QSEN: Patient-centered care.

■ = Independent   ▲ = Interprofessional Collaboration

Neurological Care Plans

Actions/Interventions

- Assess the skin color, turgor, and muscle mass.

- Assess the rate and quality of wound healing.

- Monitor daily weights.

▲ Consult with a speech therapist to evaluate for dysphagia.

Rationales

Dry, flaky skin, tenting, and decreased muscle mass indicate decreased nutritional intake.

Extra calories are needed to maintain basic metabolism plus wound healing.

Changes in weight will occur with nutritional changes. Daily fluctuations occur with shifts in fluid balance. Sustained changes over a week are reflections of nutritional status.

Swallowing and gag reflexes may be impaired as a result of head trauma. Evaluation of swallowing by the speech therapist needs to be done before initiating oral intake. This assessment is done to reduce the risk for aspiration with oral intake. QSEN: Teamwork and collaboration; Safety.

Therapeutic Interventions

Actions/Interventions

▲ Administer tube feedings.

- Maintain the head of the bed at 30 degrees.

- Avoid the insertion of a feeding tube through the nose in a patient with head injury unless the possibility of a basal skull fracture has been excluded.

Rationales

Patients with head injury need about 2000 kcal/day. Patients with multiple trauma may need two to three times that (or more). The enteral route of nutritional support is preferred over the IV route. IV nutritional support requires the placement of a central venous catheter. The central line increases the risk for infection. Hyperglycemia is a complication of total parenteral nutrition that requires frequent blood glucose monitoring and insulin administration.

This nursing action reduces the risk for aspiration with tube feedings. QSEN: Safety.

Basilar fractures often traverse the paranasal sinuses. A feeding tube could penetrate brain tissue through the fracture site.

NANDA-I
NDx Deficient Knowledge

Common Related Factors

Alteration in cognitive functioning
Insufficient information
Insufficient interest in learning
Insufficient knowledge of resources
Alteration in memory
Misinformation presented by others

Defining Characteristics

Insufficient knowledge
Inaccurate follow-through of instruction
Inaccurate performance on a test
Inappropriate behavior

Common Expected Outcome

Patient verbalizes understanding of desired content about traumatic brain injury and performs desired skills.

NOC Outcomes
Knowledge: Disease Process; Knowledge: Treatment Regimen
NIC Interventions
Learning Facilitation; Teaching: Disease Process; Teaching: Procedure/Treatment

---

Ⓔvolve **For additional care plans, go to http://evolve.elsevier.com/Gulanick/.**

Ongoing Assessment

Actions/Interventions	Rationales
■ Assess the patient's knowledge of injury, treatment, and the expected outcome.	Adults bring many life experiences to each learning session. Adults learn best when teaching builds on previous knowledge or experience. This experience is the foundation for an individualized teaching plan. Because most traumatic brain injuries occur as an unexpected accident, the patient and family have no previous experience with this type of injury. QSEN: Patient-centered care.
■ Assess the patient's cognitive function.	Traumatic brain injury can cause impaired short-term memory, decreased attention span, and decreased concentration. These changes can limit the patient's ability to learn new information.

Therapeutic Interventions

Actions/Interventions	Rationales
■ Teach the family about the intensive care unit (ICU) environment.	Traumatic brain injury can result in a life-threatening situation that will produce high levels of anxiety. In addition, the ICU environment may be stressful at first visit. The presence of high-tech equipment is a source of anxiety to most patients and families. A brief explanation of the positive features of these monitoring devices and treatments may reduce their anxiety.
■ Explain treatments or procedures and the equipment used, such as the following: • ICP monitor • IV lines and medications • Cardiopulmonary and oximetry monitors • Feeding tubes and pumps • Mechanical ventilator	The patient with cognitive impairment may have distorted perceptions of the therapeutic equipment. The patient who is disoriented may perceive the equipment as threatening and attempt to remove it. Frequent explanations in simple terms may calm anxiety and promote reality orientation. QSEN: Pateint-centered care.
■ Reinforce information given to the patient or family about the following: • Type of head injury and what brain functions will be affected by the injury • Results of computed tomography (CT) scan, radiographs, magnetic resonance imaging (MRI)	Repetition may be beneficial in retaining new information. Daily updates and explanations can help the patient and family cope with the uncertainty they experience with the long-term rehabilitation.
■ Keep the family up to date with any new changes in condition.	Regular conferences with family caregivers help them become members of the interprofessional rehabilitation team. They can provide insights about the patient's personality and behavior before the injury. QSEN: Patient-centered care.
■ Discuss the role of the physical, occupational, or speech therapist.	Specialized services may be required for recovery. Patient and family members need to understand the roles of members of the health care team.
■ Discuss the need for rehabilitation and home care support, if necessary.	Parents or spouses often become the primary caregivers when the patient is discharged from the rehabilitation setting. They need ongoing support to adapt to the changes in roles and responsibilities.

Neurological Care Plans

■ = Independent   ▲ = Interprofessional Collaboration

Actions/Interventions

- Prepare the patient and family for changes in personality and behavior.
- Provide the family with names and numbers of local support groups, if available.

- Refer the family to social services or financial counselors, as appropriate.

Rationales

It may take months for the patient to recover; some personality changes may be permanent.

Groups that come together for mutual support can be beneficial. These groups often provide best practices for managing care at home and maintaining positive family relationships.

The patient and family may need ongoing support for decisions about financial resources, guardianship, powers of attorney, and living wills. Resources for respite care may help families cope more effectively with responsibilities for patient care. QSEN: Teamwork and collaboration.

Related Care Plans

Decreased intracranial adaptive capacity, Chapter 2
Ineffective airway clearance, Chapter 2
Impaired physical mobility, Chapter 2
Self-care deficit, Chapter 2

Neurological Care Plans

Gastrointestinal and Digestive Care Plans

Bariatric Surgery

Overweight; Obesity; Gastric Banding; Gastric Bypass

Overweight and obesity are major health problems in the United States, and their prevalence is growing globally. Bariatric surgical procedures are usually used for those patients considered morbidly obese with a body mass index (BMI) greater than 40. Patients with a BMI between 35 and 40 may be candidates for this type of surgery if they have other chronic health problems related to their obesity, such as diabetes mellitus, sleep apnea, hypertension, or heart failure. Evidence indicates that these surgical approaches to weight management provide the patient with more long-lasting weight loss compared to nonsurgical approaches such as diet and exercise. In addition, patients usually experience significant improvement in their obesity-related health problems. Gastric banding or stapling surgical techniques restrict the volume of the stomach and therefore decrease the amount of food the patient consumes. Gastric bypass procedures reroute the passage of food through the small intestine to reduce the absorption of food intake. Most bariatric surgery programs include a long-term postoperative program of lifestyle modifications such as eating habits, physical activity, and psychological support.

NANDA-I
NDx **Deficient Knowledge**

Common Related Factors
Insufficient information
Insufficient interest in learning
Insufficient knowledge of resources
Misinformation presented by others

Defining Characteristics
Insufficient knowledge about bariatric surgery
Inappropriate behavior

Common Expected Outcomes
Patient verbalizes understanding of benefits and risks of bariatric surgery.
Patient verbalizes health consequences of continued obesity.

NOC Outcomes
Knowledge: Treatment Procedure; Information Processing
NIC Interventions
Health Literacy Enhancement; Learning Facilitation; Health Education; Teaching: Procedure/Treatment; Teaching: Preoperative

Ongoing Assessment	
Actions/Interventions	**Rationales**
■ Assess the patient's knowledge regarding bariatric surgical procedures.	An individualized teaching plan begins with the patient's understanding of the various surgical procedures for weight loss. Teaching standardized content that the patient already knows wastes valuable time and hinders critical learning. QSEN: Patient-centered care.
■ Assess the patient's motivation for considering bariatric surgery.	A positive motivation for change will enhance the patient's learning of new information. Many patients who seek surgical options are frustrated with repeated failures to sustain weight loss through diet and exercise. These patients may have significant obesity-related health problems. In addition, the patient may be motivated by problems with employment, social interactions, and body image.
■ Determine the patient's self-efficacy to learn and apply new knowledge.	Self-efficacy refers to a person's confidence in his or her ability to perform a behavior. Some lifestyle changes associated with the long-term postoperative care can be difficult for the patient to sustain for the required period of time to achieve successful recovery and weight loss.

Therapeutic Interventions	
Actions/Interventions	**Rationales**
■ Include the family and caregiver in teaching sessions about bariatric surgery.	The patient will be more likely to adhere to the long-term postoperative eating and lifestyle changes when family members are involved in those changes.
■ Teach the patient about the criteria to be a candidate for bariatric surgery.	Most bariatric surgery programs require that candidates have a body mass index (BMI) of 40 or greater than 35 with one or more obesity-related health problems. The patient needs to have been obese for at least 5 years with repeated failures to lose weight by diet and exercise. Patients considered for bariatric surgery need to have stable mental health and social health. Patients need to be willing to adhere to a long-term postoperative program of follow-up care and counseling. If obesity is the result of a treatable endocrine problem, the patient is not a candidate for bariatric surgery. Patients with problems related to substance abuse or major psychiatric disorders may not be suitable candidates for bariatric surgery.
■ Provide the patient with information about bariatric surgical procedures. Information may include:	This information provides the patient with a foundation for making decisions about bariatric surgery and the commitment to long-term follow-up care requirements for weight loss. Surgical options depend on the patient's appropriateness for a procedure and usually according to extensive criteria, such as the extent of obesity, existing complications of obesity, and the likelihood of postprocedure compliance. Patients should be referred to their physicians to discuss the appropriateness of such procedures. The obese patient is at an increased risk for cardiovascular and pulmonary complications with surgical procedures. Many procedures are done using minimally invasive surgery (MIS) techniques. QSEN: Patient-centered care.

Gastrointestinal and Digestive Care Plans

Actions/Interventions	**Rationales**
• Types of procedures:	
• Lipectomy and/or liposuction	These procedures involve the removal of body fat and are considered cosmetic, body-shaping surgeries. The patient needs to understand that removing body fat does not result in long-term weight loss. If eating habits continue after this procedure, the patient will restore the fat that was removed.
• Roux-en-Y gastric bypass	The Roux-en-Y procedure is a type of gastric bypass surgery. The volume capacity of the stomach is reduced. An anastomosis is created directly between the smaller stomach pouch and the jejunum. Weight loss occurs by decreased gastric capacity and some reduced intestinal absorption.
• Biliopancreatic diversion	The biliopancreatic diversion is another type of gastric bypass surgery recommended for patients with a BMI of 50 or higher. A variety of specific surgical techniques are used for this procedure. Approximately 70% of the stomach is removed. The remaining gastric tissue is formed into a sleeve or tube and anastomosed to a portion of the small intestine. Surgical channels are created to allow for the passage of biliary and pancreatic secretions into the intestines. Weight loss occurs by decreased gastric capacity and the significant reduction of intestinal absorption.
• Sleeve gastrectomy	Sleeve gastrectomy is the first part of the biliopancreatic diversion. Most of the stomach is removed, and the remaining tissue is shaped into a sleeve or tube. This procedure may be performed to allow the patient to lose some weight before the biliopancreatic diversion is performed. Weight loss occurs through reduced gastric capacity.
• Gastric banding	Gastric banding uses techniques to partition the stomach into a small upper portion and the larger lower portion. Techniques include inflated, adjustable gastric bands and vertical gastric stapling. Weight loss occurs through reduced gastric capacity. Weight loss tends to be less and occur at a slower rate than with gastric bypass procedures.
• Risks of weight loss surgery	The general risks with bariatric surgery are the same as with any major surgical procedure. Specific risks associated with bariatric surgery include vitamin and mineral deficiencies, fluid volume deficit, gastric ulcers, dumping syndrome, increased risk for cholelithiasis and renal calculi, food intolerances, and hypoglycemia. QSEN: Safety.
■ Teach the patient about the postoperative diet plan.	After surgery, the patient will need to follow a very specific diet and eating plan for about 3 months before he or she begins eating solid foods. The purpose of this diet plan is threefold: to promote healing of the stomach and intestinal suture lines; to help the patient learn to eat smaller amounts of food without distending the smaller stomach pouch; and to promote weight loss. In addition, the diet plan helps the patient learn to avoid the side effects of the bariatric surgery (e.g., dehydration, dumping syndrome, vomiting, blockage of the stomach pouch).

Gastrointestinal and Digestive Care Plans

■ = Independent   ▲ = Interprofessional Collaboration

NANDA-I NDx Risk for Imbalanced Nutrition: Less Than Body Requirements (Postoperative)

Common Risk Factors

Insufficient dietary intake of vitamins, folate, and iron, preoperatively

Inability to absorb nutrients, postoperatively

Common Expected Outcomes

Patient demonstrates understanding of and participates in planned vitamin and iron supplementation.

Patient does not exhibit signs of anemia.

NOC Outcomes

Nutritional Status: Nutrient Intake; Knowledge: Medication

NIC Interventions

Medication Management; Nutritional Monitoring

Ongoing Assessment

Actions/Interventions	**Rationales**
■ Assess the patient for signs of anemia.	Bariatric surgery procedures restrict the volume of food the patient consumes and may alter the absorption of nutrients from the intestine. The patient with a nutritional deficiency anemia may develop fatigue, weakness, shortness of breath, paresthesia, pale skin and mucous membranes, cold extremities, changes in the surface of the tongue, oral lesions, and altered nail growth. QSEN: Safety.
■ Monitor laboratory values for red blood cell (RBC) count, hemoglobin, hematocrit, serum iron, serum ferritin, serum folate, and vitamin B_{12}.	The diagnosis of nutritional deficiency anemia is based on characteristic changes in RBCs, iron, folate, and vitamin B_{12}. The serum values for these indicators will be decreased with nutritional deficiency anemia. QSEN: Safety.
■ Assess the patient for a history of anemia before surgery.	Many obese patients have nutritional deficiency anemias before surgery. These anemias are usually corrected with vitamin and iron replacement therapy before surgery.

Therapeutic Interventions

Actions/Interventions	**Rationales**
■ Teach the patient and family about vitamin and iron supplementation.	Oral vitamin and iron supplementation is part of the dietary plan after bariatric surgery. Vitamin and iron absorption may be decreased if the patient has a malabsorptive type of bariatric surgery. Because food intake is restricted in the first few months after surgery regardless of the type of surgery, the patient is not able to include sufficient food sources for iron, vitamin B_{12}, and folic acid. These nutrients are necessary to support the formation of normal RBCs.
■ Encourage the patient to keep follow-up appointments to monitor for anemia.	Periodic blood work is done during the first year after bariatric surgery to evaluate the patient for anemia.
■ Teach the patient about the symptoms to report to the health care provider.	The patient needs to report the symptoms associated with anemia to ensure prompt treatment. These symptoms include fatigue, weakness, dizziness, pale skin and mucous membranes, shortness of breath, and changes in the hands or feet such as numbness, tingling, or coldness. QSEN: Safety.

Gastrointestinal and Digestive Care Plans

 evolve For additional care plans, go to http://evolve.elsevier.com/Gulanick/.

Risk for Disturbed Body Image

Common Risk Factors

Alteration in self-perception (change in appearance as weight loss begins)

Alteration in body function (due to loose and hanging skin following significant weight loss)

Common Expected Outcome

Patient demonstrates enhanced body image and self-esteem as evidenced by ability to talk about the role weight loss plays in body image disturbance.

NOC Outcomes
Body Image; Self-Esteem

NIC Intervention
Body Image Enhancement

Ongoing Assessment

Action/Intervention	Rationale
■ Assess the patient's perceptions of the changes in body size and shape after surgery.	Most patients experience positive changes in body image and self-esteem as they lose weight after surgery. Evidence suggests that these improvements occur early in the postoperative period and remain stable during the first 2 years after surgery. Areas of dissatisfaction with body image are most often related to loose and hanging skin that occurs with significant weight loss. QSEN: Patient-centered care; Evidence-based practice.

Therapeutic Interventions

Actions/Interventions	Rationales
■ Encourage the patient to explore options to manage skin changes:	Self-esteem is enhanced when the patient feels a sense of control in making decisions about options for managing skin changes. QSEN: Patient-centered care.
• Plastic surgery	Many patients choose plastic and/or reconstructive surgery following weight loss to modify body contours and tighten loose skin. The patient needs to understand that this type of cosmetic surgery may not be covered by health insurance.
• Counseling	The patient may benefit from professional therapy to address body image concerns if plastic surgery is not a realistic option. QSEN: Teamwork and collaboration.
• Clothing	The patient should select clothing that is an appropriate size and does not draw attention to loose, hanging skin.
■ Include significant others in education, planning, and goal setting.	These people will be important sources of ongoing support for the patient as he or she adjusts to changes in body size and shape.
■ Refer the patient to support groups, if desired.	Support groups provide opportunities for sharing concerns and may offer solutions to common problems after bariatric surgery.

Gastrointestinal and Digestive Care Plans

■ = Independent   ▲ = Interprofessional Collaboration

NANDA-I NDx **Risk for Deficient Fluid Volume**

Common Risk Factor

Inadequate fluid intake

Common Expected Outcome

Patient is normovolemic as evidenced by systolic BP 90 mm Hg or greater (or patient's baseline), absence of orthostasis, HR 60 to 100 beats/min, urine output greater than 30 mL/hr, and normal skin turgor.

NOC Outcomes
Fluid Balance; Hydration

NIC Interventions
Fluid Monitoring; Fluid Management

Ongoing Assessment

Actions/Interventions	**Rationales**
■ Assess the patient's fluid intake.	The dietary guidelines most patients follow during the first several weeks after bariatric surgery restrict fluid intake at mealtime to prevent nausea, vomiting, and dumping syndrome. Fluids taken with meals may contribute to feeling full and limit the intake of nutrient-rich foods. Because the stomach pouch is smaller, patients are taught to take about 30 to 60 minutes to consume 1 cup of liquid. The patient is encouraged to wait about 30 minutes after each meal before drinking additional liquids. The patient may be eating up to six small meals of pureed or very soft foods each day. These dietary guidelines may make it challenging for the patient to drink sufficient fluid to maintain hydration.
■ Assess skin turgor and mucous membranes for signs of dehydration.	A loss of interstitial fluid causes the loss of skin turgor. Changes in skin turgor in the extremities may be difficult to assess as the patient begins to experience weight loss after surgery. Therefore skin turgor assessed over the sternum or the forehead is best. Several longitudinal furrows and coating may be noted along the tongue. Weight loss, as a measure of deficient fluid volume, will not be a reliable assessment because the patient is experiencing intentional weight loss.
■ Assess the color and amount of urine.	A decrease in urine volume and increased concentrated urine, as evidenced by a darker urine color, denotes fluid deficit.
■ Monitor and document the patient's HR and BP.	A reduction in circulating blood volume can cause hypotension and tachycardia. The change in HR is a compensatory mechanism to maintain cardiac output. Usually the pulse is weak and may be irregular if electrolyte imbalance also occurs. Hypotension is evident in hypovolemia.
■ Monitor the patient's BP for orthostatic changes (seen when changing from a supine to a standing position).	Postural hypotension is a common manifestation in fluid loss. Note the following orthostatic hypotension significances: • Greater than 10 mm Hg drop: circulating blood volume is decreased by 20%. • Greater than 20 to 30 mm Hg drop: circulating blood volume is decreased by 40%. QSEN: Safety.

Gastrointestinal and Digestive Care Plans

 evolve For additional care plans, go to http://evolve.elsevier.com/Gulanick/.

Therapeutic Interventions

Actions/Interventions	Rationales
■ Encourage the patient to sip 6 to 8 cups of water or low-calorie, noncarbonated, and/or caffeine-free fluid between meals, throughout the day.	Drinking additional fluid throughout the day will maintain hydration. Timing this fluid intake between meals will reduce feelings of fullness at mealtime and promote the intake of nutrient-rich foods with meals. Carbonated or caffeinated beverages are discouraged initially after bariatric surgery because they may contribute to nausea, vomiting, or abdominal pain.
■ Encourage regular oral hygiene.	Fluid deficit can cause a dry, sticky mouth. Attention to mouth care promotes an interest in drinking and reduces the discomfort of dry mucous membranes.
■ For the patient who is unable to take sufficient oral fluids, consider the need for hospitalization and the administration of parenteral fluids as ordered.	Fluids are needed to maintain hydration status. Determination of the type and amount of fluid to be replaced and infusion rates will vary depending on the patient's clinical status.

NANDA-I NDx Risk for Ineffective Health Management

Common Risk Factors

Complex postoperative dietary regimen
Insufficient social support

Common Expected Outcomes

Patient demonstrates ongoing adherence to postoperative treatment program.
Patient identifies appropriate resources.
Patient demonstrates required competencies.

NOC Outcomes
Compliance Behavior; Knowledge: Treatment Regimen

NIC Interventions
Self-Modification Assistance; Teaching: Prescribed Diet; Teaching: Prescribed Exercise

Ongoing Assessment

Actions/Interventions	Rationales
■ Assess the patient's prior efforts to follow a regimen.	This knowledge provides an important starting point in understanding any complexities in implementing the postoperative dietary plan. For the obese patient, bariatric surgery may be a final attempt at weight loss after years of failed efforts at following other diet and exercise plans to lose weight. The patient may have a history of limited success with long-term adherence to a diet plan. QSEN: Patient-centered care.
■ Assess the patient's confidence in his or her ability to follow the postoperative diet plan.	According to the self-efficacy theory, positive conviction that one can successfully execute a behavior is correlated with performance and a successful outcome.
■ Assess the patient's social support system.	Effective support from family and friends will help the patient's motivation to adhere to the lifestyle modifications.

Gastrointestinal and Digestive Care Plans

■ = Independent ▲ = Interprofessional Collaboration

Gastrointestinal and Digestive
Care Plans

Therapeutic Interventions

Actions/Interventions	Rationales
■ Inform the patient of the benefits of adhering to the prescribed dietary program:	Patients who believe in the efficacy of the dietary program to lose weight and promote health are more likely to engage in it. The diet program following bariatric surgery requires the patient to adhere strictly to a very specific eating plan. Understanding the benefits of the postoperative plan will provide the patient with a foundation of knowledge to support decisions needed to achieve the desired outcomes of surgery. QSEN: Patient-centered care; Evidence-based practice; Safety.
• Long-term weight loss	Evidence indicates that bariatric surgery results in more long-term weight loss than other types of weight loss programs the patient may have tried in the past. Patients who do not follow the diet plan after bariatric surgery may actually gain weight and over time increase the size of the gastric pouch.
• Healing of incisions	One of the goals of the diet program after bariatric surgery is to promote the healing of gastric incisions. Stretching of the staple line may occur if the patient consumes more than the prescribed food volume in the early phases of the diet plan. During the first few days of the diet plan the patient is sipping small volumes (2 to 3 ounces) of liquids frequently during the day. These foods may include broth, juice, and milk. For the next several weeks, the patient will be eating pureed foods as 4 to 6 small meals a day. After this phase, the patient gradually includes soft foods at mealtimes and reduces the number of meals per day. Eating solid foods may not begin until 2 months after the surgery. The patient may be able to follow a regular, healthy diet and meal plan within 3 to 4 months after bariatric surgery.
• Improvement of chronic, obesity-related health problems	Many patients will see an improvement in chronic health problems such as type 2 diabetes mellitus, hypertension, or sleep apnea as they begin losing weight. They may be able to reduce the amount of medication taken to control these problems. The patient may notice a significant improvement in the quality of sleep.
• Prevention of complications	Patients need to understand that the diet program after bariatric surgery is designed to not only provide for weight loss but also to prevent complications such as nausea, vomiting, dumping syndrome, and intestinal obstruction. Patients who eat too much food or too quickly at mealtime, or drink liquids too close to mealtime are at risk to experience nausea, vomiting, diarrhea, and dizziness. Patients are taught to chew solid foods thoroughly. The opening from the gastric pouch to the intestines is small and may be obstructed by any but the smallest food particle.

Actions/Interventions

■ Inform the patient about the benefit of progressive exercise after bariatric surgery.

■ Teach the patient's support system about the lifestyle modification program.

■ Encourage the patient to identify meaningful rewards for following the lifestyle modification program after surgery.

■ Refer the patient to bariatric surgery support groups.

Rationales

Exercise after bariatric surgery has the same benefits as any exercise program. The patient will increase calorie expenditure, improve muscle tone and bone density, increase energy levels, promote cardiopulmonary endurance with activity, and enhance self-esteem. Bariatric surgery programs often refer the patient to a physical therapist for guidance in starting an exercise program before surgery. Many obese patients may have become very sedentary prior to surgery. Musculoskeletal pain and exertional dyspnea related to their obesity may have limited their activity level. They may feel challenged to initiate the habit of regular exercise as part of their daily routine. In the hospital the patient will be encouraged to walk as part of the immediate recovery from surgery. During the first month at home the patient needs to continue increased incidental activity by walking around the house or using stairs. Some activity restrictions may be prescribed as part of the healing process. At about 5 to 6 weeks after surgery, the patient should begin to add low-impact aerobic exercise such as housework, riding a stationary bicycle, or walking for longer periods of time. The patient's long-term goal is to engage in a moderate level of activity for 30 minutes a day, 5 or 6 days per week.

To provide positive support, the patient's family and friends need to understand the rigors of the diet plan and the importance of progressive activity. For example, the family may need to explore ways to shift the main focus at mealtime and other family gatherings away from food to other activities and conversations. The patient needs to feel comfortable having different foods than the rest of the family. The family can join the patient in exercise activities. Current research suggests that family members of the patient who has had bariatric surgery also experience weight loss once the patient returns home. QSEN: Evidence-based practice.

A system of rewards will provide the patient with positive feedback for success and offer incentives to adhere to the program. Patients who have used food as rewards in the past will need to identify nonfood rewards as part of this positive feedback.

Sharing experiences with others in the same situation may help the patient to cope with the challenges of adhering to the postoperative regimen and lifestyle modifications.

Related Care Plans

Acute pain, Chapter 2
Diarrhea, Chapter 2
Noncompliance, Chapter 2
Surgical experience: Preoperative and postoperative care, Chapter 4

Gastrointestinal and Digestive Care Plans

■ = Independent ▲ = Interprofessional Collaboration

Bowel Diversion Surgery: Colostomy, Ileostomy

Fecal Diversion; Stoma

Bowel diversion surgery creates an opening into the small or large intestine that is brought to the external surface of the abdominal wall (stoma). These surgeries are done for the purpose of diverting the fecal stream past an area of obstruction or disease, protecting a distal surgical anastomosis, or providing an outlet for stool in the absence of a functioning intact rectum. The procedures may be performed to promote wound healing of an intestinal injury such as a gunshot wound. Diverted fecal material is directed away from the wound to promote wound healing. Depending on the purpose of the surgery and the integrity and function of anatomical structures, stomas may be temporary or permanent. Peristomal skin irritation, body image, self-care, and deficient knowledge are important nursing concerns. This care plan focuses primarily on the person with a new stoma who is being cared for in the hospital environment.

NANDA-I NDx Deficient Knowledge: Surgical Procedure

Common Related Factors
Insufficient information
Insufficient interest in learning
Insufficient knowledge of resources
Misinformation presented by others

Defining Characteristics
Insufficient knowledge
Inaccurate follow-through of instruction
Inaccurate performance on a test
Inappropriate behavior

Common Expected Outcomes
Patient verbalizes understanding that loss or bypass of anal sphincter will result in the need to surgically create a stoma and wear a collection pouch.
Patient demonstrates correct techniques for care of stoma and collection pouch.

NOC Outcomes
Knowledge: Treatment Regimen; Knowledge: Treatment Procedure

NIC Interventions
Health Literacy Enhancement; Learning Facilitation; Teaching: Procedure/Treatment; Teaching: Preoperative

Ongoing Assessment

Actions/Interventions	Rationales
■ Assess the patient's understanding about ostomy formation (e.g., purpose, site) and if the stoma will be permanent or temporary.	The patient needs to understand the purpose of the surgical procedure in relation to the underlying gastrointestinal (GI) problem. Adults must see a need or purpose for learning. Some patients are ready to learn soon after they are diagnosed; others cope better by denying or delaying the need for instruction. Learning readiness is often delayed in patients with temporary stomas. Individuals with temporary stomas often may feel that learning ostomy management is not necessary.
■ Identify the priority of learning needs within the overall care plan.	This information provides the starting base for educational sessions. During the immediate postoperative period, the family or significant others may require the most teaching. QSEN: Patient-centered care.
■ Explore any previous contact that the patient has had with people with a stoma.	Previous experience, whether positive or negative, will have an impact on the patient's expectations and fears regarding this surgery and postoperative stoma care.

Gastrointestinal and Digestive Care Plans

Actions/Interventions

- Identify any misinformation and misconceptions the patient has about the ostomy.

Rationales

Providing factual information can ease the patient's anxiety and provide a basis for learning new knowledge and self-care skills that achieve optimal learning outcomes. QSEN: Patient-centered care.

Therapeutic Interventions

Actions/Interventions

- Reinforce the information the patient has received previously about the proposed procedure.

- Use diagrams, pictures, and audiovisual equipment to explain the anatomy and physiology of the GI tract, the pathophysiology necessitating the ostomy, and the proposed location of the stoma. Show the patient the actual pouch or one similar to the one that the patient will wear after surgery.

- Explain the need for a pouch in terms of loss of the sphincter.

- Offer a visit from a person with an ostomy (ostomate) who has been successful in mastering ostomy management care.

Rationales

Patients may have received ostomy management information during preoperative teaching sessions. Anxiety often makes it necessary to repeat instructions or explanations several times before patients are able to comprehend.

The visualization of information reinforces and enhances learning. Ileostomy stomas are located in the right lower quadrant; colostomy stomas may be in the upper right quadrant, mid-abdomen at the waistline, or the left upper or lower quadrant. Understanding the purpose and need for a pouch encourages the patient to participate in ostomy management. QSEN: Patient-centered care.

Patients should be told that preoperative bowel habits may return after surgery but that control of defecation is lost, and therefore a pouch is necessary to collect or contain stool and gas. The location of the stoma in the GI tract determines stool frequency and consistency. Output from a sigmoid colostomy is soft to solid, frequency is similar to preoperative patterns, and output may be regulated by irrigation. With a transverse colostomy, the output is mushy, occurs after meals, and cannot be regulated. Output from an ileostomy is liquid.

Contact with another individual who has undergone the same procedure reinforces factual information from health care personnel.

Risk for Toileting Self-Care Deficit

Common Risk Factors

Presence of new stoma
Presence of poorly placed stoma
Presence of pouch
Poor hand-eye coordination

Common Expected Outcome

Patient performs self-care needs (emptying and changing pouch) independently or with minimal assistance.

NOC Outcome
Self-Care: Toileting
NIC Intervention
Ostomy Care

Gastrointestinal and Digestive Care Plans

■ = Independent ▲ = Interprofessional Collaboration

Ongoing Assessment

Actions/Interventions	Rationales
■ Assess for the following: presence of old abdominal scars, presence of bony prominences on the anterior abdomen, presence of creases or skin folds on the abdomen, extreme obesity, scaphoid abdomen, pendulous breasts, and the ability to see and handle equipment.	Stoma placement is easier for a patient who has a flat abdomen with no scars, bony prominences, or obesity. The stoma should be placed in a site that is visible and easily reached by the patient in a sitting position.
■ Assess for patient concerns about caring for the stoma and the collection pouch.	Patients may have many concerns that will influence their ability to successfully manage changes in toileting self-care associated with a stoma. These concerns may include the visibility of the stoma and collection pouch, handling the fecal-filled pouch, or a noticeable smell. QSEN: Patient-centered care.

Therapeutic Interventions

Actions/Interventions	Rationales
▲ Consult an enterostomal therapy (ET) nurse or surgeon to indelibly mark the proposed stoma site that the patient can easily see and reach; scars, bony prominences, and skin folds are avoided; hip flexion should not change the contour.	Stoma location is a key factor in self-care. A poorly located stoma can delay or preclude self-care. ET nurses are commonly asked by surgeons to preoperatively mark stoma areas. The stoma location is determined ideally with the patient in a sitting position. QSEN: Teamwork and collaboration.
■ If possible, have the patient wear a pouch over the proposed site; evaluate its effectiveness 12 to 24 hours after applying the pouch.	Stoma site selection is facilitated when the nurse and the patient can observe the appliance faceplate on the person's body under normal wearing conditions (e.g., dressed in normal clothing, moving about). QSEN: Patient-centered care.

NDx Risk for Ineffective Stoma Tissue Perfusion

Common Risk Factor

Interruption in blood flow to stoma (e.g. surgical manipulation of bowel, postoperative edema, tightly fitting faceplate, pressure on stoma from rod or other support device)

Common Expected Outcome

Patient's stoma remains pink and moist.

NOC Outcome
Tissue Perfusion: Abdominal Organs
NIC Interventions
Ostomy Care; Surveillance

Gastrointestinal and Digestive Care Plans

Ongoing Assessment

Actions/Interventions	Rationales
■ Assess the following at least every 4 hours for the first 24 hours after surgery, and notify the physician of any changes:	Frequent assessment of the stoma in the early postoperative hours allows for prompt identification of impaired stoma tissue perfusion. Immediate intervention is necessary to restore tissue perfusion and preserve stoma integrity. QSEN: Safety.
• Color of the stoma	The stoma (a piece of intestine) should be pink and moist, indicating good perfusion and adequate venous drainage. A dusky or blue appearance may indicate venous congestion or poor blood supply, either of which could result in a necrotic stoma.
• Moist appearance of the stoma	Healthy intestine continuously secretes mucus, which maintains the moisture of the stoma.
• Stomal edema	Edema is caused by preoperative pathology or by the manipulation of the bowel during surgery; the stoma can be quite swollen.
• Presence of rods or support devices	Rods or other support devices are used for transverse or loop stomas. The support device usually is removed several days after surgery; patients may be discharged with the support device in place. The placement of the support device may create pressure on the stoma.
• Correctly fitted faceplate	The opening of the ostomy appliance should be ⅛ inch larger than the stoma itself. A faceplate that is too tight can constrict the venous return of the stomal circulation and result in edema or damage to the stoma.
• Abdominal distention	Abdominal distention may decrease blood flow to the distal bowel and stoma.

Therapeutic Interventions

Actions/Interventions	Rationales
■ Fit the patient with a correctly sized faceplate.	A proper fit protects the surrounding skin from contact with drainage and ensures adequate blood flow to the stoma.
■ Anticipate and prepare the patient for possible surgical stoma revision if signs or symptoms of compromised circulation are present.	Necrosis extending to the fascia may represent a surgical emergency because of the threat of perforation and peritonitis. QSEN: Safety.

NANDA-I
NDx Risk for Impaired Skin Integrity

Common Related Factors
Continuous contact of bowel secretions with skin
Fungal infection

Common Expected Outcomes
Patient's skin is free of irritation caused by contact with fecal output from ostomy.
Patient's skin is free of infection.

Defining Characteristics
Patient complains of burning and itching
Skin is red and tender
Skin is excoriated

NOC Outcomes
Tissue Integrity: Skin and Mucous Membranes; Bowel Continence

NIC Interventions
Skin Care: Topical Treatments; Ostomy Care

Gastrointestinal and Digestive Care Plans

■ = Independent ▲ = Interprofessional Collaboration

Ongoing Assessment

Action/Intervention

■ Assess the peristomal skin for redness, excoriation, tenderness, vesicles, papular rashes, or drainage.

Rationale

A loss of peristomal skin integrity is associated with allergies, mechanical trauma, chemical reactions, and infection. Small bowel effluent contains proteolytic enzymes. Exposure of the skin to the effluent can cause skin irritation within hours. *Candida albicans* is a common cause of peristomal skin infection.

Therapeutic Interventions

Actions/Interventions

■ Maintain intact peristomal skin using the following method:
  • Choose the appropriate pouch by evaluating the skin's condition (pouch adhesives will not adhere to wet or moist skin), size and shape of the abdomen, presence of current or recent sutures, stoma site, and characteristics of ostomy effluent.
  • Clean and prepare the skin with mild soap and water.

  • Prepare a pattern as a guide to customize the fit of the pouch; apply a hydrocolloid skin barrier. Apply the collection pouch over the skin barrier according to the manufacturer's directions.
  • Empty the pouch when it is one third to one half full. Keep the pouch emptied routinely. Change the skin barrier every 3 or 4 days.

Rationales

The pouch opening should be no more than ⅛ inch larger in diameter than the stoma. A minimal gap between the pouch opening and the stoma prevents the leakage of effluent onto peristomal skin.

Skin preparation is the most important step in pouching the stoma to prevent leakage.
A correctly fitted pouch used with a skin barrier will promote skin integrity.

More frequent changes of the skin barrier can cause mechanical trauma to the skin. Emptying the pouch when it is one third to one half full reduces the risk for leakage and odor. The weight of a full pouch can pull it away from the skin barrier.

NANDA-I
NDx   **Risk for Disturbed Body Image**

Common Risk Factors

Alteration in body function (due to presence of stoma; loss of fecal continence, presence of pouch)
Alteration in self-perception (due to fear of offensive odor, fear of appearing "different")

Common Expected Outcome

Patient demonstrates enhanced body image and self-esteem, as evidenced by ability to look at, touch, talk about, and care for the stoma and ostomy pouch.

NOC Outcomes
Body Image; Psychosocial Adjustment: Life Change
NIC Interventions
Ostomy Care; Body Image Enhancement; Self-Esteem Enhancement; Coping Enhancement; Grief Work Facilitation

Gastrointestinal and Digestive Care Plans

Ongoing Assessment

Actions/Interventions	Rationales
■ Assess the patient's perception of the change in body structure and function.	The patient may experience a period of grief about the loss of normal bowel elimination. The patient needs to recognize these feelings before they can be dealt with effectively.
■ Assess the patient's perceived impact of the change.	Changes in body image can have an impact on the person's ability to carry out daily roles and responsibilities. The patient's response to real or perceived changes in body structure and function is related to the importance that the patient places on the structure or function (e.g., a very fastidious person may experience the visual presence of a stool-filled pouch on the anterior abdomen as intolerable). QSEN: Patient-centered care.
■ Note any verbal and nonverbal references to the stoma.	Negative statements about the stoma may indicate a limited ability to integrate the change into the patient's self-concept. Patients often "name" stomas as an attempt to separate the stoma from themselves. Others may look away or totally deny the presence of the stoma until they are able to cope.
■ Note the patient's ability and readiness to look at, touch, and care for the stoma and ostomy equipment.	Looking at the stoma is often the first indication that the patient is ready to participate in stoma care.

Therapeutic Interventions

Actions/Interventions	Rationales
■ Acknowledge the normalcy of the patient's emotional response to the perceived change in body structure and function.	The loss of control over bowel elimination may threaten the patient's developmental level. Because the control of elimination is a skill or task of early childhood and is a socially private function, a loss of control precipitates body image change and possible self-concept change. The patient needs to understand that grief is a normal response. QSEN: Patient-centered care.
■ Provide stoma care in a matter of fact manner.	The verbal response and facial reactions of the nurse, while caring for the stoma, will guide the patient in his or her acceptance of the change in body image.
■ Assist the patient in looking at, touching, and caring for the stoma when ready.	The patient's readiness to learn may be judged by his or her willingness to look at the stoma and ask questions. Some patients acknowledge the stoma with minimal emotional difficulty, whereas others have a more difficult time adjusting.
■ Assist the patient in identifying specific actions that could be helpful in managing the perceived loss or problems related to the stoma.	The most common concern is odor; helping patients gain control over odor will facilitate an acceptable body image. QSEN: Patient-centered care.

NANDA-I
NDx Deficient Knowledge: Stoma Care

Common Related Factors	Defining Characteristics
Insufficient information	Insufficient knowledge of stoma care
Insufficient interest in learning	Inaccurate follow-through of instruction
Insufficient knowledge of resources	Inaccurate performance of stoma care
Misinformation presented by others	Inappropriate behavior

Gastrointestinal and Digestive Care Plans

■ = Independent   ▲ = Interprofessional Collaboration

Common Expected Outcomes

Patient or significant other verbalizes understanding of ostomy care.

Patient or significant other demonstrates ostomy care on discharge.

NOC Outcomes

Knowledge: Treatment Regimen; Knowledge: Prescribed Diet; Knowledge: Health Resources

NIC Interventions

Health Literacy Enhancement; Learning Facilitation; Ostomy Care; Teaching: Psychomotor Skill; Teaching: Prescribed Diet

Ongoing Assessment

Actions/Interventions	Rationales
■ Assess the patient's ability to empty and change the pouch.	Most patients will be independent in emptying the pouch by the time of discharge; some may still need assistance with pouch changing and may require outpatient follow-up care by a home health nurse. QSEN: Patient-centered care.
■ Assess the patient's ability to care for peristomal skin, and identify any problems.	The patient needs to be able to maintain pouch integrity to prevent fecal material from coming into contact with the skin and causing breakdown. QSEN: Safety.
■ Assess the patient's concerns about diet, activity, hygiene, and clothing.	The teaching plan needs to provide information to allay patient concerns about how the presence of the stoma may affect the diet, activity, hygiene, and clothing selection. This information provides the starting base for educational sessions. QSEN: Patient-centered care.

Therapeutic Interventions

Actions/Interventions	Rationales
■ Provide psychomotor teaching during the first and subsequent applications of the pouch. Include at least one caregiver as approved or desired by the patient.	Even before patients are able to participate actively, they can observe and discuss ostomy care. It is beneficial to teach others alongside the patient, as long as all realize that the goal is for the patient to become independent in ostomy self-care. QSEN: Patient-centered care.
■ Gradually transfer the responsibility for pouch emptying and changing to the patient.	Repeated practice by the patient with positive feedback from the nurse will help the patient gain confidence in self-care ability.
■ Allow at least one opportunity for a supervised return demonstration of pouch changing before discharge.	Ostomy care requires both cognitive and psychomotor skills. Postoperatively, learning ability may be decreased, requiring repetition and the need for return demonstrations.
■ Teach the patient about resuming activity.	The patient should understand that activity should not be altered by the presence of the stoma or pouch.
■ Teach about bathing and showering.	Normal bathing or showering is acceptable; the patient should be prepared for the possibility that small amounts of stool may pass during bathing and showering. Some patients purchase small, disposable pouches for bathing and showering; others prefer removing the pouch for bathing and showering.
■ Teach about selecting clothing.	No special clothing or alterations in existing clothing should be required by the presence of the stoma or pouch.

Gastrointestinal and Digestive Care Plans

Actions/Interventions

- Teach the patient the following regarding diet:
  - *For ileostomy:* Eat a balanced diet; use special care in chewing high-fiber foods (e.g., popcorn, peanuts, coconut, vegetables, string beans, olives); increase fluid intake during hot weather or vigorous exercise.
  - *For colostomy:* Eat a balanced diet; no foods are specifically contraindicated; certain foods (e.g., eggs, fish, green onions, cheese, asparagus, broccoli, leafy vegetables, carbonated beverages) may increase flatus and fecal odor.
- Discuss odor control, and acknowledge that odor (or fear of odor) can impair social functioning.

- Teach the patient to report a lack of stool output from the stoma.
- Discuss the availability of ostomy support groups (e.g., United Ostomy Association, National Foundation for Ileitis and Colitis).
- Instruct the patient to maintain contact with an enterostomal therapy (ET) nurse.

Rationales

Dietary intake will influence the consistency and frequency of fecal output from the stoma. Patients need to learn individual responses to foods. The patient must understand that not eating to minimize fecal output is detrimental and that the stoma will have output regardless. QSEN: Patient-centered care.

Odor control is best achieved by eliminating odor-causing foods from the diet. Green leafy vegetables, eggs, fish, and onions are primary odor-causing foods. Oral deodorants and pouch deodorants may also help. Pouch filters help muffle sounds and deodorize flatus.

An absence of ostomy output may be a sign of intestinal obstruction. QSEN: Safety.

Contact with other people who have ostomies increases the perception of the ostomy being manageable and enhances the patient's sense of control. QSEN: Patient-centered care.

Contacting this member of the interprofessional health team provides the patient with an opportunity for follow-up care and guidance with problem-solving. QSEN: Teamwork and collaboration.

Related Care Plans

Risk for infection, Chapter 2
Ineffective sexuality pattern, Chapter 2
Surgical experience: Preoperative and postoperative care, Chapter 4

Cholecystectomy

Laparoscopic/Open, Postoperative Care

Cholecystitis is an inflammation of the gallbladder. Most patients who develop cholecystitis have cholelithiasis or gallstones. The most common manifestation of acute cholecystitis is right upper quadrant pain that occurs after eating a high-fat meal. Although eating a fat-free diet will decrease the patient's symptoms temporarily, surgical removal of the gallbladder and gallstones (cholecystectomy) is usually recommended. The preferred method for cholecystectomy is laparoscopic surgery, a minimally invasive surgery (MIS) technique, using small abdominal incisions in combination with endoscopic visualization of the abdominal cavity. The abdominal cavity is inflated with carbon dioxide to facilitate visualization of the abdominal organs generally and the gallbladder specifically. Once the gallbladder is dissected away from surrounding tissue, it is removed through one of the abdominal incisions. The carbon dioxide is evacuated, and the multiple incisions are closed. If the surgeon is not able to successfully remove the gallbladder using a laparoscopic approach, a larger open incision is made in the right upper quadrant for direct visualization and removal of the gallbladder.

Gastrointestinal and Digestive Care Plans

■ = Independent   ▲ = Interprofessional Collaboration

Risk for Infection

Common Risk Factor

Invasive procedure (abdominal incisions; presence of tubes and drains)

Common Expected Outcomes

Patient remains free of infection, as evidenced by normal vital signs and absence of purulent drainage from wounds, incisions, and tubes.

Infection is recognized early to allow for prompt treatment.

NOC Outcomes

Infection Severity; Tissue Integrity: Skin and Mucous Membranes; Wound Healing: Primary Intention

NIC Interventions

Infection Control; Teaching: Prescribed Medication; Wound Care

Ongoing Assessment

Actions/Interventions	Rationales
■ Monitor the patient's temperature.	For the first 48 to 72 hours postoperatively, temperatures of up to 38.5°C (101.3°F) are expected as a normal stress response to surgery. Beyond 72 hours, temperature should return to the patient's baseline. Temperature spikes, usually occurring in late afternoon or at night, are often indications of infection.
■ Assess the incisions for redness, drainage, swelling, and increased pain.	Incisions that have been closed with sutures or staples should be free of redness, swelling, and drainage. Some incisional discomfort is expected. An incision for an open cholecystecomy is usually kept covered by a large adhesive bandage for 24 to 48 hours; beyond 48 hours, there is no need for a dressing. Laparoscopic incisions may be covered with smaller adhesive bandages. QSEN: Safety.
■ Assess the stability of tubes and drains.	If an open cholecystectomy was performed, a wound drain may be placed and removed before discharge. The in-and-out motion of improperly secured tubes and drains allows access by pathogens through stab wounds where tubes and drains are placed.
▲ Monitor white blood cell (WBC) count.	An increasing WBC count indicates the body's efforts to combat pathogens. Normal values are 4000 to 11,000/mm^3. In older patients, infection may be present without an increased WBC count. QSEN: Evidence-based practice.

Therapeutic Interventions

Actions/Interventions	Rationales
■ Implement the following nursing actions:	These nursing actions reduce the risk of infection. QSEN: Safety.
• Wash hands before contact with the postoperative patient.	Handwashing remains the most effective method of infection control.
• Use aseptic technique during dressing changes, wound care, or the handling or manipulating of tubes and drains.	Aseptic technique prevents transmission of pathogens to the area.

Gastrointestinal and Digestive Care Plans

Actions/Interventions

- Ensure that surgical tubes and drains are not inadvertently interrupted (opened). Securely tape connectors, and pin extensions or drainage tubing to the patient's clothing.

■ Instruct the patient and caregiver in the administration of antibiotics and antipyretics as prescribed.

Rationales

Opening sterile systems allows access by pathogens and puts the patient at risk for infection. Drains may be left in place until the first return visit to the surgeon (about 7 days), if not removed at the time of discharge.

Antibiotics are necessary for the treatment of abscess and infection. Antipyretics will reduce fever and promote comfort.

NANDA-I NDx Risk for Ineffective Breathing Pattern

Common Risk Factor

Pain (right upper quadrant abdominal incision)

Common Expected Outcome

Patient maintains effective breathing pattern as evidenced by relaxed breathing at normal rate and depth and absence of dyspnea.

NOC Outcomes
Respiratory Status: Ventilation; Comfort Status

NIC Interventions
Respiratory Monitoring; Pain Management; Cough Enhancement

Ongoing Assessment

Actions/Interventions

■ Assess the rate, rhythm, and depth of respirations.

■ Auscultate the patient's breath sounds.

■ Observe for splinting.

■ Assess the patient's ability to use incentive spirometry.

■ Assess for abdominal distention.

■ Assess the patient's temperature according to postoperative policy.

■ Assess the amount and characteristics of sputum.

■ Monitor the patient's pain level and the use of analgesics.

Rationales

The right upper quadrant incision from an open cholecystectomy and postoperative abdominal pain may limit the patient's ability to take a deep breath. Shallow breathing puts the patient at risk for atelectasis and pneumonia. QSEN: Safety.

The lung bases are least likely to be ventilated; therefore breath sounds may be diminished over the bases.

Splinting refers to the conscious minimization of an inspiration to reduce the amount of discomfort caused by full expansion of the lungs. The location of the incision may cause the patient to limit deep inspiration.

In incentive spirometry, the patient takes and holds a deep breath for a few seconds. Incentive spirometry encourages deep breathing, and holding the breath allows for the full expansion of alveoli.

Distention can impair thoracic excursion and result in an ineffective breathing pattern. The distention may be a result of retained carbon dioxide used to inflate the abdomen during laparoscopic surgery.

An elevated temperature in the first 48 hours postoperatively may indicate atelectasis, which can lead to pneumonia.

Increased amounts of sputum as well as changes in color and a thicker consistency may indicate pneumonia.

Pain inhibits the ability to cough and deep breathe and use the incentive spirometer correctly.

Gastrointestinal and Digestive Care Plans

■ = Independent ▲ = Interprofessional Collaboration

Therapeutic Interventions

Actions/Interventions	Rationales
■ Encourage deep breathing, coughing, and the use of incentive spirometry every hour while the patient is awake.	Increasing deep breathing will expand the alveoli and decrease the development of atelectasis. QSEN: Safety.
■ Encourage the patient to splint the incision area when coughing and deep breathing.	Providing external support to the operative site will decrease the discomfort associated with increased respiratory effort. Some patients may use a pillow to splint the incision, whereas others may use their hands.
▲ Administer analgesics at regular intervals.	Controlling pain will help the patient feel more comfortable with deep breathing.

NANDA-I
NDx Deficient Knowledge

Common Related Factors
Insufficient information
Insufficient interest in learning
Insufficient knowledge of resources
Misinformation presented by others

Defining Characteristics
Insufficient knowledge
Inaccurate follow-through of instruction
Inaccurate performance on a test
Inappropriate behavior

Common Expected Outcome
Patient verbalizes understanding of and demonstrates ability to perform postoperative care after discharge.

NOC Outcomes
Knowledge: Treatment Regimen; Knowledge: Prescribed Activity

NIC Interventions
Health Literacy Enhancement; Learning Facilitation; Wound Care; Teaching: Prescribed Exercise; Teaching: Psychomotor Skill

---

Ongoing Assessment

Actions/Interventions	Rationales
■ Assess the patient's ability to perform wound care, verbalize appropriate activities, and describe an appropriate diet.	This information is the foundation for an individualized teaching plan. Teaching standardized content that the patient already knows wastes valuable time and hinders critical learning. QSEN: Patient-centered care.
■ Assess the patient's understanding of the need for close follow-up observation.	Patients who leave the hospital with sutures, staples, or drains in place need to return for removal, usually about 1 week after surgery.

Therapeutic Interventions

Actions/Interventions	Rationales
■ Teach the patient to perform appropriate wound care: • Abdominal incisions	Staples or sutures and dressings may be present at the time of discharge. If a dressing is not used at the time of discharge, the patient may be able to clean the incision during normal showering activities.

Gastrointestinal and Digestive Care Plans

Actions/Interventions	Rationales
• Dressings	Dressings are usually adhesive bandages. Most bandages can be removed within 1 to 2 days following laparoscopic surgery.
■ Teach the patient appropriate activities: no lifting more than 10 pounds for 6 weeks, return to work in 3 or 4 days, showering and bathing are acceptable.	Activity restrictions reduce strain on abdominal muscles and promote healing. These restrictions reduce the risk for wound dehiscence. QSEN: Safety.
■ Teach the patient about eating a well-balanced, high-calorie, high-protein diet.	Many patients can eat their usual diet after laparoscopic surgery. Eating the prescribed diet promotes healing. A high-fat meal may result in diarrhea because of the reduced availability of bile for fat digestion.
■ Teach the patient that bowel function will return to pre-operative baseline in 2 to 3 days.	Bowel sounds will be hypoactive initially but should return to normal within the first 2 to 3 days postoperatively. The presence of flatus or stool signals the return of peristalsis.
■ Instruct the patient to seek medical attention for any of the following: temperature higher than 38°C (100.4°F), foul-smelling wound drainage, redness or unusual pain in any incision, or the absence of bowel movements.	Signs and symptoms of wound infection should be reported to the physician. Delayed return of bowel movements may indicate constipation, or paralytic ileus. Prompt interventions to treat infection or constipation are necessary to promote postoperative recovery. QSEN: Safety.
■ Teach the patient that minor abdominal pain and shoulder pain are expected after laparoscopic surgery and may be managed with oral analgesic agents.	During abdominal laparoscopic surgery, the peritoneal cavity is filled with carbon dioxide; this facilitates the visualization of structures by the surgeon. Until the gas is completely absorbed, some discomfort is typical in the shoulder area; this referred pain is caused by irritation of the nerves by the unabsorbed carbon dioxide gas.
■ Teach the patient to empty the drainage collection devices.	With open cholecystectomy and common bile duct exploration, drains may be left in place until the drainage is less than 30 mL/24 hr; this usually occurs 3 to 7 days postoperatively. Patients may be discharged with the drains in place. Patients should prepare a clean surface (e.g., clean paper towels) to work on and should wash hands with soap under running water before emptying the collection device. These measures reduce the risk for infection. QSEN: Safety.

Related Care Plans

Acute pain, Chapter 2
Surgical experience: Preoperative and postoperative care, Chapter 4

Cirrhosis

Laënnec's Cirrhosis; Hepatic Encephalopathy; Ascites; Liver Failure

Cirrhosis is a chronic and progressive inflammatory disease of the liver. The inflammatory process results in irreversible fibrosis and scarring of hepatic tissue. The scarring produces changes not only in the size and shape of the liver but also in its function and blood flow. Worldwide the most common cause of cirrhosis is viral infection such as hepatitis B and C. Alcohol abuse is the primary cause of Laënnec's cirrhosis. Other causes include biliary obstruction, prolonged right-sided heart failure, and metabolic defects such as alpha-1 antitrypsin deficiency. The incidence of cirrhosis is highest in men between 40 and 60 years old. The development of cirrhosis occurs over many years before the person presents with characteristic symptoms. Malnutrition contributes to the development of cirrhosis in people who abuse alcohol. The disruption of hepatic function in cirrhosis can lead to the development of end-stage liver disease with ascites, portal hypertension, hepatic encephalopathy, and liver failure.

Gastrointestinal and Digestive Care Plans

■ = Independent   ▲ = Interprofessional Collaboration

NANDA-I NDx Imbalanced Nutrition: Less Than Body Requirements

Common Related Factors

Insufficient dietary intake
Biological factors (excess alcohol intake)
Economically disadvantaged
Altered hepatic metabolic function
Inability to digest foods (inadequate bile production)
Inability to ingest foods (nausea, vomiting, anorexia)

Common Expected Outcomes

Patient or caregiver verbalizes and demonstrates selection of foods or meals that will achieve a cessation of weight loss.
Patient weighs within 10% of ideal weight range.

Defining Characteristics

Body weight 20% or more below ideal weight range
Food intake less than recommended dietary allowance (RDA)
Excessive hair loss
Pale mucous membranes
Muscle wasting, especially in extremities
Signs and symptoms consistent with vitamin deficiencies

NOC Outcome
Nutritional Status: Nutrient Intake
NIC Interventions
Nutrition Therapy; Nutritional Monitoring; Teaching: Prescribed Diet

Ongoing Assessment

Actions/Interventions	Rationales
■ Assess for changes in body weight and muscle mass.	Actual weight may remain steady while muscle mass deteriorates and ascitic fluid accumulates in the peritoneal space. Muscle wasting and weight loss are common in advanced cirrhosis.
■ Obtain a nutritional history; include the family, significant others, or the caregiver in the assessment.	The patient's perception of actual intake may differ from his or her actual intake. Family members may provide a more accurate estimate of the patient's eating habits and food intake. A diary kept by the patient or caregiver may facilitate nutritional assessment in the home. Patients with a history of alcohol abuse often have coexisting problems with protein malnutrition. QSEN: Patient-centered care.
▲ Monitor albumin and/or protein levels and potassium levels.	Serum albumin and protein levels are decreased secondary to the decreased hepatic production of protein and the loss of protein molecules to the peritoneal space. Hypokalemia is common in cirrhosis as a result of increased aldosterone levels, which increase K^+ excretion. QSEN: Safety.
▲ Monitor glucose levels.	Patients with cirrhosis may be hypoglycemic, because the liver fails to perform glycolysis (breakdown of stored glycogen) and gluconeogenesis (formation of glucose from amino acids).
▲ Monitor the coagulation profile.	Several coagulation factors made by the liver require adequate amounts of vitamin K. Patients with cirrhosis commonly have hypovitaminosis that is severe enough to precipitate coagulopathy that increase the risk for bleeding. QSEN: Safety.

Gastrointestinal and Digestive Care Plans

Therapeutic Interventions

Actions/Interventions	Rationales
■ Instruct the patient in the need for a diet high in calories from carbohydrate sources. Instruct the patient to have protein in the diet up to 75 to 100 g/day. Protein restriction is needed in the later stages of cirrhosis.	Aberrant protein metabolism in the failing liver can cause hepatic encephalopathy because ammonia, which is normally metabolized into urea (which can be excreted by the kidney), passes through the damaged liver unchanged and goes on to become a cerebral toxin in the blood. QSEN: Safety.
■ Suggest small, frequent meals and assistance with meals as needed.	Fatigue is a common symptom in cirrhosis that can limit the energy for eating. Meals should be planned for times when the patient is least fatigued. QSEN: Patient-centered care.
▲ Collaborate with members of the interprofessional health team about dietary and pharmacological vitamin supplementation.	The dietitian may provide guidance in selection of nutrition supplements to promote adequate nutrient intake. If bile production is impaired, the absorption of fat-soluble vitamins A, D, E, and K will be inadequate. B vitamin supplements are needed for patients with alcoholic cirrhosis. The pharmacist can provide vitamin supplements in an appropriate form for the patient's needs. QSEN: Teamwork and collaboration.
▲ Provide enteral or parenteral nutritional support as ordered, using carbohydrates as the calorie source.	The patient in advanced stages of cirrhosis may require nutritional support. The patient may need total parenteral nutrition (TPN) if bleeding complications make the intestines unsuitable for enteral nutrition.
▲ Administer prescribed medications: • Acid-suppressing agents • Antiemetics	Medications alleviate gastric distress and promote increased appetite and food intake.

NANDA-I NDx Excess Fluid Volume, Extravascular (Ascites)

Common Related Factors

Compromised regulatory mechanisms (increased portal venous pressure; hypoalbuminemia; low serum oncotic pressure; aldosterone imbalance)
Low protein intake or malnutrition

Defining Characteristics

Weight gain over a short period of time
Edema
Increasing abdominal girth
Ballottement
Taut abdomen, dull to percussion
Dehydration
Adventitious breath sounds: crackles
Change in respiratory pattern
Jugular vein distention
Increased central venous pressure (CVP)

Common Expected Outcomes

Patient experiences a decrease in ascites formation and accumulation as evidenced by decreased abdominal girth.
Patient is normovolemic as evidenced by urine output greater than or equal to 30 mL/hr, balanced intake and output, stable weight (or loss attributed to fluid loss), absence or reduction of edema, HR 60 to 100 beats/min, and absence of pulmonary crackles.

NOC Outcomes

Fluid Balance; Knowledge: Treatment Regimen; Nutritional Status: Food and Fluid Intake

NIC Interventions

Fluid Monitoring; Fluid/Electrolyte Management

Gastrointestinal and Digestive Care Plans

■ = Independent   ▲ = Interprofessional Collaboration

Ongoing Assessment

Actions/Interventions	Rationales
■ Assess for the presence of ascites:	Ascites is a third space collection of protein-rich fluid in the peritoneal cavity. Its volume may be so severe as to impair respiratory and digestive functions, as well as mobility.
• Measure the abdominal girth, taking care to measure at the same point consistently.	An accumulation of fluid in the peritoneal cavity results in an increased abdominal girth. Measuring changes in abdominal girth can help assess the progression of ascites.
• Percuss the abdomen for dullness.	Fluid in the peritoneal cavity will produce a dull percussion sound.
▲ Monitor serum albumin, serum protein, and globulin levels.	Protein molecules act as fluid "magnets" that help maintain body fluid in the correct compartments; low serum protein levels allow a shift of fluid to the extravascular space of the abdominal cavity from vascular and interstitial spaces. QSEN: Safety.
■ Assess for the signs of portal hypertension: a history of upper gastrointestinal (GI) bleeding from esophageal varices, hemorrhoids, and visible superficial veins.	Portal hypertension is high pressure within the portal vein and mesenteric vascular bed, which is usually a high-flow, low-resistance vascular system. As cirrhosis progresses, normally distensible hepatic tissue is replaced by nonelastic scar tissue; blood flowing through the hepatic vasculature is subjected to higher pressures, called portal hypertension. The higher pressure in this venous system leads to the distention of superficial abdominal veins. The patient may develop prominent internal hemorrhoids. Esophageal varices may develop and rupture, leading to upper GI bleeding.
■ Monitor the patient's fluid intake, urinary output, and body weight.	Although overall intake of fluid may be adequate, a shifting of fluid out of the intravascular space and into the extravascular spaces may result in dehydration. The risk for fluid imbalance occurring increases when diuretics are given. Weight gain occurs with fluid retention.
■ Assess breathing patterns.	Ascites may limit the excursion of the diaphragm on inspiration. The patient may hypoventilate in a supine position. QSEN: Safety.

Therapeutic Interventions

Actions/Interventions	Rationales
■ Instruct the patient and caregiver to:	
• Restrict fluid and sodium intake as ordered.	Increased aldosterone levels contribute to aggressive sodium reabsorption, which enhances the accumulation of ascitic fluid.
• Take or administer spironolactone as prescribed.	Spironolactone, a diuretic, antagonizes aldosterone. It causes the excretion of sodium and water but spares potassium.
• Take or administer diuretics cautiously.	Excess fluid is extravascular; aggressive diuresis can lead to dehydration and acute tubular necrosis or hepatorenal syndrome.
▲ For patients unresponsive to the aforementioned measures, consult with members of the interprofessional health team about performing a paracentesis as needed.	A paracentesis is a bedside procedure to remove ascitic fluid from the peritoneal cavity. A trocar catheter is inserted into the abdomen using sterile technique and local anesthesia. The procedure is done to obtain fluid for laboratory analysis or as a temporary measure to relieve abdominal pressure. The rapid removal of ascitic fluid may be necessary to improve breathing, appetite, mobility, and comfort; reaccumulation of the fluid is common. QSEN: Teamwork and collaboration.

Gastrointestinal and Digestive Care Plans

Actions/Interventions

- For patients with a peritoneovenous shunt (LeVeen shunt, Denver shunt):

  - Apply an abdominal binder.
  - Encourage the use of incentive spirometry.

Rationales

Although paracentesis effectively removes ascitic fluid, it also wastes protein and is only a temporary measure. Peritoneovenous shunting returns ascitic fluid to the vascular space.

Inspiring against resistance and the use of an abdominal binder increase intraperitoneal pressures, causing the valve in the shunt to open and allowing ascitic fluid to shunt into the vascular space.

NANDA-I NDx **Risk for Deficient Fluid Volume**

Common Risk Factors

Active fluid loss (diuresis; gastrointestinal [GI] bleeding; coagulopathies)

Fluid shifts (ascites)

Common Expected Outcome

Patient maintains normal fluid volume as evidenced by systolic BP 90 mm Hg or greater (or patient's baseline), absence of orthostasis, HR 60 to 100 beats/min, urine specific gravity less than 1.030, urinary output greater than 30 mL/hr, and moist mucous membranes.

NOC Outcomes
Fluid Balance; Hydration

NIC Interventions
Fluid Monitoring; Fluid Management; Fluid Resuscitation

Ongoing Assessment

Actions/Interventions

- Monitor the patient's BP and HR; check for orthostatic changes.

- Measure the urine specific gravity, amount, and color.

- Check for moisture of the mucous membranes.
- Assess for hematemesis (vomited blood), hematochezia (bright red blood per rectum), and melena (dark, tarry stool). Test any emesis, gastric aspirate, or stool for blood.

Rationales

Changes from the patient's baseline vital signs can indicate shifts in fluid balance. Decreased BP and an elevated HR may occur with decreased circulatory blood volume. Orthostatic changes in BP may be an early indicator of decreasing circulatory blood volume. QSEN: Safety.

Decreased fluid volume is associated with decreased urine volume, an increased urine specific gravity, and a darker urine color.

Dry mucous membranes indicate dehydration.

As portal hypertension worsens and possible coagulopathies develop, patients with cirrhosis are at risk for bleeding. Esophageal varices, because of the close proximity of the hepatic vasculature and the venous drainage of the esophagus, are common among patients with cirrhosis. QSEN: Safety.

Therapeutic Interventions

Actions/Interventions

- ▲ For signs of fluid volume deficit:
  - Hold diuretics
  - Administer intravenous (IV) fluids as prescribed.

Rationales

These drugs may deplete intravascular volume.

IV fluids may be administered at home, or the patient may require hospital admission for severe dehydration.

■ = Independent ▲ = Interprofessional Collaboration

Gastrointestinal and Digestive Care Plans

Actions/Interventions

▲ If GI bleeding occurs, administer IV fluids, volume expanders, or blood products.

Rationales

If bleeding occurs, IV fluids and volume expanders expand intravascular fluid volume and prevent complications of hypovolemia (e.g., acute tubular necrosis, shock). Transfusion with blood products may be necessary.

NANDA-I
NDx **Risk for Acute Confusion**

Common Risk Factors

Hepatic encephalopathy
Delirium tremens
Acute alcohol intoxication
Hepatic metabolic insufficiency

Common Expected Outcome

Patient remains arousable, oriented, able to follow directions, and free from injury caused by neurosensory changes.

NOC Outcomes
Cognitive Orientation; Delirium Level
NIC Interventions
Environmental Management: Safety; Medication Management; Delusion Management; Delirium Management

---

Ongoing Assessment

Actions/Interventions

■ Monitor or instruct the caregiver to monitor for the following signs and symptoms: altered attention span; inability to give an accurate history; inability to follow commands; disorientation to person, place, or time; delusions; inappropriate behavior; self-directed or other-directed violence; and inappropriate affect.

▲ For patients requiring hospitalization, monitor the blood alcohol level on admission. Note the time since the last ingestion of alcohol.

▲ Monitor blood ammonia levels.

Rationales

All signs and symptoms may be caused by alcohol intoxication, delirium tremens, or hepatic encephalopathy. Hepatic encephalopathy typically occurs in end-stage liver disease. The accumulation of ammonia and other neurological toxins can impair thinking and neuromuscular function. QSEN: Safety.

Patients with cirrhosis from alcohol abuse may still be actively using alcohol. It is important to determine whether changes in the level of consciousness are related to acute alcohol intoxication or to hepatic encephalopathy. Delirium tremens can occur up to 7 days after the last alcohol intake.

Normally, ammonia is produced in the colon by the interaction of amino acids and colonic bacteria, metabolized by the liver, and excreted. Patients with cirrhosis may lack the hepatic ability to metabolize ammonia, which accumulates and acts as a cerebral toxin.

Gastrointestinal and Digestive Care Plans

Actions/Interventions

■ Assess for the signs and symptoms of hepatic encephalopathy; note the stage:
  - *Stage I:* mild confusion, mood changes, inability to concentrate, sleep disturbances, and mild asterixis (rapid wrist flapping or liver flap)
  - *Stage II:* confusion, apathy, aberrant behavior, asterixis, and apraxia (loss of the ability to carry out familiar, purposeful movements)
  - *Stage III:* severe confusion, incoherence, diminished responsiveness to verbal stimuli, and hyperactive deep tendon reflexes
  - *Stage IV:* no reaction to stimuli, no corneal reflex, dilated pupils, and flexion or extension posturing

Rationales

In the early stages, hepatic encephalopathy can be reversed with early intervention. Symptoms of encephalopathy may progress slowly. The patient may fluctuate among the four stages. QSEN: Safety.

Therapeutic Interventions

Actions/Interventions

▲ Protect the patient from physical harm:
  - Keep the bed in a low position.
  - Assist the patient with ambulation.
  - Restrain the patient if necessary.
  - Administer sedatives that require nonhepatic metabolism as prescribed, document their effectiveness, and notify the physician if the dosage needs adjustment.
  - Orient the patient to time, place, and person; place a calendar and clock in the room, provide environmental stimulation (television, radio, newspaper, visitors).
  - Provide emotional support by reassuring the patient and family of the physiological cause of confusion.

▲ Decrease the intestinal bacteria content:
  - Administer nonabsorbable antibiotics (neomycin, kanamycin) as prescribed.

  - Administer lactulose as prescribed.

▲ Consult with members of the interprofessional health team about measures to decrease the sources of dietary ammonia.

Rationales

Acute confusion increases the patient's risk for injury and falls. Physical restraints and sedatives should be used only when all other interventions prove ineffective. Overmedication may precipitate coma. QSEN: Safety.

Because ammonia is produced by the interaction of the colonic bacteria and amino acids, reduction of the bacteria colonies normally present in the colon will result in the reduced production of ammonia.

This laxative alters colonic pH and stimulates evacuation. An acidic pH in the colon inhibits bacteria production; the evacuation of colonic contents reduces the absorption of ammonia into the bloodstream and therefore improves encephalopathic states.

The dietitian can provide guidance in ordering a diet that is low in protein (0 to 40 g/day) and other dietary sources of ammonia such as foods containing gelatin, onions, and string beans. Protein makes amino acids available in the colon, which in turn enhances the production of ammonia. QSEN: Teamwork and collaboration.

Risk for Impaired Skin Integrity (Itching)

Common Risk Factors

Dermatitis/pruritus or itching (e.g., jaundice; elevated serum bilirubin levels)

■ = Independent ▲ = Interprofessional Collaboration

Common Expected Outcomes

Patient's skin remain intact.

Patient verbalizes decreased itching or ability to tolerate itching without scratching.

NOC Outcomes

Risk Control; Risk Detection; Tissue Integrity: Skin and Mucous Membranes; Self-Care: Hygiene

NIC Interventions

Skin Surveillance; Skin Care: Topical Treatments; Medication Administration

---

Ongoing Assessment

Actions/Interventions	Rationales
■ Assess the general condition of the skin.	Healthy skin varies among individuals but should have good turgor (an indication of moisture), feel warm and dry to the touch, be free of impairment (scratches, bruises, excoriation, rashes), and have quick capillary refill (less than 6 seconds). Older patients' skin is normally less elastic, has less moisture, and has thinning of the epidermis, making for higher risk for skin impairment. QSEN: Patient-centered care.
■ Monitor serum bilirubin levels	The patient with cirrhosis and hepatic failure will have elevated serum bilirubin levels. Normal adult total serum bilirubin is 0.1 to 1.2 mg/dL. When the serum bilirubin is greater than 3.0 mg/dL, jaundice is more likely to develop.
■ Assess for the presence of jaundice, patient complaints of itching, and scratching.	In hepatic failure, bilirubin cannot be excreted, and accumulates in the skin and other tissues (sclerae of the eyes). Unexcreted bilirubin moves by diffusion into subcutaneous and cutaneous structures and irritates the tissue, causing histamine release and itching. Excessive scratching can disrupt skin integrity and reduce its barrier function.

Therapeutic Interventions

Actions/Interventions	Rationales

■ Emphasize the importance of keeping the skin clean and well moisturized:
  • Use tepid water.
  • Avoid alkaline soaps.
  • Apply emollient lotions.
	Keeping the skin clean and moisturized reduces the drying that can contribute to itching.

■ Discourage scratching; keep the fingernails short. Suggest that the patient wear hand mitts if scratching cannot be discouraged by other means.	Nails can introduce pathogens and cause localized infection. Long fingernails may cause skin trauma from repeated scratching.
■ Keep the room temperature cool. Encourage the patient to wear loose-fitting, soft cotton clothing.	Cotton clothing allows for the evaporation of perspiration and adds to the patient's comfort.
▲ Administer antihistamines as ordered.	These medications can reduce itching by blocking the histamine at tissue receptors.

Related Care Plans

Disturbed body image, Chapter 2

Ineffective coping, Chapter 2

Ineffective health maintenance, Chapter 2

Risk for bleeding, Chapter 2

Gastrointestinal and Digestive Care Plans

ⓔvolve **For additional care plans, go to http://evolve.elsevier.com/Gulanick/.**

Colorectal Cancer

Colon Cancer; Rectal Cancer; Bowel Resection; Hemicolectomy; Colectomy

Colorectal cancer is the second most common fatal cancer in the United States. Colon cancer occurs more often than rectal cancer. Risk factors for colorectal cancer include familial polyposis, family history of colorectal cancer, and a personal history of colorectal cancer, colorectal polyps, or chronic bowel inflammatory disease. Other risk factors include physical inactivity, obesity, smoking, alcohol consumption, and a diet that is high in fat and low in fiber. Overall, men and women are affected about equally. Early colorectal cancer often has no symptoms, which is why screening is so important. Most colorectal cancers begin as a polyp, a small growth in the wall of the colon. However, over time some polyps grow and become malignant. Signs of colorectal cancer include bleeding from the rectum, blood in the stool or in the toilet after having a bowel movement, a change in the shape of the stool, cramping pain in the lower stomach, and a feeling of discomfort or an urge to have a bowel movement when there is no need to have one. The tumor, node, metastasis (TNM) staging system indicates tumor depth, node involvement, and presence of tumor metastasis, which have been shown to be the most significant variables in determining the prognosis of colon cancer. Colorectal cancer may metastasize through direct extension to adjacent tissues or by hematological-lymphatic spread. Surgical removal is the preferred treatment for colorectal cancer, although irradiation may be used preoperatively. Postoperative chemotherapy has proved to be beneficial in treatment of colon cancer. Irradiation and immunotherapy are used, but with limited success. This care plan addresses the preoperative stage, care of the patient who has undergone colon resection, and self-care teaching.

Deficient Knowledge: Preoperative

Common Related Factors
Insufficient information about colorectal cancer
Insufficient interest in learning
Insufficient knowledge of resources
Misinformation presented by others

Defining Characteristics
Insufficient knowledge
Inaccurate follow-through of instruction
Inaccurate performance on a test
Inappropriate behavior

Common Expected Outcomes
Patient verbalizes understanding of disease process for colorectal cancer.
Patient verbalizes understanding of proposed diagnostic and surgical procedures.

NOC Outcomes
Knowledge: Disease Process; Knowledge: Treatment Procedure
NIC Interventions
Health Literacy Enhancement; Learning Facilitation; Teaching: Disease Process; Teaching: Preoperative; Teaching: Procedure/Treatment

Ongoing Assessment

Actions/Interventions
- Assess the motivation and willingness of the patient and caregivers to learn.

Rationales
Some patients are ready to learn soon after they are diagnosed; others cope better by denying or delaying the need for instruction. Learning also requires energy, which patients may not be ready to use.

Gastrointestinal and Digestive Care Plans

■ = Independent   ▲ = Interprofessional Collaboration

Actions/Interventions

■ Assess the patient's knowledge of the following topics:

- Common signs and symptoms of colon cancer

- Necessary diagnostic procedures

- Proposed method of treatment and possible outcomes

Rationales

This information provides the starting base for educational sessions. Teaching standardized content that the patient already knows wastes valuable time and hinders critical learning. QSEN: Patient-centered. care

Because many colon cancers are advanced by the time of diagnosis, patients may feel guilty about not having sought treatment sooner.

The patient may have had multiple diagnostic examinations at this point and may not understand the importance of repeating procedures or undergoing further diagnostic studies. Diagnostic tests may be repeated to determine the exact size and location of tumors before surgery. Scans of distant tissues may be done to identify possible metastasis at the time of surgery.

As with other cancers, patients may feel hopeless that "nothing can be done." Patients may have previous experience with people who had cancer. This knowledge may influence the patient's attitude and anxiety about learning. Knowledge serves to correct the patient's misperceptions and faulty ideas about colorectal cancer treatment.

Therapeutic Interventions

Actions/Interventions

■ Teach patient the following about colon cancer:

- Risk factors

- Signs and symptoms

- Method of spread and its relationship to treatment

Rationales

This information may help the patient understand the process of colon cancer development, diagnosis of the cancer, and methods of treatment. Patients are better able to ask questions when they have basic information about what to expect. Accurate, clear information provides rationale for treatment and aids the patient in assuming responsibility for care at a later time. QSEN: Patient-centered care.

Family history and a personal history of colorectal cancer, colorectal polyps, or chronic inflammatory bowel disease is the greatest risk for cancer. Other risk factors include the American diet (high calorie, high fat, low fiber) and a history of other cancers, especially breast cancer in women.

Because the right side of the colon is distensible, tumors on the right side are usually asymptomatic until the disease is widespread. Symptoms at that time include weight loss, anemia, weakness, and fatigue. Tumors on the left side of the colon usually result in bleeding, constipation and diarrhea, increased abdominal cramping, decreased caliber of the stool (i.e., pencil or ribbon shaped), a feeling of incomplete evacuation, and sometimes complete obstruction.

Colon cancer spreads by direct extension into the surrounding tissue, by lymphatic channels, and by seeding into the peritoneal cavity. Excision of the tumor and surrounding tissue is the only curative treatment, although radiation therapy, chemotherapy, and immunotherapy may help reduce the tumor and check the spread. Biopsies done by colonoscopy may indicate the stage of a colon tumor. The full extent of the disease may be known only after biopsy of the tissue removed at the time of surgery.

Actions/Interventions

Rationales

■ Teach the patient about the following diagnostic procedures, as appropriate:

This information may help the patient understand tests and procedures done to diagnosis of the cancer. Patients are better able to ask questions when they have basic information about what to expect. Accurate, clear information provides rationale for treatment and aids the patient in assuming responsibility for care at a later time. QSEN: Patient-centered care.

• Colonoscopy with biopsy of lesions to confirm a diagnosis

Colonoscopy is a procedure that uses a flexible scope instrument to visualize the entire colon directly. Although a tumor may have been identified by digital examination, the entire colon should be examined before surgery; the presence of more than one tumor is possible.

• Carcinoembryonic antigen (CEA)

CEA is a blood test that gives an indication of ongoing cancer activity. Blood is drawn preoperatively so that progress can be monitored postoperatively.

• Chest x-ray examination

A preoperative chest x-ray study may be done to evaluate the lung for evidence of metastatic disease.

• Computed tomography (CT) scans

CT scans are done to determine distant metastatic spread. This information helps the surgeon decide how extensive a procedure is necessary.

• Complete blood count (CBC)

CBC is determined to assess for anemia. Colon tumors, particularly advanced colon tumors, bleed; bleeding may result in significant anemia, which is corrected before surgery.

• Endoscopic ultrasound

An ultrasound identifies lesions within the layers of the bowel wall and distinguishes involved lymph nodes.

■ Teach the patient about the types of surgical treatment.

This information may help the patient understand the surgical procedures done to treat cancer. Patients are better able to ask questions and provide informed consent when they have basic information about what to expect. Accurate, clear information provides rationale for treatment and aids the patient in assuming responsibility for care at a later time. The type of surgery will be determined by the location of the tumor and whether or not there is metastasis. Right or left hemicolectomy (removal of the right or left half of the colon or large intestine) is done to remove tumors of the ascending, transverse, descending, and sigmoid colon. Tumors that are too close to the anus are treated with abdominoperineal resection (resection of a portion of the colon, along with the rectum); this procedure results in a permanent colostomy because the rectum is gone. Tumors that are in the lower rectosigmoid colon or in the rectum may be treated with a low anterior resection, in which the tumor and surrounding colon are removed and the colon is then anastomosed (no colostomy). QSEN: Patient-centered care.

■ Teach the patient about the steps taken to prepare the bowel for surgery:

Decreasing the amount of fecal material in the colon before surgery is necessary to reduce the risk for postoperative peritonitis and wound infection. QSEN: Safety.

• Clear liquid diet

This diet reduces the residue in the bowel.

• Antibiotics

These drugs are not absorbed from the intestine and therefore reduce bacteria normally present in the colon to prevent postoperative peritonitis.

• Colyte, GoLYTELY, or other osmotic agents

These laxatives induce diarrhea and clean the bowel before surgery; they may also be used before colonoscopy.

Gastrointestinal and Digestive Care Plans

■ = Independent   ▲ = Interprofessional Collaboration

Actions/Interventions

■ Prepare the patient for what to expect after surgery:
- Incisions, drains

- IV lines

- Activity

- Pain management

- Thromboembolism precaution

Rationales

After a colectomy, most patients have one midline incision. Patients who have had an abdominoperineal resection have an anterior midline incision, a perineal incision where the rectum was removed, and a colostomy. Anterior incisions are typically sutured or stapled closed; perineal incisions may be closed or may be packed and left to heal by secondary intention. All patients have small drains in the lower abdomen to drain lymphatic fluid from the operative area.

Patients resume oral feedings when peristalsis resumes; therefore administration of IV fluids is necessary and continues until the patient can tolerate oral fluids.

Patients should expect to get out of bed on the first postoperative day to prevent complications of immobility (e.g., deep vein thrombosis, atelectasis). QSEN: Safety.

Patients should be involved in the choice of postoperative pain management. Options include medications given via IV patient-controlled analgesia, or bolus or continuous-infusion epidural analgesics. Oral administration of analgesics will begin when the patient is able to resume oral intake. QSEN: Patient-centered care.

Patients undergoing colon resection for cancer have a high incidence of venous thromboembolism, including deep vein thrombosis and pulmonary embolism. There is strong evidence that the use of low-molecular-weight heparin (e.g., enoxaparin) reduces the risk. Intermittent pneumatic calf compression has been shown to be effective in reducing the risk for thromboembolism. Whether there is an additive effect by using more than one mode of prophylaxis for patients undergoing colonic resection is yet to be determined. QSEN: Safety; Evidence-based practice.

NANDA-I
NDx **Risk for Constipation (Postoperative Ileus)**

Common Risk Factors

Postsurgical bowel obstruction (general anesthesia; manipulation of bowel during surgery)
Pharmacological agent (opioid analgesics)

Common Expected Outcome

Patient passes flatus and stool 48 to 72 hours postoperatively.

NOC Outcome
Bowel Elimination
NIC Interventions
Flatulence Reduction; Bowel Management

Ongoing Assessment

Actions/Interventions	Rationales
■ Assess for bowel sounds, abdominal distention, the presence of flatus or stool, and nausea.	Bowel sounds will be hypoactive initially, but should return to normal 48 to 72 hours after surgery. The presence of flatus or stool indicates the return of peristalsis. The absence of bowel sounds, flatus, and stool with abdominal distention may indicate a postoperative paralytic ileus. Nausea may occur as a result of the accumulation of intestinal content.
■ Monitor use of opioid analgesics for postoperative pain management.	The opioid analgesics act by binding to mu receptors through the body. Peristalsis decreases when these analgesics bind to mu receptors in the intestines.

Therapeutic Interventions

Actions/Interventions	Rationales
■ Maintain nothing by mouth (NPO) status until bowel sounds return and the patient begins to pass flatus. Fluids will be administered intravenously.	Until peristaltic activity returns, oral intake puts the patient at risk for nausea and vomiting. QSEN: Safety.
■ Ensure patency of the nasogastric tube, and provide good oral care.	Keeping the stomach empty reduces the risk for nausea, vomiting, and aspiration.
■ Encourage and assist with ambulation beginning the first postoperative day.	Increasing ambulation hastens resolution of the ileus by stimulating peristalsis.
■ Assist the patient with initial food and fluid selection.	Low-fiber foods and easily digestible foods produce less gas and distention.

 NANDA-I NDx **Risk for Infection**

Common Risk Factors
Invasive procedures (intraoperative leakage of bowel contents; insertion of circular staple gun through rectum to abdominal cavity)

Common Expected Outcomes
Patient remains free of infection, as evidenced by normal vital signs and absence of purulent drainage from wounds, incisions, and tubes.
Infection is recognized early to allow for prompt treatment.

NOC Outcomes
Risk Control; Wound Healing: Primary Intention; Infection Severity
NIC Interventions
Infection Control; Infection Precautions; Wound Care

Ongoing Assessment

Actions/Interventions	Rationales
■ Assess the length of the surgical procedure.	The longer the patient is in surgery, the greater the risk for postoperative infection.
■ Assess the wound for redness, warmth, drainage, pain, swelling, or dehiscence.	These assessment findings are signs of wound infection. QSEN: Safety.

■ = Independent   ▲ = Interprofessional Collaboration

Gastrointestinal and Digestive Care Plans

Actions/Interventions

▲ Obtain a culture of any suspicious drainage.

■ Monitor the patient's temperature.

▲ Monitor the white blood cell (WBC) count.

Rationales

Normal drainage is clear, yellow, and odorless. Identifying infecting microorganisms is necessary to select the appropriate antibiotic therapy. QSEN: Safety.

A temperature above 38.5°C (101.3°F) should arouse suspicion of infection. QSEN: Safety.

An elevated WBC count is an indication of infection. QSEN: Safety.

Therapeutic Interventions

Actions/Interventions

■ Wash hands on entering the room.

■ Use aseptic technique for dressing changes.

▲ Administer antibiotics and antipyretics as prescribed.

■ If a stoma is present, maintain a good skin seal.

Rationales

Handwashing remains the most effective means of infection control. QSEN: Safety.

Aseptic technique prevents the transmission of bacterial infections to the surgical wound. QSEN: Safety.

These drugs treat infections and the fever associated with infections.

Whereas many patients will have a colon resection with end-to-end anastomosis, some patients may have extensive removal of the large intestine that requires the creation of a colostomy. A minimal gap between the stoma and collection pouch opening contains fecal drainage and prevents possible contamination of the incision.

NANDA-I
NDx Deficient Knowledge: Postoperative

Common Related Factors

Insufficient information about postoperative care
Insufficient interest in learning
Insufficient knowledge of resources
Misinformation presented by others

Defining Characteristics

Insufficient knowledge
Inaccurate follow-through of instruction
Inaccurate performance on a test
Inappropriate behavior

Common Expected Outcome

Patient or caregiver verbalizes knowledge and demonstrates ability to perform wound care, select appropriate diet, plan activity, report complications, and receive necessary follow-up care.

NOC Outcomes

Knowledge: Prescribed Diet; Knowledge: Disease Process; Knowledge: Treatment Regimen

NIC Interventions

Health Literacy Enhancement; Learning Facilitation; Teaching: Disease Process; Teaching: Psychomotor Skill; Teaching: Prescribed Exercise; Teaching: Prescribed Diet

---

Ongoing Assessment

Actions/Interventions

■ Assess the patient's ability to perform wound care, verbalize appropriate activity, and describe an appropriate diet.

Rationales

This information provides the starting base for educational sessions. Teaching standardized content that the patient already knows wastes valuable time and hinders critical learning. QSEN: Patient-centered care.

---

evolve **For additional care plans, go to http://evolve.elsevier.com/Gulanick/.**

Actions/Interventions

- Assess the patient's understanding of expected bowel function.
- Assess the patient's understanding of the need for further cancer therapy and regular follow-up care.

- Determine the patient's or the caregiver's self-efficacy to learn and apply new knowledge.

Rationales

Patients should understand that their usual bowel pattern might not return until 2 to 3 weeks postoperatively.

Patients who have abdominal surgery for malignancies may require further therapy such as chemotherapy, irradiation, or immunotherapy. Ongoing surveillance is needed to detect the recurrence of cancer.

A first step in teaching may be to foster increased self-efficacy in the patient's ability to learn the desired information or skills. Some lifestyle changes can be difficult to make.

Therapeutic Interventions

Actions/Interventions

- Teach the patient or caregiver to perform appropriate wound care:
  - Anterior abdominal wound

  - Perineal wound

- If the patient has a colostomy:
  - Teach the patient or caregiver how to apply a skin barrier around the stoma.
  - Inform the patient or caregiver that the barrier can remain on the skin for 3 to 4 days. It should be removed after the fourth day, and the skin around the stoma should be inspected.
  - Clean the skin with warm water and mild soap. Dry the skin completely before applying a new barrier.
  - Apply a clean collection bag (appliance) and empty the bag when it is about half full of stool.
  - Note the amount, color, and consistency of stool.

  - If there is no stool from the colostomy, check the stoma with a gloved, lubricated finger. If there is still no stool or flatus, notify the physician.
- Teach the patient that bowel function may not return to preoperative baseline for several weeks.

- Teach the patient appropriate activity guidelines:
  - No lifting more than 10 pounds for 6 weeks

  - Mild exercise (e.g., walking)

  - Showering
  - Bathing unless an open perineal wound exists

  - No driving until the anterior abdominal wound has healed

Rationales

Teaching the patient and caregiver about wound care is important to reduce the risk of infection. QSEN: Safety.

Staples or sutures and dressings usually have been removed by the time of discharge, and Steri-Strips have been placed to maintain wound approximation. Steri-Strips should be left in place until they fall off.

The patient can take sitz baths twice daily for cleansing and comfort, after which the wound is repacked with saline solution–moistened gauze. Usually clean technique (hands washed; clean but not sterile gloves) is used.

This barrier promotes peristomal skin integrity and prevents the irritation of skin from fecal output. QSEN: Safety.

Skin infections, irritation, and allergic reactions to the barrier material can occur around the stoma.

These measures promote skin integrity and reduce infection.

Emptying the bag before it gets too full reduces the risk for leakage of fecal material and odor.

Changes in the diet and infections can produce changes in the fecal output from the stoma.

An absence of colostomy output may be a sign of intestinal obstruction.

The more colon that is resected, the longer the period of adaptation. During this time stool may be loose and bowel movements more frequent.

This activity restriction reduces strain on the abdominal muscles and the risk for stoma prolapse. QSEN: Safety.

Exercise increases stamina and prevents deep vein thrombosis and pneumonia.

The patient can usually shower once the incisions have healed.

It may take up to 8 weeks to heal completely. Using a hand-held shower head is a good way to clean the wound.

Operating foot pedals while driving, especially the brake pedal, increases the strain on abdominal muscles.

Gastrointestinal and Digestive Care Plans

■ = Independent ▲ = Interprofessional Collaboration

Actions/Interventions

- Teach the patient the following about diet:
  - Consume a well-balanced, high-calorie, high-protein diet.
  - Fiber should be added to the diet.

- Teach the patient the rationale for any further cancer therapy planned (e.g., chemotherapy, radiation therapy, immunotherapy).

- Teach the patient the importance of follow-up colonoscopies.

- Discuss family risk with the patient.

- Teach patients who have had removal of the rectum that phantom rectum sensations and a feeling of needing to have a bowel movement are normal and will subside over time.

- Instruct the patient to seek medical attention for any of the following: a temperature higher than 38°C (100.4°F), foul-smelling wound drainage, redness or unusual pain in any incision, or the absence of bowel movements.

Rationales

This type of diet should continue over a period of weeks to promote effective healing.

Because the patient has already had colon cancer, the risk for future tumors is high. A high-fiber diet is associated with more frequent bowel movements and less time for suspected carcinogenic food by-products to be in contact with the colonic mucosa. Foods high in fiber include grains, fruits, and vegetables.

These therapies are typically offered if the pathology report indicates that the tumor was not confined to the bowel or bowel wall.

These procedures allow for early detection of any recurrent tumors. They are usually scheduled every 6 months for people with a history of colon cancer. QSEN: Safety.

Parents, siblings, and adult children older than 40 years should be screened yearly for colon cancer.

These situations are related to the remaining nerve fibers in the perineum.

These signs and symptoms are indicative of an infection or possible bowel obstruction. QSEN: Safety.

Related Care Plans

Acute pain, Chapter 2
Grieving, Chapter 2
Ineffective coping, Chapter 2
Surgical experience: Preoperative and postoperative care, Chapter 4
Bowel diversion surgery: Colostomy, ileostomy, Chapter 8

Gastrointestinal Bleeding

Lower Gastrointestinal Bleed; Upper Gastrointestinal Bleed; Esophageal Varices; Ulcers

Loss of blood from the gastrointestinal (GI) tract is most often the result of erosion or ulceration of the mucosa, but it may also be the result of arteriovenous (AV) malformation or malignancies, increased pressure in the portal venous bed, or direct trauma to the GI tract. Alcohol abuse is a major etiological factor in GI bleeding. Varices, usually located in the distal third of the submucosal tissue of the esophagus or the fundus of the stomach, can also cause life-threatening GI hemorrhage. Upper GI bleeding may manifest as blood-tinged, bright red, or coffee grounds emesis.

The patient with upper GI bleeding may also experience dark, tarry stools. Lower GI bleeding may occur as bright red blood from the rectum. This type of bleeding is often associated with the presence of hemorrhoids. Tumors of the colon may cause bleeding detected as occult blood in the feces rather than visible bleeding. Inflammatory bowel disease may cause lower GI bleeding characterized as bloody diarrhea. Factors that alter coagulation or cause generalized inflammation of the intestinal mucosa can contribute to bleeding anywhere in the GI tract. Treatment may be medical or surgical or may involve mechanical tamponade. Acute GI bleeding may be life threatening without prompt treatment. In patients with GI bleeding, stabilization of BP and restoration of intravascular volume are the highest priority. The focus of this care plan is the acute hospital management phase of a patient with active GI bleeding.

NANDA-I
NDx Deficient Fluid Volume

Common Related Factors
Active fluid loss from bleeding in the esophagus, stomach, small intestine or large intestine
Inadequate fluid intake

Defining Characteristics
Decrease in urine output (less than 30 mL/hr)
Increase in urine concentration (urine specific gravity > 0.125)
Sudden weight loss
Decreased venous filling pressures (preload)
Increase in hemoglobin
Decrease in BP/orthostasis
Thirst
Tachycardia/weak, rapid HR
Decreased skin turgor
Dry mucous membranes
Weakness
Altered mental state

Common Expected Outcome
Patient is normovolemic as evidenced by no signs of active bleeding, systolic BP greater than 90 mm Hg (or patient's baseline), absence of orthostasis, HR 60 to 100 beats/min, urine output greater than 30 mL/hr, and normal skin turgor.

NOC Outcomes
Blood Coagulation; Fluid Balance; Hydration
NIC Interventions
Bleeding Reduction: Gastrointestinal; Fluid Monitoring; Fluid Management; Fluid Resuscitation

Ongoing Assessment

Actions/Interventions

- Monitor the color, amount, and consistency of hematemesis, melena, or rectal bleeding; encourage the patient to describe unwitnessed blood loss accurately using common household measures (e.g., a cupful, a spoonful, a pint).
- Obtain a history of the use or abuse of substances known to predispose to GI bleeding: aspirin, aspirin-containing drugs, nonsteroidal anti-inflammatory drugs, alcohol, steroids.
- Monitor BP for orthostatic changes (changes seen when changing from a supine to a standing position).

Rationales

Careful assessment of GI bleeding can help determine the exact site of the bleeding.

Drugs that cause ulceration of the GI mucosa contribute to the development of bleeding. QSEN: Patient-centered care.

Early identification of orthostatic changes in blood pressure guides specific interventions to reduce harm from injury or falls. Postural hypotension is a common manifestation in fluid loss. The incidence increases with age. Note the following orthostatic hypotension significances:
- Greater than 10 mm Hg drop: circulating blood volume is decreased by 20%.
- Greater than 20 to 30 mm Hg drop: circulating blood volume is decreased by 40%. QSEN: Safety.

Gastrointestinal and Digestive Care Plans

■ = Independent   ▲ = Interprofessional Collaboration

Actions/Interventions

▲ Monitor the coagulation profile, hemoglobin (Hgb), and hematocrit (Hct).

■ Monitor the patient's urine output.

Rationales

Many individuals with GI bleeding have long-standing nutritional deficits that result in an altered coagulation profile because of the liver's inability to produce adequate amounts of vitamin K, a precursor to many coagulation factors. Hgb and Hct are monitored as indicators of both blood loss and hydration status. Initially, Hgb and Hct will drop because of blood loss; as fluid resuscitation proceeds, hemodilution may result in further drop in Hgb and Hct. QSEN: Safety.

Urine output of at least 30 mL/hr is an indication of adequate renal perfusion.

Therapeutic Interventions

Actions/Interventions

▲ Provide volume resuscitation with crystalloids or blood products as ordered through one or more large-bore IV lines.

■ Monitor the cardiopulmonary response to volume expansion through changes in the HR and heart rhythm, BP, and the auscultation of breath sounds.

▲ Insert a nasogastric (NG) tube for stomach lavage.

▲ Assist members of the interprofessional health team with diagnostic procedures performed to identify the bleeding site:
• Endoscopy

• Sigmoidoscopy, proctoscopy, and colonoscopy

• Barium studies:
  • Barium swallow

  • Barium enema
• Small bowel follow-through

Rationales

Crystalloids are more commonly used, whereas blood products are selectively used to replace specific coagulation factors (e.g., platelets only, fresh-frozen plasma). Rapid volume expansion is necessary to prevent or treat hypovolemia complications; IV medication and/or blood component administration is likely.

The amount of fluid administered will depend on the rate of bleeding and the patient's hemodynamic status. A poor response to fluid resuscitation may result in an increased HR or dysrhythmias. The patient may become hypotensive. Respiratory crackles may occur as a result of left-sided heart failure. Patients with a history of alcohol abuse may have alcohol-related cardiomyopathies. Elderly patients may experience cardiovascular difficulty with rapid fluid volume resuscitation because of diminished cardiac function, a normal phenomenon of aging. QSEN: Safety.

The NG tube provides a way to monitor continuing blood loss closely and for medication administration. Lavage of the stomach is done using room-temperature saline solution until clots are no longer present and the return is clear. Iced saline solution may cause undesirable ischemic changes in the gastric mucosa.

The nurse collaborates with endoscopic specialists and radiologists to ensure that the patient is prepared appropriately for these procedures. QSEN: Teamwork and collaboration.

This procedure provides direct visualization of the esophagus, stomach, and duodenum. The procedure must precede x-ray films requiring barium ingestion to maximize visualization by the endoscopist.

These procedures provide direct visualization of the rectum and colon.

This x-ray procedure is an indirect visualization of the esophagus, stomach, and small intestine.

This x-ray procedure is an indirect visualization of the colon.

This x-ray procedure is an indirect visualization of the small intestine.

Gastrointestinal and Digestive Care Plans

Actions/Interventions

- Angiography
  - After angiography: dress the site with pressure dressing; connect the arterial line to pressure or flush the system.
- ▲ Administer a vasopressin drip as ordered.

- ■ Monitor for the side effects of vasopressin.

- ▲ Administer vitamin K as ordered.
- ▲ Administer antacids and histamine-2–receptor antagonists.
- ■ Avoid the administration of drugs that may potentiate further bleeding.

- ▲ For the patient who is bleeding from esophageal or gastric varices and who is in a critical care area, prepare for the insertion of a Sengstaken-Blakemore tube.

- ▲ Assist members of the interprofessional health team with preparation of the patient for surgical procedures.

Rationales

This procedure may be diagnostic or performed for arterial line placement to infuse vasoconstrictive medications locally. A conclusive diagnosis is made only if bleeding is more than 0.5 mL/min.

Vasopressin is a commercial preparation of antidiuretic hormone that promotes vasoconstriction and reduces bleeding. The drug may be given as IV continuous drip, piggyback bolus, or intra-arterially if a line was placed during an angiographic procedure to a specific area (e.g., celiac artery for esophageal bleeding).

Side effects of vasopressin may include anginal pain, ST-segment changes on electrocardiogram, sinus bradycardia, tremors, sweating, vertigo, pounding in the head, abdominal cramps, circumoral pallor, nausea and vomiting, flatus, urticaria, and fluid retention. Elevated BP can be the result of vasoconstriction from vasopressin. QSEN: Safety.

This drug allows coagulation factor production.

These drugs suppress gastric and duodenal secretions.

Aspirin-containing compounds and anticoagulants interfere with the coagulation mechanisms and increase the risk for bleeding. QSEN: Safety.

The Sengstaken-Blakemore tube has balloons that inflate in the esophagus and upper portion of the stomach to provide tamponade (pressure) against the vessels that are bleeding.

If esophageal varices are the source of the bleeding, surgical measures may be used to control the bleeding. These surgical procedures may include sclerotherapy, endoscopic varicose ligation, or thermal coagulation. QSEN: Teamwork and collaboration.

NANDA-I
NDx **Deficient Knowledge**

Common Related Factors

Insufficient information
Insufficient interest in learning
Insufficient knowledge of resources
Misinformation presented by others

Defining Characteristics

Insufficient knowledge
Inaccurate follow-through of instruction
Inappropriate behavior

Common Expected Outcome

Patient or significant other verbalizes understanding of causes and management of GI bleeding.

NOC Outcomes

Knowledge: Treatment Regimen; Knowledge: Treatment Procedure

NIC Interventions

Health Literacy Enhancement; Learning Facilitation; Teaching: Procedure/Treatment; Teaching: Medication Management; Substance Use Treatment

Gastrointestinal and Digestive Care Plans

■ = Independent   ▲ = Interprofessional Collaboration

Ongoing Assessment

Actions/Interventions	Rationales
■ Assess the patient's understanding of the cause and treatment of GI bleeding.	This information provides the starting base for educational sessions. During the acute stages, the family or significant others may require the most teaching. QSEN: Patient-centered care.
■ Determine the patient's self-efficacy to learn and apply new knowledge needed for follow-up care.	Self-efficacy refers to a person's confidence in his or her ability to perform a behavior. Prevention of the recurrence of bleeding may require health behavior changes by the patient. Some lifestyle changes can be difficult to make.

Therapeutic Interventions

Actions/Interventions	Rationales
■ Explain the procedures necessary for diagnosis or treatment before they are performed.	Understanding the need for unpleasant procedures may help the patient participate in and increase the effectiveness of the treatment or procedure. QSEN: Patient-centered care.
■ Explain the importance of avoiding substances containing aspirin, alcohol, nonsteroidal anti-inflammatory drugs, and steroids.	The use of these products is known to damage the mucosal barrier and predispose to bleeding. The patient will need to make health behavior changes to limit use of these substances. QSEN: Safety.
■ Teach the patient the dose, administration schedule, expected actions, and possible adverse effects of medications that may be prescribed for long periods.	Drugs given to decrease gastric acid production may be prescribed indefinitely; patients must understand that the cessation of bleeding or other symptoms does not mean the need for medication has ended.
▲ Refer the patient to an alcohol rehabilitation program if indicated.	The patient may benefit from a formal treatment program to control alcohol use and prevent future bleeding episodes.

Related Care Plans

Diarrhea, Chapter 2
Fear, Chapter 2
Ineffective health management, Chapter 2
Risk for bleeding, Chapter 2
Risk for impaired skin integrity, Chapter 2

Inflammatory Bowel Disease

Crohn's Disease; Ulcerative Colitis; Diverticulitis

Inflammatory bowel disease (IBD) refers to a cluster of specific bowel abnormalities for which symptoms are often so similar as to make diagnosis difficult and treatment empirical. Crohn's disease is associated with involvement of all four layers of the bowel and may occur anywhere in the gastrointestinal (GI) tract, although it is most common in the small bowel at the terminal ileum. Ulcerative colitis occurs only in the colon bond involves the mucosal and submucosal layers. Cause is unknown for both diseases, but a familial history of IBD is found in patients who develop Crohn's disease and ulcerative colitis. Specific genetic mutations have been identified in people with Crohn's disease. The incidence of Crohn's disease is higher in people of Ashkenazi Jewish heritage than in other ethnic groups. Incidence is usually in the 15- to 30-year-old age group. Both Crohn's disease and ulcerative colitis are associated

Gastrointestinal and Digestive Care Plans

with the development of diarrhea and nutritional deficiencies. Systemic manifestations can involve the liver, joints, skin, and eyes. Diverticulitis is inflammation of a diverticulum in the colon. The diverticulum is a herniation of the mucosal layer of the colon through the muscle layer. Obstruction of the diverticulum with hardened fecal material or undigested food particles causes the inflammation.

Diverticular disease often occurs in people older than 40 years of age; it seems to be etiologically related to high-fat, low-fiber diets and occurs almost exclusively in the colon. IBD is treated medically. Bowel diversion surgery may be indicated if medical management fails or if the patient develops complications. This care plan focuses on chronic, ambulatory care.

NANDA-I
NDx Acute Pain: Abdominal, Joint

Common Related Factor

Biological injury agent (bowel inflammation and contractions of diseased bowel or colon; systemic inflammation)

Defining Characteristics

Self-report of intensity using standardized pain scale
Self-report of pain characteristics using standardized pain instrument
Diaphoresis
Self-focused
Facial expression of pain
Positioning to ease pain
Change in physiological parameter (e.g., BP, HR, respiratory rate, and oxygen saturation)

Common Expected Outcomes

Patient reports satisfactory pain control and a decreased intensity using a standardized pain scale.
Patient uses pharmacological and nonpharmacological pain management strategies.
Patient exhibits increased comfort such as baseline levels for pulse, BP, respirations, and relaxed muscle tone or body posture.

NOC Outcomes

Comfort Status; Medication Response; Pain Control; Pain Level

NIC Interventions

Medication Administration: Oral; Medication Administration: Rectal; Pain Management

---

Ongoing Assessment

Actions/Interventions

■ Assess the patient's pain: intermittent, colicky abdominal pain; abdominal pain and cramping associated with eating; joint pain.

■ Assess the patient's perception of the intensity of the pain using a standardized rating scale.
■ Auscultate bowel sounds.

Rationales

The patient is the most reliable source of information about his or her pain. Although the exact mechanism is unclear, a strong autoimmune etiology is believed to exist in Crohn's disease and ulcerative colitis; systemic manifestations often include arthritis-like symptoms. The patient with diverticulitis may report dull pain in the left lower quadrant of the abdomen. Changes in the severity and nature of the abdominal pain may indicate a life-threatening condition such as perforation of the GI tract. QSEN: Patient-centered care.
A numeric rating scale or other descriptive scales can be used to identify the intensity of pain.
Inflammation of the intestines contributes to increased peristalsis and diarrhea. The intestinal hypermotility combined with the inflammation causes cramping abdominal pain. Hyperactive bowel sounds are typical with this type of pain.

Gastrointestinal and Digestive Care Plans

■ = Independent   ▲ = Interprofessional Collaboration

Actions/Interventions

- Evaluate the patient's perception of dietary intake on abdominal pain.

- Assess the presence of changes in bowel habits, such as diarrhea.

- Determine any measures the patient has successfully used to control pain.

Rationales

Many patients with IBD cannot tolerate dairy products and may not tolerate many other foods. Pain and diarrhea may intensify with the consumption of these foods.

Cramping abdominal pain often increases with diarrhea. Patients with diverticular disease may have a history of constipation alternating with diarrhea.

This information can be helpful in developing an effective pain management program. Incorporating pain management strategies that the patient has found successful allows the patient to be a full partner in providing effective pain management care. QSEN: Patient-centered care.

Therapeutic Interventions

Actions/Interventions

- Instruct the patient to take medications as prescribed:

  - Sulfasalazine

  - Corticosteroids

  - Immunosuppressants and immunomodulators

  - Anticholinergics and/or antidiarrheals

- Encourage the patient to engage in usual diversional activities, hobbies, relaxation techniques, and psychosocial support systems as tolerated.

- Recommend necessary alterations in the diet.

Rationales

The goal of medical treatment is to induce clinical remission while avoiding toxic medications. Pain diminishes with remission of the inflammation. QSEN: Evidence-based practice.

Sulfasalazine (Azulfidine) is an aminosalicylate (5-ASA) that decreases inflammation and is typically used to bring the disease to remission.

Corticosteroids are given to decrease inflammation. These drugs may be administered by a variety of routes including oral, IV, and rectal.

Drugs that suppress or modify immune system activity are initiated when patients do not respond to sulfasalazine and corticosteroids. The effectiveness of this group of drugs is often enhanced when they are given in combination with corticosteroids.

Anticholinergics and antidiarrheal drugs are given to manage diarrhea by decreasing smooth muscle spasms and reducing intestinal motility and secretions. These drugs help manage symptoms of inflammatory bowel disease but do not address the underlying inflammation of the intestines.

Distraction heightens the patient's concentration on non-painful stimuli to decrease the awareness and experience of pain. Relaxation techniques bring about a state of physical and mental awareness and tranquility to reduce tension and pain. The patient's social support network can reduce the burden of suffering associated with pain.

Small frequent meals tend to be better tolerated and cause less GI distress. An increase in dietary fiber reduces constipation and abdominal discomfort for the patient with diverticular disease. These modifications may reduce the pain and discomfort experienced by the patient.

Imbalanced Nutrition: Less Than Body Requirements

Common Related Factors

Inability to absorb nutrients
Insufficient dietary intake
Inability to ingest foods (anorexia and nausea)

Defining Characteristics

Body weight 20% or more below ideal weight range
Food intake less than recommended dietary allowance (RDA)
Excessive hair loss
Pale mucous membranes
Insufficient interest in food
Sore buccal cavity

Common Expected Outcomes

Patient or caregiver verbalizes and demonstrates selection of foods or meals that will achieve a cessation of weight loss.
Patient weighs within 10% of ideal weight range.

NOC Outcomes
Nutritional Status: Nutrient Intake; Nutritional Status: Food and Fluid Intake
NIC Interventions
Nutritional Monitoring; Nutrition Management

Ongoing Assessment

Actions/Interventions	Rationales
■ Document the patient's actual weight and height (do not estimate).	Decreased body weight is a sign of poor nutrition. These anthropomorphic assessments are used to determine the patient's caloric and nutrient requirements.
■ Obtain the patient's nutritional history; monitor the patient's dietary intake.	This assessment information provides the basis for initiating diet therapy. The patient's perception of actual intake may differ from his or her actual intake. Family members may provide a more accurate estimate of the patient's eating habits and food intake. QSEN: Patient-centered care.
■ Assess for skin lesions, skin breaks, tears, decreased skin integrity, and edema of the extremities.	Protein malnutrition causes impaired skin integrity and tissue edema.
▲ Assess serum electrolytes, calcium, vitamins K and B_{12}, folic acid, and zinc levels to determine actual or potential deficiencies.	Patients may experience deficiencies related to altered food intake or the inability of the bowel mucosa to absorb nutrients.
■ Assess the patterns of bowel elimination: color, amount, consistency, frequency, odor, and the presence of steatorrhea (stools high in undigested fat).	Diarrhea and steatorrhea are indications of nutrient malabsorption.

Therapeutic Interventions

Actions/Interventions	Rationales
▲ Consult with members of the interprofessional health team about strategies to improve nutrient intake.	Dietitians can analyze the patient's nutritional history and provide guidance in selecting foods to improve the patient's nutritional status. High-calorie, high-protein, low-residue diets are recommended to maximize calorie and nutrient absorption and reduce diarrhea. QSEN: Teamwork and collaboration.
■ Encourage the patient or caregiver to evaluate factors that enhance appetite, and adjust the environment accordingly.	An environment free of distractions and unpleasant odors can promote increased intake.

Gastrointestinal and Digestive Care Plans

■ = Independent   ▲ = Interprofessional Collaboration

Actions/Interventions

▲ Administer vitamin and mineral supplements as ordered.

▲ Anticipate the need for total parenteral nutrition (TPN) as prescribed.

▲ Administer medications to control diarrhea.

Rationales

These replacements compensate for deficiencies that are the result of malabsorption in the inflamed intestines.

This therapy is for patients who cannot tolerate oral intake or require bowel rest during an acute exacerbation of the disease.

Antidiarrheals can reduce loose stools, urgency, and fecal soiling. Controlling diarrhea can contribute to increased nutrient absorption and improve the patient's appetite.

NANDA-I
NDx **Risk for Deficient Fluid Volume**

Common Risk Factors

Active fluid loss (excessive diarrhea; blood loss from inflamed bowel mucosa)
Insufficient fluid intake

Common Expected Outcome

Patient is normovolemic as evidenced by systolic BP greater than or equal to 90 mm Hg (or patient's baseline), absence of orthostasis, HR 60 to 100 beats/min, urine output greater than 30 mL/hr, and normal skin turgor.

NOC Outcomes
Fluid Balance; Blood Coagulation; Hydration
NIC Interventions
Bleeding Reduction: Gastrointestinal; Fluid Monitoring; Fluid Management; Fluid Resuscitation

---

Ongoing Assessment

Actions/Interventions

■ Assess the patient's hydration status: skin turgor, mucous membranes, fluid intake and urine output, weight, BP, and HR.
■ Monitor BP for orthostatic changes (changes seen when changing from supine to standing position). Monitor HR for orthostatic changes.

■ Determine the patient's fluid preferences: type, temperature (hot or cold).
▲ Document hemoccult-positive stools or the obvious presence of bloody diarrhea. Monitor hemoglobin and hematocrit if the patient is bleeding.

Rationales

Tenting of the skin, dry mucous membranes, reduced urine output, weight loss, increased HR, and hypotension are signs of fluid deficit. QSEN: Safety.

Postural hypotension is a common manifestation in fluid loss as reflected by a 20 mm Hg drop in systolic BP and a 10 mm Hg drop in diastolic BP. The incidence increases with age. Note the following orthostatic hypotension significance:
- Greater than 10 mm Hg drop: circulating blood volume is decreased by 20%.
- Greater than 20 to 30 mm Hg drop: circulating blood volume is decreased by 40%.
- Orthostatic hypotension caused by volume depletion is associated with a compensatory increase in HR (more than 20 beats/min). QSEN: Safety.

Selecting those fluids that the patient enjoys drinking can facilitate replacement therapy. QSEN: Patient-centered care.

Bleeding leads to decreased circulatory volume and fluid deficit. Blood loss is typically most severe in patients with ulcerative colitis, but patients with Crohn's disease also may have bloody diarrhea. Decreased hemoglobin and hematocrit occur with bleeding.

Gastrointestinal and Digestive Care Plans

⊖volve **For additional care plans, go to http://evolve.elsevier.com/Gulanick/.**

Therapeutic Interventions

Actions/Interventions	Rationales
■ Encourage the patient to drink at least 8 to 10 glasses of fluid daily.	Oral fluid intake is the preferred method to maintain hydration and fluid balance.
■ Instruct the patient to take medications as ordered.	A variety of drugs are used to reduce intestinal inflammation and control diarrhea. Decreasing diarrhea will limit the fluid lost with stools.
■ Provide oral hygiene.	Fluid deficit can cause a dry, sticky mouth. Attention to mouth care promotes interest in drinking and reduces discomfort of dry mucous membranes.
▲ Anticipate the need for IV therapy.	IV fluids are used if the patient's oral intake is inadequate to maintain a normal fluid volume status.

NANDA-I NDx Deficient Knowledge

Common Related Factors
Insufficient information about inflammatory bowel disease and its management
Insufficient interest in learning
Insufficient knowledge of resources
Misinformation presented by others

Defining Characteristics
Insufficient knowledge
Inaccurate follow-through of instruction
Inappropriate behavior

Common Expected Outcome
Patient or caregiver verbalizes understanding of inflammatory bowel disease and the importance of compliance with medical regimen.

NOC Outcomes
Knowledge: Disease Process; Knowledge: Treatment Regimen
NIC Interventions
Health Literacy Enhancement; Learning Facilitation; Teaching: Disease Process; Teaching: Prescribed Diet; Teaching: Prescribed Medication

Ongoing Assessment

Actions/Interventions	Rationales
■ Assess the patient's understanding of inflammatory bowel disease (IBD) and its necessary management.	This information provides the starting base for educational sessions. Patients need to understand that IBD differs from individual to individual; some cases are managed successfully throughout the course of the disease on medications alone, whereas others progress to needing surgical intervention. QSEN: Patient-centered care.
■ Assess the motivation and willingness of the patient and caregivers to learn.	Adults must see a need or purpose for learning. Some patients are ready to learn soon after they are diagnosed; others cope better by denying or delaying the need for instruction.

Gastrointestinal and Digestive Care Plans

■ = Independent   ▲ = Interprofessional Collaboration

Therapeutic Interventions

Actions/Interventions	Rationales
■ Discuss the disease process and its management.	The chronic nature of IBD requires that the patient understand that remissions and exacerbations are the expected course of the disease. Medication and dietary management are typically ongoing, although adjustments may be required, depending on the stage of the disease. Careful medical management may eliminate or postpone the need for surgical intervention. QSEN: Patient-centered care.
■ Discuss the surgical interventions for IBD.	Bowel resection with either anastomosis or bowel diversion with an ostomy may be done for patients with severe IBD. A total colectomy with an ileostomy can cure ulcerative colitis. Crohn's disease cannot be cured with surgery but bowel resections with anastomosis may be done to manage complications and severe symptoms of the disease. Colon resection may be indicated for management of severe diverticular disease.
■ Encourage contact with the Crohn's & Colitis Foundation of America.	Community resources provide the patient and caregiver with ongoing support and information about best practices for managing the disease.

Related Care Plans

Deficient fluid volume, Chapter 2
Diarrhea, Chapter 2
Ineffective health management, Chapter 2
Risk for impaired skin integrity, Chapter 2
Parenteral nutrition, Chapter 4
Bowel diversion surgery: Colostomy, ileostomy, Chapter 8

Peptic Ulcer Disease

Duodenal Ulcers; Gastric Ulcers; Stress-Induced Ulcers

Peptic ulcer disease (PUD) develops from a weakening in the lining of the mucosa that surrounds the upper gastrointestinal (GI) tract. The result of this weakness is erosion and eventual ulceration of the mucosa. These ulcerations may develop in the lower esophagus, stomach, or duodenum. Factors that contribute to the development of PUD include hyperacidity, pepsin, bile salts, ischemia, aspirin, and nonsteroidal anti-inflammatory drugs (NSAIDs). NSAIDs cause a weakening in the lining of the GI tract by decreasing the protective function of the mucosal layer. This decrease in the protective layer is attributed to the inhibition of cyclooxygenase-1 (COX-1) by the NSAIDs. Prostaglandins stimulate the secretion of mucus and bicarbonate, which helps in making the mucosa more resistant to acid penetration. Prostaglandins also increase mucosal blood flow and play a role in healing. *Helicobacter pylori* is a common cause of duodenal ulcers, although the mechanism is not fully understood. Current evidence suggests that the bacteria produce enzymes that cause direct injury to the mucosal lining. Indirectly, the bacteria stimulate release of hydrogen ions that increase acidity and further contribute to mucosal erosion. Gastric ulcers develop when the protective mucosal layer becomes more permeable to hydrogen ions. This type of ulcer is associated with bile reflux and use of NSAIDs. Other factors that contribute to the development of PUD include altered gastric emptying (delayed or too rapid), bile reflux through an incompetent pyloric sphincter, or increased stress associated with critical illness, surgery, or acute trauma. Stress-induced ulcers may be the result of elevated cortisol levels as part of the normal stress response. Increased serum cortisol impairs the rate of mucosal cell replacement. Ulcerative or erosive diseases in the upper GI tract can cause GI bleeding, abdominal pain, anorexia, nausea and vomiting, or diarrhea.

Gastrointestinal and Digestive Care Plans

NANDA-I NDx Imbalanced Nutrition: Less Than Body Requirements

Common Related Factors

Inability to ingest foods (nausea, vomiting, abdominal pain)
Inability to digest foods
Biological factors (alcohol intake)

Defining Characteristics

Body weight 20% or more below ideal weight range
Food intake less than recommended dietary allowance (RDA)

Common Expected Outcomes

Patient or caregiver verbalizes and demonstrates selection of foods or meals that will achieve a cessation of weight loss.
Patient weighs within 10% of ideal weight range.

NOC Outcomes
Nutritional Status: Nutrient Intake; Knowledge: Healthy Diet
NIC Interventions
Nutritional Monitoring; Nutrition Therapy

Ongoing Assessment

Actions/Interventions	Rationales
■ Measure weight and height; do not estimate.	Weight loss is an indication of inadequate nutritional intake. Gastric ulcers are more likely to be associated with loss of appetite, vomiting, and weight loss than duodenal ulcers. A patient's estimate of his or her actual weight and height or weight loss may be inaccurate. These anthropomorphic assessments are used to determine the patient's caloric and nutrient requirements.
■ Obtain a nutritional history; include the family, significant others, or the caregiver in the assessment.	Patients may often overestimate the amount of food eaten. Family members may provide a more accurate estimate of the patient's eating habits and food intake. The patient may not eat sufficient calories or essential nutrients as a way to reduce pain episodes with peptic ulcer disease. Because of this, patients are at risk for malnutrition. QSEN: Patient-centered care.
▲ Monitor laboratory values for serum albumin.	This test indicates the degree of protein depletion (2.5 g/dL indicates severe depletion; 3.8 to 4.5 g/dL is normal). QSEN: Safety.

Therapeutic Interventions

Actions/Interventions	Rationales
■ Teach about the importance of eating a balanced diet with meals at regular intervals.	Specific dietary restrictions are no longer part of the treatment for PUD. During the symptomatic phase of an ulcer the patient may obtain some pain relief from eating small meals at more frequent intervals.
■ Assist the patient with identifying foods that cause gastric irritation.	Patients need to learn what foods they can tolerate without gastric pain. Soft, bland, nonacidic foods cause less gastric irritation. The patient is more likely to increase food intake if the foods are not associated with pain. Foods that may contribute to mucosal irritation include spicy foods, pepper, and raw fruits and vegetables. QSEN: Patient-centered care.

Gastrointestinal and Digestive Care Plans

■ = Independent   ▲ = Interprofessional Collaboration

Actions/Interventions

- Encourage the patient to limit the intake of coffee and other dietary sources of caffeine.

- Instruct in the importance of abstaining from excessive alcohol.
- ▲ Consult a dietitian for recommendations regarding methods for nutritional support.

Rationales

Caffeine stimulates the secretion of gastric acid. Coffee, even if decaffeinated, contains a peptide that stimulates the release of gastrin and increases acid production. Other dietary sources of caffeine include cola beverages, non-cola flavors of soda, energy drinks, tea, and chocolate. QSEN: Safety.

Alcohol causes gastric irritation and increases gastric pain.

The dietitian can calculate the patient's daily requirements of specific nutrients to promote adequate nutritional intake. Based on the patient's nutritional requirements, the dietitian will recommend the most appropriate method to increase nutritional intake that is consistent with the patient's food and eating preferences. QSEN: Teamwork and collaboration.

NANDA-I NDx Acute Pain

Common Related Factors

Biological injury agent (e.g., *Helicobacter pylori* infection, mucosal inflammation)
Chemical injury agent (e.g., excess gastric acid)

Defining Characteristics

Self-report of intensity using standardized pain scale
Self-report of pain characteristics using standardized pain instrument
Positioning to ease pain
Change in physiological parameter (e.g., BP, HR, respiratory rate, and oxygen saturation)

Common Expected Outcomes

Patient reports satisfactory pain control and a decreased intensity using a standardized pain scale.
Patient uses pharmacological and nonpharmacological pain management strategies.
Patient exhibits increased comfort such as baseline levels for pulse, BP, respirations, and relaxed muscle tone or body posture.

NOC Outcomes

Pain Control; Comfort Status; Medication Response; Pain Level

NIC Intervention

Pain Management

Ongoing Assessment

Actions/Interventions

- Assess the patient's pain, including the location, characteristics, precipitating factors, onset, duration, frequency, quality, intensity, and severity.

Rationales

The patient is the most reliable source of information about his or her pain. Patients with gastric ulcers typically demonstrate pain 1 to 2 hours after eating. The patient with duodenal ulcers demonstrates pain 2 to 4 hours after eating or in the middle of the night. With both gastric and duodenal ulcers the pain is located in the upper abdomen and is intermittent. Patients may report relief after eating or taking an antacid. QSEN: Patient-centered care.

Gastrointestinal and Digestive Care Plans

Actions/Interventions

■ Assess for signs and symptoms associated with pain.

Rationales

Some people deny the experience of pain when it is present. Attention to associated signs may help the nurse in evaluating pain. The patient in acute pain may have elevated BP, HR, and temperature. The patient's skin may be pale and cool to touch. The patient may be restless and have difficulty concentrating. Patients with PUD may also experience nausea, vomiting, and indigestion with the abdominal pain.

Therapeutic Interventions

Actions/Interventions

▲ Administer the prescribed drug therapy:
  • Proton pump inhibitors
  • Antibiotics such as metronidazole, tetracycline, clarithromycin, or amoxicillin
  • Histamine-2 (H2)-receptor antagonists
  • Prostaglandin analogues
  • Antacids
  • Sucralfate

■ Teach the use of nonpharmacological pain relief strategies such as guided imagery, relaxation, distraction, music therapy, or acupressure.

Rationales

Proton pump inhibitors block the production and secretion of gastric acid and thereby reduce gastric pain. Antibiotics treat the *Helicobacter pylori* infection and promote healing of the ulcer. As the ulcer heals, the patient experiences less pain. H2 antagonists block the secretion of gastric acid. Prostaglandin analogues reduce acid secretion and enhance the integrity of the gastric mucosa to resist injury. Antacids buffer gastric acid and prevent the formation of pepsin. This mechanism of action promotes healing of the ulcer. Sucralfate forms a barrier at the base of the ulcer crater to protect the healing ulcer from gastric acid. QSEN: Evidence-based practice.

Nonpharmacological relaxation techniques will decrease the production of gastric acid, which in turn will reduce pain.

NANDA-I NDx Risk for Deficient Fluid Volume

Common Risk Factors

Active fluid loss (GI bleeding; vomiting)
Inadequate fluid intake

Common Expected Outcome

Patient is normovolemic as evidenced by systolic BP greater than or equal to 90 mm Hg (or patient's baseline), absence of orthostasis, HR 60 to 100 beats/min, urine output greater than 30 mL/hr, and normal skin turgor.

NOC Outcomes
Fluid Balance; Hydration; Tissue Integrity: Skin and Mucous Membranes
NIC Interventions
Fluid Monitoring; Fluid Management; Fluid Resuscitation

Ongoing Assessment

Actions/Interventions

■ Monitor the patient's vital signs

Rationales

The erosion of an ulcer through the gastric or duodenal mucosal layer may cause GI bleeding. The patient may develop anemia. If bleeding is brisk, a decrease in BP with an increase in HR may develop rapidly.

Gastrointestinal and Digestive Care Plans

■ = Independent   ▲ = Interprofessional Collaboration

Actions/Interventions

- Monitor BP for orthostatic changes (changes seen when changing from supine to standing position). Monitor HR for orthostatic changes.

Rationales

Postural hypotension is a common manifestation in fluid loss as reflected by a 20 mm Hg drop in systolic BP and a 10 mm Hg drop in diastolic BP. The incidence increases with age. Note the following orthostatic hypotension significance:

- Greater than 10 mm Hg drop: circulating blood volume is decreased by 20%.
- Greater than 20 to 30 mm Hg drop: circulating blood volume is decreased by 40%.
- Orthostatic hypotension caused by volume depletion is associated with a compensatory increase in HR (more than 20 beats/min). QSEN: Safety.

- Monitor the patient's fluid intake and urine output.

The kidney will reabsorb water into circulation to support a decrease in blood volume. This compensatory mechanism results in decreased urine output. A decrease in circulatory blood volume leads to decreased renal perfusion and decreased urine output.

- ▲ Monitor hemoglobin (Hgb) and hematocrit (Hct) laboratory values.

Erosion of the gastric mucosa by an ulcer results in GI bleeding. A decrease in Hgb and Hct occurs with bleeding.

- Assess for the signs of hematemesis or melena.

The patient with a bleeding ulcer may vomit bright red blood or coffee grounds emesis. Melena occurs when there is bleeding in the upper GI tract. QSEN: Safety.

Therapeutic Interventions

Actions/Interventions

- Instruct the patient to report symptoms of nausea, vomiting, dizziness, shortness of breath, or dark tarry stool immediately.
- ▲ Encourage the patient to drink prescribed fluid amounts.

Rationales

These assessment findings are signs of GI bleeding and should be reported immediately. These symptoms may occur before obvious signs of bleeding are present. QSEN: Safety.

Oral fluid replacement is indicated for mild fluid deficit and is a cost-effective method for replacement treatment. Older patients have a decreased sense of thirst and may need ongoing reminders to drink. Being creative in selecting fluid sources (e.g., flavored gelatin, frozen juice bars, sports drink) can facilitate fluid replacement. Oral rehydration solutions (e.g., Rehydralyte, Gatorade, Pedialyte) can be considered as needed.

- ▲ Administer IV fluids, volume expanders, and blood products as ordered.

Isotonic fluids, blood products, and volume expanders such as albumin can restore or expand intravascular volume.

NANDA-I NDx Deficient Knowledge

Common Related Factors

Insufficient information about peptic ulcer disease
Insufficient interest in learning
Insufficient knowledge of resources
Misinformation presented by others

Defining Characteristics

Insufficient knowledge
Inaccurate follow-through of instructions
Inappropriate behavior

Common Expected Outcome

Patient verbalizes understanding of importance of compliance with medical regimen, knowledge of peptic ulcer disease, and commitment to self-care management.

NOC Outcomes

Knowledge: Disease Process; Knowledge: Healthy Diet; Knowledge: Medication; Information Processing

NIC Interventions

Health Literacy Enhancement; Learning Facilitation; Teaching: Individual

Ongoing Assessment

Actions/Interventions	Rationales
■ Assess the patient's knowledge about peptic ulcer disease, lifestyle behaviors, and the treatment regimen.	This information provides the starting base for educational sessions. Teaching standardized content that the patient already knows wastes valuable time and hinders critical learning. QSEN: Patient-centered care.
■ Determine the patient's self-efficacy to learn and apply new knowledge.	A first step in teaching may be to foster increased self-efficacy in the patient's ability to learn the desired information or skills. Some lifestyle changes, as part of the treatment for peptic ulcer disease, can be difficult to make.

Therapeutic Interventions

Actions/Interventions	Rationales
■ Explain the process of peptic ulcer disease and how it relates to the functioning of the body.	An understanding of the disease process helps to foster willingness to follow the recommended treatment plan and modify behaviors to prevent recurrent ulcer episodes or related complications, such as GI bleeding.
■ Discuss the lifestyle changes required to prevent further complications or episodes of peptic ulcer disease.	The modification of lifestyle behaviors such as alcohol use, coffee and other caffeinated beverages, and the overuse of aspirin or other nonsteroidal anti-inflammatory drugs is necessary to prevent recurrent ulcer development and prevent complications during the healing phase. QSEN: Safety.
■ Instruct the patient in what signs and symptoms to report to the health care provider.	Recognizing the signs and symptoms can help ensure the early initiation of treatment. QSEN: Safety.
■ Discuss the therapy options and the rationales for using these options.	The patient needs accurate information to ensure correct use of antibiotics and acid suppression medications that promote rapid healing of an ulcer.

Related Care Plans

Acute pain, Chapter 2
Ineffective health management, Chapter 2
Gastrointestinal bleeding, Chapter 8

Gastrointestinal and Digestive Care Plans

■ = Independent ▲ = Interprofessional Collaboration

CHAPTER

9

Musculoskeletal Care Plans

Amputation, Lower Extremity

Generally there are about 11 lower limb amputations for every upper limb amputation performed. The level of the amputation depends on the amount of affected tissue, the ability of the blood supply to promote healing, and the prognosis for fitting a functional prosthesis. The leading cause of amputation is vascular disease, with an equal prevalence rate in men and women, who are usually in the 61- to 70-year-old age range. Clinical conditions that predispose the patient to amputation include peripheral arterial disease, diabetes mellitus, and Buerger's disease. The second leading cause of amputation is trauma, in which the accident itself may sever the limb or in which the limb is so damaged that it must be removed after the accident. Primary bone tumors account for less than 5% of all amputations, with about one third of these occurring in the 16- to 20-year-old age range.

The surgical procedure for an uncomplicated amputation rarely requires hospitalization for more than 5 days, but often the clinical situations surrounding amputation make these patients medically unstable and requiring longer lengths of stay. The portion of the limb that remains intact after the surgery is referred to as the *residual limb* or *stump* and may be fitted with an artificial device called a *prosthesis* that takes the place of the severed limb. The vast majority of recovery takes place out of the hospital, either in a rehabilitation center or on an outpatient basis. This care plan primarily covers information about patient care before and immediately after lower extremity amputation. Because nurses will encounter patients in various stages of recovery and rehabilitation, references are made about rehabilitation after discharge from the hospital.

NANDA-I NDx Anxiety, Preoperative

Common Related Factors
Major change in health status
Stressors associated with surgery
Situational crisis: surgery

Defining Characteristics
Worried about amputation of wrong extremity
Restlessness, insomnia
Fear
Diminished ability to learn or problem-solve
Increased BP, pulse, respirations

Common Expected Outcomes
Patient uses effective coping mechanisms.
Patient describes a reduction in the level of anxiety experienced.
Patient maintains desired level of role function and problem-solving.

NOC Outcomes
Anxiety Level; Anxiety Self-Control; Coping
NIC Interventions
Anxiety Reduction; Coping Enhancement; Presence; Relaxation Therapy; Emotional Support

Ongoing Assessment

Actions/Interventions	Rationales
■ Assess the patient's level of anxiety.	The level of preoperative anxiety will vary based on the patient's understanding of the surgery, perception of surgical outcomes, previous surgery experience, and personality. The reason for the amputation (vascular disease versus trauma) may be a factor in the level of anxiety experienced by the patient. Reactions to anxiety may range from mild to severe. The patient may appear calm but express nervousness with mild anxiety. As the level of anxiety increases, the patient may experience increased vital signs and report feeling overwhelmed by the anticipated surgery.
■ Determine the patient's concerns about the anticipated amputation.	Patients facing extremity amputation may express fear about the wrong extremity being amputated. Other concerns may include postoperative pain, body image changes, and changes in role function. QSEN: Patient-centered care.
■ Determine how the patient uses defense mechanisms to cope with anxiety.	The assessment of defense mechanisms helps determine the effectiveness of coping strategies used by the patient. Some defense mechanisms may be highly adaptive in managing anxiety. Other defense mechanisms may lead to less adaptive behavior with long-term use. QSEN: Patient-centered care.

Therapeutic Interventions

Actions/Interventions	Rationales
■ Acknowledge awareness of the patient's anxiety.	Acknowledgment of the patient's feelings validates the feelings and communicates acceptance of those feelings.
■ Stay with the patient as necessary during preoperative visits by members of the surgical team.	The presence of a trusted person may help the patient feel less threatened.
■ Assist the patient in verbalizing anxious feelings and assessing the situation realistically.	Talking about anxiety-producing situations and anxious feelings can help the patient perceive the surgical procedure in a less threatening manner.
■ Support the patient's use of coping strategies that the patient has found effective in the past.	Using anxiety-reduction strategies enhances the patient's sense of personal mastery and confidence. QSEN: Patient-centered care.
■ Use simple language and brief statements when teaching the patient about what to expect before surgery.	Patients experiencing moderate to severe anxiety may be unable to comprehend anything more than simple, clear, and brief explanations.
▲ Collaborate with the surgeon to accurately mark the extremity to be amputated before the patient is moved to the operating room.	Being present with the patient during the marking of the extremity may lessen the patient's concern of the wrong extremity being amputated. The Joint Commission developed patient safety goals for hospital staff to mark the surgical site without ambiguity. This marking should take place while the patient is awake and aware. QSEN: Teamwork and collaboration; Safety.
■ Review with the patient all surgical consent forms to ensure that the extremity to be amputated is accurately reported.	Including the patient in the record review allows the patient to have a sense of control for ensuring that the correct extremity is amputated. QSEN: Patient-centered care; Safety.

■ = Independent ▲ = Interprofessional Collaboration

Actions/Interventions

■ Teach the patient about measures used by the surgical team in the operating room, such as a time-out, to ensure that the correct extremity is amputated.

Rationales

Teaching the patient about expectations to promote safety during the procedure may reduce the patient's level of anxiety. The Joint Commission patient safety goals include performance standards to promote communication among all members of the surgical team at all stages of preparation for the procedure. These standards include a time-out before the start of the procedure to conduct a final assessment that the correct patient, site for amputation, and positioning are identified and that all consents, relevant information, and equipment are available. QSEN: Safety; Evidence-based practice.

NANDA-I NDx **Risk for Impaired Skin Integrity**

Common Risk Factors

Mechanical trauma (surgical incision)
Mechanical factors (poorly fitting prosthesis)

Common Expected Outcome

Patient's skin remains intact as evidenced by healing of incision, no redness over bony prominences, and a properly fitting prosthesis.

NOC Outcomes

Risk Control; Risk Detection; Tissue Integrity: Skin and Mucous Membranes; Wound Healing: Primary Intention

NIC Interventions

Amputation Care; Incision Site Care; Skin Surveillance

Ongoing Assessment

Actions/Interventions

■ Assess the wound for:
  • Normal healing

  • Bleeding and hemorrhage

  • Proper fit of postsurgical cast or pressure dressing

Rationales

The wound should be clean and dry, with edges of the incision approximated and intact. Patients with diabetes or with poor circulation, such as the elderly, may face considerable obstacles in healing, and the course of wound healing may be prolonged.

As with other surgical dressings, there should be no frank bleeding from the incisional site. A small amount of oozing from the incision is normal. Documenting drainage characteristics helps other caregivers assess status changes. Initially most postamputation dressings are pressure or pressure cast dressings. A surgical drain may be placed to remove fluid or blood that might interfere with granulation.

A rigid dressing or a cast may be applied to the residual limb immediately after the surgery and will remain in place for 7 to 10 days, until the sutures are removed. This type of dressing contributes to shaping of the residual limb for proper fitting of the prosthesis. After removal of the sutures, a new cast or rigid dressing may be applied. Occasionally these casts are fitted with a basic prosthetic device that allows for early ambulation.

Actions/Interventions

■ Monitor the residual limb every hour for the first 24 hours; observe for symptoms indicative of infection.

■ Check the residual limb for signs of impaired circulation. Check the pulses above the amputation site.

■ Assess for prolonged pressure on the tissues associated with immobility.

■ Monitor vital signs, including temperature, according to postoperative protocol.

Rationales

Signs of inflammation may be present. Edema, redness, pain, and tenderness should decrease over the first 3 to 5 postoperative days. QSEN: Safety.

The residual limb should be warm and dry with no discoloration reflective of impaired circulation. Many patients experience circulatory compromise before the amputation; this problem may continue to represent a threat to the residual and unaffected limb. Preserving the health in the residual limb is of the utmost importance. The patient's adaptation to the prosthesis depends on having an adequate residual limb remaining for a good prosthetic fit and stability of the joints above the residual limb. QSEN: Safety.

Nonblanching redness over areas of pressure is an early indicator of impaired skin integrity. Early ambulation will prevent the development of pressure ulcers and contractures from prolonged inactivity. During the early postoperative phase, the patient may have some weight-bearing limitations with ambulation. QSEN: Safety.

Tachycardia, tachypnea, and fever are early signs of infection. It is normal for the temperature and HR to be elevated in the first few days after surgery. Temperature should not exceed 38.3°C (101°F), and the HR should not exceed 120 beats/min. Unusual pain in the residual limb may reflect the development of a postoperative infection. QSEN: Safety.

Therapeutic Interventions

Actions/Interventions

■ Elevate the residual limb for the first 24 hours.

■ Reinforce or change the dressing as needed; use aseptic technique. Note any drainage. If a rigid dressing is not used, remove the bandage on the residual limb, cleanse the wound frequently, and reapply dressings using a smooth figure-eight wrap.

■ Instruct the patient in how to wrap the residual limb with compression bandages.

■ Discuss weight-bearing limitations and their importance.

Rationales

Elevation of the residual limb for the first 24 hours reduces edema and promotes venous return. Prolonged elevation of the residual limb increases the risk for hip flexion contractures that may delay or interfere with rehabilitation and mobility.

Daily cleansing helps prevent infection. The proper application of elastic bandages using the figure eight technique helps reduce edema and helps shape the residual limb. QSEN: Safety.

Compression bandages aid in shaping the residual limb in preparation for prosthesis fitting. Wrapping the compression dressing around the waist seems to be essential in keeping the bandage firmly in place, and compressing the medial thigh encourages the residual limb to shrink in a fashion that will promote good interface with the prosthetic socket. Patients may need time to adjust to seeing their residual limb and may balk at assuming responsibility for its care until they are ready. QSEN: Patient-centered care.

These activity restrictions prevent skin breakdown and facilitate proper wound healing. The patient's limb may be non–weight bearing for 4 to 6 weeks after surgery; other patients will begin partial weight bearing on the residual limb soon after the surgery. Factors that influence how soon weight bearing takes place include the indications for the amputation, the level and the type of the amputation, and the repair and preparation of the residual limb.

■ = Independent ▲ = Interprofessional Collaboration

Actions/Interventions

- Teach the signs and symptoms of residual limb breakdown.

Rationales

Early detection of residual limb breakdown allows for prompt treatment. Slippage of the cast or rigid dressing may reflect underlying pathology such as infection or incomplete closure of the skin flap, which would interrupt healing. Complications may jeopardize the patient's rehabilitation plan and make further amputation necessary. QSEN: Safety.

NANDA-I NDx Impaired Physical Mobility

Common Related Factors

Musculoskeletal impairment (loss of body part)
Insufficient muscle strength
Imposed restrictions of movement, including change in center of gravity creating balance problems
Insufficient knowledge of mobility strategies

Defining Characteristics

Impaired ability to reposition self in bed
Impaired ability to turn from side to side
Impaired ability to move between sitting and supine positions
Impaired ability to move between long sitting and supine positions
Impaired ability to move between prone and supine positions

Common Expected Outcomes

Patient performs physical activity independently or within limits of amputation.
Patient is free of complications of immobility, as evidenced by intact skin, absence of thrombophlebitis, normal bowel pattern, and clear breath sounds.
Patient demonstrates use of adaptive techniques that promote ambulation and transferring.

NOC Outcomes

Mobility; Ambulation: Wheelchair; Coordinated Movement; Transfer Performance

NIC Interventions

Self-Care Assistance: Transfer; Exercise Therapy: Ambulation; Energy Management; Exercise Therapy: Balance

Ongoing Assessment

Actions/Interventions

- Assess the patient's bed positioning and transfer skills.

- Assess the patient's nutritional status.

- Assess the patient's understanding of postoperative activity and the exercise program.

Rationales

Learning transfer techniques helps reestablish the patient's independence and promotes a feeling of security when moving in bed and ambulating. A patient who had normal mobility before the amputation may find crutch walking or walking with a prosthesis more tiring. The patient may require exercises that strengthen appropriate muscle groups to support ambulation. QSEN: Safety; Patient-centered care.

Adequate calories and protein are needed for healing and energy for ambulation and transfer techniques. Performing transfer techniques and performing activities with a prosthetic device consume more calories and take a greater physical effort than normal ambulation.

Postoperatively, range of motion (ROM) exercises will be encouraged in all unaffected extremities. Some patients will begin to ambulate soon after surgery. Other patients will remain non–weight bearing until the temporary prosthesis is made 4 to 6 weeks after surgery. At that time physical therapists will implement a program of functional training with the patient and the prosthesis. QSEN: Patient-centered care.

Actions/Interventions

■ Assess the patient's knowledge of ambulating and moving with assistive devices.

▲ Determine whether the patient is a candidate for a prosthesis.

■ Assess the impact of the loss of sensory information that was perceived via the amputated part.

Rationales

Patients may already know how to crutch walk, but balance is significantly affected after an amputation. Attention must be paid to developing an awareness of new physical boundaries after the amputation.

This decision involves consideration of the type and level of amputation, age and strength of the patient, type of function the patient is attempting to regain, and perhaps most of all the motivation of the patient. Older or debilitated patients may not be able to handle a prosthesis; a wheelchair may be more appropriate. On the other hand, no assumptions should be made about older patients being too old to adapt to a prosthesis. QSEN: Patient-centered care.

The lack of sensory feedback may be a major limitation in the effective use of a prosthesis. Other factors that may exaggerate the effect of the sensory loss are the age of the patient and the existence of other sensory deficits (e.g., vision or hearing deficits, bilateral amputations).

Therapeutic Interventions

Actions/Interventions

■ Reinforce and teach proper positioning:

- Have the patient lie on his or her back, keeping the pelvis level and the hip joint extended.

- Teach the patient to use a trochanter roll to prevent external rotation.
- Teach the patient to lie prone with the lower extremity in extension for 30 minutes three or four times a day.

■ Instruct the patient to perform ROM exercises:
- Adduction exercises of the lower extremity 10 times every 4 hours after the first 24 hours
- Hamstring tightening exercises in the prone position 10 times every 4 hours after the first 24 hours

■ Provide a trapeze bar in bed.

■ Encourage early ambulation with assistive devices. Encourage the patient to ask for needed assistance.

Rationales

Patients often develop contractures of the affected extremity, which complicates rehabilitation and the use of a prosthesis. QSEN: Safety.

This positioning prevents flexion or abduction contractures. The patient should avoid the use of pillows under the residual limb.

The residual limb will have the tendency to externally rotate the hip on the affected limb.

This activity prevents flexion contracture, especially in the patient who is in a sitting position for long periods of the day.

Exercise therapy maintains and strengthens muscle groups. ROM exercises are directed toward maintaining normal joint mobility. Disuse can cause permanent shortening of the muscle, resulting in contractures. Quadriceps settings are performed for above- and below-the-knee amputations. Straight leg raises are performed with the knee fully extended for below-the-knee amputations. Hip adductions are done for above-the-knee amputations. Patients will need to continue the muscle-strengthening program throughout the rehabilitation program and beyond.

A trapeze bar increases mobility in bed and allows the patient to be more independent with transfers. QSEN: Patient-centered care.

Early ambulation promotes confidence about regaining independence. The patient may use a walker, crutches, or wheelchair as appropriate. These activities help the patient develop strength and skill with transfer techniques. Assistance may be required to prevent new injuries that would complicate recovery. Muscle weakness and impaired balance after a lower extremity amputation may result in an injury. The patient's center of gravity changes after a lower extremity amputation. Adjustment to the change in the center of gravity initially requires a conscious effort to maintain balance during transfer and ambulation. QSEN: Safety.

■ = Independent ▲ = Interprofessional Collaboration

Actions/Interventions

- Instruct patients in the use of crutches, wheelchairs, walkers, support bars, and a trapeze.

- Teach the patient not to bend the knee over the bed or edge of the chair if the patient had a below-the-knee amputation.

▲ Collaborate with members of the interprofessional health care team.

- Instruct the patient awaiting a prosthesis regarding the need for a long-term functional training program.

Rationales

Learning correct technique with assistive devices promotes safety and reduces the risk for falls. Even patients with previous experience using crutches may find that the change in the center of gravity presents a challenge in using crutches safely and effectively after an amputation. QSEN: Safety.

Allowing the residual limb to hang in a dependent position decreases venous return and increases edema. Flexion contractures may occur if the residual limb remains bent.

The nurse will coordinate activities of different disciplines to maximize the patient's return to an optimal level of mobility. The disciplines involved may include occupational therapy, vocational rehabilitation, physical therapy, work of the prosthetic maker, ongoing medical care, social services, and psychological support services. QSEN: Teamwork and collaboration.

It may take several months for the lower extremity to reach a point at which a final device may be fitted. This period allows for the patient to adapt progressively to wearing a prosthesis and to work toward regaining function of the remaining limb.

NANDA-I NDx   Disturbed Body Image

Common Related Factors

Alteration in body function (due to amputation)
Alteration in self-perception

Common Expected Outcome

Patient demonstrates enhanced body image and self-esteem, as evidenced by ability to look at residual limb and talk about amputation and the ability to provide self-care to the residual limb (as appropriate).

Defining Characteristics

Avoids looking at or touching residual limb
Preoccupation with changed body and loss of limb
Refusal to discuss change
Change in social involvement

NOC Outcomes

Body Image; Self-Esteem; Adaptation to Physical Disability

NIC Interventions

Amputation Care; Body Image Enhancement; Grief Work Facilitation; Self-Esteem Enhancement; Coping Enhancement

---

Ongoing Assessment

Actions/Interventions

- Assess the patient's perception of change in structure or function from the loss of the body part.

Rationales

The acute (versus chronic) nature of the factors requiring amputation, the patient's prior health and age, the feelings and responses of significant others, and the patient's lifestyle and work affect the patient's adjustment to amputation. The extent of the patient's response is more related to the value or importance the patient places on the extremity or its function than the actual value or importance. Even when an alteration improves the overall health of the patient, the alteration may result in a body image disturbance. QSEN: Patient-centered care.

Actions/Interventions

■ Assess the patient's feelings about using a mechanical part to replace or substitute for a missing body part.

■ Note the patient's behavior regarding the actual or perceived changed body part or function. Assess the patient's ability to use effective coping mechanisms.

■ Assess the patient's perception of the impact of the amputation on his or her ability to perform self-care measures and on his or her social behavior, personal relationships, and occupational activities.

■ Note the frequency of the patient's self-critical remarks.

■ Assess the need for a support group.

Rationales

Artificial limbs are clearly mechanical devices that never feel or perform like a real body part. There is always some loss of function, and sensory changes are massive and may include some low-level noise that may draw further attention to the operation of the prosthesis. Patients may be dependent on a prosthesis, but they may also despise the experience of wearing and using one.

At the heart of the adaptive process for the patient with an amputation is the need to accept the loss of the limb and to realize that the loss is permanent. Patients will express a wide range of feelings in response to their loss, including anger, rage, sadness, helplessness, and hopelessness. Patients will be likely to fall back on known coping skills, including humor, denial, distraction, and expression of thoughts and feelings in talk and writing. Previously successful coping skills may not be effective in the present situation. QSEN: Patient-centered care.

For some patients who have undergone an amputation, the psychological and social aspects of amputation are experienced as far greater consequences of the surgical procedure. QSEN: Patient-centered care.

Negative statements about the affected body part indicate a limited ability to integrate the change into the patient's self-concept.

Support groups are usually a component of most formal rehabilitation programs; however, patients may require this kind of intervention earlier, in the immediate postoperative period.

Therapeutic Interventions

Actions/Interventions

■ Encourage the verbalization of feelings.

■ Allow the patient time to work through grief stages.

■ Listen and support verbalized feelings about body and lifestyle changes.

■ Encourage the patient to participate fully in the design of the therapeutic regimen.

■ Encourage family members to support the patient and allow independence.

Rationales

Loss of a limb requires significant psychological adjustment. It is worthwhile to encourage the patient to separate feelings about changes in body structure and function from feelings about self-worth. The expression of feelings can enhance the patient's coping strategies.

Working through stages of grief over the loss of a leg is normal and typically involves a period of denial, the length of which varies among individuals. Patients will do this at their own pace and in their own way. Accommodation to amputation is a lifetime process for some patients. QSEN: Patient-centered care.

These changes will be massive. There is no way to prepare patients for the impact this will have on their lives. The health care provider should not minimize or negate the patient's experiences.

This approach to planning care fosters in the patient a sense of still being in control of his or her own life. QSEN: Patient-centered care.

The family may have a need to take care of the patient. This response communicates the concept of the patient as damaged. The patient may develop an unhealthy dependence on family members, setting a precedent that is difficult to disrupt later in the recovery period.

■ = Independent ▲ = Interprofessional Collaboration

Actions/Interventions	Rationales
■ Encourage the patient to participate in the care of the residual limb.	Such activity promotes independence and helps the patient's adjustment to a new body image.
■ Encourage the use of clothing to enhance the patient's appearance.	Amputation is a very public disability. It may be the first thing people notice about an individual. Shock and embarrassment are often initial responses of the public to seeing an individual with an amputation. Attractive clothing can enhance a patient's self-image and confidence.
■ Discuss the use of a prosthesis for both cosmetic and functional purposes.	Both are equally acceptable reasons to use a prosthesis. Some people have more than one device, one for cosmetic use and one for functional use.
▲ Consult with members of the interprofessional health team for referrals to support groups.	Occupational therapists, physical therapists, social workers, and rehabilitation specialists may be able to provide the patient and family with connections to support groups for people who have had an amputation. People who have themselves experienced an amputation can offer a unique type of support that is perceived as helpful by patients. It is often possible to match up individuals by age, sex, and education; in some situations, career matches can be made. Opportunities for positive feedback and success in social situations may hasten adaptation. QSEN: Teamwork and collaboration.

NANDA-I NDx Acute Pain and Chronic Pain

Common Related Factors

Physical injury agent (amputation, prosthesis fit)
Damage to nervous system (phantom sensation, phantom pain)

Defining Characteristics

Self-report of intensity using standardized pain scale
Self-report of pain characteristics using standardized pain instrument
Restlessness
Withdrawal, irritability
Altered ability to continue previous activities

Common Expected Outcomes

Patient reports satisfactory pain control at a decreased intensity using a standardized pain scale.
Patient uses pharmacological and nonpharmacological pain management strategies.
Patient engages in desired activities without an increase in pain intensity.

NOC Outcomes

Pain Control; Medication Response; Pain: Disruptive Effects; Pain: Adverse Psychological Response

NIC Interventions

Medication Management; Pain Management; Acupressure; Heat/Cold Application; Progressive Muscle Relaxation; Transcutaneous Electrical Nerve Stimulation (TENS); Massage

ⓔvolve For additional care plans, go to http://evolve.elsevier.com/Gulanick/.

Ongoing Assessment

Actions/Interventions	Rationales
■ Assess the patient's description of pain. Have the patient rate the pain on a standardized pain scale.	A thorough assessment of pain characteristics will assist the nurse in differentiating phantom limb sensations from incision pain. The nurse needs to understand the type of pain the patient is experiencing to select the appropriate pain management interventions. Pain is what the patient states it is. Early detection and intervention promote patient comfort. QSEN: Patient-centered care.
■ Assess for nonverbal signs of pain.	Tense posture, tightening fists, diaphoresis, and increased HR may be the only indications of acute pain.
■ Assess the patient's understanding of the occurrence and management of phantom limb sensations.	Phantom limb sensations are the painless awareness of the presence of the amputated part and are often experienced as a tingling sensation caused by nerve stimulation proximal to the level of amputation but perceived as coming from the amputated limb. In a lower limb amputation, sensations in the foot will be experienced more strongly than the leg and the great toe more strongly than the other toes.
■ Assess the patient's understanding of phantom pain.	When phantom limb sensations become disagreeable and painful, they are called *phantom pain*. Phantom limb pain may be continuous or occasional, with a wide range in the intensity experienced by the patient. Patients may experience the pain as a cramping or squeezing sensation; a burning sensation; or a sharp, shooting pain. Phantom limb pain tends to disappear over time, but phantom limb sensation may remain indefinitely.
▲ Collaborate with members of the interprofessional health team to assess the fit of the prosthesis and determine whether the fit is resulting in the development of pressure points and pain.	A prosthetic device is frequently experienced as uncomfortable by the patient. Prosthetic devices are fitted over tissues that would not normally bear weight. Patients may experience significant discomfort until these tissues become adjusted to the prosthesis. The prosthesis maker is the person best able to assess the proper fit of the prosthetic device. QSEN: Teamwork and collaboration.

Therapeutic Interventions

Actions/Interventions	Rationales
▲ Provide medications as prescribed for surgical pain relief; evaluate their effectiveness and modify doses as needed.	Patients have a right to adequate pain relief. Bone surgery is extremely painful. Phantom limb pain is real pain, and the patient requires appropriate analgesics as part of a total pain management program.
▲ Use additional comfort measures as appropriate to relieve phantom sensations.	Long-term management of phantom limb sensations includes the use of nonpharmacological measures such as diversional activities; relaxation techniques; position changes; exercise; range of motion of the residual limb; application of pressure to the residual limb; and transcutaneous electrical nerve stimulation. Current research indicates that these measures are effective. QSEN: Evidence-based practice.

■ = Independent   ▲ = Interprofessional Collaboration

NANDA-I NDx Deficient Knowledge

Common Related Factors

Insufficient information about amputation and prosthesis
Insufficient interest in learning
Insufficient knowledge of resources
Misinformation presented by others

Common Expected Outcomes

Patient verbalizes understanding of residual limb care.
Patient verbalizes understanding of the rehabilitation program and prosthetic fitting.

Defining Characteristics

Insufficient knowledge
Inaccurate follow-through of instruction
Inappropriate behavior

NOC Outcomes

Knowledge: Disease Process; Knowledge: Treatment Regimen

NIC Interventions

Health Literacy Enhancement; Learning Facilitation; Teaching: Disease Process; Teaching: Psychomotor Skill

---

Ongoing Assessment

Actions/Interventions	Rationales
■ Assess the patient's knowledge of care of the residual limb, phantom limb pain management, signs and symptoms of circulatory problems, prosthetic care, follow-up appointments, and community resources.	This information provides the starting base for educational sessions. An accurate understanding of self-care following an amputation facilitates a smooth transition from the hospital to home. QSEN: Patient-centered care.
■ Assess the motivation and willingness of the patient and caregivers to learn.	Some patients are ready to learn soon after they consent to the amputation; others cope better by denying or delaying the need for instruction. Learning also requires energy, which patients may not be ready to use.
■ Determine the patient's and the caregiver's self-efficacy to learn and apply new knowledge.	Self-efficacy refers to a person's confidence in his or her ability to perform care of the residual limb and prosthesis. Some lifestyle changes associated with the amputation and prosthesis can be difficult to make for both the patient and caregiver.

Therapeutic Interventions

Actions/Interventions	Rationales
■ Reinforce teaching for the care of the residual limb (e.g., wrapping the residual limb, skin care, and weight-bearing limitations).	Accurate self-care measures promote optimal rehabilitation. The patient may need to continue wrapping the residual limb to promote the effective shaping and successful fit of the prosthesis.
■ Provide information for phantom limb pain or sensation management.	Phantom limb sensations may continue for several months or longer. The patient may need to continue using techniques begun in the hospital to manage these sensations.
■ Discuss the signs and symptoms of circulatory problems. Reinforce the need for the patient to protect the residual limb from infection and circulatory compromise or damage.	Signs of infection, circulatory compromise, or skin breakdown should be reported to the physician immediately. QSEN: Safety.
■ Reinforce teaching about the care of the prosthesis if applicable.	Some patients may go home with a temporary prosthesis. The patient needs to understand how to maintain the prosthesis in proper working order.

---

 evolve **For additional care plans, go to http://evolve.elsevier.com/Gulanick/.**

Actions/Interventions

- Provide the patient with information about community resources and support groups.

Rationales

These groups offer support and best practice information to help the patient adapt to the amputation.

Related Care Plans

Ineffective coping, Chapter 2
Risks for falls, Chapter 2
Risk for infection, Chapter 2
Ineffective peripheral tissue perfusion, Chapter 2
Surgical experience: Preoperative and postoperative care, Chapter 4

Arthritis, Rheumatoid

Rheumatoid arthritis (RA) is a chronic, systemic, inflammatory disease. RA is classified as an autoimmune disorder that develops as a result of interactions between autoantibodies and immunoglobulins. Rheumatoid factor (RF) is the primary autoantibody that acts against immunoglobulin G (IgG). The disorder usually presents as symmetrical synovitis primarily of the small joints of the body. The diagnosis of RA is based on the presence of criteria established by the American Rheumatism Association. These criteria include morning joint stiffness lasting at least 1 hour, soft tissue swelling of three or more joint areas, simultaneous symmetrical joint swelling, subcutaneous rheumatoid nodules, presence of RF in the serum, and radiographic evidence of joint erosion or periarticular osteopenia. Synovial fluid analysis may be done to confirm the diagnosis of RA. Extra-articular manifestations may include rheumatoid nodules, pericarditis, scleritis, and arteritis. RA is characterized by periods of remission and prolonged exacerbation of the disease, during which the joints can become damaged. In the initial phase of RA, the synovial membrane becomes inflamed and thickens, associated with an increased production of synovial fluid. As this tissue develops, it causes erosion and destruction of the joint capsule and subchondral bone. These processes result in decreased joint motion, deformity, and finally ankylosis, or joint immobilization. Anyone can develop RA, including children and older adults, but it usually occurs in people in the young to middle years. RA strikes women at a 3:1 ratio compared with men and occurs in all ethnic groups worldwide. The specific cause of RA is unknown, but the tendency to develop it may be inherited. The gene that seems to control RA is one of the genes that control the immune system, but not everyone who has this gene goes on to develop RA. Factors that may influence gene expression in the development of RA include Epstein-Barr virus, increased estrogen concentrations, and emotional stressors. The disease behaves differently in each person who contracts it. In some people the joint inflammation that marks RA will be mild, with long periods of remission between "exacerbations," or increased periods of disease activity. For others the activity of the disease may seem continuous and worsening as time passes. The goals of treatment are to relieve pain and inflammation and reduce joint damage. The long-term goal of treatment is to maintain or restore use in the joints damaged by RA. This care plan focuses on the outpatient management of patients who are affected by RA.

NANDA-I
NDx Deficient Knowledge

Common Related Factors

Insufficient information
Insufficient interest in learning
Insufficient knowledge of resources
Misinformation presented by others

Defining Characteristics

Insufficient knowledge
Inaccurate follow-through of instruction
Inaccurate performance on a test
Inappropriate behavior

■ = Independent   ▲ = Interprofessional Collaboration

Common Expected Outcome

Patient verbalizes understanding of rheumatoid arthritis (RA) and treatment.

NOC Outcomes
Knowledge: Disease Process; Knowledge: Medication; Knowledge: Treatment Regimen

NIC Interventions
Health Literacy Enhancement; Learning Facilitation; Teaching: Disease Process; Teaching: Prescribed Medication

---

Ongoing Assessment

Actions/Interventions	Rationales
■ Assess the patient's level of knowledge of RA and its treatment.	This information provides the starting base for educational sessions. Patients will be responsible for evaluating their RA on a daily basis to make determinations about exercise, the use of analgesics, and seeking medical intervention. QSEN: Patient-centered care.
■ Determine the patient's self-efficacy to learn and apply new knowledge.	A first step in teaching may be to foster increased self-efficacy in the patient's ability to learn the desired information or skills. Some lifestyle changes associated with RA and its management can be difficult for the patient to make.
■ Identify any existing misconceptions regarding material to be taught.	Many patients may have the misconception that RA is a normal part of the aging process. Some may think it is the same thing as osteoarthritis.

Therapeutic Interventions

Actions/Interventions	Rationales
■ Introduce or reinforce disease process information: unknown cause, chronicity of RA, process of inflammation, joint and other organ involvement, remissions and exacerbations, and control versus cure.	Patients must have accurate and comprehensive information as a foundation for their active participation in disease management. QSEN: Patient-centered care.
Initial presentation with symptoms of joint inflammation:	
• Patients may feel systemically ill, with additional symptoms of fever, chills, loss of appetite, decreased energy, and weight loss.	Simultaneous, symmetrical joint inflammation differentiates RA from other forms of arthritis. This inflammatory process is not limited to the joints; progressive changes occur in the heart, with pericarditis, congestive heart failure, and cardiomyopathies developing; in the skin; in the kidneys, with chronic renal failure developing; and in the lungs, with chronic restrictive pulmonary disease and repeated infections occurring.
• The synovial lining of the joints and tendons becomes inflamed, with a progressive proliferation of the synovium within and outside the joint capsule itself (pannus formation).	
• Joint inflammation may affect more than one joint at a time, and usually the inflammation affects the same joint bilaterally.	
• Cartilage eventually becomes involved; the inflammatory process erodes the surface between the bone ends, leaving the surfaces exposed.	
• Further inflammation results in the development of bone fissures, cysts on the bones, spurs, fibrosis, and shortening of the tendons.	

Actions/Interventions	Rationales
Diagnosis:	
• Laboratory tests:	No single laboratory test is capable of ruling out RA.
• Anti–cyclic citrullinated peptide (anti-CCP) antibodies	Anti-CCP is a predictive diagnostic marker for the development of RA.
• Rheumatoid factor (or the RA antibody)	It is important to note that not all people with RA will have a positive antibody titer.
• Hemoglobin and hematocrit	Patients with RA may develop normocytic, hypochromic anemia. Iron deficiency anemia may be present.
• Serum complement	This laboratory value is decreased during periods of exacerbation.
• Erythrocyte sedimentation rate (ESR)	Laboratory tests may include acute phase reactors (ESR and C-reactive protein). These two tests are good indicators of the inflammatory activity of the disease.
• C-reactive protein	
• Liver function tests and kidney function tests	These tests help facilitate RA monitoring, the early detection of disease complications, and the presence of treatment side effects.
• X-ray films of the hands, feet, and chest are recommended initially, and x-ray films of the feet and hands should be repeated annually for the first 3 years of the disease.	X-ray films should be examined for the presence of bony erosions, which are more frequent at the beginning of the disease process. Erosions of the hands or feet develop in about 70% of patients by the end of the first 2 to 3 years. Their presence and the speed of onset are associated with poorer outcomes. A chest x-ray film is recommended for initial evaluation and to identify the appearance of possible problems during the course of the disease and its treatment.
• Joint arthroscopy	Arthroscopic examinations are used to evaluate for characteristic changes in synovial fluid. Cartilage destruction and pannus formation may be identified.
General treatment and management guidelines:	
• Adequate sleep, at least 8 to 10 hours each night with periods of rest during the day	Sleep enhances immune system function to reduce inflammation. Fatigue contributes to increased joint pain.
• Rest of the affected joints with splinting	Splinting is sometimes helpful in protecting joints, which can become overused during the course of daily activities. QSEN: Safety.
• Application of hot or cold packs on painful, inflamed joints	Alternating the use of hot and cold is sometimes helpful in reducing the local inflammatory process in the joints. Individual patients may prefer heat over cold or vice versa.
• Collaboration with members of the interprofessional health team.	The physical therapist can design a therapy plan that provides a balance between maintaining function in a threatened joint while respecting the inflammatory nature of the disease. The occupational therapist can evaluate the patient's needs and provide devices that can be adjusted to fit the individual patient and preserve independence with ADLs. QSEN: Teamwork and collaboration.
• Relearning how to perform activities of daily living (ADLs)	As joint deformity progresses and joint mobility decreases, the patient may benefit from using assistive devices to complete ADLs, such as using long-handled eating utensils.
• Prescribed medications:	Patients usually benefit from a combination drug plan that includes a nonsteroidal anti-inflammatory drug (NSAID) and a disease-modifying antirheumatic drug (DMARD) or a biological response modifier. Short-term therapy with corticosteroids may be included during exacerbations. QSEN: Evidence-based practice.

■ = Independent   ▲ = Interprofessional Collaboration

Actions/Interventions

- • DMARDs: hydroxychloroquine (Plaquenil), methotrexate (Rheumatrex), gold salts (Ridaura, Solganal), sulfasalazine (Azulfidine), azathioprine (Imuran), leflunomide (Arava), and cyclosporine (Sandimmune, Neoral)

- • NSAIDs

- • Corticosteroids

- • Biological response modifiers: etanercept (Enbrel), adalimumab (Humira), infliximab (Remicade), anakinra (Kineret), abatacept (Orencia)

■ Stress the importance of long-term follow-up.

■ Encourage the patient to discuss new or over-the-counter treatments with members of the interprofessional health care team.

■ Inform the patient of resources such as the Arthritis Foundation.
▲ Suggest a referral to an arthritis specialist for optimal treatment.

Rationales

This group of drugs is recommended as the first line of treatment for a patient diagnosed with RA. Because of its efficacy and toxicity profile, methotrexate is the recommended initial treatment in all patients who have not previously received DMARDs. These drugs substantially reduce the inflammation of RA. Studies suggest that DMARDs can reduce or prevent joint damage, preserve structure and function, and enable a person to continue his or her daily activities. Several weeks to months of treatment are often necessary before the effects of DMARDs become evident.

These drugs relieve mild to moderate pain and have an anti-inflammatory effect. The anti-inflammatory effect is not strong enough to alter the long-term damaging effects of RA on the joints. The selective NSAIDs (cyclooxgenase [COX]-2 inhibitors) act by reducing prostaglandin synthesis via inhibition of cyclooxygenase-2. As a result, this class of NSAIDs has fewer gastrointestinal side effects than nonselective NSAIDs. These drugs may be used in combination with DMARDs.

Steroids have strong anti-inflammatory effects. However, if used alone, steroids have only a modest effect on decreasing arthritis damage.

This class of drugs treats RA by interfering with the signaling pathways involved in inflammation. The onset of action of these medications is more rapid than that of DMARDs. Because of the cost of these medications and uncertainty about their long-term effects, they are often reserved for people who have not responded fully to DMARDs and for people who cannot tolerate DMARDs in doses large enough to control inflammation. These drugs interfere with the ability to fight infection and should not be used in people with serious infections.

Patients with RA should be monitored for an indefinite period. Patients in complete remission should be seen every 6 months or yearly; patients with recent disease onset, frequent exacerbations, or persistent activity should be seen more often depending on the treatment used and disease activity until control is achieved. Aging may alter hepatic function, thus decreasing the metabolism of drugs that are broken down in the liver. The possibility of adverse effects and drug interactions should be monitored in older patients. QSEN: Safety.

The patient may be vulnerable to fads or advertisements claiming the curative effects of high-dose vitamins, special health foods, or copper bracelets. QSEN: Safety; Teamwork and Collaboration.

This organization is a comprehensive resource center for patients suffering with RA.

This practitioner may be in the best position to understand the nuances of an individual's disease, because so much of it is seen within the practice. In addition, the rheumatologist will be aware of the latest treatment regimens. QSEN: Teamwork and collaboration.

NANDA-I NDx   Chronic Joint Pain

Common Related Factors

Chronic musculoskeletal condition
Emotional stress

Defining Characteristics

Self-report of intensity using standardized pain scale
Self-report of pain characteristics using standardized pain instrument

Common Expected Outcomes

Patient reports satisfactory pain control at a decreased intensity using a standardized pain scale.
Patient uses pharmacological and nonpharmacological pain management strategies.
Patient engages in desired activities without an increase in pain intensity.

NOC Outcomes

Pain Control; Pain: Disruptive Effects; Pain: Adverse Psychological Response

NIC Interventions

Pain Management; Medication Management; Acupressure; Heat/Cold Application; Progressive Muscle Relaxation; Transcutaneous Electrical Nerve Stimulation (TENS); Massage

Ongoing Assessment

Actions/Interventions	Rationales
■ Assess for the signs of joint inflammation (redness, warmth, swelling, decreased motion).	Local signs of inflammation may be the first to manifest. Joint swelling usually accompanies joint pain.
■ Evaluate the location and the patient's description of the pain.	Pain occurs primarily in small joints, such as the hands, wrists, fingers, and ankles. Assessment includes a "joint count" of the number of joints affected by pain and swelling. The most reliable source of information about the chronic pain experience is the patient's self-report. QSEN: Patient-centered care.
■ Assess for interference with the patient's lifestyle.	Joint pain and decreased range of motion (ROM) can limit the fine motor and gross motor movements required for completing ADLs. QSEN: Patient-centered care.

Therapeutic Interventions

Actions/Interventions	Rationales
■ Instruct the patient to take anti-inflammatory medications as prescribed.	Nonselective COX inhibitors (e.g., ibuprofen, naproxen) and selective COX-2 inhibitors (celecoxib) are useful in managing arthritic pain and inflammation through inhibition of prostaglandins. Anti-inflammatory drugs should not be taken on an empty stomach (they can irritate the stomach lining and lead to ulcer disease).
■ Encourage the patient to continue with DMARD and/or biological response modifier therapy.	Drug therapy to manage the autoimmune basis of RA can reduce episodes of joint pain and swelling. Some drugs may take weeks or months for a full therapeutic effect to be evident.
▲ Suggest the use of nonopioid analgesics as necessary.	Central-acting analgesics such as opioids are not as effective in relieving inflammatory pain.

■ = Independent   ▲ = Interprofessional Collaboration

Actions/Interventions

- Encourage the patient to monitor his or her position and to always maintain an anatomically correct alignment of the body. Instruct the patient to:
  - Not use pillows to prop the knees.

  - Use a small, flat pillow under the head.

  - Wear splints as prescribed.

- Recommend the use of hot (e.g., heating pad) or cold packs on painful, inflamed joints.

- Encourage the use of ambulation aids when pain is related to weight bearing.

- Suggest that the patient apply a bed cradle.

- Encourage the use of alternative methods of pain control such as relaxation, guided imagery, or distraction.

Rationales

Muscle spasms can result from nonfunctional body alignment and result in pain and predispose to deformity formation. QSEN: Safety.

Prolonged knee flexion can lead to decreased ROM and increased pain.

It is important not to increase the flexion of the neck, which could lead to further deformity and neck strain.

Splints provide rest to inflamed joints and may reduce muscle spasms. These periods of joint rest can help in pain management.

Alternating the use of hot and cold is sometimes helpful in reducing the inflammatory response in the joints. Individual patients may prefer heat over cold or vice versa.

Relief of weight bearing on an inflamed joint can help reduce pain. Some of the weight normally transferred to the affected extremity can be shifted to the ambulation device; the device may also improve balance.

Protective devices keep the pressure of bed covers off the inflamed lower extremities and prevent the development of contractures. QSEN: Safety.

These measures may augment medications to diminish pain and relieve muscle spasms.

NDx Joint Stiffness

Common Related Factors

Inflammation associated with increased disease activity
Degenerative changes secondary to long-standing inflammation

Common Expected Outcomes

Patient verbalizes decrease in stiffness.
Patient is able to participate in self-care activities.

Defining Characteristics

Patient's complaint of joint stiffness
Guarding on motion of affected joints
Refusal to participate in usual self-care activities
Decreased functional ability

NOC Outcomes
Pain Control; Coordinated Movement
NIC Interventions
Pain Management; Heat/Cold Application

Ongoing Assessment

Actions/Interventions

- Assess the patient's description of stiffness:

  - Location: What specific joints are affected?
  - Timing (morning, night, all day)
  - Length of time the stiffness persists

Rationales

Joint stiffness is a common problem for the patient with RA. The patient is the best source of information about his or her stiffness. QSEN: Patient-centered care.

Stiffness may rotate among various joints involved in RA.
Stiffness characteristically occurs on awaking in the morning.
Stiffness usually lasts 30 minutes; it may last longer as the disease progresses.

Actions/Interventions

- Relationship to activities (aggravate or alleviate stiffness)
- Measures used to alleviate stiffness

■ Assess how stiffness interferes with the patient's lifestyle.

Rationales

Stiffness is usually aggravated by prolonged inactivity; it may be precipitated by joint motion.

Most patients will have rituals that they perform to reduce stiffness (e.g., taking a warm bath, foot soaks).

Joint stiffness may interfere with the patient's ability to complete desired activities and maintain independence with activities of daily living.

Therapeutic Interventions

Actions/Interventions

■ Encourage the patient to take a 15-minute warm shower or bath on arising. Localized heat (hand soaking) is also useful. Encourage the patient to perform ROM exercises after the shower or bath, two repetitions per joint.

■ Suggest that the patient plan sufficient time for performing activities and avoid scheduling tasks or therapy when stiffness is present.

■ Instruct the patient to take anti-inflammatory medications in the morning. Remind the patient that anti-inflammatory drugs should not be taken on an empty stomach.

■ Suggest the use of elastic gloves (e.g., Isotoner) at night.

■ Remind the patient to avoid prolonged periods of inactivity.

Rationales

Warm water reduces stiffness and relieves pain and muscle spasms. ROM is important to maintain joint mobility.

Performing tasks while joints are stiff depletes energy, because the functional capacity of the joints may be reduced. Performing simple tasks may take longer. Excessive movement at these times may increase the inflammatory response.

The first dose of the day should be taken as early in the morning as possible, with a small snack. The earlier in the day that the patient takes the medication, the sooner stiffness will abate. Anti-inflammatory agents cause irritation of the gastric mucosa as a side effect.

Supportive gloves that provide mild compression may decrease hand stiffness.

Muscle activity must be balanced with rest, or the joint will become frozen and muscles will atrophy.

NANDA-I NDx ## Impaired Physical Mobility

Common Related Factors

Physical deconditioning
Musculoskeletal impairment
Insufficient muscle strength
Insufficient knowledge of mobility strategies
Pain

Defining Characteristics

Impaired ability to reposition self in bed
Impaired ability to turn from side to side
Impaired ability to move between sitting and supine positions
Impaired ability to move between long sitting and supine positions
Impaired ability to move between prone and supine positions

Common Expected Outcomes

Patient performs physical activity independently within limits of RA.
Patient demonstrates use of adaptive techniques that promote ambulation and transfer.

NOC Outcomes

Joint Movement; Ambulation; Self-Care: Activities of Daily Living (ADLs)

NIC Interventions

Exercise Therapy: Ambulation; Exercise Therapy: Joint Mobility; Self-Care Assistance

---

■ = Independent ▲ = Interprofessional Collaboration

Ongoing Assessment

Actions/Interventions	Rationales
■ Assess the patient's ability to perform ADLs effectively and safely on a daily basis using an appropriate assessment tool, such as the Functional Independence Measures (FIM).	Joint pain and stiffness interfere with performing ADLs. A variety of assessment tools are available, depending on the clinical setting. Such tools provide objective data for baselines. For example, the FIM measures 18 self-care items related to eating, bathing, grooming, dressing, toileting, bladder and bowel management, transfer, ambulation, and stair climbing. QSEN: Patient-centered care; Evidence-based practice.
■ Observe the patient's ability to ambulate and to move all joints functionally.	Pain and fatigue may cause a progressive loss of function.
■ Evaluate the need for ambulatory aids (e.g., single point cane, quad cane, crutches, walker).	Proper use of canes, walkers, and other assistance can promote activity and reduce dangers of falls. The specific aid required depends on the amount of weight bearing that is tolerated, and the ability of the patient to balance safely. QSEN: Safety.
▲ Evaluate the need for home assistance (e.g., physical therapy, home care nurse).	Obtaining appropriate assistance for the patient can ensure safe and proper progression of activity. QSEN: Teamwork and collaboration; Safety.

Therapeutic Interventions

Actions/Interventions	Rationales
■ Reinforce the need for adequate time to perform activities.	The patient may need more time than others to complete the same tasks.
■ Reinforce the proper use of ambulation devices as taught by the physical therapist.	Proper use of assistive ambulation devices conserves energy and provides more protection and support to the patient. These devices reduce the weight-bearing load on joints. QSEN: Teamwork and collaboration.
■ Encourage the patient to wear proper footwear (properly fitting, with good support and nonskid bottoms) when ambulating, and to avoid wearing house slippers.	Patients may select floppy shoes because of pain or because of deformities in the foot. This type of footwear may be easier to put on if the patient has limited ROM in the hands to manage better supportive shoes. It is important for the patient's safety with ambulation that footwear fit correctly to provide support for the foot. QSEN: Safety.
■ Assist with ambulation as necessary.	The first few minutes of weight bearing may be difficult on a joint; support to the standing or sitting position may be helpful to the patient.
■ Reinforce the techniques of therapeutic exercise taught by the physical therapist.	ROM, muscle strengthening, and endurance exercise within a prescribed regimen promote joint function and increase physical stamina.
■ Instruct the patient to avoid excessive exercise during acute inflammatory exacerbations.	Exercise during this time may exacerbate the inflammatory process and contribute to additional joint injury.
■ Reinforce the principles of joint protection taught by the occupational therapist.	Joint protection preserves joint mobility and prevents injury that increases inflammation. QSEN: Teamwork and collaboration.
■ Reinforce proper body alignment when sitting, standing, walking, and lying down.	Improper body alignment can lead to unnecessary pain and contracture. Poor body alignment with ambulation may contribute to falls. QSEN: Safety.
■ Encourage family members to promote independence by:	The patient's self-image improves when he or she can perform personal care independently.
• Assisting the patient only as necessary	During times of exacerbations, patients need more assistance than at other times; the family needs to be sensitive to this.
• Providing necessary adaptive equipment (e.g., raised toilet seat, dressing aids, eating aids)	Such aids promote independence and may enhance safety.

Related Care Plans

Chronic pain, Chapter 2
Fatigue, Chapter 2
Self-care deficit, Chapter 2
Risk for infection, Chapter 2

Fractures: Extremity and Pelvic

Closed Reduction; Open Reduction; Internal Fixation; External Fixation

A fracture is a break or disruption in the continuity of a bone. Fractures occur when a bone is subjected to more stress than it can absorb. Fractures are treated by one or a combination of the following methods: closed reduction—alignment of bone fragments by manual manipulation without surgery; open reduction—alignment of bone fragments by surgery; internal fixation—immobilization of fracture site during surgery with rods, pins, plates, screws, wires, or other hardware or immobilization through use of casts, splints, traction, or posterior molds; external fixation—immobilization of bone fragments with the use of rods and pins that extend from the incision externally and are fixed. This care plan covers the management of patients with fractures and cast immobilization and contains occasional references to more complicated fractures.

NANDA-I
NDx **Acute Pain**

Common Related Factor

Biological injury agent (fracture, soft tissue injury)

Defining Characteristics

Self-report of intensity using standardized pain scale
Self-report of pain characteristics using standardized pain instrument
Guarding behavior
Increased pulse rate
Increased BP
Crying, moaning, grimacing

Common Expected Outcomes

Patient reports satisfactory pain control and a decreased intensity using a standardized pain scale.
Patient uses pharmacological and nonpharmacological pain management strategies.
Patient exhibits increased comfort such as baseline levels for pulse, BP, respirations, and relaxed muscle tone or body posture.

NOC Outcomes
Comfort Status; Pain Level; Pain Control; Medication Response
NIC Interventions
Pain Management; Analgesic Administration

■ = Independent   **▲** = Interprofessional Collaboration

Ongoing Assessment

Actions/Interventions	Rationales
■ Assess for pain or discomfort.	Immediately after the fracture, there may be a period of 15 to 20 minutes in which no pain is apparent. This period of transient anesthesia may be related to the immediate response of nerves that are damaged by the trauma of the fracture. Eventually, sensation is returned and the traumatized area becomes painful enough for the patient to guard the affected area. Subsequent pain from a fracture is associated with muscle spasms and soft tissue injury. The patient may experience pain that is aggravated by movement of the affected area. QSEN: Patient-centered care.
■ Assess the patient's description of pain.	A numeric rating scale or other descriptive scales can be used to identify the intensity of pain. Patients with pelvic fractures may have intense pain from secondary injuries associated with the fracture. These injuries include trauma to pelvic blood vessels, the intestines, or the urinary bladder. Intense pain that persists or pain that returns to previous levels of intensity may indicate a developing complication such as infection or compartment syndrome.
■ Assess the effectiveness of pain-relieving interventions.	Patients have a right to effective pain relief. Pain relief is not determined to be effective until the patient indicates that it is acceptable. It is important to help patients express as factually as possible (i.e., without the effect of mood, emotion, or anxiety) the effect of pain relief measures. Discrepancies between behavior or appearance and what the patient says about pain relief (or lack of it) may be more a reflection of other methods the patient is using to cope with the pain rather than pain relief itself. QSEN: Patient-centered care.

Therapeutic Interventions

Actions/Interventions	Rationales
■ Explain analgesic therapy, including medication and schedule; instruct the patient to take pain medications as needed. Instruct the patient to request pain medication before the pain becomes severe.	Discomfort will be directly related to the type of fracture and the amount of soft tissue damage. Pain with simple fractures may be effectively managed with nonsteroidal anti-inflammatory drugs. Pain related to more serious fractures with complicated types of tissue damage and a need for surgical reduction requires opioid analgesics. Care providers often assume that the patient will request pain medication when needed. The patient may think it is his or her duty or responsibility to tolerate pain until it can no longer be tolerated and may be waiting for the nurse to offer pain medication when it is available. If pain is too severe before analgesics or therapy is instituted, relief takes longer. QSEN: Patient-centered care.
■ If the patient is a candidate for IV patient-controlled analgesia (PCA) (inpatients only), explain its concept and use.	PCA refers to a method that allows the patient to control pain by using an IV drug delivery system. This method allows the patient to self-administer a prescribed opioid analgesic in controlled doses at a frequency necessary to effectively manage the pain. Successful use of PCA requires the patient to have knowledge of its use and the manual dexterity to operate it.

Actions/Interventions

▲ Administer opioid analgesics every 3 to 4 hours around the clock for the first 24 hours after surgical reduction or pin placement.

■ Encourage the use of analgesics 30 to 45 minutes before physical therapy.

■ Encourage the patient to change positions every 2 hours or more often for comfort.

■ Maintain immobilization and support of the affected part. Elevate the affected extremity.

■ Reposition and support the unaffected parts as permitted.

■ Apply ice packs for 20 to 30 minutes every 1 to 2 hours.

■ Teach relaxation techniques.

▲ Administer muscle relaxants as necessary.

Rationales

Manipulation, nerve trauma, and tissue damage result from the fracture and the surgical procedure. Assume that the patient requires analgesia. The patient's ability to fall asleep between pain assessments is not a good indicator of the patient's level of comfort. Adjusting to pain depletes the patient's energy levels and leads to fatigue.

Unrelieved pain hinders the patient's active participation in the therapeutic program.

Repositioning reduces pressure and pain on bony prominences.

Immobility prevents further tissue damage and muscle spasm. Elevation decreases edema. These actions contribute to the reduction of pain.

These techniques promote general comfort and maintain good body alignment.

Cold therapy decreases swelling (first 24 to 48 hours) and reduces pain.

Complementary therapies can enhance the effects of analgesic agents.

These medications prevent muscle spasms, which may be painful.

NANDA-I
NDx Impaired Physical Mobility

Common Related Factors

Musculoskeletal impairment

Insufficient muscle strength

Imposed restrictions of movement, including casts, fixation devices, and immobilizer devices

Insufficient knowledge of mobility strategies

Pain

Defining Characteristics

Impaired ability to reposition self in bed

Impaired ability to turn from side to side

Impaired ability to move between sitting and supine positions

Impaired ability to move between long sitting and supine positions

Impaired ability to move between prone and supine positions

Common Expected Outcomes

Patient performs physical activity independently or within limits of activity restrictions.

Patient demonstrates use of adaptive techniques that promote ambulation and transferring.

Patient is free of complications of immobility, as evidenced by intact skin, absence of thrombophlebitis, normal bowel pattern, and clear breath sounds.

NOC Outcomes

Ambulation; Mobility; Balance; Bone Healing; Transfer Performance

NIC Interventions

Exercise Therapy: Joint Mobility; Exercise Therapy: Ambulation; Self-Care Assistance: Transfer

---

Ongoing Assessment

Actions/Interventions

■ Assess ROM of unaffected joints proximal and distal to the immobilization device.

Rationales

Patients with casts, external fixators, or other immobilizer devices will experience some degree of limited ROM to the affected area. Optimal ROM is critical for movement and necessary for rehabilitation.

■ = Independent   ▲ = Interprofessional Collaboration

Actions/Interventions

- Determine the type of assistive devices the patient will require for ambulation in anticipation of discharge.
- Assess muscle strength in all extremities.

Rationales

Patients may require a cane, walker, or crutches to enhance ambulation.

The rehabilitation program will be geared toward maximizing strength in the unaffected extremities and maintaining as much strength as possible in the affected or immobilized extremity. QSEN: Patient-centered care.

Therapeutic Interventions

Actions/Interventions

- Encourage isometric, active, and resistive ROM exercises to all unaffected joints on a schedule consistent with the rehabilitation program and as tolerated.
- Perform flexion and extension exercises to proximal and distal joints of the affected extremity, when indicated.
- Assist the patient up to the chair when ordered; teach transfer technique. Lift the extremity by the external fixation frame if stable; avoid the handling of injured soft tissue.
- ▲ Consult with the physical therapist, about appropriate weight-bearing techniques and mobility aids as prescribed.

Rationales

Exercise prevents muscle atrophy and maintains adequate muscle strength required for mobility.

These exercises serve to maintain mobility.

Early mobility reduces the complication of immobility. Learning the correct way to transfer is important to maintain optimal mobility and patient safety. QSEN: Safety.

The physical therapist will teach the patient about use of appropriate mobility aids. Some patients will have limited or no weight bearing on the affected extremity to allow the fracture adequate time to begin healing. QSEN: Teamwork and collaboration.

NANDA-I
NDx Risk for Ineffective Peripheral Tissue Perfusion

Common Risk Factors

Interruption in blood flow (cast, inflammatory process and edema, mobilization of a fat embolism)
Insufficient knowledge of aggravating factors (immobility)

Common Expected Outcome

Patient maintains optimal peripheral tissue perfusion as evidenced by strong palpable peripheral pulses, reduction in or absence of pain, warm and dry extremities, adequate capillary refill (less than 2 seconds), and prevention of ulceration.

NOC Outcomes

Tissue Perfusion: Peripheral; Risk Control; Risk Detection

NIC Interventions

Circulatory Care: Arterial Insufficiency; Circulatory Care: Venous Insufficiency; Circulatory Precautions

---

Ongoing Assessment

Actions/Interventions	Rationales
■ Assess and compare the neurovascular status of all extremities before and after the application of a cast or surgical reduction of a fracture. This assessment should continue at intervals of 1 to 2 hours and include the following parameters:	Changes in neurovascular assessment findings may indicate the onset of compartment syndrome. Assessment must include the unaffected and affected extremities to establish a baseline and monitor for changes in neurovascular status. QSEN: Safety.
• Skin temperature	Injured tissues are usually cooler than those on the nonaffected side. Normal temperature indicates adequate perfusion.
• Capillary refill of nail beds	Normal refill is 2 to 4 seconds. In the first hours after injury, capillary refill may be sluggish, but refill that exceeds 4 to 6 seconds should be reported to a member of the interprofessional health team.
• Skin color	Color should be pink, not pale or white. The affected area may be paler than the unaffected area. In patients with darker skin color, the loss of underlying red tones may indicate impaired perfusion.
• Peripheral pulses	All peripheral pulses will be felt; however, the posterior tibialis and the dorsalis pedis in the lower extremities and the radial and ulnar pulses in the upper extremities may be weaker than in the unaffected area.
• Paresthesias	Reports of numbness, tingling, or a "pins and needles" feeling may indicate pressure on nerves and should be investigated.
• Range of motion (ROM)	ROM indicates the amount and degree of limitation. Injured tissues will have decreased ROM. The opposite side should have normal ROM. A decreased ability to wiggle the fingers or toes occurs with nerve damage from compartment syndrome.
• Pain	Pain indicates injury, trauma, or pressure. The surgical site will normally be painful. Intense pain that is unrelieved by analgesics may be an indicator of compartment syndrome.
▲ Monitor the results of lung scans, chest films, and films of the extremity fracture.	These tests may be used to identify a nonhealing fracture or respiratory complications, such as a pulmonary embolus or a fat embolus.
■ Assess for the symptoms of fat embolism.	This complication occurs most often within 2 to 4 days after long bone or pelvic fractures. It may occur because fat molecules are mobilized into general circulation from the bone marrow during a fracture. Fat emboli represent a fatal risk to patients as much as 40% of the time and must be regarded as a potential life-threatening risk.
	The patient may experience a sense of impending doom; chest pain; and signs and symptoms of shock, including tachypnea, tachycardia, hypoxia confusion, or disorientation. The patient may manifest a rash over the chest from below the nipple line up to the neck (may also include the conjunctivae). QSEN: Safety.

■ = Independent   ▲ = Interprofessional Collaboration

Therapeutic Interventions

Actions/Interventions	Rationales
▲ Notify the interprofessional health team immediately if signs of altered circulation are noted.	Venous pressures in the interstitial area surrounding an operative site can be measured through a small catheter inserted into the compartment. A surgical fasciotomy can be performed, which would release constriction and increase arterial inflow, restoring adequate circulation. The best indicators of developing compartment syndrome are patient reports of excessive pain, peripheral pulses becoming weaker or absent, and an increase in pain on passive movement of the distal part. QSEN: Safety; Teamwork and collaboration.
■ Elevate the extremity, and apply ice packs after the surgical reduction (open reduction with internal fixation [ORIF]) or cast application.	These measures reduce edema formation and decrease the risk for compartment syndrome. QSEN: Safety.
▲ Administer anticoagulants as ordered.	These drugs may be given prophylactically to reduce the risk for deep vein thrombosis (DVT).
▲ Apply antiembolic hose or sequential compression devices as indicated.	These devices decrease venous pooling and may enhance venous return, thereby reducing the risk for thrombus formation. QSEN: Safety.
▲ Split or bivalve the cast as needed.	This technique may be done on an emergency basis to reduce restriction and improve impaired circulation resulting from compression and edema of the injured extremity.
▲ Implement emergency measures in the presence of symptoms of a fat embolism:	
• Administer oxygen to keep the saturation level greater than 90%.	Impaired gas exchange is a priority concern. Supplemental oxygen will improve gas exchange and promote effective breathing. QSEN: Safety.
• Titrate IV fluids closely.	Fluid overload can lead to pulmonary edema.
• Transfer the patient to the intensive care unit.	Significantly compromised or unstable patients require critical care management.

NANDA-I
NDx **Deficient Knowledge**

Common Related Factors
Insufficient information
Insufficient interest in learning
Insufficient knowledge of resources
Misinformation presented by others

Defining Characteristics
Insufficient knowledge of care or use of immobilization device, mobility limitations, complications, and follow-up care
Inaccurate follow-through of instruction
Inaccurate performance on a test
Inappropriate behavior

Common Expected Outcome
Patient or caregiver verbalizes understanding of care and use of immobilization device, mobility limitations, complications, and follow-up care.

NOC Outcomes
Knowledge: Treatment Regimen; Safe Home Environment
NIC Interventions
Health Literacy Enhancement; Learning Facilitation; Cast Care: Maintenance; Teaching: Psychomotor Skill; Teaching: Prescribed Exercise

⊖volve   For additional care plans, go to http://evolve.elsevier.com/Gulanick/.

Ongoing Assessment

Actions/Interventions

- Assess the patient's understanding of the factors that facilitate bone healing:
  - The bone ends or fragments must be brought into anatomical alignment.
  - Fracture site is immobilized.
  - Weight bearing is reduced or prohibited.
  - Joints above and below the injury may be immobilized to prevent movement that might dislodge bone ends.
- Determine the patient's and the caregiver's self-efficacy to learn and apply new knowledge about the treatment, follow-up care, and readiness and ability to assume self-care and ADLs.

- Determine the patient's recognition of hazards in the home that will compromise the patient's ability to be effectively mobile at home.
- ▲ Assess the availability of people on whom the patient may rely for support and assistance while mobility is impaired. Consult with members of the interprofessional health care team.

Rationales

Knowledge about fractures and the treatment procedures can help the patient be an active participant in making decisions about his or her care. The patient needs to understand that limited weight bearing on the affected extremity is a necessary component of the healing process for a fracture. QSEN: Patient-centered care.

Effective discharge planning is based on a clear understanding of the needs of the patient and family members who will assume caregiver roles. A first step in teaching may be to foster increased self-efficacy in the patient's ability to learn the desired information or skills necessary to assume responsibility for care at a later time.

Stairs, areas rugs, and so on can limit the patient's progressive mobility and increase the risk for falls. QSEN: Safety.

A social support network can help the patient cooperate with mobility restrictions during the healing process. Referral to a home care agency may be necessary to determine what is needed for a safe transition from the hospital to home for the patient and family caregivers. QSEN: Teamwork and collaboration.

Therapeutic Interventions

Actions/Interventions

- Instruct the patient/caregiver to:
  - Perform prescribed exercises several times a day.

  - Use the appropriate assistive device (walker, crutches), and maintain the prescribed weight-bearing status.
  - Identify and report to the physician signs of neurovascular compromise of the extremity: pain, numbness, tingling, burning, swelling, or discoloration.
  - Use pain relief measures as ordered.

  - Obtain proper nutrition.

  - Keep all follow-up and physical therapy appointments.

- Instruct the patient in cast care:

  - Keep the cast clean and dry; tub bathe only if the cast is protected, not immersed.
  - Inspect the skin around the cast edges for irritation.

  - Do not put anything under the cast, poke under the cast, or put powder or lotion under the cast.

Rationales

Regular exercise is necessary to maintain muscle tone and promote bone healing.

Assistive devices help the patient maintain mobility and comply with weight-bearing restrictions.

Early assessment reduces the risk for injury or complications. QSEN: Safety.

Knowledge helps the patient make decisions about measures to achieve effective pain management. QSEN: Patient-centered care.

A diet with sufficient protein, vitamin D, calcium, and fiber promotes bone and wound healing and prevents constipation.

The rehabilitation program will be modified regularly as the fracture heals.

These measures will ensure stability of the cast and reduce the risk of skin irritation. QSEN: Safety.

Moisture can break down the cast and limits the cast's ability to stabilize the fracture during healing.

Rough edges of the cast can lead to skin irritation and breakdown.

These actions may abrade the skin and cause infection.

■ = Independent   ▲ = Interprofessional Collaboration

Actions/Interventions

- Notify the physician if the cast cracks or breaks, if foul odor under the cast is detected, if fresh drainage through the cast occurs, if anything gets inside the cast, if areas of skin breakdown around the cast occur, if pain or burning inside the cast is present, or if warm areas on the cast are noted.
- Instruct the patient with a surgical incision to observe for signs of infection and to notify the physician if they develop.
- Instruct the patient with an external fixation device to perform pin care, perform wound care, and observe for the loosening of pins.

Rationales

The cast may need to be removed and reapplied if infection or skin breakdown occurs.

Prompt treatment of infection is necessary to prevent osteomyelitis. QSEN: Safety.

The patient needs to implement measures that reduce the risk for infection at pin insertion sites. The external fixation device serves to keep the fracture immobilized during the healing process. Changes in the alignment of the device or the loosening of pins needs to be reported immediately. Corrective action is needed to reestablish appropriate immobilization. QSEN: Safety.

NANDA-I
NDx   Risk for Impaired Urinary Elimination

Common Risk Factors

Urinary tract injuries (e.g., pelvic fracture; urethral tear secondary to high-velocity trauma)
Bladder rupture secondary to punctures from bony fragments
Immobility
Infection

Common Expected Outcome

Patient maintains urine output greater than 30 mL/hr with normal color and negative urine culture.

NOC Outcome
Urinary Elimination
NIC Interventions
Urinary Retention Care; Urinary Catheterization

Ongoing Assessment

Actions/Interventions

- Assess the frequency, amount, and character of urine and for any signs of incontinence.
- Observe for gross hematuria, pelvic hematoma, and an edematous and ecchymotic scrotum.

- Record intake and output.

- Palpate the suprapubic area of the abdomen for bladder distention or suprapubic pain.

Rationales

Bladder trauma may occur with pelvic fractures and result in changes in urinary elimination.

Blood-tinged urine may reflect trauma or damage of the urinary tract system. Excessive bruising or hematoma formation in the pelvic or perineal area may indicate bladder trauma has occurred.

Hourly output should not fall below 30 mL/hr. A Foley catheter may be required to assess output.

Urinary retention may indicate edema or nerve damage secondary to the trauma. Pelvic injuries frequently cause internal injury to the urinary tract; IV pyelogram, cystogram, and a kidney and ureter bladder examination may be required for diagnosis.

Actions/Interventions

■ Assess for the signs and symptoms of urinary tract infection: frequency, burning on urination, elevated temperature, and elevated white blood cell count.

Rationales

Urinary tract infection may be a complication of bladder trauma. QSEN: Safety.

Therapeutic Interventions

Actions/Interventions

■ Encourage oral fluids.

▲ Insert a Foley catheter, or institute intermittent catheterization using aseptic technique, as prescribed.

▲ Administer antibiotics, as prescribed.

■ Notify the physician immediately of any abnormalities in the urine or the process of voiding.

Rationales

If the urine is kept dilute, urinary stasis with resultant infection is less likely. If the patient is unable to maintain adequate oral fluid intake, IV fluids may be necessary. QSEN: Safety.

Catheterization prevents bladder distention and further trauma to the bladder.

Antibiotics may be given to reduce the risk for urinary tract infection from bladder trauma.

Bladder trauma may not be immediately apparent after pelvic fracture.

NANDA-I
NDx Risk for Injury

Common Risk Factors

Improper positioning of immobilization device—sling, external fixator
If cast is in place, loss of continuity of cast
Pelvic fracture

Common Expected Outcomes

Patient maintains correct body position and alignment.
Patient maintains intact cast.

NOC Outcomes
Risk Control; Risk Detection; Bone Healing
NIC Interventions
Cast Care: Wet; Cast Care: Maintenance; Traction/Immobilization Care

---

Ongoing Assessment

Actions/Interventions

■ Assess the stabilization device for the pelvic fracture.

■ Assess the patient's position in the immobilization apparatus.

Rationales

The application of an external compression device is indicated for an unstable pelvic fracture. For pelvic stabilization to be effective, the device must be properly applied. The patient's own movement may result in subtle changes in the apparatus, which can result in malalignment. This would result in patient discomfort and poor healing of the fracture. QSEN: Safety.

The patient should be in an anatomically correct body alignment. If not, painful muscle spasms, muscle fatigue, and malalignment of the healing pelvic bones can occur.

■ = Independent   ▲ = Interprofessional Collaboration

Actions/Interventions

■ Assess the cast for cracks; weakened, softened, or wet areas; indentations; or odors.

Rationales

A weakened cast cannot adequately hold the patient's limbs in the positions necessary for correct healing. It may also indicate that there is bleeding or an infective process going on within the cast. QSEN: Safety.

Therapeutic Interventions

Actions/Interventions

Pelvic stabilization:

■ Maintain the proper alignment of the pelvis and of the affected extremity.

▲ Verify with the physician how much lifting and turning the patient is allowed.

Cast:

■ Leave the cast open to air until completely dry. Do not cover it with blankets or sheets or balance it on the edge of a hard surface.

■ Prevent indenting of the wet cast by moving and supporting it with the palms of your hands.
■ Reposition the patient in a cast every 2 hours.
■ Instruct the patient not to insert anything into the cast (such as an object that might be used to scratch an itch).

■ Petal the edges of the cast with tape.

Rationales

Only in this position will it be possible for the fracture to be reduced (the edge of the fracture will be properly aligned and juxtaposed).
Activity limitations are necessary to enhance healing and recovery.
These nursing actions are necessary to ensure effective immobilization with the cast and reduce the risk for injury. QSEN: Safety.
Coverings may retain moisture and prevent the proper drying of the cast. Resting the cast on the edge of a hard surface will cause indentation. The drying time for the cast depends on the casting material. Most synthetic cast materials may be completely dry within 1 hour of application. Plaster casts may take 2 to 3 days to dry completely.
Indentations will contribute to skin irritation under the cast.

Changing positions allows for complete drying.
Objects may damage the underlying tissue and result in infection or may become trapped within the cast and cause constriction and nerve damage.
This procedure reduces or prevents tissue trauma to the skin underlying the edges of the cast.

Related Care Plans

Deficient fluid volume, Chapter 2
Disturbed body image, Chapter 2
Risk for impaired skin integrity, Chapter 2

Joint Arthroplasty/Replacement: Total Hip, Knee, Shoulder

Total hip arthroplasty/replacement is a total joint replacement by surgical removal of the diseased hip joint, including the femoral neck and head, as well as the acetabulum. The femoral canal is reamed to accept a metal component placed into the femoral shaft, which replaces the femoral head and neck. A polyethylene cup replaces the reamed acetabulum. The prosthesis is either cemented into place or a porous coated prosthesis is used, which allows bio-ingrowth, resulting in retention and stability of the joint. Some arthroplasty procedures are done using a minimally invasive approach. These techniques use multiple small incisions compared to the more traditional approach that uses a single, long incision. A less invasive surgical technique for joint arthroplasty is associated with earlier ambulation, decreased incidence of joint dislocation, and shorter length of stay postoperatively.

Knee hemiarthroplasty is replacement of deteriorated femoral, tibial, and patellar articular surfaces with prosthetic metal and plastic components. The prosthetic devices are held in place through the use of cement or the device is porous, allowing for bio-ingrowth, which eventually secures the replacement. Total knee replacement is the preferred treatment for the older patient with advanced osteoarthritis and for the young and elderly with rheumatoid arthritis (RA). Although knee implants are thought to be durable over time and result in a degree of predictable pain relief, which makes them desirable for all patients, younger patients will almost certainly require revision at some point after the device becomes worn. The hospitalization for total knee replacement rarely exceeds 5 days, with rehabilitation and recovery expected to take from 6 weeks to 3 months. Elderly patients may require additional care in a rehabilitation setting.

Shoulder hemiarthroplasty is the surgical removal of the head of the humerus with replacement by a prosthesis. Total shoulder arthroplasty is the surgical removal of the head of the humerus and the glenoid cavity of the scapula, with replacement by an articulating prosthesis. A metallic humerus is inserted into the shaft, and a high-density polyethylene cup is cemented into place. Patients most likely to undergo this procedure (many of whom are older) have experienced joint damage and functional limitations secondary to osteoarthritis or rheumatoid arthritis. Full recovery takes 3 to 6 months to achieve optimal movement.

NANDA-I NDx **Acute Pain**

Common Related Factor

Physical injury agent (bone and soft tissue trauma caused by surgery)

Defining Characteristics

Self-report of intensity using standardized pain scale
Self-report of pain characteristics using standardized pain instrument
Guarding behavior
Narrowed focus (e.g., time perception, interaction with people and environment)
Expressive behavior (e.g., crying, restlessness, vigilance)
Facial expression of pain
Positioning to ease pain
Change in physiological parameter (e.g., BP, HR, respiratory rate, and oxygen saturation)

Common Expected Outcomes

Patient reports satisfactory pain control and a decreased intensity using a standardized pain scale.
Patient uses pharmacological and nonpharmacological pain management strategies.
Patient exhibits increased comfort such as baseline levels for pulse, BP, respirations, and relaxed muscle tone or body posture.

NOC Outcomes

Comfort Status; Pain Level; Pain Control; Medication Response; Self-Care: Parenteral Medication

NIC Interventions

Pain Management; Analgesic Administration; Patient-Controlled Analgesia (PCA); Sedation Management

■ = Independent   ▲ = Interprofessional Collaboration

Ongoing Assessment

Actions/Interventions	**Rationales**
■ Assess the patient's description of pain.	Postoperative pain is usually localized to the affected joint. It will be acute and sharp. The pain should decrease in intensity over the 5 days after surgery. Intense pain that persists or pain that returns to previous levels of intensity may indicate a developing complication such as infection or compartment syndrome. Compartment syndrome is a condition that results from the unyielding nature of fascial coverings over muscles. The inflammatory process is the result of injury to tissues during surgery causing increased venous pressure, reduced venous return, and subsequent decreased arterial perfusion. If tissue ischemia persists for longer than 6 hours, permanent tissue damage may result. QSEN: Patient-centered care; Safety.
■ Assess the effectiveness of pain-relieving interventions.	Under treatment of pain may limit the patient's postoperative mobility and ability to participate actively in the rehabilitation program. QSEN: Patient-centered care.

Therapeutic Interventions

Actions/Interventions	**Rationales**
■ Explain analgesic therapy, including the medication and schedule. If the patient is a candidate for patient-controlled analgesia (PCA), explain the concept and routine. Instruct the patient to request pain medication before the pain becomes severe.	Care providers often assume that the patient will request pain medication when needed. The patient may be waiting for the nurse to offer it when it is available. Successful use of PCA requires the patient to have knowledge of its use and the manual dexterity to operate it. If pain is too severe before analgesics or therapy is instituted, relief takes longer. QSEN: Patient-centered care.
▲ Administer opioid analgesics every 3 to 4 hours around the clock for the first 24 hours.	A massive amount of manipulation, nerve trauma, and tissue damage occurs during the surgical procedure. The best approach by the nurse is to assume that the patient requires analgesia. The patient's ability to fall asleep between pain assessments is not a good indicator of the patient's level of comfort. Coping with unrelieved pain depletes energy reserves and contributes to fatigue. The patient may sleep and still be in pain.
■ Encourage the use of analgesics 30 to 45 minutes before physical therapy.	Adequate pain relief will enhance the patient's level of participation in physical therapy activities.
■ Change the patient's position (within hip precautions) every 2 hours or more often for comfort.	The patient's inability to move freely and independently may result in pressure and pain on bony prominences.
▲ Apply ice packs as ordered.	Cold reduces pain, inflammation, and muscle spasticity by decreasing the release of pain-inducing chemicals and slowing the conduction of pain impulses.
■ Encourage the use of nonpharmacological measures (e.g., massage, back rubs, diversional activities, guided imagery, progressive relaxation).	These measures reduce muscle tension, refocus attention, promote a sense of control, and may enhance the patient's coping abilities in relation to pain. QSEN: Patient-centered care.
■ Maintain the proper position of the affected extremity.	Correct alignment and anatomical positioning reduces muscle spasms and undue tension on the new prosthesis and surrounding tissue. This action will contribute to effective pain management.
■ Investigate patient reports of sudden severe joint pain with muscle spasms and changes in joint mobility, and of sudden severe chest pain with dyspnea and restlessness.	Early recognition of developing problems such as dislocation of the prosthesis or pulmonary emboli provides for the prompt intervention and treatment of more serious complications. QSEN: Safety.

Impaired Physical Mobility

Common Related Factors

Physical deconditioning
Musculoskeletal impairment
Insufficient muscle strength
Imposed restrictions of movement, including mechanical and medical protocol
Insufficient knowledge of mobility strategies
Pain

Defining Characteristics

Impaired ability to reposition self in bed
Impaired ability to turn from side to side
Impaired ability to move between sitting and supine positions
Impaired ability to move between long sitting and supine positions
Impaired ability to move between prone and supine positions

Common Expected Outcomes

Patient performs physical activity within limitations of prescribed mobility restrictions.
Patient demonstrates use of adaptive techniques that promote ambulation and transferring.
Patient is free of complications of immobility, as evidenced by intact skin, absence of thrombophlebitis, normal bowel pattern, and clear breath sounds.

NOC Outcomes
Bone Healing; Ambulation; Joint Movement; Mobility; Transfer Performance
NIC Interventions
Positioning; Exercise Therapy: Joint Mobility; Exercise Therapy: Ambulation; Self-Care Assistance: Transfer

---

Ongoing Assessment

Actions/Interventions	Rationales
■ Assess the patient's fear and anxiety about transferring or ambulating.	The patient may be fearful of injuring the joint replacement. Allaying anxiety or fear will allow the patient to concentrate on correct techniques for transfer and mobility. QSEN: Patient-centered care.
■ Assess the patient's level of understanding of postoperative restrictions.	The degree of mobility restrictions depends on the involved joint. Initially, the patient may be non–weight bearing on the prosthetic joint. Progressive weight bearing will be implemented as the prosthetic joint becomes more stable. Postoperative mobility restrictions must be maintained at all times to prevent dislocation. QSEN: Safety.
■ Assess the postoperative ROM; document improvement and the failure to progress compared with the preoperative status.	ROM of joints must be maintained during periods of decreased activity. Arthritic joints lose function more rapidly when activity is restricted.

Therapeutic Interventions

Actions/Interventions	Rationales
Hip:	
■ Encourage active ROM with all unaffected extremities.	Decreased mobility results in the loss of muscle tone in all muscle groups. Active ROM promotes muscle tone.
■ Encourage exercise as prescribed to the affected joint.	Exercise aids in increasing muscle strength and tone in the affected extremity.
■ Encourage the use of analgesics before position changes.	Effective pain management allows the patient to participate more fully with prescribed therapy.
■ Use a trapeze bar in bed to assist in mobility.	This device facilitates movement in bed and increases the patient's independence and safety with transfers. QSEN: Patient-centered care; Safety.

■ = Independent   ▲ = Interprofessional Collaboration

Actions/Interventions

■ Instruct the patient in maintaining total hip arthroplasty precautions during position changes.

▲ Maintain weight-bearing status on the affected extremity as prescribed.

Knee:

▲ If prescribed, apply a continuous passive motion (CPM) machine to the affected leg at the prescribed degrees.

▲ Maintain the proper position in CPM: maintain the leg in a neutral position; adjust CPM so the knee joint corresponds to the bend in the CPM machine; adjust the footplate so the foot is in a neutral position in the boot; instruct the patient to keep the opposite leg away from the machine.

■ Assist and encourage the patient to perform quad sets, gluteal sets, and ROM to both legs.

▲ Reinforce muscle-strengthening exercises taught by the physical therapist.

■ Elevate the leg on a pillow when not in CPM. Place the pillow under the calf.

■ Assist the patient with sitting in a chair with the legs dependent several times per day. Initiate weight bearing as prescribed.

■ Encourage ambulation with a walker or canes after initiated by the physical therapist.

Shoulder:

■ Maintain the arm in a shoulder immobilizer as prescribed. After the immobilizer is removed, maintain the arm in a sling.

■ Encourage and assist the patient in performing basic ADLs: self-feeding, brushing teeth, and combing hair. Provide extra time for the performance of these activities.

Rationales

These precautions prevent hip dislocation by limiting ROM of the hip joint. The precautions need to be maintained for up to 6 weeks during the healing process. These precautions may include the use of an abductor wedge while in bed to prevent adduction of the joint. The patient should not flex the hip more than 90 degrees, and should not bend from the waist. QSEN: Safety.

Excessive weight bearing on the new hip increases the risk for dislocation until healing occurs. Patients will begin physical therapy within 24 hours postoperatively.

CPM facilitates joint ROM, promotes wound healing, maintains mobility of the knee, and prevents the formation of adhesions to the operative knee. Evidence suggests that use of a CPM device may not improve knee ROM during postoperative recovery. QSEN: Evidence-based practice.

Proper positioning is imperative to prevent injury from moving parts. QSEN: Safety.

These exercises increase muscle strength and tone. Maintenance of optimal function in all unaffected joints is critical to overall recovery, because collateral extremities will be responsible for weight bearing during transfers and ambulation until recovery is completed.

These exercises optimize the return of full knee extension. QSEN: Teamwork and collaboration.

This position promotes full leg extension.

Patients will progress from a walker to crutches and finally to a cane. Progressive weight bearing will occur as the prosthesis becomes stable.

Progressive daily ambulation promotes the patient's safety and a return to increased physical activity.

The immobilizer may consist of a sling or a sling and a strap that is applied around the body to restrain the arm and maintain proper body alignment.

The patient may be performing ADLs using the nondominant arm, if the surgical site is located in the dominant arm.

NANDA-I

NDx **Risk for Ineffective Peripheral Tissue Perfusion**

Common Risk Factors

Interruption in blood flow
Immobility

Common Expected Outcomes

Patient maintains optimal peripheral tissue perfusion as evidenced by strong palpable peripheral pulses, reduction in or absence of pain, warm and dry extremities, adequate capillary refill (less than 2 seconds), and prevention of ulceration.

NOC Outcome
Tissue Perfusion: Peripheral
NIC Interventions
Circulatory Care: Arterial Insufficiency; Circulatory Care: Venous Insufficiency; Circulatory Precautions

Ongoing Assessment

Actions/Interventions	Rationales
■ Assess the affected extremity every 1 to 2 hours for signs of neurovascular compromise and damage:	Changes in neurovascular assessment findings may indicate the onset of compartment syndrome, peripheral arterial embolism, or deep vein thrombosis (DVT). QSEN: Safety.
• Skin temperature	Injured tissues are usually cooler than on the nonoperative side. Normal temperature indicates adequate perfusion.
• Capillary refill of nail beds	Normal refill time is 2 to 4 seconds. In the first hours after surgery, capillary refill may be sluggish, but refill that exceeds 4 to 6 seconds should be reported to the physician.
• Skin color	Skin color in the operative extremity should be consistent with the other extremities. The affected extremity may be paler than the unaffected extremity if the patient experiences impaired tissue perfusion.
• Peripheral pulses	All peripheral pulses will be felt; however, the posterior tibialis and the dorsalis pedis in the lower extremities and the radial and ulnar pulses in the upper extremities may be weaker than in the unaffected area.
• Paresthesias	Reports of numbness, tingling, or a "pins and needles" feeling may indicate pressure on nerves from impaired perfusion or the presence of compartment syndrome.
• ROM	This evaluation indicates the amount and degree of limitations. Injured tissues will have decreased ROM. A decreased ability to wiggle the fingers or toes occurs with nerve damage from compartment syndrome.
• Pain	Pain indicates injury, trauma, or pressure. The surgical site will normally be painful. Monitor and report excessive reports of pain as an indication of compartment syndrome.
▲ Check the sequential compression device and thromboembolic disease (TED) support stocking for extreme tightness.	Excessive compression may result in neurovascular compromise. QSEN: Safety.
■ Assess for the signs and symptoms of DVT:	DVT is a serious complication after joint replacement surgery. QSEN: Safety.
• Positive Homans' sign (the examiner dorsiflexes the patient's foot toward the tibia, and the patient experiences pain in the calf muscles)	Research indicates that assessment for Homans' sign may not be a reliable indicator of DVT. Homans' sign may be absent with a DVT. Some patients without a DVT may report calf pain with dorsiflexion. QSEN: Evidence-based practice.
• Increased leg circumference	The leg affected by a DVT will develop edema and result in increased leg circumference compared to the unaffected leg.
• Abnormal blood flow study findings (if prescribed)	A Doppler ultrasound examination may be performed to diagnose a DVT.

■ = Independent ▲ = Interprofessional Collaboration

Actions/Interventions

- Assess for the signs and symptoms of PE: tachypnea, chest pain, dyspnea, tachycardia, hemoptysis, cyanosis, anxiety, abnormal arterial blood gas values, and abnormal ventilation-perfusion scan result.

- Assess for the signs and symptoms of a fat embolism: pulmonary (dyspnea, tachypnea, cyanosis); cerebral (headache, irritability, delirium, coma); cardiac (tachycardia, decreased BP, petechial hemorrhage of upper chest, axillae, and conjunctivae); fat globules in the urine.

Rationales

The onset of symptoms can be sudden and overwhelming and can constitute a life-threatening situation for the patient. QSEN: Safety.

Fat embolism is usually seen the second day after surgery. The fat globules released from the bone marrow during surgery gain access to the circulatory system. Symptoms may be sudden and precipitous and represent an immediate threat to the patient's life. QSEN: Safety.

Therapeutic Interventions

Actions/Interventions

▲ Notify the physician immediately if signs of compartment syndrome are noted.

- Encourage leg exercises, including quad sets, gluteal sets, and active ankle ROM.

▲ Institute antiembolic devices as prescribed (sequential compression device or TED stockings).

▲ Administer anticoagulant agents as ordered.

- Encourage the patient to be out of bed as soon as prescribed.

Rationales

Venous pressures in the interstitial area surrounding an operative site can be measured through a small catheter inserted into the compartment. A surgical fasciotomy can be performed, which would release constriction and increase arterial inflow, restoring adequate circulation. The best indicators of developing compartment syndrome are patient reports of excessive pain, peripheral pulses becoming weaker or absent, and an increase in pain on passive movement of the part distal to the surgery. QSEN: Safety.

These exercises not only improve muscle tone but also promote venous return from the legs. Venous stasis may predispose the patient to DVT.

Antiembolic devices increase venous blood flow to the heart and decrease venous stasis, thereby decreasing the risk for DVT and PE. These devices are often applied in the post-anesthesia recovery unit and continued until the patient is discharged. The devices can be removed when the patient is ambulatory but are reapplied when the patient is in bed.

Prophylactic anticoagulants reduce the risk for DVT. The patient must be monitored closely because these medications may cause bleeding.

Mobility restores normal circulatory function and decreases the risk for venous stasis.

NANDA-I NDx Deficient Knowledge

Common Related Factors

Insufficient information
Insufficient interest in learning
Insufficient knowledge of resources
Misinformation presented by others

Defining Characteristics

Insufficient knowledge of discharge and rehabilitation plan
Inaccurate follow-through of instruction for mobility and arthroplasty precautions
Inappropriate behavior

 Evolve **For additional care plans, go to http://evolve.elsevier.com/Gulanick/.**

Common Expected Outcome

Patient verbalizes understanding of discharge instructions; arthroplasty precautions, and follow-up rehabilitation regimen.

NOC Outcomes

Knowledge: Disease Process; Knowledge: Treatment Regimen; Knowledge: Prescribed Activity

NIC Interventions

Health Literacy Enhancement; Learning Facilitation; Teaching: Disease Process; Teaching: Prescribed Exercise

Ongoing Assessment

Actions/Interventions	Rationales
■ Assess the patient's understanding of the discharge instructions and follow-up regimen.	This information provides the starting base for educational sessions. The patient will be responsible for continuing mobility restrictions, exercises, and medications after discharge. QSEN: Patient-centered care.
■ Determine the patient's self-efficacy to learn and apply new knowledge.	A first step in teaching may be to foster increased self-efficacy in the patient's ability to learn the desired information and skills for arthroplasty precautions and progressive ambulation.

Therapeutic Interventions

Actions/Interventions	Rationales
■ Review the total hip arthroplasty precautions: • Maintain abduction with an abductor device when at rest. • Always keep the legs externally or neutrally rotated. • Avoid hip flexion of greater than 90 degrees. • Avoid bending from the waist. • Do not cross the legs. • Ambulate (weight bearing as instructed) with an assistive device (walker or crutches). • Call the physician immediately if sharp pain or "popping" is felt in the affected extremity or if there is a feeling of the hip being "out of socket." • Instruct the patient not to drive until directed by the physician.	The patient needs to understand how to prevent hip dislocation. Extremes of joint flexion and adduction during the healing process place stress on the prosthesis and increase the risk for dislocation. QSEN: Safety. Bending causes hip flexion of greater than 90 degrees. This position causes adduction, which can lead to dislocation. Protected ambulation promotes healing of the affected hip. Dislocation of the prosthesis requires immediate attention and possible surgical intervention. Muscle contraction and joint movement associated with operating the accelerator and brake pedals puts stress on the healing prosthetic joint.
■ Review the knee arthroplasty precautions: • Use a walker or crutches to ambulate with prescribed weight bearing on the operative knee. • Do not participate in sports until the physician indicates that it is permissible. • Notify the physician of knee pain that returns to a previous level of discomfort, excessive swelling, leaking of fluid from the incision, chest pain, shortness of breath, or pain and swelling in the calf of either leg.	These nursing actions reduce harm to the patient from stressors on the prosthesis during the healing process. QSEN: Safety. Assistive devices reduce stress on the affected joint during the healing process. The patient needs to limit activities that put stress on the affected joint during healing. These symptoms indicate complications of joint replacement and require immediate attention.

Actions/Interventions

- Review the shoulder arthroplasty precautions:
  - Initially, perform only passive ROM exercises, gradually adding active exercises as instructed.
  - Avoid using the affected arm for heavy lifting (more than 5 pounds), pulling, or pushing. Follow weight-bearing precautions as instructed.
  - Avoid activities that involve exaggerated external rotation and abduction of the affected shoulder.
- Reinforce the need to continue prescribed ROM exercises. This may require home physical therapy.

- Emphasize the importance of removing environmental hazards (e.g., throw rugs, low tables, pets, electrical cords, toys).

Rationales

Gradual increase in ROM and weight bearing as necessary allows healing of the affected joint and prevents dislocation of the prosthesis. QSEN: Safety.

Physical therapy at home helps the patient gain strength in muscle groups to support the integrity of the prosthetic joint. QSEN: Teamwork and collaboration.

The patient needs to understand how to maintain a safe home environment to promote progressive ambulation and prevent falls. QSEN: Safety.

Related Care Plans

Risk for falls, Chapter 2
Surgical experience: Preoperative and postoperative care, Chapter 4

Osteoarthritis

Osteoarthritis (OA) is a progressive degeneration of articular cartilage in synovial joints. Weight-bearing joints, the hands, and the spine are affected most often. This disorder was formerly known as degenerative joint disease (DJD). Although the disease occurs more often in older adults, OA is not part of the normal aging process. Idiopathic (primary) OA is more likely to affect women older than age 65. People with this type of OA usually have a family history of the disorder but no direct history of joint disease or injury. Secondary OA occurs more often in men. People with this type of OA are likely to have a history of joint trauma or repetitive joint injury related to the person's occupation or sports activity. OA is characterized by a progressive degeneration of the cartilage in a joint. The changes in articular cartilage represent an imbalance between lysosomal enzyme destruction of and chrondrocyte production of cartilage matrix. This imbalance leads to an inability of the cartilage to withstand the normal weight-bearing stress in the joint. Cartilage becomes thin, rough, and uneven, with areas that soften, eventually allowing bone ends to come closer together. X-ray examination of the affected joint may show a narrowed and uneven joint space. Small fragments of the cartilage may float about freely within the joint space, initiating an inflammatory process. True to the progressive nature of the disease, the cartilage continues to degenerate, and bone spurs called osteophytes develop at the joint margins and at the attachment sites of the tendons and ligaments. Over time these changes have an effect on the mobility and size of the joint. As joint cartilage becomes fissured, synovial fluid leaks out of the subchondral bone and cysts develop on the bone. Treatment is aimed at relieving pain, maintaining optimal joint function, and preventing progressive disability. Guidelines from the Osteoarthritis Research Society International (OARSI) recommend core treatments that include land-based and water-based exercise, weight management, and strength training. This care plan focuses on the outpatient nursing management for this group of patients.

Acute Pain/Chronic Pain

Common Related Factors
Biological injury agent (joint degeneration, muscle spasm, bone deformities)
Physical injury agent (weight bearing)
Chronic musculoskeletal condition

Defining Characteristics
Self-report of intensity using standardized pain scale
Self-report of pain characteristics using standardized pain instrument
Self-focused
Alteration in sleep pattern
Altered ability to continue previous activities

Common Expected Outcomes
Patient reports satisfactory pain control and a decreased intensity using a standardized pain scale.
Patient uses pharmacological and nonpharmacological pain relief strategies.
Patient exhibits increased comfort such as baseline levels for HR, BP, respirations, and relaxed muscle tone or body posture.
Patient engages in desired activities without an increase in pain level.

NOC Outcomes
Comfort Status; Pain Level; Pain Control; Medication Response
NIC Interventions
Pain: Disruptive Effects; Pain: Adverse Psychological Response; Medication Administration; Analgesic Administration; Heat/Cold Application

Ongoing Assessment

Actions/Interventions	Rationales
■ Assess the patient's description of pain.	Systematic assessment and documentation of the chronic pain experience provides direction for a pain management plan. The patient may report pain in the fingers, hips, knees, lower lumbar spine, and cervical vertebrae. The patient may experience sharp, painful muscle spasms and paresthesias. QSEN: Patient-centered care.
■ Identify factors or activities that seem to precipitate acute episodes or aggravate a chronic condition.	Pain may be associated with specific movements, especially repetitive movements of the involved joints. Pain is usually provoked by activity and relieved by rest; joint pain and aching may also be present when the patient is at rest. Pain may manifest as an ache, progressing to sharp pain when the affected area is brought to full weight bearing or full ROM.
■ Assess the patient's previous experiences with pain and pain relief.	The patient may have a tried-and-true plan to implement when osteoarthritis (OA) becomes exacerbated. An effective pain management plan will be based on the patient's previous experience with pain relief measures. Consideration should be given to implementing this plan, with modifications if necessary, when pain becomes acute. QSEN: Patient-centered care.
■ Determine the patient's emotional reaction to chronic pain.	The patient may find coping with a progressive, debilitating disease difficult. Coping with chronic pain can deplete the patient's energy for other activities. The patient often looks tired, with a drawn facial expression that lacks animation.
■ Determine whether the patient is reporting all of the pain he or she is experiencing.	Patients who have become accustomed to living with chronic pain may learn to tolerate basal levels of discomfort and only report those discomforts that exceed these "normal" levels. The care provider is not getting an accurate picture of the patient's status if this pain is not reported. The nurse may need to be sensitive to nonverbal cues that pain is present.

■ = Independent ▲ = Interprofessional Collaboration

Therapeutic Interventions

Actions/Interventions	Rationales
■ Instruct the patient to implement the following pain management interventions:	A pain relief regimen is based on the patient's identified aggravating and relieving factors. QSEN: Patient-centered care.
• Change positions frequently while maintaining functional alignment.	Muscle spasms may result from poor body alignment, resulting in increased discomfort. Frequent position changes can reduce stress on joints and muscles.
• Support joints with correctly fitted biomechanical devices.	The use of biomechanical devices such as braces, sleeves for knees, and foot orthotics have been shown to be effective in decreasing pain and joint stiffness. QSEN: Evidence-based practice.
• Apply a hot or cold pack.	Heat reduces pain through improved blood flow to the area and through the reduction of pain reflexes. Special attention needs to be given to preventing burns with this intervention. Heat may be provided by warm baths or showers or by direct application of warm packs to the affected joint. Cold reduces pain, inflammation, and muscle spasticity by decreasing the release of pain-inducing chemicals and slowing the conduction of pain impulses. These interventions require no special equipment and can be cost-effective. Hot or cold applications should last about 20 to 30 min/hr. QSEN: Safety.
• Provide for adequate rest periods.	Resting painful joints reduces the stressors on the joint that stimulate inflammation and cartilage destruction. Fatigue impairs the patient's ability to cope with discomfort.
• Use adaptive equipment (e.g., cane, walker), as necessary.	These aids assist in ambulation and reduce joint stress from weight-bearing activity. Evidence suggests that a walking cane compared to crutches is effective in reducing joint pain for patients with OA of the knee. QSEN: Evidence-based practice.
• Medicate for pain before activity and exercise therapy.	Exercise is necessary to maintain joint mobility, but patients may be reluctant to participate in exercise if they are in too much pain.
• Eliminate additional stressors.	Chronic pain takes an enormous emotional toll on patients. Reducing other factors that cause stress may make it possible for the patient to have greater reserves of emotional energy for effective coping.
■ Instruct the patient to take prescribed analgesics and/or anti-inflammatory medications. Provide instruction in important side effects.	The OARSI guidelines provide suggestions for implementing drug therapy to manage pain and minimize side effects. QSEN: Evidence-based practice; Safety.
• Acetaminophen	This drug relieves pain but has no effect on inflammation. Current OARSI guidelines suggest conservative dosing and limited duration of use for acetaminophen because of an increased risk for adverse effects.
• Nonselective NSAIDs	These drugs are anti-inflammatory, antipyretic, and analgesic agents. They are usually used for their anti-inflammatory action to relieve mild to moderate pain. Side effects include mild GI disturbances and fluid retention. OARSI guidelines recommend this class of drugs for patients with OA and no other co-morbid conditions such as hypertension, cardiovascular disease, chronic kidney disease, GI bleeding, depression, or obesity.

Actions/Interventions

- Selective NSAIDs

- Corticosteroids

Rationales

This class of drugs acts by reducing prostaglandin synthesis via the inhibition of cyclooxygenase-2 (COX-2). These drugs are used with caution in people with a history of gastric ulcers, liver disease, stroke, or cardiovascular disease. OARSI guidelines recommend these drugs as appropriate for patients with OA and moderate co-morbidity risk.

These drugs are anti-inflammatory and usually used for the treatment of acute episodes of joint inflammation to provide short-term pain relief. The drug is injected directly into the inflamed joint. The injections may be repeated at 3- to 4-month intervals to manage recurring joint inflammation.

NANDA-I NDx Impaired Physical Mobility

Common Related Factors

Physical deconditioning
Musculoskeletal impairment
Insufficient muscle strength
Insufficient knowledge of mobility strategies
Pain

Defining Characteristics

Impaired ability to reposition self in bed
Impaired ability to turn from side to side
Impaired ability to move between sitting and supine positions
Impaired ability to move between long sitting and supine positions
Impaired ability to move between prone and supine positions

Common Expected Outcomes

Patient performs physical activity independently or within limits of joint mobility and weight bearing.
Patient demonstrates use of adaptive techniques that promote ambulation and transferring.
Patient is free of complications of immobility, as evidenced by intact skin, absence of thrombophlebitis, normal bowel pattern, and clear breath sounds.

NOC Outcomes

Ambulation; Knowledge: Prescribed Activity; Transfer Performance

NIC Interventions

Exercise Therapy: Joint Mobility; Exercise Therapy: Ambulation; Teaching: Prescribed Exercise; Self-Care Assistance: Transfer

Ongoing Assessment

Actions/Interventions

- Assess ROM in all joints, comparing passive and active ROM.
- Assess the patient's posture and gait.

- Assess the patient's ability to perform ADLs. Determine what adaptive measures the patient has already taken to be able to perform self-care measures.

Rationales

Pain or joint deformity may cause a progressive loss of ROM.

It is important to assess for indicators of a decreased ability to ambulate and move purposefully: shorter, shuffling steps, unstable gait, uneven weight bearing, an observable limp, change in posture such as rounding of the back or hunching of the shoulders.

Joint deformity, especially in the hands, that occurs with OA may limit certain self-care activities by the patient. A spouse may assist in buttoning clothes or picking up dropped objects. The patient may have had assistive devices installed in the shower or near the toilet (e.g., handlebars, raised toilet seat). This information gives the nurse a sense of the measures the patient has had to take to remain functional. QSEN: Patient-centered care.

■ = Independent   ▲ = Interprofessional Collaboration

Actions/Interventions	Rationales
■ Assess the patient's comfort with and knowledge of how to use assistive devices.	The correct use of assistive devices for ambulation can improve mobility and reduce the risk for falls. Some patients refuse to use assistive devices because they attract attention to their impaired mobility. QSEN: Safety.
■ Assess the patient's weight.	Excessive weight may add stress to painful joints and contribute to degeneration of joint cartilage.
■ Assess the patient's vital signs after physical activity.	Elevations in HR, respiratory rate, and BP may be a function of increased effort and discomfort during ambulation and ADLs.

Therapeutic Interventions

Actions/Interventions	Rationales
■ Instruct the patient in how to perform isometric, and active and passive ROM exercises to all extremities.	Muscular exertion through exercise promotes circulation and free joint mobility, strengthens muscle tone, develops coordination, and prevents nonfunctional contracture.
■ Encourage the patient to increase activity as indicated.	Increasing activity at home can be effective in maintaining joint function and independence. A balance must exist between the patient performing enough activity to keep joints mobile and stressors to the joint that increase joint inflammation.
▲ Consult physical therapy staff to prescribe an exercise program.	The physical therapist can help the patient with exercises to promote muscle strength and joint ROM and therapies to promote the relaxation of tense muscles. Evidence supports land-based exercise for improved physical functioning for patients with OA. Water-based exercise has short-term benefits for improved joint function and quality of life. These interventions also may contribute to effective pain management. The therapist can teach the patient about effective use of mobility aids to reduce stress on affected joints from weight bearing. QSEN: Teamwork and collaboration.
■ Encourage the patient to ambulate with assistive devices (e.g., crutches, walker, cane).	Using mobility aids reduces the weight-bearing load on the joint and promotes safety. OARSI guidelines recommend cane walking over crutches for the patient with knee OA. QSEN: Evidence-based practice; Safety.
■ Encourage sitting in a chair with a raised seat and firm support.	This adaptive technique facilitates getting in and out of a chair safely.
■ Encourage the patient to rest between activities that are tiring. Suggest strategies for getting out of bed, rising from chairs, and picking up objects from the floor to conserve energy.	Rest periods are necessary to conserve energy. The patient must learn to respect the limitations of his or her joints; pushing beyond the point of pain will only increase the stress on the joint. The patient needs to recognize and accept the limitations of his or her joints. Rushing is likely to be frustrating and self-defeating and may result in unsafe conditions for the patient.
■ Discuss the environmental barriers to mobility.	It may no longer be reasonable for the patient to continue to live in a home or apartment with multiple flights of stairs or to continue to try to take care of a large home. If the patient is using a cane or walker, carpets must be tacked down or removed. Items that are used often should be kept within reach. Ambulation pathways need to be clear of clutter and obstructions. QSEN: Safety.

Actions/Interventions

- Provide the patient with access to and support during weight-reduction programs.

- Suggest a referral to community resources such as the Arthritis Foundation.

Rationales

Weight reduction results in decreased trauma to bones, muscles, and joints. OARSI guidelines recommend weight management as part of the core treatment plan for patient with OA. QSEN: Evidence-based practice.

Community resources can provide the patient with peer support and additional information about resources (e.g., assistive devices).

Related Care Plans

Chronic pain, Chapter 2
Disturbed body image, Chapter 2
Self-care deficit, Chapter 2

Osteoporosis

Brittle Bone

Osteoporosis is a metabolic bone disease characterized by a decrease in bone mass, resulting in porosity and brittleness. Bone resorption occurs at a rate that is faster than the process of new bone formation. Primary causes are a decrease in dietary intake of calcium or a decrease in calcium absorption and estrogen deficiency. Secondary causes may include steroid use, tobacco and alcohol use, and endocrine and liver diseases. Osteoporosis occurs most commonly in women who are menopausal, although it may also be present in women who exercise to such an extent that menstruation and resultant estrogen production are suppressed. Estrogen has been demonstrated to have a protective effect against the development and progression of bone changes that result in osteoporosis. Men and African-American women have denser bones than Caucasian women. Men develop osteoporosis much later in life than women. These factors together with a decrease in physical activity and weight-bearing activities result in bones that are brittle and

fragile. Even normal physical activity can result in fracture. Common fractures include compression fractures of the vertebrae and fractures of the femur, hip, and wrist. Vertebral compression fractures result in a progressive decrease in height and development of kyphosis. Osteoporosis combined with an increased incidence of falls in the elderly puts the older adult at higher risk for fractures. The National Osteoporosis Foundation (NOF) has published evidence-based clinician guidelines for the prevention and treatment of osteoporosis. Universal recommendations for all patients include adequate calcium and vitamin D intake, treatment of vitamin D deficiency, regular muscle-strengthening and weight-bearing exercises, fall prevention, and cessation of tobacco use and excessive alcohol intake. Bisphosphonates (Fosamax, Actonel), salmon calcitonin, and raloxifene are medications used to prevent and treat osteoporosis. They act by reducing bone resorption. This care plan focuses on early identification and prevention of the disease.

NANDA-I NDx Deficient Knowledge

Common Related Factors

Insufficient information
Insufficient interest in learning
Insufficient knowledge of resources
Misinformation presented by others

Defining Characteristics

Insufficient knowledge of dietary intake of calcium and vitamin D, fall prevention, bone density
Inaccurate follow-through of instruction
Inappropriate behavior

■ = Independent ▲ = Interprofessional Collaboration

Common Expected Outcomes

Patient verbalizes an understanding of osteoporosis and fall prevention measures.

Patient verbalizes understanding of the osteoporosis and treatment.

NOC Outcomes

Knowledge: Disease Process; Knowledge: Medication; Knowledge: Prescribed Diet; Fall Prevention Behavior

NIC Interventions

Health Literacy Enhancement; Learning Facilitation; Teaching: Disease Process; Teaching: Prescribed Diet; Teaching: Prescribed Medication

---

Ongoing Assessment

Actions/Interventions	Rationales
■ Assess the patient's knowledge of osteoporosis and treatment.	This information provides the starting base for educational sessions. As people live longer, the risk for osteoporosis increases. However, many people do not believe they are susceptible to it, do not understand the life-threatening injuries that may occur secondary to it, and do not realize that it can be prevented. Men may believe that only women develop osteoporosis. Patients may have the misconception that osteoporosis is part of the normal aging process. QSEN: Patient-centered care.
■ Assess the patient's dietary intake of calcium and the use of calcium supplementation.	Daily dietary intake of 1000 to 1200 mg of calcium is necessary. Calcium supplements are necessary if dietary intake is inadequate. Some people stop taking calcium supplements because of gastrointestinal (GI) upset, constipation, or cost.
■ Assess whether a woman is postmenopausal or has had a hysterectomy with bilateral oophorectomy.	Resorption of the bone is accelerated with natural or surgically induced menopause. The normal balance of bone resorption and new bone formation is a function of the RANKL/RANK/OPG system. The receptor activator of nuclear factor κβ ligand (RANKL) is a cytokine that binds to the RANK receptor and stimulates maturation of osteoclasts. Osteoprotegerin (OPG) is a decoy receptor that decreases expression of RANKL on osteoclast cells. Estrogen stimulates the secretion of OPG. Loss of estrogen allows for increased osteoclast activity and increased bone resorption.
■ Assess tobacco, alcohol, and exercise history, and if the patient is taking medications that decrease calcium absorption.	Smoking, excessive alcohol intake, and having only minimal weight-bearing exercise are risk factors for the development of osteoporosis. Medications such as cortisone, antacids, tetracycline, and laxatives may inhibit calcium absorption from the intestines.
■ Assess the patient's height.	The patient's height should be measured using a wall-mounted stadiometer. A decrease in the patient's height is associated with vertebral compression fractures. The NOF suggests that an historical height difference of 1.5 inches or more between the patient's current height and self-reported peak height at age 20 years is diagnostic for osteoporosis. A prospective height loss of 0.8 inch between the patient's current height and a previously documented height is diagnostic for osteoporosis. QSEN: Evidence-based practice.

Musculoskeletal Care Plans

Actions/Interventions

▲ Monitor the patient's calcium levels.

Rationales

Elevated calcium levels indicate calcium malabsorption. This may indicate the need for vitamin D supplementation to aid in calcium absorption. The usual dose is 200 to 400 international units daily.

Therapeutic Interventions

Actions/Interventions

■ Provide the patient with information about the risk factors for osteoporosis.

Rationales

This knowledge allows the patient to make decisions about lifestyle modifications to prevent the development of osteoporosis. Risk factors are an inadequate dietary calcium intake, family history, and an inactive lifestyle. Also at risk are people who use cigarettes, caffeine, and alcohol and are older than 45 years, with or without endocrine disease. Estrogen deficiency is the primary risk factor for women. QSEN: Patient-centered care; Safety.

■ Describe the diagnostic tests available for osteoporosis:

NOF clinician guidelines recommend bone mineral density (BMD) testing in women age 65 and older and men age 70 and older. Patients, regardless of gender, who have a positive risk factor profile for osteoporosis, should begin BMD testing at ages 50 to 69. Postmenopausal women and men age 50 or older with an adult age fracture should have BMD testing. Medicare Part B (medical insurance) currently covers the cost of BMD once every 24 months. QSEN: Evidence-based practice.

• Dual-energy x-ray absorptiometry (DXA)

This test is used for early detection of the disease. Dual photons are used to measure bone density. This type of screening can be done for the hip, wrist, or spinal column. Patients at risk for osteoporosis should begin bone density screening in their 40s.

• Quantitative computed tomography (QCT)

QCT measures the density of bone.

• Ultrasound

Ultrasound measurements of bone density of the heel have been found to reliably detect osteoporosis and the risk for subsequent fractures of the hip.

• Biochemical assessment

Tests such as serum osteocalcin provide information on osteoblastic activity. Low levels of alkaline phosphatase are present in patients with osteoporosis.

■ Provide information about increased calcium intake.

Natural sources of calcium may provide more elemental or useful forms of calcium. Calcium-rich foods include skim milk, cheeses, yogurt, ice cream; whole-grain cereals; green, leafy vegetables; almonds and hazelnuts.

▲ Consult a dietitian when appropriate.

A registered dietitian can provide specific dietary guidelines for calcium and vitamin D intake based on an analysis of the patient's dietary history. QSEN: Teamwork and collaboration.

■ = Independent   ▲ = Interprofessional Collaboration

Actions/Interventions

▲ Instruct the patient in taking calcium supplementation therapy as ordered.

■ Provide information about exercise and fall prevention:

- Physical activity, at least 30 minutes most days of the week

- Use of assistive devices (e.g., canes, walkers)

- Consultation with an occupational therapist

■ Provide information on medications used in the prevention and treatment of osteoporosis:

- Bisphosphonates given in conjunction with calcitonin

Rationales

The patient needs to understand that calcium supplements are available as calcium compounds. Calcium carbonate has the highest concentration of elemental calcium. This compound is often the least expensive. The patient should read labels and look for the word "purified" or "USP" (United States Pharmacopeia). Supplements without these words may be less reliable and may contain high levels of lead. Calcium supplements are better absorbed when taken with meals. If flatulence or constipation occurs with taking calcium supplements, the patient can increase his or her fluid and dietary fiber intake. However, eating large amounts of dietary fiber can interfere with calcium absorption. Foods high in oxalates such as spinach may also interfere with calcium absorption.

Weight-bearing exercise and muscle-strengthening exercise at a moderate level aids in the development and maintenance of bone mass, posture, balance, and agility. The benefits of these activities are essential to fall prevention. QSEN: Evidence-based practice; Safety.

This activity may include walking, running, dancing, skipping rope, tai chi, yoga, circuit-resistance training, or stair climbing,

These devices assist in balance and provide partial weight bearing. They can help prevent falls and associated fractures in the patient with osteoporosis.

The occupational therapist, as a member of the interprofessional health team, can provide the patient with a home safety assessment and direction for home modifications as needed. Until bone density is enhanced and stabilized, falls will constitute a grave risk to the patient manifesting symptoms of osteoporosis. Severe hip fractures can be fatal in certain debilitated populations. QSEN: Teamwork and collaboration.

The NOF guidelines suggest FDA-approved treatments for osteoporosis for patients who have a vertebral or hip fracture; documented hip or lumbar DXA results of osteoporosis; or low bone mass and a WHO Fracture Algorithm (FRAX) probability of a major osteoporosis related fracture. QSEN: Evidence-based practice; Safety.

These compounds inhibit bone breakdown and slow bone removal. Bisphosphonates increase bone density and decrease the risk for fractures. Patients taking oral bisphosphonates need to learn the correct method of administration. These drugs are best taken in the morning, 30 to 60 minutes before breakfast. The patient needs to remain upright during this time to reduce the risk for esophageal reflux. IV forms of these drugs are available for patients who do not tolerate the oral preparations. The IV bisphosphonates are administered once per year to four times per year, depending on the specific drug.

Actions/Interventions

- Calcitonin subcutaneous injection or nasal spray

- Estrogen agonist/antagonist (formerly known as selective estrogen receptor modulators [SERMs])

- Teriparatide

Rationales

Calcitonin is a naturally occurring hormone involved in calcium regulation and bone metabolism. This drug is recommended for women who are at least 5 years post-menopause. Calcitonin prevents further bone loss by slowing the removal of bone and may be helpful in relieving the pain associated with osteoporosis. The drug has been shown to decrease the risk of vertebral fracture.

This drug activates estrogen receptors in target organs to produce effects on estrogen-responsive tissues. Raloxifene (Evista) is given for the prevention and treatment of post-menopausal osteoporosis.

Teriparatide is a recombinant human parathyroid hormone used for the treatment of postmenopausal osteoporosis and in men with idiopathic or hypogonadal osteoporosis who are at high risk for fractures or who failed or are intolerant to prior osteoporosis therapy.

NANDA-I
NDx   Risk for Falls

Common Risk Factors

History of falls
Age above 65 years
Use of assistive devices (e.g., walker, cane)
Impaired mobility
Difficulty with gait
Impaired balance

Common Expected Outcomes

Patient will not sustain a fall.
Patient and caregiver will implement strategies to increase safety and prevent falls in the home.

NOC Outcomes

Fall Prevention Behavior; Knowledge: Fall Prevention; Risk Control; Risk Detection

NIC Interventions

Fall Prevention; Environmental Management; Safety

Ongoing Assessment

Actions/Interventions

- Observe the patient's ability to ambulate and to move all body parts functionally.

- Assess the environment for safety.

Rationales

Walking or getting up from a chair or bed may present difficulty to the patient because of balance or gait problems. Because fractures can occur spontaneously with normal activity, protective measures must be taken until bone density has increased sufficiently to tolerate exercise. QSEN: Safety.

A safe environment reduces the risk for falls and potential fractures. Anything that blocks or limits a clear, straight path for ambulation can contribute to a person's fall risk. QSEN: Safety.

■ = Independent   ▲ = Interprofessional Collaboration

Therapeutic Interventions

Actions/Interventions	Rationales
▲ Collaborate with the interprofessional health team to promote the patient's safety with mobility.	The physical therapist can develop an exercise program that includes muscle strengthening and weight bearing. Weight bearing stimulates osteoblast activity and new bone growth. Muscle strengthening improves balance and posture with activity. The exercise program will require modification on an ongoing basis as the patient's condition improves and bone strength is enhanced. QSEN: Teamwork and collaboration.
■ Encourage the patient to request assistance with ambulation as necessary. Recommend low, comfortable shoes for walking. Provide adaptive equipment (e.g., cane, walker) as necessary.	Fractures are a complication of falls. Assistive devices promote safety with ambulation. QSEN: Safety.
■ Teach the patient to create a safe environment at home: remove or tack down throw rugs, wear firm-soled shoes, install grab bars in the bathroom, do not carry heavy objects.	A safe home environment is necessary to prevent falls and potential fractures. QSEN: Safety.
■ If a patient is hospitalized, provide a safe environment: bed rails up, bed in the lowest position, necessary items (e.g., telephone, call light, walker, cane) within reach, adequate lighting, grab bars in the bathroom (if available).	These measures may decrease the risk for falls. QSEN: Safety.

NANDA-I
NDx **Disturbed Body Image**

Common Related Factors

Alteration in body function (due to kyphosis from vertebral fractures)
Alteration in self-perception (due to use of assistive devices)

Common Expected Outcome

Patient demonstrates enhanced body image and self-esteem, as evidenced by ability to look at, touch, talk about, and care for actual or perceived change in posture and height.

Defining Characteristics

Focusing behavior on changed body part/function
Preoccupation with change or loss
Alteration in body structure or body function
Refusal to acknowledge change

NOC Outcomes
Body Image; Self-Esteem
NIC Interventions
Body Image Enhancement; Self-Esteem Enhancement

Ongoing Assessment

Actions/Interventions	Rationales
■ Assess the patient's perception of the change in posture and height.	Bone loss causes a loss of height and the appearance of kyphosis. This increased anteroposterior curve of the thoracic vertebrae is the result of vertebral fractures. Kyphosis and lordosis (increase in the inward curvature of the lumbar spine) are deformities often found in osteoporosis. QSEN: Patient-centered care.

---

 volve **For additional care plans, go to http://evolve.elsevier.com/Gulanick/.**

Musculoskeletal Care Plans

Actions/Interventions

■ Assess the patient's perception of how physical changes associated with osteoporosis change the patient's ability to perform ADLs, interact with others, and continue to be involved in occupational and diversional activities.

Rationales

Patients may isolate themselves for fear of falling, difficulty in getting around, or self-consciousness about their changed appearance. The patient may find it challenging to wear clothing that fits properly. QSEN: Patient-centered care.

Therapeutic Interventions

Actions/Interventions

■ Acknowledge the patient's emotional response to actual or perceived changes in posture or height.

■ Encourage a positive attitude that some of the physical disabilities experienced will respond to adequate treatment and be abolished, reduced, or controlled.

■ Remind the patient to allow adequate time for self-care activities.

▲ Collaborate with members of the interprofessional team to help the patient learn self-care techniques.

■ Provide the patient with community resources that can be helpful in supporting special needs in the home.

■ Encourage participation in support groups.

Rationales

Once these changes have been acknowledged, ways can be found to reenter social life, interpersonal relationships, and occupational activities that enhance body image and self-esteem. QSEN: Patient-centered care.

The therapeutic regimen can be effective in reversing some of the early changes of osteoporosis. Realistic hope may enhance the patient's self-esteem.

The patient's self-image improves when he or she can perform personal care independently.

The occupational therapist can provide opportunities for the patient to learn new ways to perform self-care activities. Success with these adaptive skills increases the patient's sense of independence and contributes to enhanced body image and self-esteem. QSEN: Teamwork and collaboration.

Such resources can increase independence and foster enhanced self-image. Community agencies may offer best practices for managing osteoporosis in the home.

This allows for open, nonthreatening discussion of feelings with others with similar experiences. Groups can give a realistic picture of the condition and suggestions for problem-solving and coping.

■ = Independent   ▲ = Interprofessional Collaboration

Hematolymphatic, Immunological, and Oncological Care Plans

Anemia

Iron Deficiency; Cobalamin (Vitamin B$_{12}$) Deficiency; Pernicious Anemia; Aplastic Anemia

Anemia is a general diagnostic term referring to a decrease in number or derangement in function of erythrocytes (red blood cells [RBCs]), and is the most common hematological disorder. Classification of the type of anemia begins with the complete blood count, with subsequent stepwise testing providing the actual diagnosis that guides treatment and prognosis. Three anemia classification strategies exist: cytometric, which measures the RBC mass and hemoglobin concentration; erythrokinetic, which measures RBC destruction and production; and biochemical, which looks at DNA. Cytometric measurements are easily performed and begin with evaluation of the mean corpuscular hemoglobin concentration (MCHC) and mean corpuscular volume (MCV). MCHC may be normocytic or hypochromic. MCV may be normocytic, macrocytic, or microcytic. The pattern of combination of these indexes classifies the anemia, directing the next sequence of blood work to assist in determining the cause of the anemia and thus the diagnosis.

Normocytic/normochromic anemia (normal MCHC, normal MCV)	Anemia of chronic disease Sickle cell anemia Pregnancy Acute hemorrhage Hemolytic anemias Aplastic anemia
Microcytic/hypochromic anemia (low MCHC, low MCV)	Iron deficiency anemia Thalassemia major and minor Liver disease
Macrocytic/normochromic anemia (normal MCHC, high MCV)	Vitamin B$_{12}$ deficiency Folate deficiency

Iron deficiency anemia is a hypochromic, microcytic anemia usually occurring over time, resulting from dietary deficiencies, poor absorption, chronic blood loss as seen in younger women with heavy menses or older persons with gastrointestinal (GI) loss from an ulcer, use of nonsteroidal medications, or GI malignancy. Cobalamin, or vitamin B$_{12}$, deficiency and pernicious anemia are both caused by deficiency of vitamin B$_{12}$. Pernicious anemia impedes vitamin B$_{12}$ absorption by lack of intrinsic factor in the stomach. Poor diet intake (e.g., vegan diets or diets lacking dairy products), certain medications, alcoholism, and some bowel disorders can cause cobalamin deficiency, resulting in this macrocytic anemia. Nutritional anemia is a significant problem in older adults.

Aplastic anemia is a disease of diverse causes characterized by a decrease in precursor cells in the bone marrow and replacement of the marrow with fat. Aplastic anemia is characterized by pancytopenia, depression of all blood elements: white blood cells (leukopenia), RBCs (anemia), and platelets (thrombocytopenia). The underlying cause of aplastic anemia remains unknown. Possible pathophysiological mechanisms include certain infections, toxic dosages of chemicals and drugs, radiation damage, and impairment of cellular interactions necessary to sustain hematopoiesis. Treatment focuses on removing the causative factors, preventing complications, and providing supportive care until the condition resolves. For severe cases, advances in bone marrow transplantation and immunosuppressive therapy have significantly improved outcomes. This care plan focuses on ongoing care in the ambulatory care setting.

NANDA-I **NDx** **Deficient Knowledge**

Common Related Factors

Insufficient information
Insufficient interest in learning
Misinformation presented by others
Insufficient knowledge of resources

Defining Characteristics

Insufficient knowledge
Inaccurate follow-through of instruction
Inappropriate behavior

Common Expected Outcome

Patient verbalizes understanding of own type of anemia and its treatment plan.

NOC Outcomes
Knowledge: Disease Process; Knowledge: Treatment Procedure

NIC Interventions
Health Literacy Enhancement; Learning Facilitation; Teaching: Disease Process; Teaching: Procedure/Treatment

Ongoing Assessment

Actions/Interventions

- Assess the patient's and family's understanding of the new medical vocabulary.

- Assess current knowledge of the diagnosis, possible causative factors, disease process, and treatment.

Rationales

Most people have little exposure to hematological diseases and therefore have not heard or do not understand terms commonly used by health professionals.

Appropriate and individualized teaching can begin only after the patient's current knowledge and perceptions are determined. Patients may have a general understanding of anemia related to iron deficiency but lack knowledge of other types of anemia. QSEN: Patient-centered care.

Therapeutic Interventions

Actions/Interventions

- Explain the hematological vocabulary and the functions of blood elements, such as red blood cells (RBCs), white blood cells (WBCs), and platelets.
- Instruct the patient to avoid causative factors if known (e.g., certain chemicals).

- Explain the necessity for diagnostic procedures, including a possible referral to a hematology specialist and bone marrow aspiration.

Rationales

Patients commonly have only a basic understanding of the hematological system.

Numerous causes are possible, including dietary deficiencies, medication side effects, alcoholism, and a variety of toxic chemicals. The anemia may be acute or chronic, depending on the cause. QSEN: Safety.

A diagnosis of anemia is based on characteristic changes in RBC indexes and bone marrow. Often, stepwise testing is necessary to make the diagnosis. QSEN: Teamwork and collaboration.

Hematolymphatic, Immunological, and Oncological Care Plans

■ = Independent ▲ = Interprofessional Collaboration

Actions/Interventions

For nutritional deficiency anemias:

- Explain the use of diet therapy, medications, and supplements.

- Teach the patient and family about food sources of iron, folic acid, and vitamin B_{12}.

- Teach the patient and family about replacement therapy with iron and folic acid.

- Explain the need for vitamin B_{12} replacement.

For blood loss anemia:

- Instruct the patient regarding medications that may stimulate RBC production in the bone marrow.

- Explain that a transfusion of packed RBCs may be needed.

For aplastic anemia:

- Explain that allogeneic hematopoetic stem cell transplantation is the recommended treatment for patients younger than 55 years of age who have human leukocyte antigen (HLA)-identical related donors.
- Explain the need for rapid HLA typing.
- Explain that blood transfusions from prospective marrow donors should be avoided.
- Explain that immunosuppressive therapy is the treatment of choice in patients without HLA-matched donors and/ or older than 55 years of age.

Rationales

A balanced diet that includes a variety of foods from each food group usually contains adequate nutrients to support RBC formation. Dietary replacement may not be sufficient to correct nutritional deficiency anemia. Supplementation is often necessary to support the formation of normal RBCs. Parenteral injections or intranasal sprays are the primary therapy for vitamin B_{12} deficiency. QSEN: Patient-centered care.

Patients need to have an adequate intake of dark green, leafy vegetables; red meat; organ meat; eggs; raisins; fish; nuts; citrus foods; and whole grain, enriched, and fortified breads and cereals.

The dosage and frequency of administration will depend on the severity of the anemia. Folic acid is given orally. Iron supplements may be given orally, preferably 1 hour before meals when the duodenal mucosa is most acidic. Intramuscular injections of iron may be given using the Z-track method to prevent leakage of the solution into subcutaneous tissue along the needle track. For severe cases, a parenteral intravenous (IV) solution can be given.

The injections may need to be given monthly for the remainder of the patient's life. High doses of oral and sublingual vitamin B_{12} have been shown to be effective for those with intact GI absorption.

Medications such as colony-stimulating factors (e.g., filgrastim, sargramostim, and pedfilgrastim) and epoetin alfa may stimulate the bone marrow to produce new blood cells, increase hemoglobin, and reduce the need for blood transfusion.

Blood transfusion may be indicated to control bleeding and relieve anemic symptoms. Packed RBCs can be transfused to increase the amount of hemoglobin in the blood that can carry oxygen. One unit of packed RBCs typically will raise the hemoglobin concentration by 1 g/dL.

Aplastic anemia sometimes occurs because the immune system attacks its own cells in error. For severe cases, advances in bone marrow transplantation and immunosuppressive therapy have significantly improved outcomes. QSEN: Evidence-based practice.

Hematopoetic stem cell transplantation has a high success rate. In allogenic transplant, stem cells are removed from a donor with the same HLA genetic makeup as the patient.

This typing is performed to identify possible marrow donors.
Histocompatibility antigens could lead to the rejection of donor marrow.
Immunosuppressive therapy has become standard therapy for patients who do not have an HLA-identical donor. Autologous transplantation is not an option, because the patient's own marrow is defective. Immunosuppressive therapy includes antithymocyte globulin, cyclosporine, and corticosteroids.

Actions/Interventions

- Explain the potential complications associated with immunosuppressive therapy:

  • Rejection of donor marrow

  • Acute graft-versus-host disease (GVHD)

  • Chronic GVHD

Rationales

Providing information about complications allows the patient to be a full partner in making decisions and reducing the risk of harm from this type of therapy. QSEN: Safety.

Rejection results from sensitization to histocompatibility antigens acquired during previous blood transfusions and carries a high mortality rate. Conditioning regimens using cyclophosphamide (Cytoxan) and total lymphoid irradiation show a reduction in the risk for graft failure.

A red maculopapular rash within 3 months after transplantation signals acute GVHD and carries a high mortality rate.

This can be manifested by many symptoms. Mucosal degeneration leading to guaiac-positive diarrhea, vomiting, and malnutrition is one manifestation.

NANDA-I NDx **Fatigue**

Common Related Factor

Reduced oxygen-carrying capacity of blood from decreased number of red blood cells (RBCs)

Defining Characteristics

Nonrestorative sleep patterns
Insufficient energy/Tiredness
Inability to maintain usual level of physical activity and/or usual routines
Increase in rest requirements

Common Expected Outcomes

Patient verbalizes reduction in fatigue, as evidenced by reports of increased energy and ability to perform desired activities.
Patient verbalizes use of energy-conservation principles.

NOC Outcomes

Fatigue Level; Fatigue: Disruptive Effects; Energy Conservation; Activity Tolerance

NIC Intervention

Energy Management

Hematolymphatic, Immunological, and Oncological Care Plans

Ongoing Assessment

Actions/Interventions

- Assess the patient's ability to perform activities of daily living (ADLs), instrumental ADLs (IADLs), and the demands of daily living.

- Assess the specific cause of fatigue.

- ▲ Monitor hemoglobin, hematocrit, RBC counts, and reticulocyte counts.

Rationales

Fatigue can limit the patient's ability to participate in self-care and perform his or her role responsibilities in family and society, such as working outside the home. Specific information about the patient's ability to function can help the nurse to develop an individualized approach to care. QSEN: Patient-centered care.

Symptoms of nutritional types of anemia are frequently overlooked and mistaken for normal consequences of aging. Besides tissue hypoxia from normocytic anemia, the patient may have associated depression or related medical problems that can compromise activity tolerance.

Decreased RBC indexes are associated with decreased oxygen-carrying capacity of the blood. It is critical to compare serial laboratory values to evaluate progression or deterioration in the patient and to identify changes before they become potentially life-threatening. QSEN: Safety.

■ = Independent ▲ = Interprofessional Collaboration

Therapeutic Interventions

Actions/Interventions	Rationales
■ Teach energy-conservation techniques.	Patients and caregivers may need to learn skills for delegating tasks to others, setting priorities, and clustering care to use available energy to complete desired activities. Organization and time management can help the patient conserve energy and reduce fatigue.
■ Assist the patient in planning ADLs. Guide the patient in prioritizing activities for the day.	Setting priorities is one example of an energy-conservation technique that allows the patient to use available energy to accomplish important activities. Not all self-care and hygiene activities need to be completed in the morning. Likewise, not all housework needs to be completed in 1 day. QSEN: Patient-centered care.
■ Assist the patient in developing a schedule for daily activity and rest. Stress the importance of frequent rest periods.	Energy reserves may be depleted unless the patient respects the body's need for increased rest. A plan that balances periods of activity with periods of rest can help the patient complete desired activities without adding to levels of fatigue.
▲ Refer the patient and family to an occupational therapist.	The occupational therapist can teach the patient about using assistive devices. The therapist also can help the patient and family evaluate the need for additional energy-conservation measures in the home setting. QSEN: Teamwork and collaboration.
■ Instruct the patient about medications that may stimulate RBC production in the bone marrow.	Recombinant human erythropoietin (e.g., epoetin alfa and darbepoetin), a hematological growth factor, increases hemoglobin and decreases the need for RBC transfusions.
▲ Anticipate the need for the transfusion of packed RBCs.	Packed RBCs increase oxygen-carrying capacity of the blood.
▲ Institute supplemental oxygen therapy, as needed.	Oxygen saturation should be kept at 90% or greater.

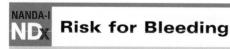

NANDA-I
NDx Risk for Bleeding

Common Risk Factors
Bone marrow malfunction
Marrow replacement with fat in aplastic anemia

Common Expected Outcome
Patient has reduced risk for bleeding, as evidenced by normal or adequate platelet levels and absence of bruises and petechiae.

NOC Outcome
Blood Coagulation
NIC Interventions
Bleeding Reduction; Bleeding Precautions

Ongoing Assessment

Actions/Interventions	Rationales
▲ Monitor the patient's platelet count.	Thrombocytopenia, or a low platelet count, is due to bone marrow malfunction caused by nutritional deficiencies, drugs, certain viral causes, or aplastic anemia. Some causes may result in temporary platelet abnormalities, whereas others are permanent. The risk for bleeding is increased as platelet counts are decreased. QSEN: Safety.

Actions/Interventions

- Assess the skin for evidence of petechiae or bruising.

- Assess for frank bleeding from the nose, gums, vagina, or urinary or gastrointestinal tract.
- Monitor stool (guaiac) and urine (Hemastix) for occult blood.

Rationales

Petechiae or bruising is usually seen when the platelet count falls below 20,000/mm^3. QSEN: Safety.

Early assessment facilitates prompt treatment. These sites are most common for spontaneous bleeding. QSEN: Safety.

These tests help identify the site of bleeding. QSEN: Safety.

Therapeutic Interventions

Actions/Interventions

- Consolidate laboratory blood sampling tests.

- Instruct the patient regarding bleeding precautions, also known as platelet precautions:
  - Avoid rectal procedures such as enemas, suppositories, and temperature readings.
  - Avoid douching, vaginal suppositories, and tampons.
  - During sexual intercourse the patient and his or her partner should avoid vigorous thrusting and use water-based lubricant to reduce friction and potential tissue tearing.
  - Instruct the patient to shave with an electric razor and to use a soft toothbrush.
- Instruct the patient in dietary modifications to reduce constipation.

▲ If platelet counts are very low, anticipate the need for platelet transfusions and premedication with antipyretics and antihistamines.

Rationales

Frequent blood sampling over time can contribute to anemia. Consolidation reduces the number of venipunctures and optimizes blood volume.

Precautions are necessary when the platelet count falls below 50,000/mm^3. Trauma should be avoided to reduce the risk for bleeding. At 20,000/mm^3 spontaneous bleeding can occur. Teaching content on bleeding precautions serves to reduce the risk of harm to the patient. QSEN: Safety.

Constipation results in the passage of hard stools that can irritate the rectal mucosa and stimulate bleeding. Modifications include increased water intake to soften stool and avoiding rough foods. Stool softeners may be needed.

Platelet replacement may be required to reduce the risk of bleeding. Premedication may reduce transfusion reaction effects.

NANDA-I
NDx Risk for Infection

Common Risk Factors

Bone marrow malfunction
Marrow replacement with fat in aplastic anemia

Common Expected Outcome

Patient has reduced risk for infection, as evidenced by normal white blood cell (WBC) count, absence of fever, and implementation of preventive measures.

NOC Outcome
Immune Status
NIC Intervention
Infection Protection

Hematolymphatic, Immunological, and Oncological Care Plans

Ongoing Assessment

Actions/Interventions

▲ Monitor for trends in WBC laboratory values.

Rationales

A low WBC count, or leukopenia, is a decrease in disease-fighting cells circulating in the body. A low WBC count in adults is generally fewer than 3500/mm^3. QSEN: Safety.

■ = Independent   ▲ = Interprofessional Collaboration

Actions/Interventions	Rationales
■ Assess for local or systemic signs of infection, such as fever, chills, malaise, swelling, and pain.	Opportunistic infections can easily develop, especially in immunosuppressed patients. Early assessment is key. QSEN: Safety.

Therapeutic Interventions

Actions/Interventions	Rationales
■ Stress the importance of thorough handwashing by the patient, caregiver, and visitors.	Meticulous handwashing is a priority in both the hospital and the outpatient or home setting to prevent the transmission of pathogens. QSEN: Safety.
■ Reinforce the need for daily hygiene, mouth care, and perineal care.	These measures prevent skin breakdown and reduce the risk for infection. QSEN: Safety.
■ Instruct the patient to avoid contact with people with colds or infections.	These people are sources of infection for the compromised patient. Children 12 years of age or younger put the patient at particular risk because they can be "carriers" of infection, especially upper respiratory infections. QSEN: Safety.
■ Instruct the patient to follow a low-microbial diet as indicated (well-cooked meat, poultry, and seafood; fresh fruits and vegetables that can be well washed and peeled; pasteurized milk and dairy products; well-cooked eggs and egg products).	These precautions reduce the microbial level in foods; microbes could colonize and infect the gastrointestinal tract. QSEN: Safety; Patient-centered care.
▲ Administer WBC growth factor to stimulate the production of neutrophils.	Granulocyte colony-stimulating factor (G-CSF), granulocyte-macrophage colony-stimulating factor (GM-CSF), filgrastim, and long-acting pegfilgrastim are effective as mobilizers of peripheral blood progenitor cells. QSEN: Evidence-based practice.
■ Instruct the patient to report the signs and symptoms of infection immediately.	Any fever is significant. Antibiotics may be indicated. QSEN: Safety.
▲ Anticipate the need for antibiotic, antifungal, and antiviral IV agents.	These agents counteract opportunistic infections.
■ If the patient is hospitalized, provide a private room for protective isolation.	Environmental changes may be necessary if the absolute neutrophil count is less than 500/mm^3. Protective isolation precautions may include placing the patient in a private room, limiting visitors, and having all people who come in contact with the patient use masks, gloves, and gowns. These patients are at a significant risk for infection. QSEN: Safety.

Related Care Plans

Hematopoietic stem cell transplantation, Chapter 10
Neutropenia, Chapter 10

Cancer Chemotherapy

Cancer chemotherapy is the administration of cytotoxic drugs by various routes for the purpose of destroying malignant cells. Chemotherapeutic drugs are commonly classified according to their antineoplastic action: alkylating agents, antitumor antibiotics, antimetabolites, vinca alkaloids, and hormonal agents. Another way of classifying cancer chemotherapeutic agents is based on where in the cancer cell's life cycle the drug has its effect. Cell cycle–specific drugs exert their cytotoxic effect at a specific point in the cell cycle. Drugs that affect the cancer cell at any point in its cycle are called cell cycle–nonspecific drugs. These drugs are dose dependent in their therapeutic effect. Typically a combination of chemotherapeutic agents is administered to destroy the greatest number of tumor cells at different stages of cell replication. Cancer chemotherapy may be administered in the hospital, in the ambulatory care setting, or even in the home setting. It is recommended by the Oncology Nursing Society that chemotherapy, biotherapy, and targeted therapies be administered by a qualified chemotherapy-competent nurse. Depending on the specific cancer, cell type, cellular mutations, and stage of disease, newer targeted therapies or biotherapies may be administered along with chemotherapy. The goal of systemic treatment is cure, control, or palliation. It is often used as an adjunct to surgery and radiation. Because chemotherapy drugs are highly toxic and are given systemically, they affect normal cells as well as cancer cells. Most of the side effects of cancer chemotherapy are the result of the drugs' effects on rapidly dividing normal cells in the hair follicles, the gastrointestinal tract, and the bone marrow. The Oncology Nursing Society has developed evidence-based resources for patients experiencing chemotherapy-related side effects.

NANDA-I
NDx **Deficient Knowledge**

Common Related Factors
Insufficient information
Insufficient interest in learning
Misinformation presented by others
Insufficient knowledge of resources

Defining Characteristics
Insufficient knowledge
Inaccurate follow-through of instruction
Inappropriate behavior

Common Expected Outcome
Patient or caregiver verbalizes understanding of chemotherapy treatment, including rationale for treatment, self-management of interventions to prevent or control side effects, and follow-up care.

NOC Outcome
Knowledge: Cancer Management
NIC Interventions
Health Literacy Enhancement; Learning Facilitation; Teaching: Procedure/Treatment; Chemotherapy Management

Hematolymphatic, Immunological, and Oncological Care Plans

Ongoing Assessment

Actions/Interventions	Rationales
■ Assess the patient's and family's prior experiences with chemotherapy.	An individual's beliefs and expectations regarding treatment may be influenced by past experiences and hearsay.
■ Assess the patient's understanding of the rationale for chemotherapy and the type and goal of treatment.	The patient and family need information based on their understanding of the treatment plan using chemotherapeutic agents. A successful treatment plan requires the cooperation of the patient and support of the patient's family members. QSEN: Patient-centered care.

Therapeutic Interventions

Actions/Interventions	Rationales
■ Instruct the patient and caregiver as needed:	Providing information allows the patient to be a full partner in making decisions regarding his/her role in implementing the treatment plan. QSEN: Patient-centered care; Evidence-based practice.

■ = Independent ▲ = Interprofessional Collaboration

Actions/Interventions

Treatment plan:

- Need and schedule for laboratory tests before and during treatment

- Chemotherapy agents to be used

- Method of administration

- Schedule of administration

- Setting for administration

Chemotherapy side effects:

- Potential short- and long-term side effects and toxicities

- Period of anticipated side effects and toxicities

- Preventive measures to minimize or alleviate potential side effects and toxicities

Discharge planning and teaching:

- Catheter care (central venous, arterial, intraperitoneal catheters and devices)
- Signs and symptoms to report to health care professionals (e.g., bleeding, fever/chills, acute pain, shortness of breath, intractable nausea and vomiting, inability to eat or drink, diarrhea)
- Measures to prevent infection:
  - Avoid exposure to anyone with an infection and anyone recently immunized with live vaccines.
  - Avoid sharing drinking and eating utensils.
  - Avoid crowds. Wear a mask as appropriate.
  - Wash hands meticulously.
  - Maintain meticulous oral hygiene.
  - Restrict exposure to plants and gardening soil.
  - Avoid contact with cat litter boxes, fish tanks, and human or animal excreta.
  - Institute a low-microbial diet as described later under Risk for Infection.

Rationales

Regular laboratory tests are done to assess for electrolyte and metabolic changes; cardiac, pulmonary, liver, and renal alterations; bone marrow function; the need for blood component transfusions; and the presence of infection.

Single agents are rarely used. Instead, combination therapies are used for their synergistic effects and to capitalize on their different mechanisms of action and side effect profiles. Many chemotherapy agents in combination with targeted therapies or monoclonal antibody regimens are approved and are in wide use.

Oral and IV routes are most common, although regional delivery directly to the tumor site may be selected, such as instillation into the bladder, abdominal cavity, or ventricles in the brain. Topical preparations and intra-arterial infusions may also be indicated, depending on the specific cancer type.

Each drug protocol has a preferred time for administration followed by a rest period. Therapy is usually given in cycles.

Although therapy may be initially started in the hospital setting, over 90% of systemic treatment is given in the outpatient setting.

Teaching content on early identification and management of chemotherapy side effects serves to reduce the risk of harm to the patient. QSEN: Safety.

A variety of serious and distressing side effects occur with aggressive chemotherapy. They may include nausea, vomiting, diarrhea, constipation, fatigue, mucositis, alopecia, and peripheral neuropathy.

Patients need to be informed of the side effect profile for their specific agents.

Patients need to be informed that most side effects can be managed to some degree.

Providing information regarding home care responsibilities allows the patient to be a full partner in providing care, making decisions, and achieving optimal recovery outcomes. QSEN: Patient-centered care; Safety.

Ongoing care is an important responsibility. Refer to the care plan for Central Venous Access Devices, Chapter 4.

Patients and family caregivers need to be able to recognize early indications of drug side effects. Early interventions to control side effects can minimize the impact on the patient's daily routines. QSEN: Safety.

The patient's immune function is usually impaired by chemotherapy-induced bone marrow suppression. Patient must understand strategies and measures by which they can protect themselves during times of compromised defense. QSEN: Safety.

Actions/Interventions

- Importance of a balanced diet and adequate fluid intake

- Medications after discharge
- ADLs

- Follow-up care

- Community resources and support systems

- Chemotherapy precautions at home

Rationales

The patient and family caregivers need to understand how adequate nutrition can promote improvement in the patient's quality of life, but patients should not be forced to eat.

Patients will be assuming responsibility for care.

Fatigue, neutropenia, and other side effects will determine the patient's rate of return to ADLs.

Periodic evaluation of the patient's response to therapy will need to be closely monitored.

Advocates are available for information, support, and even caregiving.

Drugs are excreted in the urine and bodily fluids for up to 48 hours.

NANDA-I NDx Nausea

Common Related Factors

Treatment related:
- Side effects of chemotherapy (inability to taste and smell foods, loss of appetite, nausea, vomiting, mucositis, dry mouth, diarrhea)
- Medications (e.g., opioids, antibiotics, vitamins)

Disease effects:
- Primary malignancy or metastasis

Psychogenic effects:
- Conditioning to adverse stimuli (e.g., anticipatory nausea and vomiting; tension, anxiety, stress)
- Depression

Defining Characteristics

Reports "nausea" or "sick to stomach"

Increase in salivation

Increase in swallowing

Gagging sensation

Sour taste

Aversion toward food

Common Expected Outcome

Patient reports diminished severity or elimination of nausea.

NOC Outcomes

Medication Response; Nutritional Status: Food and Fluid Intake; Comfort Status; Symptom Severity

NIC Interventions

Chemotherapy Management; Nutrition Therapy; Oral Health Maintenance; Medication Administration

Hematolymphatic, Immunological, and Oncological Care Plans

Ongoing Assessment

Actions/Interventions

■ Assess the patient's description of nausea and vomiting patterns before each cycle of chemotherapy.

Rationales

Patient responses are individualized, depending on the type and dosage of chemotherapy. Ongoing assessment is important so that treatment plans can be revised as needed. Nausea and vomiting may be acute, may be delayed, and for some patients may appear even before ("anticipatory") the chemotherapy treatment. QSEN: Patient-centered care.

■ = Independent   ▲ = Interprofessional Collaboration

Actions/Interventions

- Evaluate the effectiveness of the antiemetic and comfort measure regimens.

- Observe the patient for potential complications of prolonged nausea and vomiting.

- Weigh the patient at each clinic visit and always prior to each treatment with the same scale. If the patient is at home, stress the importance of maintaining a log.
- Encourage the patient to record any food intake using a daily log.

Rationales

Patient responses to antiemetic medications are highly variable and must be explored with each patient. Newer antiemetic medications have improved this condition for many patients.

Nausea and vomiting can alter a patient's hydration status because of fluid loss and effect electrolyte imbalance (hypokalemia; decreased sodium and chloride). Persistent vomiting and reduced nutritional intake can result in weight loss, decreased activity level, and lethargy. QSEN: Safety.

Consistent weighing ensures accuracy. Without monitoring, the patient may be unaware of actual weight loss resulting from imbalanced nutrition.

Determination of the type, amount, and pattern of food intake (if any) is facilitated by accurate documentation, which provides data as to whether oral intake meets daily nutritional requirements.

Therapeutic Interventions

Actions/Interventions

▲ Administer antiemetics according to protocol.

- Explain that the selection of antiemetic agents should be based on the emetic risk of the therapy and risk factors in the patient.

▲ Administer antiemetics around the clock rather than as needed during periods of high incidence of nausea and vomiting.
- Institute or teach measures to reduce or prevent nausea and vomiting:

- Small dietary intake before treatments

Rationales

Symptoms of chemotherapy-induced nausea and vomiting (CINV) can have an acute, delayed, anticipatory, or breakthrough onset. Often a combination of antiemetic medications is needed to effectively control nausea and vomiting and must correlate appropriately to the emetogenic potential of chemotherapy agents given. Serotonin 5-HT$_3$ receptor antagonists (i.e., ondansetron and palonosetron), neurokinin-1 receptor antagonists (i.e., aprepitant), and corticosteroids (i.e., dexamethasone) are the most common drug classes used for CINV. Other drug classes include phenothiazines (i.e., prochlorperazine), benzodiazepines (i.e., lorazepam), cannabinoids (i.e., dronabinal), and the dopamine 2 receptor antagonist, metoclopramide. QSEN: Evidence-based practice.

The Oncology Nursing Society provides resources for recommended antiemetic regimens for high, moderately high, low, and minimal emetogenic chemotherapy. Administration of optimal antiemetic therapy during every cycle of chemotherapy will reduce the risk for the development of anticipatory nausea and vomiting. QSEN: Evidence-based practice.

The effectiveness of antiemetic therapy is increased when adequate plasma levels are maintained.

Behavioral and dietary interventions seem to be most effective in the management of anticipatory nausea and vomiting, in which the patient develops nausea and vomiting in response to stimuli associated with the administration of chemotherapeutic drugs. Patients may try a variety of interventions to find those that best control this type of nausea and vomiting before drug administration. Antiemetic medications are less effective in the management of anticipatory nausea and vomiting. However, antianxiety medications such as lorazepam may be effective. QSEN: Evidence-based practice.

Having some food in the stomach before chemotherapy may reduce emesis. Eating small amounts reduces gastric overstimulation, thus reducing the vomiting risk.

Actions/Interventions

- Antiemetic half an hour before meals as prescribed

- Foods with a low potential to cause nausea and vomiting (e.g., dry toast, crackers, ginger ale, cola, popsicles, gelatin, baked or boiled potatoes, fresh and canned fruit, bland foods)
- Avoidance of spices, gravy, greasy fried foods, and foods with strong odors
- Meals at room temperature; serve foods cold if odors cause aversions
- Avoidance of coaxing, bribing, or threatening in relation to intake (help the family to avoid being "food pushers")
- Sucking on hard candy (e.g., peppermint) while receiving chemotherapeutic drugs with a "metallic taste"
- Drinking fluids at a different time than when eating solid snacks or meals
- Offering meat dishes in the morning

- Minimal physical activity and no sudden rapid movements during times of increased nausea
- Relaxation and distraction techniques, guided imagery

- Use of acupuncture or acupressure

- Cannabis

Rationales

Appropriate timing of medications can reduce the onset and severity of nausea.
These foods are easily digested and provide a measure of success to augment nutrition.

Fats are difficult to digest and may exacerbate nausea and can stimulate gastric motility.
The smell of cooking foods may aggravate feelings of nausea. Hot foods can stimulate peristalsis.
Such behaviors tend to only aggravate the situation.

Hard candies can reduce the metallic or bitter taste.

Separating fluids from solids will help in not "filling" the stomach quickly. This may help prevent nausea as well.
Aversions tend to increase during the day; chicken, cheese, and eggs are usually well-tolerated protein sources.
Activity or sudden movements may potentiate nausea and vomiting.
These techniques, especially guided imagery, are useful adjuncts to antiemetic drug therapy. They can be helpful if used before nausea occurs or increases.
Several small studies report acupuncture and acupressure to be useful measures in reducing nausea and vomiting risk.
Medical cannabis is somewhat effective in CINV and may be a reasonable option for patients who do not improve with standard treatment. The FDA has approved two cannabinoids (dronabinol and nabilone) for prevention and treatment of CINV.

Hematolymphatic, Immunological, and Oncological Care Plans

NANDA-I
NDx **Cancer-Related Fatigue**

Common Related Factors	Defining Characteristics
Tumor and metastatic disease Chemotherapy and/or targeted therapy Radiation Pain Distress (spiritual or emotional) Anxiety and/or fear Malnutrition Anemia	A sense of physical or emotional tiredness that is not proportional to recent activity or treatment and interferes with the individual's daily functioning Inability to restore energy, even after sleep Verbalization of an overwhelming lack of energy

■ = Independent   ▲ = Interprofessional Collaboration

Common Expected Outcomes

Patient reports reduction in fatigue, as evidenced by reports of increased energy and ability to perform desired activities.

Patient reports use of energy-conservation principles.

NOC Outcomes
Fatigue Level; Fatigue: Disruptive Effects; Activity Tolerance; Energy Conservation; Self-Care: Activities of Daily Living (ADLs)

NIC Interventions
Energy Management; Nutrition Management; Sleep Enhancement; Exercise Promotion

Ongoing Assessment

Actions/Interventions	Rationale
■ Assess for fatigue regularly using a scale of 0 to 10 and defining characteristics.	Fatigue has become the most common and distressing complaint for cancer patients, especially during treatment. Regular assessment allows the nurse to evaluate the fatigue and response to interventions and to develop and alter the plan accordingly. QSEN: Patient-centered care.
■ Refer to Fatigue (Chapter 2).	

Therapeutic Interventions

Actions/Interventions	Rationales
In addition to the interventions in the Fatigue care plan, consider the following:	Providing information allows the patient to be a full partner in making decisions and assuming responsibility for care at a later time. QSEN: Patient-centered care.
■ Educate the patient regarding these treatments:	
• Assigning priorities to activities to accommodate energy levels	Setting priorities while conserving energy will allow the patient to achieve most desired goals and feel a sense of accomplishment.
• Energy-conservation strategies, such as: • Sitting to do tasks • Pushing rather than pulling • Working at an even pace • Placing frequently used items within easy reach • Using wheeled carts for laundry, shopping, cleaning needs (see Fatigue, Chapter 2)	Energy conservation techniques reduce oxygen consumption, allowing for more prolonged activity.
• Limiting naps to 20 to 30 minutes	Limiting the amount of sleep during naps will help the individual to sleep at night.
• Use of psychostimulants (e.g., Ritalin) after ruling out other causes	These medications have been used cautiously and demonstrate improved symptoms of fatigue in some patients.
• Treatment for anemia as indicated	Cancer patients' anemia results from the disease itself and treatment. Correcting the anemia may improve the patient's energy level.
• Cognitive behavioral therapy	Fear and anxiety associated with the patient's response to cancer and its treatment requires the expenditure of energy. This type of psychotherapy facilitates psychological adjustment to the cancer experience by helping certain patients recognize and change maladaptive thoughts.
• Nutrition consultation	Protein caloric malnutrition can contribute to weakness and fatigue. A dietitian can counsel the patient and family on how to maximize the patient's intake during treatment for optimal nutritional needs. QSEN: Teamwork and collaboration.

NDx Risk for Infection

Common Risk Factors

Immunosuppression secondary to high-dose chemotherapy
Cancer, resulting in altered immunological responses

Common Expected Outcome

Patient is at reduced risk for local and systemic infection,
as evidenced by negative blood surveillance culture
findings, compliance with preventive measures, normal
chest radiograph, intact mucous membranes and skin,
and prompt reporting of early signs of infection.

NOC Outcomes

Infection Severity; Medication Response

NIC Interventions

Infection Protection; Chemotherapy
Management; Medication Administration;
Teaching: Individual

Ongoing Assessment

Actions/Interventions	Rationales
■ Inspect the body sites with a high potential for infection (mouth, throat, axilla, perineum, rectum).	Opportunist infections are often the first type of infection to develop in immunosuppressed patients. Early detection facilitates prompt treatment. QSEN: Safety.
■ Inspect the peripheral IV, central venous catheter and port sites for redness and tenderness.	These are frequent sites of infection. QSEN: Safety.
■ Monitor temperature as indicated. Observe closely for fever and chills.	A temperature greater than 37°C (98.6°F) may indicate a systemic infection. This may be the initial presentation of infection because, in the absence of granulocytes, the locus of infection may develop without characteristic inflammation or pus formation at the site. QSEN: Safety.
■ Auscultate the lung field for crackles, rhonchi, and breath sounds.	Pneumonia infections are common and can be fatal in this population. QSEN: Safety.
■ Observe for changes in the color, character, and frequency of urine and stool.	These observations provide data on a possible urinary tract infection or intestinal infection. QSEN: Safety.
▲ Obtain cultures for temperature elevation per institutional protocol.	Cultures provide data on which microorganisms are causing infection and antibiotic drug sensitivity. QSEN: Safety.

Therapeutic Interventions

Actions/Interventions	Rationales
■ Explain the effects of chemotherapy on the immune system.	This information provides a basis for ongoing education.

■ Instruct the patient to maintain personal hygiene, especially at home:
  • Bathe with chlorhexidine.
  • Wash hands well before eating and after using the bathroom.
  • Wipe the perineal area from front to back.
	Handwashing removes transient and resident bacteria from hands. The perineal area is a source of pathogens and a frequent entry port for microorganisms. QSEN: Safety.

■ Instruct the patient regarding a meticulous oral hygiene regimen.	Oral hygiene is important in the prevention of periodontal disease as a locus of infection. QSEN: Safety.

■ = Independent   ▲ = Interprofessional Collaboration

Actions/Interventions

▲ Instruct on the importance of a low-microbial diet. Refer the patient to a dietitian as needed.

■ Instruct to avoid herbal supplements (homeopathic remedies or herbal products, such as Chinese medicines).

▲ Instruct the patient to take prescribed anti-infective drugs for prophylaxis or treatment, as prescribed.

■ Instruct in measures to prevent infection:
- Avoid exposure to anyone with an infection and anyone recently immunized with live vaccines.
- Avoid sharing drinking and eating utensils.
- Avoid crowds. Wear a mask as appropriate.
- Wash hands meticulously.
- Maintain meticulous oral hygiene.
- Restrict exposure to plants and gardening soil.
- Avoid contact with cat litter boxes, fish tanks, and human or animal excreta.
- Refer to Neutropenia Care Plan for additional information.

Rationales

A low-microbial diet protects the patient from exposure to pathogens from foods at a time when host defenses are greatly compromised. Refer to Neutropenia in Chapter 10 for more detailed instruction. QSEN: Teamwork and collaboration; Safety.

There are no federal standards for these products in the United States. Moreover, they may be processed or stored in a risky way. The products themselves could interfere with some prescription medications.

Prophylactic anti-infective administration may be indicated to prevent viral, fungal, and bacterial infections through immune reconstitution.

The patient's immune function is usually impaired by chemotherapy-induced bone marrow suppression. Patients must understand strategies and measures by which they can protect themselves during times of compromised defense. QSEN: Evidence-based practice; Safety.

NANDA-I NDx Risk for Bleeding

Common Risk Factors

Bone marrow toxicity of chemotherapy
Disease of bone marrow
Invasion of bone marrow by malignant cells
Genetically transmitted platelet deficiency coagulopathies (tumor related or other)
Abnormal hepatic or renal function
Exposure to toxic substances (e.g., benzene, antibiotics)

Common Expected Outcome

Patient has reduced risk for bleeding, as evidenced by platelets, coagulation factors and fibrinogen within acceptable limits; compliance with preventive measures; and prompt reporting of early signs and symptoms.

NOC Outcome
Blood Coagulation
NIC Interventions
Bleeding Precautions; Chemotherapy Management; Blood Products Administration

Ongoing Assessment

Actions/Interventions	Rationales
▲ Monitor platelet counts. Anticipate the platelet count nadir.	The risk for bleeding increases as the platelet count drops: Nadir is when platelets are at their lowest point and can vary with type of chemotherapy regimen received. • Less than 20,000/mm³= severe risk • 20,000 to 50,000/mm³= moderate risk; may note prolonged bleeding at invasive sites • 50,000 to 100,000/mm³= mild risk; does not usually require treatment • Greater than 100,000/mm³= no significant risk QSEN: Safety.
▲ Monitor coagulation parameters (fibrinogen, thrombin time, bleeding time, fibrin degradation products) if indicated.	The blood-clotting cascade is an integrated system requiring intrinsic and extrinsic factors. Derangements in any factors can affect clotting ability. These laboratory tests provide important information on clotting ability and bleeding potential. QSEN: Safety.
■ Evaluate for any medications that can interfere with hemostasis (e.g., salicylates, anticoagulants, nonsteroidal anti-inflammatory drugs).	Drugs that interfere with clotting mechanisms or platelet activity increase the risk for bleeding. QSEN: Safety.
■ Assess the patient regularly for evidence of the following: • Spontaneous petechiae (all skin surfaces, including oral mucosa) • Prolonged bleeding or new areas of ecchymoses or hematoma from invasive procedures (venipuncture, injection, and bone marrow sites) • Oozing of blood from nose or gums • Rectal bleeding, vaginal bleeding, or increased menstruation • Neurological status	Changes in the coagulation profile may be marked by ecchymoses, hematomas, petechiae, blood in body excretions, bleeding from body orifices, and a change in neurological status (including headache, visual disturbances, or change in level of consciousness). QSEN: Safety.
▲ If any significant bleeding occurs, monitor vital signs closely until the bleeding is controlled.	Sinus tachycardia and increased arterial blood pressure (BP) are seen in the early stages to maintain an adequate cardiac output. BP drops as the condition deteriorates. QSEN: Safety.

Therapeutic Interventions

Actions/Interventions	Rationales
■ Instruct the patient or significant others of the effects of chemotherapy on bone marrow function and platelet count, and the relationship between platelets and bleeding.	Most individuals are not familiar with the complexities of the hematological system. A successful treatment plan requires the knowledge and cooperation of the patient and family members. QSEN: Patient-centered care.
■ Implement bleeding precautions for a platelet count of less than 20,000/mm³.	An understanding of precautionary measures reduces the risk for bleeding. At platelet counts less than 20,000/mm³ spontaneous bleeding can occur. QSEN: Safety.
■ Avoid nonessential invasive procedures, punctures, and injections.	This practice reduces bleeding at vascular access sites. QSEN: Safety.
■ Avoid rectal thermometers, suppositories, and enemas.	Their use increases the chance of rectal bleeding. QSEN: Safety.
▲ Communicate the anticipated need for platelet support to a transfusion center. Transfuse single or random donor platelets, as ordered.	It is important to have platelets available when needed (e.g., when platelet counts are less than 10,000/mm³ or in the presence of active bleeding). Platelet thresholds need to be individualized. Prophylactic platelet transfusions may be administered. QSEN: Safety.

Hematolymphatic, Immunological, and Oncological Care Plans

■ = Independent ▲ = Interprofessional Collaboration

Actions/Interventions

▲ Administer fresh frozen plasma or coagulation factors, as prescribed.

■ See additional bleeding precautions and nursing interventions, in Leukemia, Chapter 10.

Rationales

These therapies provide all the needed clotting factors, except platelets.

NANDA-I NDx   Risk for Injury

Common Risk Factors

Hypersensitivity to drugs
Potential side effects
Extravasation
Infiltration of drug from vein

Common Expected Outcome

Patient has reduced risk for injury from drug therapy, as evidenced by normal vital signs, absence of reaction, no pain at infusion site, adequate blood return from IV catheter, and prompt reporting of adverse signs and symptoms.

NOC Outcomes
Medication Response; Risk Control; Risk Detection

NIC Interventions
Allergy Management; Medication Administration; Emergency Care; Intravenous (IV) Therapy; Central Venous Access Device Management

---

Ongoing Assessment

Actions/Interventions

■ Note the patient's allergy history.

■ Monitor for potential hypersensitivity to chemotherapeutic drugs.

■ Monitor for side effects to the chemotherapeutic drugs.

■ Monitor for hypersensitivity to the drug.

Rationales

Drug hypersensitivity is an immune-mediated reaction to a drug. Symptoms range from mild to severe. This information guides the selection of prescribed medications. Patient safety is a priority. QSEN: Safety.

Patients, family, and staff need to be vigilant when the patient is starting any new agent. Common reactions can include wheezing, bronchospasm, hypertension, hypotension, tachycardia, increased or decreased BP, fever, rigors, rash, and hives. Most reactions occur during or shortly after the infusion. QSEN: Safety.

A variety of responses to chemotherapy are possible. Most of the side effects of cancer chemotherapy are the result of the drug's effects on rapidly dividing normal cells in the hair follicles, the gastrointestinal tract, and the bone marrow. Examples include alopecia, nausea/vomiting, mucositis, bone marrow suppression, peripheral neuropathy, and cognitive changes. The Oncology Nursing Society has developed evidence-based resources for patients experiencing chemotherapy-related side effects. QSEN: Safety.

Symptoms such as wheezing, high or low BP, fever, and hives can signal a reaction to the chemotherapeutic agent, requiring prompt treatment. QSEN: Safety.

Actions/Interventions

- Assess the IV insertion site at frequent intervals according to established hospital policy and procedure: blood return, patency of vein and catheter, signs of infiltration.

- Determine whether the chemotherapeutic agent has vesicant properties. Observe the injection or infusion site closely during chemotherapy administration. Instruct patient to report to nurse pain, redness, burning, or swelling at or above insertion site.
- ▲ Monitor relevant laboratory data.

Rationales

A defective or malpositioned indwelling central venous catheter or access device can cause extravasation into local subcutaneous tissue surrounding the administration site. QSEN: Safety.

Chemotherapy can cause tissue damage if it leaks outside the vein; however, not all agents have the same likelihood of causing tissue damage if infiltrated. Refer to the hospital policy and procedure manual for guidelines. QSEN: Safety.

A complete blood count, differential, metabolic panel, and electrocardiogram provide baseline and response data. QSEN: Safety.

Therapeutic Interventions

Actions/Interventions

- Ensure that two chemotherapy-competent registered nurses perform an independent double check of the written order for each agent for the specific drug name, dose, route, time, and frequency of the antiemetic or chemotherapy drugs to be administered, based on the patient's body surface area and treatment regimen.
- Know the immediate and delayed side effects of the drugs to be administered.

- Inform the patient or significant others to report adverse effects. Delineate which changes indicate emergencies that must be reported immediately.
- Maintain or restore adequate fluid balance.

- ▲ When an adverse drug reaction is suspected, stop the infusion; administer emergency drugs as prescribed; notify the physician; take and record vital signs; maintain a patent IV line with normal saline solution; reassure the patient.
- Select veins most suitable for administration of chemotherapeutic agents.

- Avoid veins in the antecubital fossa, near the wrist, or on the dorsal surface of the hand.
- Instruct the patient to report tenderness, stinging, burning, or other unusual sensations at the IV site immediately. Evaluate patient reports of "painful infusion."

- ▲ Keep an extravasation kit and chemotherapy spill kits available.

Rationales

Patient safety is a priority. Double-checking provides a measure of safety. QSEN: Safety; Evidence-based practice.

Each nurse has a responsibility to be familiar with potential side effects or complications associated with each agent being administered, whether a standard or experimental drug treatment. QSEN: Safety.

Changes that a patient perceives as minor may be highly significant.

Fluid therapy reduces potential drug toxicity in that fluids help clear the body of accumulated metabolic by-products. Older patients with reduced blood volumes and functional deterioration are especially at risk.

Prompt treatment reduces complications and provides reassurance to the patient. QSEN: Safety.

These are the cephalic, median brachial, and basilic veins in the mid-forearm area. Venous access devices may also be used. *Note:* Only nurses specially trained and with appropriate competencies can administer chemotherapy. QSEN: Safety.

Damage to underlying tendons and nerves may occur in the event of drug extravasation of a vesicant. QSEN: Safety.

The infiltration of chemicals (vesicants) causes tissue damage on direct contact, with pain as the most frequent complaint. Accurate assessment guides treatment. It is important to rule out the source of extravasation versus other causes of pain (which may include chemical composition of drug, venous spasm, phlebitis, and/or psychogenic factors). QSEN: Safety.

Contents vary according to hospital policy. Kits and procedures for treating extravasation must also be available in the home if chemotherapy is being administered in that setting. Chemotherapy spill kits should also be available in the home. QSEN: Safety.

Hematolymphatic, Immunological, and Oncological Care Plans

■ = Independent ▲ = Interprofessional Collaboration

Actions/Interventions

▲ When drug extravasation is suspected, stop the infusion, initiate the extravasation management appropriate for the chemotherapeutic drug being infiltrated, notify the physician, reassure the patient, and document the incident according to institutional policy and procedure.

Rationales

Management of the site after extravasation remains a controversial issue in chemotherapy administration. However, most hospitals and agencies have developed care standards in management of extravasation of drugs classified as "vesicants." These agents potentially cause cellular damage, ulceration, and tissue necrosis. A plastic surgeon may be consulted for debridement or skin grafting, depending on the extent of injury.

NANDA-I
NDx Disturbed Body Image

Common Related Factors

Loss of hair (scalp, eyebrows, eyelashes, pubic and body hair)
Discoloration of fingernails, veins
Breakage or loss of fingernails
Changes in skin color and texture
Generalized wasting
Presence of externalized or implanted venous access device
Concurrent surgical changes (mastectomy, colostomy)

Defining Characteristics

Negative feeling about body
Preoccupation with change
Avoids looking at one's body
Hiding of body part (compensatory use of makeup, concealing makeup, clothing, devices)
Change in social involvement

Common Expected Outcomes

Patient demonstrates enhanced body image as evidenced by ability to look at, touch, talk about, and care for altered body part.
Patient verbalizes understanding of temporary nature of side effects.
Patient engages in meaningful social interactions.

NOC Outcomes
Body Image; Self-Esteem
NIC Interventions
Body Image Enhancement; Hope Inspiration; Coping Enhancement

Ongoing Assessment

Actions/Interventions

■ Assess any perception of change in the structure or function of the body part.

■ Note the frequency of the patient's self-critical remarks.

■ Note the patient's behavior regarding the actual or perceived changed body part.

Rationales

The extent of the response is more related to the value or importance the patient places on the part than the actual value.
Negative statements about the affected body part indicate a limited ability to integrate the change into the patient's self-concept. QSEN: Patient-centered care.
A broad range of behaviors are associated with body image disturbance, ranging from totally ignoring the altered structure or function to preoccupation with it.

Therapeutic Interventions

Actions/Interventions

■ Acknowledge the normalcy of the emotional response to the actual or perceived changes in physical appearance.
■ Encourage the verbalization of feelings; listen to concerns.

Rationales

For some patients, the fear of treatment side effects can feel worse than the disease.
This may open lines of communication and help relieve anxiety. The expression of feelings can enhance the patient's coping strategies. QSEN: Patient-centered care.

Hematolymphatic, Immunological, and Oncological Care Plans

Actions/Interventions

- Convey feelings of acceptance and understanding.

- Provide anticipatory guidance on hair alternatives for alopecia (e.g., suggest the purchase of a wig or turbans before chemotherapy), on makeup and skin care for changes in skin color and texture, and on clothing to camouflage the venous access device.

- Offer realistic assurance of the temporary nature of some physical changes.

- Refer to a support group composed of individuals with similar alterations.

Rationales

The nurse is in an ideal position to promote acceptance of the situation.

Adaptive behaviors can compensate for the changed body structure and function. Patients need to understand that hair loss may occur over a short period of time. Some patients begin wearing wigs, scarves, or other types of head coverings before the hair loss occurs. This approach decreases the dramatic changes in their appearance. QSEN: Patient-centered care.

It is important that the patient understand that hair and nails will begin to regrow, usually within 1 to 2 months after chemotherapy is completed, and that external or implanted venous access devices will eventually be removed.

Groups that come together for mutual support and information can be a valuable resource. Although family and friends can be great allies, often a formal support group or communication with a cancer survivor is most helpful.

NANDA-I NDx Risk for Injury

Common Risk Factor
Improper handling or disposal of waste material in the home

Common Expected Outcome
Nurse, patient, or caregiver maintains safe handling and disposal of waste material according to institutional procedures and policies.

NOC Outcome
Safe Home Environment
NIC Interventions
Surveillance; Home Maintenance Assistance

Ongoing Assessment

Actions/Interventions

If chemotherapy is administered in the home:
- Determine that chemotherapy medications are clearly labeled and safely transported to the home.

- Determine that an adequate area is available for the safe preparation of the medication.
- Ensure that waste materials are disposed of in accordance with established policies (e.g., not flushing unused medication or fluids down the toilet; always placing contaminated needles, tubing, and syringes in biohazard containers).

Rationales

Safety is a priority. Special heavy duty plastic bags are used that are leak resistant when being transported. Bags should include a chemotherapy biohazard warning. QSEN: Safety.
This area should be at a bathroom or kitchen counter but away from food items that could become contaminated.
Waste materials are usually returned to the health care facility for appropriate disposal. QSEN: Safety.

Therapeutic Interventions

Actions/Interventions
- Instruct the family and caregiver to avoid contact with the patient's excreta (i.e., urine, stool, vomitus).

Rationales
The patient may need to use a private bathroom. Contaminated linen should be cared for according to established procedure. QSEN: Safety.

■ = Independent ▲ = Interprofessional Collaboration

Actions/Interventions

- Reassure the patient that kissing is safe, and that sexual intercourse is safe with condoms.
- If a spill occurs, institute safety precautions according to established procedures (e.g., use of gloves, gown, goggles, plastic disposal bags).

Rationales

Patients are frequently concerned that kissing and intercourse put their partners at risk.

These measures should be rehearsed in the home environment so the patient and caregivers are prepared to act. QSEN: Safety.

Related Care Plans

Anxiety, Chapter 2
Deficient fluid volume, Chapter 2
Diarrhea, Chapter 2
Fatigue, Chapter 2
Fear, Chapter 2
Imbalanced nutrition: Less than body requirements, Chapter 2
Risk for infection, Chapter 2
Neutropenia, Chapter 10
Hematopoietic stem cell collection, ⊖volve

Cancer Radiation Therapy

External Beam; Brachytherapy; Teletherapy; Radiotherapy

Radiation therapy is the use of ionizing radiation delivered in prescribed doses to a malignancy. Ionizing radiation interacts with the atoms and molecules of malignant cells, interfering with mitotic activity, thereby causing DNA damage. This damage interferes with the malignant cell's ability to reproduce. Adjacent healthy cells experience the same detrimental effects, however, resulting in untoward side effects from radiation therapy. Radiation therapy may be curative of some cancers, or it may be used as a palliative treatment to reduce the pain and pressure from large tumors. Radiation may be used alone or in combination with other treatment modalities such as surgery, chemotherapy, and/or biotherapy.

Radiation therapy can be divided into two broad categories: external radiation, also known as *teletherapy,* and internal radiation, commonly known as *brachytherapy.* Teletherapy administers a prescribed dosage of radiation at a distance from the patient using a machine, such as a linear accelerator. The patient does not become radioactive. Brachytherapy is the implantation of either sealed (solid) or unsealed (fluid) radioactive sources. The sealed radioactive implant may be contained within an applicator, needle, or seed, and is placed in or near the malignancy. The unsealed radioactive isotope can be administered through the intravenous or oral route or by instillation into a specific body cavity. With each of these methods the patient does emit radiation for a period of time.

The radiation oncologist prescribes the treatment modality and amount of treatment necessary. This treatment plan is based on the location, size, and biological characteristics of the malignancy. The patient's health history, current health status, and previous cancer treatments are taken into consideration in treatment planning. All health care providers need to implement principles of radiation safety when caring for patients undergoing radiation therapy.

NANDA-I NDx Deficient Knowledge

Common Related Factors	Defining Characteristics
Insufficient information	Insufficient knowledge
Insufficient interest in learning	Inaccurate follow-through of instruction
Misinformation presented by others	Inappropriate behavior
Insufficient knowledge of resources	

⊖volve　For additional care plans, go to http://evolve.elsevier.com/Gulanick/.

Common Expected Outcome

Patient verbalizes accurate knowledge about radiation therapy.

NOC Outcomes
Knowledge: Treatment Procedure; Anxiety Self-Control

NIC Interventions
Health Literacy Enhancement; Learning Facilitation; Teaching: Procedure/Treatment; Radiation Therapy Management; Anxiety Reduction

Ongoing Assessment

Actions/Interventions

- Assess the patient's knowledge of and previous experience with radiation therapy.

- Assess any fears, myths, or misconceptions that the patient has about radiation therapy.

Rationales

Appropriate and individualized teaching is based on the patient's current knowledge and perceptions. QSEN: Patient-centered care.

Patients and families may have anxiety and fear about the radioactivity of the patient during therapy. These misconceptions need to be clarified and corrected to promote the patient's cooperation with the treatment plan. QSEN: Patient-centered care.

Therapeutic Interventions

Actions/Interventions

- Explain the purpose of radiation therapy.

- Teach the patient and family what to expect during the treatment procedure:
  - Planning simulation
  - External beam treatment
  - Insertion of internal radiation

- Explain all site-specific care to the patient and family.

Rationales

The patient and family need to understand the role that radiation therapy has in the treatment of the patient's cancer. They need to understand whether the treatment goal is curative or palliative and how it may work with other treatment procedures. QSEN: Patient-centered care.

The process of preparation for therapy can be more anxiety producing than the actual procedure itself. Patients having external beam therapy will undergo an extensive and time-consuming planning process that includes a simulation of the treatment. During this simulation, the treatment area is located and marked on the skin. Adjacent tissue areas that will be shielded or blocked during therapy are identified. The procedure for implanting internal radiation will depend on the location of the malignancy.

For the patient undergoing external beam therapy, maintaining skin integrity and reporting side effects will facilitate prompt intervention and reduce complications. The generalized side effects associated with radiation therapy are fatigue and anorexia. QSEN: Safety.

Hematolymphatic, Immunological, and Oncological Care Plans

■ = Independent   ▲ = Interprofessional Collaboration

Actions/Interventions

■ Correct any misconceptions the patient and family have about radioactivity.

■ Provide information about the common side effects.

Rationales

The patient undergoing external beam therapy is never radio-active. The patient and family do not need to take any special safety precautions. The patient with a temporary implant emits radioactivity during the time the implant is in place. These patients are usually hospitalized, and specific precautions are taken to reduce radiation exposure to staff and visitors. The patient with a permanent sealed implant has a low level of radiation outside the body and the risk to others is minimal. The patient and family will be taught specific precautions to be taken at home depending on the location of the implant and the half-life of the isotope. QSEN: Patient-centered care; Safety.

Side effects depend on the treatment dose and the part of the body that is treated. Fatigue and skin reactions are commonly experienced during radiation to any site. Fatigue can be debilitating. Site-specific side effects may include dry mouth, difficulty swallowing, and bone changes. Anorexia is likewise commonly experienced.

NANDA-I NDx Risk for Impaired Skin Integrity

Common Risk Factor

External beam radiation

Common Expected Outcome

The patient's skin will remain intact and free of irritation or breakdown.

NOC Outcome
Tissue Integrity: Skin and Mucous Membranes

NIC Interventions
Skin Surveillance; Radiation Therapy Management; Skin Care: Topical Treatments

---

Ongoing Assessment

Actions/Interventions

■ Assess the patient's skin in the treatment area for the signs of radiation effects:

- Erythema and darkening

- Dry desquamation

- Wet desquamation

Rationales

Every effort is made in planning external beam treatment to implement skin-sparing approaches that minimize the effect on healthy skin.

Redness of the skin may develop within the first 24 hours after the first treatment. As the melanocytes in the skin are stimulated during treatment, the skin may appear darker.

When basal cells of the epidermis are affected by radiation, they begin to shed from the skin and allow new cells to develop.

If the rate of epidermal cell sloughing exceeds the rate of new cell replacement, the skin becomes moist and begins to break down.

Actions/Interventions

■ Assess the skin for the long-term effects of radiation therapy.

Rationales

Long-term changes in the skin are related to the total amount of radiation the patient received during therapy. The epidermis may be thinner, with less hair and fewer sweat glands in the treatment area. The skin will be less resistant to trauma and may take longer to heal. Fibrosis of the dermis and hyperplasia of the blood vessels may lead to the development of telangiectasia and spider veins.

Therapeutic Interventions

Actions/Interventions

■ Clean the skin in the treatment area with a mild, nonperfumed soap and tepid water. Use one's hand or a soft cloth, and avoid rubbing the skin. Dry thoroughly. Do not apply any skin care products within 4 hours before treatment.

■ Apply lubricating lotions or creams that do not contain metals, alcohol, fragrances, or additives that irritate the skin. This includes antiperspirants containing aluminum.

■ Instruct the patient to avoid scratching dry, itchy skin.

■ Teach the patient to avoid exposing the skin to pressure, sunlight, rough clothing, shaving, and extremes of temperature. Avoid tape or other products that may cause tearing or scratching of the skin.

▲ Consult with the radiation oncologist or wound care specialist for recommendations. Implement skin care protocols for wet desquamation. For example:
  • A standard treatment protocol may include irrigation of the area with a solution of one part hydrogen peroxide with three parts normal saline.
  • Dry the area thoroughly, and leave it open to air.
  • If drainage is present or if the area comes in contact with clothing, a nonadherent dressing may be applied. Use nontape methods to secure the dressing.

Rationales

Keeping the skin clean, dry, and free of irritants will promote skin integrity and reduce the risk for wet desquamation. Any markings used as treatment guidelines should not be removed from the skin until therapy is completed. QSEN: Safety.

Intervention protocols may vary among treatment centers. The radiation oncologist may recommend particular brands of moisturizers to relieve dry skin. QSEN: Teamwork and collaboration.

Scratching increases skin trauma in the treatment area. Cornstarch, sprinkled on the skin, may provide some relief from itching.

Pressure from tight or irritating clothing will increase skin irritation and the risk for skin breakdown in the treatment area. Soft, lightweight cotton clothing is best. The skin in the treatment area is more vulnerable to the effects of heat, cold, and ultraviolet light from sunlight or artificial sources such as tanning lamps. The use of protective clothing and sunscreens is recommended for the treatment area even after therapy is completed. QSEN: Safety.

Treatment of wet desquamation varies among treatment centers. QSEN: Teamwork and collaboration.

NANDA-I
NDx   Risk for Injury (Radiation Exposure)

Common Risk Factors

Internal radiation
Dislodged radiation implant
Lack of knowledge of radiation safety principles

■ = Independent   ▲ = Interprofessional Collaboration

Hematolymphatic, Immunological, and Oncological Care Plans

Common Expected Outcome

Health care providers and visitors will have minimal radiation exposure.

NOC Outcomes
Knowledge: Personal Safety; Risk Control; Risk Detection
NIC Interventions
Radiation Therapy Management; Environmental Management: Worker Safety

Ongoing Assessment

Action/Intervention	Rationale
■ Review the radiation treatment plan: • Type of radiation • Isotope half-life • Method of delivery • Duration of treatment	Implementation of radiation safety precautions will depend on the amount of energy emitted by the isotope, the half-life of the isotope, and the method used to deliver the radiation. With a sealed implant, the patient's excreta are not radioactive, but the actual implant is. If a systemic unsealed delivery method is used, the patient's secretions and excretions will be radioactive for a time based on the isotope's half-life. QSEN: Safety.

Therapeutic Interventions

Actions/Interventions	Rationales
■ Provide the patient with a private room and a private bathroom.	This type of room placement reduces the risk for radiation exposure to other patients.
▲ Consult with the hospital's radiation safety officer about appropriate radiation safety protocols.	The radiation safety officer will provide appropriate safety guidelines based on the type of internal radiation to be used. QSEN: Teamwork and collaboration; Evidence-based practice; Safety.
■ Post signs outside the patient's room. Many hospitals have specialized rooms or units designated for this purpose.	Health care providers and visitors at risk for the effects of radiation need to be warned before entering the patient's room. Signs should indicate the precautions to be used when entering the patient's room. Women who are pregnant should avoid all direct contact with the patient until radiation treatment is completed. QSEN: Safety.
■ Provide film badges to staff members who are responsible for the direct care of the patient.	Film badges record the amount of exposure to a radiation source. The badge should be worn outside the clothing during all direct contact activities with the patient. The radiation safety officer will periodically review all film badges and quantify the staff member's amount of radiation exposure. QSEN: Safety.
■ For patients with encapsulated forms of internal radiation, keep appropriate lead-lined containers in the patient's room.	When an implanted radiation source becomes dislodged, most institutions require nurses not to touch the source but to call a radiation safety officer to handle the source. The nurse should never pick up a radiation source with bare hands. QSEN: Safety.

Actions/Interventions

- Implement all direct patient care activities using principles of time and distance.
  - Organize care activities to minimize the amount of time at the patient's bedside.
  - Provide only essential care to promote patient comfort.
  - Prepare meal trays outside the room.
  - Keep bedside tables, call lights, and personal care items within easy reach of the patient at all times to reduce return trips to the bedside.

Rationales

Radiation exposure is based on the law of inverse squares. The amount of radiation exposure is inversely related to the square of the distance from the radiation source. A nurse standing 2 feet from the patient has one quarter the exposure of someone standing next to the patient ($2^2 = 4$; the inverse of 4 is $\frac{1}{4}$).

Related Care Plan

Fatigue, Chapter 2

Disseminated Intravascular Coagulation

Coagulopathy; Defibrination Syndrome; DIC

Disseminated intravascular coagulation (DIC) is a coagulation disorder that prompts overstimulation of the normal clotting cascade and results in simultaneous thrombosis and hemorrhage. The formation of microclots affects tissue perfusion in the major organs, causing hypoxia, ischemia, and tissue damage. Coagulation occurs in two different pathways: intrinsic and extrinsic. These pathways are responsible for formation of fibrin clots and blood clotting, which maintains hemostasis. In the intrinsic pathway, endothelial cell damage commonly occurs because of sepsis or infection. The extrinsic pathway is initiated by tissue injury such as from malignancy, trauma, or obstetrical complications. DIC may present as an acute or chronic condition. The medical management of DIC is primarily aimed at: (1) treating the underlying cause, (2) managing complications from both primary and secondary causes, (3) supporting organ function, and (4) stopping abnormal coagulation and controlling bleeding. Morbidity and mortality risks depend on underlying cause and severity of the coagulopathy.

Hematolymphatic, Immunological, and Oncological Care Plans

NANDA-I NDx Risk for Bleeding

Common Risk Factors

Abnormal blood profiles (depleted coagulation factors)
Drug therapy (adverse effects of heparin)

Common Expected Outcomes

Patient experiences reduced episodes of bleeding and hematomas.
Patient maintains therapeutic levels of coagulation laboratory profiles (prothrombin time [PT], partial prothrombin time [PPT], fibrinogen, fibrin split products, bleeding time).
Patient's side effects of medication therapy are reduced through ongoing assessment and early intervention.

NOC Outcomes
Blood Coagulation; Circulation Status
NIC Interventions
Bleeding Precautions; Bleeding Reduction; Blood Products Administration; Medication Administration

■ = Independent   ▲ = Interprofessional Collaboration

Ongoing Assessment

Actions/Interventions

- Assess for the underlying cause of DIC.

▲ Monitor serial coagulation profiles.

▲ Monitor hematocrit (Hct) and hemoglobin (Hgb) levels.

- Examine the skin surface for signs of bleeding. Note petechiae; purpura; hematomas; oozing of blood from IV sites, drains, and wounds; and bleeding from the mucous membranes.
- Observe for signs of external bleeding from the gastrointestinal (GI) and genitourinary (GU) tracts.

- Note any hemoptysis or blood obtained during suctioning.
- Observe for signs of internal bleeding, such as pain or changes in the level of consciousness. Institute a neurological checklist.
- Monitor the patient's heart rate (HR) and BP. Observe for signs of orthostatic hypotension.

- If heparin therapy is initiated, observe for:
  - Any increase in bleeding from IV sites, GI/GU tracts, respiratory tract, or wounds
  - New purpura, petechiae, or hematomas

Rationales

DIC is not a primary disease but occurs in response to a precipitating factor such as an infection or tumor. Successful treatment of DIC includes management of the underlying disorder. QSEN: Patient-centered care.

Initially, accelerated clotting is noted. As the clotting then stimulates the fibrinolytic system, clotting factors become depleted and large quantities of proteins are produced as part of the fibrin degradation process. Common laboratory values in DIC are PT greater than 15 seconds, PTT greater than 60 to 90 seconds, hypofibrinogenemia, thrombocytopenia, elevated fibrin split products (FSPs), elevated D-dimers (a type of FSP), and prolonged bleeding time. All put the patient at risk for increased bleeding. Specific deficiencies guide treatment therapy. QSEN: Safety.

Decreased Hgb and Hct levels are associated with bleeding from DIC. Early assessment guides treatment. QSEN: Safety.

Prolonged oozing of blood from injection sites or venipuncture sites could be the first indication of DIC. QSEN: Safety.

One of the diagnostic hallmarks of acute DIC can be manifested as bleeding simultaneously from at least three unrelated sites associated with shock, respiratory failure, or renal failure. For example, the patient may have increased skin bruising, hemoptysis, and hematuria. QSEN: Safety.

These are common manifestations of acute DIC. QSEN: Safety.

Changes in the level of consciousness may occur with the decreased fluid volume or with decreasing Hgb. QSEN: Safety.

Tachycardia and hypotension are signs of decreased cardiac output. Orthostasis (a drop of more than 15 mm Hg when changing from a supine to a sitting position) indicates reduced circulating fluids. QSEN: Safety.

Heparin is used for milder cases when clotting is more of a problem than bleeding. It aborts the clotting process by blocking thrombin production. QSEN: Safety.

Therapeutic Interventions

Actions/Interventions	Rationales

■ Institute precautionary measures:
  • Avoid unnecessary venipunctures; draw all laboratory specimens through an existing line.
  • Use only compressible vessels for IV sites.
  • Apply pressure to any oozing site.
  • Avoid intramuscular injections.
  • Prevent trauma to the catheters and tubes by proper taping; minimize pulling.
  • Minimize the number of cuff BPs.
  • Use gentle suctioning.
  • Use gentle chest physiotherapy.
  • Provide gentle oral care, using saline and water rinses instead of toothbrushes.
  • Use an electric razor for shaving.
  • If the patient is confused or agitated, pad the side rails.
	Nursing interventions should be planned and implemented to eliminate potential sources of bleeding and to control the amount of potential bleeding and tissue injury. QSEN: Safety.

▲ Administer blood products as prescribed: red blood cells (RBCs), fresh frozen plasma (FFP), cryoprecipitate, and platelets.	Blood products are cautiously given based on specific component deficiencies for patients with significant hemorrhage. Blood and plasma transfusions replace blood-clotting factors. RBCs increase oxygen-carrying capacity; FFP replaces clotting factors and inhibitors; platelets and cryoprecipitate provide proteins for coagulation.
▲ Administer heparin therapy as prescribed. The dose may be titrated based on laboratory values and the clinical situation. If bleeding is increased, notify the physician of the possible need to decrease the IV drip.	Heparin is used for milder cases when clotting is more of a problem than bleeding. Heparin augments antithrombin III activity that interrupts the clotting cycle and conversion of fibrinogen to fibrin. It also blocks the intrinsic and extrinsic pathways by inhibiting factor X, which slows clot formation. As the clinical situation improves, the need for heparin decreases. The challenge lies in differentiating the blood loss as an untoward effect of heparin therapy from a worsening of DIC.
▲ Administer parenteral fluids as prescribed. Anticipate the need for an IV fluid challenge with the immediate infusion of fluids for patients with hypotension.	Maintenance of an adequate blood volume is vital for maintaining cardiac output and systemic perfusion.
▲ Administer additional medications or investigational drugs as ordered:	A hematologist can guide medical treatment. These medications are based on recommendations from national organizations. QSEN: Teamwork and collaboration; Evidence-based practice; Safety.
• Antithrombin III concentration	This is a cofactor of heparin used for more severe cases. The anti-inflammatory properties may be of benefit when sepsis is the causative factor.
• Recombinant human activated protein C	This inhibits factors Va and VIIIa of the coagulation cascade.
• Epsilon aminocaproic acid (Amicar)	This antifibrinolytic agent is reserved for when other measures have failed. Its use can lead to organ failure from large vessel thrombosis, and thus its use is controversial.

Hematolymphatic, Immunological, and Oncological Care Plans

■ = Independent   ▲ = Interprofessional Collaboration

NANDA-I NDx Impaired Gas Exchange

Common Related Factor

Altered oxygen-carrying capacity of blood

Defining Characteristics

Confusion
Somnolence
Restlessness
Irritability
Hypercapnia
Hypoxia/hypoxemia
Abnormal breathing (rate, rhythm, depth)
Dyspnea
Abnormal arterial blood gases (ABGs)

Common Expected Outcome

Patient maintains optimal gas exchange, as evidenced by ABGs within patient's usual range; oxygen saturation of 90% or greater; alert, responsive mentation or no further reduction in level of consciousness; and relaxed breathing and baseline HR for patient.

NOC Outcome
Respiratory Status: Gas Exchange
NIC Interventions
Respiratory Monitoring; Oxygen Therapy; Ventilation Assistance

---

Ongoing Assessment

Actions/Interventions	Rationales
■ Assess the respiratory rate, rhythm, and depth.	The patient will adapt breathing patterns over time to facilitate gas exchange. Rapid, shallow respirations may result from hypoxia or from the acidosis with the shock state. The development of hypoventilation indicates that immediate ventilator support is needed. QSEN: Safety.
■ Assess for tachycardia, shortness of breath, and use of accessory muscles.	With initial hypoxia, HR increases. The use of accessory muscles increases chest excursion to facilitate effective breathing. These signs signify an increased work of breathing. QSEN: Safety.
■ Assess the patient's breath sounds. Assess cough for signs of bloody sputum.	Changes in breath sounds may reveal the cause of impaired gas exchange. Hemoptysis is an indication of bleeding in the respiratory tract. QSEN: Safety.
■ Assess for changes in the level of consciousness.	Early signs of cerebral hypoxia are restlessness and irritability; later signs are confusion and somnolence. QSEN: Safety.
▲ Use pulse oximetry to monitor oxygen saturation; assess ABGs.	Pulse oximetry is a useful tool to detect early changes in oxygen saturation. Oxygen saturation should be kept at 90% or greater. Increasing $Paco_2$ and decreasing Pao_2 are signs of hypoxemia and respiratory acidosis. QSEN: Safety.

Therapeutic Interventions

Actions/Interventions	Rationales
■ Position the patient in a high-Fowler's position (if hemodynamically stable).	An upright position allows for adequate diaphramatic and lung excursion and promotes optimal lung expansion.
■ Change the patient's position every 2 hours, and perform chest physiotherapy.	These maneuvers facilitate the movement and drainage of secretions.

---

 evolve For additional care plans, go to http://evolve.elsevier.com/Gulanick/.

Actions/Interventions

- Assist with coughing or suction as needed.

- Provide reassurance and allay anxiety by staying with the patient during acute episodes of respiratory distress.

- ▲ Maintain an oxygen administration device as ordered.

- ▲ Anticipate the need for intubation and mechanical ventilation.

Rationales

Productive coughing is the most effective way to remove most secretions. If the patient is unable to perform independently, suctioning may be needed to promote airway patency and reduce the work of breathing.

Anxiety increases dyspnea, the work of breathing, and the respiratory rate. The patient's feeling of stability increases in a calm environment. QSEN: Patient-centered care.

The appropriate amount of oxygen must be delivered continuously so that the patient maintains an oxygen saturation of 90% or greater.

Early intubation and mechanical ventilation are recommended to prevent full decompensation of the patient. Mechanical ventilation provides supportive care to maintain adequate oxygenation and ventilation to the patient. QSEN: Safety.

NANDA-I
NDx ## Deficient Knowledge

Common Related Factors

Insufficient information
Insufficient interest in learning
Misinformation presented by others
Insufficient knowledge of resources

Defining Characteristics

Insufficient knowledge
Inaccurate follow-through of instruction
Inappropriate behavior

Common Expected Outcome

Patient and/or significant others verbalize basic understanding of disseminated intravascular coagulation (DIC) and its management.

NOC Outcomes

Knowledge: Disease Process; Knowledge: Treatment Procedure

NIC Interventions

Health Literacy Enhancement; Learning Facilitation; Teaching: Disease Process; Bleeding Precautions

Hematolymphatic, Immunological, and Oncological Care Plans

Ongoing Assessment

Action/Intervention

- Assess the patient's knowledge of DIC.

Rationale

DIC usually occurs acutely, so the patient and family have no prior knowledge of it. Assessment provides a baseline for teaching. QSEN: Patient-centered care.

Therapeutic Interventions

Actions/Interventions

- Carefully explain the underlying cause that precipitated DIC.
- Instruct the patient or significant others to notify the nurse of new bleeding from wounds or IV sites.

Rationales

Patients are better able to ask questions when they have basic information about what to expect.

This notification can aid in achieving early intervention at bleeding sites. However, any new episodes of bleeding may have a traumatic impact on the patient and family. QSEN: Safety.

■ = Independent ▲ = Interprofessional Collaboration

Actions/Interventions

- Explain the purpose of drug and transfusion therapy.

Rationales

The challenging nature of treatment may be difficult for the patient or significant others to understand in the acute setting. In addition, the frequent use of blood components may cause fear regarding the transmission of infectious diseases such as hepatitis or human immunodeficiency virus (HIV).

Related Care Plans

Acute pain, Chapter 2
Anxiety, Chapter 2
Deficient fluid volume, Chapter 2
Ineffective peripheral tissue perfusion, Chapter 2
Mechanical ventilation, Chapter 6
Acute respiratory distress syndrome (ARDS),
   Chapter 6

Hematopoietic Stem Cell Transplantation

Bone Marrow Transplant; Peripheral Blood Stem Cell Transplant

Hematopoietic stem cell transplantation (HSCT) is used as both a curative and investigational treatment for both malignant and nonmalignant conditions (e.g., leukemia, lymphomas, multiple myeloma, sickle cell disease, and aplastic anemia). HSCT should not be confused with the controversial field of embryonic stem cells. Embryonic stem cells, derived from fertilized embryos, are undifferentiated cells that have the ability to form any adult cell. Hematopoietic stem cells are the "mother" cells that differentiate only into the cells of the blood system (e.g., white blood cells [WBCs], red blood cells [RBCs], platelets).

HSCT is used to replace diseased bone marrow as a hematopoietic rescue after high-dose therapy (radiation or chemotherapy), as a form of immunotherapy, and as a vehicle for gene therapy. HSCT is an intensive procedure that can be lifesaving, but it also has many serious complications (pancytopenia, graft versus host disease) that can result in death. Patients need to talk extensively with the health care team to weigh the chances for remission or cure against the risk of treatment failure or death.

There are three sources of hematopoietic stem cells:

- *Peripheral stem cell apheresis:* The stem cells that normally reside in the bone marrow can be moved or mobilized into the bloodstream (peripheral circulation) and collected in an outpatient procedure via a cell separator or apheresis machine. This procedure does not require anesthesia. The majority of all transplants performed today use peripheral blood stem cells rather than bone marrow stem cells. Drugs such as plerixafor (Mozobil), hematopoietic growth factors

(e.g., granulocyte-macrophage colony-stimulating factor [GM-CSF]), and chemotherapy are given days ahead of time to "mobilize" or boost the number of peripheral stem cells prior to harvesting.
- *Bone marrow harvest:* These cells are collected from the pelvic bones through a series of aspirations. Bone marrow harvesting is a surgical procedure done under general anesthesia.
- *Umbilical cord, blood stem cell banking:* This is a rich source of stem cells that are collected at the time of delivery from tissue that is normally discarded.

There are three major types of transplants:

- *Allogeneic:* The donor can be related (from a matched sibling) or unrelated (from a volunteer in the Be The Match Registry). This type is also referred to as a HLA (human leukocyte antigen) matched stem cell transplant or a matched unrelated donor (MUD) transplant.
- *Syngeneic:* Donor is an HLA-identical twin.
- *Autologous:* Transplant is taken directly from the patient.

There is one other classification of transplant based on the amount and type of pretransplant therapy that is administered. Standard transplants use strong treatment (chemotherapy and/or radiation therapy) administered before transplantation to destroy the host's diseased cells and suppress the host's immune system. This therapy is referred to as *ablative therapy,* because it eliminates all host blood and immune cells. Reduced-intensity transplants—also called *nonmyeloablative transplants* or *minitransplants*—are transplants that use less intense

Hematolymphatic, Immunological, and Oncological Care Plans

treatment to prepare for transplantation than a standard transplant does. Thus the doses of chemotherapy given before transplantation are much lower and do not necessarily eliminate all diseased cells. This type of transplant is only used in the allogeneic setting, because this method relies on the donor's immune cells to fight disease. This care plan focuses on inpatient care. Emotional issues related to HSCT are not addressed here.

NANDA-I NDx

Deficient Knowledge

Common Related Factors

Insufficient information
Insufficient interest in learning
Misinformation presented by others
Insufficient knowledge of resources

Defining Characteristics

Insufficient knowledge
Inaccurate follow-through of instruction
Inappropriate behavior

Common Expected Outcome

Patient or significant others verbalize understanding of procedures, treatments, possible complications, and follow-up care pertaining to HSC transplantation.

NOC Outcomes

Knowledge: Disease Process; Knowledge: Treatment Procedure

NIC Interventions

Health Literacy Enhancement; Learning Facilitation; Teaching: Disease Process; Teaching: Preoperative; Teaching: Prescribed Medication; Teaching: Procedure/Treatment

Ongoing Assessment

Action/Intervention

■ Assess the patient's and significant others' understanding of procedures, treatment protocol, potential side effects and complications, schedule of overall treatment plan, and follow-up care after discharge.

Rationale

The patient and family need information based on their understanding of the treatment care plan. A successful treatment plan requires the cooperation of the patient and support of the patient's family. QSEN: Patient-centered care.

Therapeutic Interventions

Actions/Interventions

■ Share with the patient a written calendar or schedule of the overall treatment plan.

■ Instruct the patient (and significant others as needed) about the central venous access device if not already in place.

Rationales

This schedule helps the patient process the timeline for treatment. The transplantation process includes several phases (i.e., mobilization, collection of hematopoietic stem cells [HSCs], conditioning, regimen, transplantation, engraftment, and post-transplant recovery) depending on the type of transplant.

Accurate information provides the rationale for treatment. The device is used for the administration of chemotherapy, collection of peripheral blood stem cells, stem cell infusion, antibiotic treatment, blood draws, blood component replacement, and parenteral nutrition as appropriate. These catheters may remain in place for several months or longer.

Hematolymphatic, Immunological, and Oncological Care Plans

■ = Independent ▲ = Interprofessional Collaboration

Actions/Interventions	Rationales
■ Explain bone marrow or peripheral stem cell harvesting, storage, and its potential complications.	If bone marrow is used, the patient will require preoperative and postoperative teaching. In the operating room, multiple aspirations are taken from the iliac crest to obtain the stem cells. If peripheral blood stem cells are used, the patient will require mobilization therapy with chemotherapy or hematopoietic growth factors, and/or plerixafor (Mozobil), an immunostimulant to increase the number of available stem cells. Next, the collection of peripheral blood stem cells via apheresis is performed (see Hematopoietic Stem Cell Collection care plan on the ⊜volve website).
■ Discuss the preparative or conditioning regimen, potential short- and long-term side effects, and preventive measures to minimize or alleviate toxicities (e.g., antiemetic, oral regimens, pain control).	The conditioning regimen using chemotherapy and/or total body irradiation is used to both deplete the patient's bone marrow to prevent rejection of the transplanted cells and to eradicate the cancer cells. The conditioning regimen is individualized based on the patient's specific cancer, the type of transplant, and any chemotherapy or radiation in the past. The conditioning regimen can be ablative (high-dose) or nonmyeloablative (reduced-intensity). Potential side effects will vary (e.g., nausea and vomiting and loss of appetite are generally less with the nonmyeloablative conditioning protocols).
■ Discuss the hematopoietic stem cell transplantation (HSCT) procedure for peripheral stem cell infusion and its potential complications.	The procedure and potential complications for stem cell infusion depend on whether the stem cell product is fresh or frozen. Allogeneic transplants generally mean that the stem cell product is collected from the donor and infused to the recipient on the same day (i.e., "fresh"). In this case, the stem cell infusion is similar to a blood transfusion. Autologous transplants use frozen stem cells, in that stem cells from the donor (i.e., the patient) have been collected and stored ahead of time. Infusion of frozen or cryopreserved stem cells is more involved, with more potential complications related to the infusion of the cryopreservative (dimethyl sulfoxide [DMSO]), which can cause side effects in the recipient.
■ Discuss the time frame for marrow engraftment.	After infusion, stem cells travel to the bone marrow and stimulate the production of new blood cells (RBCs, WBCs, and platelets). This process is referred to as *engraftment*. The time after transplantation until engraftment depends on many factors but usually takes between 2 and 6 weeks.
■ Discuss the administration of neutrophil growth factors (i.e., granulocyte colony-stimulating factor [G-CSF]).	Growth factors are sometimes administered after stem cell infusion to accelerate engraftment.
■ Discuss the need to maintain a protective environment (e.g., private room, negative pressure airflow room). Provide information about isolation techniques and procedures.	Environmental changes protect the patient from contagions during the myelosuppression period. QSEN: Safety.
■ Discuss anti-infective drugs for prophylaxis or treatment, as prescribed.	Medications may be given before and after transplant for prophylactic, empiric, or actual treatment. Prophylactic anti-infective administration is given to prevent viral, fungal, and bacterial infections through immune reconstitution. QSEN: Evidence-based practice; Safety.

Hematolymphatic, Immunological, and Oncological Care Plans

Actions/Interventions

■ Instruct on the importance of a low-microbial diet. Refer the patient to a dietitian as needed.

■ Instruct to avoid herbal supplements (homeopathic remedies or herbal products, such as Chinese medicines).

■ Explain the need for frequent blood sampling.

■ Explain the need for the frequent inspection and culturing of all orifices and potential infection sites.

■ Discuss discharge planning and teaching:

• Timing of discharge

• Importance of follow-up visits for blood studies and monitoring for potential complications
• ADLs

• Medications after discharge

• Importance of balanced diet and adequate fluid intake
• Central venous catheter care (e.g., Hickman, Permcath)
• Measures to prevent infection (e.g., avoiding children with infections or who have recently been immunized, avoiding crowds)

• Recognition and reporting of signs and symptoms of bleeding, low RBC count, and infection
• Sexual relations and contraception

• Return to work or school

Rationales

This diet protects the patient from exposure to pathogens from foods at a time when host defenses are greatly compromised. Refer to institutional guidelines. Refer to Neutropenia in Chapter 10 for more detailed information.

There are no federal standards for these products in the United States. Moreover, they may be processed or stored in a risky way. The products themselves could interfere with some prescription medications.

Sampling is indicated to assess for electrolyte and metabolic changes; cardiac, pulmonary, and renal alterations; bone marrow function; the need for blood component transfusions; and the presence of infection. Cultures provide data to identify the microorganisms causing infection and determine antibiotic drug sensitivity.

This assessment is required for the surveillance of opportunistic microorganisms, early detection, and the prompt treatment of infection.

Providing information regarding home care responsibilities allows the patient to be a full partner in providing care, making decisions, and achieving optimal recovery outcomes. QSEN: Patient-centered care.

Timing depends on the type of transplant and course of the postengraftment period. Discharge criteria include an absolute granulocyte count above 500 to 1000/mm^3, no fever, oral food intake, no evidence of infection or bleeding, adequate oral fluid intake and hydration, and psychological readiness to return home.

This information aids the patient in assuming responsibility for ongoing care.

The patient should gradually resume activities, because fatigue and reduced endurance will be a problem.

Patients are better able to ask questions and seek assistance when they know basic information about all medications prescribed.

This information provides a rationale for therapy.

The risk for complications is associated with long-term use. Aseptic techniques need to be taught.

The patient's immune function is not fully restored until about 6 to 12 months after transplantation; many patients are fearful of leaving the hospital's protective isolation environment and thus need information to optimize their self-care regimen. QSEN: Safety.

Early assessment facilitates prompt treatment. QSEN: Safety.

Libido may be decreased. Women may need vaginal lubrication. Men may need medical management for erectile dysfunction.

The timing for return is related to the risk for infection and the patient's performance status.

Hematolymphatic, Immunological, and Oncological Care Plans

■ = Independent   ▲ = Interprofessional Collaboration

NANDA-I NDx **Risk for Infection**

Common Risk Factors

Immunosuppression secondary to high-dose chemotherapy or radiation therapy
Antimicrobial therapy (i.e., superimposed infection)
Prolonged bone marrow regeneration
Failure of bone marrow graft
Cytomegalovirus (CMV)/herpes simplex virus seropositivity

Common Expected Outcome

Patient is at reduced risk for local and systemic infection, as evidenced by negative blood surveillance culture findings, compliance with preventive measures, normal chest radiograph, intact mucous membranes and skin, and prompt reporting of early signs of infection.

NOC Outcomes
Infection Severity; Medication Response

NIC Interventions
Infection Protection; Chemotherapy Management; Medication Administration; Teaching: Individual

Hematolymphatic, Immunological, and Oncological Care Plans

Ongoing Assessment

Actions/Interventions	Rationales
■ Inspect the body sites with a high potential for infection (mouth, throat, axilla, perineum, rectum).	Opportunist infections are often the first type of infection to develop in immunosuppressed patients. Early detection facilitates prompt treatment. QSEN: Safety.
■ Inspect the peripheral IV, central venous catheter and port sites for redness and tenderness.	These are frequent sites of infection. QSEN: Safety.
■ Observe closely for fever and chills.	A temperature greater than 37°C (98.6°F) may indicate a systemic infection. This may be the initial presentation of infection because, in the absence of granulocytes, the locus of infection may develop without characteristic inflammation or pus formation at the site. QSEN: Safety.
■ Auscultate the lung field for crackles, rhonchi, and breath sounds.	Pneumonia infections are common and can be fatal in this population. QSEN: Safety.
■ Assess for risk factors predisposing the patient to CMV infection.	Infections are common after transplant, especially with CMV. Specific risk factors in this population include allogenic transplants, CMV seropositivity, total body irradiation, and acute graft-versus-host disease (GVHD). QSEN: Safety.
▲ Monitor the WBC count with differential and the absolute neutrophil count daily for evidence of rising or falling counts.	Neutropenia puts patients at increased risk, especially before engraftment. Even a slight rise in the WBC count may signal an infection because of the patient's impaired immune system. QSEN: Safety.
▲ Monitor cultures and sensitivities and CMV titers of blood, sputum, and urine.	Cultures provide data on which microorganisms are causing infection and antibiotic drug sensitivity. QSEN: Safety.

Therapeutic Interventions

Actions/Interventions	Rationales
▲ Place the patient in protective isolation according to transplant protocol.	Protective isolation precautions may include placing the patient in a private room, limiting visitors, and having all people who come in contact with the patient use masks, gloves, and gowns. Some hospitals may place patients in special sterile laminar airflow rooms. These precautions reduce the risk for patient exposure to opportunistic infections. QSEN: Safety; Evidence-based practice.
■ Ensure thorough handwashing (using vigorous friction) by the staff and visitors before physical contact with the patient.	Handwashing removes transient and resident bacteria from hands, thus minimizing or preventing transmission to the patient. QSEN: Safety.
■ Teach or provide meticulous total body hygiene with special attention to the frequent sites of infection (e.g., anal area, groin, breast folds, skin folds).	The perineal area is a source of many pathogens and a frequent portal of entry for microorganisms. Skin fold areas can also harbor pathogens. QSEN: Safety.
■ Implement a meticulous oral hygiene regimen.	Oral hygiene is important in the prevention of periodontal disease as a locus of infection. QSEN: Safety.
▲ Institute a low-microbial diet.	This diet emphasizes the need for well-cooked foods (meat, fish, poultry), pasteurized milk and dairy products, well-cooked eggs, well-washed and peeled raw fruits and vegetables. It protects the patient from exposure to pathogens from foods at a time when host defenses are greatly compromised. QSEN: Safety.
▲ Administer anti-infective drugs for prophylaxis or treatment, as prescribed.	Medications may be given before and after transplant for prophylactic, empiric, or actual treatment. Prophylactic anti-infective administration is given to prevent viral, fungal, and bacterial infections through immune reconstitution. QSEN: Safety.
■ Explain the effects of chemotherapy and radiation therapy on the immune system.	This information provides a basis for ongoing education.

■ Explain to the patient or significant others the role of WBCs in infection prevention:
• Normal range of WBCs
• Function of leukocytes and neutrophils
• Meaning or importance of the absolute neutrophil count (ANC):
  • Greater than 2000/mm^3= no risk
  • 1500 to 2000/mm^3= mild risk
  • 1000 to 1499/mm^3= moderate risk
  • 500 to 999/mm^3= high risk
  • Less than 500/mm^3= life-threatening risk
	Patients need to be co-managers of their treatment plan. Adequate knowledge is necessary for the ongoing monitoring of potential complications. Patients may be unaware of the many medical terms used to guide therapy. QSEN: Safety; Evidence-based practice.

■ Teach the patient or significant others the measures to prevent infection after discharge until immune function is fully restored (about 9 to 12 months after transplantation).	Patients and family members are more likely to implement infection control measures at home when they understand the risks and benefits to the patient. Animal excreta, soil, and people with known infections are sources of opportunistic infections for the immunocompromised patient after transplantation. QSEN: Safety; Evidence-based practice.

Hematolymphatic, Immunological, and Oncological Care Plans

NANDA-I NDx Ineffective Protection

Common Related Factors

Bone marrow suppression secondary to chemotherapy and radiation therapy
Prolonged bone marrow regeneration
Failure of bone marrow graft
Invasion of bone marrow by malignant cells
Sinusoidal occlusive disease
Graft-versus-host disease (GVHD)
Drug injury (chemotherapy or antimicrobial therapy)
Hepatic malignancy
Immunosuppressive therapy (e.g., cyclosporine, tacrolimus, sirolimus, methotrexate, steroids, antithymocyte globulins)
Drug or transfusion reactions

Defining Characteristics

Pancytopenia: reduced platelets, reduced red blood cells (RBCs), reduced white blood cells (WBCs)
Liver dysfunction or failure
Renal dysfunction
Facial edema and flushing
Wheezing
Skin rashes

Common Expected Outcomes

Patient maintains reduced risk for bleeding, as evidenced by normal platelet count, absence of signs of bleeding, and early report of any signs of bleeding.
Patient maintains optimal liver function, as evidenced by serum and urine laboratory values within normal limits, absence of ascites, balanced intake and output, and normal weight for patient.
Patient maintains optimal renal function, as evidenced by balanced intake and output (I&O), weight within normal limits, normal vital signs, and normal level of consciousness.
Patient maintains optimal skin integrity.
Patient is free of injury from drug or blood therapy as evidenced by normal vital signs, absence of pain, and absence of nausea and vomiting.

NOC Outcomes
Circulation Status; Blood Coagulation; Vital Signs
NIC Interventions
Chemotherapy Management; Bleeding Precautions; Hemodynamic Regulation; Vital Signs Monitoring

Hematolymphatic, Immunological, and Oncological Care Plans

Ongoing Assessment

Actions/Interventions

For risk for bleeding:

- Assess for any signs of bleeding. Signs may be obvious (e.g., epistaxis, bleeding gums, petechiae, bruising hematemesis, hemoptysis, hematuria,) or occult (e.g., neurological changes, dizziness).
- Monitor the patient's vital signs as needed.
- ▲ Monitor platelet counts, including nadir.

Rationales

Early assessment facilitates prompt treatment and a reduced risk for complications. QSEN: Safety.
Signs of bleeding are most commonly seen during the first 4 weeks after transplant.

Increased HR and orthostatic BP changes accompany bleeding.
The risk for bleeding increases as the platelet count drops:
- Mild thrombocytopenia: platelets 50,000 to 100,000/mm^3
- Moderate risk: platelets 20,000 to 50,000/mm^3
- Severe: platelets 20,000/mm^3 or less
- Transfusion threshold: platelet count less than 10,000/mm^3 or signs of active bleeding

---

Actions/Interventions

For risk for liver dysfunction:

■ Assess for risk factors predisposing the patient to the development of hepatic sinusoidal obstructive syndrome (HSOS):
  • Intense toxic conditioning regimen
  • Total body irradiation
  • Liver abnormalities before transplantation (hepatitis)
  • Allogeneic stem cell transplant or hematopoietic stem cell transplantation (HSCT)
  • Patients with malignant diseases (leukemia, lymphoma, solid tumors)
  • Second stem cell transplant or HSCT

■ Assess for the signs of liver dysfunction: sudden weight gain, enlarged liver, right upper quadrant pain, ascites, jaundice, tea-colored urine, labored and shallow respirations, dyspnea, confusion, and lethargy and fatigue.

▲ Monitor laboratory values daily for:
  • Increased alkaline phosphatase, bilirubin, serum aspartate aminotransferase, alanine aminotransferase, lactic dehydrogenase, and ammonia levels
  • Decreased serum albumin level
  • Electrolyte imbalance
  • Abnormal coagulation profile

For risk for renal dysfunction:

■ Monitor the patient's urine output.

▲ Monitor laboratory data: sodium, potassium, blood urea nitrogen (BUN), creatinine, osmolality.

■ Monitor fluid balance (at minimum, I&O every 8 hours and daily weight).

■ Observe for the presence of peripheral or dependent edema.

■ Monitor for changes in the level of consciousness.

■ Monitor the drug profile for medications potentially contributing to renal insufficiency or changes in the level of consciousness.

For risk for drug or transfusion reactions:

■ Assess for reactions from chemotherapeutic drugs: restlessness, facial edema and flushing, wheezing, skin rash, tachycardia, hypotension, hematuria (and increased uric acid levels.

■ Test the urine for blood.

Rationales

Attention to early changes followed by prompt treatment reduces the risk of harm to the patient. QSEN: Safety.

Chemotherapy or radiation therapy can cause deposits of fibrous materials to form in the small veins of the liver, obstructing blood flow from it. HSOS is the occlusion of these vessels; there is no proven preventive therapy.

Classic signs of HSOS include right upper quadrant pain, jaundice, ascites, and hepatomegaly. Typically, symptoms develop 1 to 4 weeks after transplantation. Patients usually present with some but not all of these symptoms.

These laboratory tests provide data on liver function. Specific deficiencies guide treatment.

Attention to early changes followed by prompt treatment reduces the risk for harm to the patient. QSEN: Safety.

A decreased urine volume less than 30 mL/hr suggests renal insufficiency.

Increased potassium, BUN, and creatinine are associated with decreased renal function. Chemotherapy, radiation therapy, antibiotics, and immunosuppressive drugs may cause renal failure.

Close monitoring of fluid balance is necessary to determine adequate replacement needs and to prevent excessive administration of oral or IV fluids during decreased renal function. Body weight is a more sensitive indicator of fluid retention than I&O.

Edema occurs when fluid accumulates in the extravascular spaces. These changes reflect fluid imbalance.

BUN and other waste products can build up in the blood and can cause uremic encephalopathy.

A drug dosage adjustment or discontinuation may be necessary to prevent toxic side effects of poorly excreted drugs.

Attention to early changes followed by prompt treatment reduces the risk for harm to the patient. QSEN: Safety.

Careful monitoring for potential adverse effects is required both during and after administration.

Hematuria may be caused by irritation of the bladder lining secondary to the conditioning regimen or infection. High urine flow, alkalinization of urine, and frequent voiding help prevent the concentration of metabolites in the bladder, thus reducing the risk for hemorrhagic cystitis.

Hematolymphatic, Immunological, and Oncological Care Plans

■ = Independent   ▲ = Interprofessional Collaboration

Actions/Interventions	Rationales
■ Assess for reactions from immunoglobulins: urticaria, pain (local erythema), headache, muscle stiffness, fever and malaise, nephrotic syndrome, angioedema, and anaphylaxis.	Reactions can be serious and even life threatening.
■ Assess for reactions to immunosuppressive therapy: mucositis, nausea and vomiting, bone marrow suppression, fluid retention, hypertension, headache, hypomagnesemia, renal toxicity, tingling in extremities, tremors, and anaphylaxis-like reactions.	A variety of reactions may occur, depending on the agent administered.
For risk for GVHD:	Attention to early changes followed by prompt treatment reduces the risk for harm to the patient. QSEN: Safety.
■ Assess for risk factors predisposing the patient to the development of GVHD: • Older age of either donor or recipient • Donor/recipient HLA mismatch • Female donor who has been pregnant in the past • Type of GVHD prophylaxis • Myeloablative conditioning regimen	GVHD is one of the most serious complications of allogeneic HSCT. It occurs when T cells from the donated marrow (the "graft") identify the recipient body (the "host") as foreign and attack it. However, the presence of some level of GVHD does indicate adequate or successful engraftment.
■ Assess for the signs of acute GVHD: skin rash or scaling, elevated bilirubin levels, aminotransferases, alkaline phosphates, gastrointestinal (GI) changes (diarrhea, abdominal cramps).	Symptoms can occur within weeks of transplant. The first and most common clinical manifestation is a maculopapular rash. GVHD can affect the eyes, GI tract, and liver. Inflammation and sensitivity on the palms of the hands, neck, ears, shoulders, and plantar surfaces of the feet are early signs of GVHD.

Therapeutic Interventions

Actions/Interventions	Rationales
For risk for bleeding:	
▲ Implement bleeding precautions for a platelet count less than 50,000/mm³:	Understanding the importance of precautionary measures reduces the risk for bleeding. At 20,000/mm³, spontaneous bleeding can occur. QSEN: Safety.
• Avoid nonessential invasive procedures, punctures, and injections.	This precaution reduces bleeding at vascular access sites.
• Avoid rectal thermometers, suppositories, and enemas.	This reduces mucosal injury.
• Maintain appropriate fall precautions.	Safety measures reduce the risk for trauma.
▲ Communicate the anticipated need for platelet support to the transfusion center. Transfuse platelets as prescribed.	This measure ensures the availability and readiness of platelets when needed to prevent spontaneous or excessive bleeding. Platelet transfusion is indicated for counts less than or equal to 10,000/mm³ unless the patient is actively bleeding; this decreases the risk for the patient becoming refractory to platelet transfusions.
▲ Maintain a current blood sample for "type and screen" in the transfusion center. If a significant drop in hemoglobin (Hgb) and hematocrit (Hct) is noted, transfuse packed RBCs as prescribed.	This ensures the availability and readiness of packed RBCs. Packed RBCs are used to restore Hgb and Hct to levels at which the patient experiences minimal symptoms. All products transfused should be leukocyte-reduced, cytomegalovirus (CMV)-negative, and irradiated products.
For risk for liver dysfunction:	
▲ Restrict fluids and sodium as prescribed.	Restrictions reduce fluid buildup. Fluid management is key.
▲ Consult a dietitian about dietary modifications in enteral or parenteral nutrition.	Oral protein may need to be restricted; parenteral nutrition solutions may need to be concentrated. The dietitian can provide specialized care. QSEN: Teamwork and collaboration.

Actions/Interventions	Rationales
▲ Administer Actigall as ordered.	This medication is used routinely for patients at high risk for or exhibiting signs and symptoms of potential hepatic sinusoidal obstructive syndrome (HSOS). QSEN: Safety.
▲ Administer IV medications with a minimal amount of solution. Consult a pharmacist.	This measure decreases unnecessary fluids. QSEN: Teamwork and collaboration.
▲ Administer diuretics as prescribed.	Diuretics decrease the amount of ascites and help maintain adequate renal perfusion.
▲ Transfuse packed RBCs as prescribed.	Packed RBCs maintain intravascular fluid volume. The goal of hypertransfusion of packed RBCs is to attain an Hct of 40 or greater, which helps maintain high osmotic pressure within the vascular space. This in turn draws extravascular interstitial fluid back into the vessels.
▲ Administer analgesics as prescribed.	Analgesics are used to reduce patient discomfort with ascites and related problems. Opioids and sedatives with shorter half-lives and fewer metabolites given in reduced doses should be considered to prevent compounding of hepatic encephalopathy.
For risk for renal dysfunction:	
▲ Administer IV fluids and diuretics as prescribed.	These therapies are used to correct vascular volume disequilibrium.
▲ Administer electrolytes in IV fluids.	Replacement is necessary to match any calculated loss and correct any deficit.
▲ Administer low-dose ("renal dose") dopamine.	This medication is indicated to maintain urine flow. However, it does not offer renoprotective effects.
▲ Consult a dietitian about dietary modifications in enteral or parenteral nutrition.	Specialty expertise may be needed to balance fluid and nutritional needs. QSEN: Teamwork and collaboration.
For risk for drug or blood reactions:	
▲ Keep emergency drugs (IV diphenhydramine [Benadryl], albuterol, hydrocortisone, epinephrine 1:1000) readily available.	Patient safety is a priority. Being prepared reduces complications. QSEN: Safety.
▲ Administer IV fluids and diuretics before, during, and after the conditioning regimen, as prescribed.	These are used to maintain good urine output and counteract the antidiuretic effect of medications. As chemotherapy destroys tumor cells, uric acid is liberated and accumulates in the blood. High urine flow prevents uric acid deposits in the kidneys. QSEN: Safety.
▲ Premedicate the patient with antiemetics and antihistamines as prescribed before infusion.	These medications are used to reduce the incidence of nausea and vomiting and allergic reactions. Allergic reactions, including shortness of breath, are possibly the result of the liberation of histamines from broken marrow cells.
■ Provide warm blankets if chills occur during reinfusion.	Chills usually are secondary to the cool temperature of thawed marrow or peripheral stem cell concentrate.
▲ Do the following when a drug or transfusion reaction is suspected: stop the infusion, notify the physician, administer emergency drugs as prescribed, and reassure the patient.	Rapid, efficient intervention is critical to saving life. QSEN: Safety.
For GVHD:	
▲ Administer immunosuppressive drugs and topical steroids as prescribed.	These drugs are used to prevent or treat acute GVHD (drugs include cyclosporine, tacrolimus, methotrexate, steroids, immunoglobulins). GVHD results when the T lymphocytes in the transplanted donor bone marrow recognize the marrow recipient as foreign and mount an immunological attack against the host. GVHD generally is seen in patients receiving allogeneic HSCT. It remains one of the major causes of transplantation-related death. QSEN: Safety.

Hematolymphatic, Immunological, and Oncological Care Plans

■ = Independent   ▲ = Interprofessional Collaboration

Actions/Interventions	Rationales
▲ Implement the following once the signs of GVHD skin changes are present:	
• Use a mild soap and oatmeal bath preparation daily.	These soothe dry, flaky, irritated skin.
• Administer antipruritic agents (i.e., antihistamines) and topical steroid medications.	Both systemic and topical agents can be effective in relieving itching and promoting comfort.
• Trim the patient's nails, and discourage him or her from scratching; consider the use of mittens.	This measure reduces skin trauma.
• Lubricate the skin well with frequent applications of a mixture of half-and-half mineral oil and ointment.	Lubrication provides relief to the skin.
• Provide pain control as prescribed.	Pain medications are individualized depending on the source of pain, and acute versus chronic setting.

NANDA-I NDx Diarrhea

Common Related Factors

Intestinal graft-versus-host disease (GVHD)
Side effects of high-dose chemotherapy or radiation therapy
Oral magnesium
Medication use: antacids, antibiotic therapy
Infection

Defining Characteristics

Abdominal pain
Cramping
Frequency of stools
Loose or liquid stools
Urgency
Hyperactive bowel sounds

Common Expected Outcomes

Patient passes soft, formed stool no more than three times per day.
Patient has negative stool cultures.

NOC Outcomes

Bowel Elimination; Fluid Balance; Medication Response

NIC Interventions

Diarrhea Management; Nutrition Therapy; Medication Administration; Perineal Care

Ongoing Assessment

Actions/Interventions	Rationales
■ Check the patient's bowel sounds; observe for abdominal distention, rigidity, and discomfort.	Hyperactive bowel sounds and abdominal pain and cramping are associated with diarrhea.
■ Monitor the patient's stool pattern; record the frequency, character, and volume.	Diarrhea can be the first manifestation of GVHD; it is usually high volume (500 to 1500 mL/day), watery, and green and contains mucus strands, protein, and cellular debris.
▲ Obtain a stool specimen for culture and sensitivity, as prescribed.	A specimen provides evidence of a causative organism, such as *Clostridium difficile.* QSEN: Safety.
■ Hematest all watery stools.	A hematest aids in detecting possible GI mucosal sloughing caused by chemotherapy or radiation therapy or by GVHD-related mucosal injury.
▲ Monitor serum electrolytes.	Sodium, potassium, and chloride may be low because of electrolyte losses with diarrhea. QSEN: Safety.

⊜volve **For additional care plans, go to http://evolve.elsevier.com/Gulanick/.**

Therapeutic Interventions

Actions/Interventions	Rationales
▲ Administer antidiarrheal, and antispasmodic medications as prescribed; document their effectiveness.	Most antidiarrheal drugs suppress gastrointestinal (GI) motility, thus allowing for more fluid absorption. Antispasmotic drugs relieve cramps or spasms of the stomach or intestines.
▲ Administer IV analgesics.	These medications may be needed to relieve abdominal pain and cramping.
■ Implement a meticulous perianal care regimen.	Perianal care prevents mucosal irritation/breakdown. QSEN: Safety.
▲ Administer IV hydration and parenteral nutrition as prescribed.	Increased fluid intake replaces fluid lost in the liquid stools. Optimal nutritional support is important in view of inadequate oral intake and decreased absorption secondary to diarrhea and intestinal GVHD.
▲ Consult a dietitian for diet advancement based on symptoms: NPO (nothing by mouth, for bowel rest), clear liquid, full liquid, soft foods, and regular diet.	A specialist may be able to tailor an optimal meal plan for the patient. QSEN: Teamwork and collaboration.

Hematolymphatic, Immunological, and Oncological Care Plans

NANDA-I NDx   Risk for Imbalanced Nutrition: Less Than Body Requirements

Common Risk Factors

Side effects of chemotherapy or radiation therapy (inability to taste and smell foods, loss of appetite, nausea and vomiting, mucositis, mouth and throat lesions, xerostomia, diarrhea)

Intestinal graft-versus-host disease (GVHD): abdominal cramping, diarrhea, and malabsorption of nutrients

Increased metabolic rate secondary to fever or infection and other metabolic alterations

Common Expected Outcome

Patient maintains optimal nutritional status and protein stores as evidenced by caloric intake adequate to meet body requirements, balanced intake and output, and absence of nausea and vomiting or other GI symptoms.

NOC Outcomes

Nutritional Status: Food and Fluid Intake; Nutritional Status: Nutrient Intake

NIC Interventions

Nutrition Therapy; Total Parenteral Nutrition (TPN); Chemotherapy Management

Ongoing Assessment

Actions/Interventions	Rationales
■ Determine the specific cause or causes for imbalanced nutrition.	A specific cause guides the treatment plan. These may include side effects of chemotherapy or radiation therapy, GVHD, and infection.
■ Obtain a history of the side effects of previous chemotherapy or radiation therapy and treatment measures used in the past.	Patients may have had adverse side effects in the past. However, newer antiemetic agents have improved the management of nausea and vomiting for many patients. QSEN: Patient-centered care.
■ Review the patient's description of the current nausea and vomiting pattern, if present.	The pattern may guide treatment because not all patients experience the same response. QSEN: Patient-centered care.

■ = Independent   ▲ = Interprofessional Collaboration

Actions/Interventions

- Evaluate the effectiveness of the current antiemetic regimen.

- Monitor daily calorie counts and intake and output.

- Weigh the patient daily on the same scale and at the same time.

▲ Monitor laboratory values: red and white blood cell counts; serum electrolytes; transferrin, and serum albumin.

- If receiving parenteral nutrition, monitor closely for a tolerance to the solution and for any potential adverse complications.

Rationales

Ongoing nausea and vomiting can significantly affect the quality of one's life. Patient responses to antiemetic and comfort medications are highly variable and must be explored with each patient. Newer antiemetics may be effective. QSEN: Patient-centered care.

These assessments are important to determine whether the patient's oral intake meets daily nutritional requirements.

Consistent weighing is important to ensure the accuracy of weight. Without monitoring, the patient may be unaware of small weight changes.

Laboratory values provide information on nutrition and electrolyte status. Albumin indicates the degree of protein depletion; transferrin is important for iron transfer and typically decreases as the serum protein decreases. Anemia and leukopenia occur in malnutrition. Sodium and potassium are typically decreased in malabsorption. QSEN: Safety.

Common problems include hyperglycemia or hypoglycemia, hypophosphatemia, electrolyte disorders, hyperosmolarity, dislodgement of the catheter or infiltration, and catheter sepsis.

Therapeutic Interventions

Actions/Interventions

- Identify and provide the patient's favorite foods; avoid serving them during periods of nausea and vomiting.
▲ Administer supplemental feedings or fluids, as prescribed.
- Implement an appropriate GVHD diet or nothing by mouth status ("gut rest") in the presence of abdominal cramps, pain, or diarrhea.

- Teach methods to minimize or prevent nausea and vomiting and maintain adequate nutritional intake:

  • Small dietary intake before treatments

  • Foods with a low potential for nausea (e.g., dry toast, crackers, ginger ale, cola, popsicles, gelatin, baked or boiled potatoes)
  • Avoidance of spices, gravy, greasy foods, and foods with strong odors
  • Modification of food consistency or type, as needed
  • Oral hygiene measures before, after, and between meals

  • Relaxation therapy, guided imagery

▲ Administer an antiemetic around the clock rather than as needed. Schedule antiemetics before, during, and after chemotherapy or radiation therapy.

Rationales

The patient may develop an aversion to specific foods as a result of drug side effects.

Such supplements can be used to increase calories and protein.

These symptoms generally indicate an injury to intestinal mucosal surfaces, resulting in nutrient malabsorption. Parenteral support may be necessary to maintain balanced nutrition.

Modifications in dietary intake may reduce the stimulus for nausea and vomiting. Interventions to stimulate appetite and reduce noxious environmental stimuli may enhance nutrient intake. QSEN: Patient-centered care.

Limited intake reduces gastric overdistention. Having some food in the stomach before treatment may reduce emesis.

These foods are easily digested and provide a measure of success to augment nutrition.

Fats are difficult to digest, may exacerbate nausea, and can stimulate gastric motility.

Bland foods may be better tolerated.

Nausea is often associated with anorexia and increased salivation. Oral hygiene will help promote comfort.

These techniques can be helpful if used before nausea occurs or increases.

Antiemetics relieve nausea and vomiting. The selection of antiemetic agents should be based on the risk factors of the patient for nausea or vomiting. The effectiveness of therapy is increased when adequate plasma levels are maintained. QSEN: Patient-centered care.

Related Care Plans

Central venous access devices, Chapter 4
Leukemia, Chapter 10
Neutropenia, Chapter 10

Human Immunodeficiency Virus (HIV) Disease

Acquired Immunodeficiency Syndrome (AIDS)

Human immunodeficiency virus (HIV) causes acquired immunodeficiency syndrome (AIDS). Transmission of HIV occurs in situations that allow contact with body fluids that are infected with the virus. The primary body fluids associated with transmission are blood, vaginal fluids, semen and pre-seminal fluids, rectal fluids, and breast milk. Transmission of HIV can occur during sexual intercourse with an infected partner. Transmission through blood and blood product administration occurred early in the history of HIV in the United States. With current methods for screening blood donors and testing donated blood before transfusion, this is no longer considered a route of infection transmission. However, contact with infected blood through shared IV equipment and accidental needle sticks is still possible. Perinatal transmission of the virus from mother to baby is thought to occur during pregnancy, during delivery, or through breastfeeding. Most of the early victims of the syndrome were homosexual men; however, in many cities today, infected IV drug users, their sexual partners, and their children outnumber infected homosexual men. Despite efforts to increase routine, voluntary testing and counseling for HIV, many patients first learn that they are infected after their disease is advanced.

The first signs of HIV infection occur when the body produces HIV antibodies. Flulike signs and symptoms that may last 1 to 3 weeks characterize this stage of the infection. After this stage, the patient may be asymptomatic for acute infection, depending on his or her general state of health. This asymptomatic stage can last 10 years or longer. When the immune system begins to fail, the patient exhibits signs of immune system incompetence. The patient begins to develop clinical conditions such as cancers and opportunistic infections. When the patient's CD4 lymphocyte count falls below 200 cells/mm^3, AIDS is diagnosed. Patients present at various stages of the disease. Antiretroviral therapy is prescribed for everyone with HIV. While it does not cure HIV, it does prolong life and reduce the risk of transmission. People who don't have HIV but who are at high risk (e.g., unprotected high-risk sex or injection drug exposures) should receive pre-exposure prophylaxis (PrEP). Patients are treated in hospital, ambulatory care, and home care settings. The nursing diagnosis list of problems for various stages of HIV infection and AIDS is extensive. Some are highlighted here.

Hematolymphatic, Immunological, and Oncological Care Plans

NANDA-I NDx Deficient Knowledge: Disease and Transmission

Common Related Factors

Emotional state affecting learning (e.g., fear of AIDS)
Insufficient information
Insufficient interest in learning
Misinformation presented by others
Insufficient knowledge of resources

Defining Characteristics

Insufficient knowledge
Inaccurate follow-through of instruction
Inappropriate behavior

 = Independent   ▲ = Interprofessional Collaboration

Common Expected Outcome

Patient verbalizes understanding of desired content and performs desired skills.

NOC Outcomes

Knowledge: Disease Process; Knowledge: Infection Management; Knowledge: Sexual Functioning

NIC Interventions

Health Literacy Enhancement; Learning Facilitation; Teaching: Disease Process; Teaching: Prescribed Medication; Teaching: Safe Sex; Teaching: Individual; Infection Protection

Ongoing Assessment

Actions/Interventions	Rationales
■ Assess the patient's knowledge of the disease process, routes of transmission, complications, and treatment modalities.	Because of the chronic nature of HIV infection, the patient needs information about the disease and its treatment to make appropriate decisions about his or her health behaviors. QSEN: Patient-centered care.
■ Determine the patient's or significant others' concerns about HIV infection.	Patients, family members, and significant others may have a fear of rejection or retaliation when disclosing a patient's HIV infection. Lack of accurate information about the disease and its transmission may interfere with interpersonal relationships and social support for the patient.
■ Determine at-risk behaviors, including sexual activities and IV drug use.	HIV is spread primarily through unprotected sexual activity and by sharing contaminated needles and syringes for IV drug use. Anal sex is the most risky for HIV transmission. QSEN: Safety.

Therapeutic Interventions

Actions/Interventions	Rationales
■ Instruct the patient in the signs and symptoms of disease, opportunistic infections, and neoplasms, as well as the person to whom information should be reported.	Patients are better able to ask questions when they have basic information about what to expect. Collaborative management of this disease focuses on monitoring for the progression of disease, the effectiveness of drug therapy, side effects experienced, and the occurrence of complications. QSEN: Patient-centered care; Safety.
■ Instruct the patient regarding interventions to prevent opportunistic infections:	Appropriate prophylaxis can reduce risks of morbidity and mortality. QSEN: Evidence-based care; Safety.
• Vaccines	Vaccines may include hepatitis B virus (HBV) vaccine, as well as annual influenza and pneumococcal vaccines.
• Medications	Patients with a lymphocyte count of less than 200 CD4 cells need medications to prevent *Pneumocystis* pneumonia (PCP). Patients with a lymphocyte count of less than 100 CD4 cells who are infected with *Toxoplasma gondii* need medication to prevent reactivation. Patients with a lymphocyte count of less than 50 CD4 cells need medication to prevent *Mycobacterium avium* complex (MAC) infection. Patients with a history of cryptococcal meningitis or end-organ cytomegalovirus disease need ongoing medication to prevent recurrence. Patients with tuberculosis (TB) skin test results that indicate latent TB infection need treatment to prevent progression to TB.

Actions/Interventions	**Rationales**
• Other:	These foods harbor bacteria and protozoa that may cause infection in severely compromised people.
• Avoid raw or undercooked meat, poultry, seafood; unpasteurized milk and dairy products; unwashed and unpeeled fruits and vegetables.	
• Avoid changing the cat's litter box.	*T. gondii* may be transmitted from the stool of an infected cat.
■ Instruct the patient in the methods of preventing HIV transmission sexually:	Activities in which there is no contact with a partner's blood, semen, or vaginal secretions are safe. When properly used, latex condoms reduce the risk for HIV transmission for both partners. Both male and female condoms are available. These instructions are based on recommendations from national organizations and support evidence-based practice. QSEN: Safety; Evidence-based practice; Patient-centered care.
• Safe sex: closed-mouth kissing, touching, mutual masturbation	
• Using latex condoms correctly every time having vaginal, anal or oral sex. Male condoms considered safer than female ones.	
• Have less risky sex.	
• Oral sex is less risky than anal or vaginal sex, especially if condom is used.	
• Anal sex is the most risky for HIV transmission.	
• Avoid any sexual activities that cause bleeding.	
■ Explore ways to express physical intimacy that do not lead to infection.	Patients need to have open communication with their sexual partners to negotiate risk-reduction methods. QSEN: Patient-centered care; Safety.
■ Explore the patient's sexual partner's perception of personal risk for HIV infection.	It is important to assess knowledge rather than make assumptions. Pre-exposure prophylaxis (PrEP) is an important prevention option for people who don't have HIV but who are at risk of being infected. It involves taking a specific HIV medication every day (e.g., emtricitabine and tenofovir). Prevention meds need to be combined with safe sex practices with correct condom use, risk reduction counseling and HIV testing. QSEN: Patient-centered care; Safety.
■ Role-play to practice new behaviors (e.g., saying "no" or negotiating condom use) in situations that may lead to transmission.	Practice instills the confidence to perform the desired behavior. Older adults may be reluctant to use condoms because they are past childbearing age.
■ Explore the benefits and drawbacks of HIV testing of sexual partners and needle-sharing partners.	If the test is positive, benefits include initiation of antiviral therapy; drawbacks include possible discrimination and emotional depression.
■ Instruct the patient and partners to prevent pregnancy. Instruct in birth control methods, including condom use.	HIV can be easily transmitted to the baby unless treatment has been initiated. Women with HIV who take antiretroviral medications can reduce the risk of transmission of HIV to less than 1%. QSEN: Safety.
■ Encourage the use of clean IV equipment when recreational drugs are used. Refer patients to drug rehabilitation programs as appropriate.	HIV is quickly killed by 10% hypochlorite solution. Flush syringes and needles with household bleach diluted ninefold with water; rinse with tap water. QSEN: Safety.
■ Explain the importance of the following:	These are established modes of transmission.
• Refraining from donating blood, semen, or organs	
• Cleaning blood or excreta containing blood with 10% hypochlorite solution	This solution should be used on blood and stool (carriers of HIV), but it is not necessary to use bleach to wash the patient's dishes, clothes, or personal items.
■ Instruct the patient to avoid exposure to infectious diseases:	Immunocompromised patients are especially vulnerable to viral infections (e.g., herpes or genital warts). Syphilis is more difficult to diagnose and treat in HIV-infected patients and progresses more rapidly. Normally nonpathogenic intestinal flora may cause disease in HIV-infected patients; therefore such people should refrain from anal-oral sexual activities. Used properly, condoms can help prevent STI spread during vaginal or anal intercourse. QSEN: Safety.
• Avoid sexual practices that lead to sexually transmitted infections (STIs).	
• Avoid contact with people who have infectious diseases.	

Hematolymphatic, Immunological, and Oncological Care Plans

■ = Independent   ▲ = Interprofessional Collaboration

NDx Infection

Common Related Factor

HIV infection

Defining Characteristics

Decreased number of CD4 cells
Positive HIV antibody with confirmatory Western blot
Detectable HIV viral load (HIV-1 RNA)

Common Expected Outcomes

Patient does not experience opportunistic infections.
The number of CD4 cells stabilizes or increases.

NOC Outcomes

Medication Response; Infection Severity

NIC Interventions

Infection Protection; Medication Administration

Hematolymphatic, Immunological, and Oncological Care Plans

Ongoing Assessment

Action/Intervention	Rationale
■ Monitor the CD4 level and viral load.	Patients need to have regular laboratory testing of CD4 levels and viral load to monitor the status of HIV. Decreasing CD4 levels and increasing viral load indicate progression of the infection and an increasing risk for opportunistic infections. QSEN: Safety.

Therapeutic Interventions

Actions/Interventions	Rationales

■ Instruct in the terminology commonly used in treatments:
  • CD4 cell count
  • Viral load
  • Antiretroviral agent
	CD4 cells (T cells) are white blood cells that fight infection.
	Viral load is the amount of HIV in a sample of blood.
	Antiretroviral agents are medications that interfere with the replication of retroviruses such as HIV.

■ Instruct the patient about antiretroviral medications and the potential therapeutic effects and side effects to monitor:	There are several classes of FDA-approved medications. Typically the drug regimen consists of three HIV medications from at least two different drug classes. Antiretrovirals are usually used in combinations; however, each regimen is tailored to the individual patient. Regimens may include fixed-dose combinations of medication. Additional experimental medications may be available through clinical trials. The patient and health care provider need to discuss the choice of HIV medications to include in the regimen. This decision depends on a person's individual needs and factors such as chronic conditions, such as renal failure, hepatic dysfunction, diabetes, tuberculosis (TB), or cardiovascular disease. Patient compliance is key in selecting medications. QSEN: Patient-centered care; Evidence-based practice.
• Treatment effects	Successful treatment usually results in at least a 10-fold reduction in HIV-1 RNA copies/mL during the first month and a further drop to 50 copies/mL by 6 months, depending on the baseline value of viral load. To evaluate treatment, viral load tests are usually repeated every 3 or 4 months.

Actions/Interventions

- Drug-specific categories and actions:

  - Nucleoside reverse transcriptase inhibitors (NRTIs), such as emtricitabine, lamivudine, zalcitabine, zidovudine, azidothymidine, didanosine enteric-coated, tenofovir disoproxil fumarate, stavudine, abacavir sulfate
  - Non-nucleoside reverse transcriptase inhibitors (NNRTIs), such as etravirine, delavirdine, efavirenz, nevirapine, and rilpivirine
  - Protease inhibitors, such as tipranavir, indinavir, saquinavir mesylate, ritonavir, fosamprenavir calcium, ritonavir, darunavir, atazanavir sulfate, nelfinavir mesylate

  - Entry inhibitors (CCR5 antagonists), such as maraviroc

  - Integrase strand transfer inhibitors (INSTIs), such as raltegravir, dolutegravir, and elvitegravir

  - Fusion inhibitors, such as enfuvirtide
  - Pharmacokinetic enhancers, such as cobicistat

- ■ Encourage the adherence to therapy, and avoid interruptions of therapy.

- ▲ Follow local regulations for obtaining a separate consent to be tested for HIV and for reporting results to the health department.

Rationales

These medications are based on recommendations from national organizations. QSEN: Evidence-based practice.

NRTIs block reverse transcriptase, an enzyme that HIV needs to make more copies of itself. Most of these drugs cause gastrointestinal (GI) problems, rash, and sleep disturbances.

NNRTIs block reverse transcriptase, an enzyme that HIV needs to make more copies of itself. Most of these drugs cause GI problems, rash, and sleep disturbances.

Protease inhibitors block protease, an enzyme that HIV needs to make more copies of itself. Because ritonavir inhibits metabolism of other protease inhibitors, it is often used to boost and maintain the plasma concentrations of other protease inhibitors for longer periods. Ritonavir-boost regimens alter the dose and frequency of other medications.

CCR5 antagonists work by blocking one of the receptors needed by HIV to enter cells. They are effective only for patients with CCR5-tropic variants of HIV-1. Over time, HIV-1 may adapt to use an alternative CXCR4 receptor, which renders this drug class ineffective.

Integrase inhibitors block integrase, a protein that HIV needs to put its genetic material in the genetic material of an infected cell.

Fusion inhibitors block HIV from entering cells.

Pharmacokinetic enhancers are used to increase the effectiveness of an HIV medication included in the treatment regimen.

Strict adherence is needed to stall the emergence of drug-resistant HIV strains. Antiretrovirals are taken throughout the course of infection unless the toxicities outweigh the potential benefits.

All pregnant women should be screened for HIV as early as possible during pregnancy so antiretroviral therapy can be initiated to reduce any risk of transmitting HIV to the baby.

Hematolymphatic, Immunological, and Oncological Care Plans

Imbalanced Nutrition: Less Than Body Requirements

NANDA-I NDx

Common Related Factors	Defining Characteristics
Biological factors (e.g., increased metabolic demands; infections) Insufficient dietary intake Inability to absorb food Adverse drug reactions	Body weight 20% or more below ideal weight range Food intake less than recommended daily allowance Insufficient interest in food Food aversion Insufficient muscle tone Sore buccal cavity Diarrhea Decreased body mass index (BMI)

■ = Independent   ▲ = Interprofessional Collaboration

Common Expected Outcomes

Patient regains weight or does not lose additional weight. Patient verbalizes understanding of necessary caloric intake to achieve a cessation of weight loss.

NOC Outcomes

Nutritional Status: Food and Fluid Intake; Nutritional Status: Nutrient Intake

NIC Interventions

Nutritional Monitoring; Nutrition Therapy; Medication Administration; Total Parenteral Nutrition (TPN); Oral Health Restoration

Ongoing Assessment

Actions/Interventions	Rationales
■ Assess any changes in weight.	HIV wasting syndrome is one of the clinical conditions that occur with AIDS. This condition is defined as an involuntary loss of more than 10% of total body weight. Persistent diarrhea and recurrent fevers are associated with the syndrome. Other factors contributing to weight loss include reduced food intake from anorexia, oral or esophageal lesions from candidiasis, and drug side effects. Inflammatory bowel disease from HIV may lead to malabsorption syndromes. Chronic HIV infection increases metabolic demands. QSEN: Patient-centered care.
▲ Obtain a nutritional history: intake, difficulty in swallowing, weight loss. Consult with a dietitian.	Attention to individual factors helps in designing an appropriate plan. Routine evaluations of changes in weight and caloric intake are useful to prevent weight loss and malnutrition. QSEN: Patient-centered care; Teamwork and collaboration.
▲ Inspect the mouth for candidal infection.	This infection causes difficulty in swallowing.
■ Evaluate for possible adverse reactions to medications.	Many drugs used to treat HIV can cause anorexia, nausea and vomiting, and weight loss.
▲ If the patient receives parenteral nutrition, monitor serum glucose and electrolyte levels.	The high glucose content of parenteral solutions can cause short-term hyperglycemia that may require insulin administration. QSEN: Safety.

Therapeutic Interventions

Actions/Interventions	Rationales
■ Provide dietary planning to encourage the intake of high-calorie, high-protein foods and dietary supplements.	Patients may not easily understand what is involved in a special dietary plan. They are better able to ask questions and seek assistance when they know basic information. QSEN: Patient-centered care.
▲ Provide antiemetics before meals.	Antiemetics can reduce nausea and improve intake.
■ Assist with meals as needed.	Fatigue and weakness may prevent the patient from eating.
■ Encourage exercise as tolerated.	Metabolism and the utilization of nutrients are enhanced by activity.
▲ Administer dietary supplements or parenteral nutrition, as ordered.	HIV may cause wasting syndrome. Oral nutritional supplements should be tried first. Parenteral nutrition should be reserved for severe intestinal dysfunction.
▲ Administer antimonilial medication, as prescribed.	Oral and esophageal candidiasis can cause a sore throat, which may cause a lack of appetite.
▲ Administer medications for opportunistic pathogens affecting the gastrointestinal tract.	Bowel inflammation from opportunistic infections causes malabsorption of nutrients.

ⓔvolve **For additional care plans, go to http://evolve.elsevier.com/Gulanick/.**

Related Care Plans

Diarrhea, Chapter 2
Disturbed body image, Chapter 2
Fatigue, Chapter 2
Spiritual distress, Chapter 2
Ineffective coping, Chapter 2
Hepatitis, Chapter 8
Acute kidney injury/Chronic kidney disease,
    Chapter 11
Diabetes mellitus, Chapter 13

Leukemia, Adult

Acute Lymphocytic Leukemia; Acute Myelocytic Leukemia; Chronic Lymphocytic Leukemia;
Lymphocytic Leukemia; Chronic Myelocytic Leukemia; Nonlymphocytic Leukemia;
Myelogenous Leukemia; Granulocytic Leukemia

Leukemia is a malignant disorder of the blood-forming system, including the bone marrow and spleen. The proliferation of immature white blood cells (WBCs) interferes with the production and function of the red blood cells (RBCs) and platelets. Leukemia can be characterized by identification of the type of leukocyte involved: myelogenous or lymphocytic. In acute lymphocytic leukemia there is a proliferation of lymphoblasts (most commonly seen in children); in acute myelocytic leukemia (most common after 60 years of age), there is a proliferation of myeloblasts. In chronic lymphocytic leukemia, there are increased lymphocytes (more common in men, especially after 50 years of age); in chronic myelocytic leukemia, granulocytes are increased (common in middle age).

Depending on the type of leukemia, therapeutic management may consist of combined chemotherapeutic agents, radiation therapy, and/or stem cell transplantation. Chemotherapeutic treatment consists of several stages: induction therapy, intensification, consolidation therapy, and maintenance therapy. The goals of nursing care are to prevent complications and provide educational and emotional support. This care plan addresses ongoing care of a patient in an ambulatory setting receiving maintenance therapy.

Hematolymphatic, Immunological, and Oncological Care Plans

NANDA-I NDx **Deficient Knowledge**

Common Related Factors

Insufficient information
Insufficient interest in learning
Misinformation presented by others
Insufficient knowledge of resources

Common Expected Outcome

Patient verbalizes understanding of the diagnosis of leukemia, its treatment strategies, and prognosis.

Defining Characteristics

Insufficient knowledge
Inaccurate follow-through of instruction
Inappropriate behavior

NOC Outcomes

Knowledge: Cancer Management; Knowledge: Disease Process; Knowledge: Treatment Procedure

NIC Interventions

Health Literacy Enhancement; Learning Facilitation; Teaching: Disease Process

■ = Independent   ▲ = Interprofessional Collaboration

Ongoing Assessment

Action/Intervention

■ Assess the patient's knowledge of the disease, treatment strategies, and prognosis.

Rationale

Several types of leukemia occur, which can be confusing. Each has its own treatment approach and prognosis. QSEN: Patient-centered care.

Therapeutic Interventions

Actions/Interventions

■ Describe the cause of leukemia:
  • Multifactorial involving genetic and environmental factors
  • May be related to exposure to radiation or chemical agents, viruses, immunological deficiencies, or antineoplastic drugs

■ Explain the blood-forming changes that occur with all types of leukemia:
  • Bone marrow failure; leukemic infiltrates
  • Granulocytopenia from reduced number of WBCs
  • Anemia from reduced RBC production
  • Thrombocytopenia from decreased platelet production

■ Clarify the difference between acute and chronic leukemia:
  • Acute leukemia is an abnormal proliferation of *immature* leukocytes or blasts with a rapid onset of symptoms.
  • Chronic leukemia is characterized as a disease of *mature* WBCs with a progressive, gradual onset of symptoms.

■ Describe the patient's specific type of leukemia.

■ Explain the diagnostic process:
  • Peripheral blood analysis
  • Bone marrow examination/biopsy

  • Lumbar puncture and computed tomography scan

■ Describe the common approaches to treatment:

  • Combination chemotherapy/biological therapies

  • Targeted therapy

  • Radiation therapy

Rationales

The exact cause of leukemia is unknown. Many causative factors seem to play a role in the development of both the acute and chronic forms of the disease. A group of preleukemic or myelodysplastic syndromes has been identified as significant in the development of leukemia in older adults.

Most people are unfamiliar with the various components of normal blood and marrow and the respective functions of the different blood cells.

Knowing the type will guide the treatment. Acute leukemia is treated immediately, whereas in chronic leukemia symptoms may be "watched" until they worsen. Leukemias may be further classified as lymphocytic or myelocytic according to the type of WBC involved in the disease.

Four major types of leukemia are known, as described in the introductory paragraph. Distinguishing the specific subtypes is important to guide appropriate therapy. QSEN: Patient-centered care.

Analysis is necessary to detect immature blood cells.

This is the key diagnostic tool and assists in the staging of the disease.

These tests are done to determine the presence of leukemic cells throughout the body.

Treatment is guided by current research findings and definitive protocols for the specific types of leukemia. Initial chemotherapy doses may be given in the hospital. However, follow-up courses may be administered in an outpatient or even in a home setting. QSEN: Evidence-based practice.

Chemotherapy is the primary treatment. Combination therapy has reduced side effects and an improved response. A variety of drugs are available depending on the leukemia type. Several types of biological therapies can treat leukemia. This type of therapy improves the body's natural defenses against cancer. Examples include monoclonal antibodies for chronic lymphocytic leukemia and interferon for chronic myelocytic leukemia.

Targeted therapy blocks cancer cells but not normal cells. For example, Gleevec is used for chronic myeloid leukemia.

Radiation therapy may be used as an adjunct to chemotherapy to keep acute leukemia from spreading or to relieve pain in chronic leukemia. Total body radiation is used (along with high-dose chemotherapy) for patients undergoing hematopoietic stem cell transplant.

Actions/Interventions

- Stem cell transplantation, especially with acute myelocytic leukemia
- Clinical trials

■ Explain the common complications of therapy.

■ Discuss the prognosis:
- The prognosis is hopeful, with the treatment goal being a curative attempt, although at times the treatment may only result in prolonged remission.
- Patients may be in remission for a long time, especially with chronic leukemia.

Rationales

Transplantation is a standard treatment for leukemia.

Ongoing research continues to explore improved treatments. Some are indicated for patients *before* any treatment, others for patients with refractory disease.

A variety of serious and distressing side effects occur with aggressive treatment. These may include pancytopenia from radiation and chemotherapy (anemia, bleeding, infection); nausea and vomiting from chemotherapy; fatigue and weakness.

The patient's adjustment to any form of leukemia and its treatment requires an understanding of the expected course of exacerbations and remissions.

NANDA-I NDx **Risk for Ineffective Coping**

Common Risk Factors

Situational crisis
Inadequate support system
Inadequate coping methods

Common Expected Outcomes

Patient demonstrates positive coping strategies.
Patient uses available resources and support systems.
Patient verbalizes realistic goal setting for future.

NOC Outcomes
Coping; Social Support; Family Coping

NIC Interventions
Coping Enhancement; Hope Inspiration; Grief Work Facilitation; Support System Enhancement

Hematolymphatic, Immunological, and Oncological Care Plans

Ongoing Assessment

Actions/Interventions

■ Assess the patient's knowledge of the disease and its treatment plan.
■ Assess for the coping mechanisms used in previous illnesses and any hospitalization experiences.

■ Evaluate the resources and support systems available to the patient in the home and community.

Rationales

Because leukemia is cancer, patients may expect to die. Realistic but positive information may be indicated.

Successful coping is influenced by previous success. Patients with a history of maladaptive coping may require additional resources. Likewise, previously successful coping skills may be inadequate in the present situation. QSEN: Patient-centered care.

Leukemia treatment may include months and years of ongoing chemotherapy, depending on the length of remission. The demands of managing therapy and preventing complications in the home setting can disrupt the lives of both the patient and family members. The availability of support systems may change over time. QSEN: Patient-centered care.

■ = Independent   ▲ = Interprofessional Collaboration

Actions/Interventions

- Assess the financial resources required for expensive long-term therapy.

Rationales

The financial aspects of acute care and long-term follow-up can be overwhelming, especially when the patient is dealing with a new diagnosis.

Therapeutic Interventions

Actions/Interventions

- Establish open lines of communication; establish a working relationship with the patient through the continuity of care.
- Provide opportunities for the patient and significant others to openly express feelings, fears, and concerns. Provide hope but avoid false reassurances.

- Assist the patient and significant others in redefining the hopes and components of individuality (e.g., roles, values, and attitudes).
- Encourage the patient to seek information that will improve his or her coping skills.
- Introduce new information about the disease's treatment as available.

- Assist the patient in becoming involved as a co-manager of the treatment plan.

- Describe community resources available to meet the unique demands of leukemia, its treatment, and survival (e.g., Leukemia and Lymphoma Society, American Cancer Society, National Coalition for Cancer Survivorship).
- ▲ Refer to a social worker for financial assistance, as indicated.

- Assist in the development of an alternative support system, as indicated. Encourage participation in self-help groups as available.

- Assist the patient in grieving and working through the losses from life-threatening illness and a change in body function.

Rationales

The nurse may be the first source of support for the patient and family. An ongoing relationship establishes trust, reduces the feeling of isolation, and may facilitate coping.

Verbalization of actual or perceived threats can help reduce anxiety and open doors for ongoing communication. An honest relationship facilitates problem-solving and successful coping. False reassurances are never helpful to the patient and only serve to relieve the discomfort of the care provider. QSEN: Patient-centered care.

Emphasizing the patient's intrinsic worth and viewing the immediate situation as manageable in time may provide support.

Patients who are not coping well may need more guidance initially.

Chronic leukemia is seldom cured. However, remission is possible, and long-term survival is feasible. Acute leukemia is treated to the remission stage, with maintenance therapy given to prevent relapse.

Involvement helps the patient regain control over the situation. Many patients become educated about their chemotherapeutic agents, using abbreviations fluently. Others become knowledgeable about blood components and vigilantly record daily or weekly laboratory results. QSEN: Patient-centered care.

It is helpful for patients to have more than one resource for helping them in this process. Reliable websites may likewise offer information and support.

The social worker can assist the patient and family with decisions about finances, living arrangements, wills, advance directives, and power of attorney. QSEN: Teamwork and collaboration.

Relationships with people with common interests and goals can be beneficial. Participation in support groups may allow the patient to realize that others have the same problem, and the patient may use this as an aid for coping. QSEN: Patient-centered care.

Grief is a universal experience; people who have successfully undergone grief over loss can be enormously helpful to others undergoing the same feelings. QSEN: Patient-centered care.

NANDA-I NDx Risk for Infection

Common Risk Factors
Cancer, resulting in altered immunological responses
Immunosuppression secondary to chemotherapy or radiation therapy

Common Expected Outcome
Patient is at reduced risk for local or systemic infection, as evidenced by afebrile state, normal vital signs, chest x-ray film results within normal limits, negative results of blood and surveillance cultures, compliance with preventive measures, and prompt reporting of early signs of infection.

NOC Outcomes
Immune Status; Knowledge: Infection Management; Tissue Integrity: Skin and Mucous Membranes

NIC Interventions
Infection Protection; Teaching: Disease Process; Oral Health Maintenance

---

Ongoing Assessment

Actions/Interventions	Rationales
■ Auscultate the lung fields for crackles, rhonchi, and decreased breath sounds.	Pulmonary infections are common, especially in immunosuppressed patients. QSEN: Safety.
■ Observe the patient for coughing spells and the character of sputum.	Increased sputum production and a change in color from clear or white to yellow or green may indicate respiratory infection. QSEN: Safety.
■ Inspect body sites with a high infection potential (mouth, throat, axilla, perineum, rectum).	Many infections that occur in patients with leukemia are opportunistic because of the patients' immunocompromised status. Opportunistic infections of the mucous membrane surfaces of the body are often the first type of infection to develop in immunosuppressed patients. QSEN: Safety.
■ Inspect the peripheral IV, central venous catheter or port sites for redness, tenderness, pain, and itching.	In the absence of granulocytes, a site of infection may develop without characteristic pus formation. QSEN: Safety.
■ Observe for changes in the color, character, and frequency of urine and stool.	These observations provide data on a possible urinary tract infection or intestinal infection. QSEN: Safety.
■ Monitor temperature as indicated.	Fever may be the only sign of infection. Patients need to be instructed to record serial temperatures at home. QSEN: Safety.
▲ Obtain cultures for temperature elevation per institutional protocol.	Cultures are required to determine the organism causing the infection and antibiotic sensitivity. QSEN: Safety.

Therapeutic Interventions

Actions/Interventions	Rationales
■ Explain the cause and effects of leukopenia.	Leukemic cells replace normal cells. Also, chemotherapy causes bone marrow suppression and a reduced number of neutrophils needed to fight infection.
■ Instruct the patient to maintain personal hygiene, especially at home: • Bathe with chlorhexidine (Hibiclens) • Wash hands well before eating and after using the bathroom • Wipe the perineal area from front to back	Handwashing removes transient and residual bacteria from the hands. The perineal area is a source of pathogens and a frequent entry port for microorganisms. Providing information allows the patient to be a full partner in assuming responsibility for care at home. QSEN: Safety.

■ = Independent   ▲ = Interprofessional Collaboration

Actions/Interventions

- Instruct the patient to brush teeth with a soft toothbrush four times a day and as necessary, to remove dentures at night, and to rinse the mouth after each emesis or when expectorating phlegm.

- Teach the patient to inspect the oropharyngeal area daily for white patches in the mouth, coated or encrusted oral ulcerations, a swollen and erythematous tongue with a white or brown coating, an infected throat and pain on swallowing, debris on the teeth, ill-fitting dentures.

- Teach the patient to avoid mouthwashes that contain alcohol and to avoid irritating foods and acidic drinks.

- Teach the patient to use prescribed topical medications (e.g., nystatin [Nilstat] and lidocaine [Xylocaine]).

- Instruct the patient and caregiver to maintain strict aseptic technique when changing dressings and to avoid wetting central catheter dressings.

- Instruct the patient to observe for fever spikes and flulike symptoms (e.g., malaise, weakness, myalgia) and to notify the nurse or physician if they occur.

- Instruct the patient and caregiver regarding the importance of eliminating potential sources of infection at home (especially when neutrophil counts are low):
  - Avoiding contact with visitors and family, especially children with colds or infections, or persons recently immunized with live vaccine
  - Avoiding shared drinking and eating utensils
  - Avoiding contact with cat litter boxes, fish tanks, and human or animal excreta
  - Avoiding swimming in private or public pools
  - Restricting contact with live plants

- ▲ Instruct on the importance of a low-microbial diet. Refer the patient to a dietitian as needed.

- Instruct to avoid herbal supplements (homeopathic remedies or herbal products, such as Chinese medicines).

- Instruct the patient regarding protective isolation if laboratory results indicate neutropenia (absolute neutrophil count [ANC] less than 500 to 1000/mm³):
  - Implement thorough handwashing for staff and visitors before physical contact with the patient.

- Instruct the patient to take prescribed antibiotic, antifungal, or antiviral drugs on time.

- ▲ Refer the patient to a dietitian for instructions on the maintenance of a well-balanced diet.

Rationales

Keeping oral mucous membranes intact reduces a possible site for opportunistic infection to develop. Periodontal disease is a locus of infection. QSEN: Safety.

The oral cavity and upper respiratory tract are common infection sites in patients with leukemia and neutropenia. Candidiasis is a common opportunistic infection in the immunocompromised patient. QSEN: Safety.

Alcohol has a drying effect on mucous membranes that can impair their integrity.

These agents may require specific instruction.

Information about aseptic technique helps the patient and caregiver assume responsibility for care and reduce the risk of harm. These aseptic measures help prevent bacterial growth. QSEN: Safety.

Early assessment facilitates prompt treatment and reduces the risk of harm to the patient. QSEN: Safety.

Patients must understand strategies and measures by which they can protect themselves during times of compromised defense. Animal excreta, soil, and people with known infections are sources of opportunistic infection for the immunocompromised patient. QSEN: Safety.

This diet protects the patient from exposure to pathogens from foods at a time when host defenses are greatly compromised. See the Neutropenia care plan in Chapter 10 for a more detailed listing of foods. QSEN: Patient-centered care; Teamwork and collaboration; Safety.

There are no federal standards for these products in the United States. Moreover, they may be processed or stored in a risky way. The products themselves could interfere with some prescription medications.

Institutional protocols may vary. Recommendations are based on national guidelines. QSEN: Safety; Evidence-based practice.

Handwashing removes transient and resident bacteria from the hands, thus minimizing or preventing transmission to the patient.

A regular schedule is needed to maintain therapeutic drug levels.

A specialist may provide additional help. This diet is for the maintenance of optimal health status, which promotes the improvement of host resistance and bone marrow recovery. QSEN: Teamwork and collaboration.

NANDA-I NDx **Risk for Bleeding**

Common Risk Factors

Bone marrow depression secondary to chemotherapy
Proliferation of leukemic cells

Common Expected Outcome

Patient's risk for bleeding is reduced, as evidenced by platelet count within acceptable limits, compliance with preventive measures, and prompt reporting of early signs and symptoms.

NOC Outcomes

Blood Coagulation; Knowledge: Treatment Regimen

NIC Interventions

Bleeding Precautions; Teaching: Disease Process

Ongoing Assessment

Actions/Interventions

▲ Monitor platelet counts, including nadir.

Rationales

Nadir is when platelets are at their lowest point. The risk for bleeding increases as the platelet count drops:

- Mild thrombocytopenia: platelets 50,000 to 100,000/mm^3
- Moderate risk: platelets 20,000 to 50,000/mm^3
- Severe risk: platelets 20,000/mm^3 or less
- Transfusion threshold: platelet count less than 10,000/mm^3 or signs of active bleeding

Attention to changes in platelet counts reduces the risk of harm. QSEN: Safety.

■ Assess for signs and symptoms of bleeding. These may include petechiae and bruising; hemoptysis; epistaxis; bleeding in oral mucosa; hematemesis; hematochezia; melena; vaginal bleeding; dizziness; orthostatic changes; decreased BP; headaches; changes in mental and visual acuity; and increased HR.

Early assessment facilitates prompt treatment and a reduced risk for complications. QSEN: Safety.

■ Note bleeding from any recent puncture site (e.g., venipuncture, bone marrow aspiration site).

The prolonged oozing of blood from puncture sites may be the first sign of a coagulation problem.

Therapeutic Interventions

Actions/Interventions

■ Explain to the patient and significant others the symptoms of thrombocytopenia and the functions of platelets:
- Normal range of platelet count
- Effects of thrombocytopenia
- Rationale of bleeding precautions

■ Instruct the patient in precautionary measures. Initiate bleeding precautions for a platelet count less than 50,000/mm^3:

- Use a soft toothbrush and nonabrasive toothpaste.
- Inspect the gums for oozing.
- Avoid the use of toothpicks and dental floss.
- Avoid rectal suppositories, thermometers, enemas, vaginal douches, and tampons.

Rationales

Most individuals are not familiar with the complexities of the hematological system. A successful plan requires the knowledge and cooperation of the patient and family members. QSEN: Patient-centered care.

An understanding of precautionary measures reduces the risk for bleeding. At platelet counts of <20,000/mm^3 spontaneous bleeding can occur. QSEN: Safety; Evidence-based practice.

This method reduces the risk for bleeding.

Oozing can be an early sign of bleeding.

This measure reduces mucosal trauma.

This measure reduces mucosal trauma.

■ = Independent   ▲ = Interprofessional Collaboration

Hematolymphatic, Immunological, and Oncological Care Plans

Actions/Interventions	Rationales
• Avoid aspirin or aspirin-containing products, nonsteroidal anti-inflammatory drugs (NSAIDs), and anticoagulants.	These medications interfere with platelet function.
• Avoid straining with bowel movements, forceful nose blowing, coughing, or sneezing.	This measure reduces the risk for bleeding.
• Count used sanitary pads during menstruation. Report any menstrual cycle changes.	This measure provides data on bleeding status.
• Avoid sharp objects such as scissors and knives. Use an electric razor for shaving (not razor blades).	It is important to prevent cuts, which would not only bleed but also become portals of entry for microorganisms, leading to infection in the presence of neutropenia.
• Lubricate the nostrils with saline solution drops as necessary and lips with petroleum jelly as needed.	Lubrication prevents drying and cracking.
• Practice gentle sex; use water-based lubricant before sexual intercourse.	These measures prevent mucosal trauma.
• Protect self from injury and trauma (e.g., falls, bumps, strenuous exercise, contact sports).	Patient safety is a priority.
• Give the patient and family at least two telephone numbers to call in case of bleeding.	Prearranged contact information facilitates early treatment.
• Instruct the patient to take antacids as prescribed when taking steroids, nonsteroidal anti-inflammatory drugs (NSAIDs), or aspirin.	Antacids reduce gastric irritation that can lead to bleeding.
In the health care setting:	These nursing actions reduce the risk of harm to the patient from bleeding. QSEN: Safety.
■ Avoid finger sticks if possible. Coordinate laboratory work so all tests are done at one time.	This precaution reduces bleeding potential.
■ Avoid intramuscular and subcutaneous injections. If necessary, use small-bore needles for injections and apply ice to the injection site for 5 minutes. Observe the site for oozing.	These measures reduce bleeding potential at the injection sites.
■ Apply pressure, a dressing, or sandbag to the bone marrow aspiration site.	This procedure prevents excessive pressure when compressing soft tissues and deeper structures of the arm, because this may lead to bruising or hematomas.
▲ Apply ice or topical thrombin promptly as prescribed for bleeding mucous membranes.	Thrombin promotes clot formation.
■ Discuss the possibility of platelet transfusions. Teach the patient the purpose and possible reactions to transfusions.	Knowledge reduces anxiety. Transfusions may be needed to maintain an adequate platelet count to prevent spontaneous or excessive bleeding.
▲ Ensure the availability and readiness of platelets for transfusion.	It is important to have platelets available when needed to prevent spontaneous or excessive bleeding (generally for platelet count less than 10,000/mm^3, unless active bleeding is present, or according to institutional protocol).

NANDA-I NDx Cancer-Related Fatigue

Common Related Factors	Defining Characteristics
Tumor and metastatic disease	A sense of physical or emotional tiredness that is not proportional to recent activity or treatment and interferes with the individual's daily functioning.
Chemotherapy and/or targeted therapy	Inability to restore energy, even after sleep
Radiation	Verbalization of an overwhelming lack of energy
Pain	
Distress (spiritual or emotional)	
Anxiety and/or fear	
Malnutrition	
Anemia	

Common Expected Outcomes

Patient reports reduction in fatigue, as evidenced by reports of increased energy and ability to perform desired activities.

Patient reports use of energy-conservation principles.

NOC Outcomes
Activity Tolerance; Endurance; Energy Conservation; Self-Care: Activities of Daily Living (ADLs)

NIC Interventions
Energy Management; Nutrition Management; Sleep Enhancement; Exercise Promotion

Ongoing Assessment

Actions/Interventions

■ Assess for fatigue regularly using a scale of 0 to 10 and defining characteristics.

■ Refer to Fatigue (Chapter 2).

Rationale

Fatigue has become the most common and distressing complaint for patients with cancer, especially during treatment. Regular assessment allows the nurse to evaluate fatigue and the patient's response to interventions and to develop and alter the plan accordingly. QSEN: Patient-centered care.

Therapeutic Interventions

Actions/Interventions

In addition to the Fatigue care plan, consider interventions in the following:

■ Educate the patient regarding these treatments:

• Assigning priorities to activities to accommodate energy levels

• Energy-conservation strategies, such as:
  • Sitting to do tasks
  • Pushing rather than pulling
  • Working at an even pace
  • Placing frequently used items within easy reach
  • Using wheeled carts for laundry, shopping, cleaning needs (see Fatigue, Chapter 2)
• Limiting naps to 20 to 30 minutes

• Use of psychostimulants (e.g., Ritalin) after ruling out other causes
• Treatment for anemia as indicated

• Cognitive behavioral therapy

• Nutrition consultation

Rationales

Providing information regarding home care responsibilities allows the patient to be a full partner in providing care, making decisions, and achieving optimal recovery outcomes. QSEN: Patient-centered care.

Setting priorities while conserving energy will allow the patient to achieve most desired goals and feel a sense of accomplishment.

Energy-conservation techniques reduce oxygen consumption, allowing more prolonged activity.

Limiting the amount of sleep during naps will help the individual sleep at night.

These medications have been used cautiously and demonstrate improved symptoms of fatigue in some patients.

Cancer patients' anemia results from the disease itself and treatment. Correcting the anemia may improve the patient's energy level.

This type of psychotherapy facilitates psychological adjustment to the cancer experience by helping certain patients recognize and change maladaptive thoughts.

A dietitian can counsel the patient and family on how to maximize the patient's intake during treatment for optimal nutritional needs. QSEN: Teamwork and collaboration.

Hematolymphatic, Immunological, and Oncological Care Plans

■ = Independent   ▲ = Interprofessional Collaboration

NANDA-I NDx Nausea

Common Related Factors

Treatment effects:
- Side effects of chemotherapy (inability to taste and smell foods, loss of appetite, nausea, vomiting, mucositis, dry mouth, diarrhea)
- Medications (e.g., opioids, antibiotics, vitamins)

Disease effects:
- Primary malignancy or metastasis
- Tumor waste products

Psychogenic effects:
- Conditioning to adverse stimuli (e.g., anticipatory nausea and vomiting, tension, anxiety, stress)
- Depression

Defining Characteristics

Reports "nausea" or "sick to stomach"
Increased salivation
Increased swallowing
Gagging sensation
Sour taste
Aversion toward food

Common Expected Outcome

Patient reports diminished severity or elimination of nausea.

NOC Outcomes

Nutritional Status: Food and Fluid Intake; Nutritional Status; Symptom Severity

NIC Interventions

Chemotherapy Management; Nutrition Therapy; Oral Health Maintenance; Medication Administration

Ongoing Assessment

Actions/Interventions

- Assess the patient's description of his or her nausea and vomiting pattern before each cycle of chemotherapy.

- Evaluate the effectiveness of the antiemetic and comfort measure regimens.

- Observe for the potential complications of prolonged nausea and vomiting.

- Weigh the patient at each clinic visit and always prior to each treatment. If the patient is at home, stress the importance of maintaining a daily log.
- Encourage the patient to record any food intake using a daily log.

Rationales

Patient responses are individualized, depending on the type and dosage of chemotherapy. Ongoing assessment is important so that treatment plans can be revised as needed. Assessment data should include the number of episodes of nausea or vomiting, timing of nausea and vomiting, ability to eat after chemotherapy, antiemetics taken, and other related symptoms. QSEN: Patient-centered care.

The patient response to antiemetic and comfort medications is highly variable and must be explored with each patient. Newer antiemetic medications have improved this condition for many patients. QSEN: Patient-centered care.

Nausea and vomiting can alter a patient's hydration status because of fluid loss and effect electrolyte imbalance (hypokalemia; decreased sodium and chloride). Persistent vomiting and reduced nutritional intake can result in weight loss, a decreased activity level, and lethargy.

Consistent weighing is important to ensure accuracy. Without monitoring, the patient may be unaware of small changes in weight resulting from imbalanced nutrition.

Determining the type, amount, and pattern of food intake (if any) is facilitated by accurate documentation, which provides information as to whether oral intake meets daily nutritional requirements.

Therapeutic Interventions

Actions/Interventions	Rationales
▲ Administer antiemetics according to protocol.	Symptoms of chemotherapy-induced nausea and vomiting (CINV) can have an acute, delayed, anticipatory, or breakthrough onset. Often a combination of antiemetic medications is needed to effectively control nausea and vomiting and must correlate appropriately to the emetogenic potential of chemotherapy agents given. Serotonin 5-HT$_3$ receptor antagonists (i.e., ondansetron and palonosetron), neurokinin-1 receptor antagonists (i.e., aprepitant), and corticosteroids (i.e., dexamethasone) are the most common drug classes used for CINV. Other drug classes include phenothiazines (i.e., prochlorperazine), benzodiazepines (i.e., lorazepam), cannabinoids (i.e., dronabinal), and the dopamine 2 receptor antagonist, metoclopramide. QSEN: Evidence-based practice.
■ Explain that the selection of antiemetic agents should be based on the emetic risk of the therapy and risk factors in the patient.	The Oncology Nursing Society provides resources for the recommended antiemetic regimens for high, moderately high, low, and minimal emetogenic chemotherapy. The administration of optimal antiemetic therapy during every cycle of chemotherapy will reduce the development of anticipatory nausea and vomiting. QSEN: Patient-centered care; Evidence-based practice.
▲ Administer antiemetics around the clock rather than as needed during periods of high incidence of nausea and vomiting.	The effectiveness of antiemetic therapy is increased when adequate plasma levels are maintained.
■ Institute or teach measures to reduce or prevent nausea and vomiting:	Behavioral and dietary interventions seem to be most effective in the management of anticipatory nausea and vomiting. This pattern of nausea and vomiting is related to classic conditioning. The patient develops nausea and vomiting in response to stimuli associated with the administration of chemotherapeutic drugs. Patients may try a variety of interventions to find those that best control this type of nausea and vomiting before drug administration. Antiemetic medications have been found to be less effective in managing anticipatory nausea and vomiting. However, antianxiety medications such as lorazepam may be effective. QSEN: Patient-centered care; Evidence-based practice.
• Small dietary intake before treatment	Eating small amounts reduces gastric overstimulation, thus reducing vomiting risk.
• Antiemetic half an hour before meals as prescribed	The appropriate timing of medications can reduce the onset and severity of nausea.
• Foods with low potential to cause nausea and vomiting (e.g., dry toast, crackers, ginger ale, cola, popsicles, gelatin, baked or boiled potatoes, fresh or canned fruit)	These foods are easily digested and provide a measure of success to augment nutrition.
• Avoidance of spices, gravy, greasy fried foods, and foods with strong odors	Fats are difficult to digest and may exacerbate nausea, and stimulate gastric motility.
• Meals at room temperature; serve foods cold if odors cause aversions	Hot foods can stimulate peristalsis. The smell of cooking food may aggravate feelings of nausea.
• Avoidance of coaxing, bribing, or threatening in relation to intake (help the family avoid being "food pushers")	Such behaviors tend to only aggravate the situation.
• Sucking on hard candy (e.g., peppermint) while receiving chemotherapeutic drugs with a "metallic taste"	Hard candies can reduce the metallic or bitter taste.

Hematolymphatic, Immunological, and Oncological Care Plans

■ = Independent   ▲ = Interprofessional Collaboration

Actions/Interventions	**Rationales**
• Drinking fluids at a different time than when eating solid snacks or meals	Separating fluids from solids will help in not filling the stomach quickly. This may help prevent nausea as well.
• Offering meat dishes in the morning	Aversions tend to increase during the day: chicken, cheese, eggs, and fish are usually well-tolerated protein sources.
• Minimal physical activity and no sudden rapid movements during times of increased nausea	Activity or sudden movements may potentiate nausea and vomiting.
• Relaxation and distraction techniques; guided imagery	These techniques, especially guided imagery, are useful adjuncts to antiemetic drug therapy. They can be helpful if used before nausea occurs or increases.
• Use of acupressure or acupuncture	Several small studies report acupressure and acupuncture to be useful measures in reducing nausea and vomiting risk.
• Cannabis	Medical cannabis is somewhat effective in CINV and may be a reasonable option for patients who do not improve with standard treatment. The FDA has approved two cannabinoids (dronabinol and nabilone) for prevention and treatment of CINV. QSEN: Patient-centered care; Evidence-based practice.

Related Care Plans

Caregiver role strain, Chapter 2
Deficient fluid volume, Chapter 2
Disturbed body image, Chapter 2
Fear, Chapter 2
Cancer chemotherapy, Chapter 10
Cancer radiation therapy, Chapter 10
Hematopoietic stem cell transplantation, Chapter 10

Lymphoma

Hodgkin's Lymphoma; Non-Hodgkin's Lymphoma

Lymphoma is a malignant disorder of the lymph nodes, spleen, and other lymphoid tissue. It is not a single disease but rather a group of diseases. Lymphomas include related diseases with a variety of symptoms, treatment options, and outcomes depending on the lymphocyte type and stage of disease. Lymphomas are classified as either Hodgkin's lymphoma or non-Hodgkin's lymphoma. A specific cause has not been identified, although associations with viral disease such as Epstein-Barr and mononucleosis, genetic predisposition, and environmental exposure to toxins have been noted. The Centers for Disease Control and Prevention has included lymphoma in the list of clinical conditions that are part of the case definition for AIDS.

Hodgkin's lymphoma is a disorder of the lymph nodes, usually presenting with painless node enlargement in the earlier stages. It is seen more frequently in men than women,

first between the ages of 20 and 40, and then again after 55 years of age. Hodgkin's and Reed-Sternberg cells are the hallmark marker for Hodgkin's lymphoma. Non-Hodgkin's lymphoma is a disorder of the lymphocytes that involves many different histological variations; it does not have the Reed-Sternberg cell, differentiating it from the Hodgkin's lymphoma. It is seen more frequently in middle-aged men.

Depending on the type of lymphoma, therapeutic management may consist of combination chemotherapy, radiation therapy, and/or stem cell transplantation. The prognosis is usually poorer for non-Hodgkin's lymphoma because of its later stage at diagnosis.

The goals of nursing care are to provide educational and emotional support and to prevent complications. This care plan addresses ongoing care of a patient in an ambulatory setting receiving maintenance therapy.

Hematolymphatic, Immunological, and Oncological Care Plans

Deficient Knowledge

Common Related Factors

Insufficient information
Insufficient interest in learning
Misinformation presented by others
Insufficient knowledge of resources

Defining Characteristics

Insufficient knowledge
Inaccurate follow-through of instruction
Inappropriate behavior

Common Expected Outcome

Patient verbalizes understanding of diagnosis, treatment strategies, and prognosis.

NOC Outcomes
Knowledge: Cancer Management; Knowledge: Disease Process; Knowledge: Treatment Procedure

NIC Interventions
Health Literacy Enhancement; Learning Facilitation; Teaching: Disease Process; Teaching: Procedure/Treatment

Ongoing Assessment

Action/Intervention

■ Assess the patient's knowledge of the disease, its treatment strategies, and prognosis.

Rationale

Several types of lymphoma occur, each with its own treatment approach and prognosis; this can be confusing. QSEN: Patient-centered care.

Therapeutic Interventions

Actions/Interventions

■ Describe the function of the lymphatic system and the abnormalities associated with lymphoma.
■ Clarify the diagnostic process:
  • Peripheral blood analysis

  • Lymph node biopsy

  • Bone marrow biopsy
  • Computed tomography (CT) scan/magnetic resonance imaging (MRI)
  • X-ray study

  • Positron emission tomography (PET) scan

Rationales

Most individuals are not familiar with the complexities of the hematological system unless an illness strikes.

Analysis may reveal a microcytic hypochromic anemia, lymphopenia (neutrophilic leukocytosis), and elevated platelet count.
Lymph node biopsy provides tissue for histological examination that is needed in diagnosing cell types and staging the disease. Knowing the stage of the disease determines treatment and aids in the estimation of prognosis. Biopsy may be performed either as an open biopsy (in the operating room) or a closed needle biopsy (at the bedside or as an outpatient procedure).
Bone marrow biopsy can assist with the staging of the disease.
These scans are used to assess abdominal lymph nodes and liver, spleen, bone, and brain infiltrates.
An x-ray study is used to detect lymphoma in the chest area as well as additional sites of disease.
A PET scan provides information on the site of the tumor using increased metabolic activity as a marker.

Hematolymphatic, Immunological, and Oncological Care Plans

■ = Independent   ▲ = Interprofessional Collaboration

Actions/Interventions	Rationales
■ Clarify the similarities and differences between Hodgkin's lymphoma and non-Hodgkin's lymphoma. 　• Common presenting symptoms include fever, weight loss, night sweats, pruritus, nontender enlarged lymph nodes, and possibly an enlarged spleen and liver.	Although both have similar presenting symptoms and treatment approaches, significant differences in actual treatment therapies and response to therapy do exist. Non-Hodgkin's lymphoma has a poorer prognosis because of its later stage at diagnosis.
■ Discuss common treatment approaches:	Providing information about treatment approaches allows the patient to be a full partner in making decisions regarding care. QSEN: Evidence-based practice; Patient-centered care.
• Radiation therapy	Radiation therapy is indicated for stages 1 and 2 in Hodgkin's lymphoma and for localized non-Hodgkin's lymphoma. Radiation therapy is most useful when the lymphoma is in one part of the body, e.g., the chest. It is often given after chemotherapy, as combined treatment is more effective. A newer type of radiation, involved site radiation therapy (ISRT), is now used because of its ability to focus directly on the diseased lymph nodes while sparing nearby tissues. Patients getting stem cell transplants may get total body irradiation along with chemotherapy.
• Combined chemotherapy/biological therapy (immunotherapy)	Combined chemotherapy, which includes monoclonal antibodies, is common for stages 3 and 4 in Hodgkin's lymphoma. Chemotherapy is also indicated for generalized non-Hodgkin's lymphoma. Many protocols exist depending on the type of lymphoma. *NOTE:* Older patients have significant problems dealing with the adverse side effects of these aggressive treatments. Initial chemotherapy is performed in the hospital. However, follow-up courses may be administered in an outpatient or sometimes a home setting.
• Stem cell transplantation	Transplantation is indicated when patients have not shown remission with radiation and/or chemotherapy or have relapsed after chemotherapy. Autologous (patient is the donor) transplantations are most frequently used. Allogenic (matched donor) transplantation is used if the disease has spread to the bone marrow.
• Participating in a clinical trial	Clinical trials may be an option for patients before starting standard treatment or for those who are nonresponsive to treatment.
■ Explain common complications of the therapy.	Complications include pancytopenia from radiation and chemotherapy (anemia, bleeding, infection), nausea and vomiting from chemotherapy, fatigue and weakness.
■ Discuss the prognosis.	Prognosis depends on the type of disease, the stage at which the diagnosis was made, and the response to the treatment plan. Generally complete remissions are possible in about 80% of patients with Hodgkin's lymphoma. Patients with non-Hodgkin's lymphoma usually have a poorer prognosis because of its later stage at diagnosis. QSEN: Patient-centered care.

Hematolymphatic, Immunological, and Oncological Care Plans

NANDA-I NDx **Cancer-Related Fatigue**

Common Related Factors

Tumor and metastatic disease
Chemotherapy or targeted therapy
Radiation
Pain
Distress (spiritual or emotional)
Anxiety and/or fear
Malnutrition
Anemia

Defining Characteristics

A sense of physical or emotional tiredness that is not proportional to recent activity or treatment and interferes with the individual's daily functioning
Inability to restore energy, even after sleep
Verbalization of an overwhelming lack of energy

Common Expected Outcomes

Patient reports reduction in fatigue, as evidenced by reports of increased energy and ability to perform desired activities.
Patient reports use of energy-conservation principles.

NOC Outcomes

Fatigue Level; Fatigue: Disruptive Effects; Activity Tolerance; Endurance; Energy Conservation; Self-Care: Activities of Daily Living (ADLs)

NIC Interventions

Energy Management; Nutrition Management; Sleep Enhancement; Exercise Promotion

Ongoing Assessment

Actions/Interventions

■ Assess for fatigue regularly using a scale of 0 to 10 and defining characteristics.

■ Refer to Fatigue (Chapter 2).

Rationale

Fatigue has become the most common and distressing complaint for patients with cancer, especially during treatment. Regular assessment allows the nurse to evaluate the fatigue and the response to interventions and develop and alter the plan accordingly. QSEN: Patient-centered care.

Therapeutic Interventions

Actions/Interventions

In addition to the interventions in the Fatigue care plan, consider the following:
■ Educate the patient regarding these treatments:

• Assigning priorities to activities to accommodate energy levels

• Energy-conservation strategies, such as:
  • Sitting to do tasks
  • Pushing rather than pulling
  • Working at an even pace
  • Placing frequently used items within easy reach
  • Using wheeled carts for laundry, shopping, cleaning needs
• Limiting naps to 20 to 30 minutes

Rationales

Providing information regarding home care treatments allows the patient to be a full partner in providing care, making decisions, and achieving optimal recovery outcomes. QSEN: Patient-centered care.
Setting priorities while conserving energy will allow the patient to achieve most desired goals and feel a sense of accomplishment.
Energy-conservation techniques reduce oxygen consumption, allowing more prolonged activity

Limiting the amount of sleep during naps will help the patient to sleep at night.

■ = Independent ▲ = Interprofessional Collaboration

Hematolymphatic, Immunological, and Oncological Care Plans

Actions/Interventions

- Use of psychostimulants (e.g., Ritalin) after ruling out other causes
- Treatment for anemia as indicated

- Cognitive behavioral therapy

- Nutrition consultation

Rationales

These medications have been used cautiously and demonstrate improved symptoms of fatigue in some patients.

Cancer patients' anemia results from the disease itself and treatment. Correcting the anemia may improve the patient's energy level.

This type of psychotherapy facilitates psychological adjustment to the cancer experience by helping certain patients recognize and change maladaptive thoughts.

A dietitian can counsel the patient and family on how to maximize the patient's intake during treatment for optimal nutritional needs. QSEN: Teamwork and collaboration.

NANDA-I NDx **Risk for Ineffective Coping**

Common Risk Factors

Situational crisis
Inadequate support system
Inadequate coping methods

Common Expected Outcome

Patient demonstrates positive coping strategies, as evidenced by expression of feelings and hopes, realistic goal setting for future, and use of available resources and support systems.

NOC Outcomes
Coping; Social Support; Family Coping
NIC Interventions
Coping Enhancement; Hope Inspiration; Grief Work Facilitation; Support System Enhancement

---

Ongoing Assessment

Actions/Interventions

- Assess the patient's knowledge of the disease and its treatment plan.
- Assess for the coping mechanisms used in previous illnesses or prior hospitalizations.

- Evaluate the resources and support systems available to the patient at home and in the community.

- Assess the financial resources required for extensive long-term therapy.

Rationales

Because lymphoma is a cancer, the patient may expect to die. Realistic but positive information may be indicated.

Successful coping is influenced by previous successes. Patients with a history of maladaptive coping may require additional resources. Likewise, previously successful coping skills may be inadequate in the present situation. QSEN: Patient-centered care.

Lymphoma treatment may require months and years of ongoing chemotherapy, depending on the length of remission. Available support systems may change over time. QSEN: Patient-centered care.

The financial aspects of acute care and long-term follow-up can be overwhelming, especially when the patient is dealing with a new diagnosis.

---

evolve For additional care plans, go to http://evolve.elsevier.com/Gulanick/.

Therapeutic Interventions

Actions/Interventions	Rationales
■ Establish open lines of communication; establish a working relationship with the patient through continuity of care.	The nurse may be the first person the patient and family turn to as a source of support. An ongoing relationship establishes trust, reduces the feeling of isolation, and may facilitate coping.
■ Provide opportunities for the patient and significant others to openly express feelings, fears, and concerns. Provide hope but avoid false reassurances.	The verbalization of actual or perceived threats can help reduce anxiety and open doors for ongoing communication. An honest relationship facilitates problem-solving and successful coping. False reassurances are never helpful to the patient and only serve to relieve the discomfort of the care provider. QSEN: Patient-centered care.
■ Assist the patient in grieving and working through the losses associated with life-threatening illness, if appropriate.	Grief is a universal experience; people who have successfully undergone grief over a loss can be enormously helpful to others undergoing the same feelings. QSEN: Patient-centered care.
■ Assist the patient and significant others in redefining hopes and components of individuality (e.g., roles, values, and attitudes).	Emphasizing the patient's intrinsic worth and viewing the immediate situation as manageable in time may provide support. QSEN: Patient-centered care.
■ Introduce new information about disease treatment, as available.	Chemotherapy agents may change. The patient may become a candidate for stem cell transplantation. Clinical trials are also available for these patients.
■ Assist the patient in becoming involved as a co-manager of the treatment plan.	This helps the patient regain control over the situation. Many patients become educated about their chemotherapeutic agents and possible side effects. QSEN: Patient-centered care.
■ Assist in the development of an alternative support system. Encourage participation in self-help groups as available.	Relationships with people with common interests and goals can be beneficial. Participation in support groups may allow the patient to realize that others have the same problem, and they may use this as an aid for coping. QSEN: Patient-centered care.
■ Describe the community resources available to meet the unique demands of lymphoma, its treatment, and survival.	It is helpful for patients to have more than one resource for assisting them in this process. Reliable websites may likewise offer information and support.
▲ Refer to a social worker for financial assistance as indicated.	The social worker can assist the patient and family with decisions about finances, living arrangements, wills, advance directives, and power of attorney. QSEN: Teamwork and collaboration.

Hematolymphatic, Immunological, and Oncological Care Plans

Risk for Infection

Common Risk Factors

Cancer resulting in altered immunological responses
Immunosuppression secondary to chemotherapy and radiation therapy

Common Expected Outcome

Patient is at reduced risk for local or systemic infection, as evidenced by afebrile state, normal vital signs, chest x-ray film results within normal limits, negative results of blood and surveillance cultures, compliance with preventive measures, and prompt reporting of early signs of infection.

NOC Outcomes

Immune Status; Knowledge: Infection Management; Tissue Integrity: Skin and Mucous Membranes

NIC Interventions

Infection Protection; Teaching: Disease Process; Oral Health Maintenance

---

■ = Independent   ▲ = Interprofessional Collaboration

Ongoing Assessment

Actions/Interventions	Rationales
■ Auscultate the lung fields for crackles, rhonchi, and decreased breath sounds.	Pulmonary infections are common in immunocompromised patients. QSEN: Safety.
■ Observe the patient for coughing spells and the character of sputum.	An increase in the amount of sputum and changes in its color from clear or white to yellow or green may indicate a respiratory infection. QSEN: Safety.
■ Inspect the body sites with a high infection potential (mouth, throat, axilla, skin folds, perineum, rectum).	Opportunistic infections of the mucous membrane surfaces of the body are often the first type of infection to develop in the immunocompromised patient. QSEN: Safety.
■ Inspect the peripheral IV, central venous catheter and port sites for redness, tenderness, pain, and itching.	In the absence of granulocytes, a site of infection may develop without characteristic pus formation. Careful assessment is key. QSEN: Safety.
■ Observe for changes in the color, character, and frequency of urine and stool.	These observations provide data on a possible urinary tract infection or intestinal infection. QSEN: Safety.
■ Monitor the patient's temperature as indicated. Report elevations per protocol.	Fever may be the only sign of infection. Patients need to be instructed to record serial temperatures at home. QSEN: Safety.
▲ Obtain culture for temperature elevation per institutional protocol.	Cultures are required to determine the organism causing the infection and antibiotic sensitivity. QSEN: Safety.

Therapeutic Interventions

Actions/Interventions	Rationales
■ Explain the cause and effects of leukopenia.	Leukopenic cells replace normal cells. Also, chemotherapy causes bone marrow suppression and a reduced number of neutrophils needed to fight infection.
■ Instruct the patient to maintain personal hygiene, especially at home: • Encourage a daily shower with a mild antimicrobial soap • Wash hands well before eating and after using the bathroom • Wipe the perineal area from front to back	Handwashing removes transient and residual bacteria from the hands. The perineal area is a source of pathogens and a frequent entry port for microorganisms. Providing information allows the patient to be a full partner in assuming responsibility for care at home. QSEN: Safety; Patient-centered care.
■ Instruct the patient to brush teeth with a soft toothbrush four times per day and as necessary, to remove dentures at night, and to rinse the mouth after each emesis or when expectorating phlegm.	Intact oral mucous membranes are the first line of defense in controlling the development of oral infections. Periodontal disease is a locus of infection. QSEN: Safety.
■ Teach the patient to inspect the oropharyngeal area daily for white patches in the mouth, coated or encrusted oral ulcerations, a swollen and erythematous tongue with a white or brown coating, an infected throat and pain on swallowing, debris on the teeth, ill-fitting dentures, and the amount and viscosity of saliva.	The oral cavity and upper respiratory tract are common infection sites in patients with lymphoma and neutropenia. Candidiasis is a common opportunistic infection of the oral and esophageal mucous membranes. QSEN: Safety.
■ Teach the patient to avoid mouthwashes that contain alcohol and avoid irritating foods and acidic drinks.	Alcohol has a drying effect on mucous membranes.
■ Teach the patient to use prescribed topical medications (e.g., nystatin [Nilstat] and lidocaine [Xylocaine]).	These agents may require specific instructions.
■ Instruct the patient and caregiver to maintain strict aseptic technique when changing dressings and to avoid wetting central catheter dressings.	These measures help prevent bacterial growth. Information about aseptic technique helps the patient and caregiver assume responsibility for care and reduce the risk of harm to the patient. QSEN: Safety.
■ Instruct the patient to observe for fever spikes and flulike symptoms (e.g., malaise, weakness, myalgia) and to notify the nurse or physician if they occur.	Early assessment facilitates prompt treatment and reduces the risk of harm to the patient. QSEN: Safety.

Actions/Interventions

- Instruct the patient and caregiver regarding the importance of eliminating potential sources of infection at home (especially when neutrophil counts are low):
  - Avoid contact with visitors or family, especially children with colds or infections and those who attend daycare, preschool, or elementary school.
  - Restrict contact with a person recently immunized with a live vaccine.
  - Avoid sharing drinking and eating utensils.
  - Avoid contact with cat litter boxes, fish tanks, and human or animal excreta.
  - Avoid swimming in private or public pools.
  - Restrict contact with live plants.
- Instruct the patient regarding protective isolation if laboratory results indicate neutropenia (absolute neutrophil count [ANC] <500 to 1000/mm³).
- Implement thorough handwashing for staff and visitors before physical contact with the patient.

- Instruct the patient to take prescribed antibiotic, antifungal, or antiviral drugs on time.
- ▲ Refer the patient to a dietitian for instructions on the maintenance of a well-balanced diet.

Rationales

Patients must understand the strategies and measures by which they can protect themselves during times of compromised defense. Animal excreta, soil, and people with known infections are sources of opportunistic infection for the immunocompromised patient. QSEN: Safety.

Institutional protocols may vary, but are based on national guidelines. QSEN: Safety; Evidence-based practice.

Handwashing removes transient and resident bacteria from hands, thus minimizing or preventing transmission to the patient. QSEN: Safety.

A regular schedule is needed to maintain therapeutic drug levels.

A specialist may provide additional help. This diet is for the maintenance of optimal health status, which promotes the improvement of host resistance and bone marrow recovery. QSEN: Teamwork and collaboration.

NANDA-I NDx Risk for Bleeding

Common Risk Factor

Bone marrow depression secondary to chemotherapy or radiation therapy

Common Expected Outcome

Patient's risk for bleeding is reduced, as evidenced by platelet count within acceptable limits, compliance with preventive measures, and prompt reporting of early signs and symptoms.

NOC Outcomes
Blood Coagulation; Knowledge: Disease Process

NIC Interventions
Bleeding Precautions; Teaching: Disease Process

Hematolymphatic, Immunological, and Oncological Care Plans

Ongoing Assessment

Actions/Interventions

- ▲ Monitor the patient's platelet count, including nadir.

Rationales

Nadir is when platelets are at their lowest point. The risk for bleeding increases as the platelet count drops:
- Mild thrombocytopenia: platelets 50,000 to 100,000/mm³
- Moderate risk: platelets 20,000 to 50,000/mm³
- Severe risk: platelets 20,000/mm³ or less
- Transfusion threshold: platelet count less than 10,000/mm³ or signs of active bleeding

Early assessment reduces risk. QSEN: Safety.

■ = Independent ▲ = Interprofessional Collaboration

Actions/Interventions

- Assess for signs and symptoms of bleeding. These may include petechiae and bruising, hemoptysis, epistaxis, bleeding in oral mucosa, hematemesis, hematochezia, melena, vaginal bleeding, dizziness, orthostatic changes, decreased BP, headaches, changes in mental and visual acuity, and an increased pulse rate.
- Note bleeding from any recent puncture site (e.g., venipuncture, bone marrow aspiration site).

Rationales

Early assessment facilitates prompt treatment and the reduced risk for complications. QSEN: Safety.

Prolonged oozing from puncture sites may be the first sign of bleeding problems. QSEN: Safety.

Therapeutic Interventions

Actions/Interventions

- Explain to the patient and significant others the symptoms of thrombocytopenia and the functions of platelets:
  - Normal range of platelet count
  - Effects of thrombocytopenia
  - Rationale of bleeding precautions
- Instruct the patient in precautionary measures. Initiate bleeding precautions for a platelet count less than 50,000/mm³:

  - Use a soft toothbrush and nonabrasive toothpaste.
  - Inspect the gums for oozing.
  - Avoid using toothpicks and dental floss.
  - Avoid rectal suppositories, thermometers, enemas, vaginal douches, and tampons.
  - Avoid aspirin or aspirin-containing products, nonsteroidal anti-inflammatory drugs (NSAIDs), and anticoagulants.

  - Avoid straining with bowel movements, forceful nose blowing, coughing, or sneezing.
  - Count used sanitary pads during menstruation. Report any menstrual cycle changes.
  - Avoid sharp objects such as scissors and knives. Use an electric razor for shaving (not razor blades).

  - Lubricate the nostrils with saline solution drops as necessary and lips with petroleum jelly as needed.
  - Practice gentle sex; use a water-based lubricant before sexual intercourse.
  - Protect self from injury and trauma (e.g., falls, bumps, strenuous exercise, contact sports).
  - Give the patient and family at least two telephone numbers to call in case of bleeding.
  - Instruct the patient to take antacids as prescribed when taking steroids, NSAIDs, or aspirin.

In the health care setting:

- Avoid finger sticks if possible. Coordinate laboratory work so all tests are done at one time.
- Avoid intramuscular and subcutaneous injections. If necessary, use small-bore needles for injections and apply ice to the injection site for 5 minutes. Observe the site for oozing.

Rationales

Most individuals are not familiar with the complexities of the hematological system. A successful plan requires the knowledge and cooperation of the patient and family members. QSEN: Patient-centered care.

An understanding of precautionary measures reduces the risk for bleeding. At platelet counts less than 20,000/mm³, spontaneous bleeding can occur. QSEN: Safety; Evidence-based practice.

This method reduces the risk for bleeding.

Oozing can be an early sign of bleeding.

These items stimulate bleeding.

This measure reduces mucosal trauma.

These medications interfere with platelet function.

This measure reduces the risk for bleeding.

This measure provides data on bleeding status.

It is important to prevent cuts, which would not only bleed but also become portals of entry for microorganisms, leading to infection in the presence of neutropenia.

Lubrication prevents drying and cracking.

These measures prevent mucosal trauma.

Patient safety is a priority.

Prearranged contact information facilitates early treatment.

Antacids reduce gastric irritation.

These nursing actions reduce the risk of harm to the patient from bleeding. QSEN: Safety.

This precaution reduces bleeding risk.

These measures reduce bleeding potential at the injection site.

Actions/Interventions

■ Apply pressure, a dressing, or sandbag to the bone marrow aspiration site.

▲ Apply ice or a topical thrombin promptly as prescribed for bleeding mucous membranes.

■ Discuss the possibility of platelet transfusions. Teach the patient the purpose and possible reactions to transfusions.

▲ Ensure the availability and readiness of platelets for transfusion.

Rationales

This procedure prevents excessive pressure when compressing soft tissues and deeper structures of the arm, because this may lead to bruising or hematomas.

Thrombin promotes clot formation.

Knowledge reduces anxiety. Transfusions may be needed to maintain an adequate platelet count to prevent spontaneous or excessive bleeding.

It is important to have platelets available when needed to prevent spontaneous or excessive bleeding (generally for a platelet count less than 20,000/mm^3 or according to institutional protocol).

NANDA-I
ND$_X$ Nausea

Common Related Factors

Treatment effects:
- Side effects of chemotherapy (inability to taste and smell foods, loss of appetite, nausea, vomiting, mucositis, dry mouth, diarrhea)
- Medications (e.g., narcotics, antibiotics, vitamins)

Disease effects:
- Primary malignancy or metastasis
- Tumor waste products

Psychogenic effects:
- Conditioning to adverse stimuli (e.g., anticipatory nausea and vomiting, tension, anxiety, stress)
- Depression

Defining Characteristics

Reports "nausea" or "sick to stomach"
Increased salivation
Increased swallowing
Gagging sensation
Sour taste
Aversion toward food

Common Expected Outcome

Patient reports diminished severity or elimination of nausea.

NOC Outcomes

Nutritional Status: Food and Fluid Intake; Comfort Status; Symptom Severity

NIC Interventions

Chemotherapy Management; Nutrition Therapy; Oral Health Maintenance; Medication Administration

---

Ongoing Assessment

Actions/Interventions

■ Assess the patient's description of the nausea and vomiting pattern before each cycle of chemotherapy.

Rationales

Patient responses are individualized, depending on the type and dosage of chemotherapy. Ongoing assessment is important so that treatment plans can be revised as needed. Assessment data should include the number of episodes of nausea or vomiting after therapy; the timing of nausea or vomiting; the ability to eat after therapy; antiemetics taken; and other related symptoms. Nausea and vomiting may be acute, delayed, and for some patients even before ("anticipatory") the chemotherapy treatment. QSEN: Patient-centered care.

■ = Independent   ▲ = Interprofessional Collaboration

Hematolymphatic, Immunological, and Oncological Care Plans

Actions/Interventions

■ Evaluate the effectiveness of the antiemetic and comfort measure regimens.

■ Observe the patient for potential complications of prolonged nausea and vomiting.

■ Weigh the patient at each clinic visit and always prior to each treatment. If the patient is at home, stress the importance of maintaining a daily log.

■ Encourage the patient to record any food intake using a daily log.

Rationales

A patient's response to antiemetic and comfort medications is highly variable and must be explored with each patient. Newer antiemetic medications have improved this condition for many patients. Anticipatory nausea can be difficult to overcome. QSEN: Patient-centered care.

Nausea and vomiting can alter a patient's hydration status because of fluid loss and effect electrolyte imbalance (hypokalemia; decreased sodium and chloride). Persistent vomiting and reduced nutritional intake can result in weight loss, a decreased activity level, and lethargy. QSEN: Safety.

Consistent weighing is important to ensure accuracy. Without monitoring, the patient may be unaware of small changes in weight.

Determination of the type, amount, and pattern of food intake (if any) is facilitated by accurate documentation, which provides information as to whether oral intake meets daily nutritional requirements.

Therapeutic Interventions

Actions/Interventions

▲ Administer antiemetics according to protocol.

■ Explain that the selection of antiemetic agents should be based on the emetic risk of the therapy and risk factors in the patient.

▲ Administer antiemetics around the clock rather than as needed during periods of high incidence of nausea and vomiting.

Rationales

Symptoms of chemotherapy-induced nausea and vomiting (CINV) can have an acute, delayed, anticipatory, or breakthrough onset. Often a combination of antiemetic medications is needed to effectively control nausea and vomiting and must correlate appropriately to the emetogenic potential of chemotherapy agents given. Serotonin 5-HT$_3$ receptor antagonists (i.e., ondansetron and palonosetron), neurokinin-1 receptor antagonists (i.e., aprepitant), and corticosteroids (i.e., dexamethasone) are the most common drug classes used for CINV. Other drug classes include phenothiazines (i.e., prochlorperazine), benzodiazepines (i.e., lorazepam), cannabinoids (i.e., dronabinal), and the dopamine 2 receptor antagonist, metoclopramide. QSEN: Evidence-based practice.

The Oncology Nursing Society provides resources for recommended antiemetic regimens for high, moderately high, low, and minimal emetogenic chemotherapy. The administration of optimal antiemetic therapy during every cycle of chemotherapy will reduce the development of anticipatory nausea and vomiting. QSEN: Evidence-based practice; Patient-centered care.

The effectiveness of antiemetic therapy is increased when adequate plasma levels are maintained.

Actions/Interventions

■ Institute or teach measures to reduce or prevent nausea and vomiting:

- Small dietary intake before treatment

- An antiemetic half an hour before meals as prescribed

- Foods with a low potential to cause nausea and vomiting (e.g., dry toast, crackers, ginger ale, cola, popsicles, gelatin, baked or boiled potatoes, fresh or canned fruit, bland foods)
- Avoidance of spices, gravy, greasy fried foods, and foods with strong odors
- Meals at room temperature; serve foods cold if odors cause aversions
- Avoidance of coaxing, bribing, or threatening in relation to intake (help the family avoid being "food pushers")
- Sucking on hard candy (e.g., peppermint) while receiving chemotherapeutic drugs with a "metallic taste"
- Drinking fluids at a different time than when eating solid snacks or meals
- Offering meat dishes in the morning

- Minimal physical activity and no sudden rapid movements during times of increased nausea
- Relaxation and distraction techniques; guided imagery

- Use of acupuncture or acupressure.

- Cannabis

Rationales

Behavioral and dietary interventions seem to be most effective in the management of anticipatory nausea and vomiting. This pattern of nausea and vomiting is related to classic conditioning. The patient develops nausea and vomiting in response to stimuli associated with the administration of chemotherapeutic drugs. Patients may try a variety of interventions to find those that best control this type of nausea and vomiting before drug administration. Antiemetic medications have been found less effective in the management of anticipatory nausea and vomiting. However, antianxiety medications (e.g., lorazepam) may be effective. QSEN: Evidence-based practice; Patient-centered care.

Eating small amounts reduces gastric overstimulation, thus reducing vomiting risk.

Antiemetics relieve nausea and vomiting. The appropriate timing of medications can reduce the onset and severity of nausea.

These foods are easily digested and provide a measure of success to augment nutrition.

Fats are difficult to digest and may exacerbate nausea and can stimulate gastric motility.

Hot foods can stimulate peristalsis. The smell of cooking foods may aggravate feelings of nausea.

Such behaviors tend to only aggravate the situation.

Hard candies can reduce the metallic or bitter taste.

Separating fluids from solids will help with not "filling" the stomach quickly. This may help prevent nausea as well.

Aversions tend to increase during the day: chicken, cheese, eggs, and fish are usually well-tolerated protein sources.

Activity or sudden movements may potentiate nausea and vomiting.

These techniques, especially guided imagery, are useful adjuncts to antiemetic drug therapy. They can be helpful if used before nausea occurs or increases.

Several small studies report acupuncture and acupressure to be useful measures in reducing nausea and vomiting risk.

Medical cannabis is somewhat effective in CINV and may be a reasonable option for patients who do not improve with standard treatment. The FDA has approved two cannabinoids (dronabinol and nabilone) for prevention and treatment of CINV. QSEN: Evidence-based practice; Patient-centered care.

Related Care Plans

Caregiver role strain, Chapter 2
Deficient fluid volume, Chapter 2
Disturbed body image, Chapter 2
Fear, Chapter 2
Cancer chemotherapy, Chapter 10
Cancer radiation therapy, Chapter 10
Hematopoietic stem cell transplantation, Chapter 10

Hematolymphatic, Immunological, and Oncological Care Plans

■ = Independent ▲ = Interprofessional Collaboration

Multiple Myeloma

Plasma Cell Myeloma; Monoclonal Gammopathy of Undetermined Significance (MGUS)

Multiple myeloma is a plasma B-cell malignancy that is characterized by the overproduction of immunoglobulins (abnormal antibodies known as monoclonal proteins or M proteins). This pathophysiology results in disruption of normal red blood cells, leukocytes, and platelets, resulting in anemia, infection, and bleeding problems. The excess immunoglobins also produce excess cytokines resulting in progressive bone destruction. The cause of multiple myeloma is unknown, with no clear risk factors identified beyond age (mid 60s), male sex, and black race. Multiple myeloma usually starts out as a benign condition called monoclonal gammopathy of undetermined significance (MGUS) characterized by the presence of abnormal M proteins. Only about 1% of people with MGUS go on to develop multiple myeloma. Multiple myeloma develops slowly with no specific symptoms. Clinically, it may present itself as destruction of bone, infiltration of bone marrow, the presence of immunoglobulins in the urine or serum, recurrent infections, pain, fatigue, or symptoms of renal failure. While previously considered to be incurable, newer therapies, especially stem cell transplant, are significantly prolonging lives.

NANDA-I
NDx Deficient Knowledge

Common Related Factors
Insufficient information
Insufficient interest in learning
Misinformation presented by others
Insufficient knowledge of resources

Defining Characteristics
Insufficient knowledge
Inaccurate follow-through of instruction
Inappropriate behavior

Common Expected Outcome
Patient and significant others verbalize understanding of the diagnosis and treatment plan for multiple myeloma, side effects of medications, and follow-up care.

NOC Outcomes
Knowledge: Disease Process; Knowledge: Treatment Procedure

NIC Interventions
Health Literacy Enhancement; Learning Facilitation; Teaching: Disease Process; Support System Enhancement

---

Ongoing Assessment

Action/Intervention	Rationale
■ Assess the patient's knowledge of the disease, its treatment plan, and prognosis.	The patient and family need information based on their understanding of the disease. This type of cancer is less publicized in the media than lung, breast, and colon cancers, so patients may have had little exposure to this hematological cancer. QSEN: Patient-centered care.

Therapeutic Interventions

Actions/Interventions	Rationales
■ Provide information on the following:	
• Nature of the disease	Malignant plasma cells infiltrate the bone marrow and disrupt blood cells.
• Diagnosis	A diagnosis of multiple myeloma requires the consideration of several factors: physical examination, laboratory tests, and symptoms.
• Bone marrow analysis	Large numbers of immature plasma cells are noted with this diagnosis.
• Computed tomography (CT) bone scans, x-ray studies, magnetic resonance imaging (MRI)	These tests show the degree of demineralization and osteoporosis.
• Laboratory studies (chemistry, complete blood count, serum protein electrophoresis, C-reactive protein [CRP], monoclonal immunoglobulin levels, beta 2-albumin)	An abnormal globulin (Bence Jones protein) is seen in serum and urine; increased serum calcium is noted. Because of the increased number of plasma cells producing immunoglobulins, plasma electrophoresis is performed to quantify amounts.
• Twenty-four–hour urine protein and urine protein electrophoresis	These tests show the presence of M proteins (Bence Jones proteins) in the urine and help stage the disease.
• Treatment plan—medical treatment of signs and symptoms:	Treatment is focused on managing both the disease and its symptoms. For some patients without symptoms, treatment may not be necessary. For most, chemotherapy with corticosteroids is usually the first-line agents. Many combinations are available depending on the type of myeloma and stage of the disease. Drug selection is determined by whether the patient is a candidate for stem cell transplant. Targeted therapy blocks the action of a substance in myeloma cells that breaks down proteins, causing myeloma cells to die. QSEN: Evidence-based practice.
• Watchful waiting for asymptomatic patients	
• Targeted therapy (bortezomib and carfilzomib)	
• Biological therapy (thalidomide, lenalidomide, pomalidomide)	
• Chemotherapy (many possible agents can be used), with high dose indicated prior to hematopoietic stem cell transplantation	
• Hematopoietic stem cell transplantation	
• Radiation therapy	
• Pain management strategies	An analgesic combination is required for relief. Radiation therapy may be required to help control bone pain.
• Diet and fluid therapy	Therapy is required to prevent or treat hypercalcemia, hyperuricemia, and renal impairment.
• Importance of mobility	Weight bearing prevents further bone demineralization.
• Safety precautions	Great care must be taken to prevent falls and pathological fractures in this high-risk population.
■ Involve the family and caregivers so they can effectively provide support in the home environment.	Because most patients are older, a variety of support services may be required.

Acute Pain

NANDA-I NDx

Common Related Factors	Defining Characteristics
Pain resulting from medical problem (invasion of marrow and bone by plasma cells)	Self-report of pain using a standardized pain scale
Pathological fractures	Facial expression of pain
	Change in physiological parameters (e.g., BP, HR, respiratory rate)

■ = Independent ▲ = Interprofessional Collaboration

Common Expected Outcomes

Patient reports satisfactory pain control at a decreased intensity using a standardized pain scale.

Patient uses pharmacological and nonpharmacological pain relief measures.

Patient exhibits increased comfort such as baseline levels for BP, HR, respirations, and relaxed muscle tone or body posture.

NOC Outcomes

Pain Control; Comfort Status; Medication Response

NIC Interventions

Pain Management; Analgesic Administration; Distraction

Ongoing Assessment

Actions/Interventions

■ Assess the location of pain and its characteristics.

■ Assess the effectiveness of relief measures.

Rationales

Assessment of the pain experience is the first step in planning pain management strategies. Skeletal pain, especially in the lower back and ribs, occurs most commonly and is often the presenting symptom. Pain may be constant and severe, and may increase with movement. QSEN: Patient-centered care.

It is important to help patients express as factually as possible the effect of pain relief measures. During terminal stages, pain management is extremely challenging. QSEN: Patient-centered care.

Therapeutic Interventions

Actions/Interventions

▲ Provide analgesics in the dosage, route, and frequency best suited to the individual patient. Consider an around-the-clock schedule, continuous infusion, fentanyl (Duragesic) patch, or patient-controlled analgesia. Consider combination analgesics.

■ Instruct the patient to take analgesics early and regularly to prevent severe pain. Schedule pain-inducing procedures and activities during the peak analgesic effect.

■ Suggest nonpharmacological measures for comfort: acupuncture, aromatherapy, massage, relaxation techniques unless contraindicated (e.g., because of spinal lesions).

▲ Notify the physician if pain medications are ineffective.

Rationales

The patient with multiple myeloma responds to a combination of interventions for effective pain management. Drug therapy that combines nonsteroidal anti-inflammatory drugs (NSAIDs) with low doses of opioid analgesics is often more effective in decreasing bone pain. QSEN: Patient-centered care.

The timing of administration is crucial to prevent peak pain periods. Unless contraindicated, all patients with acute pain should receive around-the-clock analgesics. Each patient must be evaluated individually as to the optimal regimen.

Patients may not be aware of the effectiveness of nonpharmacological therapies. A trial-and-error period may be required to match therapies to patient preferences. The immobilization of painful areas with braces and splints may enhance pain relief.

A pain service may need to be consulted. Radiation therapy may be required to decrease the size of the lesions causing pain. QSEN: Teamwork and collaboration.

NANDA-I NDx **Impaired Physical Mobility**

Common Related Factors
Bone weakness and osteoporosis
Generalized weakness caused by chemotherapy
Pain or discomfort
Depression
Deconditioning
Decreased endurance
Decreased muscle strength or control
Restricted movement and impaired coordination

Defining Characteristics
Inability to move purposefully within physical environment
Decrease in ability to perform ADLs
Reluctance to attempt movement
Limited range of motion (ROM)

Common Expected Outcomes
Patient performs physical activity independently or within limits of disease.
Patient demonstrates adaptive techniques that promote ambulation and transfer.

NOC Outcomes
Ambulation; Mobility
NIC Interventions
Exercise Therapy: Joint Mobility; Exercise Therapy: Muscle Control; Exercise Therapy: Ambulation

Ongoing Assessment

Actions/Interventions	Rationales
■ Assess the patient's ability to carry out ADLs effectively and safely.	Osteoporosis, progressive weakness, skeletal muscle pain, and malaise are common symptoms of this disease and reduce mobility. Assessing causative factors is key. QSEN: Patient-centered care; Safety.
■ Assess the ability to perform ROM and the level of muscle strength.	Assessment provides data on the extent of physical problems. Decreases in ROM and muscle strength occur as a result of decreased mobility. QSEN: Patient-centered care.

Therapeutic Interventions

Actions/Interventions	Rationales
■ Instruct regarding the importance of ambulation.	Weight bearing stimulates reabsorption and helps prevent further bone demineralization.
■ Stress the importance of maintaining an uncluttered environment.	Attention to environmental factors helps prevent falls and bumping into objects. Bone weakening can readily result in fractures. QSEN: Safety.
■ Encourage the patient to perform ROM exercises.	Exercises promote an increased venous return, prevent stiffness, and maintain muscle strength and endurance. To be most effective, all joints should be exercised to prevent contractures.
■ Instruct the patient to change position every 1 to 2 hours and to get up and sit in a chair as tolerated.	Position changes optimize circulation to all tissues and relieve pressure. Activity and movement reduce the risk for pneumonia, a complication of immobility, especially in older patients.
■ Encourage caregivers to assist the patient with ADLs as indicated.	Help may be required for safety and comfort, but it needs to be balanced with not making the patient unnecessarily dependent.

Hematolymphatic, Immunological, and Oncological Care Plans

■ = Independent   ▲ = Interprofessional Collaboration

Actions/Interventions

- Provide assistive devices (e.g., walker, cane, back brace) as needed.
- Teach energy-saving techniques, and stress the importance of rest periods after ambulation.

Rationales

These devices assist the patient with mobility and enhance patient safety. QSEN: Safety.

Rest periods are necessary to conserve energy. The patient must learn to respect the limits of his or her restrictions. QSEN: Patient-centered care.

NANDA-I
NDx **Risk for Impaired Urinary Elimination**

Common Risk Factors

Immunoglobulin precipitates
Hypercalcemia, hypercalciuria
Hyperuricemia
Pyelonephritis
Myeloma kidney or renal failure
Renal vein thrombosis
Spinal cord compression

Common Expected Outcome

Patient maintains optimal renal function, as evidenced by serum and urine laboratory values within normal limits, and balanced intake and output.

NOC Outcome
Electrolyte and Acid/Base Balance
NIC Interventions
Electrolyte Management: Hypercalcemia; Fluid Management

Ongoing Assessment

Actions/Interventions

▲ Monitor serum laboratory values.

- Assess for signs of hypercalcemia: nausea, vomiting, anorexia, confusion, weakness, constipation, ileus, or abdominal pain.
- Monitor for signs of decreased urine output related to impaired renal function.
- Assess for signs of fluid overload: dyspnea, tachycardia, crackles, distended neck veins, and peripheral edema.

- Monitor the urine for specific gravity, pH, color, odor, and blood.
- Palpate the abdomen for bladder distention.

Rationales

Hypercalcemia and increased uric acid levels occur from bone destruction. Crystallization leads to renal impairment, as seen by increased blood urea nitrogen and creatinine levels. QSEN: Safety.

Gastrointestinal and neurological changes are common manifestations and need to be identified early. QSEN: Safety.

Hyperuricemia may cause renal tubular obstruction and interstitial nephritis from uric acid buildup. QSEN: Safety.

Hydration is used to counterbalance the effects of calcium and protein buildup. Overhydration needs to be prevented. QSEN: Safety.

These tests provide data on fluid balance, as well as evidence of bleeding. QSEN: Safety.

Bladder distention may indicate spinal cord compression from bone damage. QSEN: Safety.

Therapeutic Interventions

Actions/Interventions

- Promote calcium excretion; prevent dehydration.

Rationales

The effects of hypercalcemia are reduced when urine output is maintained at a level of 1.5 to 2 L/24 hr.

---

evolve **For additional care plans, go to http://evolve.elsevier.com/Gulanick/.**

Actions/Interventions

▲ If hypercalcemia is present, increase fluids to 2500 to 3000 mL/day as prescribed.

▲ Provide a low-calcium, low-purine diet, if prescribed.

▲ Administer medications as ordered: biphosphonates such as etidronate (Didronel), pamidronate (Aredia), and zoledronic acid (Zometa).

■ If the patient is confused secondary to increased calcium, provide a safe environment.

■ Prepare for dialysis or plasmapheresis for ongoing renal problems.

Rationales

Hydration dilutes calcium and prevents renal tubular obstruction from protein buildup.

Hypercalcemia is a clinical manifestation of multiple myeloma.

These drugs may be used for hypercalcemia to inhibit the resorption of bone. *NOTE:* Some are given intravenously and require aggressive IV hydration with 0.9% normal saline; allopurinol is given for hyperuricemia; oral phosphates are given for hypophosphatemia.

Safety is a priority. QSEN: Safety.

These therapies may be indicated to prevent or treat impending renal failure.

NANDA-I
NDx Ineffective Protection

Common Related Factors

Bone marrow depression or failure

Replacement or invasion of bone marrow by neoplastic plasma cells

Decrease in synthesis of immunoglobulin by plasma cells secondary to decrease in normal circulating antibodies

Decreased autoimmune response

Chemotherapy

Bone marrow transplantation

Defining Characteristics

Bleeding

Thrombocytopenia

Anemia

Infection

Common Expected Outcomes

Patient maintains hemoglobin (Hgb), hematocrit (Hct), and platelets within normal limits.

Patient's risk for infection is reduced or prevented, as evidenced by normal temperature and absence of active infection.

NOC Outcomes

Immune Status; Blood Coagulation; Infection Severity

NIC Interventions

Chemotherapy Management; Bleeding Precautions; Infection Protection

Hematolymphatic, Immunological, and Oncological Care Plans

Ongoing Assessment

Actions/Interventions

▲ Monitor Hgb, Hct, red blood cells (RBCs), and platelet count.

■ If on chemotherapy, evaluate regimens for potential myelosuppression.

■ If the patient is a candidate for stem cell transplantation, monitor closely for signs of anemia, bleeding, and infection.

■ Observe for signs and symptoms of bleeding.

■ Monitor for signs of infection.

Rationales

Impaired bone marrow function caused by infiltration by plasma cells can predispose the patient to bleeding. QSEN: Safety.

Chemotherapy may aggravate an already existing problem. QSEN: Safety.

Pretreatment with high-dose chemotherapy to eradicate disease may cause significant problems. QSEN: Safety.

Abnormal platelet production increases the risk for bleeding. QSEN: Safety.

Infection is a frequent complication secondary to deficient antibody production and reduced granulocytes from bone marrow depression. QSEN: Safety.

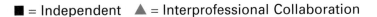

■ = Independent   ▲ = Interprofessional Collaboration

Actions/Interventions

- Observe for coughing (productive and nonproductive) and changes in the color and odor of sputum.
- Review medications.

- ▲ Obtain urine, sputum, and blood for culture and sensitivity testing for temperature elevation per institutional protocol.

Rationales

Bronchopneumonia is a common complication, especially in immunocompromised patients. QSEN: Safety.

The patient taking steroids may not have overt infection symptoms. QSEN: Safety.

Culture and sensitivity results guide antibiotic therapy. QSEN: Safety.

Therapeutic Interventions

Actions/Interventions

- Instruct the patient to avoid unnecessary trauma.

- ▲ Avoid unnecessary IV and intramuscular (IM) injections; if necessary, use the smallest needle possible; apply direct pressure for 3 to 5 minutes after IM injection, venipuncture, and bone marrow aspiration.
- Instruct the patient to:
  - Prevent constipation by increasing oral fluid, increasing fiber intake, and using stool softeners, as prescribed.
  - Use soft toothbrushes.
  - Use an electric razor, not blades.
  - Avoid rectal temperatures and enemas.
- Instruct the patient to avoid aspirin and aspirin-containing compounds.
- ▲ Administer hormones (steroids and androgens) and erythropoietin agents as ordered (e.g., epoetin alfa).

- ▲ Consider platelet and packed RBC transfusion for a platelet count below 10,000/mm^3 and/or Hgb below 7 to 8 g/dL per patient protocol, or for signs of active bleeding.
- ▲ If granulocyte counts are low:
  - Institute a low-microbial diet (well-cooked meat, poultry, and seafood; fresh fruits and vegetables that can be well-washed and peeled; pasteurized milk and dairy products; well-cooked eggs).
  - Instruct the patient to:
    - Avoid exposure to anyone with an infection and anyone recently immunized with live vaccines
    - Avoid sharing drinking and eating utensils
    - Avoid crowds; wear a mask as appropriate
    - Wash hands meticulously
    - Maintain meticulous oral hygiene
    - Restrict exposure to plants and gardening soil
    - Avoid contact with cat litter boxes, fish tanks, and human or animal excreta
- ▲ Maintain a normal or near-normal body temperature with medications as prescribed, a tepid bath, a cooling blanket, and ice packs.

Rationales

Platelet abnormalities increase the risk for bleeding. QSEN: Safety.

This measure reduces the potential for bleeding from injection sites. QSEN: Safety.

Precautions reduce the risk for trauma. Straining causes the breakage of small blood vessels around the anus. Rectal procedures can traumatize the intestinal mucosa. QSEN: Safety.

These drugs interfere with hemostatic platelet function. QSEN: Safety.

These agents stimulate RBC production.

Replacement therapy is indicated to correct deficiencies.

These measures reduce exposure to microbes in food and the environment, which could colonize and increase the risk for infection. The patient's immune function is usually impaired by chemotherapy-induced bone marrow suppression. Patients must understand strategies and measures by which they can protect themselves during times of compromised defense. QSEN: Safety; Patient-centered care; Evidence-based practice.

Normothermia prevents stress on the body and promotes comfort.

Hematolymphatic, Immunological, and Oncological Care Plans

Related Care Plans

Grieving, Chapter 2
Ineffective coping, Chapter 2
Risk for falls, Chapter 2
Cancer chemotherapy, Chapter 10
Hematopoietic stem cell transplantation, Chapter 10
Neutropenia, Chapter 10

Neutropenia

Granulocytopenia

Neutropenia is a deficiency in granulocytes, a type of white blood cell (WBC). There are three types of granulocytes: basophils, eosinophils, and neutrophils. Neutropenia and its complications center around the neutrophilic granulocyte. Neutropenia is a below-normal number of circulating neutrophils that may result in overwhelming, potentially life-threatening infection. Neutrophils constitute 45% to 75% of all WBCs. Their primary function is phagocytosis, the digestion and subsequent destruction of microorganisms; as such, they are one of the body's most powerful first lines of defense against infection. The chance of developing a serious infection is related not only to the absolute level of circulating neutrophils but also to the length of time the patient is neutropenic. A rapid drop and prolonged duration predispose the patient to a higher risk for infection. Neutropenia not only predisposes one to infection but also causes it to be more severe when an infection occurs. Neutropenia is usually associated with another medical condition being treated. It can be acute or chronic. It also occurs as a side effect of taking certain drugs (e.g., chemotherapy and immunosuppressive therapy). Primary diagnosis is by complete blood cell count and bone marrow aspiration. Treatment depends on cause and severity. This care plan focuses on outpatient management.

Hematolymphatic, Immunological, and Oncological Care Plans

NANDA-I NDx Risk for Infection

Common Risk Factors
Neutropenia, secondary to:
- Cancer or similar diseases that destroy bone marrow
- Radiation therapy that damages bone marrow
- Chemotherapy that damages bone marrow
- Hypersplenism that destroys blood cells
- Autoimmune disorders that destroy neutrophils
- Overwhelming infections that destroy neutrophils
- Drugs that impair bone marrow production

Common Expected Outcome
Patient is at reduced risk for local or systemic infection, as evidenced by normal temperature and vital signs, chest x-ray film results within normal limits, negative results of blood and surveillance cultures, compliance with preventive measures, and prompt reporting of early signs of infection.

NOC Outcomes
Infection Severity; Risk Control
NIC Interventions
Infection Protection; Infection Control; Self-Care Assistance; Home Maintenance Assistance; Support System Enhancement

 = Independent   ▲ = Interprofessional Collaboration

Ongoing Assessment

Actions/Interventions

▲ Monitor the WBC with differential count (especially neutrophils and bands).

■ Identify the sources of the low WBC count.

■ Inspect the body sites with a high potential for infection (e.g., orifices, catheter sites, implanted ports, central venous catheters, skin folds).

■ Note any abnormalities in the color and character of sputum, urine, wounds, and stool that might indicate the presence of infection.

■ Monitor for an increased temperature, tachycardia, tachypnea, and hypotension.

■ Assess for local or systemic infection signs and symptoms (e.g., fever, chills, diaphoresis, local redness, warmth, pain, tenderness, excessive malaise, sore throat, dysphagia, retrosternal burning, cellulitis).

■ Identify the medication that the patient may have taken that would mask infection signs and symptoms (e.g., steroids, antipyretics).

▲ Send and evaluate cultures as prescribed for temperature elevation per institution protocol.

Rationales

This laboratory test is used to determine relative risk for bacterial infections associated with absolute neutrophil count (ANC).
- Neutropenia: ANC less than 1500 cells/mm^3
- Mild neutropenia: 1000 to 1500 cells/mm^3
- Moderate neutropenia: 500 to 999 cells/mm^3
- Severe neutropenia: less than 500 cells/mm^3

Early assessment reduces risk for harm. QSEN: Safety.

Several cytotoxic and immunosuppressive medications and therapies can potentially cause neutropenia. QSEN: Safety.

These are frequent sites for infection. Patients with neutropenia do not have the ability to fight infections. QSEN: Safety.

Early detection facilitates prompt intervention for what could be a life-threatening infection. QSEN: Safety.

Neutropenia reduces the body's ability to fight an infection, so signs and symptoms are often subtle. A low-grade fever may be the only predominant warning sign. QSEN: Safety.

Fever and chills may be the initial presentation of infection because in the absence of granulocytes, a locus of infection may develop without the characteristic inflammation or pus formation. A lack of physical signs and symptoms does not exclude the possibility of infection. QSEN: Safety.

This knowledge may lead to more aggressive assessments. QSEN: Safety.

Blood cultures are required to determine the organism causing the infection and antibiotic sensitivity. In severely low counts, antibiotics are started before the source of infection is known. QSEN: Safety; Evidence-based practice.

Therapeutic Interventions

Actions/Interventions

▲ Observe the neutropenic protocol.

■ Wash hands thoroughly with antimicrobial cleanser before physical contact with the patient and between patient care activities (e.g., central line dressing change, mouth care, perineal care).

■ Encourage a daily shower with a mild antimicrobial soap (e.g., chlorhexidine cloths). Explain the need for perineal care (with soap and water) after urination and defecation.

■ Apply lotion to the body after bathing and as needed.

Rationales

The neutropenic protocol protects the patient from exposure to environmental contagions. QSEN: Safety; Evidence-based practice.

Meticulous handwashing is a priority both in the hospital and in the home or ambulatory care setting. Handwashing removes transient and residual bacteria from the hands and prevents transmission to the high-risk patient. QSEN: Safety.

Research continues to determine the best antimicrobial soaps and wipes for bathing. The perineal area is a source of many pathogens and a frequent portal of entry for microorganisms. QSEN: Safety; Evidence-based practice.

The skin and mucous membranes are the first line of defense for the body; when this barrier is weakened or interrupted (e.g., dryness, cracking, abrasions), the site becomes a potential portal of entry for microorganisms and a source of infection. QSEN: Safety.

Actions/Interventions

- Encourage meticulous oral hygiene before and after each meal and at bedtime.
- Encourage oral fluids.

- Instruct on the importance of a low-microbial diet. Refer the patient to a dietitian as needed. Refer to Knowledge Deficit below for more detailed listing of instructions.

- Instruct to avoid herbal supplements (homeopathic remedies or herbal products, such as Chinese medicines).

- ▲ Assist the patient in the selection of a high-protein, high-vitamin, high-calorie diet (refer to a dietitian as needed).

- ▲ Administer stool softeners and high-fiber foods.

- Avoid rectal temperatures, suppositories, and enemas.

- Encourage women to use sanitary napkins instead of tampons.
- Use sterile technique with dressing changes and catheter care.
- Restrict contact with live plants.
- Limit visitors to healthy adults. Discourage anyone with a current or recent infection from visiting the patient either in the hospital or the home. Avoid contact with children of school age. Restrict contact with a person recently immunized with a live virus vaccine.
- If hospitalized, avoid unnecessary invasive procedures. Limit intramuscular and subcutaneous injections.
- ▲ Initiate IV broad-spectrum antibiotic therapy as prescribed, followed by culture-specific antibiotics.

- Instruct the patient regarding the possible addition of granulocyte colony-stimulating factor (G-CSF) and granulocyte-macrophage colony-stimulating factor (GM-CSF) to the medical regimen.

- Anticipate corticosteroid treatment.

Rationales

Oral hygiene is important in the prevention of periodontal disease as a locus of infection. QSEN: Safety.

Fluids assist in meeting hydration requirements (particularly during fever episodes).

This diet protects the patient from exposure to pathogens from foods at a time when host defenses are greatly compromised. Dietary expertise may be needed. QSEN: Safety; Teamwork and collaboration.

There are no federal standards for these products in the United States. Moreover, they may be processed or stored in a risky way. The products themselves could interfere with some prescription medications.

This diet is for the maintenance of optimal health status, which promotes the improvement of host resistance and provides the nutrients necessary to meet energy demands for bone marrow recovery and tissue repair. QSEN: Safety.

Stool softeners prevent constipation, which could traumatize the intestinal mucosa and increase the risk for perirectal abscess or fistula formation. QSEN: Safety.

These objects can traumatize the intestinal mucosa. QSEN: Safety.

The use of napkins avoids trauma to the vaginal mucosa. QSEN: Safety.

This technique also applies to home health nurses and caregivers. QSEN: Safety.

Plants could harbor infective organisms. QSEN: Safety.

People with known infections are sources of opportunistic infections for the immunocompromised patient. Children are commonly exposed to sick playmates. Live attenuated vaccines use an active germ/bacteria and could potentially infect a person who is immunocompromised. QSEN: Safety.

This precaution minimizes the risk for infection. QSEN: Safety.

Broad-spectrum therapy prevents the early dissemination of suspected infection. Once the infection-causing organism is determined, antimicrobial therapy may be adjusted to the type of organism and infection and to the clinical response. QSEN: Safety.

These growth factors can enhance granulocyte recovery secondary to chemotherapy and potentiate the phagocytic activity of neutrophils. Typical medications include filgrastim, pegfilgrastim, and sargramostim. QSEN: Evidence-based practice.

Steroids are indicated to treat neutropenia caused by autoimmune reactions.

Hematolymphatic, Immunological, and Oncological Care Plans

■ = Independent ▲ = Interprofessional Collaboration

NANDA-I NDx Deficient Knowledge

Common Related Factors

Insufficient information
Insufficient interest in learning
Misinformation presented by others
Insufficient knowledge of resources

Defining Characteristics

Insufficient knowledge
Inaccurate follow-through of instruction
Inappropriate behavior

Common Expected Outcome

Patient or caregiver verbalizes understanding of medical diagnosis, treatment plan, safety measures, and follow-up care.

NOC Outcomes

Knowledge: Disease Process; Knowledge: Infection Management

NIC Interventions

Health Literacy Enhancement; Learning Facilitation; Teaching: Disease Process; Teaching: Prescribed Medication; Infection Protection

---

Ongoing Assessment

Action/Intervention	Rationale
■ Assess the patient's knowledge of neutropenia.	Understanding may vary among patients exhibiting their first episode versus patients who experience this side effect more routinely. QSEN: Safety; Patient-centered care.

Therapeutic Interventions

Actions/Interventions	Rationales
■ Explain the factors that contribute to a low neutrophil count (e.g., chemotherapy, drug sensitivity).	Information enables the patient to understand the cause of the problem.
■ Explain that low neutrophil counts produce a high susceptibility to infection.	Infection and sepsis in a neutropenic patient can be fatal. Patients must understand the significance of these counts and their own role in prevention.
■ Explain the signs and symptoms of infection; instruct the patient to contact the appropriate health team member immediately if any signs or symptoms occur or are suspected.	Vigilant monitoring helps reduce the consequences of infection. QSEN: Safety.
■ Instruct the patient regarding: • Use of prescribed medications (indications, dosages, side effects)	Both antimicrobial medications and colony-stimulating factors are prescribed. The choice of antimicrobial depends on the type of infection present: viral, fungal, or bacterial. Colony-stimulating factors are growth factors that stimulate the bone marrow to produce granulocytes.
• Need for frequent blood draws	Blood draws are required to monitor the neutrophil white blood cell status.
■ Instruct the patient regarding: • Importance of good handwashing • Importance of meticulous body and oral hygiene • Avoidance of shared drinking and eating utensils. • Importance of keeping all household surfaces clean • Avoidance of crowds and people with current or recent infection • Need to wear a mask in public	Most infections result from organisms residing in the local environment. Patients must understand strategies and measures by which they can protect themselves during times of compromised defense. QSEN: Safety.
• Avoidance of contact with cat litter boxes, fish tanks, and human and animal excreta	These are possible sources of parasites that can cause infection in the immune-compromised patient.

 evolve For additional care plans, go to http://evolve.elsevier.com/Gulanick/.

Hematolymphatic, Immunological, and Oncological Care Plans

Actions/Interventions

Rationales

■ Instruct in the specifics of a low-microbial diet, including the following foods to avoid:
  • Uncooked eggs (including salad dressings containing raw eggs, such as Caesar salad dressing)
  • Unpasteurized milk and dairy products; cheeses from delis
  • Raw or undercooked meats and poultry
  • Raw and undercooked fish, shellfish, clams, oysters, sushi, etc.
  • Unwashed and unpeeled raw fruits, vegetables, or herbs
  • All salads from delis or salad bars
  • Unpasteurized eggnog or apple cider and other unpasteurized fruit or vegetable juices
  • Unpasteurized beer (e.g., microbrewery beer), wine, fountain beverages
  • All nuts or dried fruits that are sold open and in bulk; raw nuts
  • Unrefrigerated cream-filled pastry products
  • Pump serve condiments (e.g., ketchup)
  • Fast food and take-out not freshly made to order

These precautions reduce the microbial level in foods, which could colonize and infect the gastrointestinal tract. QSEN: Safety.

■ Instruct to eat the following foods:
  • Well-cooked foods, meat, poultry, seafood
  • Any breads, grains, and cereals (unless they have raw or undercooked grains or brewer's yeast)
  • Pasteurized milk and dairy products, including grade A commercially available products, yogurts, sour cream, prepackaged ice cream and sherbet, freshly made milkshakes, processed cheese slices and spreads, commercially packaged hard and semi-soft cheese, cooked soft cheeses such as brie and feta
  • Well-cooked eggs, pasteurized eggs and egg substitutes
  • Well-cooked meats, bacon, fish and other seafood, canned meats, commercially prepared deli meats sold in sealed packages
  • Well-washed and peeled raw fruits and vegetables; cooked frozen or canned fruits and vegetables
  • Factory-packaged nuts and dried fruits; nuts in baked goods; commercially packaged nut butters
  • Packaged or canned condiments that are refrigerated after opening
  • Refrigerated, commercially made, and homemade cakes, pies, pastries, and pudding

These precautions reduce the microbial level in foods, which could colonize and infect the gastrointestinal tract. QSEN: Safety.

■ Instruct to adhere to the following guidelines when eating out.
  • Ask that all foods be fully cooked and meats to be well done.
  • Don't order foods that may have raw eggs (hollandaise sauce, Caesar salad dressing).
  • Avoid foods from salad bars and buffets.
  • Don't order or take food served from steam tables or stored under heat lamps, including individual pizza slices.
  • Only use single-serving condiments not shared by others.
  • Don't eat soft-serve ice cream or yogurt from dispensers that may not be clean.

These precautions reduce the microbial level in foods, which could colonize and infect the gastrointestinal tract. QSEN: Safety.

Hematolymphatic, Immunological, and Oncological Care Plans

■ = Independent ▲ = Interprofessional Collaboration

Actions/Interventions	Rationales
■ Instruct to avoid herbal supplements (homeopathic remedies or herbal products, such as Chinese medicines).	There are no federal standards for these products in the United States. Moreover, they may be processed or stored in a risky way. The products themselves could interfere with some prescription medications.
■ Instruct the patient regarding avoidance of activities that may result in trauma to the mucosa and alternatives where appropriate: (e.g., oral and axillary temperatures instead of rectal, electric razors instead of razor blades, sanitary napkins instead of tampons, tooth sponge instead of toothbrush); limited sexual intercourse with condoms if white blood cells (WBCs) and platelets are low.	Trauma sites can easily become infected. Providing information about ways to reduce the risk for injury and infection allows the patient to be a full partner in making decisions and reducing the risk of harm from these activities. QSEN: Safety.
■ Instruct the patient to make routine dental visits when WBC counts are not compromised (e.g., before starting chemotherapy treatment or bone marrow transplantation).	Dental care reduces the opportunity for infection to begin in the oral cavity.

Related Care Plan

Impaired oral mucous membrane, Chapter 2

Hematolymphatic, Immunological, and Oncological Care Plans

Systemic Lupus Erythematosus

SLE; Lupus

Systemic lupus erythematosus (SLE) is a chronic, autoimmune disease that causes a systemic inflammatory response in various parts of the body. The cause of SLE is unknown, but genetics and hormonal and environmental factors are involved. Under normal circumstances the body's immune system produces antibodies against invading disease antigens to protect itself. In individuals with SLE the body loses its ability to discriminate between antigens and its own cells and tissues. It produces antibodies against itself, called *autoantibodies,* and these antibodies react with the antigens and result in the development of immune complexes. Immune complexes proliferate in the tissues of the patient with SLE and result in inflammation, tissue damage, and pain. Mild disease can affect joints and skin. More severe disease can affect kidneys, heart, lung, blood vessels, central nervous system, joints, and skin.

There are three types of lupus. The discoid type is limited to the skin and only rarely involves other organs. Systemic lupus is more common and usually more severe

than discoid; it can affect any organ system in the body. With systemic lupus there may be periods of remission and flares. The third type of lupus is transient, drug induced, and can be triggered by certain types of antiseizure, antihypertensive, and antibiotic medications. Symptoms usually do not present until after months or years of continued administration. The symptoms are usually abolished when the drugs are discontinued.

Women are affected by SLE ten times more often than men, most commonly between 15 and 40 years of age. It is also more common among African Americans, Hispanics, and Asians. The fact that the symptoms occur more frequently in women, especially before menstrual periods and during pregnancy, may suggest that hormonal factors influence development and progression of the disease. For some individuals, the disease remains mild and affects only a few organ systems; for others, the disease can cause life-threatening complications that can result in death. This care plan addresses the nursing management of patients with systemic lupus in an ambulatory setting.

Deficient Knowledge

Common Related Factors

Insufficient information
Insufficient interest in learning
Misinformation presented by others
Insufficient knowledge of resources

Defining Characteristics

Insufficient knowledge
Inaccurate follow-through of instruction
Inappropriate behavior

Common Expected Outcome

Patient verbalizes understanding of disease process and its treatment.

NOC Outcomes

Self-Management: Chronic Disease; Knowledge: Disease Process; Knowledge: Medication; Knowledge: Treatment Regimen

NIC Interventions

Health Literacy Enhancement; Learning Facilitation; Teaching: Disease Process; Teaching: Prescribed Medication

---

Ongoing Assessment

Action/Intervention	Rationale
■ Assess the patient's knowledge of systemic lupus erythematosus (SLE) and its treatment.	Lack of knowledge about SLE and its chronic and progressive nature can compromise the patient's ability to care for self and cope effectively. QSEN: Patient-centered care.

Therapeutic Interventions

Actions/Interventions	Rationales
■ Introduce or reinforce the disease process information: unknown cause, chronicity of SLE, processes of inflammation and fibrosis, remissions and exacerbations, control versus cure.	The goal of treatment is to reduce inflammation, minimize symptoms, and maintain normal body functions. The incidence of flares can be reduced by maintaining good nutrition and engaging in exercise habits.
■ Discuss common diagnostic tests.	There is no one specific test for SLE. A variety of tests commonly used to diagnose rheumatoid arthritis are used here. These include immunologically based tests (e.g., antinuclear antibody [ANA], erythrocyte sedimentation rate [ESR], serum protein electrophoresis, rheumatoid factor, serum complement [especially C3 and C4]). Additional tests may also be indicated to assess for major organ or systemic involvement, such as kidney and liver assessments.
■ Introduce or reinforce information on drug therapy. Instruct the patient in the potential effects of steroids, immunosuppressant medication, and other drugs used to treat SLE.	Patients are better able to ask questions when they have basic information about what to expect. QSEN: Patient-centered care; Evidence-based practice.
• Nonsteroidal anti-inflammatory drugs	These drugs are used for their anti-inflammatory actions to treat pain, swelling, and fever. Side effects include gastrointestinal (GI) distress.

■ = Independent ▲ = Interprofessional Collaboration

Hematolymphatic, Immunological, and Oncological Care Plans

Hematolymphatic, Immunological, and Oncological Care Plans

Actions/Interventions	Rationales
• Antimalarials (hydroxychloroquine, chloroquine)	These medications are used in the treatment of skin and joint symptoms of SLE. It may take months to see treatment effects. Side effects are rare, but patients are cautioned to see their eye physician several times a year to rule out the development of irreversible retinopathy. Patients may also experience mild GI disturbances.
• Corticosteroids	This classification of drugs is used for their anti-inflammatory and immunoregulatory properties (they suppress the activity of the immune system). Topical preparations are effective for skin problems. Oral prednisone may be indicated for minor disease effects. Common side effects include facial puffiness, buffalo hump, diabetes mellitus, osteoporosis, avascular necrosis of the hip, increased appetite, cataracts, and an increased risk for infection.
• Stress to the patient the importance of not altering the steroid dose or suddenly stopping the medication.	Steroids must be tapered slowly after high-dose or long-term use. The body produces the hormone cortisol in the adrenal glands. After high-dose or long-term use of exogenous forms of steroids, the body no longer produces adequate cortisol levels. Increased cortisol levels are needed in times of stress. Without supplementation, a steroid-dependent patient will enter addisonian crisis. The nurse must stress the importance of wearing a medical alert tag at all times that states the patient uses steroids and immunosuppressants. QSEN: Safety.
• Immunosuppressants (azathioprine, cyclophosphamide, methotrexate, leflunomide, and mycophenolate mofetil)	This classification of drug is used to suppress the activity of the immune system, thereby decreasing the proliferation of the disease, especially during severe flares and in renal or central nervous system (CNS) involvement. Side effects include an increased infection risk caused by bone marrow suppression, nausea and vomiting, liver disease, sterility, hemorrhagic cystitis, and cancer.
• Topical immunomodulators (tacrolimus, pimecrolimus)	These medications suppress immune activity in the skin. They serve as an alternative to steroids for treating skin conditions.
• Biologicals (belimumab [Benlysta])	This drug is a human monoclonal antibody and the first new drug approved for SLE since 1955. B cells are responsible for part of the normal immune response, and for the over-aggressive immune response in autoimmune diseases like SLE. In SLE, abnormal B cells contribute to autoantibodies. Belimumab prevents B lymphocyte–stimulating protein from binding to B-cell receptor sites, thus decreasing B-cell survival. This drug is quite expensive. QSEN: Evidence-based practice.
■ Provide information on appropriate clinical trials.	New therapies for lupus are being researched all the time investigating the role of biological and targeted therapy agents that interfere with the immune response. Qualified patients may find hope and even relief from symptoms and complications.
■ Instruct the patient to monitor for the signs of fever.	Fever is a common manifestation of SLE in the active phase of the disease. Patients should also report accompanying chills, shaking, and diaphoresis. Patients taking aspirin as an antipyretic should have frequent liver studies performed, because aspirin use by patients with SLE has been demonstrated to cause transient liver toxicity. QSEN: Safety.

ℯvolve **For additional care plans, go to http://evolve.elsevier.com/Gulanick/.**

Actions/Interventions

■ Instruct in the opportunities for support groups in the community or on reputable Internet websites.

■ Instruct in lifestyle activities that can help reduce flare-ups: rest, avoiding sun exposure, engaging in regular exercise, and eating a balanced diet of grains, fruits, and vegetables.

Rationales

Members of groups that come together for specialized problems can be helpful to each other. The Lupus Foundation and the Arthritis Foundation are national websites that offer excellent resources.

A positive approach to useful therapies allows the patient to be an active partner in treating this chronic condition. QSEN: Patient-centered care; Safety.

NANDA-I NDx **Impaired Skin Integrity**

Common Related Factors

Inflammation
Vasoconstriction
Exacerbation of disease process
High-dose corticosteroid use
Use of immunosuppressant drugs

Defining Characteristics

Redness
Pain and tenderness
Itching
Skin breakdown
Oral and nasal ulcers
Skin rash
Diffuse areas of hair loss
Loss of discrete patches of scalp hair
Scalp hair loss possibly accompanied by lesions, scarring, or dry, scaling skin tissue

Common Expected Outcomes

Patient maintains optimal skin integrity, as evidenced by absence of rashes and skin lesions.
Skin lesions are identified early so that treatment can be implemented.
Patient verbalizes ability to cope with hair loss.
Patient identifies ways to conceal scalp loss as required by personal preference.

NOC Outcomes

Tissue Integrity: Skin and Mucous Membranes; Knowledge: Treatment Regimen; Body Image

NIC Interventions

Teaching: Disease Process; Skin Care: Topical Treatments; Skin Surveillance; Body Image Enhancement

---

Ongoing Assessment

Actions/Interventions

■ Assess for an erythematous rash, which may be present on the face, neck, or extremities.

■ Assess the skin for integrity.

■ Assess for photosensitivity.

■ Assess the patient's description of pain.

■ Assess the degree to which symptoms interfere with the patient's lifestyle and body image.

Rationales

The classic "butterfly" rash may appear across the bridge of the nose and on the cheeks and is characteristically displayed in the configuration of a butterfly. This is evident in about 50% of patients.

Small lesions may appear on the oral and nasal mucous membranes. Disklike lesions that appear as a dense maculopapular rash may occur on the patient's face or chest.

Patients may respond violently to ultraviolet light or to sunlight. Disease flares or outbreaks of severe rash may occur in response to exposure.

Gathering information about pain can guide treatment. Each patient may exhibit slightly different presentations.

A broad range of behaviors are associated with body image changes, ranging from totally ignoring the change to a preoccupation with it. QSEN: Patient-centered care.

■ = Independent   ▲ = Interprofessional Collaboration

Hematolymphatic, Immunological, and Oncological Care Plans

Therapeutic Interventions

Actions/Interventions

- Instruct the patient to clean, dry, and moisturize intact skin; use warm (not hot) water, especially over bony prominences; use unscented lotion (e.g., Eucerin or Lubriderm). Use mild shampoo.
- Encourage adequate nutrition and hydration.

- Recommend prophylactic pressure-relieving devices (e.g., special mattress, elbow pads).
- Instruct the patient to avoid contact with harsh chemicals (e.g., household cleaners, detergents) and to wear appropriate protective gloves, as needed. Avoid hair dye, permanent solution, and curl relaxers.

For skin rash:
- Instruct the patient to:
  - Avoid ultraviolet light.
  - Wear maximum protection sunscreen (SPF 15 or above) in the sun. Sunbathing is contraindicated.
  - Wear a wide-brimmed hat and carry an umbrella.
  - Wear protective eyewear.
- Introduce or reinforce information about the use of hydroxychloroquine (Plaquenil).

- Inform the patient of the availability of special makeup (at large department stores) to cover rashes, especially facial rashes (e.g., Covermark [Lydia O'Leary], Dermablend, Marilyn Miglin).

For oral ulcers:
- Instruct the patient to rinse the mouth with half-strength hydrogen peroxide three times per day.
- Instruct the patient to avoid spicy or citrusy foods.

- Instruct the patient to keep ulcerated skin clean and dry. Apply dressings as needed.
- Instruct the patient to apply topical ointments as prescribed.

For hair loss:
- Instruct the patient that scalp hair loss occurs during the exacerbation of disease activity.

- Instruct the patient that scalp hair loss may be caused by high-dose corticosteroids (prednisone) and immunosuppressant drugs.
- Encourage the patient to investigate ways (e.g., scarves, hats, wigs) to conceal hair loss.

Rationales

Scented lotions may contain alcohol, which dries skin. Prescribed solutions reduce dryness of the scalp and maintain skin integrity.

These measures promote healthy skin and healing in the presence of wounds.

Such devices aid in the prevention of skin breakdown. QSEN: Safety.

Chemicals aggravate this condition and avoiding them can reduce the risk of harm. QSEN: Safety.

The sun can exacerbate a skin rash or precipitate a disease flare. Special lotions, glasses, and other items may be required to protect the skin from exposure to sunlight. QSEN: Safety.

This antimalarial drug is a slow-acting medicine used to relieve or reduce inflammation and rash. It may take 8 to 12 weeks for effect. A potential side effect is retinal toxicity. The patient must follow up with an ophthalmologist every 6 months. Topical cortisone medication may likewise be used. QSEN: Teamwork and collaboration.

These preparations are especially formulated to completely cover rashes, birthmarks, and darkly pigmented areas. This will help the patient who is having problems adjusting to body image changes.

Hydrogen peroxide helps keep oral ulcers clean.

These foods might irritate fissures or ulcers in the mucous membranes.

Skin care is necessary to prevent infection and promote healing.

Vitamins A and E may be useful in maintaining skin health.

Scalp hair loss may be the first sign of impending disease exacerbation. Scalp hair loss may not be permanent. As disease activity subsides, scalp hair begins to regrow.

Hair will regrow as the dose decreases.

Hair loss may interfere with lifestyle and self-image.

NANDA-I NDx Joint Pain/Stiffness

Common Related Factor

Inflammation associated with increased disease activity

Defining Characteristics

Verbalized complaint of joint pain or stiffness
Guarding on motion of affected joints
Facial mask of pain
Moaning or other pain-associated sounds

Common Expected Outcomes

Patient reports pain or stiffness at a level less than 3 or 4 on a scale of 0 to 10.
Patient implements a pain management plan that includes pharmacological and nonpharmacological strategies.
Patient is able to participate in self-care activities.

NOC Outcomes

Pain Control; Medication Response; Mobility

NIC Interventions

Analgesic Administration; Pain Management; Exercise Therapy: Joint Mobility

---

Ongoing Assessment

Actions/Interventions	Rationales
■ Assess for the signs of joint inflammation (redness, warmth, swelling) or decreased motion.	Usual signs of inflammation may not be present with this disease.
■ Assess the patient's description of pain.	Patients with SLE often experience arthralgias of many joints with morning stiffness. Joint stiffness related to systemic lupus erythematosus (SLE) may not be related to activity or overuse; it is instead a response to immune complexes proliferating and setting up an inflammatory response in that particular body part. Patients with SLE may also have arthritis; thus stiffness and discomfort are multifactorial.
■ Determine the past measures used to alleviate pain.	Patients may not know of or may not have tried all currently available treatments. Pain management is directed at the resolution of discomfort as it is presenting at that specific moment in time, because relief measures may change with the joints affected. QSEN: Patient-centered care.
■ Assess the impact of pain or stiffness on the patient's ability to perform interpersonally, socially, and professionally.	SLE-related arthritis usually does not result in deformity as in rheumatoid arthritis, but physical activity may still be severely limited at times. Strategies may have to be developed so that the patient is able to maintain a maximum level of function in each of these areas. QSEN: Patient-centered care.

Therapeutic Interventions

Actions/Interventions	Rationales
■ Instruct the patient to take anti-inflammatory medications as prescribed. Explain the need for taking the first dose of the day as early in the morning as possible with a small snack.	The sooner the patient takes the medication, the sooner the stiffness will abate. Anti-inflammatory drugs should not be taken on an empty stomach.
■ Suggest nonopioid analgesics as necessary.	Opioid analgesia appears to work better on mechanical pain and is not particularly effective in dealing with pain associated with inflammation. Opioids can be habit forming.
■ If the patient is hospitalized, ask about the normal home medication schedule and try to continue it.	Patients often develop effective regimens for dealing with their disease, and this should be respected.

■ = Independent ▲ = Interprofessional Collaboration

Hematolymphatic, Immunological, and Oncological Care Plans

Hematolymphatic, Immunological, and Oncological Care Plans

Actions/Interventions

- Encourage the patient to assume an anatomically correct position with all joints. Suggest that the patient use a small flat pillow under the head and not use a knee gatch or pillow to prop the knee.
- Encourage the use of ambulation aids when pain is related to weight bearing.
- Suggest that the patient apply a bed cradle.

- ▲ Consult an occupational therapist for the proper splinting of affected joints.

- ▲ Encourage the patient to wear splints, as ordered.

- Encourage the use of alternative methods of pain control such as relaxation, guided imagery, or distraction.
- Encourage the patient to take a 15-minute warm shower or bath on arising.
- Encourage the patient to perform range-of-motion exercises after the shower or bath, two repetitions per joint.
- Remind the patient to allow sufficient time for all activities.
- Remind the patient to avoid prolonged periods of inactivity.

Rationales

Such measures assist in preventing the development of contractures.

Crutches, walkers, and canes can be used to absorb some of the weight from the inflamed extremity.

Protective devices keep the pressure of bed covers off the inflamed lower extremities.

Specialty expertise may be required to ensure optimal joint function and relief of pain. QSEN: Teamwork and collaboration.

Splints provide rest to inflamed joints and may reduce muscle spasms

These measures may augment other medications used to diminish pain.

Warmth reduces stiffness and relieves pain. Water should be warm. Excessive heat may promote skin breakdown.

These exercises help reduce stiffness and maintain joint mobility.

Performing even simple activities in the presence of significant joint stiffness can take longer.

Activity is required to prevent further stiffness and to prevent joints from freezing and muscles from becoming atrophied.

NANDA-I NDx Fatigue

Common Related Factors

Physiologic condition
Physical deeconditioning
Depression

Defining Characteristics

Tiredness
Insufficient energy
Impaired ability to maintain usual physical activity and routines
Nonrestorative sleep pattern
Increase in rest requirement
Alteration in concentration

Common Expected Outcomes

Patient verbalizes reduction in fatigue level, as evidenced by reports of increased energy and ability to perform desired activities.
Patient demonstrates use of energy-conservation principles.

NOC Outcomes

Fatigue Level; Fatigue: Disruptive Effects; Activity Tolerance; Endurance; Energy Conservation; Sleep

NIC Interventions

Energy Management; Relaxation Therapy

Ongoing Assessment

Actions/Interventions	Rationales
■ Assess the patient's description of fatigue: timing (afternoon or all day), relationship to activities, and aggravating and alleviating factors.	This information may be helpful in developing and organizing patterns of activity that optimize the times when the patient has the greatest energy reserve. QSEN: Patient-centered care.
■ Determine the patient's nighttime sleep pattern.	The discomfort associated with systemic lupus erythematosus (SLE) may obstruct sleep.
■ Determine whether fatigue is related to psychological factors (e.g., stress, depression).	Fatigue is best treated by determining the causative factor. Depression is a common problem for people suffering from chronic disease, especially when discomfort is an accompanying problem. Medications are available that are successful in treating clinical depression.

Therapeutic Interventions

Actions/Interventions	Rationales
■ Reinforce energy-conservation principles:	
• Pacing of activities (alternating activity with rest)	The patient often needs more energy than others to complete the same tasks.
• Adequate rest periods (throughout the day and night)	Energy reserves may be depleted unless the patient respects the body's need for increased rest.
• Organization of activities and environment	Organization can help the patient conserve energy and reduce fatigue.
• Proper use of assistive and adaptive devices	Adequately used, these devices can support movement and activity, resulting in the conservation of energy.
If fatigue is related to interrupted sleep:	
■ Encourage a warm shower or bath immediately before bedtime.	Warm water relaxes muscles, facilitating total body relaxation; excessive heat may promote skin breakdown.
■ Encourage gentle range-of-motion (ROM) exercises (after a shower or bath).	These exercises maximize the muscle-relaxing benefits of the warm shower or bath.
■ Encourage the patient to sleep in an anatomically correct position and not to prop up affected joints.	Good body alignment will result in muscle relaxation and comfort.
■ Encourage the patient to change position frequently during the night.	Repositioning promotes comfort.
■ Instruct the patient to avoid stimulating foods (caffeine) or activities before bedtime.	Environmental stimuli can inhibit relaxation, interrupt sleep, and contribute to fatigue.
■ Encourage the use of progressive muscle-relaxation techniques.	These techniques promote relaxation and rest.
▲ Suggest a nighttime analgesic and/or a long-acting anti-inflammatory drug as ordered.	The relief of pain can facilitate rest and sleep.

Related Care Plans

Acute pain, Chapter 2
Chronic pain, Chapter 2
Disturbed body image, Chapter 2
Grieving, Chapter 2
Insomnia, Chapter 2
Ineffective coping, Chapter 2
Self-care deficit, Chapter 2

Hematolymphatic, Immunological, and Oncological Care Plans

■ = Independent   ▲ = Interprofessional Collaboration

CHAPTER

11

Renal and Urinary Tract Care Plans

Acute Kidney Injury

Acute Tubular Necrosis (ATN); Renal Insufficiency; Acute Renal Failure

Acute kidney injury (AKI) is the abrupt loss of kidney function that renders the kidneys incapable of adequately clearing the blood of the waste products of metabolism. It is usually associated with another medical condition or event. AKI may occur as a single event, with return of normal renal function, or may progress to chronic kidney disease or kidney failure. Severity of AKI is based on the degree of increases in serum creatinine clearance and reduced urine output. The causes of AKI can be divided into three major types: prerenal, resulting from a decrease in renal perfusion; intrarenal, caused by a direct injury to the glomeruli, nephrons, or tubules from ischemia or renal toxins; and postrenal, as a result of urinary tract obstruction that leads to the backflow of urine into the kidney. Hospital-acquired AKI is most likely a result of acute tubular necrosis (ATN), which results from the administration of nephrotoxins or an acute episode of renal ischemia. Because of declines in renal function as part of the normal aging process, older patients are more at risk when receiving nephrotoxic agents, such as intravenous (IV) contrast media or certain medications. Treatment is focused on addressing any underlying or precipitating cause for the kidney injury, and treating any complications while the kidney is recovering. During the period of loss of renal function, renal replacement therapy (e.g., hemodialysis, peritoneal dialysis, or continuous ultrafiltration therapy) may be required to clear the accumulated metabolic waste produces from the blood. This care plan focuses on the patient with AKI during hospitalization.

NDx Impaired Renal Function

Common Related Factors

Severe renal ischemia secondary to sepsis, shock, or severe hypovolemia with hypotension (usually after surgery or trauma)
Nephrotoxic drugs (including antibiotics such as amphotericin B or aminoglycosides)
Renal vascular occlusion
Hemolytic blood transfusion reaction

Defining Characteristics

Increased blood urea nitrogen (BUN) and serum creatinine
Reduced creatinine clearance
Urine specific gravity fixed at or near 1.010
Hematuria, proteinuria
Urine output <400 mL/24 hr (in absence of inadequate fluid intake or fluid losses by other route)
Weight gain
Hyperkalemia, hyperphosphatemia, hypocalcemia, metabolic acidosis, hyponatremia, and hypermagnesemia
Decreased hemoglobin (Hgb) and hematocrit (Hct)

Common Expected Outcome

Patient achieves optimal urinary elimination, as evidenced by urine output >30 mL/hr; electrolytes, BUN, creatinine within or near normal levels; and normal urine specific gravity.

NOC Outcomes
Urinary Elimination; Fluid Balance; Vital Signs
NIC Interventions
Urinary Elimination Management; Fluid/
Electrolyte Management

Ongoing Assessment

Actions/Interventions	Rationales
■ Monitor and record the patient's intake and output; include all fluid losses (e.g., stool, emesis, and wound drainage). Report an output of <30 mL/hr.	Patients may exhibit oliguria (<400 mL/day) or anuria (<100 mL/day) in the early phases of AKI. Fluid status also changes as the patient transitions from an oliguric to a diuretic phase. The diuretic phase of AKI indicates a gradual return of glomerular function. The diuretic phase places the patient at risk for dehydration and hypokalemia. Fluid replacement therapy is calculated to replace fluid losses from all sources.
■ Monitor the urine specific gravity.	The ability to concentrate urine is lost in intrarenal failure and the urine specific gravity may remain as low as 1.010.
▲ Monitor blood and urine laboratory tests as prescribed:	
• BUN, creatinine	Both BUN and creatinine are elevated in renal failure; however, creatinine is more specific and reliable because it is not affected by diet, blood in the gut, hydration, or metabolism.
• Sodium	Hyponatremia is caused by the dilutional effect of hypervolemia because water excretion is impaired.
• Potassium	Levels rise in AKI because the kidneys are unable to filter and excrete potassium.
• Calcium, phosphate	In AKI, the ability to excrete phosphate and to activate vitamin D needed for calcium absorption in the gut is impaired. The serum calcium level falls to less than 8.5 mg/100 mL and serum phosphate is increased to greater than 4.5 mg/100 mL.
• Magnesium	Hypermagnesemia occurs as a result of the decreased excretion of magnesium resulting from the kidney injury.
• pH	Metabolic acidosis develops because acid cannot be excreted from the kidneys, and the production and retention of bicarbonate is decreased.
• Urinalysis (especially for protein, sodium, and blood), osmolality, specific gravity, 24 hr creatinine clearance	Urine osmolality, specific gravity, and sodium content can help differentiate various causes for AKI. The presence of sediment, casts, protein, or blood in urine indicates an abnormal state and can suggest an intrarenal cause. The 24-hour creatinine clearance test provides evidence of the kidney's ability to clear creatinine. Older patients will normally have a somewhat reduced creatinine clearance. A creatinine clearance of less than 10 mL/min indicates kidney failure. Urine sodium concentrations are high with intrarenal injury, yet low with prerenal causes of AKI.
• Hgb/Hct	Anemia occurs as a result of insufficient erythropoietin production. Erythropoietin is a hormone produced by the kidney that promotes the maturation and differentiation of erythrocyte stem cells in the bone marrow. The accumulation of nitrogenous wastes decreases the normal life span of circulating red blood cells and contributes to anemia. Preexisting nutritional deficiencies may be a factor in the development of anemia.

Renal and Urinary Tract Care Plans

■ = Independent   ▲ = Interprofessional Collaboration

Actions/Interventions	Rationales
■ Monitor daily weights with the same scale and preferably at the same time of day with the patient wearing the same amount of clothing.	Changes in daily body weight reflect changes in fluid balance. Sudden weight gains indicate fluid retention. QSEN: Safety.
■ Monitor for the signs and symptoms of excess fluid volume:	Early identification of signs and symptoms of excess fluid volume will guide therapeutic interventions to reduce the risk of fluid volume deficit. QSEN: Safety.
• Edema (degree and location)	Water excretion is impaired. Fluid is retained and moves from the vascular space into interstitial spaces as a result of increased serum hydrostatic pressure.
• Jugular vein distention	Engorgement of the neck veins with the head of the bed at 30 to 45 degrees indicates excess fluid volume.
• Hypertension	Excess circulatory volume contributes to an increase in blood pressure (BP).
• Crackles	Movement of fluid from pulmonary circulation into the alveolar spaces causes adventitious lung sounds.
• Increased respiratory rate	Presence of fluid in the alveoli impairs gas exchange and causes a compensatory increase in respiratory rate.
▲ Anticipate diagnostic testing with ultrasound, computed tomography (CT), or x-rays as indicated.	Ultrasound images can show the size of the kidneys and patency of the ureters. CT scans (without contrast agent) can determine adequacy of blood flow and identify possible obstructions. X-ray studies of the renal system may help identify any contributing factors to AKI.

Therapeutic Interventions

Actions/Interventions	Rationales
▲ Evaluate the cause of the renal failure: prerenal, intrarenal, or postrenal.	AKI is reversible if it is detected and treated in a timely manner. Medical therapy is directed at supporting renal function and relieving the cause of renal failure. QSEN: Safety.
▲ Administer fluids and diuretics as prescribed.	The kidney's ability to regulate fluid balance is lost in AKI, and hypervolemia can easily occur. Close fluid management is important. Volume replacement and fluid challenges may be especially important in prerenal causes. Central venous pressure monitoring may be indicated in higher risk patients. Diuretics are used cautiously in AKI. Loop diuretics, such as furosemide, and osmotic diuretics are used most often.
▲ When administering medications (e.g., antibiotics) metabolized by the kidneys, anticipate that dosages, frequency, or both may require adjustment.	Drug excretion will be affected by impaired renal function leading to elevated, and possibly toxic, levels. QSEN: Safety.
▲ Anticipate renal replacement therapy if conservative management is ineffective.	Hemodialysis is the most commonly used renal replacement therapy for the patient with AKI. Renal replacement therapies are used to clear excess fluid and metabolic waste products.

Renal and Urinary Tract Care Plans

⊝volve   **For additional care plans, go to http://evolve.elsevier.com/Gulanick/.**

Excess Fluid Volume

Common Related Factors

Compromised regulatory mechanisms
Excess fluid intake
Excess sodium intake

Defining Characteristics

Weight gain over a short period of time
Edema
Urine specific gravity less than 1.010
Tachycardia
Oliguria
Orthopnea/dyspnea
Adventitious breath sounds: crackles
Presence of third heart sound (S_3)
Alteration in BP
Jugular vein distention
Change in mental status
Azotemia
Electrolyte imbalance
Decreased Hgb or Hct

Common Expected Outcome

Patient is normovolemic as evidenced by urine output greater than or equal to 30 mL/hr, balanced intake and output, stable weight (or loss attributed to fluid loss), absence or reduction of edema, HR 60 to 100 beats/min, and absence of pulmonary crackles.

NOC Outcomes

Fluid Balance; Cardiopulmonary Status

NIC Interventions

Fluid Management; Fluid Monitoring

Ongoing Assessment

Actions/Interventions

- Weigh the patient daily on the same scale and with the same clothing.

- Monitor and record intake and output. Include all stool, emesis, and wound drainage amounts.

- Monitor the patient's HR, BP, and respiratory rate. Inspect the jugular veins.
- Auscultate breath sounds and heart sounds for signs of fluid overload.

Rationales

Patient weight is the best indicator of fluid status. Weight gains of 1 to 2 pounds in 24 hours are associated with fluid volume excess.

Close monitoring of all fluid losses and urine output is necessary to determine adequate replacement needs and to prevent excessive administration of oral or IV fluids during decreased renal function. The insertion of a Foley catheter may facilitate accurate measurement of urine output. QSEN: Safety.

Fluid volume excess causes increased BP, tachycardia, and tachypnea. Jugular veins may be distended.

The patient may have crackles and an S_3 gallop. The kidney's ability to regulate fluid balance is lost in AKI, and hypervolemia can easily occur, resulting in heart failure. QSEN: Safety.

Therapeutic Interventions

Actions/Interventions

▲ Administer oral and IV fluids as prescribed. Administer IV medications in the least amount of fluid possible.

Rationales

During the oliguric phase of AKI the patient may have fluid intake restricted to manage the excess fluid volume. The diuretic phase of renal failure requires fluid replacement as well as close monitoring of sodium and potassium levels. With tubular patency partially restored, sodium and potassium losses may occur.

■ = Independent   ▲ = Interprofessional Collaboration

Renal and Urinary Tract Care Plans

Actions/Interventions

▲ Administer medications (e.g., diuretics) as prescribed.

■ If peripheral edema is present, move the patient gently and reposition often.

▲ Prepare the patient for renal replacement therapy if indicated.

Rationales

Diuretic therapy requires close monitoring of vital signs and serum BUN and creatinine levels because reduced blood volume can result in inadequate renal perfusion. Furosemide can be nephrotoxic and may further nephron injury. QSEN: Safety.

Edematous tissue is at greater risk for injury and breakdown. QSEN: Safety.

Renal replacement therapies such as ultrafiltration, peritoneal dialysis, or hemodialysis clear the body of excess fluid and waste products.

NANDA-I NDx

Risk for Decreased Cardiac Output

Common Risk Factors

Increased or decreased ventricular filling (preload)
Increased afterload
Impaired contractility
Alteration in heart rate (HR), rhythm, and conduction
Decreased oxygenation

Common Expected Outcome

Patient maintains adequate cardiac output, as evidenced by systolic BP within 20 mm Hg of baseline; HR 60 to 100 beats/min with regular rhythm; urine output 30 mL/hr or greater; strong peripheral pulses; warm and dry skin; eupnea with absence of pulmonary crackles; orientation to time, place, person.

NOC Outcomes

Cardiopulmonary Status; Circulation Status; Vital Signs; Electrolyte and Acid/Base Balance

NIC Interventions

Hemodynamic Regulation; Electrolyte Management

Ongoing Assessment

Actions/Interventions

■ Assess for the signs of decreased cardiac output: change in BP, HR, central venous pressure (CVP), peripheral pulses; jugular venous distention (JVD); decreased urine output; abnormal heart sounds; dysrhythmias; anxiety or restlessness.

▲ Monitor serum electrolytes.

Rationales

These signs may indicate decreased cardiac output. Fluid volume excess and electrolyte imbalances can reduce myocardial contractility and lead to decreased cardiac output, especially in older adults and patients with a history of cardiac disease. QSEN: Safety.

The patient experiencing AKI is most likely to develop hyperkalemia, hypocalcemia, and hyperphosphatemia. These electrolyte imbalances put the patient at risk for abnormalities in myocardial conduction and contractility. Electrolyte imbalances can be caused by very high ultrafiltration rates seen in continuous renal replacement therapies (CRRTs). High clearances of small molecules such as sodium, potassium, and bicarbonate occur as a result. Inadequate replacement of fluids and electrolytes during CRRT also may contribute to electrolyte imbalances. QSEN: Evidence-based practice; Safety.

Renal and Urinary Tract Care Plans

Actions/Interventions

- ■ Monitor the patient's cardiac rhythm.

- ■ Auscultate the patient's heart sounds for the presence of a third heart sound (S_3, indicating fluid overload, which may precede the onset of heart failure) or a pericardial friction rub (indicating uremic pericarditis).

- ▲ Monitor the chest x-ray reports.

- ▲ Monitor for the signs and symptoms of metabolic acidosis.

Rationales

The patient experiencing AKI may develop dysrhythmias as a result of the decreased renal elimination of potassium, phosphate, magnesium, and sodium. Hyperkalemia, hypocalcemia, or metabolic acidosis can cause life-threatening dysrhythmias. These dysrhythmias can contribute to a serious decrease in cardiac output. QSEN: Safety.

If either is present, the patient may require prompt renal replacement therapy. Pericarditis can occur with AKI and develop into a pericardial effusion or even cardiac tamponade. Evidence suggests that pericarditis may be caused by the presence of uremic toxins in the pericardial fluid. QSEN: Safety; Evidence-based practice.

Enlargement of the cardiac silhouette on x-ray film may indicate early signs of heart failure from excess fluid volume in AKI.

Decreasing arterial pH and bicarbonate levels indicate metabolic acidosis. In AKI, acidosis develops when the kidney is unable to excrete hydrogen ions and maintain the bicarbonate buffers through the synthesis of ammonia and reabsorption of bicarbonate.

Therapeutic Interventions

Actions/Interventions

- ▲ Administer medications as prescribed:
  - • Sodium bicarbonate

  - • Calcium gluconate

  - • IV insulin and glucose

  - • Potassium-exchange resins (e.g., Kayexelate)

- ▲ Prepare the patient for renal replacement therapy when indicated.

- ▲ If dysrhythmias occur, treat them as appropriate.

Rationales

Hyperkalemia can be a life-threatening complication of AKI. Sodium bicarbonate will temporarily shift potassium back into the cell. This action helps with the correction of acidosis or hyperkalemia in the event of seriously elevated potassium levels. However, it can result in the elevation of sodium (as sodium is pushed out of the cell) and water retention from the sodium load. QSEN: Safety.

Calcium gluconate treats hypocalcemia. Calcium may also be given to stabilize the cell membrane from depolarization in the hyperkalemic state.

Insulin is able to shift potassium back into the cells to correct hyperkalemia. The glucose is administered to prevent hypoglycemia from the effect of insulin. QSEN: Safety.

Resins exchange potassium for sodium in the gastrointestinal tract, thereby decreasing serum potassium levels. The bound potassium is then excreted in the bowel movement. These resins are used to correct hyperkalemia. They may be administered orally or rectally. There is a risk for increasing sodium levels and fluid retention. QSEN: Safety.

Hemodialysis is the most common renal replacement therapy used in AKI. This therapy removes excess fluid and corrects electrolyte imbalances. CRRT (also known as ultrafiltration) slowly removes water, electrolytes, and uremic toxins and is indicated for hemodynamically unstable patients who are not able to tolerate conventional hemodialysis.

Treating dysrhythmias helps reduce the risk for decreased cardiac output. QSEN: Safety.

Renal and Urinary Tract Care Plans

■ = Independent   ▲ = Interprofessional Collaboration

Actions/Interventions

■ Notify the physician of the presence of a pericardial friction rub.

▲ If signs of decreased cardiac output are noted:
  · Administer oral and IV fluids as prescribed. Note the effects.
  · Administer inotropic agents as prescribed.

Rationales

If pericarditis is present, the patient will need to be started on steroids or nonsteroidal anti-inflammatory drugs to reduce inflammation and discomfort. Also, heparin use should be limited to decrease the potential for bleeding into the pericardial space that may predispose the patient to develop pericardial tamponade. QSEN: Teamwork and collaboration; Safety.

The administration of fluids will help increase cardiac output by increasing circulating blood volume.
An increase in myocardial contractility will help increase cardiac output through an increase in stroke volume.

NANDA-I
NDx **Imbalanced Nutrition: Less Than Body Requirements**

Common Related Factors
Inability to ingest foods
Inability to digest foods
Inability to absorb nutrients
Biological factors
Insufficient dietary intake

Defining Characteristics
Weight loss with adequate food intake
Body weight 20% or more below ideal weight range
Food intake less than recommended dietary allowance (RDA)
Excessive hair loss
Pale mucous membranes
Insufficient interest in food
Sore buccal cavity
Weakness of muscles needed for mastication and/or swallowing

Common Expected Outcomes
Patient or caregiver verbalizes and demonstrates selection of foods or meals that will achieve a cessation of weight loss.
Patient weighs within 10% of ideal weight range.

NOC Outcomes
Knowledge: Kidney Disease; Nutritional Status: Nutrient Intake
NIC Interventions
Nutrition Management; Nutritional Monitoring; Nutritional Therapy

---

Ongoing Assessment

Actions/Interventions

■ Assess for possible causes of a decreased appetite or gastrointestinal (GI) discomfort (e.g., stomatitis, anorexia, nausea and vomiting, diarrhea, constipation, melena, or hematemesis).
■ Monitor the patient's actual oral intake; obtain calorie counts as necessary.
▲ Monitor the serum albumin level.

■ Assess the patient's weight gain pattern.

Rationales

Uremia manifestations include GI disturbances related to the accumulation of toxins and altered intestinal motility (increased or decreased).

The information provides accurate measurement of nutritional intake. QSEN: Patient-centered care.
Serum albumin indicates the degree of protein depletion (3.8 to 4.5 g/100 mL is normal).
Weight gain may be related to fluid retention. A weight increase of $\frac{1}{2}$ to 1 pound per week is associated with an increased nutritional intake.

Therapeutic Interventions

Actions/Interventions	Rationales
■ Provide the patient with small, frequent feedings as tolerated.	The patient with GI symptoms will tolerate small, frequent meals better than large meals less frequently.
■ Make meals look appetizing; try to eliminate other procedures at mealtime if possible, and focus on eating.	Decreasing distractions at mealtime allows the patient to focus attention on eating. The patient needs to use available energy to increase nutritional intake. QSEN: Patient-centered care.
■ Provide frequent oral hygiene.	Frequent oral hygiene will keep oral mucous membranes moist and stimulate saliva production, which can help increase the patient's oral intake. Oral hygiene will promote patient comfort from the dry mucous membranes associated with the fluid restrictions during the oliguric phase.
▲ Consult a dietitian.	In general, a diet high in carbohydrates and low in protein is used to reduce catabolism and prevent additional elevations of blood urea nitrogen. The dietitian is best qualified to calculate the patient's daily needs. QSEN: Teamwork and collaboration.
▲ Adjust the potassium and phosphorus restrictions as indicated.	In AKI, the kidney is unable to excrete potassium and phosphorus. Dietary restriction is needed to maintain serum levels within normal limits.
▲ Administer enteral or parenteral feedings as prescribed.	Tube feedings or total parenteral nutrition helps maintain optimal nourishment; however, patients are at an increased risk for fluid volume overload. QSEN: Safety.
▲ Offer antiemetics as prescribed.	Controlling nausea may improve the patient's appetite and food intake.
▲ Administer antacids and H₂-receptor–blocking agents.	These drugs reduce gastric acidity and prevent mucosal ulceration. Antacids should not contain aluminum or magnesium because the patient with AKI cannot excrete aluminum or magnesium, and hypermagnesemia would develop. QSEN: Safety.
▲ Provide renal replacement therapy as ordered.	Therapy removes uremic toxins and prevents GI complications that result from the accumulation of uremic toxins. QSEN: Safety.

NANDA-I NDx Risk for Infection

Common Risk Factors

Invasive procedures related to insertion of indwelling bladder catheters, dual-lumen venous catheters, or peripherally inserted central catheters

Inadequate secondary defenses: immunosuppression from uremia

Insufficient knowledge to avoid exposure to pathogens

Common Expected Outcomes

Patient remains free of infection, as evidenced by normal vital signs and absence of purulent drainage from wounds, incisions, and tubes.

Infection is recognized early to allow for prompt treatment.

NOC Outcomes
Risk Control; Risk Detection; Immune Status; Infection Severity

NIC Interventions
Infection Protection; Infection Control

Renal and Urinary Tract Care Plans

■ = Independent ▲ = Interprofessional Collaboration

Ongoing Assessment

Actions/Interventions	Rationales
■ Assess for potential sites of infection: urinary, pulmonary, wound, or IV line.	Infection must be monitored closely because of the tendency for the development of infection with AKI. Infection increases the mortality rate associated with AKI, especially in older patients. QSEN: Safety.
■ Monitor the patient's temperature.	Because of a decreased immune response, an elevated temperature may not be present with infection in the patient with AKI.
▲ Monitor the white blood cell (WBC) count.	The patient's WBC count will increase in the presence of infection.
■ Note any signs of localized or systemic infection and report them promptly.	Infection is the leading cause of death in AKI. Local signs of infection include redness, warmth, and swelling. Systemic signs of infection may include fever, elevated WBC count, and fatigue.
▲ If infection is suspected, obtain specimens of blood, urine, and sputum for culture and sensitivity, as prescribed.	Identifying the source of the infection is necessary to plan appropriate therapy.

Therapeutic Interventions

Actions/Interventions	Rationales
■ Provide meticulous skin care.	Skin is the first line of defense against infection. Skin that is clean, dry, and free of prolonged pressure is resistant to breakdown and possible infection.
■ Use aseptic technique during dressing changes, wound irrigations, catheter care, and other invasive procedures.	The patient's risk for infection is decreased when aseptic technique is used during care activity. QSEN: Safety.
■ Avoid use of indwelling bladder catheters or IV lines whenever possible.	Invasive lines increase the patient's exposure to infectious agents.
■ Protect the patient from exposure to persons demonstrating signs or symptoms of an infectious illness.	Visitors, family members, and other patients with obvious infections pose an infection risk to the patient in renal failure who may be immunocompromised. QSEN: Safety.
▲ If infection is present, administer antibiotics as prescribed.	The treatment of any infection with antibiotics is necessary to prevent further complications associated with infections.

NANDA-I
NDx Deficient Knowledge

Common Related Factors
Insufficient information
Insufficient interest in learning
Insufficient knowledge of resources
Misinformation presented by others

Defining Characteristics
Insufficient knowledge of AKI
Inaccurate follow-through of instruction
Inaccurate performance on a test
Inappropriate behavior

Common Expected Outcome
Patient and significant others verbalize understanding of AKI, the possible outcomes, and associated treatments.

NOC Outcome
Knowledge: Kidney Disease
NIC Interventions
Health Literacy Enhancement; Learning Facilitation; Teaching: Disease Process; Teaching: Procedure/Treatment

Renal and Urinary Tract Care Plans

⊘volve For additional care plans, go to http://evolve.elsevier.com/Gulanick/.

Action/Intervention

- Assess the patient's knowledge and understanding of AKI, the possible outcomes, and associated treatments.

Rationale

This information provides the starting base for educational sessions. Teaching standardized content that the patient already knows wastes valuable time and hinders critical learning. During the acute stages of AKI, the family or significant others may require the most teaching. QSEN: Patient-centered care.

Therapeutic Interventions

Actions/Interventions

- Explain all the tests and procedures before they occur. Use terms the patient can understand; be clear and direct.

- Explain the purpose of fluid restrictions.

- Discuss the need for a reduced-protein diet.

- Explain the need for renal replacement therapy as appropriate and what to expect during the procedure.
- Discuss the need for follow-up visits after discharge.

▲ Encourage family conferences with members of the patient's interprofessional health team (e.g., physicians, nurses, rehabilitation personnel, dietitians, social workers), as necessary.

Rationales

Patients are more likely to cooperate with care and experience less anxiety when they understand what to expect during tests and procedures. QSEN: Patient-centered care.

The patient needs to understand the importance of fluid restrictions during the oliguric phase to prevent fluid excess. As the patient moves from the oliguric to diuretic phase, fluid restrictions may be modified or discontinued. QSEN: Safety.

The reduced-protein diet helps prevent excessive elevations in blood urea nitrogen.

This therapy may involve hemodialysis or continuous renal replacement therapy.

The return of renal function may occur over a 12-month period, necessitating changes in medications, diet, and fluid restriction, as well as close medical supervision. Occasionally, renal function does not return and instead deteriorates to chronic kidney disease.

These conferences facilitate family involvement in interprofessional planning. The patient may recover renal function or may need long-term dialysis if there is no return of kidney function. QSEN: Teamwork and collaboration.

Related Care Plans

Anxiety, Chapter 2
Ineffective coping, Chapter 2
Hemodialysis, Chapter 11
Peritoneal dialysis, Chapter 11
Chronic kidney disease, Chapter 11

Chronic Kidney Disease (CKD)

Uremia; Renal Failure; Chronic/End-Stage Renal Disease

Chronic kidney disease (CKD) is a condition characterized by a progressive, irreversible loss of kidney function causing chronic abnormalities in the body's homeostasis and affecting every body system. It is caused primarily by diabetes and high blood pressure, accounting for two thirds of all cases. In early stages there may be only non-specific signs and symptoms of the disease, so the kidney disease goes undetected and untreated. Early detection by simple tests such as urine albumin and serum creatinine can detect CKD and help prevent the progression of kidney

Renal and Urinary Tract
Care Plans

■ = Independent   ▲ = Interprofessional Collaboration

disease to kidney failure. Despite the complexities of kidney failure, heart disease is the major cause of death for most people with CKD. The glomerular filtration rate (GFR) is the best estimate of kidney function and the best way to determine the stage of CKD. Five stages of CKD are used to guide treatment:

Stage 1 = Kidney damage with normal kidney function (GFR ≥90 mL/min/1.7 m^2). Treatment focuses on diagnosis and CVD risk reduction.

Stage 2 = Kidney damage with mild loss of kidney function (GFR 89-60 mL/min/1.7 m^2). Treatment focuses on reduction of risk factors.

Stage 3 = Kidney damage with moderate loss of kidney function (GFR 30-59 mL/min/1.7 m^2). Treatment focus is on strategies to slow disease progression.

Stage 4 = Severe loss of kidney function (GFR 29-15 mL/min/1.7 m^2). Treatment focuses on managing complications and preparing for future renal replacement therapy.

Stage 5 = Kidney failure (GFR <15 mL/min/1.7 m^2 or dialysis). Renal replacement therapy, ideally kidney transplant, is needed to prevent death from life-threatening consequences.

Treatment goals for CKD include preserving kidney function, reducing risks for cardiovascular disease, preventing complications, and providing for optimal quality of life. End-stage kidney disease (ESKD) has a high mortality rate. For eligible patients requiring dialysis therapies, Medicare will cover 80% of eligible charges. This care plan provides an overview of some of the more common complications associated with CKD treated in the outpatient setting or at-home setting.

NANDA-I
NDx Deficient Knowledge

Common Related Factors
Insufficient information
Insufficient interest in learning
Insufficient knowledge of resources
Misinformation presented by others

Common Expected Outcome
The patient verbalizes understanding of chronic kidney disease, prevention of complications, medication therapy, and necessary dietary restrictions.

Defining Characteristics
Insufficient knowledge
Inaccurate follow-through of instruction
Inaccurate performance on a test
Inappropriate behavior

NOC Outcomes
Knowledge: Chronic Kidney Disease;
Knowledge: Treatment Regimen

NIC Interventions
Health Literacy Enhancement; Learning Facilitation; Teaching: Chronic Kidney Disease; Teaching: Prescribed Diet

---

Ongoing Assessment

Actions/Interventions

■ Assess the patient's understanding of CKD, the stages of CKD, and the overall treatment approach for patient's specific stage.

■ Determine the patient's understanding of his or her specific risk factors for cardiovascular disease.

Rationales

CKD is a progressive disease that requires ongoing self-management to reduce disease progression and complications. The treatment plan includes nutrition therapy, medication compliance, and prevention of complications. An understanding of CKD will facilitate compliance with the long-term treatment plan. QSEN: Patient-centered care.

Cardiovascular disease is the major cause of death in patients with CKD. Attention to specific risk factors (e.g., diabetes, hypertension, dyslipidemia) and a prescribed risk reduction program can improve outcomes for the patient. QSEN: Safety; Patient-centered care.

Renal and Urinary Tract Care Plans

Actions/Interventions

- Determine the patient's self-efficacy to learn about CKD and apply this new knowledge to participation in treatment of the disease.

Rationales

A first step in teaching may be to foster increased self-efficacy in the patient's ability to learn the desired information or skills. Some lifestyle changes can be difficult to make for the patient with CKD.

Therapeutic Interventions

Actions/Interventions

- Instruct the patient in dietary components of the treatment plan:
  - Nutritional therapy
  - Fluid restrictions
  - Low-fat diet
  - Vitamin and mineral requirements

- Involve significant others in instruction sessions on special diets and fluid restrictions.

- Discuss the need for reading food labels for sodium, potassium, and other mineral content before using.

- Discuss the importance of taking prescribed medications (e.g., diabetes and hypertensive medications, statins for dyslipidemias, fibrates to control triglycerides, medications to treat anemia, diuretics for fluid overload, phosphate binders). Discuss thoroughly the dosages and side effects.

- Instruct the patient to notify members of the interprofessional health team of any questions or concerns regarding over-the-counter medications and food or herbal supplements.

- Instruct the patient in the recognition of complications such as fluid volume excess and electrolyte imbalances.

- If the patient has diabetes, instruct the patient to closely monitor urine for microalbuminuria and report any changes in urine.

- Discuss ESKD with the patient, including the need for dialysis or renal transplantation for survival.

Rationales

The diet needs to be individualized according to the impairment of renal function. In general, diets are high in carbohydrates (unless contraindicated by diabetes mellitus) and within allotted sodium, potassium, phosphorus, and protein limits. Daily requirements will change if the patient is receiving dialysis treatment. A lower-fat diet may be indicated for dyslipidemia. Vitamin D and calcium may require replacement. QSEN: Patient-centered care.

Significant others may be the people who buy and prepare the patient's food. They need to have this information to support the dietary needs of the patient. QSEN: Patient-centered care.

Many processed foods contain high levels of sodium. The sodium may be in forms other than salt or sodium chloride. Salt substitutes may be high in potassium.

Patients are better able to manage the complexity of their medications with sufficient knowledge. The patient needs to understand the importance of reporting side effects rather than discontinuing the medication. Adjustments in drugs and dosages may be possible to reduce unpleasant side effects. QSEN: Patient-centered care; Safety.

This measure helps prevent complications from drug and herbal interactions with prescribed medications. QSEN: Safety; Teamwork and collaboration.

Changes in fluid and electrolyte balance may indicate the need for adjustments in the treatment plan. The patient and caregivers at home need to know the early signs and symptoms to report to their health care provider such as headache, swelling of the hands and feet, weight gain of 1 to 2 pounds in 24 hours, or paresthesias. QSEN: Safety.

Persistent albuminuria is an indicator of progression of CKD associated with diabetes. Early recognition can facilitate revision of the treatment plan to preserve renal function. QSEN: Safety.

Patients need information about treatment options to make informed decisions and should be active partners in weighing the pros and cons of the types of dialysis. Ideally a transplant can occur prior to starting dialysis therapy. QSEN: Patient-centered care.

Renal and Urinary Tract Care Plans

■ = Independent ▲ = Interprofessional Collaboration

NANDA-I NDx Excess Fluid Volume

Common Related Factors

Excess fluid intake
Excess sodium intake
Compromised renal regulatory mechanisms

Defining Characteristics

Weight gain over a short period of time
Edema
Tachycardia
Orthopnea/dyspnea
Adventitious breath sounds: crackles
Presence of third heart sound (S_3)
Alteration in BP
Jugular vein distention
Change in mental status
Restlessness and anxiety

Common Expected Outcome

Patient is normovolemic as evidenced by weight gain less than 2 to 3 pounds between hemodialysis treatments, reduction of edema, HR 60 to 100 beats/min, absence of pulmonary crackles.

NOC Outcomes

Fluid Balance; Electrolyte and Acid/Base Balance; Cardiopulmonary Status

NIC Intervention

Fluid/Electrolyte Management

Ongoing Assessment

Actions/Interventions	Rationales
■ Assess vital signs for fluid volume excess.	The kidney's ability to regulate fluid balance is lost in CKD. The signs of fluid volume excess are the result of sodium and water retention leading to increased circulatory fluid volume. These signs may include elevated BP, tachycardia, and tachypnea.
■ Auscultate for crackles.	Crackles signify the presence of fluid in the alveoli. The patient may have orthopnea.
■ Assess for peripheral edema by palpating the area over the tibia, ankles, sacrum, and back and by assessing the appearance of the face.	Peripheral edema may be more noticeable in the dependent areas of the body. The patient may have periorbital edema.
■ Assess the patient's compliance with dietary and fluid restrictions at home.	Excess fluid or sodium intake can lead to fluid volume excess in the patient with CKD, especially ESKD. Maintaining fluid balance requires the patient to adhere to fluid intake and dietary sodium prescriptions. QSEN: Safety; Patient-centered care.
■ Assess the patient's weight at every visit before and after dialysis	Changes in weight are a reliable measure of fluid gains and losses. Weight gain is the best sign of fluid volume excess and should not exceed 2 to 3 pounds between visits.

Therapeutic Interventions

Actions/Interventions	Rationales
■ Have the patient sit up if he or she reports shortness of breath.	This position promotes pooling of fluid in the lung bases and makes more lung tissue available for gas exchange.
■ Advise the patient to elevate his or her feet when sitting down.	This position reduces edema in the lower extremities and increases venous return.

---

 evolve **For additional care plans, go to http://evolve.elsevier.com/Gulanick/.**

Renal and Urinary Tract Care Plans

Actions/Interventions

■ Instruct the patient in the administration of antihypertensive medications if prescribed.

■ Instruct the patient regarding restricting fluid intake as required by the patient's condition.
■ Instruct the patient regarding restricting dietary sodium.

■ Instruct the patient in methods to relieve dry mouth and maintain fluid restriction:
  • Suggest taking ice chips, as needed.

  • Suggest using sugar-free hard candy or gum.

  • Suggest frequent mouth rinses using $\frac{1}{2}$ cup of mouthwash mixed with $\frac{1}{2}$ cup of ice water.
▲ Adjust renal replacement therapy as indicated.

Rationales

Maintaining fluid balance is improved by the control of BP to preserve remaining nephron function and slow the progression of CKD. Common medications include calcium channel blockers and angiotensin-converting enzyme inhibitors. As a rule, hypertension management can be difficult in this population and may require multiple medications. QSEN: Evidence-based practice; Patient-centered care.

Patients on dialysis need to understand the importance of maintaining fluid balance between treatments.

Sodium intake produces a feeling of thirst. By restricting sodium intake, the amount of fluid a patient drinks can be reduced.

One cup of ice equals only $\frac{1}{2}$ cup of water. Sucking a cup of ice takes much longer than drinking $\frac{1}{2}$ cup of water; the patient may attain more satisfaction in relieving a dry mouth.

Sucking on hard candy or chewing gum can stimulate saliva secretion and relieve dry mouth.

Rinses can produce freshness in the mouth and temporarily alleviate thirst.

Renal replacement therapies such as peritoneal dialysis or hemodialysis are calculated to remove excess fluid and maintain a normovolemic state. QSEN: Patient-centered care.

NANDA-I NDx **Risk for Decreased Cardiac Output**

Common Risk Factors

Increased ventricular filling (fluid volume excess)
Alteration in heart rate, rhythm, and conduction
Impaired contractility from accumulated toxins or pericarditis
Increased afterload

Common Expected Outcome

Patient has adequate cardiac output as evidenced by systolic BP within 20 mm Hg of baseline; HR 60 to 100 beats/min with regular rhythm; strong peripheral pulses; warm and dry skin; eupnea with absence of pulmonary crackles; and orientation to person, time, and place.

NOC Outcomes
Circulation Status; Electrolyte and Acid/Base Balance
NIC Interventions
Hemodynamic Regulation; Hemodialysis Therapy; Electrolyte Management

Ongoing Assessment

Actions/Interventions

■ Monitor the patient's BP and HR.

Rationales

The majority of patients with CKD experience hypertension. The result of hypertension is left ventricular hypertrophy and an increased risk for heart failure and decreased cardiac output. Tachycardia may occur as a compensatory response for decreasing cardiac output. QSEN: Safety.

■ = Independent   ▲ = Interprofessional Collaboration

Actions/Interventions	Rationales
■ Assess the skin's temperature and peripheral pulses.	Peripheral vasoconstriction may occur as a compensation for decreasing cardiac output. The patient will have cool, pale, diaphoretic skin and diminished peripheral pulses.
■ Assess level of consciousness.	Decreased cardiac output leads to reduced cerebral tissue perfusion. Early signs of cerebral hypoxia are restlessness and anxiety, leading to agitation and confusion. QSEN: Safety.
■ Use pulse oximetry to monitor oxygen saturation; assess arterial blood gases as ordered.	Pulse oximetry is a useful tool to detect changes in oxygenation. Oxygen saturation should be at 90% or greater. Changes in arterial blood gases may indicate hypoxemia and metabolic acidosis associated with CKD.
■ Monitor for dysrhythmias.	Cardiac dysrhythmias may contribute to decreasing cardiac output or be the result of the low perfusion state. Patients in the later stages of CKD are at risk for dysrhythmias from metabolic acidosis, hyperkalemia, or hypocalcemia.
▲ Monitor laboratory study findings for serum potassium, calcium, phosphorus, blood urea nitrogen (BUN), and creatinine.	These tests provide data on electrolyte imbalances and accumulated toxins. BUN also may be increased from nonrenal causes such as dehydration; however, in those situations the creatinine will not be elevated. Hyperkalemia can cause the most serious life-threatening dysrhythmias. The patient with CKD will have low serum calcium and elevated serum phosphorus. QSEN: Safety.
■ Auscultate the patient's heart sounds for the presence of pericardial friction rub or distant or muffled heart sounds; assess for hypotension and jugular venous distention indicating pericardial effusion or pericardial tamponade.	Patients receiving hemodialysis are at a greater risk for the development of pericarditis, increasing the risk for pericardial effusion and pericardial tamponade. Pericarditis may be caused by accumulation of uremic toxins in the pericardial fluid. Pericarditis can develop into a pericardial effusion and even result in cardiac tamponade. QSEN: Safety.

Therapeutic Interventions

Actions/Interventions	Rationales
▲ Administer oral and IV fluids as prescribed. Use fluid restriction as appropriate.	Optimal fluid balance improves cardiac output. For the patient in ESKD, fluid balance is maintained through the careful regulation of fluid intake and dialysis treatments.
▲ Administer medications as prescribed:	Hyperkalemia can be a life-threatening complication for the patient with CKD. These medications temporarily equilibrate electrolyte disturbances and reduce the risk for dysrhythmias. QSEN: Evidence-based practice; Safety.
• Sodium bicarbonate	Sodium bicarbonate will temporarily shift potassium back into the cells to correct metabolic acidosis and hyperkalemia. However, it can result in an elevation of sodium and water retention from the sodium load.
• IV insulin and glucose	Insulin shifts potassium back into the cells to correct metabolic acidosis and hyperkalemia. Glucose is administered to prevent hypoglycemia from the effect of insulin.
• Potassium-exchange resins (e.g., Kayexelate)	These resins exchange potassium for sodium in the gastrointestinal tract, thereby decreasing serum potassium levels. The bound potassium is excreted in the bowel movement.
• Calcium gluconate	Calcium gluconate treats hypocalcemia. It also may be given to stabilize the cell membrane from depolarization in the hyperkalemic state.
▲ Administer oxygen as needed.	Oxygen improves arterial saturation.
▲ Treat dysrhythmias as appropriate.	Untreated dysrhythmias contribute to decreased cardiac output.

evolve **For additional care plans, go to http://evolve.elsevier.com/Gulanick/.**

Actions/Interventions

▲ Administer inotropic agents as prescribed.
▲ Prepare the patient for dialysis when indicated.

Rationales

These drugs increase myocardial contractility.
Dialysis is used to maintain fluid and electrolyte balance and remove metabolic wastes. This treatment reduces the patient's risk for decreased cardiac output. QSEN: Safety.

NANDA-I NDx **Risk for Electrolyte Imbalance: CKD Mineral and Bone Disorders**

Common Risk Factors

Renal dysfunction
Phosphorus retention (level >5 mg/100 mL)
Bone resorption of calcium (demineralization)
Increased parathyroid hormone
Inadequate calcium absorption
Compromised regulatory mechanisms

Common Expected Outcomes

Patient's risk for hypocalcemia is diminished through ongoing assessment and early intervention.
Patient follows appropriate ambulation and safety measures.

NOC Outcomes

Self-Management: Kidney Disease; Electrolyte and Acid/Base Balance; Medication Response

NIC Interventions

Electrolyte Management: Hypocalcemia; Electrolyte Management: Hyperphosphatemia

---

Ongoing Assessment

Actions/Interventions

■ Assess for the signs and symptoms of hypocalcemia.

▲ Monitor calcium and phosphorus levels.

■ Assess for signs or symptoms of metastatic pulmonary calcifications.

Rationales

The inability of the kidneys to excrete phosphorus leads to hyperphosphatemia with resultant hypocalcemia. The decreased activation of vitamin D by the kidney leads to a decreased intestinal absorption of calcium. The patient may exhibit tingling sensations at the ends of the fingers or around the mouth, muscle cramps, and carpopedal spasms, tetany, and seizures. CKD mineral and bone disorders (MBDs) occur when the kidneys fail to maintain the proper levels of calcium and phosphorus in the blood, leading to abnormal bone hormone levels. CKD-MBD is a common problem in people with kidney disease and affects almost all patients receiving dialysis. QSEN: Safety.

Early identification of changes in serum calcium and phosphorus levels allows for prompt interventions. Hypercalcemia can result from the calcium binders used to decrease phosphate levels. QSEN: Safety.

Metastatic pulmonary calcifications occur as part of the process of renal osteodystrophy from calcium phosphate deposits in soft tissues of the body (e.g., primarily pulmonary tissues, blood vessels, joints, muscles, myocardium, and eyes). These deposits develop as a result of increased parathyroid hormone in response to hypocalcemia. The patient may have decreased tissue perfusion in the fingers and toes, eye redness, or cardiac dysrhythmias. QSEN: Safety.

Renal and Urinary Tract Care Plans

■ = Independent ▲ = Interprofessional Collaboration

Actions/Interventions

- Assess for pruritus.

- Observe the patient's gait and ambulation.

Rationales

Pruritus can be caused by dry skin or the accumulation of calcium phosphate precipitation associated with renal osteodystrophy. Scratching by the patient to relieve pruritus increases the risk of skin trauma. QSEN: Safety.

Hypocalcemia can lead to bone pain, neuromuscular irritability, and altered mobility. Renal osteodystrophy, hypocalcemia, and increased parathyroid hormone cause demineralization of the bones. The patient is at an increased risk for fractures with minimal trauma. QSEN: Safety.

Therapeutic Interventions

Actions/Interventions

- Instruct the patient in the need to limit dietary phosphorus intake.

- ▲ Administer or instruct the patient to take phosphate-binding medications (e.g., calcium acetate, sevelamer hydrochloride, calcium carbonate) as prescribed depending on the stage of CKD. Avoid magnesium antacids, because the kidney may not be able to excrete magnesium.

- ▲ Instruct the patient to take vitamin D supplements as ordered.

- Instruct the patient about strategies to manage pruritus:
  - Wearing loose-fitting clothes
  - Avoiding scratching the skin
  - Keeping finger nails short
  - Using lotions or emollients for dry, scaling skin
  - Using tepid water for bathing
  - Taking medications such as antihistamines
- Discuss needed safety measures: an uncluttered room, orientation to surroundings, proper lighting.

- ▲ Refer to physical therapy as indicated for instruction in the use of ambulation aids and safe transfer techniques.

Rationales

Phosphorus and calcium have an inverse relationship. Hyperphosphatemia worsens hypocalcemia. The degree of dietary phosphorus restriction is related to the stage of CKD. QSEN: Patient-centered care.

The phosphate-binding medication prevents ingested phosphorus from being absorbed; instead, phosphorus will bind with the medication and then be excreted through bowel movements.

The kidney is no longer able to activate vitamin D that is needed for the intestinal absorption of calcium. There are several vitamin D supplements that promote calcium absorption.

Restrictive clothing can aggravate the problem and increase the risk for skin breakdown. Scratching can cause lesions and open sores. Lotions and emollients can provide lubrication to the skin and promote comfort. Increased warmth in bathing can increase the itch. Antihistamines can relieve itching. QSEN: Safety.

Environmental modifications may be needed to promote safety with ambulation. Bones may become fragile increasing the risk for stress fractures, even from mild trauma. QSEN: Safety.

The physical therapist, as a member of the interprofessional health team, can teach the patient about the use of assistive devices for ambulation. These ambulation aids may reduce the risk for injury. QSEN: Teamwork and collaboration.

NANDA-I
NDx **Ineffective Protection: Anemia/Thrombocytopenia**

Common Related Factors

Bone marrow suppression secondary to insufficient renal production of erythropoietic factor

Increased hemolysis leading to decreased life span of red blood cells (RBCs) secondary to abnormal chemical environment in plasma

Nutritional deficiencies

Bleeding tendencies: decreased platelets and defective platelet cohesion, inhibition of certain clotting factors

Blood loss related to hemodialysis procedure

Defining Characteristics

Decreased hemoglobin (Hgb) and hematocrit (Hct)

Fatigue or pallor

Decreased platelet count

Increase in coagulation times

Bruising tendencies

Renal and Urinary Tract Care Plans

Common Expected Outcome

Patient maintains Hgb and Hct levels and adequate platelet counts within a range acceptable for the stage of CKD.

NOC Outcome
Blood Coagulation
NIC Interventions
Bleeding Precautions; Surveillance

Ongoing Assessment

Actions/Interventions	Rationales
■ Observe for signs of anemia.	Anemia is associated with the decreased oxygen-carrying capacity of RBCs. The patient may exhibit fatigue, pallor, and decreased activity tolerance.
■ Observe for signs of thrombocytopenia.	Uremia leads to coagulopathies and increases the patient's risk for bleeding. The patient may have prolonged bleeding from minor trauma, bleeding gums, nose bleeds, and increased bruising. QSEN: Safety.
■ Use pulse oximetry to monitor oxygen saturation; assess arterial blood gases as ordered.	Pulse oximetry is a useful tool to detect changes in oxygenation. Oxygen saturation should be at 90% or greater. Decreased oxygen saturation may be a sign of anemia.
▲ Monitor the results of laboratory studies (Hgb, Hct, platelets, coagulation studies), as prescribed.	The Hct may be as low as 20% to 22% from the reduced secretion of erythropoietin by the kidney. Decreased platelet counts and alterations in clotting factors may occur with dialysis and the use of anticoagulants.
■ Test stools and emesis for occult blood if a decrease in Hct and Hgb occurs.	The presence of occult blood in the feces is an indicator of gastrointestinal (GI) bleeding. QSEN: Safety.

Therapeutic Interventions

Actions/Interventions	Rationales
■ Instruct the patient about the signs and symptoms that need to be reported to a health care provider.	Early identification of anemia or thrombocytopenia allows for prompt intervention. The patient must be aware of the signs of anemia such as increasing fatigue, shortness of breath, or pale skin. The patient must be advised to monitor for signs of bright red blood from the rectum or a change in feces to a black, tarry color and consistency. These changes are most likely to be associated with GI bleeding. QSEN: Patient-centered care.
▲ Administer or instruct the patient in the administration of epoetin alfa (Epogen), or darbepoetin alfa, as prescribed.	These medications replace the erythropoietin no longer produced by the kidney. Their use may reduce the need for frequent blood transfusions by maintaining acceptable Hgb and Hct levels. The patient needs to learn subcutaneous injection technique for administration. The drugs also may be given intravenously. QSEN: Patient-centered care.
▲ Instruct the patient to take iron supplements as ordered.	Even with the use of epoetin alfa, functional iron stores may be low related to preexisting nutritional deficiencies. Dietary supplements are preferred, especially if the patient is not able to consume adequate iron from food sources because of anorexia that occurs with the later stages of CKD.
▲ Instruct the patient in the need for folic acid, as prescribed.	Folic acid is necessary for RBC formation. Folic acid is lost during dialysis and must be given after treatments. The patient may have a preexisting nutritional deficiency.

Renal and Urinary Tract Care Plans

■ = Independent   ▲ = Interprofessional Collaboration

Actions/Interventions

▲ Administer oxygen as prescribed.

▲ Anticipate or administer blood transfusions.

■ For patients with thrombocytopenia, institute precautionary measures for all invasive procedures, and monitor heparin administration closely.

■ Instruct the patient in the use of a soft toothbrush and electric razor and in avoiding constipation, forceful blowing of the nose, and contact sports.

■ Instruct the patient to avoid aspirin products.

■ Instruct the patient about the importance of wearing a medical alert bracelet.

Rationales

Supplemental oxygen improves oxygen saturation and arterial Pao$_2$.

Blood transfusions may be required if Hct falls below 20%.

Any needle stick is a potential bleeding site. Direct pressure may need to be applied for longer periods to promote hemostasis after venipunctures or injections. Whenever possible, laboratory specimens should be collected through an existing arterial or venous access device. Heparin is used to decrease the risk for clotting in the extracorporeal circuit during hemodialysis. In patients at risk for bleeding, heparin doses may need to be carefully calculated. QSEN: Safety.

These safety measures reduce the risk for trauma and bleeding. QSEN: Safety.

Aspirin inhibits platelet aggregation and prolongs bleeding time.

It is critical to alert community members and health care workers to the patient's medical condition in case of emergency. QSEN: Safety.

NANDA-I
NDx **Risk for Situational Low Self-Esteem**

Common Risk Factors

Alteration in social role (change in perceptions as autonomous and productive individual; dependence on outpatient dialysis)

Loss of organ function

Functional impairment (financial strain related to disability status or need to seek a less physically demanding job)

Alteration in body image

Common Expected Outcome

Patient verbalizes positive self-acceptance.

NOC Outcomes
Self-Esteem; Personal Resiliency; Body Image
NIC Interventions
Self-Esteem Enhancement; Coping Enhancement; Body Image Enhancement

---

Ongoing Assessment

Actions/Interventions

■ Assess for the signs of low self-esteem.

Rationales

The patient receiving long-term renal replacement therapy is faced with significant alterations in lifestyle, occupation, and financial status. The patient's future depends on medications, dietary restrictions, and hemodialysis. The patient may grieve this loss of autonomy. Signs of low self-esteem may include self-negating verbalizations, depression, anger, and social isolation, expressions of shame or guilt, or evaluation of self as unable to deal with events.

Actions/Interventions

■ Review with the patient past and current accomplishments: emotional, social, interpersonal, intellectual, vocational, and physical.

Rationales

Patients experiencing situational stress often lose sight of their past successes in managing similar situations. QSEN: Patient-centered care.

Therapeutic Interventions

Actions/Interventions

■ Assist the patient in identifying the major areas of concern related to altered self-esteem. Use a problem-solving technique with the patient.

■ Assist the patient in incorporating changes in health status into activities of daily living, social life, interpersonal relationships, and occupational activities.

■ Talk with the patient, caregivers, and friends, if possible, about expectations regarding long-term hemodialysis or renal transplantation.

■ Allow the patient time to voice concerns and express anger related to having a chronic condition.

■ Encourage an attitude of realistic hope.

▲ Use case managers, social workers, and clergy as necessary.

■ Provide or encourage discussions with other patients with late stages of CKD.

■ Encourage the patient and family to participate in support groups.

▲ Refer to a psychiatric consultant as necessary.

Rationales

The nurse-patient relationship can provide a strong basis for implementing strategies to assist the patient and family with adaptation. QSEN: Patient-centered care.

As the patient's condition worsens with ESKD, it is more difficult to engage in even routine activities. The patient may have difficulty accepting the need to ask others for help with daily activities.

Survival depends on such treatments. The patient may resent such dependence.

Denial and anger are anticipated responses to the diagnosis of a CKD and its progression to later stages of the disease.

Hope provides a way of dealing with negative feelings.

These members of the interprofessional health team can provide psychological support and assist with strategies for problem-solving. QSEN: Teamwork and collaboration.

Patients may benefit from sharing feelings with people who have successfully adjusted to the experience with the same diagnosis.

Groups that come together for mutual goals can be most helpful. These groups may provide positive support and share best practices for coping with the disease.

Most dialysis patients experience some degree of emotional imbalance. With professional psychiatric consultation, most patients can gradually accept changed self-esteem. QSEN: Teamwork and collaboration.

NANDA-I **NDx** **Sexual Dysfunction**

Common Related Factor

Alteration in body function or structure due to effects of uremia on the endocrine system (amenorrhea, failure to ovulate, and decreased libido in females; azoospermia, atrophy of testicles, impotence, decreased libido, and gynecomastia in males)

Defining Characteristics

Undesired change in sexual function
Perceived sexual limitation
Alteration in sexual excitation
Alteration in sexual satisfaction

Common Expected Outcome

Patient verbalizes comfort with sexual expression, role changes and ability to adapt to functional limitations due to CKD.

NOC Outcomes

Sexual Functioning; Role Performance; Adaptation to Physical Disability

NIC Intervention

Sexual Counseling

Renal and Urinary Tract Care Plans

■ = Independent ▲ = Interprofessional Collaboration

Ongoing Assessment

Actions/Interventions

- Assess the patient's perception of change in or lack of sexual function. Explore the meaning of sexuality with the patient.
- Assess the impact of changes in sexual function on the patient.
- Assess the need for counseling related to the need for contraception.

Rationales

Both men and women with later stages of CKD characteristically experience infertility and a decreased libido. QSEN: Patient-centered care.

Changes in sexual function can lead to depression, low self-esteem, and impaired interpersonal relationships.

With the use of epoetin and with improvement in the female patient's Hgb and Hct levels, menses is often restored and the possibility of pregnancy increases. The patient may need help deciding about becoming pregnant. Pregnant women on hemodialysis are at risk for untoward outcomes for herself and the fetus.

Therapeutic Interventions

Actions/Interventions

- Encourage the patient to verbalize his or her feelings about the change in or lack of sexual function.

- Discuss alternative methods of sexual expression with the patient or significant others. Emphasize the importance of giving and receiving love and affection, as opposed to "performing."
- ▲ Confer with members of the interprofessional health team about treatments and procedures that may alleviate some sexual dysfunction.

Rationales

Respecting the patient and treating his or her concerns as normal and important may foster greater self-acceptance. QSEN: Patient-centered care.

Patients need to understand that intercourse is not the only method for a satisfying sexual relationship.

Patients may experience a restoration of sexual function through the use of a variety of therapeutic methods. For men, possible treatments include a penile implant or medications. If the patient has low zinc levels, replacement therapy may help improve sexual function. QSEN: Teamwork and collaboration.

Related Care Plans

Fatigue, Chapter 2
Disturbed body image, Chapter 2
Risk for infection, Chapter 2
Ineffective health management, Chapter 2
Hemodialysis, Chapter 11
Peritoneal dialysis, Chapter 11
Organ transplant, solid, ⊖volve

Hemodialysis

Internal Arteriovenous Fistula; Graft; Central Venous Catheter; Renal Replacement Therapy

Hemodialysis is one of the renal replacement therapies used to sustain life in people with no or very little kidney function. In general, dialysis is the diffusion of solute molecules and fluids across a semipermeable membrane. Dialysis may be a short-term therapy in situations such as acute kidney injury (AKI) or long-term therapy for the patient with chronic kidney disease (CKD). Hemodialysis may be used to remove drugs from the circulatory system as part of the treatment for drug overdoses. The purpose of dialysis is to remove excess fluids, toxins, and metabolic wastes from the blood. The primary mechanisms of dialysis are diffusion, osmosis, and ultrafiltration. The composition of the dialysis

⊖volve   For additional care plans, go to http://evolve.elsevier.com/Gulanick/.

solution (dialysate) establishes a concentration and/or osmotic gradient to promote diffusion and osmosis of urea, creatinine, and electrolytes from the blood to the dialysate. Ultrafiltration is used to remove excess fluid by adjusting pressures in the blood compartment and the dialysate compartment. Rapid changes in vascular volume and electrolyte concentrations during hemodialysis can result in complications such as hypotension, muscle cramping, and cerebral edema. Hemodialysis increases the patient's risk for infection. The most common source for infection is through vascular access sites. The incidence of blood-borne infections such as human immunodeficiency virus (HIV) infection and hepatitis B and C has decreased with improved screening of patients and use of dedicated equipment for patients with these infections.

Hemodialysis requires a vascular access. This can be accomplished by surgically creating an arteriovenous (AV) fistula or graft (synthetic material used to connect an artery and a vein); or by insertion of an external catheter into a large central vein. The internal AV fistula is made by surgically creating an anastomosis between an artery and a vein, thus allowing arterial blood to flow through the vein, causing engorgement and enlargement. Placement may be in either forearm, using the radial artery and cephalic vein or brachial artery and cephalic vein. The internal AV fistula is the preferred access for long-term hemodialysis and must heal and mature before it may be used for access in hemodialysis. The central venous catheter may be either single or double lumen. A single-lumen catheter serves as the arterial source, and the venous return is made through a peripheral vein or by the use of an alternating flow device. A double-lumen catheter is used for both the arterial source and the venous return. Because of their location and low durability, femoral catheters are usually used only with inpatients on a short-term basis. Central venous catheters are considered a temporary access device but may be used for weeks or even months on an outpatient basis. The settings for hemodialysis include inpatient dialysis units in hospitals, outpatient dialysis centers, and the patient's home.

NANDA-I NDx   Risk for Decreased Cardiac Output

Common Risk Factors

Increased or decreased ventricular filling (preload) related to decreased fluid volume
Alteration in heart rate, rhythm, and conduction
Decreased oxygenation related to anemia

Common Expected Outcome

Patient has adequate cardiac output, as evidenced by systolic BP within 20 mm Hg of baseline; HR 60 to 100 beats/min with regular rhythm; urine output 30 mL/hr or greater, strong peripheral pulses; warm and dry skin; eupnea with absence of pulmonary crackles; and orientation to time, place, and person.

NOC Outcomes
Cardiac Pump Effectiveness; Circulation Status; Cardiopulmonary Status
NIC Interventions
Cardiac Care; Hemodynamic Regulation

Ongoing Assessment

Actions/Interventions	Rationales
Predialysis:	Assessment data gathered before dialysis establishes a baseline for monitoring the patient after dialysis. QSEN: Patient-centered care; Safety.
Assess the patient's BP and HR.	Sinus tachycardia and hypotension are indicators of decreased cardiac output after dialysis. Orthostatic hypotension is an early indicator of deficient fluid volume after dialysis. The rapid removal of fluid volume during dialysis leads to a decreased circulatory volume and decreased cardiac output.
Assess the patient's body weight daily using the same scale and clothing.	A change in body weight is an accurate indicator of fluid losses that are expected to occur during dialysis.

■ = Independent   ▲ = Interprofessional Collaboration

Actions/Interventions

- Assess the patient's level of consciousness; peripheral pulses; capillary refill; heart sounds; respiratory rate and rhythm; skin temperature, color, and moisture.

- Assess for signs of bleeding.

Rationales

Restlessness, irritability, and decreased concentration occur with changes in cerebral perfusion after dialysis. Weak peripheral pulses with slow or absent capillary refill are indicators of decreased cardiac output. The patient may develop a gallop heart rhythm. Respirations may become rapid and shallow with reduced cardiac output. Cold, pale, clammy skin occurs as a secondary response to compensatory increases in sympathetic nervous system stimulation with decreased cardiac output.

The use of anticoagulants during dialysis increases the risk for bleeding, which can compromise cardiac output.

Therapeutic Interventions

Actions/Interventions

- ▲ Consult with the physician about withholding medications before dialysis.

- ▲ Administer IV fluids as needed.

Rationales

Vasoactive drugs may contribute to postdialysis hypotension if given before dialysis. These drugs include antihypertensives, antidysrhythmics, and vasodilators. The drugs may be withheld before dialysis. QSEN: Teamwork and collaboration; Safety.

Fluid replacement therapy may be indicated to increase circulatory volume after dialysis.

NANDA-I NDx Risk for Infection

Common Risk Factors

Inadequate primary defenses: hemodialysis access site
Inadequate secondary defenses: immunosuppression; suppressed inflammatory response
Insufficient knowledge to avoid exposure to pathogens
Invasive procedures: AV access cannulation
Chronic kidney disease
Inadequate vaccination for hepatitis B

Common Expected Outcomes

Patient is free of infection as evidenced by normal body temperature and white blood cell count and no drainage, redness, or swelling at vascular access site.
Infection is recognized early to allow for prompt treatment.

NOC Outcomes
Risk Detection; Risk Control; Infection Severity
NIC Interventions
Infection Protection; Infection Control

Ongoing Assessment

Actions/Interventions

- Assess for the signs and symptoms of infection.

- ▲ Obtain a blood culture and catheter exit site culture if there is evidence of an infection.

Rationales

The presence of infection may produce pain around the central venous catheter site or over the peripheral access site. The access site may appear red, swollen, warm to the touch, and with drainage. The patient may experience a fever. QSEN: Safety.

This culture allows for identification of the causative agent and selection of appropriate antibiotic therapy. QSEN: Evidence-based practice.

⊖volve **For additional care plans, go to http://evolve.elsevier.com/Gulanick/.**

Therapeutic Interventions

Actions/Interventions	Rationales

Central venous catheter:

■ Maintain asepsis with the catheter when initiating or discontinuing dialysis

These nursing actions reduce the risk of transmitting pathogens to the patient. QSEN: Safety.

- Clean the area with antiseptic.

The antiseptics used for site care will vary and must be compatible with the catheter material. Commonly used antiseptics include povidone-iodine, chlorhexidine, and electrolyte chloroxidizers (e.g., ExSept).

- Disinfect catheter hub caps and blood line connections before separation.

Disinfectants must be compatible with catheter materials. Catheter lumens and tips should never be left open to the air, to reduce the risk for contamination by airborne pathogens.

- Wear surgical masks for all connect and disconnect procedures and dressing changes.

It is important to prevent the spread of infectious droplets that may contaminate connection sites and catheter exit sites.

- Change the sterile dressing over the catheter exit site after each dialysis treatment.

Dialysis units develop policies on sterile dressing changes to reduce the risk for introducing pathogens through the catheter.

- Restrict the use of the catheter for no other purpose but hemodialysis.

Use of the catheter for multiple purposes increases the risk for infection. The catheter should not be used for administration of other IV fluids or medications or for obtaining blood samples.

■ Instruct the patient to keep the dressing clean and dry at all times:
- Protect the catheter dressing during bathing.
- Advise against swimming.
- If the dressing loosens, instruct the patient to reinforce it with tape.
- If the dressing comes off or becomes wet, instruct the patient to go to the dialysis unit, clinic, or emergency department, as appropriate, as soon as possible for aseptic catheter site care if he or she is incapable of performing such care at home.

Meticulous care of the catheter site and the maintenance of a dry intact dressing lessens infection risk. The patient needs to recognize when to seek professional help to maintain the access site integrity. QSEN: Patient-centered care; Safety.

AV fistula or AV graft:

■ Maintain asepsis with the AV fistula or graft during dialysis:

These nursing actions reduce the risk of transmitting pathogens to the patient. QSEN: Safety.

- Wash the access site with antibacterial soap and water before disinfection and cannulation.

Cleansing the skin first decreases the number of microorganisms present on the skin and increases the effectiveness of antiseptics.

- Disinfect the cannulation sites with an antiseptic agent.

Commonly used antiseptics include povidone-iodine, alcohol, chlorhexidine, and electrolyte chloroxidizers.

- Cover cannulation sites with sterile dressings during treatment and after fistula needle removal.

Sterile dressings protect the needle puncture site until it closes. Dressings can usually be removed 4 to 6 hours after dialysis.

- Allow only dialysis staff to cannulate AV access.

Only people trained to perform venipuncture on a fistula or graft should do so. The access is the patient's lifeline and requires expert care and use. QSEN: Teamwork and collaboration.

Renal and Urinary Tract Care Plans

■ = Independent   ▲ = Interprofessional Collaboration

NDx Risk for Ineffective Peripheral Tissue Perfusion

Common Risk Factor

Interruption in AV access blood flow

Common Expected Outcome

Patient's AV access remains patent, as evidenced by palpable thrill, bruit on auscultation, and adequate color or temperature in extremity.

NOC Outcomes

Circulation Status; Tissue Perfusion: Peripheral

NIC Interventions

Circulatory Care: Arterial Insufficiency; Circulatory Care: Venous Insufficiency; Skin Surveillance

---

Ongoing Assessment

Actions/Interventions

- Assess the AV fistula or graft for the presence of adequate blood flow:
  - Palpate for a thrill over the fistula or graft.

  - Auscultate for a bruit.

  - Assess capillary refill.
  - Check for mottling of the skin and the temperature of the affected limb.
  - Assess for pain in the extremity distal to the access.

Rationales

These nursing actions determine the presence of adequate blood flow through the fistula or graft. QSEN: Safety.

Vibrations should be palpable. This sensation is often compared to that of a purring cat. The vibrations are the result of the turbulent blood flow that is present in the fistula or graft.

A "swishing" sound should be audible with a stethoscope. When the artery is connected to the vein, blood is shunted from the artery into the vein, causing turbulence.

Refill greater than 6 seconds indicates impaired circulation.

A cool extremity and changes in skin color denote compromised perfusion.

Pain results from inadequate tissue perfusion.

Therapeutic Interventions

Actions/Interventions

- Instruct the patient to maintain proper positioning of the access limb. Consider elevating the limb postoperatively in an arm sling when the patient is ambulatory.

- As the access site heals, encourage the normal use of the access limb.

- Notify the physician when pain in the extremity is accompanied by decreased sensations and decreased temperature in the extremity with pallor or cyanosis.

- Instruct the patient regarding the following preventive measures:

  - Do not allow BP measurement in the access limb.

  - Do not allow blood to be drawn from the access limb.

Rationales

These actions reduce dependent edema during the immediate postoperative period.

This measure promotes healing and reduces edema.

These are symptoms of seriously inadequate perfusion that require surgical revision of the access to prevent permanent damage to the extremity's nerves and tissues.

Thrombosis is a common complication of vascular access. Thrombi can be caused by venipuncture; extrinsic pressure from a BP cuff, or a tourniquet. Providing information allows the patient to assume responsibility for care to maintain the adequate blood flow through the vascular access. QSEN: Patient-centered care; Safety.

Activities that constrict arterial blood flow increase the risk for obstruction of the vascular access.

Venipuncture in the access limb increases the risk for compromised circulation.

Actions/Interventions

- Instruct the patient to avoid activities that endanger access patency, including the following:
  - Sleeping on the access limb
  - Wearing tight clothing over the limb with access
  - Carrying bags, purses, or packages over the access arm
  - Participating in activities or sports that involve active use of or trauma to the access limb

Rationales

Trauma to the access limb can be related to activities such as sleeping on the limb, tight clothes, or sports that involve active use of the limb. QSEN: Safety.

NANDA-I
NDx Deficient Knowledge

Common Related Factors
Insufficient information
Insufficient interest in learning
Insufficient knowledge of resources
Misinformation presented by others

Defining Characteristics
Insufficient knowledge
Inaccurate follow-through of instruction
Inaccurate performance on a test
Inappropriate behavior

Common Expected Outcome
Patient and caregivers verbalize knowledge of hemodialysis and measures to prevent and manage complications.

NOC Outcome
Knowledge: Treatment Regimen
NIC Interventions
Health Literacy Enhancement; Learning Facilitation; Teaching: Procedure/Treatment; Teaching: Prescribed Exercise

---

Ongoing Assessment

Actions/Interventions

- Assess the patient's knowledge of dialysis, vascular access, and complications.

- Determine the patient's and the caregiver's self-efficacy to learn about hemodialysis and apply new knowledge to manage the access site and prevent complications.

Rationales

This information provides the starting base for educational sessions. Family members and significant others may need as much teaching as the patient. QSEN: Patient-centered care.

Patients receiving hemodialysis in an outpatient center may feel dependent on the nursing staff for all care and not realize their responsibility in maintaining the vascular access and preventing complications.

Therapeutic Interventions

Actions/Interventions

- Review the purpose of dialysis and the rationale for the access device.

- Demonstrate and request a return demonstration of access care before discharge. Recommend a home health nurse visit as appropriate.

Rationales

This information reinforces the need for the vascular access placement and maintenance. Patients need to understand that this is their lifeline to replace kidney function. QSEN: Safety.

This approach to teaching supports the patient's learning of new skills. The home health nurse can reinforce this learning. QSEN: Patient-centered care; Teamwork and collaboration.

Renal and Urinary Tract Care Plans

■ = Independent   ▲ = Interprofessional Collaboration

Actions/Interventions	Rationales
■ Instruct the patient to inform dialysis staff immediately of any signs and symptoms of infection: pain over the access site; fever; red, swollen, and warm access site; drainage from the access; red streaks along the access area.	Prompt intervention is necessary to prevent more serious complications. QSEN: Safety.
■ Explain the importance of maintaining asepsis with the external catheter.	Infection is almost an inevitable complication of an external vascular device. Infection may be localized cellulitis, but septicemia can occur. Meticulous daily care and avoidance of trauma to the area can lessen the risk for infection. QSEN: Safety.
• Protect the catheter dressing while bathing (tub and sponge baths only); no swimming; no showers.	
• Apply a dressing to the catheter exit site as ordered.	
• Secure the catheter to prevent tugging and pulling on the catheter exit site.	This measure prevents accidental dislodging of the catheter.
■ Teach the patient how to manage the accidental separation or dislodgement of the external access connections or accidental removal of the central venous catheter.	Information given to the patient or caregiver will increase awareness of troubleshooting measures and reduce possible anxiety.
■ Instruct the patient or caregiver in the care of dressings, if applicable. Allow for return demonstrations.	This knowledge helps reduce the risk for infection. Return demonstrations allow for the correction of mistakes and provide the patient and caregiver with feedback about their skill. This feedback may enhance the patient's confidence to carry out dressing changes without supervision. QSEN: Patient-centered care.
■ Inform the patient with an AV fistula that maturation may be hastened by exercising:	Exercises should be initiated only at the direction of the dialysis staff and physician. QSEN: Teamwork and collaboration.
• Begin resistance exercises 10 to 14 days after surgery.	Resistance exercises cause vessels to stretch and engorge with blood.
• Use a light tourniquet to the upper arm. Be careful, however, not to occlude blood flow with the tourniquet; apply it tightly enough to distend the vessels.	This method pumps arterial blood against venous resistance caused by the tourniquet. The patient's squeezing of a rubber ball, tennis ball, hand grips, or a rolled-up pair of socks helps exert pressure.
• Instruct the patient to open and close the fist.	
• Repeat these exercises for 5 to 10 minutes, four or five times daily.	
■ Teach the patient how to check for adequate blood flow through the fistula or graft:	Absence of a thrill may indicate clotting of the access with the need to inform dialysis staff immediately. Waiting to declot the access may result in the inability to "save access" and may require surgery to establish a new vascular access. QSEN: Safety.
• Designate the specific areas to feel for pulses and a thrill.	
• Demonstrate how to feel for pulses and a thrill.	
■ Discuss the dietary and fluid requirements and restrictions: low sodium, low potassium, low phosphorus, adequate protein, high calories, free fluids. Arrange a dietary consultation if necessary.	Patients receiving hemodialysis may have a less restrictive diet than they did before starting dialysis. However, some restrictions for sodium, potassium, and protein may continue with dialysis treatment. QSEN: Teamwork and collaboration.
■ Recommend the patient wear a medical alert bracelet.	The vascular access is the patient's lifeline, which must be treated carefully and used only by a trained dialysis nurse. QSEN: Safety.

Related Care Plans

Anxiety, Chapter 2
Risk for bleeding, Chapter 2
Disturbed body image, Chapter 2
Ineffective coping, Chapter 2
Central venous access devices, Chapter 4

Peritoneal Dialysis

Intermittent Peritoneal Dialysis; Continuous Ambulatory Peritoneal Dialysis; Continuous Cyclic Peritoneal Dialysis; Renal Replacement Therapy

Peritoneal dialysis is indicated for patients with kidney failure who have vascular access problems, who cannot tolerate the hemodynamic alterations of hemodialysis, or who prefer the independence of managing their own therapy in their home environment. A peritoneal catheter is placed through the anterior abdominal wall to achieve access into the peritoneum. During peritoneal dialysis, the peritoneum functions as the semipermeable membrane by which molecules flow from the side of higher concentration to the side of lower concentration. This procedure removes excess fluid and waste products from the body. Peritoneal dialysis may be performed as intermittent peritoneal dialysis, continuous ambulatory peritoneal dialysis, or continuous cyclic peritoneal dialysis. Peritoneal dialysis provides more gradual physiological changes than hemodialysis and is appropriate for the older adult patient with diabetes and cardiovascular disease. It is contraindicated in patients with peritonitis, recent abdominal surgery, or respiratory insufficiency because the fluid in the peritoneum decreases lung volume. This care plan focuses on peritoneal dialysis in the acute care setting with teaching for the ambulatory and home care setting.

NANDA-I NDx Excess Fluid Volume

Common Related Factors

Compromised regulatory mechanism (renal insufficiency)
Increased peritoneal permeability to glucose, water, and protein

Defining Characteristics

Weight gain over a short period of time
Elevated BP
Peripheral edema
Orthopnea/dyspnea
Crackles

Common Expected Outcome

Patient is normovolemic as evidenced by urine output greater than or equal to 30 mL/hr, balanced intake and output, stable weight (or loss attributed to fluid loss), absence or reduction of edema, HR 60 to 100 beats/min, and absence of pulmonary crackles.

NOC Outcomes

Fluid Balance; Systemic Toxin Clearance: Dialysis; Cardiopulmonary Status

NIC Interventions

Fluid Management; Fluid Monitoring; Peritoneal Dialysis Therapy

Ongoing Assessment

Actions/Interventions

- Obtain the patient's baseline weight when the peritoneal cavity is empty, then every day using the same scale and clothing.

- Measure the inflow and outflow of dialysate with each exchange, checking that the outflow is equal to or greater than the inflow, and maintain a record of the cumulative fluid balance.
- Monitor the patient's BP and HR.

Rationales

Body weight is a more sensitive indicator of fluid or sodium retention than intake and output. Weight gain of 2 or more pounds in 24 hours can be caused by dialysate reabsorption or fluid excess. QSEN: Patient-centered care.

The concentration of the dialysate fluid determines the rate and amount of fluid removal. The volume of dialysate outflow should equal or exceed the volume of dialysate inflow.

An increased BP and HR may be an indication of fluid retention. Sinus tachycardia and increased BP are seen in early stages. Older patients have a reduced response to catecholamines; thus their response to fluid overload may be blunted, with less increase in HR. QSEN: Safety.

Renal and Urinary Tract Care Plans

■ = Independent   ▲ = Interprofessional Collaboration

Actions/Interventions

- Monitor the peritoneal catheter for kinks, fibrin, or clots.

- Assess the work of breathing and for the presence of tachypnea, retractions, nasal flaring, orthopnea, and crackles.

- Check for sacral and peripheral edema from fluid excess or protein depletion from dialysis, especially with more hypertonic dialysates.

Rationales

An obstruction of outflow of fluid from the catheter may result in retained fluid in the abdomen.

Patients already fluid-overloaded who receive 1 to 2 L of additional fluid in the peritoneal space may be significantly compromised. If dialysate fluid is retained in the abdomen, it may cause pressure on the diaphragm, resulting in a decrease in lung expansion and possible respiratory distress. Adventitious breath sounds are caused by accumulation of fluid in the lungs as part of fluid volume excess. QSEN: Safety.

Edema may develop if adequate fluid volumes are not removed by the dialysis exchanges or the exchanges are resulting in removing protein that the patient is not nutritionally replacing.

Therapeutic Interventions

Actions/Interventions

- Instruct the patient to change positions frequently. Elevate the head of bed at 45 degrees, and turn the patient from side to side.

- ▲ Institute fluid restrictions as appropriate.

- ▲ Administer IV fluids via an infusion pump, if possible.

- Elevate edematous extremities.

- In the acute care setting, notify the physician and change the dialysate concentration when the patient reaches dry weight.
- Stop the dialysis if drainage is less than the infusion.

- Ensure proper functioning if using an automatic cycler for the peritoneal dialysis exchanges.

- For home or ambulatory care: instruct the patient and caregivers about the maintenance of fluid restriction and the maintenance of a diary monitoring the cumulative record of dialysate inflow or outflow exchange. Also, instruct the patient to obtain daily weights (dry weights) at the same time each day.

Rationales

Position changes facilitate drainage and help prevent pulmonary complications by preventing an upward displacement of the diaphragm, which can result from inadequate drainage of dialysate from the peritoneal cavity.

Fluid restrictions are individualized for peritoneal dialysis patients. QSEN: Patient-centered care.

The use of infusion pumps reduces the risk for rapid infusion of fluids into the circulatory system. QSEN: Safety.

The elevation of extremities increases venous return and lessens edema.

Modification of the dialysate concentration prevents dehydrating the patient by removing too much fluid. QSEN: Teamwork and collaboration.

Overinfusion causes pain, dyspnea, nausea, and electrolyte imbalance.

The cycler may be used to deliver continuous cyclic peritoneal dialysis (CCPD), intermittent peritoneal dialysis (IPD), or nightly peritoneal dialysis. For nightly peritoneal dialysis, the machine cycles four to eight exchanges per night with alarms built into the system to make it safe for the patient to sleep at home. QSEN: Safety.

The patient is responsible for monitoring fluid balance. Providing information will increase the patient's confidence with managing dialysis at home. QSEN: Patient-centered care.

NANDA-i
NDx **Risk for Infection**

Common Risk Factors

Invasive procedures with possible contamination of peritoneal catheter entry site
Insufficient knowledge to avoid exposure to pathogens

Renal and Urinary Tract Care Plans

Common Expected Outcomes

Patient remains free of infection, as evidenced by normal temperature and absence of purulent drainage from wounds, incisions, and tubes.

Infection is recognized early to allow for prompt treatment.

NOC Outcomes
Risk Detection; Risk Control; Infection Severity

NIC Interventions
Infection Protection; Infection Control; Peritoneal Dialysis Therapy

Ongoing Assessment

Actions/Interventions	Rationales
■ Assess the patient for signs or symptoms of infection.	Peritonitis is the primary infection associated with peritoneal dialysis. If the patient experiences repeated episodes of peritonitis, catheter removal may be necessary. The patient may need to begin hemodialysis. Signs of infection may include fever; generalized malaise; reports of abdominal pain, tenderness, warm feeling, or chills; rigid abdominal wall; the peritoneal catheter site reddened with discharge; cloudy returned dialysate; positive culture and sensitivity results; nausea; vomiting; or diarrhea. QSEN: Safety.
■ Assess the peritoneal fluid drainage:	
• Cloudiness	Normal peritoneal drainage is clear. Cloudy fluid usually indicates an increased white blood cell (WBC) count.
• Volume	A decreased volume is noted with increased peritoneal permeability.
▲ If infection is suspected, collect effluent as appropriate for the following:	
• WBC count with differential	A WBC count of 100 cells/mm^3 with 50% polymorphonucleocytes indicates peritonitis.
• Culture or sensitivity with Gram stain	Identification of the specific microorganism is needed for the appropriate antibiotic therapy. A Gram stain may reveal a fungus, which takes 5 to 7 days to grow.
▲ Assess the area around the catheter site. Collect purulent drainage for culture and sensitivity testing.	The area should be clean with no signs of inflammation. Culture and sensitivity testing will identify infecting pathogens and guide the selection of appropriate antibiotics. QSEN: Evidence-based practice.
■ Auscultate the patient's bowel sounds.	Absent bowel sounds may indicate an ileus from bacterial toxins that lead to infection.
■ Monitor the patient's temperature.	An elevated temperature occurs with infection processes.

Therapeutic Interventions

Actions/Interventions	Rationales
■ Use strict aseptic technique and apply a mask to the patient and each person in the room when setting up dialysis and connecting the patient to the peritoneal dialysis tubing set.	Improper technique during connection can lead to catheter site infection, the most common complication of peritoneal dialysis. It is critical to maintain aseptic technique in peritoneal dialysis. The patient should be thoroughly instructed in this technique for home use. Tubing connection devices are commercially available to help maintain an aseptic system. QSEN: Safety.
■ Ensure the aseptic handling of the peritoneal catheter and connections.	"Touch contamination" of the catheter and connections increases the risk for infection.

■ = Independent ▲ = Interprofessional Collaboration

Actions/Interventions	Rationales
■ Maintain the drainage receptacle below the level of the peritoneum.	Positioning to promote gravity drainage prevents the backflow of dialysate, which can contribute to the risk for infection.
■ Anchor the connections and tubing securely.	This action also prevents pulling and pressure on the catheter exit site, which can cause skin breakdown and predispose to infection.
▲ If peritonitis is suspected, administer antibiotics intraperitoneally as prescribed, using shortened dwell periods for the first 24 hours.	Peritoneal administration places medications at the source of infection. Shortened dwell periods are used so that dialysate reabsorption is decreased.
▲ Perform exit site care according to unit or agency protocol.	Exit sites are a potential source of infection. Cleansing the area and dressing changes at regular intervals reduce the risk for infection. Each unit has an established exit site care protocol.
■ Instruct the patient about the importance of notifying the dialysis staff or home health nurse of any signs of infection.	Treatment can be instituted quickly, and more serious complications can be prevented. QSEN: Safety.

NANDA-I NDx Acute Pain

Common Related Factors
Physical injury agent (rapid infusion of dialysate, infusion of cold dialysate, distended abdomen)
Biological injury agent (peritonitis)

Defining Characteristics
Self-report of intensity using standardized pain scale
Self-report of pain characteristics using standardized pain instrument
Guarding behavior (abdominal)
Positioning to ease pain
Change in physiological parameter (e.g., BP, HR, respiratory rate, and oxygen saturation)

Common Expected Outcomes
Patient reports satisfactory pain control and a decreased intensity using a standardized pain scale.
Patient uses pharmacological and nonpharmacological pain management strategies.
Patient exhibits increased comfort such as baseline levels for pulse, BP, respirations, and relaxed muscle tone or body posture.

NOC Outcomes
Pain Control; Pain Level; Comfort Status
NIC Interventions
Pain Management; Peritoneal Dialysis Therapy

Ongoing Assessment

Actions/Interventions	Rationales
■ Assess for signs of discomfort during the dialysate instillation.	The infusion of the dialysate, especially at a rapid rate, can cause abdominal pressure and discomfort or back discomfort from the additional weight of the fluid. Infusion of cool dialysate can cause abdominal cramping.
■ Assess for pain in the scapula region.	Referred pain to the scapula occurs with the rapid infusion of dialysate or when air is inadvertently infused into the peritoneal cavity.

evolve **For additional care plans, go to http://evolve.elsevier.com/Gulanick/.**

Therapeutic Interventions

Actions/Interventions	Rationales
■ Remain with the patient during the initiation of dialysis. Control the rate of inflow and slow if patient complains of pain. Do not allow air inflow with the exchange; always use warm fluids.	A typical volume of prescribed dialysate is 2 L. Inflow of this volume in less than 10 minutes may cause pain. Slowing the rate of inflow will contribute to the patient's comfort level. The accidental infusion of air contributes to pain. Dialysate that is warmed to room temperature is less likely to cause pain during inflow.
■ Change the patient's position during infusion of dialysate.	Changing the patient's position relieves discomfort during inflow of dialysate.
■ If the patient experiences scapula pain, allow adequate drain time and position the patient on his or her side with the knees to the chest.	The retention of any air from the peritoneal cavity may cause pain. Positioning facilitates the removal of dialysate and air.
■ Explain the reasons for inflow pain.	Knowledge of what to expect during inflow may help the patient cope more effectively with the discomfort and pain. Fluid with a lower pH than the pH in the tissues adjacent to the peritoneum causes discomfort until equilibration occurs; pressure on the organs and diaphragm causes discomfort until the patient becomes accustomed to the procedure. QSEN: Patient-centered care.
▲ If lower back pain is the problem, consult with members of the interprofessional health team about measures to support back muscles that are bearing the additional weight of the dialysis fluid.	The physical therapist may suggest the use of an orthopedic binder and regular low back exercises. QSEN: Teamwork and collaboration.
▲ If peritonitis is the cause of pain, administer antibiotics as prescribed.	Antibiotics are required to treat the infectious process. Antibiotics will be adjusted based on peritoneal fluid cultures. QSEN: Evidence-based practice.

NANDA-I NDx Deficient Knowledge

Common Related Factors
Insufficient information
Insufficient interest in learning
Insufficient knowledge of resources
Misinformation presented by others

Defining Characteristics
Insufficient knowledge
Inaccurate follow-through of instruction
Inaccurate performance on a test
Inappropriate behavior

Common Expected Outcomes
Patient or caregiver becomes proficient at performing peritoneal dialysis.
Patient or caregiver is able to verbalize when to contact interprofessional health team members.

NOC Outcome
Knowledge: Peritoneal Dialysis
NIC Interventions
Health Literacy Enhancement; Learning Facilitation; Teaching: Peritoneal Dialysis; Peritoneal Dialysis Therapy; Teaching: Psychomotor Skill

Ongoing Assessment

Actions/Interventions	Rationales
■ Assess the patient's knowledge of the purpose for peritoneal dialysis.	Knowledge of the purpose for therapy is the basis for teaching the patient about procedural steps, complications, and fluid management goals. QSEN: Patient-centered care.

■ = Independent   ▲ = Interprofessional Collaboration

Actions/Interventions

- Assess the patient's understanding of the types of peritoneal dialysis available for the home setting.

- Determine the patient's or the caregiver's self-efficacy to learn peritoneal dialysis and apply these skills in the home setting.

Rationales

Automated cycler machines are most often used while the patient is sleeping at night. Ambulatory techniques requiring manual exchanges (i.e., continuous ambulatory peritoneal dialysis [CAPD]) are also an option for independent patients. The patient needs to be included in decisions about the type of dialysis used in the home. QSEN: Patient-centered care.

The patient or a family member needs to be capable of performing the tasks of peritoneal dialysis to be allowed to do home dialysis. Teaching the patient and/or family members is a structured process conducted by a nurse who is experienced in educating patients about peritoneal dialysis.

Therapeutic Interventions

Actions/Interventions

- ▲ Consult with a registered dietitian to teach the patient and caregiver about the dietary and fluid requirements associated with peritoneal dialysis.

- Demonstrate and request a return demonstration of peritoneal catheter care.

- Demonstrate and have the patient perform repeat demonstrations of the dialysis procedure. Emphasize how to adapt techniques to the home environment:
  - Appropriate handwashing techniques
  - Steps to peritoneal dialysis:
    - Ensuring a clean work area
    - Using appropriate supplies
    - Checking dialysate for an expiration date, dextrose concentration, correct volume, pinhole leaks, and foreign particles
    - Wearing a mask during the procedure
    - Clamping the tubing; using sterile technique when spiking or unspiking from the dialysate
- When instructing in CAPD, review the use of commercially available devices that help maintain the sterility of the system during tubing connections.

- Work collaboratively with the patient to fine-tune the length of dialysis, diet regulations, pain management, and diversion needs.
- Provide information on securing materials for traveling and vacations.

- Describe the signs and symptoms of infection or peritonitis, including the basis of occurrence and when to call the health care provider.

Rationales

As a rule, patients receiving peritoneal dialysis have fewer dietary restrictions than those on hemodialysis because of the continuous nature of peritoneal dialysis and the loss of protein during the process. The dietitian can provide teaching about dietary intake of sodium, potassium, phosphorus, adequate protein, and calories. Fluids are generally not restricted, but intake should not be excessive. QSEN: Teamwork and collaboration.

Return demonstrations allow for the correction of mistakes and provide the patient and caregiver with feedback about their performance. Positive feedback enhances the patient's and the caregiver's confidence to manage dialysis at home.

The supervised practice of skills and positive feedback from the nurse will add to the patient's confidence about managing peritoneal dialysis at home. Return demonstrations allow the nurse to correct mistakes and reinforce knowledge of the procedure. QSEN: Patient-centered care; Safety.

The patient needs to learn how to set up the machine and correctly program it for use during the night. It is of critical importance to maintain sterile technique to prevent infection. QSEN: Safety.

Careful planning helps the patient achieve optimal benefits of the treatment. QSEN: Patient-centered care.

Patients must plan ahead when scheduled to be away from home. Supplies may need to be shipped to the destination before travel.

Early detection and treatment preserve peritoneal membrane functionality and decrease the loss of membrane surface area and function. QSEN: Safety.

Actions/Interventions	Rationales
■ Discuss return appointments, follow-up care, and emergency numbers.	Ongoing care on an outpatient basis allows for laboratory monitoring, physical examination, and treatment management discussions.
▲ Consult with members of the interprofessional health team as needed to support the patient in the home setting. Arrange for a home health nurse or a peritoneal dialysis training nurse visit, as appropriate.	Home care visits allow for the assessment of procedures in the home environment and offer support in the environment where the procedure is conducted. Patients may have financial needs related to long-term dialysis that can be addressed by the social worker. QSEN: Teamwork and collaboration.

Related Care Plans

Disturbed body image, Chapter 2
Ineffective health management, Chapter 2

Urinary Diversion

Bladder Cancer; Ileal Conduit; Koch Pouch; Nephrostomy; Sigmoidostomy; Ureterostomy; Vesicostomy

Urinary diversion is the surgical diversion of urinary flow from its usual path through the urinary tract. Urinary diversion procedures may be performed as a result of obstruction of the urinary tract; destruction of normal urinary structures by trauma; neurogenic bladder caused by disease or injury; and cancer, usually of the bladder. Urinary diversion may be temporary or permanent depending on the underlying problem. Bladder cancer occurs more often in older men than in women. When the tumors are superficial in the bladder wall, a variety of surgical procedures can be performed to remove the tumor and maintain normal urinary tract function. These procedures include transurethral resection, laser photocoagulation, and segmental cystectomy. If the bladder tumor is invasive and involves the trigone area, the preferred treatment is total cystectomy with a urinary diversion to maintain outflow of urine. Some procedures result in incontinence and necessitate the wearing of a collection system or pouch. Other procedures reroute the urinary flow to another structure (e.g., a surgically created internal reservoir, colon) from which the urine is eventually excreted (often called continent procedures). Nephrostomy may be performed under fluoroscopic control as an outpatient procedure. Other diversions require open abdominal surgery, and the patient is typically hospitalized for 4 to 7 days. This care plan addresses nursing care for new postoperative patients, as well as for individuals who have undergone urinary diversion at some point in the past.

NANDA-I NDx Deficient Knowledge: Preoperative

Common Related Factors

Insufficient information
Insufficient interest in learning
Insufficient knowledge of resources
Misinformation presented by others

Defining Characteristics

Insufficient knowledge of proposed surgery and the postoperative outcomes
Inaccurate follow-through of instruction
Inappropriate behavior

Renal and Urinary Tract Care Plans

■ = Independent   ▲ = Interprofessional Collaboration

Common Expected Outcome

Patient verbalizes understanding of proposed surgical procedure, including permanent loss of urinary continence and postoperative need for a collection system.

NOC Outcome

Knowledge: Treatment Procedure

NIC Interventions

Health Literacy Facilitation; Learning Facilitation; Teaching: Preoperative; Teaching: Procedure/ Treatment

Ongoing Assessment

Actions/Interventions	Rationales
■ Assess the patient's understanding of the proposed surgical procedure and its relationship to urinary continence:	This information provides the starting base for educational sessions. The choice of surgical procedure depends on the nature of disease or disorder that makes the urinary diversion necessary. It is important that the patient understand that the proposed surgical procedure may make him or her incontinent of urine. This incontinence necessitates wearing and maintaining an external collection device. QSEN: Patient-centered care; Evidence-based practice.
• Ileal conduit (or ileal loop)	This procedure is the most common type of urinary diversion performed. It uses a piece ("loop") of small intestine as a conduit to which the ureters are attached. One end of the conduit is brought to the anterior abdominal surface as a stoma, over which a pouch must always be worn. An ileal conduit is usually done with cystectomy (removal of the bladder) for bladder cancer.
• Nephrostomy	Percutaneous catheterization of one or both kidneys is usually done when the urinary path is obstructed distally. Nephrostomy may be performed when the patient is not a candidate (e.g., a terminally ill patient with cancer or a very poor surgical risk) for more permanent diversion. This necessitates wearing one or two bags for the collection of urine. Nephrostomy catheters may be in place as a temporary measure to divert urine flow. This short-term diversion may be necessary if the ureter is obstructed or as a means to allow for the healing of incisions in the lower urinary tract.
• Sigmoidostomy	The ureters are anastomosed to the sigmoid colon. Urine is excreted with bowel elimination. The patient may experience bowel incontinence. The patient will not have an abdominal stoma.
• Ureterostomy (unilateral or bilateral)	This procedure is the implantation of one or both ureters to the anterior abdominal wall as small stomas and is usually done when the reestablishment of normal urinary flow is anticipated.
• Vesicostomy	This procedure is usually a temporary urinary diversion performed when the lower urinary tract must be bypassed (e.g., in urethral trauma). An opening is made into the bladder wall, which is attached to the lower anterior abdomen. A pouch must be worn over the vesicostomy stoma to collect the urine. This procedure also may be used to create a continent diversion using a valve to prevent urine leakage at the stoma.

Actions/Interventions

- Continent urinary diversions (e.g., Koch, Mainz, Indiana, or Florida pouch)

- ■ Determine the patient's or the caregiver's self-efficacy to learn and apply new knowledge about care of a urinary diversion collection device.

- ■ Assess the patient's knowledge about whether the urinary diversion proposed is temporary or permanent.

- ■ Ask whether the patient has had contact with another person who has a urinary diversion.

Rationales

A continent urinary diversion uses a portion of the bowel to surgically create a reservoir that collects urine within the abdominal cavity. A stoma is created on the surface of the abdominal wall. The patient inserts a catheter through the stoma to drain urine from the reservoir.

A first step in teaching may be to foster increased self-efficacy in the patient's ability to learn the desired information or skills. Some lifestyle changes can be difficult for the patient to make.

The patient's ability to cope with changes in activities of daily living necessitated by wearing an external collection device is facilitated when the patient understands that the diversion is permanent. Patients having temporary diversion may decline involvement in self-care and defer care to a family member or outside caregiver. QSEN: Patient-centered care.

Previous contact, either positive or negative, influences the patient's perception of what his or her experience will be.

Therapeutic Interventions

Actions/Interventions

- ■ Reinforce previous information and explain the proposed procedure.

- ■ Use diagrams, pictures, and models to explain the anatomy and physiology of the genitourinary tract, pathophysiology necessitating the urinary diversion, and the proposed location of the stoma:

  - Ileal conduit

  - Nephrostomy
  - Ureterostomy

  - Vesicostomy
- ■ Show the patient the pouch or collection system that will be used postoperatively.

- ■ Offer the patient a visit with a rehabilitated ostomate.

Rationales

Preoperative anxiety often makes it necessary to repeat instructions or explanations several times for the patient to comprehend.

Teaching methods need to be adapted to the patient's learning preferences. Different people take in information in different ways. It is important to match the patient's preferred learning style with the educational approach. QSEN: Patient-centered care.

This type of stoma is usually located in the lower right quadrant of the abdomen.

Tubes exit on one or both flanks, just below the costal margin.

This type of stoma can be anywhere on the anterior abdominal surface, preferably below the waistline.

This type of stoma is on the anterior abdomen, suprapubic area.

This technique helps the patient make adjustments in daily life that will result in the desired change in behavior. Allowing the patient to wear the pouch or collection device is also helpful and may identify the need for relocation of the proposed stoma.

Sometimes contact with another individual who has experience with the condition is more beneficial than factual information given by a health professional.

Risk for Toileting Self-Care Deficit

Common Risk Factors

Presence of new stoma
Presence of poorly placed stoma
Presence of urine collection device
Poor hand-eye coordination

■ = Independent ▲ = Interprofessional Collaboration

Renal and Urinary Tract Care Plans

Renal and Urinary Tract
Care Plans

Common Expected Outcome
Patient performs self-care (emptying or changing pouch) independently.

NOC Outcome
Self-Care: Toileting

NIC Interventions
Self-Care Assistance: Toileting; Ostomy Care

Ongoing Assessment

Actions/Interventions	Rationales
■ Assess for the presence of old abdominal scars, bony prominences on the anterior abdomen, creases or skin folds on the abdomen, extreme obesity, a scaphoid abdomen, pendulous breasts, and the ability to see and reach the stoma.	The placement of the stoma is facilitated when the abdomen is flat and has no scars or bony prominences, or the patient is not obese. When these factors are present, the stoma site selection may need to be altered to locate the stoma where the patient can see and reach it and where a relatively flat surface for applying the collection pouch exists. QSEN: Patient-centered care.
■ Assess for patient concerns about caring for the stoma and collection pouch.	Patients have many concerns that will influence their ability to successfully manage changes in toileting self-care associated with a stoma. These concerns may include the visibility of the stoma and collection pouch, handling the urine-filled pouch, or a noticeable smell. This information is the basis for developing a teaching plan to incorporate the patient's concerns. QSEN: Patient-centered care.

Therapeutic Interventions

Actions/Interventions	Rationales
▲ Consult an enterostomal therapy nurse or surgeon to mark the proposed stoma site indelibly in an area that the patient can easily see and reach; where scars, bony prominences, and skin folds are avoided; and where hip flexion does not change contour.	It is best to determine site selection with the patient in a sitting position. The patient needs to be included in the final decision for stoma placement. QSEN: Teamwork and collaboration; Patient-centered care.
■ If possible, have the patient wear a collection device over the proposed site before surgery; evaluate its effectiveness in terms of the patient's ability to see and handle the equipment and to wear normal clothing.	Stoma location is a key factor in self-care. A poorly located stoma can delay or preclude self-care abilities. The patient can be shown how the collection bag works. The patient can begin to experiment with ways to cover the bag with clothing. QSEN: Patient-centered care.

NANDA-I
NDx **Risk for Disturbed Body Image**

Common Risk Factors
Alteration in body function (due to loss of urinary continence; presence of stoma)
Alteration in self-perception (due to presence of pouch or urine collection system; fear of offensive odor or urine leakage; fear of appearing different)

Common Expected Outcome

Patient demonstrates enhanced body image and self-esteem, as evidenced by ability to look at, touch, talk about, and care for stoma and urine collection device.

NOC Outcomes

Body Image; Psychosocial Adjustment: Life Change

NIC Interventions

Body Image Enhancement; Self-Esteem Enhancement; Ostomy Care

Ongoing Assessment

Actions/Interventions	Rationales
■ Assess the patient's perceptions of the impact from the change in body structure and function.	The patient's response to real or perceived changes in body structure and/or function is related to the importance the patient places on the structure or function (e.g., a fastidious patient may experience the presence of a urine-filled pouch on the anterior abdomen as intolerable, or a patient who works out or swims may find the presence of visible tubes protruding from the flanks as intolerable). However, some patients will express that such changes are "a small price to pay" for the absence of disease. QSEN: Patient-centered care.
■ Note any verbal and nonverbal references to the stoma.	Patients often "name" stomas as an attempt to separate the stoma from themselves. Others may look away or totally deny the presence of the stoma until they are able to cope.
■ Note the patient's ability or readiness to look at, touch, and care for the stoma and ostomy equipment.	Often the first sign of a patient's readiness to participate in stoma care is when he or she looks at the stoma.

Therapeutic Interventions

Actions/Interventions	Rationales
■ Acknowledge the appropriateness of the patient's emotional response to actual and perceived changes in body structure and function.	Most patients perceive the control of elimination as a skill or task of early childhood and a socially private function. The loss of control precipitates a body image change and possible self-concept change for the patient.
■ Use a calm, matter-of-fact approach when helping the patient with care of the urine collection device.	Patients look for reactions, both positive and negative, from caregivers. Positive comments by the nurse, such as, "The stoma looks pink and healthy," or "The urine is clear and yellow, as it should be," help the patient develop a sense of normalcy about the change in his or her elimination. QSEN: Patient-centered care.
■ Teach patients specific actions that could be helpful in managing their perceived loss or problems related to their stoma.	Leakage of contents from the pouch, with resulting embarrassment about odor and loss of control, is a major concern. Emptying the collection device when it is about half full reduces the risk for the device leaking. A full device can pull away from the stoma because of the weight of the urine. Assuring the patient that skill will develop and that accidents are preventable will go a long way in helping him or her adapt to the altered structure or function. The use of pouch deodorizers and regular cleaning of the pouch can minimize noticeable odor.

Renal and Urinary Tract Care Plans

■ = Independent   ▲ = Interprofessional Collaboration

NDx Risk for Ineffective Tissue Perfusion: Stoma

Common Risk Factors

Surgical manipulation of small intestine (ileal conduit),
bladder (vesicostomy), ureters (ureterostomy)
Poorly fitting faceplate

Common Expected Outcome

Patient's stoma remains pink and moist.

NOC Outcome
Tissue Perfusion: Abdominal Organs
NIC Interventions
Surveillance; Ostomy Care

Ongoing Assessment

Actions/Interventions	Rationales
■ Assess the stoma for adequate arterial tissue perfusion at least every 4 hours for the first 24 hours postoperatively:	This assessment data is important to identify early changes in the stoma that may indicate reduced tissue perfusion. QSEN: Safety.
• Color of the ileal conduit stoma	The ileal conduit stoma is a piece of rerouted small intestine with attached mesentery (blood supply). It should appear pink and moist if perfusion is adequate. Some postoperative edema is expected and will subside over a period of 2 to 6 weeks. When edema becomes severe, venous congestion, evidenced by a purplish discoloration of the stoma, may occur.
• Appearance of the ureterostomy stoma	Because the ureters have a small diameter, manipulation at surgery or edema of surrounding tissue can compress the ureters at the skin line and compromise perfusion. Ureteral stomas should appear pink and moist if perfusion is adequate.
• Vesicostomy stoma	This stoma is constructed of inverted bladder that has been surgically sewn to abdominal skin; its normal appearance is pink and moist. This stoma is the least susceptible to impaired tissue perfusion.

Therapeutic Interventions

Actions/Interventions	Rationales
■ Ensure that the faceplate of the pouch is correctly fitted.	A faceplate that is tightly fitted to the stoma can reduce blood flow to the stoma and impede venous drainage, resulting in further edema and increasing the risk for ischemia. QSEN: Safety.
■ Remove the faceplate, and notify the surgeon immediately if the stoma appears dusky blue, black, or dry.	A stoma that is dusky blue, black, or dry is receiving inadequate blood supply; usually the patient returns to surgery for stoma revision. Although this is primarily a concern during the first 24 to 48 hours postoperatively, patients should be taught to examine the stoma color each time they perform a pouch change.

Renal and Urinary Tract Care Plans

Risk for Infection

Common Risk Factors

Invasive procedures: surgical incision; small bowel anastomosis (ileal conduit); anastomosis of ureters to small bowel (ileal conduit) or abdominal wall (ureterostomy); percutaneous access to renal pelvis (nephrostomy); direct opening into bladder (vesicostomy)

Insufficient knowledge to avoid exposure to pathogens

Common Expected Outcome

Patient remains free of infection as evidenced by normal temperature, normal white blood cell (WBC) count, absence of signs of local wound infection, and absence of purulent drainage from around nephrostomy tubes and all incision sites.

NOC Outcomes
Risk Detection; Risk Control; Wound Healing: Primary Intention; Infection Severity

NIC Interventions
Wound Care; Tube Care: Urinary; Ostomy Care; Infection Protection

Ongoing Assessment

Actions/Interventions	Rationales
■ Assess the surgical incisions and areas around the percutaneous nephrostomies for redness, swelling, and suspicious drainage.	These changes may indicate wound infection. The early identification of infection allows for prompt intervention. QSEN: Safety.
■ Monitor the patient's temperature.	A temperature above 38.5°C (101.3°F) after the third postoperative day is an indication of infection.
■ Assess for signs of infection in patients who have had urinary diversion surgeries including:	
• Anastomosis of the ureters to the small bowel	As the ileal conduit is fashioned, ureters are anastomosed into the segment of small bowel designated for the conduit; breakdown of these anastomoses results in peritonitis because urine spills into the peritoneal cavity instead of traveling to the conduit and out through the stoma. The patient may report abdominal pain and distention.
• Percutaneous puncture sites	Drainage from the site where nephrostomy tubes have been placed indicates infection.
• Bladder	In patients with a vesicostomy, the bladder communicates with the outside.
■ Monitor the urine output.	Diminishing amounts of urine output in patients with an ileal conduit may indicate a spillage of urine into the peritoneal cavity.
▲ Send any suspicious drainage from incisions, stomas, or surgically placed drains to the laboratory.	Drainage is analyzed to determine if an internal urine leak is the cause of infection.
▲ Monitor the patient's WBCs.	An elevated WBC count is a sign of infection.
▲ Obtain a culture of urine.	A laboratory culture determines any pathogens present and guides antimicrobial therapy.
■ Check the pH of urine.	Urine with a pH above 6.0 (i.e., alkaline urine) is more susceptible to infection than acidic urine.

Renal and Urinary Tract Care Plans

■ = Independent   ▲ = Interprofessional Collaboration

Therapeutic Interventions

Actions/Interventions

▲ Provide wound care to the incisions and areas around the percutaneous sites, vesicostomy outlet, and ureterostomies, as prescribed, using aseptic technique.

■ Wash hands before handling any tubes or drains.

■ Maintain closed drainage systems, and change collection bags and any other urine collection systems to prevent the accumulation of pathogens.

▲ Encourage measures to acidify the urine:
  • Vitamin C (ascorbic acid), 500 to 1000 mg/day
  • Cranberry juice, four to six 8-ounce glasses per day

▲ Encourage a fluid intake of 3000 to 4000 mL daily.

■ Instruct the patient to report pain, fever, and chills.

▲ Administer antibiotics and antipyretics as prescribed.

Rationales

Standard precautions and sterile technique with dressing changes reduce the risk for wound infection. QSEN: Safety.

Handwashing combined with standard precautions reduces transmission of pathogens to the patient.

Most patients can expect to wear a single collection device for up to 5 days; keeping the system closed reduces the risk for contamination. Collection devices should be emptied at least every 8 hours to prevent urine being reintroduced into the stoma.

Acidic urine inhibits the growth of pathogenic bacteria.

Cranberry juice yields hippuric acid as it is metabolized and excreted. Hippuric acid lowers the pH of the urine but may take several weeks to produce the desired effect.

An adequate fluid intake keeps urine diluted and flushes out bacteria.

Early recognition and the reporting of signs of infection allows for prompt treatment. QSEN: Safety.

These drugs eliminate infection and lower fever.

NANDA-I NDx Deficient Knowledge: Stoma Care

Common Related Factors
Insufficient information
Insufficient interest in learning
Insufficient knowledge of resources
Misinformation presented by others

Defining Characteristics
Insufficient knowledge
Inaccurate follow-through of instruction
Inaccurate performance on a test
Inappropriate behavior

Common Expected Outcome
Patient demonstrates ability to provide care for ostomy, urine collection device, nephrostomy tubes, and skin.

NOC Outcomes
Coping; Knowledge: Treatment Regimen; Social Support

NIC Interventions
Health Literacy Enhancement; Learning Facilitation; Home Maintenance Assistance; Teaching: Psychomotor Skill; Support System Enhancement; Ostomy Care

Ongoing Assessment

Actions/Interventions

■ Assess the patient's understanding of care for the stoma, nephrostomy tubes, or urine collection device.

Rationales

This information provides the starting base for educational sessions. During the acute stages after surgery, the family or significant others may require the most teaching. QSEN: Patient-centered care.

Renal and Urinary Tract Care Plans

Actions/Interventions

- Determine the patient's or the caregiver's self-efficacy to learn and apply new knowledge for ostomy care.

- Assess the availability and willingness of family members, friends, and other caregivers to assist the patient with care after discharge.

- Assess the patient's ability to empty and change the urine collection device (pouch). Determine the need for a home health care referral.

- Assess the patient's ability to care for the peristomal skin.

- Assess the patient's ability to identify peristomal skin problems:
  - Excoriation

  - Crystal formation

  - Yeast infection

  - Contact dermatitis

- Assess the patient's knowledge about the following:

  - Diet

  - Hygiene
  - Activity

Rationales

A first step in teaching may be to foster increased self-efficacy in the patient's ability to learn the desired knowledge and skills for ostomy care.

With shorter hospitalizations and same-day surgeries, patients often do not have adequate time for learning and return demonstrations before assuming full responsibility for self-care. Also, concerned others, in addition to assisting with or providing care, are often comforted by being able "to help somehow."

Some patients will be independent in emptying their pouch by the time of discharge; many may still need assistance and benefit from outpatient follow-up or in-home care. This information provides guidance in determining the need of the patient for consultation with members of the interprofessional health team after discharge to the home setting. QSEN: Patient-centered care; Teamwork and collaboration.

The care of peristomal skin is important to promote skin integrity and reduce the risk for fungal skin infections. QSEN: Safety.

This problem appears as a sore, reddened area, most typically the result of a poorly fitted faceplate that allows urine to contact the skin, too frequent changing of the pouch, or frequent accidents in which urine comes into contact with the skin.

A collection of white crystals around the stoma or on the skin around the stoma or tubes forms when urine is highly alkaline.

This type of infection acts as an abrasive, resulting in excoriation, and appears as a beefy-red, itchy area around the stoma or tubes. Infection tends to spread by "satellite," small round extensions at the perimeter of the main area of redness.

This problem is usually the result of an allergy to some product in use around the stoma or tubes and appears as a continuous reddened area; it may itch and feel painful. Contact dermatitis can develop even after years of successful use of products. It is characterized by its size and shape, which approximate the area of contact with the offending product.

This assessment data are important to develop an individualized teaching plan for discharge. QSEN: Patient-centered care.

Patients with urinary diversion are instructed to drink 3000 to 4000 mL of fluid per day to prevent stasis and infection. This amount may need to be adjusted for patients with diminished cardiovascular, renal, or pulmonary function.

Patients may bathe or shower with the pouch on or off; patients with nephrostomy tubes should always cover gauze dressings with waterproof dressings (e.g., OpSite, Tegaderm) or with waterproof tape. Other activities are governed by the patient's desire and energy level. Patients may be afraid to engage in usual activities, such as sports or sex. The lack of confidence in abilities usually diminishes as the patient gains control over the management of the urinary diversion and the fear of an "accident" diminishes.

Renal and Urinary Tract Care Plans

■ = Independent ▲ = Interprofessional Collaboration

Therapeutic Interventions

Actions/Interventions	Rationales
■ Provide teaching with each pouch change or during care for nephrostomy tubes.	Even before patients are able to participate actively, they can observe and discuss care for urinary diversion devices. Adults learn when they feel they are personally involved in the learning process. Patients know what difficulties will be encountered in their own environments, and they must be encouraged to approach learning activities from their priority needs. QSEN: Patient-centered care.
■ Include one or more caregivers as appropriate or desired by the patient.	It is beneficial to teach others alongside the patient, as long as they all realize that the goal is for the patient to become independent with care. Patients with nephrostomy tubes cannot reach the flank and will need to rely on another person to provide care.
■ Gradually transfer responsibility for care to the patient or family.	The patient and caregivers need to gain confidence in their ability to care for the urinary diversion before discharge. Repeated practice by the patient will help him or her gain confidence in self-care ability.
■ Allow at least one opportunity for a supervised return demonstration of a pouch change before discharge from the hospital, or arrange for home nursing care.	Ostomy self-care requires both cognitive and psychomotor skills; postoperatively, learning ability may be decreased, requiring repetition and opportunity for return demonstration. Teaching in the patient's home setting helps the patient fit the routine and equipment management into his or her own setting. Problem-solving small but important issues assists the patient toward confidence with self-care. QSEN: Patient-centered care.
■ Teach the patient how to care for the peristomal skin or skin around the nephrostomy tube:	
• Wash and dry skin around the stoma and tubes using soap and water.	Initial cleaning of the skin removes pathogens and skin oils that can reduce the effectiveness of pouching adhesives.
• Apply a liquid barrier film (Bard Protective Barrier Film, Skin Prep).	These products protect the skin from moisture and any adhesives used in the area.
• Change the pouch every 3 to 6 days.	More frequent changing strips away epithelial cells and can led to excoriation.
■ Discuss odor control, and acknowledge that odor (or fear of odor) can impair social functioning.	Odor control is best achieved by attention to pouch hygiene; urinary equipment can be rinsed with a half-and-half solution of water and vinegar to reduce urinary odor. Certain foods (e.g., asparagus, coffee) cause a disagreeable urinary odor and can be eliminated from the diet to control odor. Patients should not be given "absolutes," but rather assisted in deciding what is worth eliminating versus what is really important or enjoyed. QSEN: Patient-centered care.
■ Discuss the availability of ostomy support groups.	Ongoing peer support helps the patient gain confidence with long-term ostomy care.
■ Instruct the patient to maintain contact with an enterostomal therapy nurse.	These contacts help the patient with follow-up care and problem-solving. QSEN: Teamwork and collaboration.
■ For patients who travel, provide local enterostomal therapy resources and phone numbers.	Traveling away from home poses special concerns in terms of buying equipment, managing emergencies, and adjusting to different surroundings. Having a resource to call on often eases these concerns. QSEN: Teamwork and collaboration.

Related Care Plans

Ineffective coping, Chapter 2
Self-care deficit, Chapter 2
Surgical experience: Preoperative and postoperative care, Chapter 4

evolve **For additional care plans, go to http://evolve.elsevier.com/Gulanick/.**

Urinary Tract Infection

UTI; Pyelonephritis; Cystitis; Urethritis; Nephritis

Urinary tract infection (UTI) is an invasion of all or part of the urinary tract (kidneys, bladder, urethra) by pathogens. UTIs are usually caused by bacteria, with *Escherichia coli* the most common pathogen. Viral and fungal organisms also may cause UTI. UTIs may begin as pathogens from the perineum and ascend through the urethra to the urinary bladder. UTIs are common nosocomial infections and often result following instrumentation (e.g., catheterization or diagnostic procedures) of the genitourinary tract. The Centers for Disease Control and Prevention (CDC) has prepared guidelines for prevention of catheter-associated urinary tract infection (CAUTI). These guidelines include recommendations for appropriate use of urinary catheters in hospital and long-term care settings, and alternatives to indwelling urinary catheters for management of patient problems with urination. UTIs are more common in women than men, particularly in sexually active, younger women. UTIs, which can be chronic and recurring, can lead to systemic infection such as urosepsis, which can be life-threatening. In older patients, diagnosis and treatment of UTIs may be delayed because patients are often asymptomatic or demonstrate only subtle cognitive changes and urinary incontinence rather than the typical complaints of urgency, frequency, burning, and pain on urination. If infections of the urinary tract are not treated effectively, renal damage and loss of renal function can occur. The focus of this care plan is care of any individual with a UTI in any setting.

NDx Infection

Common Related Factors
Instrumentation or catheterization
Indwelling catheter
Chronically alkaline urine
Stasis (urinary retention)

Defining Characteristics
Burning on urination
Frequency of urination
Foul-smelling urine
Fever and chills
Suprapubic tenderness
Elevated white blood cell (WBC) count
Hematuria
Bacteriuria
Low back pain or flank pain
Incontinence (older adults)
Cognitive changes (older adults)

Common Expected Outcome
Patient is free of UTI as evidenced by clear, non–foul-smelling urine; pain-free urination; normal WBC count; and absence of fever, chills, flank pain, and suprapubic pain.

NOC Outcomes
Infection Severity; Medication Response; Urinary Elimination

NIC Interventions
Urinary Elimination Management; Teaching: Prescribed Medication; Fluid Management

Ongoing Assessment

Actions/Interventions	Rationales
■ Assess for any history that would predispose the patient to UTI.	A history of UTIs, urinary tract instrumentation, sexual activity, a history of sexually transmitted infections, previous surgeries of the genitourinary tract that may have resulted in scarring, or recent antibiotic therapy may all place the patient at an increased risk for developing UTI.

Renal and Urinary Tract Care Plans

■ = Independent   ▲ = Interprofessional Collaboration

Actions/Interventions

- Assess for the signs and symptoms of UTI.

▲ Assess the patient's laboratory data:
  - Urinalysis: presence of red blood cells (RBCs) and/or WBCs in the urine
  - Bacteria in the urine

  - Urine culture and sensitivity

  - WBC count

Rationales

The classic signs of UTI are frequent urination, a sensation of urgency, and burning or pain with urination. These manifestations are the result of inflammation in the bladder or urethra. Some patients with UTI may be asymptomatic, especially those with recurrent infection. Older patients who may not be cognitively capable of describing symptoms may develop a general change in behavior or decline in overall functional ability as an early indication of UTI. Confusion and incontinence are often the only signs of UTI in the older adult. QSEN: Patient-centered care.

The inflammatory response associated with infection leads to RBCs and WBCs in the urine.

Bacterial counts of 10^5 are usually considered diagnostic for UTI, although lower counts may also indicate UTI.

A positive culture will identify the causative organism. Sensitivity information is necessary for selecting the most effective antibiotic. QSEN: Evidence-based practice.

Leukocytosis is a systemic response to infection.

Therapeutic Interventions

Actions/Interventions

- Encourage the patient to drink extra fluid.

- Instruct the patient to void often (every 2 to 3 hours during the day) and to empty the bladder completely.

- Suggest cranberry or prune juice, or vitamin C 500 to 1000 mg/day.

- Encourage the patient to finish all prescribed antibiotics; note their effectiveness.

- Limit the use of indwelling bladder catheters to manage incontinence.

Rationales

Fluid promotes urine production and flushes bacteria from the urinary tract; the minimum fluid intake is 2 to 3 L/day.

A regular pattern of urination enhances bacterial clearance, reduces urine stasis, and prevents reinfection; voiding in an upright position can facilitate bladder emptying. QSEN: Safety.

These measures acidify urine; bacteria grow poorly in an acidic environment. Ideal urine pH is around 5. Cranberry juice has been shown to decrease bacterial adherence to the bladder wall. Cranberry juice (four to six 8-ounce glasses per day) produces hippuric acid as it is metabolized and excreted in the urine. This metabolism by-product reduces urine pH. The juice may take several weeks to produce a therapeutic result.

Antibiotics may be used in combination to reduce the development of bacterial resistance. The usual length of antibiotic therapy is 5 to 10 days. Patients with pyelonephritis may require a 3- or 4-day course of parenteral antibiotics to prevent bacteremia and sepsis. Long-term antibiotic therapy may be prescribed for patients with chronic UTIs. QSEN: Evidence-based practice.

Catheters increase the risk for infection. Other measures such as regular toileting and oral fluid intake can manage incontinence and prevent infection. QSEN: Evidence-based practice.

NANDA-I NDx Acute Pain

Common Related Factor

Biological injury agent (infection)

Defining Characteristics

Self-report of intensity using standardized pain scale
Self-report of pain characteristics using standardized pain instrument
Change in physiological parameter (e.g., BP, HR, respiratory rate, and oxygen saturation)
Guarding behavior

Common Expected Outcomes

Patient reports satisfactory pain control and a decreased intensity using a standardized pain scale.
Patient uses pharmacological and nonpharmacological pain management strategies.
Patient exhibits increased comfort such as baseline levels for pulse, BP, respirations, and relaxed muscle tone or body posture.

NOC Outcomes
Comfort Status; Pain Level; Pain Control
NIC Interventions
Heat/Cold Application; Pain Management

Ongoing Assessment

Action/Intervention

■ Assess the patient's description of pain. Inquire as to the quality, nature, and severity of the pain.

Rationale

The patient is the most reliable source of information about his or her pain. Typically, pain associated with UTI is described as burning on urination. Patients may also experience lower abdominal or suprapubic pain. Patients with pyelonephritis will have back or flank pain. Some patients are asymptomatic. A numeric scale or other descriptive scales can be used to identify the intensity of pain. QSEN: Patient-centered care.

Therapeutic Interventions

Actions/Interventions

■ Apply a heating pad to the suprapubic area or lower back.

■ Instruct the patient in the use of a sitz bath.
▲ Encourage the use of analgesics (e.g., acetaminophen) and/or antispasmodics (e.g., phenazopyridine), as prescribed.
■ Use nonpharmacological techniques whenever appropriate.

Rationales

Heat reduces pain through improved blood flow to the area and through reduction of pain reflexes.
Sitz baths may reduce perineal discomfort and pain.
These drugs relieve the pain and bladder spasms caused by UTI.

Complementary and alternative therapies such as progressive relaxation, guided imagery, massage, or distraction may reduce pain and promote comfort.

■ = Independent   ▲ = Interprofessional Collaboration

NANDA-I NDx **Deficient Knowledge**

Common Related Factors

Insufficient information
Insufficient interest in learning
Insufficient knowledge of resources
Misinformation presented by others

Common Expected Outcomes

Patient verbalizes knowledge of causes and treatment of UTI, and measures to control risk factors.
Patient completes medical treatment of UTI.

Defining Characteristics

Insufficient knowledge
Inaccurate follow-through of instruction
Inaccurate performance on a test
Inappropriate behavior

NOC Outcome

Knowledge: Treatment Regimen

NIC Interventions

Health Literacy Enhancement; Learning Facilitation; Teaching: Disease Process; Teaching: Prescribed Medication

---

Ongoing Assessment

Actions/Interventions

- Assess the patient's knowledge of UTI risk factors, prevention, and treatment.

- Determine the patient's self-efficacy to learn and apply new knowledge about prevention and treatment of UTI.

Rationales

This information provides the starting base for educational sessions. Frequent recurrences of UTI may indicate that the patient does not understand the risk factors or medical management of UTI. QSEN: Patient-centered care.

Self-efficacy refers to a person's confidence in his or her ability to perform a behavior. A first step in teaching may be to foster increased self-efficacy in the patient's ability to learn the desired information or skills to treat and prevent UTI.

Therapeutic Interventions

Actions/Interventions

- Teach the patient about the importance of prevention and follow-up care:

  • Drinking 2 to 3 L of fluids daily

  • Need for follow-up urine cultures

  • Need for frequent bladder emptying

  • Hygienic measures; showering is preferable to tub bathing

Rationales

The goal of patient teaching is to resolve the current infection and prevent recurrence of UTI. The patient will need to incorporate this knowledge into establishing appropriate health behaviors. QSEN: Patient-centered care; Safety.

Adequate fluid intake is necessary to promote urine production. Sufficient urine volume has a flushing action in the urinary tract to reduce the presence of pathogens.

Periodic urine cultures determine the effectiveness of the antimicrobial therapy. QSEN: Evidence-based practice.

The patient needs to understand the importance of voiding at first urge to prevent the stasis of urine in the bladder. Stasis of urine in the bladder increases the opportunity for bacterial growth.

Good hygiene of the perineal area decreases the concentration of pathogens that may ascend the urinary tract.

 For additional care plans, go to http://evolve.elsevier.com/Gulanick/.

Actions/Interventions

- Perineal hygiene with bowel elimination

- Need for daily changing of underwear, wearing well-ventilated clothing, and avoiding tight or constricting underwear or pants.

■ Teach the patient to complete the full course of antibiotic medication, even if symptoms resolve.

■ Encourage the reporting of signs and symptoms of recurrence.

Rationales

Attention to cleaning the perineal area after bowel movements decreases the migration of enteric pathogens into the urethra.

Synthetic materials harbor moisture and provide a medium for perineal bacterial growth. Loose-fitting clothing and cotton fabric in underwear promotes the evaporation of moisture.

Urinary symptoms of burning, frequency, and urgency often resolve in the first few days of antibiotic therapy. Patients may discontinue drug therapy because they feel better. If the full course of drug therapy is not completed, the bacterial colony will grow and cause a recurrent infection. QSEN: Safety.

One to 2 weeks after completion of a course of antimicrobial therapy is a common time frame for signs and symptoms to recur.

Related Care Plans

Acute pain, Chapter 2
Risk for infection, Chapter 2

■ = Independent   ▲ = Interprofessional Collaboration

CHAPTER

12

Men's and Women's Health Care Plans

GENERAL HEALTH CARE PLANS

Gender Dysphoria

Gender Identity; Transgender; Transsexual; Transman; Transwoman; Sex Reassignment Surgery

Definition: Gender dysphoria (GD) is a condition in which a person experiences clinically significant discomfort or distress (dysphoria) because of the discrepancy/incongruity of the gender assigned to them at birth and their own gender identity, which is their deeply held conviction and strongly felt interior sense of themselves as another gender. While for the majority of individuals, gender identity and physical embodiment are well matched (cisgender), most transgender individuals have a strong, persistent feeling from early childhood that they were born in the wrong body, and are not comfortable with the gender role society expects them to play based on that body. Transgenderism is not merely a lifestyle, personal choice, or political decision, but a very real biological phenomenon. Research suggests it may occur as a result of abnormal biological development of the fetus during pregnancy, possibly as a result of genetic or hormonal factors that cause the brain to develop gender identity that is different from the developing anatomy. It is recognized as a medical condition with a specific diagnosis for which treatment is often appropriate.

Gender dysphoria often involves significant anxiety, and distress in personal, social, family, and occupational areas of functioning. Furthermore, the person with gender dysphoria experiences significant "minority stress," including fear of discrimination and ridicule, stigma, rejection, marginalization, verbal harassment, or physical violence. These individuals may use negative coping strategies such as alcohol or drug misuse, or suicidal ideation. Gender dysphoria is not related to a specific sexual preference or orientation. Transgender or gender-nonconforming persons may identify themselves as heterosexual, gay, lesbian, or bisexual. The treatment goal is to assist persons with gender dysphoria in dealing with the distress that comes with their gender discrepancy (not to change their gender identity) as well as to assist these persons to explore their gender identity to find a gender role that is genuine and comfortable for them. Treatment is individualized.

NOTE: Much of this content is directly taken from the "Standards of Care for the Health of Transsexual, Transgender, and Gender-Nonconforming People" (Version 7, 2011), a publication of the World Professional Association for Transgender Health.

NDx Personal Identity Incongruence

Common Related Factors

Alteration in self-perception (incongruity between biological sex and gender identity)
Cultural incongruence
Alteration in social role
Discrimination
Low self-esteem
"Minority stress"
Perceived prejudice
Situational crisis

Defining Characteristics

Gender confusion
Stated desire to be the opposite gender
Dresses like the opposite gender
Passing for opposite gender
Desire to be treated as opposite gender
Fluctuating feelings about self
Ineffective relationships
Ineffective role performance
Change in social involvement
Depression
Anxiety
Feels alone, withdrawn, isolated

Common Expected Outcomes

Patient reports and initiates effective strategies to reduce the stress, discomfort, anxiety, or depression associated with gender dysphoria.
Patient uses available resources and support systems to resolve gender identity questions or concerns.
Patient exhibits increased comfort with their personal gender identity.

NOC Outcomes
Self-Awareness; Physical Well-Being; Coping; Quality of Life

NIC Interventions
Anticipatory Guidance; Values Clarification; Counseling; Anxiety Reduction; Self-Esteem Enhancement; Emotional Support; Active Listening; Role Enhancement

Ongoing Assessment

Actions/Interventions	Rationales
■ Affirm the patient's gender identity. Ask the patient how he/she prefers to be addressed.	The nurse needs to avoid assumptions about any patient's gender identity. Some patients have made a transition from male to female (MtF) or female to male (FtM) using hormones or surgery. Some actualize their gender identity, role and expression without hormonal or surgical interventions. When talking with patients, use their preferred name and pronouns. QSEN: Patient-centered care.
■ Explore the patient's history and development of gender dysphoric feelings.	Some individuals are aware at a young age of the incongruence between their sex assigned at birth and their personal gender identity. They may have struggled much of their life in attempting to "adapt." QSEN: Patient-centered care.
■ Determine the major kinds of psychological distress the patient is experiencing. Help the patient identify his/her feelings.	Transgender individuals are vulnerable to developing mental health problems such as anxiety or depression as well as feelings of uncertainty, inadequacy, alienation, isolation, or suicidal ideation. Some patients may have experienced verbal harassment or physical violence. Identification of feelings in a safe place can help the patient to explore the types and levels of psychological distress he/she is experiencing. This is an important first step in moving toward acceptance of self as a worthwhile person. QSEN: Patient-centered care.

■ = Independent ▲ = Interprofessional Collaboration

Actions/Interventions	Rationales
■ Explore the major sources of distress for the patient.	Socially there has been a stigma attached to gender nonconformity, which can lead to prejudice and discrimination. Many patients describe the personal stress of fearing to tell their family and friends about struggles with their identity so as not to hurt them or be rejected. Fear of being exposed can affect the work environment. Also, patients may have limited access to primary health care, either due to fear of ridicule, or from lack of health insurance. QSEN: Patient-centered care.
■ Identify the patient's current needs and realistic goals for gender expression.	Depending on their goals, what helps one person may be very different from what helps another. For some, changes in gender role and expression are enough to relieve the dysphoria. Others may need cross-hormones or surgery. Therapy can be useful to sort out needs and goals, and to learn constructive coping methods. QSEN: Patient-centered care. See also the Nursing Diagnosis: Deficient Knowledge for more information.
■ Assess what medical treatments (e.g., hormone therapy, sex reassignment surgery) the patient may have undertaken in the past that require ongoing follow-up.	Because there are risks and potential complications associated with medical interventions for gender dysphoria, it is important that patients receive ongoing monitoring by the health care team. QSEN: Safety.
■ Determine the patient's current stage of change or transition.	Patients may present at various stages of gender transition. The Transtheoretical Model emphasizes that interventions for change should be matched with the stage of change at which patients are situated. For example, if the patient is only "contemplating" making a change such as cross dressing in public, efforts may be directed toward emphasizing the positive aspects and reducing barriers; whereas if the patient is in the "preparation stage," more specific directions regarding strategies for success can be addressed. QSEN: Evidence-based practice.
■ Identify possible barriers to making changes.	If the patient is aware of possible barriers and has formulated plans for dealing with them, success is more likely.
■ Assess how the patient will tell others about their gender identity and potential transitions, and what reactions or level of support he or she anticipates from family and friends.	Many families find it confusing and difficult to understand gender identity issues. Family members (parents and other relatives, partners, and children) may vary in their level of openness, tolerance, and support. QSEN: Patient-centered care.

Therapeutic Interventions

Actions/Interventions	Rationales
■ Provide an atmosphere of respect, openness, trust, and collaboration.	The transgender experience is a human experience. Conveying respect is especially important when interacting with patients with values and beliefs that may be different from those of the health care provider.
■ Use techniques of reflection and clarification to acknowledge and facilitate the expression of concerns.	This action helps the patient understand and accept his own feelings and learn to trust himself.
■ Promote a sense of self-worth.	Most patients suffering from gender dysphoria describe a life of struggle, confusion, isolation, rejection, and lies. Support the patient in making choices to live the life he/she wants to live. QSEN: Patient-centered care.

Actions/Interventions

- ■ Assist the patient in considering the various options and the implications of gender transition. Pose reflective, clarifying questions to promote further thinking by the patient.

- ▲ Facilitate referral to a qualified mental health professional as indicated.

- ■ Promote positive expectations for success.

- ■ Assist the patient in using realistic thinking strategies to consider possible outcomes secondary to anticipated changes.

- ■ Implement the use of modeling to assist patients.

- ■ Encourage participation of a support team of trusted friends and professionals in proposed changes.

- ■ Refer the patient and significant others to gender-specific support groups.

Rationales

The nurse needs to be unbiased as the person works through the steps of decision–making, helping each individual make the best choices for himself or herself. QSEN: Patient-centered care.

Mental health professionals assess a client's gender dysphoria in the context of an evaluation of the psychosocial adjustment. They can facilitate a coming-out process, which may include use of feminizing/masculinizing medical interventions. However, qualified professionals in this new specialty are not universally available. To serve this population, multidisciplinary gender identity clinics are being formed across the United States. Advice or counseling through online outlets (e-therapy) may prove valuable to patients without other access. QSEN: Teamwork and collaboration.

Patients with stronger self-efficacy are more likely to be successful. Strategies to enhance self-efficacy should be part of the plan of care.

Realistic thinking works by changing how one interprets potential stressful situations. It includes examining the evidence, considering how likely it is to happen, and considering alternative explanations or outcomes, along with an honest appraisal of how bad the consequences would be. Finally, it includes prediction testing to demonstrate how unlikely most feared outcomes really are. A realistic appraisal of "what would happen if …" can help put life into a more accurate perspective. QSEN: Patient-centered care.

Observing the behavior of others who have successfully achieved similar goals helps provide practical direction and possible strategies the patient may find useful. Examples of some nationally known transgender people include Christine Jorgensen, Renée Richards, Chaz Bono, and Caitlyn Jenner.

Others can play an important role in providing support in the short and long term that may enhance overall adaptation to the gender changes being made.

Patients may not be aware of resources that can be a basis of support and success. Self-help and support groups provide unique perspectives on "being there."

NANDA-I

NDx Deficient Knowledge

Common Related Factors	Defining Characteristics
Insufficient information	Insufficient knowledge
Insufficient interest in learning	Inaccurate follow-through of instruction
Misinformation presented by others	Inappropriate behavior
Insufficient knowledge of resources	

■ = Independent   ▲ = Interprofessional Collaboration

Common Expected Outcomes
Patient identifies perceived learning needs.
Patient verbalizes understanding of desired content.

NOC Outcomes
Knowledge (specify type); Anticipatory Guidance; Information Processing
NIC Interventions
Health Literacy Enhancement; Learning Facilitation; Teaching: Individual

Ongoing Assessment

Actions/Interventions	Rationales
■ Identify the priority of transgender learning needs within the overall care plan: benefits of psychological counseling; strategies for modifying one's physical appearance; modifying one's body through cosmetic changes; cross-sex hormonal treatment; hair removal treatments; gender reassignment surgery; legal rights.	Assessment provides an important starting point in education. Adults learn best when teaching builds on prior knowledge or experience. Many adults may choose to begin the gender transition path, starting with non-medical treatments. Others may choose to live in their current gender role with the aid of counseling to help mitigate the dysphoric symptoms. QSEN: Patient-centered care.
■ Determine the patient's learning style.	Some people may prefer written over visual materials, group over individual instruction, or online over in-person instruction.

Therapeutic Interventions

Actions/Interventions	Rationales
■ Use culturally sensitive transgender terminology/language when delivering educational content.	This action demonstrates respect for patients and affirms the patient's gender identity.
■ Instruct the patient about the range of treatment options and their implications.	The Standards of Care for the Health of Transsexual, Transgender and Gender-Nonconforming People (Version 7, 2011) provides clinical guidance for health professionals to assist transgender people with safe and effective pathways to achieving lasting personal comfort in their gendered selves. These Standards are based on the best available science and expert professional consensus. QSEN: Patient-centered care; Evidence-based practice; Teamwork and collaboration.
• Psychotherapy and counseling for individual	Psychotherapy can provide education about a range of treatment options that may not have been previously considered by the patients. For individuals who plan to make a social role transition, the mental health professional can be instrumental in developing an individualized plan with specific goals and timelines.
• Family or couples therapy	Decisions about changes in gender role expression and medical interventions for gender dysphoria have significant implications for the patient's family and significant others. Family therapy can include work with patients, spouses or partners, as well as children and other members of the patient's extended family. Partners may want to explore their sexuality and intimacy-related concerns that may change over time.

Actions/Interventions

- Modifying one's physical appearance
  - Biological males:
    - Cross-dressing in a feminine fashion
    - Changing the body through hair removal and minor plastic cosmetic surgical procedures
    - Increasing grooming, wardrobe, and vocal expression skills
  - Biological females:
    - Cross-dressing in a masculine fashion
    - Changing the body through breast binding, weight lifting, applying theatrical facial hair
    - Padding undergarments or wearing a penile prosthesis
- Voice and communication therapy
  - Vocal characteristics may include pitch, intonation, resonance, speech rate, phrasing patterns
  - Nonverbal communication patterns may include gestures, posture/movement, facial expressions

- Social gender role transition (Real-Life Experience)

- Hormonal therapy (including expected changes and risks):
  - Estrogen therapy (and androgen-reducing medications) for man transitioning to a woman (MtF)
  - Testosterone therapy for woman transitioning to a man (FtM)

- Sex reassignment surgery (SRS) to change primary and/or secondary sex characteristics
- Options for MtF:
  - Breast/chest surgeries (breast augmentation)
  - Genital surgery (penectomy, orchiectomy, vaginoplasty, clitoroplasty, vulvoplasty)
  - Additional options (facial feminization surgery, thyroid cartilage reduction, lipofilling, voice surgery, gluteal augmentation, hair reconstruction)
- Options for FtM:
  - Breast/chest surgery (bilateral mastectomy, creation of a male chest)
  - Genital surgery (hysterectomy/salpingo-oophorectomy, reconstruction of the urethra, which can be combined with a phalloplasty, vaginectomy, scrotoplasty, and implantation of penile erection and/or testicular prostheses)
  - Additional options: liposuction, body contouring procedures.

Rationales

Modifying one's physical appearance can aid in gender adaptation by better aligning with how one feels inside. This may also consist of using a different name.

This therapy aims to help patients develop the verbal and nonverbal communication skills that facilitate comfort in their gender identity. Speech-language pathologists and speech therapists should have special training in this competency. Voice feminization surgery may also be considered for MtFs.

The Real-Life Experience requires the patient to function full time (24 hours a day) in the desired gender role for a minimum period of 12 months. The purpose of this activity is to allow people to assess how comfortable it is to live in all aspects of daily life, socially and professionally.

Hormone therapy must be individualized based on a patient's goals, the risk-benefit ratio of medications, co-morbid conditions, and consideration of social and economic issues. Possible benefits and risks, and the impact on reproductive capacity need to be discussed, as well as the potential impact of the feminizing or masculinizing therapy on how the patient may be perceived. Most physical changes occur over 2 years.

Feminizing or masculinizing genital surgery is not an elective surgery that the patient can simply request. Surgeries for gender dysphoria are only undertaken after a comprehensive evaluation by a qualified mental health professional and with written documentation that the patient has met standard eligibility and readiness criteria. This way the patient and the gender identity healthcare team all share the responsibility for the decision to make irreversible changes to the body. These surgeries may or may not be covered by health insurance. Providing patients with actual photographs from sex reassignment surgeries to review can be helpful, as the outcomes may not look as the patient has imagined.

■ = Independent ▲ = Interprofessional Collaboration

Actions/Interventions

- Assist the patient to list and evaluate the advantages and disadvantages of each option.

- Educate patients about need for follow-up care for hormonal and surgical therapies.

- Educate patients about reproductive health issues as indicated.

- Prepare the patient for issues related to possible change in sexual orientation.

- Educate about support groups, gender networks, and communication with peers via social media that can provide more information.

- Provide information regarding changes in legal documents: driver's license; passport; Social Security card.

Rationales

It is important for patients to draw upon their information and emotions to imagine what it would be like if each of the possible options were carried out. Factors to be considered include the time required for change to be noticed, cost for procedures (surgical treatment may not be covered by health insurance), some changes are irreversible, changes may compromise intimacy with current partner; lack of social support for a given change, risk for futher discrimination in the workplace and social arena; reproductive issues; legal document changes required. Other concerns are the potential side effects and complications from hormonal and surgical therapies. QSEN: Patient-centered care.

Patients may be taking hormones for many years and thus require ongoing follow-up to monitor for possible complications. Postsurgical patients are also at risk for short- and long-term complications related to the sex reassignment surgical procedures. Patients should also be guided as to how to implement general health maintenance practices. QSEN: Safety.

Patients who may consider having children need to understand that cross-sex hormonal therapy limits fertility. Sex reassignment surgery may have involved removing/altering one's reproductive organs. Sperm banking and embryo freezing options should be discussed and considered. QSEN: Patient-centered care.

Once transition is complete, it is possible for a transman or transwoman to experience a change in sexual orientation. However, this varies greatly among people and for many people there is no change. For most patients, working out the issues related to gender identity are more pressing than sexual orientation concerns.

These resources can provide specialized and practical information as well as avenues for support and advocacy. Online groups such as the National Coalition for LGBT Health can be useful for people who have difficulty accessing local groups and who may have experienced isolation and stigma.

Some of these changes need to be undertaken during the social gender role transition. Patients have reported how fulfilling it is to finally see their true gender listed on such documents.

Related Care Plans

Readiness for enhanced decision-making, Chapter 2
Anxiety, Chapter 2
Chronic low self-esteem, Chapter 2
Risk for suicide, Chapter 2
Ineffective sexuality patterns, Chapter 2
Ineffective health maintenance, Chapter 2

Sexually Transmitted Diseases

The term sexually transmitted diseases (STDs) refers to a variety of clinical syndromes and infections caused by pathogens that can be acquired or transmitted through sexual contact. Although most cases of STDs are associated with oral or genital sexual activity, some can be transmitted through contact with infected blood, such as hepatitis B. STDs include many kinds of infections, and are caused by bacteria (*Chlamydia* infection, gonorrhea, syphilis), by viruses (genital warts [human papillomavirus], genital herpes, human immunodeficiency virus [HIV] infection), and by parasites (trichomoniasis). These serious illnesses require treatment. Herpes is a chronic condition that can be managed but not cured. The incidence of specific STDs has changed over time. Some infections have reached epidemic proportions among specific cohorts of populations, and variance occurs among regions and countries. This content will address common infections in the United States, where the prevalence of STDs is a major public health concern. Many factors have contributed to the rise in types of STDs

and number of people infected in the United States. Some of these factors include ease of travel; increased population mobility; changes in cultural and social norms regarding sexual activity, marriage, and women's roles; and more explicit sexual content in popular media. Those activities considered to place persons most at risk include having more than one sex partner; having sex with someone who has had many partners; having unprotected sex; trading sex for money or drugs; and having a history of STDs. Many times, STDs coexist with other STDs. That is, when a patient is diagnosed with one STI, there is a higher risk that he or she will have others and that patient should be screened for them. This care plan describes the most common STDs: *Chlamydia* infection, gonorrhea, syphilis, genital herpes, genital warts, and trichomoniasis. The information is based on the Centers for Disease Control and Prevention's (CDC's) 2015 Sexually Transmitted Diseases Guidelines. See also Human Immunodeficiency Virus (HIV), Chapter 10, and Pelvic Inflammatory Disease, later in this chapter.

NANDA-I
NDx Deficient Knowledge

Common Related Factors
Insufficient information
Insufficient interest in learning
Misinformation presented by others
Insufficient knowledge of resources

Defining Characteristics
Insufficient knowledge
Inaccurate follow-through of instruction
Inappropriate behavior

Common Expected Outcome
Patient verbalizes understanding of the disease process, transmission, prevention strategies, complications, and treatment modalities.

NOC Outcomes
Knowledge: Infection Management; Knowledge: Disease Process; Knowledge: Treatment Regimen; Risk Control: Infectious Process

NIC Interventions
Health Literacy Enhancement; Learning Facilitation; Crisis Intervention; Teaching: Individual

---

Ongoing Assessment

Actions/Interventions

 Determine the patient's previous knowledge of the disease process, routes of transmission, complications, and treatment modalities.

Rationales

Information is assimilated into previous assumptions and facts. Patients may have misconceptions about disease transmission and treatment. Patients may not be knowledgeable about the long-term risks and effects of STDs. QSEN: Patient-centered care.

■ = Independent ▲ = Interprofessional Collaboration

Actions/Interventions

- Determine the patient's understanding of medical terminology as well as slang or lay terms.

- Determine the patient's sexual history in a respectful, nonjudgmental manner.

Rationales

It is important to speak in terms the patient understands. Accurate information about sex and STDs is not always easily available to younger patients.

STIs are spread during homosexual and heterosexual activity. Risks increase with the number of lifetime sexual partners. Judgmental attitudes may preclude patients from following through with a treatment plan. The best approach is to be respectful, compassionate, and nonjudgmental using open-ended questions. Examples of questions:
- Tell me about any new sex partners you have had since your last visit.
- Are your sex partners men, women, or both?
- What are you doing to protect from STDs?
- What has your experience been with using condoms?

For men who have sex with men, it is necessary to ask if they participate in anal insertive sex and if a condom is used. For additional information about gaining cultural competency when working with gay, bisexual, or transgender patients, refer to the CDC's Guidelines. QSEN: Patient-centered care.

Therapeutic Interventions

Actions/Interventions

- Teach the medication regimen, which includes the name of the drug, dosage, administration, side effects, and action of the prescribed medication.
- Review basic hygiene before the topical administration of drugs (e.g., wash lesions with soap and water, keep the area dry, wear loose-fitting cotton undergarments).
- Discuss the importance of notifying all sexual partners.

- Instruct the patient about scheduling appointments and treatments.
- Instruct the female patient regarding the importance of yearly gynecological examinations with Papanicolaou (Pap) smears. Encourage male patients to have yearly testicular examinations.
- Instruct patients in safe practices to reduce the likelihood of transmission of STDs. Instruct in the use of condoms.

Rationales

Effective treatment requires that the patient take the medications as directed and complete the whole regimen to prevent reinfection. QSEN: Safety.

Basic hygiene of lesions helps prevent further contamination. Cotton products decrease perspiration.

It is necessary for patients to identify their other sexual contacts to decrease disease spread in the community. This decreases the chance of reinfection and of further spread of the disease. In all states syphilis, gonorrhea, and chlamydial infection are reportable diseases. Public health workers will contact sexual partners for testing and treatment. QSEN: Safety.

Follow-up testing is necessary to prove eradication of certain STDs.

These excellent screening tools provide a wonderful opportunity for education.

Practices include using a latex (or polyurethane if latex allergy) condom for genital and anal intercourse; using condoms or latex barriers (dental dams) over the genitals or anus during oral-genital-anal sexual contact; wearing gloves for finger or hand contact with the vagina or rectum. Male condoms, when used consistently and correctly, can reduce the risk for transmission of most STDs. Several types of female condoms are available that can provide protection from acquisition and transmission of STDs, although data are limited. QSEN: Safety.

Actions/Interventions

- Discuss the benefits of monogamous relationships.

Rationales

The surest way to avoid transmission of STDs is to abstain from sexual contact or to be in a long-term mutually monogamous relationship with a partner who has been tested and is known to be uninfected. QSEN: Safety.

NDx   Infection

Common Related Factors

Inadequate primary defenses
Tissue destruction
Extension of infection
Sexual exposure
Insufficient knowledge to avoid exposure

Common Expected Outcome

Patient has a decrease in or complete resolution of symptoms of infection.

Defining Characteristics

Urethral discharge
Genital lesions
Fever
Malaise
Dysuria
Enlarged lymph nodes

NOC Outcomes

Risk Control: Infectious Process; Risk Detection

NIC Interventions

Infection Control; Infection Protection

Ongoing Assessment

Actions/Interventions

- Assess for the signs and symptoms associated with specific sexually transmitted diseases (STDs).

- Assess for the general signs and symptoms of infection.

- Identify those at risk (e.g., sexual partners, unprotected sex).
- Assess individual risk factors for reactivation of the disease process.

Rationales

Urethral inflammation is a common symptom in men. The discharge may be purulent. Men will often report pain and burning with urination. In women, yeast infections such as trichomoniasis usually present with malodorous vaginal discharge and vulvar itching. The characteristics of genital lesions vary with specific STDs. QSEN: Safety.

Some STDs, such as genital herpes, may be associated with general symptoms of infection such as fever and malaise. Enlarged lymph nodes may occur in the inguinal area with many STDs. QSEN: Safety

Those exposed may require treatment to prevent the spread or development of the infection. QSEN: Safety.

Recurrence of genital warts or genital herpes is common.

■ = Independent   ▲ = Interprofessional Collaboration

Therapeutic Interventions

Actions/Interventions	Rationales
■ Provide information about the pertinent STD:	There is a wide range of STDs that can confuse the public. Each has its own infective organism and pattern of symptoms. Diagnosis varies depending on the specific STD. Diagnostic aids include history, physical examination, Pap smears, serologic testing, and tissue cultures and stains. For many infections a definitive diagnostic test has yet to be developed. QSEN: Safety; Evidence-based practice.
• *Chlamydia trachomatis*	*Chlamydia trachomatis* infection is the most common STD. Symptoms range from none to dysuria, to purulent vaginal or penile discharge, to pelvic inflammatory disease (PID) in women. The most common diagnostic tests include the nucleic acid amplification test (NAAT); direct fluorescent antibody (DFA) test; and enzyme immunoassay test. Treatment includes a course of antibiotics (azithromycin or doxycline), partner notification with treatment, as well as mandatory reporting to the state. Prevention may be acquired through consistent and correct condom use.
• Gonorrhea	Gonorrhea is caused by the *Neisseria gonorrhoeae* organism. Men complain of urethritis, urethral discharge, and often testicular swelling. Women can be asymptomatic or report vaginal discharge, dysuria or frequency of urination. It can affect joints and skin, causing arthralgias and skin lesions. A culture confirms the diagnosis, though diagnosis may be made by a NAAT. Treatment includes a course of antibiotics, partner notification with treatment, as well as mandatory reporting to the state. Prevention may be acquired through consistent and correct condom use.
• Syphilis	Syphilis is caused by *Treponema pallidum*. Sexual transmission occurs only in the presence of mucocutaneous lesions. Syphilis is easy to cure in its early stages, with benzathine penicillin G being the treatment of choice. If left untreated, syphilis can cause serious complications including death. Screening is usually completed with the Venereal Disease Research Laboratory (VDRL) test or the rapid plasma reagin test. Additional tests are used to confirm the diagnosis.
• Genital herpes	Genital herpes is an incurable and recurrent viral infection caused by the herpes simplex virus (HSV). HSV causes painful genital lesions that start as papules or vesicles. A diagnosis of genital herpes may be made by the viral culture of an actual lesion or by serologic testing. Treatment includes systemic antiviral therapy, which may control the signs and symptoms but does not cure the disease. Genital herpes may be transmitted even when no lesions are present, contrary to previously held beliefs. Even though condoms may help prevent some disease transmission, they are not fail-safe because of the location of the lesions.

Actions/Interventions	**Rationales**
• Genital warts	Genital warts (condylomata acuminata) are caused by certain types of human papillomavirus (HPV) infection. Clinically, genital warts are nonpainful and asymptomatic. Treatment includes removal of the warts by chemical or ablative methods by the health care provider. This may require multiple office visits, and removal may or may not reduce infectivity. Antimitotic gels or immune-enhancing cream for removal can be applied by the patient. Even though treatment may eliminate the warts, it does not erase infectivity. HPV infection is considered as the primary risk factor for developing cervical cancer.
• Trichomoniasis	Although trichomoniasis occurs in both men and women, it is one of the most common STD in women, characterized by malodorous vaginal discharge and vulvar irritation and/or itching. Often it is asymptomatic in men, or a transient dysuria or mild discharge may occur from urethritis. Polymerase chain reaction testing on a urine sample is the only reliable means of testing for trichomoniasis, and this is limited by its availability. Although trichomoniasis in men can be transient and clear on its own, to avoid reinfection concurrent therapy and abstinence from sexual activity are advised until the treatment of both partners has been completed. The offending organism is *Trichomonas vaginalis,* which responds to treatment with oral metronidazole or tinidazole. People taking this drug must be cautioned against alcohol intake during treatment and for several days after treatment.
■ Teach about the use of anti-infective agents as indicated:	Extended therapy may be indicated for reactivation of the disease process, or in the presence of other medical diseases such as HIV infection. The reader is referred to the CDC website for the most current treatment guidelines for STDs. QSEN: Evidence-based practice; Safety.
• For genital herpes: acyclovir, famciclovir, valacyclovir	These antivirals are the primary treatment for genital herpes. The treatment regimen varies for first episode vs. recurrent therapy. Medications may be given orally or be used topically for mild disease. Intravenous (IV) administration is recommended for severe disease and recurrent lesions. Long-term use at lower dosages is suggested to reduce transmission to partners.
• For syphilis: benzathine penicillin G	Penicillin is the treatment of choice for syphilis. It can be given as a single intramuscular injection in the early stages of the disease. In the later stages, multiple injections may be used or the drug may be given intravenously.
• For *Chlamydia* infection: doxycycline, or azithromycin • For gonorrhea: ceftriaxone or azithromycin	These agents are used alone or in combination for the treatment of *Chlamydia* infection and gonorrhea. Treatment regimens, combinations, and the length of therapy differ and change according to antimicrobial resistance patterns, stages of the disease, or if the patient is co-infected with HIV.
• For trichomoniasis: metronidazole or tinidazole	These drugs are the treatment of choice for trichomoniasis.
• For genital warts: antimitotic gels or immune-enhancing cream	These agents are effective in treating genital warts. Cryotherapy and other ablative methods may be indicated to remove warts.

■ = Independent   ▲ = Interprofessional Collaboration

Actions/Interventions

- Teach the patient to complete the prescribed treatment and take all medications.

- Teach about the need to abstain from sexual activity during treatment and for the prescribed number of days after.

- Notify the local health department.

- Teach about prevention.

Rationales

The recurrence and transmission of infection can occur if the patient does not take all of the medication. Patients often stop treatment prematurely when symptoms disappear. QSEN: Safety.

People with herpes should abstain from sexual activity with unaffected partners when lesions or other symptoms of herpes are present, and they should understand that about 70% of new cases are transmitted through silent viral shedding. Partners should be evaluated and treated to prevent reinfection of the patient. QSEN: Safety.

In all states, the STDs gonorrhea, syphilis, and *Chlamydia* infection must be reported to local health departments for purposes of surveillance and partner notifications. QSEN: Safety.

The most reliable way to avoid transmission of STDs is to abstain from oral, vaginal and anal sex, or to be in a long-term mutually monogamous relationship with an uninfected partner. Condoms can reduce transmission of HPV, genital herpes, and syphilis. Pre-exposure vaccination (e.g., Gardasil vaccine) is an effective method for preventing transmission of HPV for men who have sex with men. QSEN: Safety.

NANDA-I
NDx Disturbed Body Image

Common Related Factors
Lesions
Urethral discharge
Odiferous discharge
Topical medications

Defining Characteristics
Focuses behavior on change in body function and/or appearance
Verbalizes feelings of inadequacy and low self-worth
Discusses difficulty with coping with diagnosis of sexually transmitted disease (STD)
Actual change in body
Change in social behavior (withdrawal, isolation)
Refusal to discuss infection

Common Expected Outcome
Patient demonstrates enhanced body image and self-esteem as evidenced by the ability to look at, talk about, and care for the altered body part.

NOC Outcomes
Body Image; Self-Esteem
NIC Intervention
Self-Esteem Enhancement

Ongoing Assessment

Actions/Interventions

- Assess and validate the patient's feelings about changes in appearance and body function.

- Note the patient's withdrawal from social situations.

Rationales

The extent of the response is related more to the value or importance the patient places on the body part than its actual value. QSEN: Patient-centered care.

STDs are associated with a social stigma. Withdrawal may indicate feelings of social isolation or fear of rejection by others.

Actions/Interventions

- Assess the impact of body image disturbance in relation to the patient's developmental stage.

- Assess the coping mechanisms that the patient has used in the past.

Rationales

Early experience with STDs and its "social stigma" may affect developmental changes at a time when fostering social and intimate relationships is particularly important.

Previous coping strategies may not be adequate to support the patient's adjustment. QSEN: Patient-centered care.

Therapeutic Interventions

Actions/Interventions

- Encourage the verbalization of positive or negative feelings about body changes.
- Assist the patient in identifying the extent of changes in appearance.
- Provide hope within the parameters of the disease process. Do not give false reassurance.
- Refer to support groups.

- ▲ Refer for sexual counseling to help cope with sexuality issues.

Rationales

It is worthwhile to encourage the patient to separate feelings about changes in the body from feelings of self-worth.

This approach helps begin the process of looking toward the future and how sexual activity will be different.

Hope promotes a positive attitude and provides an opportunity to plan for the future. Many STDs can be cured.

Lay people in similar situations offer a different type of support, which is perceived as helpful.

The patient may need professional assistance to deal with issues and accept self. QSEN: Teamwork and collaboration.

Related Care Plans

Anxiety, Chapter 2
Ineffective health management, Chapter 2
Human immunodeficiency virus, Chapter 10
Pelvic inflammatory disease, Chapter 12

MEN'S HEALTH CARE PLANS

Benign Prostatic Hyperplasia

Benign prostatic hyperplasia (BPH) is a common urological disorder in men, and its incidence is age related. The prevalence rises from 40% to 50% in men 51 to 60 years of age, to more than 80% in men 80 years of age and older. BPH is an overgrowth of muscle and connective tissue (hyperplasia) of the prostate gland. As the glandular tissue enlarges, it causes obstruction of the urethra. Severity of symptoms may be ranked according to the International Prostate Symptom Score (I-PSS), which incorporates the American Urological Symptom Index. Early diagnosis and staging have improved with the availability of prostate ultrasound technology. Treatment options include "watchful waiting"; medications that cause either regression of overgrown tissue or relaxation of the urethral muscle tissue; minimally invasive treatments, including direct heat application, dilation, laser, and placement of stents to allow drainage; and surgical treatment to remove prostate tissue. The focus of this care plan is the patient with newly diagnosed BPH.

■ = Independent   ▲ = Interprofessional Collaboration

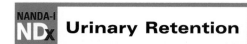

Men's and Women's Health Care Plans

NANDA-I NDx Urinary Retention

Common Related Factor
Urethral blockage

Defining Characteristics
Obstructive symptoms:
- Hesitancy
- Straining to start void
- Bladder distention
- Weak or narrowed stream
- Increased residual urine volume

Irritative symptoms:
- Frequency
- Urgency
- Nocturia

Common Expected Outcome
Patient has unobstructed flow of urine and empties bladder completely, either by medications, by catheterization, after medical or noninvasive therapies, or after surgical removal of hyperplastic prostatic tissue.

NOC Outcome
Urinary Elimination

NIC Interventions
Urinary Catheterization; Urinary Elimination Management

Ongoing Assessment

Actions/Interventions	Rationales
■ Assess urinary elimination; inquire about obstructive symptoms, which include hesitancy, difficulty starting a stream, dribbling at the end of a void, straining to void, a weak or narrow stream, and irritative symptoms such as frequency, urgency, and nocturia.	The male urethra is surrounded by the prostate gland. When the prostate gland is enlarged as a result of prostatic hyperplasia, the urethra is compressed; symptoms are a result of the decreased caliber of the urethra. Irritative symptoms occur because of obstruction that causes a hypersensitivity of the bladder.
■ Assess the history of urinary tract infections (UTIs).	Because the flow of urine is chronically obstructed, stasis of urine occurs and infections are common.
■ Assess the symptom severity of benign prostatic hyperplasia (BPH) according to the International Prostate Symptom Score (Table 12.1).	This tool provides serial objective measurements of symptom severity. It incorporates the seven symptom questions from the American Urological Association's Symptom Score for BPH, and adds one additional question on quality of life. Scoring ranges from mild (1-7), to moderate (8-19), to severe (20-35). QSEN: Evidence-based practice.
■ Assess for pain or discomfort.	Pain may be related to a concurrent UTI, residual urine, or bladder distention.
■ Assess for any over-the-counter medication use.	Over-the-counter decongestants and antihistamines can slow urinary flow and increase symptoms.
■ Percuss and palpate the abdomen for a distended bladder.	The lower abdomen becomes distended as the urine volume increases in the bladder. Urinary retention is a key symptom.
■ Assess postvoid residual urine.	These data aid in the detection of urinary stasis and impaired detrusor function. Postvoid residual urine can be assessed by postvoid catheterization, x-ray films, or most simply by ultrasound examination.
■ Assess the intake and output, noting the amount and frequency of voids.	These data give clues to the completion of bladder emptying.

evolve   For additional care plans, go to http://evolve.elsevier.com/Gulanick/.

TABLE 12.1 The International Prostate Symptom Score (I-PSS)

In the Past Month:	Not at All	Less Than 1 Time in 5 Times	Less Than Half of the Time	About Half of the Time	More Than Half of the Time	Almost Always
1. Incomplete Emptying How often have you had a sensation of not emptying your bladder?	0	1	2	3	4	5
2. Frequency How often have you had to urinate less than every two hours?	0	1	2	3	4	5
3. Intermittency How often have you found you stopped and started again several times when you urinated?	0	1	2	3	4	5
4. Urgency How often have you found it difficult to postpone urination?	0	1	2	3	4	5
5. Weak Stream How often have you had a weak urinary stream?	0	1	2	3	4	5
6. Straining How often have you had to strain to start urination?	0	1	2	3	4	5
7. Nocturia How many times do you typically get up to urinate?	0	1 (one time)	2 (two times)	3 (three times)	4 (four times)	5 (five times)

Total I-PSS Score: mild = 1 to 7 points; moderate = 8 to 19 points; severe = 20 to 35 points.

Quality of Life Due to Urinary Symptoms	Delighted	Pleasant	Mostly Satisfied	Mixed	Mostly Dissatisfied	Unhappy	Terrible
If you were to spend the rest of your life with your urinary condition just the way it is now, how would you feel about it?	0	1	2	3	4	5	6

From American Urological Association. (2010). *American Urological Association guideline: Management of benign prostatic hyperplasia (BPH). Revised, 2010.* American Urological Association Education and Research, Inc. Available at www.auanet.org/common/pdf/education/Arc-BPH-Chapter1. *See also* www.urospec.com/uro/Forms/ipss.pdf.

Actions/Interventions

■ Assess for hematuria.

▲ Review the x-ray films or ultrasound findings.

Rationales

Hematuria can result from distention of the bladder with the resultant rupture of small blood vessels. BPH is a common cause of hematuria in elderly men.

Hydroureters (distended ureters) and hydronephrosis (enlarged, overdistended kidneys) may result from long-standing obstruction caused by prostatic disease.

Therapeutic Interventions

Actions/Interventions

■ Encourage oral fluids for adequate hydration, but do not push fluids or overhydrate.

Rationales

Rapid filling of the bladder can precipitate complete urinary retention. Overhydration can aggravate the problem of residual urine and bladder distention. Coffee and other caffeinated beverages can increase the urine amount and urgency.

■ = Independent   ▲ = Interprofessional Collaboration

Men's and Women's Health Care Plans

Actions/Interventions

▲ Prepare the patient for the possible need for an indwelling catheter to restore the flow of urine. *Note:* Special catheters with curved or firm tips may be needed to accomplish catheterization in the patient with an enlarged prostate.

■ Encourage the patient to take medications as prescribed.

■ Encourage therapeutic lifestyle modifications.

■ Encourage the patient to take antibiotics as prescribed.

Rationales

Indwelling catheterization is used to allow free drainage of the bladder. Chronic urinary obstruction can result in severe damage to the kidneys and, ultimately, renal failure.

Several types of medications are available to reduce prostate size and improve urinary flow. These include 5-alpha-reductase inhibitors, alpha-blocking agents, and phosphodiesterase inhibitors. QSEN: Evidence-based practice.

These modifications may have a mild effect and include limiting fluids before bed, reducing caffeine and alcohol intake, and double voiding before bed.

Medication may be indicated to treat or prevent a UTI resulting from obstruction and stasis. QSEN: Safety.

NANDA-I NDx Deficient Knowledge

Common Related Factors

Insufficient information
Insufficient interest in learning
Misinformation presented by others
Insufficient knowledge of resources

Defining Characteristics

Insufficient knowledge
Inaccurate follow-through of instruction
Inappropriate behavior

Common Expected Outcome

Patient demonstrates understanding of diagnostic procedures and treatment options for benign prostatic hyperplasia (BPH).

NOC Outcomes

Knowledge: Disease Process; Knowledge: Treatment Regimen; Knowledge: Chronic Disease Management

NIC Interventions

Health Literacy Enhancement; Learning Facilitation; Teaching: Disease Process; Teaching: Procedure/Treatment

Ongoing Assessment

Actions/Interventions

■ Assess the patient's understanding of prostate disorders and the following commonly performed diagnostic procedures for prostate disorders:
  • Digital rectal examination (DRE)

  • Uroflowmetry

  • Cystoscopy

Rationales

Men are often embarrassed or hesitant to discuss prostate problems and often delay seeking attention for symptoms that typically have a gradual onset. QSEN: Patient-centered care.

The DRE checks for the size and firmness of the prostate gland.

Urodynamic flow studies include the determination of flow rate and evaluation of residual urine.

Visualization of the bladder and urethra through a fiberoptic scope allows the physician to see the extent of the enlargement and consequent obstruction.

ⓔvolve For additional care plans, go to http://evolve.elsevier.com/Gulanick/.

Actions/Interventions	Rationales
• Urinalysis	Examination of the urine for the presence of blood, white blood cells (WBCs), and/or bacteria is useful in the identification of urinary tract infection (UTI), which often accompanies an obstruction that causes the stasis of urine.
• Laboratory studies: blood urea nitrogen (BUN) and creatinine; prostate-specific antigen (PSA); complete blood count (CBC)	BUN and creatinine determine renal function, which can be impaired as a result of long-standing obstructive uropathy. The prostate gland normally produces PSA to liquefy semen. When the prostate is enlarged, PSA levels increase. They can also be increased because of prostate cancer, recent tests, surgery, and infection. PSA levels can be measured in total or free portions and generally are viewed over time and evaluated with other portions of the examination. An elevated PSA alone is not diagnostic of prostate cancer. The CBC is used to evaluate evidence of systemic infection.
• Transrectal ultrasound examination	This ultrasound examination is performed rectally using a wand type of ultrasound transducer to examine the prostate gland for enlargement.
■ Assess the patient's understanding of the following treatment options for prostate disorders:	These treatment options are based on recommendations from national organizations. Providing this information allows the patient to be a full partner in making decisions to achieve optimal outcomes. QSEN: Patient-centered care; Evidence-based practice.
Active surveillance	Active surveillance or "watchful waiting" is a conservative approach for patients with no or mild symptoms. Patients should be instructed to reduce fluid intake before bedtime, drink less alcohol and caffeine, and avoid over-the-counter cold and sinus medications that contain decongestants that can aggravate the prostate gland.

Medical management
• Medications
  • 5-Alpha-reductase inhibitors
  • Alpha-blocking agents
  • Combination therapy
  • Phosphodiesterase inhibitors
	Prostate size can be reduced with a 5-alpha-reductase inhibitor such as finasteride and dutasteride. These drugs inhibit production of the hormone dihydrotestosterone (DHT), which enhances prostate growth. A class of alpha-blocking agents—terazosin, doxazosin, tamsulosin, silodosin, and alfuzosin—all relax the musculature within the bladder neck and improve urinary flow. Using both classes of drugs together alleviates more symptoms and prevents the progression of BPH. More recent medications include phosphodiesterase inhibitors (e.g., Cialis) for men who also have erectile dysfunction.

Minimally invasive therapies for BPH • Transurethral microwave thermotherapy	Several techniques can be employed to heat and destroy excess prostatic tissue and reduce compression of the urethra. This procedure relieves symptoms but does not cure the problem. No incontinence or impotence has been reported.
• Transurethral needle ablation	Low-level radiofrequency energy using needles is delivered to burn away designated areas of the enlarged prostate. This procedure is used in patients with comorbid conditions and provides sustained clinical improvement in most men. No incontinence or impotence has been reported.
• Transurethral incision of the prostate	This procedure is an option for smaller enlarged prostates.

■ = Independent   ▲ = Interprofessional Collaboration

Actions/Interventions	Rationales
• Laser prostatectomy	This procedure uses a high-energy laser to destroy or remove overgrown prostatic tissue.
• Electrovaporization of the prostate	This vaporization procedure has reduced bleeding complications and has shorter recovery times but has a greater risk for urinary retention, necessitating further treatment.
• Intraprostatic urethral stents	Stents are small tubes that allow for the drainage of urine by pushing back the prostatic urethra. They were used in the past for poor-operative-risk patients but are infrequently used now because of secondary obstruction over time.
Surgical management for BPH	Several surgical approaches are available, depending on the size and location of the enlargement and patient factors such as age and comorbid conditions.
• Transurethral resection of the prostate (TURP)	This "closed" procedure is widely used to treat BPH and remains the gold standard for evaluating newer therapies. The surgeon removes the prostate by inserting a resectoscope through the urethra to remove obstructing tissue. The TURP is significantly less traumatic than open forms of surgery.
• Open prostatectomy	This "open" surgical procedure is indicated when the prostatic tissue is very enlarged, when the bladder needs repair, or when important landmarks are not visible for TURP.

Therapeutic Interventions

Actions/Interventions	Rationales
■ Discuss with the patient the advantages and disadvantages of medical and surgical treatment options.	Many factors affect the selection of optimal treatment, including the severity of symptoms, ability to tolerate medication side effects, medical contraindications to surgery, and concern for postoperative erectile dysfunction. Specific rates of sexual function, continence issues, and postsurgical complications should be referred to the surgeon. QSEN: Patient-centered care.
■ Provide the patient with postprocedure instructions about the signs and symptoms to be reported:	The nurse prepares the patient for the close monitoring required to prevent and/or treat potential complications. QSEN: Safety.
• Hematuria	In the first few weeks after TURP, some bleeding is expected. However, thick red urine or clots must be reported.
• Infection	Urinary instrumentation and surgical incisions carry a risk for sepsis.
• Unresolved incontinence or retention	Temporary incontinence is common until healing has occurred. Retention is also common after urethral catheterization.
■ Discuss PSA testing.	Controversies exist over routine PSA testing because of the number of false-positive results. Rising levels of PSA can be an indication of an enlarging prostate or prostate cancer.
■ Teach about the need for an annual prostate examination.	Existing prostatic tissue could become cancerous. One treatment does not reduce the future risk for prostate disease.
■ Teach about the behavioral methods to reduce symptom severity or reduce the occurrence or aggravation of symptoms: • Limit fluid intake after dinner.	Reducing fluids can help avoid nocturia and interrupted sleep.
• Avoid medications known to worsen urinary symptoms such as cold preparations, diuretics, antispasmodics, antihistamines, and some antidepressants.	These medications may precipitate acute urinary retention or worsen existing symptoms.

⊕volve   **For additional care plans, go to http://evolve.elsevier.com/Gulanick/.**

Actions/Interventions

■ Discuss any prior experience in taking over-the-counter herbs such as saw palmetto extract to relieve symptoms.

■ Provide Internet resources for further education.

Rationales

This extract has been tried for the longest time, but there still is no research to confirm its benefit over placebo, The American Urological Association does not recommend any herbal therapy to manage BPH. QSEN: Evidence-based practice.

The National Cancer Institute and the National Kidney and Urologic Diseases Information Clearinghouse offer excellent materials.

NANDA-I NDx   Risk for Deficient Fluid Volume

Common Risk Factors

Postoperative hemorrhage from transurethral resection of the prostate
Inadequate fluid intake (to reduce symptoms)

Common Expected Outcome

Patient is normovolemic, as evidenced by stable blood pressure (BP) and heart rate (HR) and absence of gross hematuria.

NOC Outcomes
Urinary Elimination; Fluid Balance
NIC Interventions
Bladder Irrigation; Bleeding Reduction; Tube Care: Urinary

Ongoing Assessment

Actions/Interventions

■ Monitor the patient for decreased BP, orthostatic BP, and increased HR.

■ Monitor the patient's intake and output.

▲ Monitor blood urea nitrogen (BUN) and creatinine clearance.

■ Monitor the amount and severity of hematuria and for clots in the urine.

▲ Monitor the patient's hemoglobin and hematocrit.

Rationales

Reduction in the circulatory blood volume can cause hypotension and tachycardia. Postural hypotension, especially in the elderly, is a common manifestation of a fluid deficit. QSEN: Safety.

Intake and output should include a careful record of any irrigation fluid instilled. QSEN: Safety.

An elevated BUN and creatinine suggest a fluid deficit. QSEN: Safety.

Bright red blood in the urine is expected over the first 24 hours after transurethral resection but should irrigate to clear pink without clots during that period. QSEN: Safety.

Decreases indicate significant blood loss, contributing to a fluid status problem. QSEN: Safety.

Therapeutic Interventions

Action/Intervention

■ Encourage oral fluids as prescribed or tolerated by the patient. IV fluids may be ordered.

Rationale

Oral fluid replacement is indicated for a mild fluid deficit and is a cost-effective method for replacement treatment. Older patients have a decreased sense of thirst and may need ongoing reminders. Parenteral fluid replacement may be indicated to prevent or treat hypovolemic complications.

■ = Independent   ▲ = Interprofessional Collaboration

Men's and Women's Health
Care Plans

Related Care Plans

Ineffective sexuality pattern, Chapter 2
Insomnia, Chapter 2
Urinary retention, Chapter 2
Risk for infection, Chapter 2

Prostate Cancer

Radical Prostatectomy; Localized Prostate Cancer

Prostate cancer is the most common nonskin cancer among males in the United States, and if found early it has almost a 100% cure rate. One in every seven men will be diagnosed with prostate cancer in their lifetime. It occurs mostly in older men, with 60% over 65 years of age. Prostate cancer is an androgen-dependent adenocarcinoma that is usually slow growing. The known risk factors include age, race (African Americans have highest risk), and family history. Prostate cancer can often be found early by testing the amount of prostate-specific antigen (PSA) in a man's blood, or by digital rectal examination. Specific recommendations for these screenings vary among professional organizations. Although screening can help find many prostate cancers early, there are still questions about whether this saves lives. There are clearly both pros and cons to the prostate cancer screening tests in use today. At this time, the American Cancer Society (ACS) recommends that men older than age 50 and those at high risk who are thinking about having prostate cancer screening should make informed decisions based on available information, discussion with their doctor, and their own views on the benefits and side effects of prostate cancer screening and treatment.

With prostate cancer, the patient is generally asymptomatic until obstructive symptoms of the urinary tract appear. Transrectal ultrasound examination is used to detect nonpalpable tumors and stage localized cancers. Biopsy is needed to confirm diagnosis. Medical and surgical options depend on the stage of the cancer, symptoms, and response to other therapies. Treatment may include the traditional radical prostatectomy, laparoscopic nerve-sparing procedures for more localized cancers including robotic-assisted procedures, radiation (external beam or brachytherapy [seed implant]), androgen deprivation hormonal therapy, and chemotherapy. There are two approaches for a radical prostatectomy for cancer: retropubic and perineal. The approach depends on several factors, such as coexisting bladder abnormalities, size of the prostate, and the degree of risk of the surgical candidate. Each procedure has its advantages and disadvantages. Two adverse outcomes after surgery include incontinence and erectile dysfunction. Patients and their health care providers are faced with making important decisions regarding which of the numerous treatment options are best for them. Patients presenting with early-stage cancer in which only a small amount of cancer is noted on biopsy may be considered for active surveillance (watchful waiting) as an alternative to more aggressive therapies. In addition, many clinical trials are available for patients needing additional treatments. The focus of this care plan is on the patient undergoing a radical prostatectomy.

NANDA-I NDx **Fear**

Common Related Factors

Lack of knowledge about diagnosis, treatment, and prognosis
Treatment by active surveillance (watchful waiting)
Treatments and invasive procedures
Threat of death

Defining Characteristics

Identifies object of fear
Increase in tension
Apprehensiveness
Focused narrowed to the source of fear

Common Expected Outcomes

Patient uses effective coping behaviors to reduce fear response.

Patient verbalizes a reduction or absence of fear.

NOC Outcomes
Fear Self-Control; Coping

NIC Interventions
Anxiety Reduction; Presence; Calming Technique; Emotional Support

---

Ongoing Assessment

Actions/Interventions	Rationales
■ Assess the level of fear as mild, moderate, or severe.	The threat to health, life, and role function resulting from cancer can predispose the patient to fear or anxiety. Determining the level of fear being experienced guides the appropriate treatment approach.
■ Determine the factors affecting the patient's fear.	Many misconceptions exist regarding prognosis, treatments, and potential complications such as sexual dysfunction. Patients with small, localized tumors treated by active surveillance may find "watching" over time to be more stressful than anticipated. Accurate assessment data about the source of the patient's concern guide appropriate treatments and supportive coping strategies. QSEN: Patient-centered care.
■ Determine the patient's support systems.	In some cases, there may be no readily available resources. The evaluation of supportive people from the past may provide the assistance required at this time.
■ Determine the patient's coping methods.	This information helps determine the effectiveness of coping strategies currently used by the patient. QSEN: Patient-centered care.

Therapeutic Interventions

Actions/Interventions	Rationales
■ Give the patient the opportunity to ask questions or verbalize concerns.	Men's concerns may include the fear of death, feelings of loss of control, questions regarding determination of the appropriate treatment, and how diagnosis and treatment may affect his relationship with his significant other.
■ Provide education about the diagnosis and selected treatment plan.	Education and anticipatory preparation decrease anxiety and promote cooperation. For most men diagnosed with prostate cancer, the cancer is found at an early stage. Many treatment options need to be considered, including active surveillance for older men with a slow growing tumor or those opting for a less invasive procedure. Such a complex decision can be difficult to make. Patients need to consult with health care providers, and family and friends who have faced similar issues. This care plan is focused on patients selecting a radical prostatectomy. QSEN: Patient-centered care; Evidence-based practice.
■ Provide information about resources for coping with the diagnosis.	The increased public awareness of prostate cancer has resulted in a variety of lay and professional books and Internet sites for information. Social services, support groups, and community agencies can help the patient cope with his illness and treatments. Some sources include the American Cancer Society, the National Coalition for Cancer Survivorship, and US TOO International.

■ = Independent   ▲ = Interprofessional Collaboration

Actions/Interventions	Rationales
■ Assist in identifying the strategies used in the past to deal with fearful situations.	This helps the patient focus on fear as a real and natural part of life that has been and can continue to be dealt with successfully. QSEN: Patient-centered care.
▲ Instruct in the use of physician-ordered antianxiety medications.	Short-term use of antianxiety medications can relieve unpleasant feelings.

NANDA-I NDx **Risk for Sexual Dysfunction**

Common Risk Factors

Injury to perineal nerves during surgery
Presence of indwelling urinary catheter
Dribbling and long-term incontinence
Decreased libido
Radiation side effects

Common Expected Outcomes

Patient or significant other is able to discuss concerns about sexual functioning.
Patient or significant other expresses improved satisfaction in sexual activity.
Patient adapts sexual therapies as needed to enhance performance.

NOC Outcomes
Sexual Functioning; Knowledge: Disease Process
NIC Interventions
Sexual Counseling; Teaching: Disease Process

Ongoing Assessment

Actions/Interventions	Rationales
■ Assess the patient's and significant other's expectations for sexual function.	Although many men undergoing prostatectomy are older, do not assume that sexual functioning is unimportant.
■ Assess the patient's and significant other's understanding of the potential impact that surgery may have had on sexual functioning.	A discussion of the possible negative impact of prostatectomy on sexual functioning should occur preoperatively, but often the patient is too anxious or preoccupied with other information (e.g., fear about surgery, prognosis with cancer diagnosis) to comprehend fully. If this is the case, the patient may benefit from postoperative discussion. Perineal resection carries the highest risk for sexual dysfunction. Newer nerve-sparing surgical procedures are becoming available and may be an option for some men. Radiation therapy side effects may include erectile dysfunction. Overall, most men will experience some sexual dysfunction in the first few months after treatment. QSEN: Patient-centered care.
■ Assess whether the patient and significant other need or want information during the postoperative period or if they prefer to wait a few weeks.	Timing of the patient's readiness to learn should guide the teaching plan. At a minimum, written materials can be given to the patient.
■ Assess for urinary incontinence after the removal of the catheter.	The psychological impact of urinary incontinence can negatively affect the patient's perceived ability to perform sexually. Dribbling may occur for as long as a few months after prostatectomy and catheter removal.

ⓔvolve **For additional care plans, go to http://evolve.elsevier.com/Gulanick/.**

Therapeutic Interventions

Actions/Interventions

- Teach the patient which nerves are necessary for erection and ejaculation; distinguish between sterility and impotence. Clarify all language; use diagrams and models as needed, depending on the patient's learning style.
- Offer the patient and significant other suggestions for alternatives to usual sexual practices during the postoperative period.

- Explain medications and mechanical devices available to the patient to enhance erection.

- Discuss urinary incontinence as a consequence of prostatectomy; teach Kegel exercises.

▲ Refer for sexual counseling as indicated.

Rationales

Patients may be embarrassed to ask questions that highlight a limited knowledge base; however, many misconceptions may exist.

Usual sexual activity can be resumed 4 to 6 weeks after surgery. Information about alternative ways for sexual expression may be appreciated. QSEN: Patient-centered care.

Medications such as 5-phosphodiesterase inhibitors (e.g., sildenafil) may be prescribed to maintain blood flow to the corpora cavernosa during recovery or for long-term follow-up. Mechanical devices (vacuum devices or penile prostheses) may be tried to create an erection.

Dribbling may occur for months and then resolve. Kegel exercises will increase the sphincter tone needed to achieve continence. They should be performed at each time of urination and several times throughout the day. Occasionally, incontinence after prostatectomy is permanent.

Specialty therapy may be indicated for some patients. Changes in sexual function may have adverse effects on the couple's relationship. QSEN: Teamwork and collaboration.

NANDA-I
NDx ## Deficient Knowledge: Postoperative

Common Related Factors

Insufficient information
Insufficient interest in learning
Misinformation presented by others
Insufficient knowledge of resources

Defining Characteristics

Insufficient knowledge
Inaccurate follow-through of instruction
Inappropriate behavior

Common Expected Outcome

Patient verbalizes understanding of need for follow-up care, wound care, and management of incontinence and erectile dysfunction.

NOC Outcomes
Knowledge: Disease Process; Knowledge: Treatment Procedure

NIC Interventions
Health Literacy Enhancement; Learning Facilitation; Wound Care; Teaching: Disease Process

---

Ongoing Assessment

Actions/Interventions

- Assess the patient's understanding of the need for further treatment (e.g., chemotherapy, radiation therapy) that may be required in patients who have had surgery to remove prostatic cancer.

Rationales

These treatments are part of the overall management to eliminate cancer cells that were not removed at surgery. QSEN: Patient-centered care.

■ = Independent ▲ = Interprofessional Collaboration

Actions/Interventions	Rationales
■ Assess the patient's ability to care for surgical wounds.	Infection is a common complication. Assessment provides a basis for further education. QSEN: Safety.
■ Assess the patient's understanding of potential dribbling and the methods for improving and dealing with incontinence.	The extent of the problem depends on the type of resection performed.
■ Assess the patient's knowledge of the resources for erectile dysfunction.	Erectile dysfunction may occur as a complication of prostate surgery. It may not have been a problem in the past; thus the patient may be unaware of available resources.

Therapeutic Interventions

Actions/Interventions	Rationales
■ Teach wound care.	Accurate, clear information provides a rationale for assuming responsibility for self-care at home. Patients should be instructed to shower daily for the first 2 to 3 weeks and to clean wounds with soap and water. QSEN: Safety.
■ Teach the patient the following about incontinence:	
• Instruct the patient regarding self-care and the temporary use of an indwelling catheter, if needed.	Most patients are discharged with an indwelling catheter that remains in place for several weeks. Patients are better able to ask questions when they have basic information about what to expect.
• Remind the patient that urinary incontinence may resolve up to 2 years postoperatively.	This knowledge may reduce anxiety and may help the patient with decision-making about the management of urinary elimination.
• Encourage the use of Kegel exercises.	These exercises improve perineal musculature and control over the urinary stream. They need to be performed several times throughout the day.
• Refer the patient to a urology specialist or a self-help incontinence group if chronic incontinence is a problem.	Relationships with people with common issues can be beneficial. Suggest the National Association for Continence. QSEN: Teamwork and collaboration.
■ Teach the patient to report any of the following:	For a successful recovery, the patient must know how to identify problems and what to do when problems occur. Early assessment facilitates prompt treatment. QSEN: Safety.
• Signs of infection: fever; unusual drainage from incisions; unusual drainage from the urethra, especially in patients having transurethral resection	
• Signs of urinary tract infection (cloudy, foul-smelling urine; frequency)	
• Hematuria	
• Unresolved incontinence	
■ Inform the patient of the need for a follow-up appointment to monitor PSA levels.	After successful treatment, the PSA levels should drop to near zero. The regular monitoring of these levels is important to evaluate the treatment effects and alert of possible recurrence of the cancer. QSEN: Safety.

Related Care Plans

Readiness for enhanced decision-making, Chapter 2
Ineffective coping, Chapter 2
Acute pain, Chapter 2
Risk for infection, Chapter 2
Stress urinary incontinence, Chapter 2
Erectile dysfunction, ⊖volve

Testicular Cancer

Malignant tumors of the testes are rare, accounting for only 1% of all the cancers in men reported in the United States each year. It is one of the most curable solid tumor cancers. Although the cause of testicular cancer is unknown, both congenital and acquired factors are associated with tumor development. The most common risk factors for testicular cancer are undescended testicles, family history of this cancer, white race, HIV infection, and previous cancer of one testicle. This cancer is diagnosed by physical examination, ultrasound examination, and blood tests for tumor markers (alpha-fetoprotein [AFP] and human chorionic gonadotropin [hCG]). Classification by histological types of tumors as well as clinical staging determines the treatment. Histological classification is divided into two major divisions: (1) seminoma and (2) nonseminomatous germ tumors, which include embryonal, teratoma, choriocarcinoma, and mixed tumors. The most common clinical staging system categorizes testicular cancer as stage I, a lesion confined to the testes; stage II, involving regional lymph node spread in the abdomen; and stage III, spread beyond the retroperitoneal lymph nodes. Treatment includes surgery, radiation, chemotherapy, and/or high-dose chemotherapy with stem-cell transplantation for rare conditions.

Reflecting the improvement and refinement of combination chemotherapy, survival in testicular cancer has dramatically improved, with a cure rate of more than 95% according to the American Cancer Society. Because regular testicular self-examinations have not been studied enough to show they reduce the death rate from this cancer, the ACS does not have a recommendation on regular testicular self-examinations for all men. However, some doctors recommend that all men examine their testicles monthly after puberty. Each man has to decide for himself whether or not to examine his testicles monthly.

NDx Health-Seeking Behaviors: Technique for Monthly Testicular Self-Examination

Common Related Factor
Lack of knowledge about regular testicular self-examination (TSE)

Common Expected Outcome
Patient correctly performs TSE.

Defining Characteristics
Desire for increased control of health
Expresses concern about current health status

NOC Outcome
Knowledge: Health Promotion
NIC Interventions
Self-Modification Assistance; Health Education

Ongoing Assessment

Actions/Interventions	Rationales
■ Assess the patient's knowledge of TSE.	Patients learn the material most important to them. Patients recovering from unilateral testicular cancer need to be aware that they are at an increased risk for cancer in the other testicle. QSEN: Patient-centered care.
■ Assess the patient's confidence in his ability to perform TSE.	According to self-efficacy theory, positive conviction that one can perform a behavior is correlated with its performance and successful outcome.
■ Be alert to the signs of avoidance (e.g., changing the subject or becoming withdrawn).	Denial is a defense mechanism that can block learning and the assimilation of information.

■ = Independent   ▲ = Interprofessional Collaboration

Therapeutic Interventions

Actions/Interventions

- Identify known risk factors:
  - Family history of testicular cancer
  - Cryptorchid testes (undescended testicle)
  - White race
  - Cancer of one testicle
- Instruct in the warning signs of testicular cancer:
  - Lump on the testes that is small, hard, and painless
  - Pain and/or discomfort in the testes
  - Heaviness in the testes or scrotum
  - Discomfort in the lower abdomen or groin
- Instruct in the procedure for TSE:

  - Examine the testicles monthly during a shower.
  - Examine each testicle separately by gently rolling it between the thumb and fingers while holding the penis out of the way.
  - Report any lump or swelling or any changes in size, shape, or consistency of the testes to the health care provider as soon as possible.

Rationales

These nonmodifiable risk factors need to be recognized by men, especially white men 20 to 40 years of age who are at highest risk.

Malignant tumors of the testes are rare but are the most common malignancy in males 20 to 40 years of age. Being aware of the signs facilitates early diagnosis and treatment, and saves lives.

For men deciding to examine their testicles monthly, they need accurate information regarding correct technique to be a full partner in care. QSEN: Safety.
The warmth from the water relaxes the scrotal sac.
Testicular tumors tend to appear deep in the center of the testicle.

The early detection of changes facilitates treatment and can affect the cure. The testicle can get larger for many reasons other than cancer.

NANDA-I
NDx Deficient Knowledge

Common Related Factors

Insufficient information
Insufficient interest in learning
Misinformation presented by others
Insufficient knowledge of resources

Defining Characteristics

Insufficient knowledge
Inaccurate follow-through of instruction
Inappropriate behavior

Common Expected Outcome

Patient demonstrates an understanding of the risk for and causes of testicular cancer, common diagnostic procedures, and treatment options.

NOC Outcomes

Knowledge: Cancer Management; Knowledge: Disease Process; Knowledge: Treatment Regimen

NIC Interventions

Health Literacy Enhancement; Learning Facilitation; Teaching: Disease Process; Teaching: Preoperative; Teaching: Procedure/Treatment

Ongoing Assessment

Action/Intervention

- Assess the patient's knowledge of the diagnosis and treatment options.

Rationale

This topic is difficult for many men to discuss. Men may not realize how curable testicular cancer has become.

Therapeutic Interventions

Actions/Interventions	Rationales
■ Encourage questions about the diagnosis of testicular cancer and the proposed treatment regimen.	Questions facilitate open communication between the patient and health care team and allow verification of understanding of given information and the opportunity to correct misconceptions. Often patients are embarrassed about asking questions and may need permission to ask them. QSEN: Patient-centered care.
■ Provide information on diagnostic testing:	
• Review of the TSE results	Most commonly men note a lump that is painless but uncomfortable, or they may note swelling.
• Physical examination of the testes, lymph nodes, and abdomen	Testes are evaluated for lumps and swelling. Other organs are evaluated for potential metastatic disease.
• Laboratory tests: tumor markers such as alpha fetoprotein and beta-human chorionic gonadotropin, lactate dehydrogenase	These markers are used to diagnose types of cancer, determine prognosis, evaluate response to treatment, and note recurrence.
• Diagnostic tests:	
• Ultrasound examination	Ultrasound evaluation aids in determining solid versus fluid-filled masses and benign versus malignant tumors.
• Computed tomography and magnetic resonance imaging	These scans detect metastatic lesions.
• Chest x-ray film and bone scan	These studies detect metastatic lesions.
• Radical inguinal orchiectomy (removal of one or both testes)	This procedure is used both for biopsy diagnosis and for treatment. The interval between the discovery of a scrotal lump in the testes and radical orchiectomy is often less than 1 week.
■ Provide preoperative teaching about orchiectomy.	This is a relatively uncomplicated procedure to remove the testicle. The procedure may be a same-day surgery or may require an overnight hospital stay.
■ Provide preoperative teaching about retroperitoneal lymph node dissection (RPLND).	Lymph node dissection is used for tumor staging. Treatment modalities depend on this staging process. RPLND is more commonly seen with embryonic cancer because of its high rate of metastasis. Laparoscopic surgery may be an option for some.
■ Instruct in the potential for infertility and the option for semen storage.	The removal of only one testicle does not interfere with a normal erection and the ability to produce sperm. However, more complete surgery (i.e., RPLND) and follow-up treatments may render the patient infertile. The patient may feel secure knowing there is the potential for semen storage and future access to his sperm. QSEN: Patient-centered care.
■ Explain the need to consult with both an oncologist and radiologist regarding chemotherapy or radiation therapy.	Both radiation and chemotherapy are generally coordinated by the medical oncologist. The nurse serves as the advocate by offering support, providing information, and coordinating follow-up appointments with the urologist. QSEN: Teamwork and collaboration; Evidence-based practice.
■ Provide information on follow-up therapy:	Men must realize that testicular cancer is not a death sentence. Many modalities are available to treat advanced disease. Providing information about follow-up therapy allows the patient to be a full partner in making decisions. QSEN: Patient-centered care.
• Chemotherapy	Chemotherapy is indicated for nonseminomatous tumors or for metastatic disease. Many effective therapies are available, including cisplatin, ifosfamide, etoposide, vinblastine, paclitaxel, and bleomycin.

■ = Independent   ▲ = Interprofessional Collaboration

Actions/Interventions

- Radiation therapy

- High-dose chemotherapy with stem cell transplantation

■ Provide a referral to the National Cancer Institute, the American Cancer Society, or the Lance Armstrong Foundation.

Rationales

Radiation beam therapy is indicated for patients with pure seminoma, because this tumor is radiosensitive. It is used for cancer that has spread to other organs.

Stem cell transplantation is used to treat cancer that has come back after prior chemotherapy treatment. It is a complex treatment that can have life-threatening effects that are due to the high doses of chemotherapy that are used.

Patients may be unaware of the services available for questions or problem-solving. Referral provides the patient and family with additional helpful resources, including support groups.

NANDA-I NDx Ineffective Sexuality Pattern

Common Related Factors

Lack of knowledge about alternative responses to change in sexual response
Recent orchiectomy
Infertility

Common Expected Outcome

Patient or couple verbalizes satisfaction with the way they express physical intimacy.

Defining Characteristics

Alteration in sexual activity
Difficulty with sexual activity

NOC Outcomes

Sexual Identity; Self-Esteem

NIC Interventions

Sexual Counseling: Anticipatory Guidance; Teaching: Sexuality

---

Ongoing Assessment

Actions/Interventions

■ Assess the type of surgical and/or medical treatment received.

■ Explore current and past sexual patterns, practices, and the degree of satisfaction.

■ Assess the patient's or couple's prior plans for conceiving children.

Rationales

This information guides instruction. Unilateral orchiectomy does not interfere with ejaculation and fertility, though patients with testicular cancer often have reduced sperm counts independent of treatment. Also, prior medical or psychological conditions or more advanced cancer treatment may affect sexual performance.

This information aids in developing a realistic approach to care planning. It is important for the nurse to create an environment in which the patient and/or couple feel safe and comfortable in discussing their feelings. QSEN: Patient-centered care.

The inability to conceive after surgery or treatment (unless sperm was banked) can affect the patient or couple in many ways, threatening their self-esteem, gender roles, and interactions. QSEN: Patient-centered care.

Therapeutic Interventions

Actions/Interventions	Rationales
■ Explore the patient's awareness of and comfort with a range of sexual expression and activities (not just sexual intercourse).	Patients and couples may have limited knowledge of the ways to express their sexuality. The patient may be unaware of potential options.
■ Discuss the effect of an orchiectomy on future fertility.	Removal of only one testicle does not interfere with ejaculation and fertility. Removal of lymph nodes (retroperitoneal lymph node dissection) can cause infertility. Removal of both testes does cause infertility. Cancer treatments can also affect sexual function. It is important to provide accurate information to relieve unnecessary fears.
▲ Refer to a reproductive specialist about sperm banking.	If fathering a child is an important role for the patient, and sperm banking is not an option, discuss other options such as donor insemination and adoption. QSEN: Teamwork and collaboration.
■ Encourage a discussion of feelings regarding alternative methods for reproduction.	Removing one testicle does not affect fertility or sexual function. Newer "nerve-sparing" surgical procedures are improving fertility rates.
■ Refer to support groups.	Support and self-help groups are unique sources of information and empathy. With the high cure rate among patients with advanced disease, a growing number of survivors are serving as role models and political advocates.

 NANDA-I NDx

Disturbed Body Image

Common Related Factors
Orchiectomy
Permanent alterations in structure or function

Defining Characteristics
Preoccupation with change
Avoids looking at, touching, or caring for scrotal sac
Alteration in social involvement (withdrawal or isolation)
Alteration in structure or function
Negative feelings about body

Common Expected Outcome
Patient demonstrates enhanced body image as evidenced by the ability to look at, care for, and talk about the altered appearance of the scrotal sac.

NOC Outcomes
Body Image; Self-Esteem

NIC Interventions
Body Image Enhancement; Grief Work Facilitation; Coping Enhancement

---

Ongoing Assessment

Actions/Interventions	Rationales
■ Assess and validate the patient's feelings about changes in appearance.	The extent of the response is related more to the value or importance the patient places on the body part than to the actual value or importance.
■ Assess the perceived impact on social behavior or personal relationships.	Young adult men may be particularly affected by changes in the structure or function of their bodies at a time when they are developing social and intimate relationships. QSEN: Patient-centered care.

■ = Independent   ▲ = Interprofessional Collaboration

Actions/Interventions

- Assess the patient's previous coping strategies.

- Explore options of testicular implant or prosthesis

Rationales

This helps the patient identify ways of coping that were successful in the past, although prior coping skills may not be adequate at this time. QSEN: Patient-centered care.

Testicular implants are pouches that are placed in the scrotum. They are made of solid or gel silicone and have a silicone covering. Some types are coated with polyurethane foam. Very few have Food and Drug Administration (FDA) approval. They can be considered for cosmetic reasons, but they do not make sperm or male hormones. They are associated with risks.

Therapeutic Interventions

Actions/Interventions

- Acknowledge the normalcy of the emotional response to the actual or perceived change in body structure and function.
- Teach the patient self-care activities related to body image.
- Reinforce any attempts to care for the scrotum.

- Provide information about institutional, Internet-based, political, and community resources for coping with testicular cancer.

Rationales

Acknowledging the patient's emotional response enables the patient to move through the grieving process.

These enable adaptation to the changes in body image.

Positive reinforcement allows the patient to feel good about accomplishments and gain confidence.

Social services, support groups, and community agencies can help the patient cope with this illness and treatments. As more men are being cured of this cancer, there is a growing body of "survivors" serving as role models and advocates, for example, the Lance Armstrong Foundation.

Related Care Plans

Cancer chemotherapy, Chapter 10
Cancer radiation therapy, Chapter 10
Hematopoietic stem cell transplantation, Chapter 10

WOMEN'S HEALTH CARE PLANS

Breast Cancer/Surgical Management With Breast Reconstruction Option

Breast cancer is the most commonly occurring cancer in American women (except skin cancer). It is the second leading cause of cancer death in women; lung cancer remains the most fatal of all cancers for both men and women. A woman has a 1-in-8 lifetime risk for developing this highly treatable disease. Despite its common occurrence, most women with breast cancer will not succumb to the disease; the 10-year survival rate is approximately 90%, with about 2.5 million breast cancer survivors in the United States. Complete sequencing of the human genome has led to the identification of many genes associated with the development of breast cancer and ovarian cancer. Women who carry a mutation in the *BRCA1* or *BRCA2* gene (one of the most studied genes) are known to be at increased risk for the development of breast cancer, and these cancers often develop at a much younger age than usual (age 45 or younger). The lifetime breast cancer risk for women with hereditary cancer (defined as having an inherited mutation in the *BRCA1* or *BRCA2* gene) is on average 55% to 65%. Hereditary breast cancer, however, accounts for only 5% to 10% of all breast cancer cases. The remainder of all breast cancers do not have an identified hereditary component. In other words, most women who get breast cancer have a noninherited form. In these women the incidence of the disease increases with age, with most occurring in women over 50 years of age.

Other risk factors associated with an increased risk for breast cancer include dense breast tissue, exposure to radiation (e.g., women who have received chest irradiation as prior treatment for other malignancies such as Hodgkin's lymphoma), and the period of time that the body makes estrogen. The earlier a woman begins to menstruate and the later she has her first pregnancy, or after prolonged hormone replacement therapy, the higher is her risk for breast cancer. The later menopause occurs in a woman, the higher her postmenopausal risk for breast cancer. Lifestyle risk factors such as lack of physical activity, poor diet, drinking alcohol, and being overweight/obese are also associated with an increased risk. With the use of breast self-examination and screening mammography, most breast cancer is successfully diagnosed at an early stage. Treatment recommendations are made according to the disease stage and may include surgery, radiation, chemotherapy, or a combination of these therapies. Prognosis is related to the stage and type of tumor. Adjuvant chemohormonal therapy has decreased recurrence and has improved survival rates in most subgroups of patients. Even though the treatment modalities have lengthened the survival time for metastatic breast cancer, stage IV or metastatic disease is not curable.

Surgical management of breast cancer includes two major approaches: (1) breast conservation therapy, often referred to as a lumpectomy, and (2) removal of the entire breast, which is called a modified radical or radical mastectomy. Both of these surgical approaches may include examination of the axillary lymph nodes for evidence of micrometastatic disease, usually through sentinel lymph node biopsy. The presence or absence of disease in the lymph nodes determines prognosis (and subsequent treatment) and is referred to as *nodal status.* Women with node-negative disease generally have a better prognosis than women with node-positive disease. Women undergoing mastectomy have several options for breast reconstruction, including immediate or delayed reconstruction. The timing depends on several factors, including cancer treatment protocol, gene + mutation status, other medical problems, and the woman's preference. Breast-conserving therapy (lumpectomy) with adjuvant chemotherapy, radiation therapy, or both is considered a treatment that is medically equivalent to mastectomy.

Specialized breast cancer treatment centers are available, providing an interprofessional treatment approach (e.g., medical and surgical oncologists, gynecologists, radiation oncologists, clinical nurse specialists, nurses, social workers, plastic surgeons, and genetic counselors). This care plan addresses the surgical management of breast cancer. Follow-up care and adjunct treatment would be performed in the ambulatory care setting.

NANDA-I NDx **Deficient Knowledge: Preoperative**

Common Related Factors
Insufficient information
Insufficient interest in learning
Misinformation presented by others
Insufficient knowledge of resources
Emotional state affecting learning

Defining Characteristics
Insufficient knowledge
Inaccurate follow-through of instruction
Inappropriate behavior

Common Expected Outcome
Patient verbalizes understanding of breast cancer, its diagnosis, treatment options, and prognosis.

NOC Outcomes
Knowledge: Cancer Management; Knowledge: Disease Process; Knowledge: Treatment Regimen

NIC Interventions
Health Literacy Enhancement; Learning Facilitation; Teaching: Disease Process; Teaching: Procedure/Treatment

---

■ = Independent   ▲ = Interprofessional Collaboration

Ongoing Assessment

Actions/Interventions	Rationales
■ Assess the patient's understanding of diagnostic testing.	A thorough understanding of indications for testing is necessary for informed consent to be given.
■ Assess the patient's understanding of the relationship between the disease stage and its prognosis and treatment.	Tumor size, the spread to lymph nodes, and the metastasis to distant organs are staged from 0 to IV. The lower the number, the less the cancer has spread. Tumor staging classification guides the optimal treatment plan.
■ Assess the patient's understanding of the treatment modalities: • Surgery (breast conserving/mastectomy) • Radiation (external beam/brachytherapy) • Chemotherapy • Hormonal therapy • Clinical trials	Most women want a collaborative relationship in disease management and require information about treatment rationales. They may have a preference for a specific treatment plan, but their decision-making capacity may be challenged because of the stress from the disease. QSEN: Patient-centered care; Evidence-based practice.

Therapeutic Interventions

Actions/Interventions	Rationales
■ Explain the rationale for diagnostic procedures: • Clinical examination of the breast	A lesion (lump) usually occurs in the upper outer quadrant of the breast. It is typically hard, irregularly shaped, nonmobile, and poorly delineated.
• Mammography/magnetic resonance imaging (MRI) for dense breasts	Mammography is used to locate the position and extent of a known tumor and to screen for the presence of other abnormalities not detected by clinical examination. Newer techniques such as digital mammograms and computer-aided detection and diagnosis have helped identify suspicious changes on mammograms.
• Breast ultrasound examination	The ultrasound examination can determine whether the lesion is solid or cystic (fluid-filled). Lesions larger than 1 cm can be evaluated.
• Breast biopsy	Biopsy is performed via fine-needle aspiration, needle core biopsy, excisional biopsy or lumpectomy, or needle localization for microscopic examination to confirm a benign or malignant tissue diagnosis.
• Sentinel lymph node biopsy	The presence or absence of disease in the lymph nodes determines the prognosis (and subsequent treatment). Women with node-negative disease generally have a better prognosis.
• Tumor tissue testing (hormone receptor assays, DNA, and protein markers with diagnostic and prognostic value)	Estrogen and progesterone are female hormones affecting breast and other cancer tissues. The level of hormone receptors present in the tumor indicates the tumor's dependence on these hormones. Tumors are classified as estrogen receptor (ER) or progesterone receptor (PR) positive or negative according to the amount of receptor protein present. This classification suggests tumor growth and treatment options. Tumors with positive receptors (ER/PR+, more prevalent in postmenopausal women) are associated with a better prognosis and longer survival.

Actions/Interventions

- Genetic markers (e.g., *HER2/neu*)

- Complete physical examination
- Liver function tests and scans
- Bone scan
- Computed tomography (CT) scan, MRI, positron emission tomography (PET) scan
- Explain the rationale for the suggested treatment based on the site, type, and stage of the tumor:
  - The tumor, node, metastasis (TNM) classification system

  - Clinical stages:
    - *Stage 0:* Treated by lumpectomy with radiation or mastectomy
    - *Stages I and II:* Treated with lumpectomy or mastectomy, with sentinel lymph node biopsy. The use of adjuvant radiation, chemotherapy, or hormonal or biological therapy depends on prognostic indicators (e.g., tumor size, nodal status, hormone receptor status, age, menopausal status).
    - *Stages III and IV:* Mastectomy and systemic chemotherapy; other adjuvant therapies (radiation, hormonal, or biological therapy) depend on prognostic indicators, as listed previously.
  - Chemoprevention

  - Prophylactic mastectomy

- Explain additional treatment approaches:
  - Hormonal therapy

  - Biological agent (trastuzumab [Herceptin])

  - Angiogenesis inhibitors (bevacizumab)

Rationales

This test of the biopsy sample aids in determining the prognosis and monitoring the course of the disease. The *HER2/neu* gene is associated with breast cancer; an overexpression gives the patient a poorer prognosis. Drugs such as Herceptin have significantly impacted survival for *HER2/neu*-positive patients. The best prognosis is ER/PR-positive, *HER2/neu*-negative; the worst prognosis is ER/PR-negative, *HER2/neu*-negative (triple negative!).

It is important to screen for signs of cancer in other locations.

These tests aid in identifying possible liver metastasis.

A bone scan is used in ruling out bone metastasis.

These scans are used in evaluating for tumors and distant sites of metastasis.

This system is used to stage breast cancer according to the extent of the primary tumor (T), regional lymph node metastasis (N), and distant metastasis (M).

The clinical stages range from 0 to IV. Stage 0 implies in situ (localized) cancer; stage IV implies extensive metastasis. Sentinel lymph node biopsy has replaced axillary lymph node dissection as the first-line biopsy procedure for most women.

This is the prophylactic use of antiestrogen agents (e.g., tamoxifen) in women at high risk for the development of breast cancer.

This preventive surgery consists of a total mastectomy with immediate breast reconstruction in high-risk women.

ER/PR-positive tumors respond to hormonal treatment with antiestrogens. Several antiestrogen therapies are available depending on the menopausal status of the patient, including tamoxifen and anastrozole.

Trastuzumab (Herceptin) is a monoclonal antibody that targets the *HER2/neu* protein expressed on the surface of breast cells. Approximately 20% of all women with breast cancer overexpress this protein, which leads to unregulated cell growth. The use of Herceptin can slow the growth of cancer cells.

Monoclonal antibody drugs target growth factors that normally optimize enhanced blood vessel development. When these drugs stop this growth, the tumors cannot grow.

Actions/Interventions

■ Explain the choices for breast reconstruction:
  • Timing:
    • Immediate—can be the preferred option because it avoids a second surgery and reduces the trauma of a mastectomy. A permanent implant procedure is most commonly used.
    • Delayed—often advised if immediate cancer therapies are to be started, thus avoiding the delay of incisional healing after reconstruction.
  • Procedures:
    • Permanent implant—uses a tissue expander (balloon inserted below the pectoral muscle to gradually stretch the skin with weekly saline injection before inserting the permanent implant). Indicated for smaller-breasted women, because it does not result in the typical "sag" of the natural breast.
    • Skin flap using the patient's own tissue—an abdominal or back muscle or other flap is rotated to the surgical site to create a mound to simulate a breast. It results in a more natural breast shape and feel but requires a more extensive surgical procedure.
    • Construction of the nipple (areola). This is a secondary procedure to design a projecting nipple. Nipple tattooing is also an option to help with color and appearance.

Rationales

Women vary in their response to mastectomy. Breast reconstruction is performed to provide symmetry to the breasts. It does not interfere with cancer treatments or increase the risk for future cancer. Some women may prefer to use external padding to accomplish this. More recently breast reconstruction has gained in popularity because of improved plastic surgery techniques. It is considered reconstructive, not cosmetic surgery. Providing information allows the patient to be a full partner in making decisions, and achieving optimal outcomes. QSEN: Patient-centered care.

NANDA-I
NDx **Acute Pain**

Common Related Factors

Contraction of tissue resulting from surgery and healing process
Intraoperative arm position
Possible injury to brachial plexus
Lymphedema
Infection and phlebitis

Defining Characteristics

Self-report of pain using a standardized pain scale
Facial expression of pain
Change in physiological parameters (e.g., HR, BP, respirations)

Common Expected Outcomes

Patient reports satisfactory pain control at a decreased intensity using a standardized pain scale.
Patient appears comfortable.
Patient performs range-of-motion (ROM) exercises with minimal discomfort.

NOC Outcomes

Circulation Status; Pain Level; Medication Response

NIC Interventions

Circulatory Precautions; Pain Management; Positioning

Ongoing Assessment

Actions/Interventions	Rationales
■ Note the patient's subjective reports of pain and discomfort.	Pain assessment is the basis for an individualized approach to pain management. QSEN: Patient-centered care.
■ Assess for the probable cause of pain.	Different etiological factors respond better to different therapies.
■ Assess the neurovascular status of the affected arm immediately after surgery and at regular intervals.	This assessment detects a possible brachial plexus injury. QSEN: Safety.
■ Measure biceps 2 inches above the elbow of the affected arm immediately after surgery and at every shift.	An increase in arm circumference may indicate impaired lymphatic drainage. QSEN: Safety.
■ Evaluate the range of motion of the affected arm.	Patient may refrain from certain movements to reduce pain.
■ Assess for signs of infection or phlebitis in the affected arm (e.g., pain, redness, warmth, and swelling).	Early identification of complications allows for early intervention. QSEN: Safety.

Therapeutic Interventions

Actions/Interventions	Rationales
■ Keep the arm elevated on two pillows while the patient is in bed (mastectomy).	This maneuver decreases edema and promotes lymph drainage.
■ Avoid constriction of the affected arm.	This maneuver prevents circulatory impairment and subsequent discomfort.
■ Protect the affected arm from injury. Ensure that no procedures are performed on the affected arm (e.g., BP measurement, blood drawing, IV injections). Post a notice at the bedside.	Mastectomy procedures remove lymph nodes and lymphatic vessels that drain the arm on the involved side of the body, increasing the risk for injury and infection in the involved arm. QSEN: Safety.

■ Instruct regarding postoperative exercises:
  • Straight arm extension and abduction
  • Straight elbow raises
  • Wall climbing
  • Repeated 5 to 10 times per hour as tolerated
	These exercises increase range of motion progressively in the affected arm and relieve discomfort from possible tissue contraction.

■ Administer analgesics for pain as required (e.g., before ROM exercises are performed) and determine their effectiveness.	Patients have a right to effective pain relief. Pain medications are absorbed and metabolized differently by patients, so their effectiveness must be evaluated individually by the patient. QSEN: Patient-centered care.

NANDA-I NDx **Risk for Situational Low Self-Esteem/ Disturbed Body Image**

Common Risk Factors

Permanent alterations in structure and/or function
  • Excision of breast and adjacent tissue
  • Beginning scar tissue
  • Asymmetrical breasts caused by implant or prosthesis fit or by lumpectomy
Diagnosis of cancer
History of sexual problems

■ = Independent   ▲ = Interprofessional Collaboration

Common Expected Outcome

Patient demonstrates enhanced body image, as evidenced by use of positive coping strategies, use of available resources, and absence of or decreased number of self-deprecating remarks.

NOC Outcomes

Body Image; Self-Esteem; Social Support

NIC Interventions

Body Image Enhancement; Self-Esteem Enhancement; Support System Enhancement

Ongoing Assessment

Actions/Interventions	Rationales
■ Assess and validate the patient's feelings about changes in appearance.	The extent of the response is related more to the value or importance the patient places on the breast than the actual value.
■ Assess the perceived impact on social behavior or personal relationships.	Younger women may be particularly affected by changes in their body, although elderly women may likewise be strongly affected.
■ Assess for changes in the patient's self-perceptions after (e.g., preoccupation with the altered body part, concerns about the loss of femininity and sexual identity, and negative feelings about body image).	The psychological impact of surgery may be devastating to self-esteem. Cultural and societal values about a woman's breast will influence the patient's response to surgery. QSEN: Patient-centered care.
■ Assess for any previous problems with self-esteem, body image, or sexual relations and how they were resolved.	Patients with a history of coping difficulties may need additional resources. Likewise, previously successful coping skills may be inadequate in the present situation. QSEN: Patient-centered care.

Therapeutic Interventions

Actions/Interventions	Rationales
■ Encourage the patient to look at the wound and help care for it.	Looking at the wound is often the first indication that the patient is ready to participate in self-care.
■ Encourage the patient to verbalize feelings about the effects of surgery on the ability to function as a woman and a sexual partner.	It is worthwhile to encourage women to separate feelings about changes in body structures or function from feelings about self-worth.
■ Assist the patient with wearing a prosthetic insert at discharge.	Wearing a prosthesis can provide a feeling of normalcy.
■ Provide information on shops specializing in prostheses; arrange an in-hospital consultation if possible.	Community resources provide support for the patient who is adjusting to changes in her body.
■ Encourage the family (especially significant others) to provide positive input (i.e., feelings of being loved and needed).	Limited or impaired social supports cause adjustment difficulties.
■ Refer the patient to community support resources and provide information on resources available from the American Cancer Society.	Interactions with women who have successfully dealt with breast surgery can help with adjusting to the changed body.
■ Provide the patient with information about reconstructive options.	The increased effectiveness of reconstructive surgical techniques can restore body contours in women who do not want to wear external prostheses. Some women may opt to have this procedure done during initial mastectomy surgery. Although plastic surgery procedures have made great advances, the patient must understand that the artificial breast will not be exactly like the other breast.

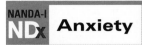

Anxiety

Common Related Factors

Major change (diagnosis of cancer, uncertain prognosis, treatments and procedures)
Threat of death
Situational crisis

Defining Characteristics

Restlessness
Expressed concern about health
Self-focused
Preoccupation
Alteration in concentration

Common Expected Outcomes

Patient describes a reduction in the level of anxiety expressed.
Patient uses effective coping mechanisms.

NOC Outcomes

Anxiety Self-Control; Social Support; Coping

NIC Interventions

Anxiety Reduction; Support System Enhancement

Ongoing Assessment

Actions/Interventions	Rationales
■ Assess the patient for signs of anxiety (e.g., withdrawal, crying, restlessness, or an inability to focus).	The threats accompanying a diagnosis of cancer can cause anxiety about health and continued productivity.
■ Assess any previous successful coping strategies and support network.	These strategies may be useful in dealing with the current crisis. QSEN: Patient-centered care.

Therapeutic Interventions

Actions/Interventions	Rationales
■ Encourage verbalizations about feelings of grief, anger, fear, and anxiety.	The verbalization of actual or perceived threats can help reduce anxiety. The initial focus may be on the threat of dying rather than on reactions to the mastectomy.
■ Reassure the patient that these feelings are normal.	Stages of fear and grief over the change or loss of a body part are normal.
■ Provide accurate information about the patient's future with breast cancer.	Most women have experience with women who have died of breast cancer. Misinformation should be corrected, and new treatment options and the prognosis explained.
■ Assist in the use of previously successful coping measures.	This helps the patient focus on anxiety as a real and natural part of life that has been and can continue to be dealt with successfully. Modification may be necessary for this specific problem. QSEN: Patient-centered care.
▲ Work collaboratively with other health care providers as indicated (social worker, psychologist, chaplain).	An interprofessional approach to patient care provides the patient with diverse support and resources. QSEN: Teamwork and collaboration.
■ Support a realistic assessment; avoid false reassurances.	This approach assists the patient in dealing with the current crisis and in gaining control over the situation. False reassurances are never helpful to the patient and only serve to relieve the discomfort of the care provider. QSEN: Patient-centered care.
▲ Administer antianxiety medications as ordered and indicated.	The short-term use of medications can relieve unpleasant feelings.

■ = Independent   ▲ = Interprofessional Collaboration

Men's and Women's Health Care Plans

NANDA-I

NDx Deficient Knowledge: Postoperative

Common Related Factors

Insufficient information
Insufficient interest in learning
Misinformation presented by others
Insufficient knowledge of resources

Common Expected Outcome

Patient verbalizes understanding of proper wound care and need for follow-up care.

Defining Characteristics

Insufficient knowledge
Inaccurate follow-through of instruction
Inappropriate behavior

NOC Outcomes

Knowledge: Cancer Management; Knowledge: Disease Process; Knowledge: Treatment Regimen

NIC Interventions

Health Literacy Enhancement; Learning Facilitation; Teaching: Disease Process; Teaching: Procedure/Treatment; Wound Care

---

Ongoing Assessment

Action/Intervention	Rationale
■ Assess the patient's knowledge level of home care and required health maintenance.	The patient may be unaware of important self-care procedures. For successful recovery the patient must know how to provide home care, how to identify problems, and what to do should problems arise. QSEN: Safety.

Therapeutic Interventions

Actions/Interventions	Rationales
■ Educate about wound care and arm care (if applicable):	This information enables the patient to assume responsibility for self-care recovery at home. QSEN: Safety.
• Check the wound drain (if in place) for the color of drainage, amount of output, and suction pressure. Empty the drainage device as needed and compress and recap it.	Wound drainage will normally decrease in volume and can be removed by the surgeon when it is less than 30 mL in 24 hours. The color will change from red and/or pink to clear. Fluid accumulation can be a source of infection. Wound drainage malfunction requires immediate intervention.
• Expect that the arm will be stiff and uncomfortable.	Exercise decreases stiffness, but numbness may remain for a prolonged time if the nodes were dissected.
• Continue range-of-motion exercises for at least 1 month.	Exercise eases tension in the arm and shoulder, maintains muscle tone, and improves lymph and blood circulation on the affected side.
• Notify the health care provider regarding fever, swelling, wound drainage, or injury.	Prompt assessment facilitates early intervention.
• Protect the arm from injury and infection.	The operative arm will remain vulnerable to lymphedema after axillary lymph node dissection.
• Use an electric razor when shaving, gloves when gardening or doing dishes, and mitts when handling hot dishes.	The patient needs to learn to protect the operative arm from any type of injury for the rest of her life.

Actions/Interventions	Rationales
• Avoid blood draws, IV lines, and injections or BP measurement in the operative arm during subsequent medical treatments.	These measures reduce the risk for injury to the blood and lymphatic vessels in the operative arm.
• Carry heavy packages or handbags with the opposite arm.	This measure reduces the risk for muscle and joint strain in the operative arm.
• Massage the incision site gently with cocoa butter and vitamin E cream.	These products promote healing and skin softness and minimize scar formation.
• Wear a temporary prosthesis or brassiere at least occasionally.	These help with adjustment to the recent loss of the breast.
■ Instruct about activity guidelines:	Each patient will progress at her own rate based on the extent of surgical intervention and the related treatment regimen.
• Resume all routine activities (e.g., driving) as tolerated.	
• Resume sexual activity as tolerated.	
■ Instruct about required follow-up care:	Providing information about follow-up care options allows the patient to be a full partner in making decisions and reducing potential risks. QSEN: Safety; Patient-centered care.
• Close surveillance of breast	Women may hesitate to examine their breasts because of difficulty viewing or touching the surgical site on the chest or fear of finding another lump.
• Annual mammogram and MRI screening (or more often)	There is an increased risk for cancer in the opposite breast. Mammography can identify breast tumors before they are palpable.
• Reconstructive surgery (if desired)	Reconstructive surgery does not influence survival rates but may improve the quality of life. It may be contraindicated in locally advanced, progressively metastatic, or inflammatory cancer.
• Importance of large-breasted women being fitted with a weighted prosthesis as soon as possible	This measure provides balance for proper posture.
■ Instruct about possible family needs. According to the American Cancer Society,	Risk is increased in daughters or sisters of women with breast cancer and is further increased in daughters or sisters of women with premenopausal bilateral breast cancer or if more than one relative has cancer. All women should be familiar with how their breasts normally look and feel and report any changes immediately to their health care provider. QSEN: Evidence-based practice.
• Women with a first-degree relative with a *BRCA1* or *BRCA2* gene mutation should consider genetic testing for themselves and get an annual MRI and mammogram.	
• Women with a lifetime risk of breast cancer of about 20% to 25% or greater (based on a tool based on family history) should get an annual MRI and mammogram.	
■ Instruct in follow-up consultations with medical and radiation specialists if required because of nodal status.	Ongoing evaluation is necessary for the development of lymphedema, metastasis, and recurrence of cancer. QSEN: Teamwork and collaboration.
■ Provide appropriate educational materials from the American Cancer Society, the National Cancer Institute, the Susan G. Komen Breast Cancer Foundation, or YWCA's ENCORE program.	Information from specialty organizations can enhance learning and compliance. Although family and friends can be great allies, often a formal support group or communication with a cancer survivor is most helpful.

Related Care Plans

Ineffective peripheral tissue perfusion, Chapter 2
Ineffective sexuality pattern, Chapter 2
Cancer chemotherapy, Chapter 10
Cancer radiation therapy, Chapter 10

■ = Independent   ▲ = Interprofessional Collaboration

Cervical Cancer

Cancer of the cervix is one of the most common cancers affecting women's reproductive organs, occurring between 35 and 55 years of age. It is more commonly seen in the Hispanic and African-American populations. Although the number of cases and deaths have significantly declined during the past 20 years, it remains a serious health risk. The human papillomavirus (HPV) infection is the major risk factor for cervical cancer, with at least 95% of the cases reported to be related to sexual exposure to HPV. The CDC recommends that the three-dose HPV vaccine (i.e., Gardasil) be given to all children who are 11 to 12 years old (before they engage in any type of sexual activity and are exposed to HPV). Young women can get HPV vaccine through age 26 and young men through age 21. Several additional factors increase one's risk for cervical cancer, including lack of regular Papanicolaou (Pap) smear screening, many sexual partners, early sexual activity, history of sexually transmitted infections, long-term use of birth control pills, having many children, weakened immune systems, and smoking habit.

The death rate from cervical cancer has significantly dropped as a result of Pap tests. When diagnosed at an early, preinvasive stage, the survival rate is nearly 100%. According to the American Cancer Society, invasive cancer that is diagnosed while still confined to the cervix has a 5-year survival rate of around 91%. Treatment options depend on the tumor stage at diagnosis. Treatment may consist of conization, loop electrosurgical excision procedure, cryosurgery, cauterization, laser surgery, hysterectomy, radiation, chemotherapy, or biological therapy.

NANDA-I NDx Deficient Knowledge

Common Related Factors
Insufficient information
Insufficient interest in learning
Misinformation presented by others
Insufficient knowledge of resources
Emotional state affecting learning

Defining Characteristics
Insufficient knowledge
Inaccurate follow-through of instruction
Inappropriate behavior

Common Expected Outcome
Patient verbalizes understanding of the risk factors and diagnosis and treatment procedures for cervical cancer.

NOC Outcomes
Knowledge: Cancer Management; Knowledge: Disease Process; Knowledge: Treatment Regimen

NIC Interventions
Health Literacy Enhancement; Learning Facilitation; Teaching: Disease Process; Teaching: Procedure/Treatment

Ongoing Assessment

Action/Intervention	Rationale
■ Assess the patient's understanding of cervical cancer. Identify any existing misconceptions.	Women may have misinformation about the types of female cancers and their causes, treatments, and prognoses. Previous experience with other women being treated for cancer or who have died of cancer will influence their beliefs; some of these may be negative or incorrect. QSEN: Patient-centered care.

Therapeutic Interventions

Actions/Interventions	Rationales
■ Explain that the cause of cervical cancer is unknown, although several risk factors have been identified: • Exposure to the human papillomavirus (HPV) and other sexually transmitted diseases (STDs) • Many sexual partners • Early sexual activity (before 18 years of age) • Smoking history • Weakened immune systems • Long-term use of birth control pills • Multiparity • Family history • Diet low in fruits and vegetables • Being overweight	Various strains of the sexually transmitted HPV account for 95% of diagnosed cases. The persistence of HPV infection in the body without treatment is what puts a woman at risk. STD viruses have been linked to atypical cell transformations that eventually convert to cancerous cells. However, not all women with HPV infections develop cancer. Studies have demonstrated higher incidences in women who have early and varied sexual habits. The mechanism between cigarette smoking and cervical cancer is unclear, although it is proposed that smoking affects the immune system's ability to respond to strains of viruses. Its effects increase with the number of cigarettes smoked daily and with pack-years of smoking. Women with weakened immune systems from HIV or immunosuppressant agents are also at higher risk. QSEN: Evidence-based practice.
■ Explain the signs and symptoms of cervical cancer.	Early cancer usually has no specific signs and is not identified without a screening Pap test. However, as the cancer progresses, abnormal bleeding is the major sign (e.g., from the vagina after intercourse, between periods, or after menopause). An increased watery, bloody vaginal discharge may also be noted. Pelvic pain and pain experienced during sexual intercourse are also common symptoms.
■ Discuss common diagnostic procedures: • Pelvic examination and Pap test (combined with HPV testing)	The Pap test allows for the detection of abnormal cells. It is only a screening test, not for diagnosis. Newer Pap smear collection procedures have enhanced diagnostic ability. A test for HPV is done using the sample of cells removed during the Pap test. Women should avoid douching or using spermicidal foams or creams for about 2 days before testing to avoid altering any abnormal cells.
• Colposcopy	Colposcopy uses a lighted magnifying instrument to examine the vagina and cervix for epithelial abnormalities.
• Biopsy	Biopsy may include a simple "punch" technique using forceps to pinch off a small piece of tissue. Another method is the loop electrosurgical excision procedure (LEEP), in which an electric wire loop slices off a thin, round area of tissue. These biopsies are performed under local anesthesia.
• Conization (cone biopsy)	Conization is surgery to remove a cone-shaped piece of tissue from the cervix and the cervical canal. It can be used for diagnosis as well as treatment.
■ Discuss the treatment options for precancerous and cancerous conditions.	Providing information about treatment options based on national recommendations allows the patient to be a full partner in making decisions. QSEN: Patient-centered care; Evidence-based practice.

■ = Independent   ▲ = Interprofessional Collaboration

Actions/Interventions

Precancerous:
- Conization and/or LEEP
- Cryosurgery (freezing)
- Laser surgery
- Hysterectomy

Cancer of the cervix:
- Surgery (hysterectomy)
- Radiation therapy (external, internal, intensity-modulated)
- Chemotherapy
- Targeted therapy

■ Discuss the common side effects related to treatments.

Rationales

Many factors determine the optimal treatment for precancerous lesions. These depend on the severity of the lesion (grade), whether the patient wants to have children in the future, the age of the patient, and her general health. Like conization and LEEP procedure, laser therapy can be performed as an office procedure in which energy from the light beam destroys the abnormal cells it contacts. Cryosurgery is a treatment that freezes a section of cervix to destroy abnormal cells. Hysterectomy may be indicated if abnormal cells are found inside the cervical opening and the patient is not interested in having children.

Treatment for cervical cancer often requires a radical hysterectomy, radiation therapy, or both. If the tumor is small, surgery may be sufficient treatment. Radiation is more effective for larger tumors or for tumors that have spread outside the cervical area but are confined to the pelvic area. The radiation may come from external sources or from an internal implant. Intensity-modulated radiation therapy uses a computer to make three-dimensional (3D) pictures of the size and shape of the tumor, so that thin beams of radiation of different intensities can be aimed at the tumor. This approach results in less damage to healthy tissue. Platinum-based chemotherapy with concurrent radiation is recommended for systemic treatment. Chemotherapy involves systemic treatment. Targeted therapy uses monoclonal antibodies such as bevacizumab to kill cancer cells, block their growth, or keep cells from spreading. Most women will benefit from seeking a second opinion to guide optimal therapy.

Minor surgery causes pelvic cramping, bleeding, or a watery discharge. Hysterectomy involves pain in the lower abdomen, some difficulty voiding or having bowel movements, and fatigue. If the uterus was removed, women will no longer have menstrual periods and may experience a change in their sexuality. Patients having external radiation therapy may experience local hair loss and drying and reddening of skin. Patients with internal implants must avoid intercourse. Both types of radiation can cause diarrhea and uncomfortable voiding. Chemotherapy effects vary with the agent used and the patient's response to it.

NANDA-I
NDx Risk for Ineffective Coping

Common Risk Factors

Threat of malignancy
Situational crisis
Inadequate support system
Inadequate coping methods
Lack of knowledge related to disease process

Common Expected Outcomes

Patient uses available resources and support systems.
Patient describes and initiates effective coping strategies.
Patient describes positive results from new behavior.

NOC Outcomes

Coping; Anxiety Self-Control; Decision-Making

NIC Interventions

Coping Enhancement; Decision-Making Support;
Anxiety Reduction; Emotional Support

Ongoing Assessment

Actions/Interventions	Rationales
■ Assess the patient's knowledge of the disease and its treatment.	Patients may hear the word "cancer" or even the words "precancerous tumor" and expect to die. Realistic information about the high survival rates with cervical cancer needs to be conveyed.
■ Assess for any coping mechanisms used in previous illnesses or prior personal problems.	Successful coping is influenced by previous successes. Patients with a history of maladaptive coping may need additional resources. Likewise, previously successful coping skills may be inadequate in the present situation. QSEN: Patient-centered care.
■ Evaluate the resources and support systems available to the patient at home and in the community.	With the diagnosis of a precancerous tumor, the patient may need only short-term support to get through the initial diagnosis and treatment period. For women with advanced disease requiring more radical surgery, radiation, or chemotherapy treatment, ongoing support will be required. Available support systems may change over time.

Therapeutic Interventions

Actions/Interventions	Rationales
■ Establish a working relationship with the patient through the continuation of care.	An ongoing relationship establishes trust, reduces the feeling of isolation, and may facilitate coping. The nurse is in an ideal position to guide women through this stressful period. QSEN: Patient-centered care.
■ Provide opportunities for the patient or significant other to openly express feelings, fears, and concerns. Avoid false reassurances.	The verbalization of actual or perceived threats can help reduce anxiety. Patients receiving radiation implant therapy may express a sense of social isolation while hospitalized, especially with staff who are required to limit their presence in the room and restrict visitors. False assurances are never helpful to the patient and serve only to relieve the discomfort of the care provider.
■ Assist the patient with becoming involved as a co-manager of her treatment plan.	It provides a way for the patient to gain some control over the situation. Many patients with advanced disease become quite educated about their treatment plan and its possible side effects. QSEN: Patient-centered care.
■ Encourage the patient to communicate feelings with her significant other.	Unexpressed feelings can increase stress.
■ Encourage participation in self-help groups as available.	Relationships with women with common interests and experiences can be beneficial. Women need to help spread the word that this cancer is easily treated if diagnosed early.

■ = Independent ▲ = Interprofessional Collaboration

Related Care Plans

Hysterectomy

Salpingectomy; Oophorectomy; Total Abdominal Hysterectomy; Cervical Cancer

Hysterectomy is a surgical procedure that involves the removal of the uterus with or without removal of the cervix. The surgery may also include removal of the ovaries (oophorectomy) and the fallopian tubes (salpingectomy). Indications for the surgery include endometriosis, uterine fibroids, gynecologic cancer, uterine prolapse or bleeding, and chronic pelvic pain. Although other, less-invasive treatments can be considered for most of these problems, hysterectomy might be the only option for cancer. Hysterectomy with oophorectomy results in surgically induced menopause. The woman may experience symptoms of menopause more severely than normal menopause because of the sudden loss of hormones.

Every attempt is usually undertaken to retain the reproductive function of women who are still of childbearing age; however, certain clinical situations, such as aggressive forms of cancer, may require aggressive surgery. A hysterectomy can be performed using an abdominal, vaginal, or laparoscopic approach. The surgical approach used depends on the surgeon and patient, as well as on the amount of visualization and area of manipulation required. The bulk of recovery takes place at home.

NANDA-I NDx Deficient Knowledge: Surgical Treatment

Common Related Factors

Insufficient information
Insufficient interest in learning
Misinformation presented by others
Insufficient knowledge of resources
Emotional state affecting learning

Defining Characteristics

Insufficient knowledge
Inaccurate follow-through of instruction
Inappropriate behavior

Common Expected Outcomes

Patient verbalizes understanding of the reason for hysterectomy, surgical procedures anticipated, postoperative recovery, discharge instructions, and follow-up care.
Patient actively participates in planning of care.

NOC Outcomes

Knowledge: Disease Process; Knowledge: Treatment Regimen

NIC Interventions

Health Literacy Enhancement; Learning Facilitation; Teaching: Disease Process; Teaching: Procedure/Treatment; Teaching: Prescribed Exercise

Ongoing Assessment

Actions/Interventions	Rationales

■ Assess the patient's understanding of the indications for surgery.
Indications include the following:
  • Severe endometriosis
  • Fibroids or nonmalignant tumors of the reproductive tract that are symptomatic
  • Unresponsive to medical management
  • Painful pelvic and abdominal adhesions
  • Malignant tumors, including cervical, endometrial, ovarian, or vaginal
Elective indications include the following:
  • Family history of reproductive malignancies
  • Menstrual irregularities
  • Severe dysmenorrhea or premenstrual syndrome
	A thorough understanding of the indications for the procedure is necessary for informed consent to be given. Providing information about indications for surgery allows the patient to be a full partner in making decisions. QSEN: Patient-centered care.

■ Assess the patient's and family's understanding of the immediate and long-term postsurgical recovery periods.	The postsurgical recovery period may be difficult and more prolonged than expected. For successful recovery, the patient must know how to provide home care, how to identify problems, and what to do when problems arise. QSEN: Safety.
■ Assess the patient's understanding of her ongoing gynecological needs after hysterectomy.	Patients may incorrectly assume that the need for yearly or regular gynecological care ceases after hysterectomy. Instruction depends on the cause for the surgery, whether the cervix was totally removed, and the presurgery Pap test status.

Therapeutic Interventions

Actions/Interventions	Rationales
■ Provide preoperative instruction, including a rationale for the planned surgical approach, an explanation of the procedures, activity restrictions, and the recovery process.	A variety of surgical approaches can be performed, with abdominal hysterectomy performed most frequently. Each approach has its own protocol that may vary among institutions. Patients are better able to ask questions when they have basic information about what to expect.
■ Provide discharge instructions:	Accurate, clear information provides a rationale for the treatment and follow-up care and assists the patient in assuming responsibility for care. For successful recovery, the patient must know how to provide home care, how to identify problems, and what to do when problems arise. QSEN: Patient-centered care; Safety.
• Wound care	Patients undergoing abdominal procedures will need to care for abdominal dressings. Those undergoing vaginal surgeries will have perineal dressings to care for.
• Abdominal support may be helpful.	This support prevents strain on the incision line.
• Avoid lifting heavy objects for about 6 to 8 weeks.	This reduces strain on the abdominal muscles and surgical incisions.
• Place nothing in the vagina; no penetrating intercourse is permitted for 4 to 6 weeks.	These restrictions facilitate healing.
• Showers, sponge bathing, light activity, and exercise are permitted.	Showers are preferred over tub baths to reduce the risk for infection. A gradual increase in exercise is encouraged within the limits of fatigue.

■ = Independent   ▲ = Interprofessional Collaboration

Actions/Interventions

- Notify the physician of any of the following: increased bleeding, pain, foul-smelling discharge, or symptoms of thrombophlebitis (e.g., leg pain; swelling of the calf during ambulation; swollen, red, hot area behind the calf).
- Instruct the patient about resuming home activities:
  - Plan brief periods of graduated activity.
  - Minimize or limit climbing stairs.

- Instruct about the need for removing sutures or staples at the postsurgical checkup.
- Stress the need to continue with routine gynecological examinations.

Rationales

Early assessment facilitates prompt treatment.

Fatigue is common after most surgeries and limits the ability to maintain usual household and work activities. The patient may need to consider the use of a bedside commode if living in a two-story house with one bathroom.

Understanding increases cooperation with routine follow-up procedures.

Periodic examination of the breasts and ovaries and Papanicolaou (Pap) tests are still recommended in case cervical cancer should ever recur. Patients on hormone therapy may be evaluated more often. Women do not need to continue having Pap smears if they had a hysterectomy for noncancer reasons (e.g., fibroids) as long as they have had a normal Pap test prior to the surgery. QSEN: Evidence-based practice; Safety.

NANDA-I NDx

Deficient Knowledge: Surgical Menopause

Common Related Factors

Insufficient information
Insufficient interest in learning
Misinformation presented by others
Insufficient knowledge of resources

Defining Characteristics

Insufficient knowledge
Inaccurate follow-through of instruction
Inappropriate behavior

Common Expected Outcome

Patient verbalizes knowledge of the effects of surgical menopause and the advantages and disadvantages of hormone therapy (HT).

NOC Outcome
Knowledge: Medication

NIC Interventions
Health Literacy Enhancement; Learning Facilitation; Teaching: Disease Process; Teaching: Prescribed Medication

---

Ongoing Assessment

Actions/Interventions

- Assess the patient's understanding of menopause.

- Assess the patient's knowledge about HT.

Rationales

Women who have both the uterus and ovaries removed undergo a menopause. Most women have some minimal information about the female climacteric, but few women understand the entire surgical process or the effects of surgical menopause.

Individual evaluation is required to determine the appropriateness of HT. All women must be given enough information to make an informed choice. Risks are present with and without the use of HT. After hysterectomy, progesterone is no longer required to offset the risk for uterine cancer. QSEN: Patient-centered care.

---

 evolve   **For additional care plans, go to http://evolve.elsevier.com/Gulanick/.**

Therapeutic Interventions

Actions/Interventions	Rationales
■ Describe surgical menopause.	With removal of the uterus or removal of the uterus, tubes, and even one ovary, the remaining ovary will continue to function until menopause, when follicular development ceases and the female body goes through a series of changes resulting from estrogen withdrawal. Removal of both ovaries (surgical menopause) results in a sudden, precipitous decrease in hormone levels. The changes that occur are more rapid. Hot flashes begin 1 to 2 days after surgery. Changes in skin and hair occur more rapidly, within months rather than over years.
■ Discuss the benefits and risks associated with estrogen therapy (ET).	The decision to take estrogen is based on each patient's personal profile. If surgical menopause results from the hysterectomy or oophorectomy, ET may be prescribed to relieve menopausal symptoms. Usually these symptoms are short-lived, and many women do not require therapy. Only short-term therapy may be needed if the outcome is symptom management with the lowest effective dose. However, there are significant risks also associated with this therapy. Evidence from the Women's Health Initiative (the largest, randomized controlled trial) reports that starting HT may be associated with an increased risk for cardiovascular events for some women. If HT is taken for more than 5 years, there is also an increased risk for breast cancer. QSEN: Safety; Evidence-based practice.
■ Describe the common HT regimens: • Cyclic HT versus continuous combined • Systemic versus local	HT needs to be "customized" to the patient, her goals, and any side effects experienced.
■ Describe the role of selective estrogen receptor modulators (SERMs).	SERMs (e.g., tamoxifen and raloxifene) exert tissue-specific effects. They exhibit some of estrogen's beneficial effects on lipid levels and bone metabolism but do not exhibit the adverse effects on breast tissue. Likewise, raloxifene has an adverse effect on endometrial tissue (i.e., cancer) and is the first SERM to be approved for osteoporosis prevention (although its effect is weaker than that of estrogen). The SERMs do increase the risk for thromboembolic events and do not relieve hot flashes (actually, they may intensify them). QSEN: Evidence-based practice.
■ Counsel the patient to discuss potential ET questions with her health care professional. Examples include the following: • "Is estrogen right for me?" • "How will it benefit my body?" • "What risk might I encounter?" • "What type of regimen is best for me?" • "How long should I take it?" • "What side effects can I expect?" • "Will I be compliant?"	Women need to be co-managers of their health. Only with proper information can they make an informed decision. QSEN: Patient-centered care.

■ = Independent   ▲ = Interprofessional Collaboration

Men's and Women's Health Care Plans

NDx Acute Pain

Common Related Factors
Incision(s)
Intraoperative positioning
Manipulation of intra-abdominal contents
Gas pains

Common Expected Outcomes
Patient reports satisfactory pain control at a decreased intensity using a standardized pain scale.
Patient uses pharmacological and nonpharmacological pain relief measures.
Patient is able to perform self-care activities and ambulate with progressive effectiveness.

Defining Characteristics
Self-report of pain using a standardized pain scale
Narrowed focus
Distraction behavior
Facial expression of pain
Change in physiological parameter

NOC Outcome
Pain Control
NIC Interventions
Analgesic Administration; Pain Management; Patient-Controlled Analgesia (PCA)

Ongoing Assessment

Actions/Interventions	Rationales
■ Assess the cause of pain:	Postsurgical pain may be a result of the incision and manipulation at the surgical site, carbon dioxide remaining in the abdominal cavity after laparoscopy, or other factors. Correct diagnosis of the cause of the pain guides the selection of an appropriate intervention.
• Intraoperative position	Intraoperative positioning may result in intense shoulder pain. This pain responds well to a heating pad or massage.
• Manipulation of intra-abdominal contents	Manipulation of the intra-abdominal contents required to visualize the uterus may cause internal pain related to organ and bowel manipulation in addition to the incisional pain. This may be alleviated with postoperative analgesia, positioning, and abdominal splinting.
• Extreme gas pains	These gas pains occur from intraoperative manipulation of bowel, intraoperative and postoperative medications, and residual gas in the abdomen from a laparoscopic procedure.
■ Assess the level of pain, the patient's expectations for pain relief, and the response to medications.	The Joint Commission mandates frequent, regular assessment of pain. Some patients may be content to have pain decreased; others will expect the complete elimination of pain. This affects their perceptions of the effectiveness of the treatment modality. Patients have a right to effective pain relief. QSEN: Evidence-based practice.
■ Assess the effectiveness of other pain-relief measures: • Position change • Back rub • Heat application • Relaxation and breathing modifications • Biofeedback	Chemical analgesia may not be effective in relieving pain; other methods may be needed. Some patients may be unaware of the effectiveness of nonpharmacological methods.

Therapeutic Interventions

Actions/Interventions	Rationales
▲ Administer pain medications every 3 to 4 hours as ordered. Ask the patient to rate her comfort level and what she feels is acceptable.	Patients have a right to effective pain relief. Pain medications are absorbed and metabolized differently by patients, so their effectiveness must be evaluated individually by the patient. Around-the-clock administration of analgesics on a regular schedule keeps the patient's pain level within a comfortable range. QSEN: Patient-centered care.
■ Anticipate periods of mobility, and administer an analgesic 20 to 30 minutes before.	Decreasing pain levels permits ambulation and improves healing.
■ Consider PCA via the epidural or IV routes.	Individual patients react to pain and analgesia differently. Epidural morphine reduces or eliminates incisional pain for 18 to 24 hours. This facilitates early ambulation and prevents many postsurgical complications. PCA provides a continuous basal dose of analgesia while allowing the patient to self-medicate up to a preprogrammed maximum dose or bolus.
■ Initiate comfort measures:	
• Position in a correct anatomical alignment. Support the position with pillows or wedges.	This position reduces pain and muscle tension.
• Use abdominal splinting during movement.	Splinting supports the incision and abdominal muscles, reducing discomfort.
• Apply heat or ice as needed.	Heat reduces pain through improved blood flow to the area and through the reduction of pain reflexes. Cold reduces pain, inflammation, and muscle spasticity by decreasing the release of pain-inducing chemicals and slowing the conduction of pain impulses.
• Encourage relaxation and breathing modification.	These techniques are used to bring about a state of physical and mental awareness and tranquility.

NANDA-I NDx Disturbed Body Image

Common Related Factors

Fears of loss of sexual identity or femininity
Loss of childbearing capacity
Effects of surgical menopause on ability to be sexually satisfied
Permanent alterations in function (removal of uterus)

Defining Characteristics

Negative feelings about surgically altered body
Preoccupation with change
Avoids looking at or caring for one's body part
Refusal to acknowledge change

Common Expected Outcomes

Patient verbalizes positive statements about body and self.
Patient identifies available resources to aid in coping.

NOC Outcomes

Body Image; Grief Resolution; Psychosocial Adjustment: Life Change

NIC Interventions

Body Image Enhancement; Grief Work Facilitation; Coping Enhancement; Teaching: Sexuality

■ = Independent   ▲ = Interprofessional Collaboration

Ongoing Assessment

Actions/Interventions	Rationales
■ Assess the patient's knowledge level about the loss of reproductive function.	Many people have misconceptions about reproduction. After hysterectomy, pregnancy cannot occur because the patient no longer has a uterus to house a developing embryo and fetus. If a woman has a whole or partial ovary remaining, ovulation continues. Reproductive ability may be maintained through cryopreservation of ova or embryos for later transplantation in a surrogate. This must be done before surgery.
■ Assess the patient's feelings about herself and her body.	The loss of reproductive ability may result in lowered feelings of femininity and sexuality. These feelings may be exaggerated by the physical and emotional changes accompanying surgical menopause. Body image changes are affected by age; the reason for surgery; religious, cultural, and childbearing expectations; previous childbearing discomfort; a history of dysmenorrhea; and any previous unpleasant physical or emotional experiences accompanying the menstrual cycle. QSEN: Patient-centered care.
■ Determine the patient's ability and comfort in discussing the effect of surgery on personal relationships.	It is important for the nurse to create an environment in which the couple feels safe and comfortable in discussing feelings. An open discussion of these issues with partners corrects misconceptions about potential changes in personal relationships. It also identifies specific problem areas to be addressed before and after surgery.
■ Assess the patient's understanding of the effect of hysterectomy on sexuality and sexual desire and functioning.	Physical and psychological effects of hysterectomy may alter sexual relations after the 4- to 6-week abstinence required by surgery. More permanent effects may result from hormonal changes, loss of hormones, vaginal changes, and dryness. Some women view sex as a means of reproduction, and if she can no longer reproduce, she may lose the desire to engage in sex.
■ Note the frequency of self-critical remarks.	Negative statements about the affected body part indicate a limited ability to integrate the change into the patient's self-concept.

Therapeutic Interventions

Actions/Interventions	Rationales
■ Provide accurate information about the effect of hysterectomy on the patient's reproductive ability, anatomy and physiology, surgical menopause, and cryopreservation of ova or embryos if desired.	It is important not to make assumptions about a patient's acceptance or willingness to permanently end her reproductive ability. This information enables the patient to take control of her life after surgery and elicits her cooperation in decision-making and postoperative treatments. QSEN: Patient-centered care.
■ Provide anticipatory guidance on the management of symptoms and physical changes resulting from the surgery.	This guidance helps the patient gain control over the situation. Exploration of the most current treatment options to decrease or alleviate symptoms enables the patient to select the options most acceptable to her and her lifestyle. QSEN: Patient-centered care.

Actions/Interventions

- Explore the physiological and emotional influences on sexual functioning:
  - Explain discomforts and fatigue.
  - Explain the process of sexual functioning and response.
  - Encourage support from her spouse or significant other.
  - Make appropriate referrals for treatments or counseling.

Rationales

A patient's response to hysterectomy may range from relief that pregnancy is no longer possible (leading to more enjoyable sexual activity) to sexual difficulties such as difficulty achieving orgasm, painful intercourse (dyspareunia), and conflicts regarding sexual identity. Hormone therapy and individual or family counseling may provide relief of these symptoms.

Related Care Plans

Constipation, Chapter 2
Fatigue, Chapter 2
Urinary retention, Chapter 2
Ineffective coping, Chapter 2
Menopause, Chapter 12

Menopause

Perimenopause; Hormone Therapy

Menopause is the point in a woman's life when menstruation stops, as does the ability to reproduce. It is usually confirmed when a woman does not have a menstrual period for 12 consecutive months, in the absence of any biological or physiological causes. It occurs naturally as a part of the aging process. The mean or median age of natural menopause ranges from 48 to 52 years of age. Cancer chemotherapy, cigarette smoking, and surgical trauma to the ovarian blood supply may contribute to the onset of menopause. There may also be a link between heredity and age at menopause.

The 2 to 8 years preceding menopause and 1 year after the final menses is often referred to as the perimenopause. Perimenopause begins with the onset of endocrinological, biological, and clinical changes often associated with menopause. Subtle hormonal changes often begin in a woman's 30s. During perimenopause, a woman's oocytes undergo accelerated depletion, which results in cessation of ovulation and changes in serum and hormone levels. The pituitary gland increases the secretion of follicle-stimulating hormone (FSH) to increase ovarian secretion of estrogen, a hormone that decreases during the perimenopause. FSH levels can fluctuate during perimenopause and may require stopping the use of oral contraceptives before a diagnosis of menopause can be made. Estradiol levels decrease, resulting in insufficient levels to maintain the endometrial lining. Menstrual cycles may become irregular, and the intervals between menses may become shorter. This irregularity may result in an unplanned pregnancy until amenorrhea has been present more than 1 year. Abnormal uterine bleeding may result from anovulation, uterine fibroids, abnormalities in the uterine lining, cancer, and blood-clotting problems. Pathological conditions must be ruled out before a diagnosis of menopause can be made.

Symptoms during the perimenopause include vasomotor symptoms (e.g., hot flashes or flushes, palpitations, anxiety, and sleep disturbances) and genitourinary effects (e.g., vulvovaginal atrophy and urinary tract conditions). The role of hormone therapy (HT), which encompasses both estrogen therapy (ET) and combined estrogen-progestogen therapy (EPT) in treating these symptoms, is well accepted. Evidence from the Women's Health Initiative, the largest randomized, controlled trial, reports that HT should not be taken for the primary prevention of coronary heart disease, stroke, or dementia. In fact, starting HT may be associated with an increased risk for cardiovascular events for some women. If EPT is taken for more than 5 years, there is also an increased risk for breast cancer. Finally, although HT can reduce the risk for osteoporosis fracture, other therapies should be considered given its associated risks.

■ = Independent ▲ = Interprofessional Collaboration

NANDA-I NDx Deficient Knowledge

Common Related Factors
Insufficient information
Insufficient interest in learning
Misinformation presented by others
Insufficient knowledge of resources
Decisional conflict

Defining Characteristics
Insufficient knowledge
Inaccurate follow-through of instruction
Inappropriate behavior

Common Expected Outcome
Patient verbalizes understanding of the process of menopause, its diagnosis, and its treatment options.

NOC Outcomes
Knowledge: Disease Process; Knowledge: Treatment Regimen
NIC Interventions
Health Literacy Enhancement; Learning Facilitation; Teaching: Disease Process; Teaching: Procedure/Treatment

Ongoing Assessment

Actions/Interventions

- Assess the patient's understanding of perimenopausal symptoms.
- Assess the patient's understanding of the relationship between the normal process of aging and perimenopausal symptoms.
- Assess the patient's understanding of the treatment options:
  - Hormone therapy (HT) (i.e., ET/EPT)
  - Complementary therapies

Rationales

Diagnosis is facilitated by the complete reporting of symptoms.
It may be important to emphasize that symptoms are related to "biological" aging, not emotional or attitudinal age.

Most patients want a collaborative relationship in the management of this normal biological process and require information about preferences for specific treatment options. QSEN: Patient-centered care.

Therapeutic Interventions

Actions/Interventions

- Explain the physiological process of menopause:
  - Cessation of ovulation
  - Hormonal fluctuations
  - Expected symptoms

- Explain the diagnostic tests commonly performed:
  - Blood test for hormone levels

  - Complete physical and pelvic examination

Rationales

Women should have accurate information about menopause before its onset. Negative images about menopause have been reinforced by the general public and in the popular media. Patients need to understand the physiological process of menopause, its effect on sexuality and reproduction, methods to manage symptoms, and treatment options to promote health and prevent postmenopausal problems such as osteoporosis and heart disease.

This test can determine the level of hormonal fluctuations for FSH and estrogen. The North American Menopause Society, however, does not recommend a single hormone test, because menopausal hormone levels fluctuate throughout the day, as well as day to day. Once a woman has not had a menstrual period for a year and her FSH levels are consistently >30 mIU/mL, menopause can be confirmed.
An examination rules out disease.

Actions/Interventions

■ Discuss the benefits and risks associated with HT (ET/EPT).

■ Describe the common HT regimens:
• Estrogen-progestogen therapy
  • Cyclic versus continuous versus intermittent

• Estrogen therapy
  • Systemic versus local

• Progestogen therapy

■ Describe the role of selective estrogen receptor modulators (SERMs) and newer selective serotonin reuptake inhibitor (e.g., paroxetine).

■ Counsel the patient to discuss potential HT questions with her health care professional. Examples include the following:
• "Is HT right for me?"
• "How will it benefit my body?"
• "What risk might I encounter?"
• "What type of regimen is best for me?"
• "How long should I take it?"
• "What side effects can I expect?"
• "Will I be compliant?"

■ Describe some nonpharmacological therapies important for maintaining health and reducing menopausal symptoms:
• Proper diet (low fat; increased fruits and vegetables, high fiber)
• Weight control

Rationales

The decision to take ET and/or EPT is based on each patient's personal profile. The primary indication for HT (ET/EPT) is for relief of menopausal symptoms. Only short-term therapy may be needed if the outcome is symptom management. However, significant risks are also associated with this therapy. Evidence from the Women's Health Initiative reports that starting hormone therapy may be associated with an increased risk for cardiovascular events for some women. If EPT is taken for more than 5 years, there is also an increased risk for breast cancer. QSEN: Evidence-based practice.

ET and/or EPT needs to be "customized" to the patient, her goals, and any experienced side effects. A patient with an intact uterus needs to take progestogen with estrogen to prevent uterine cancer. Monthly bleeding differs with the type of therapy. The current recommendation is the lowest effective dose for the shortest duration to provide symptom relief. QSEN: Evidence-based practice.

With systemic ET, a patch delivers estrogen directly through the skin into the blood, bypassing the liver. This helps reduce problems with blood clots and gallbladder disease. Vaginal creams and rings work locally, yet a small amount of estrogen can circulate in the body. Vaginal ET will not relieve hot flashes, and the risks associated with it are unclear. ET is generally prescribed for patients without a uterus.

This therapy may be indicated during perimenopause for symptomatic patients with high estrogen levels.

SERMs (e.g., tamoxifen and raloxifene) exert tissue-specific effects. They exhibit some of estrogen's beneficial effects on lipid levels and bone metabolism but do not exhibit the adverse effects on breast tissue. Likewise, raloxifene has an adverse effect on endometrial tissue (i.e., cancer) and is the first SERM to be approved for osteoporosis prevention (although its effect is weaker than that of estrogen). The SERMs do increase the risk for thromboembolic events and do not relieve hot flashes (actually, they may intensify them).

Women need to be co-managers of their health. Only with proper information can they make informed decisions. QSEN: Patient-centered care.

Menopause is not a medical disease. Regular positive health habits may be adequate to promote good health.

As the body's metabolism slows down and estrogen levels reduce, women are prone to gain weight gradually over the following years. Thus it is important to reduce daily caloric intake by 200 to 400 kcal and increase exercise.

■ = Independent ▲ = Interprofessional Collaboration

Actions/Interventions	Rationales
• Adequate calcium intake	Intake of 1200 to 1500 mg daily is required.
• Exercise	Weight-bearing exercise helps stimulate bone growth. Aerobic, strength training, and stretching exercises on a regular basis are all important.
• Smoking cessation	Cessation helps reduce hot flashes and improve high-density lipoprotein profile, as well as reduce risks for blood clotting.
• Alternative therapies	There have been a small number of clinical trials evaluating the effectiveness of phytoestrogens (plant estrogens) for the treatment of menopausal symptoms, primarily hot flashes. Soy-derived isoflavones have been shown to reduce hot flashes for some patients, depending on the product. Black cohosh has shown mixed results; it does not act like estrogen as once thought; it does have a good safety record. There is no conclusive evidence that red clover reduces hot flashes, though some women find it helpful. The evidence for the use of vitamin E for symptom relief suggests that it may be a reasonable option for a trial, but the dose should be kept at 400 IU or less. The use of therapies such as dong quai, evening primrose oil, and ginseng is not recommended by the North American Menopause Society.
■ Describe the other pharmacological therapies used for reducing menopausal symptoms.	Low-dose antidepressants such as venlafaxine (Effexor), paroxetine (Paxil), and fluoxetine (Prozac) are recommended for hot flashes for patients who are not candidates for HT, including breast cancer survivors. Nausea and sexual dysfunctions are side effects. Gabapentin (Neurontin) is also recommended as a treatment option for hot flashes. Finally, some antihypertensives (e.g., clonidine) have demonstrated moderate efficacy with high adverse effects for treatment of symptoms. QSEN: Evidence-based practice.

NANDA-I NDx Ineffective Coping

Common Related Factors
Maturational crisis (changing body image)
Inadequate confidence in ability to deal with situation
Inadequate resources

Defining Characteristics
Inability to meet role expectation
Alteration in sleep pattern
Inability to ask for help

Common Expected Outcomes
Patient uses available resources and support systems.
Patient describes and initiates effective coping strategies.
Patient describes positive results from new behaviors.

NOC Outcomes
Anxiety Self-Control; Coping; Social Support

NIC Interventions
Anxiety Reduction; Coping Enhancement; Decision-Making Support; Support System Enhancement

Ongoing Assessment

Actions/Interventions

■ Assess for the symptoms of ineffective coping.

■ Assess the patient's understanding of the relationship between hormone fluctuations and the normal process of perimenopause and menopause.

■ Assess for the feelings of optimism and value of self in the future.
■ Assess for the resources and support systems available.

■ Assess for impaired memory.

Rationales

As patients progress through menopause, they may experience mood swings, emotional upset, and irritability, which may be attributed only to hormonal fluctuations when other factors (e.g., insomnia and other life stresses) may be the cause. Although menopause itself does not cause depression, patients who have a history of psychological disorders (e.g., depression) are vulnerable to recurrent episodes at this time. QSEN: Patient-centered care.

Some patients may feel incapacitated by the thought of hormonal changes, buying into the "raging hormone" stereotype. Patients need to understand that this is a natural process. In some countries, women are revered as they go through this stage.

Not all patients view menopause as a loss of sexuality. Many feel excited about their future. QSEN: Patient-centered care.

Resources may include the family, other patients, the health care provider, community groups, and spiritual counseling.

Fatigue and labile hormone levels may disrupt the ability to remember small details, causing further frustration.

Therapeutic Interventions

Actions/Interventions

■ Provide opportunities for the patient to express fears and concerns.
■ Encourage the patient to identify her own coping strengths and abilities.

■ Identify community resources and support groups (especially women's groups).

Rationales

The verbalization of actual or perceived fears can help reduce anxiety and enhance coping ability.

Most women, by the time of menopause, have dealt successfully with many complex problems. During situational crises patients may be unable to recognize their strengths. Opportunities to highlight one's past coping skills can be useful. QSEN: Patient-centered care.

Most women rely on one another for both information and understanding. Use of support group networks can be a great source of strength. In addition, such groups can reduce any sense of isolation the patient may experience.

**NANDA-I
NDx**

Ineffective Sexuality Pattern

Common Related Factors

Knowledge of altered body function
Lack of knowledge about alternative responses to changes in sexual response related to menopause
Skill deficit related to health-related transitions

Common Expected Outcomes

Patient verbalizes relief of symptoms with correct treatment.
Patient or couple verbalizes satisfaction with the way they express physical intimacy.

Defining Characteristics

Alteration in sexual activity
Difficulty with sexual activity (e.g., painful intercourse)

NOC Outcomes

Sexual Functioning; Knowledge: Sexual Functioning

NIC Interventions

Sexual Counseling; Teaching: Sexuality

■ = Independent ▲ = Interprofessional Collaboration

Ongoing Assessment

Actions/Interventions	Rationales
■ Assess the patient's understanding of perimenopausal symptoms.	Understanding increases comfort with one's perimenopausal body.
■ Assess the severity of physical symptoms.	Some patients may just lose interest in sexual performance, whereas others may experience painful intercourse.
■ Assess the patient's understanding of possible causes of altered sexuality.	Fluctuating hormone levels contribute to vaginal dryness, sex drive changes, thinning of the vaginal mucosa, and alkalinity of the vaginal secretions. As a result of these changes, the patient may experience dyspareunia, perineal burning and itching, and an increase in vaginal infections. The patient may have concerns about her femininity, sexual attractiveness, and ability to have a satisfying sexual relationship.

Therapeutic Interventions

Actions/Interventions	Rationales
■ Explain the physiological changes affecting sexuality: • Dryness of the vaginal mucosa • Hormonal fluctuations causing hot flashes ■ Explain the treatments to reduce vaginal dryness.	Knowledge *normalizes* the process and reduces anxiety. As estrogen levels decline, tissues become thinner, drier, and less elastic. Vaginal water-based lubricants such as Astroglide, Silk-E, and Moist again, or moisturizers such as Replens and K-Y Long Lasting Vaginal Moisturizer may facilitate intercourse. Vaginal estrogen can be administered locally using a vaginal tablet, ring, or cream to reduce vaginal dryness. Ospenifine (Osphena) is a selective estrogen receptor modulator (SERM) that increases vaginal wall thickness to reduce pain during intercourse. Regular intercourse also promotes lubrication.
■ Assist in talking with the patient's partner about personal concerns and feelings.	Menopause is a natural process. Sexuality is not tied to intercourse. Starting out with other ways to show intimacy may be helpful.
■ Explain the need to discuss with the partner her slower arousal time and need for longer foreplay.	Longer foreplay is often satisfying to women, and it promotes lubrication. The patient should give herself appropriate time to be aroused.
■ Explore the use of complementary therapies.	Several homeopathic remedies may be considered to treat symptoms. They may include *Lachesis* for anxiety, sepia for vaginal dryness, and natrum muriaticum (nat mur) for emotional well-being. Supplementation with soy products has been studied, because soy contains high levels of phytoestrogens that bind to estrogen receptors. Positive results have been demonstrated in several studies, but additional research is necessary. Quality and standardization guidelines have not been established. QSEN: Evidence-based practice.

NANDA-I
NDx Insomnia

Common Related Factor	Defining Characteristics
Gender-related hormonal shifts	Difficulty maintaining sleep Nonrestorative sleep pattern Insufficient energy

Common Expected Outcome

Patient achieves optimal amounts of sleep, as evidenced by rested appearance, verbalization of feeling rested, and improvement in sleep pattern.

NOC Outcome
Sleep

NIC Intervention
Sleep Enhancement

Ongoing Assessment

Actions/Interventions	Rationales
■ Assess the severity of sleep deprivation.	Most adult women need 6 to 9 hours of sleep at night. Sleep deprivation is positively correlated with an increase in other symptoms. Hot flashes and night sweats can disrupt the usual sleep cycle. Lack of sleep can cause many patients to be unable to concentrate at work, further aggravating their response to menopause. QSEN: Patient-centered care.
■ Determine the frequency and severity of night sweats.	Night sweats are often a consequence of hot flashes. Patients commonly awaken with soaking sweats followed by chills.
■ Assess the additional factors contributing to sleep loss.	Environmental temperatures, stresses, caffeinated beverages, and vigorous exercise immediately before sleep can aggravate the situation.
■ Assess the routines that occur before sleep.	Sleep patterns are unique to each individual and knowledge may guide intervention.
■ Assess the methods used to alleviate symptoms and their level of effectiveness.	Information can guide future interventions.

Therapeutic Interventions

Actions/Interventions	Rationales
■ Explain the physiological processes resulting in sleep disruption.	Understanding reduces anxiety and fear and helps to normalize the experience.
■ Suggest methods for improving the environment and routines to facilitate sleep.	Avoiding alcohol and caffeine and emotional interactions before sleep enhances the environment and is conducive to satisfactory sleep patterns. Maintaining a regular sleep schedule and cooler room temperatures may improve sleep cycles.
■ Provide tips for dealing with night sweats.	Wearing cool cotton clothing to bed and changing bedclothes during the night may be helpful.
■ Discuss the role of hormone therapy (ET/EPT).	Hormone therapy successfully relieves vasomotor symptoms during menopause.

Related Care Plans

Osteoporosis, Chapter 9
Hysterectomy, Chapter 12

■ = Independent   ▲ = Interprofessional Collaboration

Ovarian Cancer

The cause of ovarian cancer remains unknown. This cancer accounts for only about 3% of all cancers in women, yet it causes more deaths than any other cancer of the female reproductive system because ovarian cancer is usually diagnosed in stage III or IV because the early stages are asymptomatic. Risk factors for ovarian cancer include older age (around age 63) in white women, inherited gene mutations (e.g., *BRCA1* and *BRCA2*), estrogen hormone replacement therapy for long periods, never being pregnant or childbirth after age 35, fertility treatment, family history, and obesity. Oral contraceptive use has been shown to reduce risk of ovarian cancer. About 90% of ovarian cancers develop in the epithelial layer covering the ovaries.

Increased awareness of early, nonspecific symptoms (abdominal swelling and digestive and bladder problems) can lead to earlier detection and treatment. Later signs of ovarian cancer include increased abdominal girth caused by the tumor size or ascites; abdominal, pelvic, or low back pain; urinary urgency and frequency; and constipation. Treatment depends on the stage at diagnosis. Early stages are treated with surgical removal of the uterus, ovaries, and fallopian tubes, together with the tumor and usually chemotherapy. Later stages are treated with radiation therapy, chemotherapy, and targeted therapy. A late diagnosis is associated with a poor prognosis. This care plan does not address surgical management.

NANDA-I NDx Deficient Knowledge

Common Related Factors
Insufficient information
Insufficient interest in learning
Misinformation presented by others
Insufficient knowledge of resources
Emotional state affecting learning

Defining Characteristics
Insufficient knowledge
Inaccurate follow-through of instruction
Inappropriate behavior

Common Expected Outcomes
Patient verbalizes understanding of the diagnosis and treatment procedures for ovarian cancer.
Patient freely discusses treatment options.

NOC Outcomes
Knowledge: Cancer Management; Knowledge: Disease Process; Knowledge: Treatment Regimen

NIC Interventions
Health Literacy Enhancement; Learning Facilitation; Teaching: Disease Process; Teaching: Procedure/Treatment

Ongoing Assessment

Action/Intervention

- Assess the patient's understanding of ovarian cancer and its treatment options. Identify any existing misconceptions.

Rationale

Patients may have misinformation about the types of female cancers. Previous experience with other women being treated for cancer, or who have died of it, will influence beliefs, some of which may be negative or misconceived. Ovarian cancer has a high mortality rate because of its advanced stage at diagnosis. QSEN: Patient-centered care.

Therapeutic Interventions

Actions/Interventions	Rationales
■ Explain that the cause of ovarian cancer is unknown.	Although the cause is unknown, patients should be informed of the possible risk factors. These include family history, advanced age, infertility, ovarian dysfunction, obesity, and mutations of the *BRCA* genes.
■ Discuss the clinical manifestations.	Patients need to understand why the diagnosis is challenging. No specific symptoms are recognized until the advanced stage, then abdominal swelling or pain, bloating or a feeling of fullness, vague but persistent gastrointestinal complaints, and bowel and bladder dysfunction manifest. Many of these symptoms also occur earlier, but patients tend to attribute them to other causes.
■ Discuss the common diagnostic procedures: • Pelvic examination • CA-125 blood test • Transvaginal or abdominal ultrasound examination • Computed tomography (CT) scan and/or magnetic resonance imaging (MRI) • Laparoscopy and biopsy	Unlike the Papanicolaou (Pap) test for cervical cancer, there is no specific screening test for ovarian cancer. A woman at high risk is recommended to have a pelvic examination, a CA-125 blood test, and an ultrasound examination performed twice a year beginning at 30 years of age and continuing for the rest of her life or until her ovaries are removed. Pelvic examination is used to assess for masses and growths. This examination can be challenging in obese women. CA-125 is a tumor marker for ovarian cancer; however, many false-positive results are possible. Abdominal or transvaginal ultrasound evaluates shape and size of ovaries. CT scans and MRI provide detailed cross-sectional images of any pelvic mass. Laparoscopy and biopsy are used to determine the stage and extent of the disease, guiding therapy.
■ Discuss the staging of ovarian cancer: • I—confined to one or both ovaries or fallopian tubes • II—spread to other areas within the pelvic area • III—spread beyond the pelvis to the lining of the abdomen or to the lymph nodes within the abdomen • IV—spread to organs beyond the abdomen	Staging guides the treatment options. Stage III is the most common stage at diagnosis. QSEN: Evidence-based practice.
■ Discuss the common treatment approaches: • Surgery: Total abdominal hysterectomy and bilateral salpingo-oophorectomy • Chemotherapy • Targeted therapy (e.g., bevacizumab or olaparib) • Radiation therapy (external or brachytherapy) • Clinical trials	Treatment depends on the stage and extent of the disease. For stage I, the usual treatment is total hysterectomy to remove (debulk) as much tumor as possible. In addition, chemotherapy or intraperitoneal radiation implants are usually included. At stage II, external (teletherapy) or internal (brachytherapy) radiation or systemic chemotherapy is used after tumor debulking. Stages III and IV are usually treated with chemotherapy. Common drugs include carboplatin, cisplatin, docetaxel, and paclitaxel. Overall, combination therapy is required to treat this malignant disease. Intraperitoneal chemotherapy is also used. Bevacizumab is an angiogenesis inhibitor that slows or shrinks the growth of advanced epithelial ovarian cancer. Olaparib is a type of drug known as a PARP (poly adenosine diphosphate [ADP] ribose polymerase) inhibitor. It is effective in patients with mutations of the *BRCA* genes. Patients are encouraged to participate in available trials either researching new treatments or comparing different treatments. Such participation will provide knowledge about the best way to treat this cancer. QSEN: Patient-centered care; Evidence-based practice.

■ = Independent   ▲ = Interprofessional Collaboration

NANDA-I NDx **Acute Pain**

Common Related Factors

Pain resulting from medical problems (increased abdominal pressure caused by tumor or metastasis to abdominal structures)

Pain resulting from surgical or medical treatments

Defining Characteristics

Self-report of pain using a standardized pain scale

Guarding behavior of abdominal region

Self-focused

Facial expression of pain

Distraction behavior (moaning, crying, restlessness)

Common Expected Outcomes

Patient reports satisfactory pain control at a decreased intensity using a standardized pain scale.

Patient uses pharmacological and nonpharmacological pain relief strategies.

NOC Outcomes
Pain Control; Medication Response

NIC Interventions
Pain Management; Positioning; Distraction

Ongoing Assessment

Actions/Interventions	Rationales
■ Assess the severity, quality, and location of pain.	Pain is typically abdominal but may radiate to the pelvic or low back area. Pain is caused by pressure on the abdominal structures as the tumor enlarges, or is related to surgical intervention.
■ Assess the effect of psychological factors on pain.	Pain is accentuated when the patient feels a loss of control and when her self-concept or role is threatened. The poor prognosis associated with ovarian cancer may cause grieving in anticipation of death.
■ Assess the patient's expectations for pain relief.	Some patients may be content to have pain decreased; others expect complete elimination of pain. This affects their perceptions of the effectiveness of the treatment modality and their willingness to participate in additional treatments. QSEN: Patient-centered care.
■ Assess the effect of pain on performance of activities of daily living (ADLs) and activities perceived as meaningful by the patient.	Fatigue, anxiety, or depression associated with pain can limit the patient's ability to complete self-care activities and fulfill role responsibilities. QSEN: Patient-centered care.

Therapeutic Interventions

Actions/Interventions	Rationales
■ Suggest positions for comfort.	The following positions are helpful in reducing the pain related to pressure: side-lying with the knees bent and a Fowler's position.
■ Teach alternative techniques to reduce pain:	
• Imagery	The use of a mental picture or an imagined event involving the five senses can distract the person from painful stimuli.
• Distraction techniques	These techniques heighten concentration on nonpainful stimuli to decrease awareness and experience of pain. Some methods are breathing modifications and nerve stimulation.
• Relaxation exercises	Techniques using physical and mental awareness increase muscle relaxation and reduce tension and pain.
• Massage of the back and shoulders	Massage interrupts pain transmission, increases endorphin levels, and decreases tissue edema. This intervention may require another person to provide the massage.

 evolve For additional care plans, go to http://evolve.elsevier.com/Gulanick/.

Actions/Interventions

▲ Administer analgesics as prescribed; develop a schedule for giving pain medications. Evaluate their effectiveness.

Rationales

Ongoing medication alleviates peak pain periods. Pain medications are absorbed and metabolized differently by patients, so their effectiveness must be evaluated individually by the patient. QSEN: Patient-centered care.

NANDA-I NDx **Risk for Ineffective Breathing Pattern**

Common Risk Factors

Presence of ascites (collection of protein-rich fluid in peritoneal cavity)

Pleural effusions

Common Expected Outcome

Patient maintains an effective breathing pattern, as evidenced by relaxed breathing at normal rate and depth and absence of dyspnea.

NOC Outcome

Respiratory Status: Ventilation

NIC Interventions

Respiratory Monitoring; Positioning; Medication Administration

---

Ongoing Assessment

Actions/Interventions

■ Assess for the presence of ascites:

- Measure the abdominal girth, taking care to measure at the same point consistently.
- Percuss the abdomen

- Check for ballottement.

■ Assess the breathing pattern and the position that the patient assumes for easiest breathing.

■ Monitor the effect of an ineffective breathing pattern on the ability to perform ADLs.

■ Assess for the signs of pleural effusion: decreased or absent breath sounds, a flat sound on percussion.

Rationales

Ascites is a third-space collection of protein-rich fluid in the peritoneal cavity. Its volume can be severe enough to impair respiratory function. QSEN: Safety.

This technique provides objective data regarding the progression of ascites.

Percussion over the abdomen sounds dull when fluid is present.

Ballottement is a palpation maneuver of the abdomen to detect excessive amounts of fluid. Palpation causes a fluid wave from the shifting of ascetic fluid.

Severe ascites secondary to ovarian cancer can impair breathing by limiting the full excursion of the diaphragm. Compromised breathing may present as tachypnea, shallow breathing, and complaints of dyspnea. An upright position facilitates breathing because ascetic fluid assumes a gravity-dependent position, relieving pressure on the thoracic cavity. QSEN: Safety.

Ineffective breathing reduces gas exchange and contributes to fatigue and activity intolerance.

Pleural effusions similarly compromise breathing, resulting in a shortness of breath. They are confirmed by chest x-ray film. QSEN: Safety.

■ = Independent ▲ = Interprofessional Collaboration

Therapeutic Interventions

Actions/Interventions	Rationales
■ Instruct about pacing activities.	Pacing activities reduce episodes of dyspnea from fatigue and excessive oxygen demand.
■ Assist to a Fowler's position.	This position relieves pressure from the ascitic abdomen on the thoracic cavity.
▲ Assist with paracentesis. Monitor the drainage system per protocol.	Paracentesis is a bedside procedure to remove ascitic fluid from the peritoneal cavity. A trocar catheter is inserted into the abdomen using sterile technique. The procedure is done to relieve abdominal pressure.
▲ Facilitate the shunt (LeVeen shunt, Denver shunt) function for patients with chronic ascites.	Fluid reaccumulates rapidly following paracentesis. Peritoneovenous shunting returns ascitic fluid to the vascular space and provides continuous relief of ascites.
• Apply an abdominal binder.	This binder increases intraperitoneal pressure, causing the valve in the shunt to return fluid into the vascular space.
• Encourage the use of an incentive spirometer.	Inspiring against pressure causes the valve in the shunt to open and shunt ascitic fluid into the vascular space.
• Administer diuretics as prescribed (for patients with a peritoneovenous shunt).	Diuretics facilitate the excretion of excess fluid especially in patients with a peritoneovenous shunt.
▲ Assist with thoracentesis. Monitor the drainage system per protocol.	Thoracentesis (the removal of pleural fluid by a needle) drains fluid from the pleural space to relieve dyspnea.
▲ Administer oxygen as prescribed.	Supplemental oxygen will maximize oxygen saturation, which should be 90% or greater.

NANDA-I NDx Risk for Imbalanced Nutrition: Less Than Body Requirements

Common Risk Factors

Poor appetite secondary to disease, side effects of therapies, and pressure from ascites
Depression
Fear
Pain

Common Expected Outcome

Patient maintains an adequate nutritional intake, as evidenced by calorie intake of at least 1800 kcal/day.

NOC Outcome
Nutritional Status: Food and Fluid Intake
NIC Interventions
Nutrition Therapy; Nutritional Monitoring

Ongoing Assessment

Actions/Interventions	Rationales
■ Evaluate the patient's weight history and current weight.	Ascites may cause a significant increase in overall body weight, although the body is actually cachectic.
■ Determine body weight distribution, checking the limbs for wasting.	Weight loss may appear insignificant until the weight of the ascitic abdomen is considered.
■ Assess the appetite and factors considered by the patient to influence appetite.	Appetite is a complex phenomenon involving physiological well-being and psychological, psychosocial, and environmental factors. Anorexia may result from disease, treatment modalities, complications, or the emotional turmoil of coping with a potentially terminal disease. QSEN: Patient-centered care.

Actions/Interventions

■ Assess the caloric intake.

■ Assess for presence of nausea/vomiting.

Rationales

Caloric counts quantify nourishment intake to provide accurate assessment.

Nausea/vomiting may occur secondary to the disease, the side effects of therapies, and pressure from ascites.

Therapeutic Interventions

Actions/Interventions

■ Involve the patient and caregiver in the selection of calorie-dense, high-protein, high-fiber meal plans.

▲ Consult a dietitian for dietary selections palatable to the patient.

■ Encourage small, frequent, nutrient-dense meals (at least six per day).
■ Encourage activity or exercise as tolerated.
■ Suggest mealtime companions and maintenance of a pleasant environment.
▲ Give antiemetics as prescribed.

■ Educate about oral hygiene.

Rationales

Calories and protein are necessary for strength and healing; fiber combats constipation resulting from inactivity and increased intra-abdominal pressure. Involving patients in their own nutritional care has been found to raise their intake of protein and energy levels. QSEN: Patient-centered care.

Dietitians have a greater understanding of the nutritional value of foods and may be helpful. QSEN: Teamwork and collaboration.

Small feedings reduce the work of digestion.

Activity enhances appetite by stimulating peristalsis.

Attention to the social aspects of eating is important in both the hospital and the home setting.

Antiemetics prevent or alleviate nausea and vomiting.

Often a combination of antiemetic medications is needed to effectively control nausea and vomiting and must correlate appropriately to the emetogenic potential of chemotherapy agents given. Serotonin $5-HT_3$ receptor antagonists (i.e., ondansetron and palonosetron), neurokinin-1 receptor antagonists (i.e., aprepitant), and corticosteroids (i.e., dexamethasone) are the most common drug classes used for chemotherapy-induced nausea and vomiting (CINV). Medical cannabis is somewhat effective in CINV and may be a reasonable option for patients who do not improve with standard treatment. QSEN: Evidence-based practice.

A clean, moist mouth and mucous membranes may make food more palatable.

Related Care Plans

■ = Independent   ▲ = Interprofessional Collaboration

Men's and Women's Health Care Plans

Pelvic Inflammatory Disease

Sexually Transmitted Infection (STI); Salpingitis; Oophoritis

Pelvic inflammatory disease (PID) is an infective process involving the uterus, fallopian tubes, and ovaries, as well as the peritoneum, pelvic veins, and connective tissue. It is a complication often caused by sexually transmitted diseases (STDs) such as *Chlamydia* infection and gonorrhea, but it can also occur secondary to other non-STD infections. Pelvic pain and lower abdominal pain are characteristic symptoms. Untreated PID can become a chronic condition; tissue destruction and scarring can cause the formation of abdominal and reproductive adhesions, resulting in infertility or ectopic pregnancy. If diagnosed early, PID can be treated with medications, but treatment will not undo any damage that has already affected reproductive organs. Treatment is usually completed on an outpatient basis. Both the patient and her sexual partner or partners must be treated. Many of the same factors that increase a woman's risk for STDs also place her at risk for PID. These risk factors include age younger than 26 years, multiple sex partners, history of PID, *Chlamydia* or gonorrhea infections, history of STD, and recent intrauterine device (IUD) insertion or abortion. When other STIs are present, PID must be ruled out. The most effective way to reduce the risk for PID is being in a long-term mutually monogamous relationship with a partner without an STD, and using latex condoms correctly every time having sex. The Centers for Disease Control and Prevention (CDC) recommends yearly *Chlamydia* testing of all sexually active women age 25 years or younger, pregnant women, and older women with multiple sex partners.

NANDA-I NDx Deficient Knowledge

Common Related Factors
Insufficient information
Insufficient interest in learning
Misinformation presented by others
Insufficient knowledge of resources
Embarrassment about topic, shame, fear

Defining Characteristics
Insufficient knowledge
Inaccurate follow-through of instruction
Inappropriate behavior

Common Expected Outcome
Patient verbalizes an understanding of PID infection, potential complications, medical treatment, and prevention of recurrence.

NOC Outcomes
Knowledge: Infection Management; Knowledge: Disease Process; Knowledge: Treatment Regimen

NIC Interventions
Health Literacy Enhancement; Learning Facilitation; Teaching: Disease Process; Teaching: Prescribed Medication

Ongoing Assessment

Actions/Interventions	Rationales
■ Assess the patient's knowledge of PID.	Although PID is a frequently encountered infection in women, health care providers cannot assume that all women are knowledgeable.
■ Assess the patient's knowledge of the consequences of PID.	Septic shock can be an immediate complication. Long-term infertility is a major complication. Frequent PID can result in ectopic pregnancy, cervical pathological conditions, and the resistance of organisms to antibiotics.

Actions/Interventions

- Assess the patient's past experience with STDs.

- Obtain a sexual history.

Rationales

Patients with gonorrhea or chlamydial infections are at a higher risk for PID. However, other infections can also cause PID.

The incidence of PID increases with multiple sex partners, risky sexual behaviors, and contact with an infected partner. QSEN: Patient-centered care.

Therapeutic Interventions

Actions/Interventions

- Remain supportive and nonjudgmental.

- Explain the transmission of PID.

- Teach the signs and symptoms of PID:
  - Early acute case symptoms include the following:
    - Excessive menstrual cramping
    - Bleeding or spotting outside the regular menses
    - Painful urination and sexual intercourse
    - Dull lower abdominal or pelvic pain especially with movement
    - Constipation
    - Low-grade fever
    - General malaise
  - Late symptoms include the following:
    - Pelvic pain
    - Copious, foul-smelling vaginal discharge
    - Nausea and vomiting
- Explain the common diagnostic tests:
  - Physical examination
  - Gynecological examination
  - Laboratory testing
  - Pregnancy testing
  - Pelvic ultrasound examination
  - Laparoscopy

- Explain the treatment regimens:
  - Outpatient antibiotic therapy—most common

  - Inpatient antibiotic therapy for high risk

Rationales

The moral stigma of an STD may be an obstacle for those seeking care for a real or suspected STD. Vaginal infections often result in emotional distress. Seeking medical care must not result in a negative response.

Acute or chronic PID is transmitted during or soon after sexual intercourse or pelvic surgery (e.g., abortion or childbirth). Infections may occur secondary to the use of an intrauterine device. The correct use of latex condoms reduces the infection rate. QSEN: Safety.

Symptoms may be absent in patients until late in the course of the illness. Symptoms may mimic ectopic pregnancy or appendicitis.

PID is difficult to diagnose because of the variation in signs and symptoms. Lower abdominal or pelvic tenderness or pain is a cardinal symptom. Laboratory testing may include erythrocyte sedimentation rate (ESR), C-reactive protein, white blood cell count, and cultures for *Chlamydia* and gonorrhea. Ectopic pregnancy mimics PID. Therefore pregnancy status must be determined before treatment with antibiotics. Pelvic ultrasound is used to rule out other causes such as appendicitis. Laparoscopy permits an optimal view of abdominal and pelvic organs and facilitates culture testing. It can also be used to remove an abscess if present. QSEN: Evidence-based practice.

Antibiotic treatment options are guided by culture and antibiotic sensitivity results. Most patients can manage their treatment at home.

Hospitalization may be required for patients who are pregnant, have severe symptoms, are not responding to oral medications, or have tubo-ovarian abscess.

Men's and Women's Health Care Plans

■ = Independent ▲ = Interprofessional Collaboration

Actions/Interventions

■ Treatment of sex partner(s); abstinence from sexual intercourse

Rationales

The patient can be easily reinfected by the sexual partner, who may be infected but asymptomatic. Sexual partners must be notified and treated. *Chlamydia* infection and gonorrhea are mandatory reportable STDs. Abstinence during treatment is important to prevent the spread of infection. QSEN: Safety.

NDx Infection

Common Related Factors

Gram-positive cocci:
- *Chlamydia trachomatis*
- *Neisseria gonorrhoeae*
- *Streptococcus*

Gram-negative cocci:
- *Escherichia coli*
- *Haemophilus influenzae*

Anaerobes:
- *Gardnerella vaginalis*
- *Bacteroides*

Defining Characteristics

Edematous vaginal mucosa
Copious, malodorous, greenish yellow vaginal discharge
Fever
Positive culture or screening test results
Formation of an abscess
Progression to peritonitis

Common Expected Outcome

Patient manifests signs of treated infection as evidenced by absence of fever, absence of pain, absence of vaginal discharge, and negative culture results.

NOC Outcomes

Knowledge: Infection Management; Risk Detection; Medication Response

NIC Interventions

Infection Control; Fertility Preservation; Teaching: Prescribed Medication

Ongoing Assessment

Actions/Interventions

▲ Assess for the presence of the minimum criteria for a diagnosis of PID:
- Lower abdominal tenderness on palpation
- Adnexal tenderness
- Cervical motion tenderness

▲ Assess for additional criteria to increase the specificity of diagnosis:
- Elevated temperature (>38.3°C [101°F])
- Abnormal cervical or vaginal discharge
- Elevated erythrocyte sedimentation rate or C-reactive protein
- Positive culture of cervical infection with *N. gonorrhoeae* or *C. trachomatis*

Rationales

Centers for Disease Control and Prevention (CDC) recommends using a low threshold and minimal criteria to maximize the diagnosis of PID because of its potential for serious reproductive damage to women. Treatment is thus instituted on the basis of these criteria after other competing diagnoses are ruled out. QSEN: Evidence-based practice.

According to the CDC, the presence of these additional criteria increases the specificity of the diagnosis. QSEN: Evidence-based practice.

Actions/Interventions

■ Assess the patient's pregnancy status
  • History of last menstrual period
  • Abnormal menses
■ Assess the patient's STD history.

▲ Monitor the culture results.

Rationales

The patient's pregnancy status must be known before antibiotics are administered. Certain antibiotics are not safe during pregnancy. QSEN: Safety.

More than one STD may be present at the same time. The presence of a titer elevation may represent an old or a new infection. Serial titers may be required.

Some antibiotic regimens will be implemented before culture and sensitivity results are received. Culture reports must be checked to ensure that organisms are sensitive to the current antibiotic regimen. QSEN: Safety.

Therapeutic Interventions

Actions/Interventions

▲ Institute the drug treatment as ordered. These drugs may include:
  • Cefoxitin
  • Ceftriaxone
  • Doxycycline
  • Cefotetan
  • Clindamycin
  • Metronidazole
  • Gentamicin
  • Ampicillin
■ Teach the importance of the proper administration of medications and the completion of the course of treatment.
■ Stress the importance of notifying sexual contacts.

■ Maintain blood and body fluid precautions. If the patient is hospitalized, maintain infection precautions:
  • Dispose of soiled items according to infection control policy.
  • Maintain strict handwashing for all people in contact with the patient.
  • Cleanse all equipment with disinfectant.
  • Use utensils or gloves when handling soiled materials.
■ Discourage the continuous use of perineal pads. Instruct to avoid the use of tampons.

■ Explain the importance of abstaining from sexual intercourse until after the follow-up visit.

Rationales

All patients with PID require oral or IV antibiotics, depending on the severity of the illness. Unlike specific STD organisms wherein a single treatment regimen is known, PID represents a complex syndrome that can be caused by a variety of organisms. Thus no single regimen of choice exists for PID. Therefore CDC guidelines are designed to provide broad-spectrum coverage for the most common pathogens, using at least two antibiotics. QSEN: Evidence-based practice.

This knowledge will prevent ineffective treatment, the recurrence of symptoms, and the development of antibiotic-resistant organisms. At least 14 days is usually required.

The treatment of partners prevents transmission or reinfection. This is a mandatory reportable STI. QSEN: Safety.

These precautions reduce the risk for transmitting the infection to others. QSEN: Safety.

This behavior reduces the risk for reinfection from exudates on the pad. Tampons can be a medium for further bacterial growth and may inhibit the drainage of pelvic exudates. QSEN: Safety.

The patient can be easily reinfected by the sexual partner, who may be infected but asymptomatic. Sexual partners also must be treated. QSEN: Safety.

■ = Independent   ▲ = Interprofessional Collaboration

Actions/Interventions

- Discuss contraceptive use.
  - The CDC makes the following recommendations about the proper use of male condoms:
    - Use a new condom with each act of sexual intercourse.
    - Carefully handle the condom to avoid damaging it with the fingernails, teeth, or other sharp objects.
    - Put the condom on after the penis is erect and before genital contact with the partner.
    - Ensure that no air is trapped in the tip of the condom.
    - Ensure that adequate lubrication exists during intercourse, possibly requiring the use of exogenous lubricants.
    - Use only water-based lubricants with latex condoms. Oil-based lubricants can weaken latex.
    - Hold the condom firmly against the base of the penis during withdrawal, and withdraw while the penis is still erect to prevent slippage.
  - The female condom is a lubricated polyurethane sheath or pouch with a ring on each end that is inserted into the vagina.
- Instruct the patient to notify the physician of the following:
  - Reappearance of severe symptoms
  - Lack of menstruation
  - Nonmenstrual bleeding
  - Severe abdominal cramps
  - Presence of purulent, malodorous vaginal discharge
- Refer to an STD clinic or social worker as indicated.

Rationales

Condoms may reduce the transmission of certain STIs. Spermicide-coated condoms have been associated with *E. coli* urinary tract infection. The consistent use of condoms, with or without spermicidal lubricant or vaginal application of spermicide, is recommended. QSEN: Evidence-based practice; Safety.

The female condom is an effective mechanical barrier to viruses, including HIV.

Early assessment facilitates prompt treatment. QSEN: Safety.

Risky sexual behaviors may require the implementation of a regular surveillance program (every 4 to 6 weeks or more often). QSEN: Teamwork and collaboration.

NANDA-I
NDx **Acute Pain**

Common Related Factors

Pelvic cavity inflammation
Excoriated perineal area
Development of abdominal adhesions

Defining Characteristics

Self-report of pain using a standardized pain scale
Self-focus or narrowed focus
Distraction behavior
Facial expression of pain
Change in physiological parameter (e.g., HR, BP, respiratory rate)

Common Expected Outcomes

Patient reports satisfactory pain control at a decreased intensity using a standardized pain scale.
Patient uses pharmacological and nonpharmacological pain relief measures.

NOC Outcome
Pain Control
NIC Interventions
Pain Management; Analgesic Administration

---

 evolve **For additional care plans, go to http://evolve.elsevier.com/Gulanick/.**

Ongoing Assessment

Actions/Interventions	Rationales
■ Assess for pain characteristics.	Pain may be continuous and crampy; bilateral, lower abdominal, or back pain; or increasing when the uterus is moved (e.g., during vaginal examination). Pain may increase with activity.
■ Assess bowel sounds.	Cessation of bowel sounds may indicate the progression to peritonitis.
■ Assess the response to medication effects and side effects.	Antibiotics are the treatment of choice to reduce the inflammation caused by the infection. Analgesics can be added as needed.

Therapeutic Interventions

Actions/Interventions	Rationales
▲ Administer or instruct patients in how to self-medicate with antibiotics and oral and topical analgesics, as prescribed.	Effective antibiotic management will eventually treat causative factors, subsequently relieving pain. The patient may experience extreme discomfort requiring opioid analgesia. However, aggressive antibiotic therapy may prevent tubal damage that would otherwise predispose the patient to ectopic pregnancy or infertility. QSEN: Patient-centered care.
■ Teach comfort measures: • Heat (dry or moist) • Positioning with extra pillows • Perineal care	These measures enhance the effect of pharmacological analgesia and promote comfort.
■ Encourage a semi-Fowler's position as often as possible.	This position promotes the drainage of pelvic exudates and prevents the development of pelvic abscesses.

Related Care Plans

Disturbed body image, Chapter 2
Ineffective coping, Chapter 2
Ineffective sexuality pattern, Chapter 2

■ = Independent   ▲ = Interprofessional Collaboration

Endocrine and Metabolic Care Plans

Cushing's Disease

Hypercortisolism; Cushing's Syndrome; Adrenocortical Hyperfunction

Cushing's disease reflects an excess of cortisol. Depending on the cause of the disease, mineralocorticoids and androgens also may be secreted in increased amounts. The disorder may be primary (an intrinsic adrenocortical disorder [e.g., neoplasm]), secondary (from pituitary or hypothalamic dysfunction with increased adrenocorticotropic hormone secretion resulting in glucocorticoid excess), or iatrogenic (from prolonged or excessive administration of corticosteroids). The disease results in fluid and electrolyte disturbances, suppressed immune response, altered fat distribution, and disturbances in protein metabolism. Changes in physical appearance that occur with Cushing's disease can have significant influence on the patient's body image and emotional well-being. The focus of this care plan is on the ambulatory patient with Cushing's disease.

NANDA-I
NDx Deficient Knowledge

Common Related Factors

Alteration in cognitive functioning
Insufficient information
Insufficient interest in learning
Insufficient knowledge of resources
Alteration in memory
Misinformation presented by others

Defining Characteristics

Insufficient knowledge of Cushing's disease
Inaccurate follow-through of instruction
Inaccurate performance on a test
Inappropriate behavior

Common Expected Outcomes

Patient verbalizes an understanding of Cushing's disease and guidelines for therapy.
Patient implements appropriate therapy.

NOC Outcomes
Knowledge: Cushing's Disease; Knowledge: Treatment Regimen; Knowledge: Infection Management
NIC Interventions
Health Literacy Enhancement; Learning Facilitation; Teaching: Cushing's Disease; Teaching: Prescribed Diet; Infection Protection

Ongoing Assessment

Actions/Interventions	Rationales
■ Assess the patient's level of knowledge of Cushing's disease and the guidelines for therapy.	The patient or family must understand the disease process and receive specific instructions related to treatment, methods to control symptoms, signs of infection, complications, and indicators of when to notify the physician. QSEN: Patient-centered care.
■ Assess the ability to learn, remember, or perform desired health-related care.	Cushing's disease may cause alterations in the level of consciousness because of the effects of cortisol on hippocampal neurons. The patient may have impaired memory. This change may limit the patient's ability to learn new information. QSEN: Patient-centered care.
■ Determine the patient's or the caregiver's self-efficacy to learn and apply new knowledge about the management of Cushing's disease.	A first step in teaching may be to foster increased self-efficacy in the patient's ability to learn the desired information or skills. The patient may find it difficult to make some lifestyle changes associated with the long-term treatment of Cushing's disease.

Therapeutic Interventions

Actions/Interventions	Rationales
■ Explain all tests to the patient:	The patient may undergo a variety of diagnostic tests for Cushing's disease. Many of the tests require patient cooperation in collecting urine specimens over an extended period. QSEN: Patient-centered care.
• Urine free cortisol, 17-hydroxycorticosteroids (17-OHCS), 17-ketosteroids (17-KS)	To begin the urine collection, the patient is instructed to void and discard that specimen. Then the patient needs to save all urine for 24 hours. Medications may need to be withheld for several days before urine collection. In Cushing's disease, urine free cortisol, 17-OHCS (metabolites of cortisol), and 17-KS (metabolites of androgens) levels are elevated.
• Dexamethasone suppression tests	These tests require a combination of urine collections, blood specimens, and the administration of dexamethasone. The overnight test is done as an initial screening and does not require urine collection. A prolonged version of the test may be completed over 3 days or 6 days. The results help determine the cause of the patient's Cushing's disease.
• Computed tomography, magnetic resonance imaging, and selected arteriography	These diagnostic studies are used to identify lesions of the adrenal gland, pituitary gland, or other body organs (lungs, gastrointestinal tract, pancreas) that are associated with the stimulation of cortisol secretion.
■ Anticipate the need to discuss or reinforce information about the probable treatment for correcting the hypersecretion of cortisol:	The patient will need to understand about treatment of Cushing's disease in order to make informed decisions. QSEN: Patient-centered care; Evidence-based practice.
• If an intrinsic adrenocortical disorder: probable surgery for removal of the adenoma, tumor, or adrenal glands	Adrenalectomy is the treatment of choice for the patient with an adrenal tumor or adrenal hyperplasia that is causing the increased levels of serum cortisol.
• If a disorder secondary to pituitary hypersecretion: transsphenoidal pituitary tumor resection or irradiation	The treatment of pituitary tumors is indicated for patients when the Cushing's disease is secondary to adrenocorticotropic hormone (ACTH) hypersecretion. Surgical therapy usually involves a transsphenoidal hypophysectomy. Radiation therapy may be used as part of the management of these patients.

Endocrine and Metabolic Care Plans

■ = Independent   ▲ = Interprofessional Collaboration

Endocrine and Metabolic
Care Plans

Actions/Interventions	Rationales
• If iatrogenic: gradual discontinuation of excessive administration of corticosteroids as the patient's condition permits	When Cushing's disease is secondary to the prolonged administration of glucocorticoids, treatment is focused on discontinuing the medication. This approach requires a gradual lowering of the dose over time to decrease the risk for adrenal insufficiency if the drug is stopped suddenly. If the patient's condition does not allow for discontinuing glucocorticoids, attempts will be made to adjust the dose and frequency of administration to minimize suppression of the normal hypothalamic-pituitary-adrenal function.
■ Instruct the patient to report the signs of infection.	Increased cortisol levels inhibit the immune response with a suppression of the allergic response, as well as the inhibition of inflammation. An elevated temperature may not be present with infection because of the decreased immune response. The patient needs to be aware that redness, swelling, and pain may be early indicators of skin infection. Changes in patterns of urinary elimination may indicate a urinary tract infection. A productive cough may occur with a respiratory infection. QSEN: Safety.
■ Instruct the patient to report areas of skin breakdown and inadequate wound healing.	Wound healing is prolonged in Cushing's disease. This change occurs because of impaired protein synthesis from increased cortisol levels. QSEN: Safety.
■ Teach the patient about the regular evaluation of serum glucose levels.	Increased cortisol levels contribute to impaired glucose metabolism. Hyperglycemia is a common effect. The patient may develop disease-induced diabetes mellitus. QSEN: Safety.
■ Reinforce dietary instructions. Instruct the patient in a high-calcium diet.	Cushing's disease results in weight gain and calcium and protein loss. A high-calcium diet prevents the worsening of osteoporosis.
■ Instruct the patient regarding the signs of osteoporosis such as fractures, kyphosis, or height loss.	Muscle wasting, fatigue, weakness, and osteoporosis are associated with excess cortisol. These changes put the patient at risk for fractures. Kyphosis and a decrease in height occur with spinal compression fractures. QSEN: Safety.
■ Instruct the patient regarding fat distribution.	Chronic cortisol hypersecretion redistributes body fat, with increased fat deposited on the back, shoulder, trunk, and abdomen. The patient may develop a rounding of the face (moon face) as a result of fat redistribution and edema.
■ Explain how to obtain a medical identification tag and the importance of wearing it.	The tag can inform others of the patient's condition as a warning so that appropriate treatment will occur in an emergency situation. QSEN: Safety.

NANDA-I NDx **Disturbed Body Image**

Common Related Factors	Defining Characteristics
Alteration in body function due to increased production of androgens (giving rise to virilism in women; hirsutism [abnormal growth of hair])	Preoccupation with changed body
	Hiding of body part
Disturbed protein metabolism resulting in muscle wasting, capillary fragility, and wasting of bone matrix: ecchymosis, osteoporosis, slender limbs, striae (usually purple)	Change in social involvement
Alteration in body structure due to abnormal fat distribution along with edema resulting in moon face, cervicodorsal fat (buffalo hump), trunk obesity	

evolve **For additional care plans, go to http://evolve.elsevier.com/Gulanick/.**

Common Expected Outcome

Patient demonstrates enhanced body image and self-esteem as evidenced by ability to look at, touch, talk about, and care for actual and perceived altered body parts and functions.

NOC Outcomes
Body Image; Self-Esteem
NIC Interventions
Body Image Enhancement; Self-Esteem Enhancement

Ongoing Assessment

Actions/Interventions	Rationales
■ Assess for any changes in personal appearance caused by the cortisol excess.	These changes may include obesity, thin extremities with muscle atrophy, moon face, red cheeks, buffalo hump, and increased body and facial hair. Hyperpigmentation of skin, hair, and mucous membranes occurs as a result of increased levels of melanocyte-stimulating hormones and ACTH. Acne may result from adrenal androgen excess.
■ Assess patients' feelings about their changed appearance and coping mechanisms.	The extent of the patient's response is related to the value or importance the patient places on the part or function. Negative statements about changes in appearance indicate a disturbed body image. The patient may withdraw from social interaction. Depression may occur. QSEN: Patient-centered care.
■ Assess the patient's use of coping mechanisms.	Previously successful coping skills may be inadequate in the present situation. The patient may use clothing to hide physical changes. QSEN: Patient-centered care.

Therapeutic Interventions

Actions/Interventions	Rationales
■ Encourage the expression of feelings about changes in the patient's appearance.	It is worthwhile to encourage the patient to separate feelings about changes in body structure or function from feelings about self-worth. The expression of feelings can enhance the patient's coping strategies. QSEN: Patient-centered care.
■ Reassure the patient that the physical changes are a result of the elevated hormone levels and most will resolve when those levels return to normal.	Information helps the patient develop realistic expectations about the changes in physical appearance. This information may enhance the patient's willingness to participate in recommended treatments.
■ Promote coping methods to deal with the patient's change in appearance (e.g., adequate grooming, flattering clothes).	Learning methods to compensate for changes in appearance enhances the patient's self-esteem. Helping patients remember how they managed body image issues in the past may facilitate an adjustment to the current issue.
■ Refer to local support groups.	Talking with people who have experienced similar situations provides social support. Members of a support group may offer coping strategies that have proved successful.
■ Provide an atmosphere of acceptance and positive caring.	Patients look to others for feedback about their appearance. When the nurse responds to the patient in an accepting manner, it supports the patient's adjustment to his or her appearance.

Endocrine and Metabolic Care Plans

■ = Independent   ▲ = Interprofessional Collaboration

NANDA-I NDx Risk for Injury

Common Risk Factors

Poor wound healing
Decreased bone density
Increased capillary fragility

Common Expected Outcome

Patient implements measures to prevent injury.

> **NOC Outcomes**
> Knowledge: Fall Prevention; Knowledge: Personal Safety; Risk Control; Fall Prevention Behavior
>
> **NIC Interventions**
> Fall Prevention; Surveillance; Environmental Management: Safety; Bleeding Precautions

Ongoing Assessment

Actions/Interventions	Rationales
■ Assess the skin for signs of bruising and the feces for occult blood.	Patients with Cushing's disease will experience a loss of collagen tissue that supports the superficial small blood vessels and capillaries. This change makes these blood vessels more susceptible to rupture with minimal trauma. The patient may experience easy bruising. Occult fecal blood may be an early indicator of gastrointestinal (GI) bleeding. QSEN: Safety.
■ Assess the skin for signs of breakdown.	Cushing's disease causes thinning of the skin because of a loss of collagen and stretching from increased fat deposits. The skin is more easily damaged, with resulting skin breakdown. QSEN: Safety.
■ Ask the patient about problems with slow wound healing.	Increased cortisol levels increase the catabolism of peripheral tissues. Impaired nitrogen metabolism associated with Cushing's disease contributes to impaired protein synthesis and delayed wound healing. QSEN: Safety.
■ Assess the patient for decreased height and kyphosis.	Hypercortisolism that occurs with Cushing's disease causes increased bone resorption, decreased bone formation, increased renal calcium excretion, and decreased calcium absorption from the intestines. These changes lead to decreased bone density and the development of osteoporosis. Spinal compression fractures result in decreased height and an exaggerated anteroposterior curvature of the thoracic spine (kyphosis). QSEN: Safety.
▲ Prepare the patient for a bone density evaluation.	This diagnostic procedure provides information about the loss of bone density.

Therapeutic Interventions

Actions/Interventions	Rationales
■ Instruct the patient in activities to decrease the risk for bleeding:	The patient needs to take precautions with daily activities to reduce situations that can result in skin trauma, bruising, or bleeding. QSEN: Safety.
• Use a soft toothbrush.	This device decreases trauma to the gums.
• Use an electric razor.	This type of razor reduces the risk for cutting the skin when shaving.
• Eat a high-fiber diet with adequate fluid intake.	These measures decrease the risk for developing constipation, which can result in lower GI bleeding.
■ Apply direct pressure over venipuncture sites, injection sites, or wounds for at least 1 minute or longer.	Because of capillary fragility, the patient will bleed more easily. Direct pressure helps control bleeding and reduce bruising. QSEN: Safety.
■ Instruct the patient about keeping the skin clean and moisturized.	Excessive dryness or excessive moisture increases the risk for skin breakdown. QSEN: Safety.
■ Encourage the patient to increase the dietary intake of calcium and vitamin D.	Cushing's disease is associated with loss of bone density and development of osteoporosis. The patient is at risk for pathological fractures as a result of minor stress on the weaker bones. The patient can add generous amounts of low-fat dairy products and green leafy vegetables to increase calcium intake. Vitamin D is necessary for the absorption of calcium from the intestine. Supplemental calcium and vitamin D are indicated if dietary sources are not adequate.
■ Discuss with the patient safety measures in the home environment.	The patient needs to assess the home and work environment for hazards that would contribute to falls. These hazards include loose rugs, highly waxed or wet floors, and stairs with poor lighting or inadequate handrails. QSEN: Safety.

Risk for Excess Fluid Volume

Common Risk Factor

Compromised regulatory mechanisms (cortisol excess; mineralocorticoid excess)

Common Expected Outcome

Patient is normovolemic as evidenced by urine output greater than or equal to 30 mL/hr, balanced intake and output, stable weight (or loss attributed to fluid loss), absence or reduction of edema, HR 60 to 100 beats/min, and absence of pulmonary crackles.

NOC Outcomes
Fluid Balance; Electrolyte and Acid/Base Balance; Cardiopulmonary Status

NIC Interventions
Fluid Monitoring; Fluid Management; Electrolyte Management

Ongoing Assessment

Actions/Interventions	Rationales
■ Assess the patient's HR and BP.	Cushing's disease may result in hypertension caused by expanded fluid volume from sodium and water retention. Tachycardia occurs as a compensatory response to circulatory overload.

■ = Independent ▲ = Interprofessional Collaboration

Endocrine and Metabolic Care Plans

Actions/Interventions

- Assess for the signs of circulatory overload: weight gain, edema, jugular vein distention, crackles, shortness of breath, dyspnea.

- ▲ Monitor the patient's laboratory results (especially potassium and sodium).

- Assess for cardiac dysrhythmias.

Rationales

The documentation of circulatory overload directs prompt intervention. Excessive glucocorticoid and mineralocorticoid secretion predisposes the patient to fluid and sodium retention. QSEN: Safety.

Excessive cortisol causes sodium and water retention, edema, and increased potassium excretion. Mineralocorticoids regulate sodium and potassium secretion, and excess levels cause marked sodium and water retention as well as marked hypokalemia.

Hypokalemia can result in cardiac dysrhythmias. QSEN: Safety.

Therapeutic Interventions

Actions/Interventions

- Encourage a diet low in sodium with ample potassium.

- Instruct the patient to reduce fluid intake as prescribed.

- ▲ Administer or instruct the patient to take diuretics as prescribed.

- Advise the patient to elevate his or her feet when sitting down.
- ▲ Administer or instruct the patient to take antihypertensive medications as prescribed.

Rationales

These dietary changes help control the development of fluid retention and hypokalemia. QSEN: Safety.

Regulating fluid intake is necessary to prevent circulatory overload.

Diuretics promote sodium and water excretion. Potassium-sparing diuretics may be prescribed to prevent further loss of potassium. QSEN: Evidence-based practice.

This position reduces fluid accumulation in the lower extremities.

Cortisol and mineralocorticoid excess causes hypertension as a result of sodium and water retention.

Related Care Plans

Activity intolerance, Chapter 2
Ineffective coping, Chapter 2
Risk for impaired skin integrity, Chapter 2
Diabetes mellitus, Chapter 13

Diabetes Mellitus

Type 1; Type 2

Diabetes mellitus is a disorder of metabolism in which carbohydrates, fats, and proteins cannot be used for energy. Insulin, a hormone secreted by islet cells of the pancreas, is required to facilitate movement of glucose across cell membranes. Once inside the cell, glucose is the primary metabolic fuel. Type 1 diabetes occurs when the pancreas is no longer able to secrete insulin. This condition occurs as a result of an autoimmune process with destruction of pancreatic beta cells and has its onset between ages 1 and 24 years. The autoimmune process is triggered by a combination of genetic predisposition and environmental stimuli such as a virus. The result of the insulin deficiency is hyperglycemia. It represents 5% to 10% of the cases of diabetes. Type 2 diabetes results because of resistance of peripheral tissue receptors to the effects of insulin. This type of diabetes also has a genetic predisposition for insulin resistance in skeletal muscles, fat cells, and liver cells. Type 2 diabetes is characterized by hyperinsulinemia and hyperglycemia. Over time the beta cells of the pancreas fail to produce sufficient insulin. Its onset is slow and gradual, with many individuals having had the disease 10 years before diagnosis. It represents 90% to 95% of the cases of diabetes. This is usually a condition of middle-aged to older individuals, although a recent increase in the incidence of type 2 diabetes has occurred in children. Obesity is a major factor in the development of type 2 diabetes, in both children and adults. Because obesity is a major factor, the current standards of care from the American Diabetes Association (ADA) recommend screening for diabetes should be done to adults of any age whose BMI is 25 or greater (or 23 or greater in Asian Americans) and have one or more risk factors for diabetes. Other risk factors include physical inactivity, first-degree relative who has diabetes, high-risk race/ethnicity (African American, Latino, Native American, Asian America, Pacific Islander), women who delivered a child weighing more than 9 pounds, women who had gestational diabetes, women with polycystic ovary syndrome, hypertension, high-density lipoprotein (HDL cholesterol) level above 35 mg/dL, triglyceride level above 250 mg/dL, acanthosis nigricans, and previous hemoglobin A_{1c} value of 5.7% or higher. Regardless of weight and risk factors, all adults should be screened for diabetes at least every 3 years starting at age 45. Current studies relate waist circumference of 40 inches for men and 35 inches for women to increased risk for this form of diabetes.

Diabetes is a major public health problem; in 2012, more than 29 million individuals, or 9.3% of the U.S. population, had the disease. Diabetes causes significant morbidity and death. Cardiovascular disease death rates are 1.7 times higher in adults with diabetes compared to adults without diabetes. The severity of dyslipidemia and hypertension is higher in the person with type 2 diabetes. Diabetes is the primary cause of 44% of new cases of kidney failure. Over 28% of adults aged 40 or older with diabetes have diabetic retinopathy. Diabetes is the leading cause of nontraumatic lower extremity amputations in the United States. This care plan concentrates on the care of individuals with type 2 diabetes.

NANDA-I NDx
Risk for Unstable Blood Glucose Level

Common Risk Factors
Insulin deficiency with inability to use nutrients
Excessive intake in relation to metabolic needs
Sedentary activity level

Common Expected Outcome
Patient maintains blood glucose and glycosylated hemoglobin (HbA_{1c}) levels within defined target ranges.

NOC Outcomes
Blood Glucose Level; Knowledge: Medication; Knowledge: Prescribed Diet; Knowledge: Prescribed Activity; Knowledge: Diabetes Management

NIC Interventions
Hyperglycemia Management; Teaching: Prescribed Exercise; Teaching: Prescribed Diet; Teaching: Prescribed Medication

Endocrine and Metabolic Care Plans

Ongoing Assessment

Actions/Interventions	Rationales
■ Assess for the signs of hyperglycemia.	Hyperglycemia results when there is an inadequate amount of insulin to use glucose. Excess glucose in the bloodstream creates an osmotic effect that results in increased thirst, increased hunger, and increased urination. The patient may also report nonspecific symptoms of fatigue, headache, and blurred vision.
▲ Monitor the patient's blood glucose levels at each office visit, and review the blood glucose history.	Changes in blood glucose levels, as recorded by the patient, will indicate the patient's success in managing his or her diabetes. The patient needs to notify members of the interprofessional health team if the home glucose results are higher and lower than an established goal for glucose management. QSEN: Patient-centered care; Teamwork and collaboration.

■ = Independent   ▲ = Interprofessional Collaboration

Actions/Interventions	Rationales
▲ Monitor HbA$_{1c}$ glycosylated hemoglobin.	HbA$_{1c}$ is a measure of blood glucose over the previous 2 to 3 months. Current recommendations are to have HbA$_{1c}$ measured four times each year. The goal for HbA$_{1c}$ levels varies depending on age, life expectancy, cognitive function, pregnancy, stages of comorbid conditions, and presence and severity of cardiovascular disease. Many nonpregnant adults can reasonably achieve an A$_{1c}$ of under 7%. A goal of less than 6.5% might be suggested in patients with a long life expectancy and no cardiovascular disease, as long as this can be achieved without significant hypoglycemia. A goal of less than 8% might be suggested for patients who have a limited life expectancy, have a history of severe hypoglycemia, or have advanced cardiovascular complications. QSEN: Patient-centered care; Evidence-based practice; Safety.
▲ Monitor serum insulin levels.	Hyperinsulinemia occurs early in the development of type 2 diabetes. Obesity and insulin receptor dysfunction in peripheral tissues stimulates insulin secretion from the pancreas. Over many years pancreatic cells fail to secrete sufficient insulin leading to hyperglycemia.
■ Assess the patient's current knowledge and understanding of the prescribed diet.	Nonadherence to dietary guidelines can result in hyperglycemia. Current guidelines from the American Diabetes Association recommend an individualized plan that promotes healthy eating. Too many and too few carbohydrates at meals will cause poor glycemic control; neither dietary extreme is recommended. A moderate consumption of carbohydrates at every meal (generally 45-60 g) three times a day and 15-mg carbohydrate snacks as needed is generally recommended. The patient with diabetes mellitus may experience either hyperglycemia or hypoglycemia when medication, exercise, and food intake are not balanced. QSEN: Evidence-based practice; Patient-centered care.
■ Assess the pattern of physical activity.	Physical activity has an insulin-like effect and helps lower blood glucose levels. Regular exercise is an important part of diabetes management and reduces the risk for cardiovascular complications.
■ Assess for the signs of hypoglycemia.	The patient with type 2 diabetes mellitus who uses insulin as part of the treatment plan is at increased risk for hypoglycemia. Manifestations of hypoglycemia may vary among individuals but are consistent in the same individual. The signs are the result of both increased adrenergic activity and decreased glucose delivery to the brain. The patient may experience tachycardia, diaphoresis, tremors, dizziness, headache, fatigue, hunger, and visual changes. QSEN: Safety.
■ Assess the medications that are taken regularly.	The patient with type 2 diabetes mellitus may have other chronic health problems managed by medications. Many medications cause fluctuations in blood glucose as a side effect. For example, hyperglycemia is a side effect of beta-blockers, corticosteroids, thiazide diuretics, estrogen, isoniazid, lithium, and phenytoin. Hypoglycemia is a side effect associated with the regular use of salicylates, disopyramide, insulin, sulfonylurea agents, and pentamidine. QSEN: Safety; Evidence-based practice.

Endocrine and Metabolic Care Plans

Therapeutic Interventions

Actions/Interventions

▲ Establish goals with the patient for weight loss; glucose, lipids, and HbA₁c measurements; and exercise.

■ Review the progress toward goals on each subsequent visit.

■ Assist the patient in identifying eating patterns that need changing.

▲ Refer the patient to a registered dietitian for individualized diet instruction.

■ Instruct the patient to take oral hypoglycemic medications as directed:

• Second-generation sulfonylureas: glipizide (Glucotrol), glyburide (DiaBeta), glimepiride (Amaryl)

Rationales

Weight: A moderate weight loss of 7% to 10% has been shown to improve hyperglycemia, dyslipidemia, and hypertension. *Glucose:* For intensive control in most nonpregnant adults, the range should be between 80 and 130 mg/dL before meals, less than 180 mg/dL 1 to 2 hours after the beginning of meals. *HbA₁c:* The level should be individualized depending on age, life expectancy, cognitive function, pregnancy, stages of comorbid conditions, and presence and severity of cardiovascular disease. Many nonpregnant adults can reasonably achieve an A₁c of below 7%. A goal of less than 6.5% might be suggested in patients with a long life expectancy and no cardiovascular disease, as long as this can be achieved without significant hypoglycemia. A goal of less than 8% might be suggested for patients who have a limited life expectancy, have a history of severe hypoglycemia, or have advanced cardiovascular complications. *Exercise:* The patient should perform 30 minutes of moderate physical activity on most days of the week. QSEN: Patient-centered care.

Patient involvement in the treatment plan enhances the adherence to treatment regimens that maintain glucose levels within recommended goal range. An interest in learning new health behaviors increases when the patient helps set the agenda for change and feels like an active participant. QSEN: Patient-centered care.

This information provides the basis for individualized dietary instruction. Following a recommended diet helps the patient maintain glucose levels within a recommended goal range. QSEN: Patient-centered care.

The registered dietitian will help the patient develop an individualized meal plan based on body weight, blood glucose levels, and lipid patterns. As there is no single ideal dietary distribution of calories among carbohydrates, fats, and proteins for people with diabetes, macronutrient distribution should be individualized while keeping total calorie and metabolic goals in mind. The type of carbohydrate (sugar or starch) is less important than total carbohydrate intake. Dietary fiber of 20 to 35 g/day is associated with improved glycemic control. The patient may be able to include a moderate intake of alcohol as part of the overall diet plan. Alcohol consumption, especially without carbohydrate intake, blocks the release of glycogen from the liver, causing hypoglycemia. QSEN: Teamwork and collaboration.

Each category of oral agent acts on a different site of glucose metabolism. Hypoglycemia occurs less frequently with oral agents; however, episodes of hypoglycemia can occur in patients who do not have regular eating habits. QSEN: Evidence-based practice.

These drugs stimulate insulin secretion by the pancreas. They also enhance cell receptor sensitivity to insulin and decrease the liver synthesis of glucose from amino acids and stored glycogen.

Endocrine and Metabolic Care Plans

■ = Independent ▲ = Interprofessional Collaboration

Actions/Interventions

- Meglitinides: repaglinide (Prandin)
- D-Phenylalanine derivatives: nateglinide (Starlix)

- Biguanides: metformin (Glucophage)

- Alpha-glucosidase inhibitors: acarbose (Precose), miglitol (Glyset)
- Thiazolidinediones (TZDs): pioglitazone (Actos), rosiglitazone (Avandia)
- DPP4 inhibitors: sitagliptin phosphate (Januvia), vildagliptin, saxagliptin (Onglyza), linagliptin (Tradjenta), alogliptin (Nesina)

- Bile acid sequestrants: colesevelam (Welchol)

- Dopamine-2 agonists: bromocriptine (Parlodel)

- SGLT2 inhibitors: canagliflozin (Invocana), dapagliflozin (Farxiga), empagliflozin (Jardinance)
- GLP-1 receptor agonists: exenatide (Byetta), liraglutide (Victoza), albiglutide (Tanzeum), lixisenatide (Lyxumia), dulaglutide (Trulicity)

- Amylin mimetics: pramlintide (Symlin)

■ Instruct the patient to take insulin medications as directed:

- Rapid-acting insulin analogues: lispro insulin (Humalog), insulin aspart

- Short-acting insulin: regular

- Intermediate-acting insulin: neutral protamine Hagedorn (NPH)

- Premixed insulin of intermediate and rapid insulins: 70% NPH/30% regular

- Basal insulin analogues: insulin glargine (Lantus), insulin detemir (Levemir)

Rationales

These drugs stimulate insulin secretion by the pancreas.

These drugs stimulate rapid insulin secretion to reduce the increases in blood glucose that occur soon after eating.

These drugs decrease the amount of glucose produced by the liver and improve insulin sensitivity. They enhance muscle cell receptor sensitivity to insulin. This drug group is recommended by the ADA as the first oral medication for treatment of type 2 diabetes.

These drugs delay the absorption of glucose into the blood from the intestine.

These drugs decrease insulin resistance in peripheral tissues.

These drugs inhibit DPP-4 activity and increase postprandial incretin concentrations. These drugs increase insulin secretion and decrease glucagon secretion to reduce the production of glucose.

This group of drugs decreases hepatic glucose production and increases incretin levels.

These drugs increase insulin sensitivity and modulate hypothalamic regulation of metabolism.

This group of drugs blocks glucose reabsorption by the kidney and increases excretion of glucose in the urine.

This drug group activates GLP-1 receptors and causes increased insulin secretion, causes decreased glucagon secretion, slows gastric emptying, and may help increase satiety.

This drug group activates amylin receptors, decreases glucagon secretion, slows gastric emptying, and may help increase satiety.

Insulin is required for individuals with type 1 diabetes and for many with type 2 diabetes who develop insulin deficiency over time. Beta cells begin to fail about 10 to 20 years after the development of type 2 diabetes. QSEN: Evidence-based practice.

These insulins have an onset of action within 15 minutes of administration. The duration of action is 2 to 3 hours for Humalog and 3 to 5 hours for aspart.

This insulin has an onset of action within 30 minutes of administration. The duration of action is 4 to 8 hours.

The onset of action for the intermediate-acting insulins is 1 hour after administration. The peak action is 6 to 12 hours after administration. The duration of action is 18 to 26 hours.

The premixed concentration has an onset of action similar to that of rapid-acting insulins and a duration of action similar to that of intermediate-acting insulins.

These insulins have an onset of action of 1 hour after administration. The duration of action for these long acting insulins is at least 24 hours.

Endocrine and Metabolic Care Plans

Actions/Interventions

- ■ Instruct the patient to prepare and administer insulin with accuracy.

  - • Injection procedures

  - • Rotation of injections within one anatomical site

  - • Storage of insulin

  - • Mixing of insulins: consult the manufacturer's guidelines

  - • Instruct the patient in using a continuous subcutaneous insulin infusion (CSII) pump.

- ■ Instruct the patient to exercise.
  - • Refer the patient to members of the interprofessional health team for exercise planning.

    - • 30 to 60 minutes with warm-up and cool-down periods
    - • Three to four times per week for glycemic control
    - • 5 to 7 days per week for weight loss
  - • Instruct in the methods to maintain hydration and avoid hypoglycemia during exercise.

Rationales

Inconsistencies in technique of insulin preparation and administration can result in elevated blood glucose levels. QSEN: Safety; Evidence-based practice.

The absorption of insulin is more consistent when insulin is always injected in the same anatomical site. Absorption is fastest in the abdomen, followed by the arms, thighs, and buttocks. The current American Diabetes Association recommendation is to rotate administration of insulin within the same general area (for example, the abdomen) rather than from one major site to another (for example, from the abdomen to the leg).

The injection of insulin in the same site over time will result in lipoatrophy and lipohypertrophy with reduced insulin absorption and therefore lead to decreased glycemic control.

Insulin should be refrigerated at 2° to 8°C (36° to 46°F). Unopened vials may be stored until their expiration date. To prevent irritation from the injection of cold insulin, vials of insulin may be stored at temperatures of 15° to 30°C (59° to 86°F) for 1 month. Opened vials should be discarded after that time.

The mixing of two insulins in one syringe is technically difficult for some patients. Accuracy with this technique is essential. Some insulin products cannot be mixed (glargine) or should be administered shortly after preparation (rapid-acting and long-acting, and rapid-acting and intermediate). Many patients benefit from administering insulin with a preloaded insulin cartridge device (insulin pen). The patient needs to learn the correct method for selecting the appropriate dose of insulin. For many insulin pens, a dial is turned to select the correct number of insulin units.

A CSII pump is a portable insulin pump that allows for a continuous subcutaneous infusion of a basal insulin dose. The patient can increase doses for mealtimes. Adjustments in the dose of rapid-acting insulin in the pump reservoir are based on regular capillary blood glucose monitoring results. This insulin delivery system allows the patient more flexibility in timing insulin administration to mealtimes. Insulin infusion devices provide for improved outcomes of blood glucose control compared with multiple daily injections. The use of an insulin pump requires a highly motivated patient to learn how to manage the pump.

Exercise improves glucose levels and assists with weight loss.

An exercise physiologist, physical therapist, or cardiac rehabilitation nurse can work with the patient to develop an exercise plan. Specific exercises can be prescribed for the patient with diabetes who has physical limitations. QSEN: Teamwork and collaboration.

Warm-ups before exercise and stretching after exercise help prevent muscle injury. Studies have shown sustained improvement in glucose control when a regular exercise program is maintained. QSEN: Evidence-based practice.

Dehydration can hasten hypoglycemia, especially in hot weather. Patients may need to add a snack before exercising if they experience hypoglycemia. QSEN: Safety.

Endocrine and Metabolic Care Plans

■ = Independent   ▲ = Interprofessional Collaboration

NANDA-I NDx Risk for Ineffective Health Management

Common Risk Factors

Complex therapeutic regimen
Insufficient knowledge of therapeutic regimen

Common Expected Outcomes

Patient verbalizes intention to follow prescribed regimen.
Patient describes or demonstrates required competencies.
Patient identifies appropriate resources.
Patient demonstrates ongoing adherence to treatment plan.

NOC Outcomes

Compliance Behavior; Knowledge: Diabetes Management; Blood Glucose Level; Self-Management: Diabetes

NIC Interventions

Self-Modification Assistance; Mutual Goal Setting; Teaching: Diabetes Mellitus; Teaching: Individual; Teaching: Prescribed Diet

---

Ongoing Assessment

Actions/Interventions	Rationales
■ Assess the patient's prior efforts to manage the diabetes care regimen.	This knowledge provides an important starting point in understanding any complexities the patient perceives in implementing the diabetes management regimen. The patient may report past experiences of feeling overwhelmed by attempts to manage medications, diet, exercise, blood glucose monitoring, and other measures to treat diabetes and prevent complications. QSEN: Patient-centered care.
■ Evaluate the patient's self-management skills, including the ability to perform procedures for blood glucose monitoring.	Self-management skills determine the amount and type of education that needs to be provided to promote adherence to the prescribed treatment plan.
■ Assess for factors that may negatively affect success with following the regimen.	Limited vision may impair the patient's ability to prepare and administer insulin accurately. Limited mobility and the loss of fine motor control can interfere with skills needed for insulin administration and blood glucose monitoring. QSEN: Patient-centered care; Safety.
■ Assess the patient's financial resources for health care.	The cost of medications and supplies for blood glucose monitoring may become barriers to the patient with limited financial resources.

Therapeutic Interventions

Actions/Interventions	Rationales
■ Ensure that the patient has knowledge about the symptoms, causes, treatment, and prevention of hyperglycemia.	Elevated blood glucose levels in patients previously diagnosed with diabetes indicate the need to evaluate diabetes management. QSEN: Patient-centered care; Safety.
• Symptoms: polyuria, polydipsia, polyphagia, weight loss, elevated blood glucose levels, fatigue, blurred vision, poor wound healing	The buildup of glucose in the body results in symptoms that can be identified by the patient. Ensure that the patient has been educated regarding these symptoms.
• Causes: increased food intake, decreased medications, infection, illness, stress	Increased food intake or decreased medication use for diabetes causes increased blood glucose levels. Illness, infection, and increased stress increase the counterregulatory hormones that elevate blood glucose levels.

Actions/Interventions

- Treatment: increased fluid intake, medications to reduce blood glucose levels, identification and treatment of causes

- Prevention: adherence to dietary guidelines and the medical regimen; blood glucose monitoring conducted on a regular basis to permit the early treatment of hyperglycemia

■ Ensure that the patient has knowledge about the symptoms, causes, treatment, and prevention of hypoglycemia.

- Symptoms: *autonomic*—trembling, shaking, sweating, pounding heart rate, fast pulse, tingling in the extremities, heavy breathing; *neuroglycopenic*—slow thinking, blurred vision, slurred speech, trouble concentrating, fatigue or sleepiness
- Causes: *meals*—delayed or missed meals or snacks, irregular timing of meals, irregular carbohydrate content of meals; *medications*—increased dose, medication taken at the wrong time; *activity*—increased physical activity without additional carbohydrate intake
- Treatment: 15 to 20 g of carbohydrate for blood glucose levels less than 70 mg/dL; 30 g may be needed for levels less than 50 mg/dL. Repeat treatment with an additional 15 to 20 g of carbohydrate if hypoglycemia persists 15 minutes after the first treatment.
- Prevention: adherence to medication and dietary guidelines, regular self-monitoring of blood glucose, accurate medication-taking practices, timing of exercise

▲ Refer the patient to members of the interprofessional health team for help with financial resources.

■ Review the current dietary goals for type 2 diabetes with the patient and family.

■ Review the blood glucose monitoring results on each contact with the patient.

Rationales

Dehydration causes many of the symptoms related to hyperglycemia. The patient may receive insulin to reduce blood glucose and prevent diabetic ketoacidosis (DKA) or hyperosmolar hyperglycemic nonketotic syndrome (HHNS).

Nonadherence to the medical regimen is frequently a cause of hyperglycemia. Effective long-term management of blood glucose levels reduces the risk for vascular complications of diabetes mellitus. These complications include nephropathy, neuropathy, retinopathy, cerebrovascular disease, and coronary artery disease.

Frequent episodes of hypoglycemia in individuals with previously diagnosed diabetes indicate the need to evaluate diabetes management. QSEN: Patient-centered care; Safety.

Autonomic symptoms represent the action of counterregulatory hormones, initially epinephrine, to the effects of lowered blood glucose levels. Neuroglycopenic symptoms occur because of the depletion of glucose in the central nervous system.

All cases of hypoglycemia are caused by excess insulin in relation to available nutrients.

15 to 20 g of carbohydrate should raise blood glucose levels 30 to 45 mg/dL. Examples of 15-g sources include 3 to 4 glucose tablets, 8 to 10 Lifesavers candies, and 4 to 6 ounces of fruit juice. Glucose-containing products will produce faster results than those containing fat or protein.

Hypoglycemia can largely be prevented by appropriate self-management behaviors.

Nonadherence to a treatment plan may occur because of limited resources for purchasing medications and blood glucose monitoring supplies. Some costs may not be covered by health insurance. The social worker can determine the patient's eligibility for financial assistance. QSEN: Teamwork and collaboration.

The patient and family need to recognize the goals of diet therapy, such as the following: normalize blood glucose and lipid values, improve eating habits, restrict caloric intake, achieve moderate weight loss, maintain a consistent carbohydrate intake at meals and snacks, and decrease fat intake. Successful outcomes for nutritional management require not only active participation by the patient but also participation by family members. The person responsible for meal planning and preparation needs to have a good understanding of nutritional management for diabetes.

The patient needs to participate in a periodic review of progress to achieving previously set blood glucose goals. Positive feedback on goal attainment helps motivate the patient to continue with health behaviors for effective diabetes management. QSEN: Patient-centered care.

■ = Independent   ▲ = Interprofessional Collaboration

Actions/Interventions

- Instruct the patient in how to use blood glucose results in overall diabetes management: review the basics of pattern management.

- Instruct the patient in diabetes management during illness:

  - Take all diabetes medications.

  - Self-monitor blood glucose every 2 to 4 hours.

  - Test the urine for ketones every 3 to 4 hours if blood glucose is consistently greater than 300 mg/dL in the presence of abdominal pain, nausea, or vomiting.
  - Drink 8 ounces of fluids every 4 hours: sugar-free drinks are recommended when the patient is able to maintain normal carbohydrate intake. Substitute drinks containing sugar when the individual is unable to eat solid food because of anorexia.
- Instruct the patient in how and when to take additional rapid- or short-acting insulin as directed.
- Instruct when to contact the primary care provider: blood glucose levels greater than 300 mg/dL, vomiting for more than 2 to 4 hours, failure of urinary ketones to clear within 12 hours, symptoms of dehydration, or symptoms suggesting the development of DKA or HHNS.
- Instruct the patient to carry medical identification at all times.

- Instruct the patient about planning for diabetes management when traveling, such as putting medications in carry-on luggage.

Rationales

Using blood glucose monitoring results allows the patient to make adjustments in food intake, exercise, and medication dosage to maintain therapeutic outcomes for blood glucose levels. Monitoring allows the patient to identify the onset of side effects of therapy or the onset of complications of the disease.

The patient needs to assume responsibility for managing his or her diabetes during episodes of illness. QSEN: Safety; Patient-centered care.

Insulin requirements increase with illness. The secretion of catecholamines, cortisol, and growth hormone in response to the stress of illness results in increased blood glucose levels.

An increased frequency of blood glucose testing provides information on the response of blood glucose to therapy.

Testing provides for the early detection of DKA.

Sufficient fluid intake is needed to prevent dehydration that occurs with hyperglycemia.

Administration of rapid-acting insulin may be required every 2 to 3 hours to treat hyperglycemia. QSEN: Safety.

Early treatment of hyperglycemia can prevent the occurrence of DKA or HHNS. QSEN: Safety.

It is important for medical personnel to be able to identify the patient as having diabetes to provide appropriate care in an emergency. QSEN: Safety.

Some travel may involve time changes that can disrupt the patient's usual routines. The patient needs to have easy and quick access to medications. QSEN: Safety.

NANDA-I
NDx **Risk for Injury: Feet**

Common Risk Factors

Hyperglycemia
Peripheral sensory neuropathy
Autonomic neuropathy
Immune system deficits
Vascular insufficiency

 Evolve   For additional care plans, go to http://evolve.elsevier.com/Gulanick/.

Common Expected Outcome

Patient is free of injury to feet.

NOC Outcomes

Tissue Integrity: Skin and Mucous Membranes; Self-Care: Hygiene; Knowledge: Treatment Regimen

NIC Interventions

Foot Care; Skin Surveillance; Nail Care; Teaching: Individual

Ongoing Assessment

Actions/Interventions	Rationales
■ Assess the general appearance of the foot.	Foot lesions and associated wound infections are the most common reason for hospitalization of the patient with diabetes. The patient's feet should be inspected at every visit. The patient may be unaware of injuries to the feet as a result of decreased sensation from peripheral neuropathy. Impaired vision may decrease the patient's ability to inspect the feet. QSEN: Safety.
■ Assess the status of the nails.	Fungal infections in nails serve as a portal of entry for bacteria. The patient with diabetes has an increased risk for infection because of impaired immunity. Patients with thickened, deformed, or ingrown nails should be referred to their primary care provider for appropriate treatment.
■ Assess the patient's skin integrity.	Autonomic neuropathy leads to decreased perspiration, causing excessive dryness and fissuring of the skin. Skin breakdown predisposes the patient to infection. QSEN: Safety.
■ Note the presence of callus formation or corns.	Pressure over bony prominences leads to callus formation. This condition can lead to the development of skin breakdown.
■ Assess the circulatory status of the foot by the palpation of peripheral pulses. A Doppler ultrasound transducer can be used when pulses are no longer palpable. • Dorsalis pedis • Posterior tibial	The foot is extremely vulnerable to circulatory changes from macrovascular complications of diabetes mellitus. The development of atherosclerosis is accelerated in the patient with diabetes as a result of alterations in lipid metabolism.
■ Assess for evidence of infection.	Infection may be the initiating event for eventual amputation. Symptoms of pain and tenderness may be absent because of neuropathy. Local symptoms include redness, drainage, and swelling. Systemic symptoms include fever and malaise, and loss of blood glucose control. QSEN: Safety.
■ Assess for edema.	Edema is a major predisposing factor to ulcerations. Autonomic neuropathy results in the loss of vasomotor reflexes and swelling in the foot.
■ Assess for protective sensation with a 5.07 monofilament.	The absence of protective sensation places the patient at high risk for foot injury. QSEN: Safety.
■ Examine the patient's hosiery and shoes for condition and fit.	Localized redness over bony prominences indicates the shoe is too tight.
■ Assess the patient's ability to reach his or her feet and perform self-examination and nail care.	This information provides a basis for future patient education and referrals for foot care. QSEN: Patient-centered care.

Endocrine and Metabolic Care Plans

■ = Independent ▲ = Interprofessional Collaboration

Therapeutic Interventions

Actions/Interventions	Rationales
■ Instruct the patient in the principles of hygiene: wash the feet daily in warm water using mild soap, but avoid soaking the feet. Dry carefully and gently, especially between the toes. Encourage the use of moisturizing lotion at least once daily. Avoid the area between the toes.	Maceration between the toes predisposes the patient to infection. The use of lotion replaces the moisturizing effects lost by autonomic neuropathy. The patient should select a lotion with low alcohol content to prevent further drying of the skin. QSEN: Safety.
■ Teach the patient to inspect the feet daily for cuts, scratches, and blisters. Use a mirror if necessary to examine the bottom of the foot. Instruct the patient to use both visual inspection and touch.	All surfaces of the foot need to be examined, including the skin between the toes. Touch will identify skin surface alterations that are not evident by sight. The patient may need the assistance of a family member or other caregiver to inspect the feet.
■ Report any signs of infection immediately to the primary care provider: 　• Areas of skin breakdown 　• Increase in temperature as compared with the same location on the opposite foot 　• Discharge that develops an odor	Early treatment is essential in the prevention of amputation. Clinical studies on amputations have found that as many as 85% of patients have foot ulcers before amputation. QSEN: Evidence-based practice; Safety.
■ Teach the patient to inspect shoes daily by feeling the inside of the shoe for irregularities in the lining, sharp objects in the sole of the shoe, or foreign bodies in the shoe.	Careful daily assessment reduces the risk for injury to the foot. Peripheral neuropathy and the loss of protective sensation limit the ability of the patient to feel irregularities that could precipitate an injury to the foot. QSEN: Safety.
▲ Instruct the patient in appropriate footwear. Have the foot size measured, and try shoes on before purchase.	*Width:* The widest part of the shoe must accommodate the widest part of the foot. *Length:* There should be $1\frac{1}{2}$ inches of space between the longest toe and the end of the shoe. *Toe box:* The toe box should be high with a rounded toe. *Heel height:* This should be less than 2 inches.
▲ Refer patients with structural abnormalities of the foot to a podiatrist or foot care specialist for evaluation and treatment.	These members of the interprofessional health team can help the patient manage structural foot problems. They can design custom-molded footwear for the patient. QSEN: Teamwork and collaboration.
■ Instruct the patient to wear clean, well-fitting stockings made from soft cotton, synthetic blend, or wool.	Soft cotton or wool absorbs moisture from perspiration and discourages an environment in which fungus can thrive.
■ Teach the patient to avoid thermal injuries by: 　• Testing the temperature of bathwater with the elbow, wrist, or a thermometer 　• Avoiding the use of heating pads, hot water bottles, or electric blankets 　• Maintaining a safe distance from heat sources such as the fireplace or space heater	Sensory neuropathy may result in a loss of normal pain and temperature sensation. These changes increase the risk for burns. QSEN: Safety.
■ Instruct patients to always wear protective footwear; never go barefoot.	Keeping the feet covered prevents injury to the foot. QSEN: Safety.
■ Instruct the patient to trim nails straight across and to file sharp corners to match the contour of the toe. Suggest that a family member or podiatrist trim the nails when the patient has visual impairment or has difficulty reaching his or her feet.	This technique avoids injury to the toes when self-care cannot be provided. QSEN: Safety; Teamwork and collaboration.
■ Instruct the patient to avoid self-treatment: 　• Do not use adhesive tape, wart treatments, corn plasters, or strong antiseptics.	Self-treatment of foot problems increases the patient's risk of skin ulceration, injury and infection. QSEN: Safety. Many over-the-counter agents contain salicylic acid, which can cause ulceration of the foot in the patient with diabetes.

Endocrine and Metabolic Care Plans

Actions/Interventions

- Do not use over-the-counter fungal products without the approval of the primary care provider.

- Avoid "bathroom surgery."

■ Stress the importance of maintaining normal blood glucose levels.

■ Encourage the patient to stop smoking.

Rationales

Over-the-counter products may increase microbial resistance and the risk for infection when they are used inappropriately.

Cutting away corns and calluses increases the risk for further foot injury and infection.

Elevated blood glucose or glycosylated hemoglobin levels are associated with a risk for foot ulcers. Hyperglycemia impairs wound healing. QSEN: Safety.

Chronic vasoconstriction, caused by smoking, reduces the ability of tissues to heal. QSEN: Safety.

Related Care Plans

Risk for infection, Chapter 2
Risk for impaired skin integrity, Chapter 2
Visual Impairment, Chapter 4
Peripheral arterial occlusive disease, Chronic, Chapter 5
Amputation, Lower extremity, Chapter 9
Chronic kidney disease, Chapter 11
Diabetic ketoacidosis and hyperglycemic hyperosmolar nonketotic syndrome, ⊖volve

---

Hyperthyroidism

Graves' Disease

Hyperthyroidism occurs as a result of increased circulating levels of thyroid hormones. Women are affected more often than men. The peak age for diagnosis of the disorder is 20 to 40 years. The most common cause is Graves' disease associated with Hashimoto's thyroiditis. This form of hyperthyroidism is an autoimmune disorder that contributes to a failure of the normal regulation of thyroid hormone secretion. Multiple genetic mutations transmitted as autosomal recessive traits increase susceptibility to Graves' disease. Other causes of hyperthyroidism include toxic multinodular goiter, thyroid gland tumors, and pituitary gland tumors. The clinical manifestations of

hyperthyroidism develop as a result of the hypermetabolic effects of increased thyroid hormones on all body systems. These manifestations include heat intolerance, irritability, restlessness, goiter, tachycardia, palpitations, increased blood pressure, diaphoresis, weight loss, increased appetite, diarrhea, visual changes, menstrual irregularities, and changes in libido. Thyrotoxic crisis or thyroid storm is a rare but severe form of hyperthyroidism that develops suddenly in response to excessive stress or poorly controlled hormone levels. The management of hyperthyroidism includes drug therapy, radioactive iodine therapy, and surgical removal of all or part of the thyroid gland.

Endocrine and Metabolic Care Plans

NANDA-I NDx Deficient Knowledge

Common Related Factors

Alteration in cognitive functioning
Insufficient information
Insufficient interest in learning
Insufficient knowledge of resources
Misinformation presented by others

Defining Characteristics

Insufficient knowledge of hyperthyroidism
Inaccurate follow-through of instruction
Inappropriate behavior

■ = Independent   ▲ = Interprofessional Collaboration

Common Expected Outcome

Patient and family verbalize correct information about hyperthyroidism and its treatment.

NOC Outcomes
Knowledge: Hyperthyroidism; Knowledge: Medication; Information Processing

NIC Interventions
Health Literacy Enhancement; Learning Facilitation; Teaching: Individual

---

Ongoing Assessment

Actions/Interventions	Rationales
■ Assess the patient's current knowledge of hyperthyroidism.	This information provides the starting base for educational sessions. The patient may have misconceptions about the cause of symptoms he or she is experiencing. QSEN: Patient-centered care.
■ Assess the ability to learn, remember, or perform desired health-related care.	Cognitive impairments need to be identified so an appropriate teaching plan can be designed. The patient with hyperthyroidism experiences a hypermetabolic state that leads to hyperactivity with fatigue and cyclic changes in mood. These manifestations may contribute to a decreased attention span and impaired concentration.
■ Determine the patient's or the caregiver's self-efficacy to learn and apply new knowledge about hyperthyroidism and its treatment.	A first step in teaching may be to foster increased self-efficacy in the patient's ability to learn the desired information or skills. The patient may experience difficulty with some of lifestyle changes that may be part of the management of hyperthyroidism.

Therapeutic Interventions

Actions/Interventions	Rationales
■ Teach the patient and family about hyperthyroidism.	Knowledge of the disease process and its manifestations helps the patient and family understand treatment options. This information aids the patient in assuming responsibility for care at a later time. The family may be more supportive with new understandings of the disease and its manifestations. QSEN: Patient-centered care.
■ Provide a quiet, calm atmosphere without interruptions.	Fatigue and cyclic changes in mood that occur with hyperthyroidism may contribute to a decreased attention span and impaired concentration. Teaching sessions may need to be short and planned at times when the patient can concentrate and pay attention. Learning new information requires using energy that may aggravate fatigue.
■ Teach the patient and family measures to manage symptoms, conserve energy, and promote comfort: • Environmental control • Frequent rest periods • Delegation of activities, especially those requiring fine motor control	Until hormone levels are reduced with drug or radiation therapy, the patient and family need to know how to manage symptoms associated with increased metabolic activity. The patient may have heat intolerance and diaphoresis. A cool environment with dim lighting will promote comfort and encourage rest. The patient may be hyperactive and experience fine motor tremors that interfere with activities requiring fine motor control. The family needs to support the patient by helping with these activities. Balancing periods of rest with periods of hyperactivity will help conserve the patient's energy. QSEN: Patient-centered care.

Actions/Interventions

- ■ Reinforce information the patient has received about treatment options for hyperthyroidism:

  - • Antithyroid medications such as propylthiouracil (PTU)

  - • Iodine preparations

  - • Radioactive iodine (^{131}I)

  - • Beta-adrenergic antagonists

  - • Surgical removal of all or part of the thyroid.

Rationales

Information provided by the physician may need to be repeated frequently. Written information needs to be available to reinforce verbal instructions. The patient and family can make informed decisions about treatment based on this information. QSEN: Teamwork and collaboration; Evidence-based practice; Safety.

These medications work by blocking iodide binding in the thyroid gland. This action decreases the production of thyroid hormones. PTU also interferes with the conversion of T_4 to T_3, the more potent of the two hormones. The patient needs to learn the importance of taking the drug at evenly spaced intervals during the day to achieve the maximum therapeutic benefit. Because of the chance of liver toxicity, the patient needs information about appropriate symptoms to report and follow-up care for laboratory studies of liver function.

Iodine is given most often before surgery and for a very short term of therapy. It acts to decrease the vascularity of the thyroid gland and promote the storage of hormone in the gland. The patient needs to understand that iodine may have a metallic taste.

^{131}I is taken up by the cells of the thyroid gland. This therapy is a form of local radiation that destroys a portion of the thyroid gland and thereby reduces hormone production. The therapy takes several weeks to provide the patient with significant symptom relief, so other antithyroid drugs may be given early in the therapy. The patient and family need to understand that the level of radioactivity is low and quickly clears from the body. Special safety precautions are not needed. Most patients achieve therapeutic benefit after one treatment. The patient may develop hypothyroidism after the treatment, depending of the amount of gland tissue destroyed. Thyroid replacement therapy may be required. The patient and family will need to learn the signs and symptoms of hypothyroidism.

Beta-blockers inhibit the increased sympathetic nervous system activity associated with hyperthyroidism. The drugs are given to aid in the management of symptoms such as tachycardia, palpitations, and tremors. This class of drugs has no direct effect on the thyroid gland or its hormones.

Surgery is reserved usually for patients who develop a large goiter that impairs breathing or swallowing.

NANDA-I
NDx **Imbalanced Nutrition: Less Than Body Requirements**

Common Related Factors	Defining Characteristics
Insufficient dietary intake	Weight loss with adequate food intake
Biological factors (increased metabolic demands)	Body weight 20% or more below ideal weight range

(side tab) Endocrine and Metabolic Care Plans

 = Independent   ▲ = Interprofessional Collaboration

Common Expected Outcomes

Patient or caregiver verbalizes and demonstrates selection of foods or meals that will achieve a cessation of weight loss. Patient weighs within 10% of ideal weight range.

NOC Outcomes

Nutritional Status: Nutrient Intake; Knowledge: Prescribed Diet

NIC Interventions

Nutritional Monitoring; Nutrition Management; Teaching: Prescribed Diet

Ongoing Assessment

Actions/Interventions	Rationales
■ Assess the patient's weight.	The patient with hyperthyroidism will experience an unintentional decrease in body weight because of an increased basal metabolic rate.
■ Assess the patient's appetite.	The patient is likely to report experiencing a significant increase in appetite and sensations of hunger. This inverse relationship between the person's increased appetite and decreasing weight is a characteristic finding in hyperthyroidism.
■ Assess the patient's typical food intake through a 24-hour recall.	Determining the patient's typical intake provides a basis for an individualized plan of nutrition support for the patient's increased metabolic needs. QSEN: Patient-centered care.

Therapeutic Interventions

Actions/Interventions	Rationales
■ Help the patient select foods that provide a balanced diet with increased calories in the form of carbohydrates and proteins.	The high T_3 and T_4 levels create an increased demand for calories to support the high metabolic rate of cells. The patient may need more than 3000 calories per day to support metabolic activity. Protein catabolism exceeds protein anabolism in hyperthyroidism, creating a state of negative nitrogen balance. QSEN: Patient-centered care.
■ Provide increased fluid intake.	Additional fluid intake is necessary to support the increased metabolic activity. Increased diaphoresis is a common manifestation of hyperthyroidism. This change puts the patient at risk for fluid volume deficit. QSEN: Safety.
■ Encourage the patient to eat small, frequent meals and snacks.	Eating five to six small meals throughout the day requires less energy than eating three larger meals. This approach will help the patient increase caloric intake without adding to fatigue.
■ Encourage the patient and family to have foods available that are easy to eat such as sandwiches and other "finger foods."	The patient may be too restless and hyperactive to sit down for regular meals. Foods that can be eaten while the patient is moving around will help support increased nutritional intake.
■ Teach the patient to limit foods that increase peristaltic activity.	Diarrhea is a common manifestation of hyperthyroidism. Foods that are highly seasoned or have high insoluble fiber content are more likely to aggravate the diarrhea.
▲ Provide supplemental vitamins and minerals.	The higher basal metabolic rate increases the need for additional vitamins and minerals. Supplements will correct preexisting deficiencies and prevent recurrence.
▲ Refer the patient and family to members of the interprofessional health team.	The registered dietitian can provide the patient and family with resources to increase nutritional intake. QSEN: Teamwork and collaboration.

Disturbed Body Image
NANDA-I NDx

Common Related Factor
Alteration in body function (due to goiter or exophthalmos)

Defining Characteristics
Preoccupation with change in appearance of face and neck
Refusal to acknowledge change in appearance
Wears dark glasses and clothing that conceals bulging eyes and enlarged neck

Common Expected Outcome
Patient demonstrates enhanced body image and self-esteem as evidenced by ability to talk positively about changes in appearance.

NOC Outcomes
Body Image; Self-Esteem
NIC Interventions
Body Image Enhancement; Self-Esteem Enhancement

Ongoing Assessment

Actions/Interventions

■ Assess the patient's perception of changes in appearance related to goiter or exophthalmos.

■ Assess the patient's current behavior related to goiter and exophthalmos.

■ Note the frequency of the patient's comments about his or her appearance related to an enlarged neck or bulging eyes.

Rationales

A change in appearance that is highly visible to the patient and others may create more of a threat to the patient's body image. QSEN: Patient-centered care.

The patient may ignore the changes in appearance or be preoccupied with hiding or covering the changes. The patient may use dark glasses to cover the eyes and scarves or high-necked shirts to cover the goiter. The patient may avoid public gatherings because of embarrassment.

The extent of the patient's response is more related to the value or importance the patient places on the part of the body than the actual value or importance. Negative statements by the patient about changes in appearance indicate a limited ability to integrate the change into the patient's self-concept.

Therapeutic Interventions

Actions/Interventions

■ Provide the patient with information about goiter and exophthalmos.

■ Encourage the verbalization of feelings about the changes in appearance.

Rationales

Accurate information about these changes in physical appearance will support the patient's cognitive appraisal of the changes. Goiter develops from hypertrophy and hyperplasia of the thyroid tissue as a result of increased hormone levels. The gland may be three to four times its normal size. Exophthalmos develops as a result of proptosis, eyelid retraction, muscle swelling, and orbital tissue edema. The patient has a wide-eyed stare with protruding eyes. Although goiter may regress with hyperthyroidism therapy, exophthalmos may not regress. QSEN: Patient-centered care; Evidence-based practice.

Expressions of positive and negative feelings may enhance the patient's coping strategies. QSEN: Patient-centered care.

■ = Independent ▲ = Interprofessional Collaboration

Actions/Interventions

- Help the patient identify ways of coping that have been effective in the past.

- Maintain appropriate eye contact and positive caring when interacting with the patient.

- Assist the patient with adaptive behaviors.

Rationales

Patients have experienced body image changes in the past as part of normal growth and development or other illnesses or injury. Coping strategies that were effective then may be effective in this situation.

Health care providers represent a microcosm of society, and their actions and behaviors are scrutinized as the patient develops coping strategies.

Wearing dark glasses not only promotes visual comfort for the patient with exophthalmos but also conceals the bulging eyes and startled appearance. Clothing and accessories may help cover the enlarged neck or divert attention to other parts of the body.

NANDA-I
NDx   Risk for Hyperthermia

Common Risk Factor

Increased basal metabolic rate

Common Expected Outcome

The patient maintains body temperature below 39°C (102.2°F).

NOC Outcomes
Thermoregulation; Vital Signs
NIC Interventions
Temperature Regulation; Fever Treatment

Ongoing Assessment

Actions/Interventions

- Assess the patient's body temperature.

- Assess the patient's response to environmental temperature.

- Assess for precipitating factors.

Rationales

Tympanic or rectal temperature measurement provides the most accurate indication of core body temperature.

The patient with hyperthyroidism has poor regulation of body temperature in response to environmental temperature. The patient's heat intolerance may be manifested as wearing less clothing than expected for environmental temperature or using other means of cooling such as fans or air conditioners. QSEN: Patient-centered care.

Hyperthermia may be a manifestation of thyroid storm or thyroid crisis. This condition occurs with poorly controlled hyperthyroidism or during periods of extreme physical or emotional stress. QSEN: Safety.

Therapeutic Interventions

Actions/Interventions

- Maintain a cool environmental temperature.

Rationales

Heat intolerance is a common manifestation of hyperthyroidism because of the increased basal metabolic rate. Cooler room temperatures promote patient comfort and assist in reducing stress. QSEN: Patient-centered care; Safety.

Actions/Interventions

- Encourage the patient to wear light, loose clothing. Use an electric fan to circulate room air.
- Provide an increased fluid intake.

- Encourage frequent bathing with tepid water.

- Monitor the patient's adherence to therapy for hyperthyroidism.

Rationales

These measures promote evaporative cooling of the body.

Diaphoresis is a common manifestation of hyperthyroidism. Increased fluid losses contribute to an elevated body temperature. QSEN: Safety.

This measure not only promotes the evaporative cooling of the body but also promotes patient comfort.

Patients who are inconsistent taking prescribed antithyroid medications increase the risk for developing thyroid crisis and hyperthermia. QSEN: Safety.

Related Care Plans

Anxiety, Chapter 2
Diarrhea, Chapter 2
Fatigue, Chapter 2
Insomnia, Chapter 2
Thyroidectomy, Chapter 13

Hypothyroidism

Myxedema; Goiter

Hypothyroidism occurs because of a deficiency in thyroid hormone. Almost every system in the body is affected through a general slowing of metabolic processes. The disorder is common, especially among women older than 30 years of age. In the older adult, hypothyroidism may be overlooked because many of the manifestations are similar to changes associated with the normal aging process (constipation, intolerance to cold, decreased activity tolerance, weight gain, lethargy, decreased short-term memory, depression). The most common cause of hypothyroidism is an autoimmune inflammation (Hashimoto's thyroiditis) of the thyroid gland with resulting atrophy of glandular tissue. Hypothyroidism may also develop after a thyroidectomy. Myxedema occurs in hypothyroidism as a result of hyaluronic acid accumulation in tissues. Fluid binds to the hyaluronic acid,

producing skin puffiness most noticeable around and below the eyes. Myxedema also causes enlargement of the tongue, which contributes to the impaired speech patterns of the patient with hypothyroidism. When hypothyroidism goes undiagnosed or undertreated, the patient may develop myocardial hypotonic function and ventricular dilation. The patient is at risk for developing decreased cardiac output and systemic tissue and organ hypoxia. This situation is a rare occurrence called myxedema coma and is considered life threatening. Goiter, enlargement of the thyroid gland, may occur when hypothyroidism is the result of decreased hormone synthesis. When hormone production is reduced, thyroid-stimulating hormone (TSH) secretion increases owing to lack of negative feedback. The size of the thyroid gland increases as a result of TSH stimulation.

NANDA-I
NDx Imbalanced Nutrition: More Than Body Requirements

Common Related Factors

Excessive intake in relation to metabolic need
Metabolic disorders

Defining Characteristics

Weight 20% more than ideal for height and frame
Triceps skin fold measurement greater than 15 mm in men, 25 mm in women

■ = Independent   ▲ = Interprofessional Collaboration

Endocrine and Metabolic Care Plans

Common Expected Outcomes

Patient verbalizes measures necessary to achieve beginning weight reduction.

Patient demonstrates appropriate selection of meals or menu planning toward the goal of weight reduction.

NOC Outcomes
Nutritional Status: Nutrient Intake; Knowledge: Hypothyroidism

NIC Interventions
Nutritional Monitoring; Nutrition Management; Teaching: Hypothyroidism

Ongoing Assessment

Actions/Interventions	Rationales
■ Assess the patient's weight.	Patients with hypothyroidism experience weight gain related to the slowing of metabolic processes and excess fluid volume.
■ Assess the patient's appetite.	Patients with hypothyroidism experience a decreased appetite. This inverse relationship between decreased appetite and increasing weight is a characteristic finding in hypothyroidism.
■ Assess the patient's typical food intake through a 24-hour recall.	Determining the patient's typical intake provides a basis for an individualized plan of nutrition support for the patient's changing metabolic needs. QSEN: Patient-centered care.

Therapeutic Interventions

Actions/Interventions	Rationales
■ Teach the patient to follow a low-calorie, low-cholesterol, low-saturated-fat diet.	Because of the decreased metabolic rate, the patient requires fewer calories to support metabolic activity. The patient with hypothyroidism tends to have higher cholesterol levels.
■ Teach the patient and family about the effect of hypothyroidism on body weight.	The patient and family need to understand the inverse relationship between weight gain and appetite in hypothyroidism. When thyroid hormone replacement therapy is initiated, the patient may experience weight loss. However, appetite may increase. This change may require a calorie-controlled diet to prevent additional weight gain. QSEN: Safety; Patient-centered care.
▲ Consult with members of the interprofessional health team to determine the patient caloric needs.	The registered dietitian can calculate appropriate caloric requirements to maintain nutrient intake and achieve a stable weight. QSEN: Teamwork and collaboration.
■ Provide assistance and encouragement as needed at mealtime.	Because of decreased energy levels, the patient may need help with eating to ensure the adequate intake of essential nutrients.
■ Encourage the patient to eat six small meals throughout the day.	This approach to eating may promote an adequate intake of nutrients in the patient with decreased energy levels.
■ Teach the patient about sources of dietary fiber.	Constipation is a common manifestation of hypothyroidism. Dietary fiber attracts water into the fecal mass to keep it soft and easier to pass.

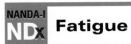

Fatigue

Common Related Factor

Hypometabolic state

Defining Characteristics

Impaired ability to maintain usual level of physical activity
Tiredness/lethargy
Drowsiness
Listlessness
Increase in rest requirements
Impaired ability to maintain usual routines
Insufficient energy
Alteration in concentration

Common Expected Outcomes

Patient verbalizes reduction of fatigue as evidenced by reports of increased energy and ability to perform desired activities.
Patient demonstrates use of energy-conservation principles.

NOC Outcomes

Fatigue Level; Fatigue: Disruptive Effects; Activity Tolerance; Endurance; Energy Conservation; Self-Care: Activities of Daily Living (ADLs)

NIC Interventions

Activity Therapy; Energy Management

Ongoing Assessment

Actions/Interventions

■ Assess the patient's ability to perform activities of daily living (ADLs).

■ Assess the patient's energy level and muscle strength and tone.

Rationales

Because of a reduced metabolic rate, the patient may experience fatigue with minimal exertion. Fatigue can limit the patient's ability to participate in self-care and perform his or her role responsibilities. QSEN: Patient-centered care.

Slowing of metabolism results in decreased energy levels. Muscles may be weaker and joints stiffer because of mucin deposits in joints and interstitial spaces. This type of cellular edema may contribute to delayed muscle contraction and relaxation. The patient may report generalized weakness and muscle aches.

Therapeutic Interventions

Actions/Interventions

■ Help the patient identify desired activities and responsibilities.

■ Encourage the patient to keep a daily log of energy levels and activities for at least 1 week.

■ Assist the patient with developing a schedule for daily activity and rest. Stress the importance of frequent rest periods.

Rationales

Activities that are important to the patient should be planned during those times of the day when the patient usually has the most energy. QSEN: Patient-centered care.

A record of energy levels and activities will help the patient identify periods of peak energy.

A plan that balances periods of activity with periods of rest can help the patient complete desired activities without adding to levels of fatigue. Not all self-care activities need to be completed at one time, such as the morning. Likewise, not all housework needs to be completed in a day.

Endocrine and Metabolic Care Plans

■ = Independent ▲ = Interprofessional Collaboration

Actions/Interventions

- Teach energy-conservation techniques.

- ▲ Refer to an occupational therapist as needed.

- Teach the patient that activity tolerance and endurance will improve in response to thyroid medication.

Rationales

Patients and caregivers may need to learn skills for delegating tasks to others, setting priorities, and clustering care to use available energy to complete desired activities. Organization and time management can help the patient conserve energy and reduce fatigue.

The occupational therapist can reinforce energy-conservation techniques and provide the patient with assistive devices as needed. QSEN: Teamwork and collaboration.

Thyroid hormone supplements will gradually increase cellular metabolism, with a resulting increased energy level. In patients with preexisting cardiac disease, increases in the metabolic rate may precipitate angina because of the increased demands on the heart. QSEN: Safety.

NANDA-I NDx Deficient Knowledge

Common Related Factors

Alteration in cognitive functioning
Insufficient information
Insufficient interest in learning
Insufficient knowledge of resources
Alteration in memory
Misinformation presented by others

Common Expected Outcome

Patient and family members verbalize correct information about hypothyroidism and taking thyroid hormone supplements.

Defining Characteristics

Insufficient knowledge of hypothyroidism and its treatment
Inaccurate follow-through of instruction
Inappropriate behavior

NOC Outcomes

Knowledge: Hypothyroidism; Knowledge: Medication

NIC Interventions

Health Literacy Enhancement; Learning Facilitation; Teaching: Hypothyroidism; Teaching: Prescribed Medication

---

Ongoing Assessment

Actions/Interventions

- Assess the patient's current knowledge of hypothyroidism and thyroid hormone replacement therapy.
- Assess the ability to learn, remember, or perform desired health-related care.

- Determine the patient's or the caregiver's self-efficacy to learn and apply new knowledge to the management of hypothyroidism.

Rationales

This information provides the starting base for educational sessions. QSEN: Patient-centered care.

Cognitive impairments need to be identified so an appropriate teaching plan can be designed. The patient with hypothyroidism may experience impaired memory, a decreased attention span, hearing loss, and confusion. These neurological changes can interfere with learning new information.

Self-efficacy refers to a person's confidence in his or her ability to perform a behavior. The patient needs to understand that taking thyroid hormone replacement medication may be a lifetime commitment to disease management.

Therapeutic Interventions

Actions/Interventions	Rationales
■ Teach the patient and family about hypothyroidism.	Impaired memory and decreased attention span that occur with hypothyroidism will influence the patient's ability to learn new information. Teaching sessions should be planned at times when the patient is best able to concentrate. Information may need to be repeated to facilitate learning. Written information reinforces verbal presentations. QSEN: Patient-centered care.
■ Teach the patient and family about taking thyroid hormones. • Review the expected benefits and possible side effects. • Encourage the patient to keep follow-up appointments for blood work. • Instruct the patient to take the dose in the morning to reduce the chances of insomnia.	Levothyroxine sodium (Synthroid) is a synthetic thyroid hormone used most often for hormone replacement therapy. Thyroid hormone should be taken on a regular schedule to achieve hormone balance. It may take several weeks or longer for a full therapeutic benefit to be noticed. The patient is usually started on a small dose that is gradually increased until a euthyroid state is achieved. Serum TSH levels will be monitored to asses for the euthyroid state. As thyroid hormone levels increase, the patient may experience weight loss and insomnia. The patient needs to report symptoms such as palpitations or chest pain. These symptoms may occur as the metabolic rate and oxygen consumption increase. Hormone replacement therapy is usually a lifelong commitment. QSEN: Evidence-based practice; Safety.
■ Encourage the patient to carry medical identification about hormone therapy and to inform all health care providers.	Medical identification provides other health care providers with information to guide decisions about care. Levothyroxine is highly protein bound in circulation. This drug characteristic contributes to many drug interactions. The patient needs to notify all health care providers about taking this drug. QSEN: Safety.

Related Care Plans

Constipation, Chapter 2
Disturbed body image, Chapter 2
Hypothermia, ⊖volve

Endocrine and Metabolic Care Plans

■ = Independent   ▲ = Interprofessional Collaboration

CHAPTER 14

Integumentary Care Plans

Burns

Partial Thickness Skin Loss; Full Thickness Skin Loss

Although the incidence of burn injury is on the decline, more than 450,000 burns still occur in the United States annually. More than half of them require hospitalization in one of the specialized burn centers across the country. Thirty-five percent of all burn injuries occur in children. Mortality rate has improved over the years because of Advanced Burn Life Support, regional burn care, and early excision; overall mortality rate is approximately 4%. The most common mechanism of injury is thermal, which can be from a flame, scald, or direct contact, but burn injuries also present because of chemical, electrical, and radiation sources. The pediatric and geriatric populations are most vulnerable because of integumentary and immunological risks. Burn care ranges from major to minor, and care ranges from the emergent through the rehabilitative phase of injury.

NANDA-I NDx Impaired Skin Integrity

Common Related Factors

Major burn
Minor burn

Defining Characteristics

Blanching of skin
Redness
Leathery appearance
Skin color changes: brown to black
Blistering, weeping skin
Pain or absence of pain
Skin loss

Common Expected Outcomes

Patient receives appropriate wound care for degree of burn.
Patient exhibits satisfactory wound healing at burn sites.
Unburned skin remains intact and free of infection.

NOC Outcomes

Burn Healing; Burn Recovery; Wound Healing: Secondary Intention

NIC Interventions

Wound Care: Burns; Wound Irrigation

Ongoing Assessment

Actions/Interventions	Rationales
■ Assess the percentage of body surface burned. Use the Lund-Browder chart (age-appropriate body surface chart).	Assessment is commonly used to determine the total body surface area (TBSA) involved. TBSA estimation should include only partial- and full-thickness injury, not superficial. For quick assessment, the "rule of nines" is commonly used to estimate the extent of burns. Another method is that the patient's palm represents 1% TBSA, which is a helpful measuring tool when burns are scattered. The more precise calculation can be achieved using laser Doppler imaging that determines the amount of perfusion of the injured tissue. Accurate calculation of TBSA is critical in determining fluid replacement therapy. QSEN: Evidence-based practice.
■ Identify and document the location of burns.	Treatment is determined by the TBSA involved and location of burns.
■ Assess the depth of the wounds: • Epidermal and/or superficial: painful, pink, not blistered • Partial-thickness: painful, red or pink, often blistered • Full-thickness: anesthetic (not painful because of destruction of the nerves), charred, gray, white	The deeper the wound, the greater the risk for infection, complications, and wound contractures.
■ Note areas where the skin is intact.	These areas must be cared for and preserved; they may serve as graft donor sites later.
■ Assess the degree of pain.	Full-thickness burns are anesthetic (painless) as a result of nerve destruction. Partial-thickness burns can cause severe pain because of exposed nerve endings. The patient may have deeper pain sensations from muscle ischemia.
■ Assess for adherent debris or hair.	Wound debris and any remaining surface hair can be sources of contamination. Epithelial migration in the healing wound is delayed if the wound is not clear of devitalized tissue.

Therapeutic Interventions

Actions/Interventions	Rationales
Major burns: ■ Provide a clean sheet.	The burn wound is not a sterile wound, so a sterile field is not required.
▲ Clean the burn wound with antimicrobial soap and water.	The wound must be cleansed with antibacterial soap to remove nonviable skin and rinsed thoroughly with water after cleansing to remove soap. This reduces the risk for infection. QSEN: Safety.
▲ Use hydrotherapy as prescribed.	Hydrotherapy aids in cleansing and loosening slough, exudate, and eschar. Wound debridement is necessary to provide a clean area for healing. A shower cart is often used to assist with this procedure.

Integumentary Care Plans

■ = Independent   ▲ = Interprofessional Collaboration

Actions/Interventions

▲ Apply topical bacteriostatic substances (e.g., silver sulfa-diazine if the patient is not allergic to sulfa, bacitracin [Neosporin], silver-coated dressings, mafenide [Sulfamylon]), as ordered.

■ Elevate the extremities, if possible.
■ Dress the wounds.

■ Keep the body and limbs in a correct anatomical position.
▲ Administer analgesics before wound care, debridement, or dressing changes.

▲ Treat facial wounds as ordered.

Minor burns:
■ Clean the burn wound with antimicrobial soap and water.

▲ Apply topical bacteriostatic and antimicrobial medications as ordered. Cover the wound with a dry, sterile dressing.
▲ Treat blisters as ordered.

■ Instruct the patient and caregiver in necessary medical follow-up care.

■ Teach the patient and caregiver about the appearance of a clean, noninfected burn wound.

Rationales

Topical agents may be applied directly to the wound or impregnated into the bandage. These substances prevent the removal of granulating skin and reduce the risk for infection. Topical agents provide some protection to the wound surface. This is a closed method that provides comfort and prevents wound desiccation. If an open method of wound care is used, the area is left open to air after ointment application. The risk with this method is increased heat loss. Some topical ointments/creams need to be changed daily. Others such as Acticoat, Mepilex Ag, and Aquacel Ag contain slower release antimicrobials within the dressing and can stay in place for up to a week. QSEN: Safety.

Elevation reduces swelling.

Dressings prevent burn-to-burn contact. The closed method of wound care uses gauze dressings to cover burn surfaces. The dressings may be soaked with antimicrobial solutions.

Correct positioning prevents contractures.

Patient comfort and cooperation with wound care are promoted with the administration of analgesics. Patients must have procedural, background, and breakthrough pain medications.

Facial burns may require an open or closed dressing depending on the depth of the burn (more superficial burns may be left open to air). Use caution when wrapping over the ears to minimize pressure. Place dry gauze in the ear to prevent the accumulation of topical agents. Avoid placing undue pressure on the ears; do not put a pillow under the head of a patient with ear burns.

This removes debris and reduces the risk for infection. The wound must be cleansed with antibacterial soap to remove nonviable skin and rinsed thoroughly with water after cleansing to remove soap. QSEN: Safety.

Topical applications prevent the removal of granulating skin and reduce the risk for infection. QSEN: Safety.

If blisters are located on an area that is not limiting mobility and not at risk for breaking, leave them intact; otherwise, debride the wound because blister fluid can be an excellent medium for bacteria.

The healing of burn wounds varies depending on the depth of the burn. A partial-thickness burn takes 3 to 4 weeks for healing. Full-thickness burns require surgical intervention for healing. Scar maturation occurs during the rehabilitative phase, which is 1 year after injury in adults. QSEN: Patient-centered care.

Clean, noninfected burn wounds are pink and moist; produce clear yellow (serous) drainage; and are odor-free. Any deviation from this should be reported to the health care provider. QSEN: Safety.

Integumentary Care Plans

NANDA-I NDx Risk for Infection

Common Risk Factors

Impaired skin integrity
Damage to respiratory mucosa
Presence of dead skin
Poor nutrition

Common Expected Outcome

Patient remains free of infection, as evidenced by normal temperature, normal white blood cell (WBC) count, and healing wounds.

NOC Outcomes
Risk Control; Risk Detection; Immune Status
NIC Interventions
Environmental Management; Surveillance; Infection Protection

Ongoing Assessment

Actions/Interventions	Rationales
■ Monitor temperature, and notify the physician if it exceeds 38.5°C (101.3°F).	Patients with burn injury are at an increased risk for infection because of the wounds and compromised immune function. An elevated temperature should arouse suspicion of infection. QSEN: Safety.
▲ With each dressing change, monitor the wound for erythema surrounding the burn, a change in the exudate color or amount, or the presence of odor from the dressing. Obtain a wound culture as indicated. Notify the physician if any change is noted.	The burn patient is at risk for infection. Appropriate topical or systemic agents can be customized after culture results are obtained. QSEN: Safety.
▲ Monitor the WBC count.	An increasing WBC count indicates the body's efforts to combat pathogens. However, in older patients, infection can be present without an increased WBC count. QSEN: Safety.
■ Monitor endotracheal secretions, and obtain a bronchial alveolar lavage specimen if the patient is febrile.	This technique provides the optimal specimen for culture analysis.
▲ Monitor all invasive lines; use antimicrobial-coated catheters when appropriate. When catheters are removed, send the tips for culture if the patient is febrile.	Indwelling catheters represent a break in the body's normal first line of defense, are a source of infection, and require meticulous care. QSEN: Safety.
▲ Monitor the effectiveness of the topical agent by culturing the wound, as prescribed.	Vigilant monitoring helps reduce the consequences of infection.

Therapeutic Interventions

Actions/Interventions	Rationales
■ Maintain aseptic technique in caring for wounds.	To prevent nosocomial contamination, the nurse should wear protective coverings when caring for the patient. Gowns, gloves, masks, shoe covers, and hair covers may be needed. QSEN: Safety.
■ Trim or shave hair around the wound (except eyebrows, because this area never grows back).	Hair removal decreases contamination.

■ = Independent ▲ = Interprofessional Collaboration

Integumentary Care Plans

Actions/Interventions	Rationales
▲ Treat blisters as ordered.	Blisters are left intact if they are not impairing mobility and have little risk for breaking. Blister fluid acts as a natural barrier and facilitates healing. However, when a blister is broken, blister fluid is an excellent medium for bacterial growth.
▲ Apply topical agents (e.g., silver sulfadiazine if not allergic to sulfa, bacitracin [Neosporin], mafenide [Sulfamylon], silver-coated dressing), as prescribed.	Topical agents provide some protection to the wound surface. They may be applied directly to the wound or impregnated into the bandage. QSEN: Safety.
■ Implement isolation precautions if needed.	Strict isolation may be necessary to prevent infection in the immunocompromised burn patient. Methicillin-resistant *Staphylococcus aureus* (MRSA) surveillance screening should be performed on admission for all patients and appropriate isolation instituted as needed. QSEN: Safety.
▲ Administer intravenous (IV) antibiotics, which may be prescribed prophylactically but should be specific to the cultured organism when identified.	IV antibiotics may be useful in treating systemic infection. However, wound infections, especially those near eschar, may be treated more easily with topical agents and debridement. QSEN: Safety.
■ Provide frequent perineal care, using diversion catheters as needed.	A Foley catheter or a bowel management system (e.g., Zassi) may be required to divert fecal material for large body surface area burns. Contamination of wounds can lead to infection and impaired wound healing. QSEN: Safety.
▲ Cover wounds with graft material or dressings as prescribed:	Covering burn wounds reduces fluid loss and protects the wound from invasion by bacteria. Early excision and grafting are desirable. Infection is the greatest threat to survival for the burned patient; covering wounds decreases the opportunity for contamination and therefore decreases the risk for infection. QSEN: Safety; Evidence-based practice.
• Biological dressings: • Xenografts	Xenografts are temporary grafts and generally are skin from another species, typically porcine (pig) skin.
• Homograft	Homograft is skin from another human, typically cadaver skin or banked frozen skin. This temporary skin is used to provide coverage in preparation for autograft.
• Autograft	Healthy skin is taken from elsewhere on the patient's body; grafting is carried out in an operating room.
• Synthetic dressings	Synthetic dressings are temporary dressings to cover wounds. Many products are available for use on partial-thickness burns or as temporary skin substitutes for full-thickness burns. Many of these dressings are transparent, allowing easier visualization of the wound status.
• Biosynthetic dressings	These dressings consist of nylon fabric that is partially embedded into a silicone film. Collagen is incorporated into both materials. It is the nylon fabric that comes into direct contact with the skin.
■ Before discharge, teach the patient or caregiver to monitor the wound's appearance and drainage.	A change in the drainage color or amount may indicate infection. Patients need to be able to recognize important signs and changes in their condition so early treatment can be initiated. QSEN: Safety.
■ Before discharge, teach the patient or caregiver to monitor his or her body temperature.	A temperature greater than 38.5°C (101.3°F) may indicate infection. Vigilant monitoring helps reduce the consequences of infection. QSEN: Safety.

Actions/Interventions

▲ On ventilated patients, elevate the head of the bed 30 degrees, provide oral care, and administer histamine-2 blockers and antacids, as ordered. Suction without the use of instilled saline.

Rationales

More compromised patients require mechanical ventilation that offers additional infection risks. The Centers for Disease Control and Prevention (CDC) provides these guidelines for the prevention of nosocomial pneumonia in ventilated patients. QSEN: Evidence-based practice.

NANDA-I NDx — Risk for Deficient Fluid Volume

Common Risk Factors

Inflammatory response to burn with protein and fluid shifts
Massive fluid shifting and circulating volume loss
Hemorrhage; stress ulcer (Curling's ulcer)
Extremes of age

Common Expected Outcomes

Patient maintains normal fluid volume, as evidenced by systolic blood pressure (BP) 90 mm Hg or greater (or patient's baseline), urine output greater than 30 mL/hr, and heart rate (HR) 60 to 100 beats/min.
Burn shock is prevented.

NOC Outcomes

Fluid Balance; Hydration; Electrolyte and Acid/Base Balance

NIC Interventions

Intravenous (IV) Insertion; Fluid/Electrolyte Management; Electrolyte Management: Hyperkalemia; Shock Prevention; Medication Administration

---

Ongoing Assessment

Actions/Interventions

■ Assess for the signs and symptoms of fluid volume deficit.

▲ Monitor laboratory results for alterations in acid-base balance, catabolism (outpouring of potassium and nitrogen), and altered electrolyte levels.

■ Monitor urine specific gravity.

Rationales

With burns, fluid shifts from the intravascular to extravascular space because of an increased capillary permeability; the first 24 to 48 hours are the most critical. Also, insensible loss from areas of lost skin are dramatically increased, adding to fluid volume deficit. *Note:* Restlessness, tachycardia, hypotension, thirst (thirst is a sensitive indicator of fluid deficit and hemoconcentration), pale and cool skin, oliguria (urine output < 30 mL/hr, indicating inadequate renal perfusion), and hypoxia (as interstitial spaces fill with fluid, alveolar oxygen exchange is impaired) are common signs and symptoms. Fluid volume deficit is directly proportional to the extent and depth of the burn injury. QSEN: Safety.

Decreased tissue perfusion leads to a buildup of lactic acid and metabolic acidosis. Tissue destruction initially causes hyperkalemia. When capillary integrity is restored, excess potassium is eliminated and may lead to hypokalemia.

Very concentrated urine (specific gravity > 1.020) indicates fluid volume deficit; a urine output of 30 to 50 mL/hr indicates adequate perfusion.

Integumentary Care Plans

■ = Independent   ▲ = Interprofessional Collaboration

Actions/Interventions

▲ Evaluate hemoglobin and hematocrit.

■ Weigh the patient daily, taking care to use the same scale and bedding.

Rationales

Elevated hemoglobin and hematocrit occur with fluid volume deficit and hemoconcentration.

Changes in body weight may be better indicators of fluid balance than intake and output records.

Therapeutic Interventions

Actions/Interventions

▲ Assist with IV and central line placements.

▲ Administer crystalloid solutions as prescribed.

▲ Administer colloid solutions as prescribed.

▲ Administer tube feedings.

Rationales

These IV lines are used for rapid fluid resuscitation to prevent circulatory collapse. Multiple large-bore lines or a central line may be required.

The amount and rate are calculated on the basis of total body surface area (TBSA) and depth of the wound, using the Parkland formula. Over the first 24 hours according to the Parkland formula, give 4 mL of lactated Ringer's solution per percentage TBSA burn per kilogram body weight as follows: half in the first 8 hours, one fourth in the second 8 hours, and one fourth in the third 8 hours. The Parkland formula is a resuscitation guideline. Patients may require more or less fluid based on their response to resuscitation. Patients with delayed presentation, dehydration, full-thickness injury, and inhalation injury may require more fluid than indicated by the Parkland formula. QSEN: Evidence-based practice.

As capillary permeability is decreased, colloid solutions may be used to restore and maintain vascular volume and correct sodium imbalances.

Feedings minimize the potential for gastric bleeding and paralytic ileus, which can further add to fluid volume deficit.

NANDA-I
NDx Risk for Ineffective Breathing Pattern

Common Risk Factors

Burns to head and neck
Circumferential chest burns
Massive edema
Inhalation of smoke or heated air

Common Expected Outcome

Patient maintains an effective breathing pattern, as evidenced by relaxed breathing at normal rate and depth, absence of dyspnea, and normal values for arterial blood gases (ABGs).

NOC Outcome
Respiratory Status: Ventilation
NIC Interventions
Airway Management; Respiratory Monitoring

Integumentary Care Plans

Ongoing Assessment

Actions/Interventions	Rationales
■ Assess for the presence of burns to the face and neck.	Facial burns may indicate that smoke inhalation and possible airway injury have occurred.
■ Assess for edema of the head, face, and neck.	As fluid shift begins to occur, the oral airway and trachea become constricted, decreasing the patient's ability to breathe.
■ Assess for a history and evidence of smoke inhalation.	Inhalation injury usually occurs when the fire was in a closed space. It can lead to respiratory failure or carbon monoxide poisoning (see Risk for Poisoning: Carbon Monoxide, later in this care plan).
■ Assess the respiratory rate, rhythm, and depth; assess breath sounds.	Respiratory rate and rhythm changes are early warning signs of impending respiratory difficulties. Crackles may be heard if fluid is accumulating from a direct burn injury or as a result of fluid shifts associated with fluid resuscitation. QSEN: Safety.
■ Assess for dyspnea, shortness of breath, the use of accessory muscles, cough, and the presence of cyanosis.	As moving air in and out of the lungs becomes more difficult, the breathing pattern alters to include use of accessory muscles to move the air. These manifestations suggest progressive hypoxia. QSEN: Safety.
▲ Monitor ABGs.	The combined effect of airway edema and the accumulation of interstitial fluid results in decreased alveolar ventilation. The patient may be hypoxemic (decreased Pao_2) or have metabolic or respiratory acidosis. QSEN: Safety.
▲ Use pulse oximetry to monitor oxygen saturation.	Pulse oximetry is a useful tool to detect changes in oxygenation. Oxygen saturation should be at 90% or greater.
■ Assess for changes in the level of consciousness.	Restlessness, confusion, or irritability can be early signs indicative of hypoxia. Lethargy and somnolence are late signs of hypoxia. QSEN: Safety.
▲ Review the chest x-ray study results.	Chest x-ray studies will reflect changing lung status.

Therapeutic Interventions

Actions/Interventions	Rationales
■ Raise the head of the bed, and maintain good body alignment.	This position promotes optimal diaphragmatic and lung excursion and chest expansion to facilitate breathing efforts.
▲ Maintain a humidified oxygen delivery system.	Initially patients may receive 100% oxygen to maintain oxygen saturation. Humidity decreases the viscosity of secretions.
▲ Provide chest physical therapy if burns are not to the chest.	Chest physical therapy loosens the secretions caused by stasis.
■ Encourage the use of incentive spirometry.	Incentive spirometry promotes deep inspiration, which increases oxygenation and prevents alveolar collapse.
▲ Be prepared for intubation and mechanical ventilation.	When edema is severe, an artificial airway may be the only means of ventilating the severely burned patient. QSEN: Safety.
▲ Be prepared for escharotomy.	Burns of the chest may cause restriction and constriction that decreases chest expansion; escharotomy (cutting through or removing eschar) will be needed to alleviate constricted movement.

■ = Independent   ▲ = Interprofessional Collaboration

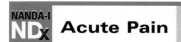 **Acute Pain**

Common Related Factors

Burn injury
Wound cleansings and dressings

Defining Characteristics

Self-report of pain using a standardized pain scale
Facial expression of pain
Protective behavior
Self-focused
Narrowed focus
Change in physiological parameter (e.g., BP, HR, respiratory rate)

Common Expected Outcomes

Patient reports satisfactory pain control at a decreased level using a standardized pain scale.
Patient uses pharmacological and nonpharmacological pain relief strategies.
Patient exhibits increased comfort such as relaxed muscle tone and baseline levels for BP, HR, and respirations.

NOC Outcomes

Comfort Status; Medication Response; Pain Control

NIC Interventions

Analgesic Administration; Pain Management; Patient-Controlled Analgesia (PCA); Distraction

---

Ongoing Assessment

Actions/Interventions

- Assess the type, location, quality, and severity of the pain or discomfort.

- Monitor the patient's HR, BP, restlessness, and ability to focus.

Rationales

The pain experience varies with the extent of the burn injury. Partial-thickness burns are very painful; pain will decrease over time and with healing. Full-thickness burns do not cause pain because of nerve destruction, but as nerves regenerate, pain will increase. As wound healing begins, the patient may report pruritus. Relief of this discomfort is important because scratching can disrupt fragile new skin or grafts. QSEN: Patient-centered care.

Increasing pain can cause transient increases in respiratory and cardiac rates and BP. Many burn patients are intubated and therefore are unable to make their needs known. Attention to associated signs may help the nurse in evaluating pain.

Therapeutic Interventions

Actions/Interventions

- ▲ Administer sedatives and analgesics prescribed for pain, evaluating their effectiveness.
- Provide background, procedural, and breakthrough pain control.
- ▲ Consider the use of patient-controlled analgesia.

- Avoid pressure on injured tissues; use a bed cradle.
- Alleviate all unnecessary stressors or sources of discomfort.

Rationales

Opioids are the drug of choice. Adjuvant drugs such as sedatives, hypnotics, and psychotropics may be added.

Many burn patients have pain all the time, so they require three types of control.

This method of analgesic administration allows the patient to manage pain relief within prescribed limits and increases the patient's sense of control over pain. QSEN: Patient-centered care.

A bed cradle keeps linens off the legs.

A quiet, relaxed environment aids in promoting comfort.

Integumentary Care Plans

Actions/Interventions

- Allay fears and anxiety.
- Turn the patient; obtain a pressure-relieving mattress or bed, as needed.
- ▲ Premedicate the patient for dressing changes; allow sufficient time for the medication to take effect.
- Moisten dressings with water to allow for trauma-free removal of dressings.
- Use distraction and relaxation techniques as indicated.

Rationales

Fear may intensify the perception of pain.

These interventions help relieve pressure points and improve circulation to painful areas.

The manipulation of burn surfaces increases the patient's pain.

This technique eases dressing removal by loosening adherents and decreasing pain.

These complementary therapies can be effective. Distraction heightens one's concentration on nonpainful stimuli to reduce the awareness and experience of pain. Relaxation techniques bring about a state of physical and mental awareness and tranquility.

NANDA-I NDx **Risk for Ineffective Peripheral Tissue Perfusion**

Common Risk Factors

Blockage of microcirculation
Blood loss
Compartment syndrome (edema restricting circulation)
Circumferential eschar

Common Expected Outcome

Patient maintains optimal tissue perfusion to extremities, as evidenced by strong palpable pulses, reduction in absence of pain, warm dry extremities, and normal sensation in extremity.

NOC Outcomes
Circulation Status; Tissue Perfusion: Peripheral
NIC Interventions
Circulatory Care: Arterial Insufficiency; Circulatory Care: Venous Insufficiency; Vital Signs Monitoring

---

Ongoing Assessment

Actions/Interventions

- Check the pulses of all extremities; use Doppler ultrasound if necessary. Notify the physician immediately of any noted alteration in perfusion.

- Monitor the patient's BP and HR for abrupt changes.

- Assess the color and temperature of the extremities.

- Check for pain, numbness, or swelling of the extremities.

Rationales

Weak, thready pulses may not be palpable. Also, feeling pulses through extremely edematous tissue or skin covered with eschar may be difficult. Doppler ultrasound is a noninvasive way to more accurately measure BP. QSEN: Safety.

Stable BP is necessary to maintain adequate tissue perfusion. An abrupt drop in BP and change in HR can indicate decreased blood flow secondary to severe third-spacing (movement of fluid into spaces normally without fluid), which impedes venous return. QSEN: Safety.

Cool, discolored extremities indicate compromised tissue perfusion. This situation, if untreated, can result in limb loss. QSEN: Safety.

Circumferential burns with eschar are most likely to cause altered tissue perfusion to the extremities, because as fluid shift occurs and eschar cannot stretch, pressure is exerted on the tissue, vessels, and nerves. QSEN: Safety.

Integumentary Care Plans

■ = Independent   ▲ = Interprofessional Collaboration

Therapeutic Interventions

Actions/Interventions

- Maintain good alignment of the extremities. Elevate the extremities on pillows or in a specially made sling.
- ▲ Apply a sequential compression device on the nonburned extremities.
- Perform passive range of motion if needed.

- ▲ Prepare for and assist with fasciotomy or escharotomy to treat full-thickness circumferential burns.

Rationales

Careful positioning allows for adequate blood flow without compression on the arteries, also reducing edema.

Compression devices improve venous return, thereby reducing the risk for clot formation in the legs of at-risk patients.

Exercise reduces venous stasis and further circulatory compromise.

Escharotomy (incision through the burn crust) or fasciotomy (incision through eschar and fascia) are indicated when the circulation is compromised as a result of increased pressure in the burned limb. This procedure relieves the compression of nerves or blood vessels.

NANDA-I NDx **Risk for Poisoning: Carbon Monoxide**

Common Risk Factor

Smoke inhalation

Common Expected Outcome

Patient maintains normal oxygen and carboxyhemoglobin levels.

NOC Outcome
Respiratory Status: Gas Exchange
NIC Intervention
Oxygen Therapy

Ongoing Assessment

Actions/Interventions

- Monitor for carbon monoxide poisoning in any burn patient.
- ▲ Measure carboxyhemoglobin levels on admission to the emergency department.

- Monitor for dyspnea, headache, and confusion, which may accompany carbon monoxide poisoning.

Rationales

Poisoning is seen especially in patients with other signs and symptoms of smoke inhalation or facial burns. QSEN: Safety.

Carbon monoxide has a high affinity for the hemoglobin molecule; when hemoglobin molecules are bound to carbon monoxide, they are not available to transport oxygen. QSEN: Safety.

At low carboxyhemoglobin levels (<10%), the patient may be asymptomatic or report a headache. Dizziness, nausea, and syncope occur at carboxyhemoglobin levels above 20%. Seizures and coma develop in patients with carboxyhemoglobin levels above 40%. QSEN: Safety.

Therapeutic Interventions

Action/Intervention

- ▲ Administer 100% humidified oxygen. Anticipate the administration of hyperbaric oxygen in some cases.

Rationale

The patient may require airway intubation and mechanical ventilation to support an effective airway and gas exchange. According to the American Burn Association's clinical practice guidelines, hyperbaric oxygen is indicated if carbon monoxide poisoning is the only injury, because increasing the delivery of 100% oxygen at increased pressure is theorized to reduce the half-life of carboxyhemoglobin. QSEN: Evidence-based practice.

Integumentary Care Plans

ⓔvolve   For additional care plans, go to http://evolve.elsevier.com/Gulanick/.

NANDA-I NDx   Risk for Imbalanced Nutrition: Less Than Body Requirements

Common Risk Factors

Prolonged interference in ability to ingest or digest food
Increased basal metabolic rate
Loss of protein from dermal wounds

Common Expected Outcome

Patient maintains an adequate nutritional intake, as evidenced by stable weight.

NOC Outcomes
Nutritional Status: Biochemical Measures;
Nutritional Status: Food and Fluid Intake
NIC Interventions
Nutrition Therapy; Nutritional Monitoring

Ongoing Assessment

Actions/Interventions	Rationales
■ Obtain the patient's base weight; weigh daily if possible, using the same scale and linens.	Such consistency facilitates accurate measurement and evaluation. Weight gain is an indicator of improved nutritional status. However, a sudden gain of more than 2 pounds in a 24-hour period usually indicates fluid retention.
■ Measure fluid intake and output, including oral and IV intake.	Changes in fluid balance can be reflected in daily weight changes. All snacks, foods from home, and items that are liquid at room temperature (gelatin, sherbet) should be included as oral intake.
■ Closely monitor the patient's caloric intake.	Patients with major burns may require a 50% to 100% increase in calorie intake to keep up with their hypermetabolic state and wound protein loss. QSEN: Patient-centered care.
▲ Monitor the skin test results for cellular immunity.	Anergic patients (those unable to muster a cellular immune response) are seriously nutritionally depleted.
▲ Monitor the patient's serum albumin levels.	Serum albumin gives an indication of protein reserve. Levels less than 2.5 g/dL indicate serious protein depletion and are linked to higher morbidity and mortality risks.
■ Monitor the residuals of enteral feeding.	Early enteral feeding may be started upon admission to prevent paralytic ileus. Continuous feedings may be held if residual volume is greater than 50% of the amount delivered in 1 hour.
▲ Monitor the patient's nitrogen balance.	If nitrogen output is greater than nitrogen intake, the patient will become nutritionally depleted.
■ Determine the environmental or situational factors (pain, odors, unpleasant sounds) that may affect eating.	These factors can diminish appetite. QSEN: Patient-centered care.

Therapeutic Interventions

Actions/Interventions	Rationales
▲ Consult a dietitian to assist in meeting the patient's nutritional needs.	Dietitians have a greater expertise in calculating caloric needs. The Curreri formula is used to calculate the caloric needs for the burn patient to support homeostasis and wound healing: (25 kcal × Usual body weight [in kg]) + (40 kcal × %TBSA) = Calories. The patient may need 1.5 to 3 g/kg per day of protein to maintain nitrogen balance. QSEN: Teamwork and collaboration.

■ = Independent   ▲ = Interprofessional Collaboration

Integumentary Care Plans

Actions/Interventions

▲ Provide nutritional supplementation and replacement as needed.

■ Plan dressing changes or other unpleasant situations away from mealtime.
■ Involve the patient in the selection of the menu to the extent possible.

▲ Administer tube feedings as ordered.

Rationales

Multivitamins, zinc, vitamin C, phosphorus, magnesium, and calcium are often provided daily or as needed based on laboratory results. Such supplements can be used to optimize balanced nutritional intake.

Comfort enhances the patient's interest in eating.

Involving patients in their own nutritional care has been found to raise the intake of protein and energy levels. QSEN: Patient-centered care.

The gastrointestinal tract is the most efficacious route for the absorption and use of nutrients. Feedings may be continuous or intermittent. See also Enteral Nutrition in Chapter 4.

NANDA-I
NDx Deficient Knowledge

Common Related Factors

Insufficient information
Insufficient interest in learning
Misinformation presented by others
Insufficient knowledge of resources

Defining Characteristics

Insufficient knowledge
Inaccurate follow-through of instruction
Inappropriate behavior

Common Expected Outcome

Patient or caregiver verbalizes understanding and ability to care for wound, mobilize resources, get follow-up care, and report signs of complication.

NOC Outcomes

Knowledge: Treatment Regimen; Coping; Family Participation in Professional Care

NIC Interventions

Health Literacy Enhancement; Learning Facilitation; Discharge Planning; Support System Enhancement; Teaching: Disease Process; Teaching: Psychomotor Skill

---

Ongoing Assessment

Actions/Interventions

■ Assess the need for ongoing wound or graft site care.

■ Assess the patient's perceived ability to care for self after discharge.

■ Assess resources (environmental and human) in the home that can be tapped for assistance.

■ Assess the need for continued rehabilitation (occupational therapy [OT], physical therapy [PT], psychosocial support).

Rationales

Grafted skin is delicate and at a continued risk for breakdown and infection. Patients must have a comprehensive understanding of the physical care required after discharge.

Patients will be responsible for evaluating their condition on a daily basis to make determinations about preventive strategies and therapeutic interventions. This information may give some perspective on home care needs. QSEN: Patient-centered care.

Although family and friends can be great allies, they sometimes may have trouble dealing with the complexities of long-term follow-up.

A variety of factors (e.g., inability to cope with body image changes; guilt about the injury or the cause of fire or accident; need for further reconstructive surgery; use of scar prevention garments) may require care for months beyond hospital discharge. QSEN: Patient-centered care.

---

evolve   For additional care plans, go to http://evolve.elsevier.com/Gulanick/.

Therapeutic Interventions

Actions/Interventions	Rationales
▲ Involve a social worker or case manager early in the course of hospitalization.	Discharge planning may be a complicated process requiring a long period of planning. QSEN: Teamwork and collaboration.
■ Instruct the patient or caregiver in wound care of graft sites and donor sites: continue to use aseptic technique until the wound is completely healed; cover open wounds with gauze; keep wounds clean and moisturized with a lanolin-based cream; avoid sun exposure of newly grafted skin.	Careful wound care is essential because infection and contractures can occur during the rehabilitative phase of burn recovery. QSEN: Safety.
■ Instruct the patient in the care and use of scar-prevention garments, which are usually worn at all times (removed for bathing and wound care) up to 18 months after injury.	The use of pressure garments and dressings can control the development of hypertrophic scarring. These may need to be replaced often to maintain the elasticity sufficient for their purpose.
■ Instruct the patient or caregiver to report any of the following: signs or symptoms of wound infection; limitation of movement, which can result from delayed contracture formation; the inability to cope with disfigurement, role change.	Early identification of signs of infection or contractures facilitates needed treatment. Difficulty adjusting to the home and loss after a burn injury is common. Additional support with coping will be necessary with integration back into society during the rehabilitative phase. QSEN: Safety.
■ Instruct the patient about pruritus, which is commonly present during the rehabilitative phase.	Patients can manage pruritus better if they are educated. Antihistamines, increased lotion, and oatmeal baths may help alleviate symptoms. Patients should avoid caffeine, nicotine, and chocolate because they can increase pruritus.
■ Encourage the patient or caregiver to maintain a follow-up schedule with the physician, registered nurse, PT, and OT, as well as social services.	Patients who become co-managers of their care have a greater stake in achieving a positive outcome. QSEN: Patient-centered care; Teamwork and collaboration.

NANDA-I NDx Disturbed Body Image

Common Related Factors
Massive edema
Visible burns
Dressings
Loss of function secondary to burns or burn treatment
Scarring or contractures
Loss of normal skin color
Use of scar-prevention garments

Defining Characteristics
Avoids looking at or caring for altered body part
Negative feeling about body
Nonverbal response to change in body part
Preoccupation with change

Common Expected Outcome
Patient demonstrates enhanced body image, as evidenced by ability to verbalize feelings, participate in self-care, and reintegrate into activities of daily living (ADLs) as capable.

NOC Outcomes
Body Image; Social Involvement; Social Support

NIC Interventions
Grief Work Facilitation; Body Image Enhancement; Coping Enhancement; Active Listening; Presence

Ongoing Assessment

Actions/Interventions	Rationales
■ Note the patient's ability to look at burns or dressings and his or her reactions to them.	Denial, looking away, or refusing to participate may indicate body image disturbance or may represent a normal stage of the grieving process.

■ = Independent   ▲ = Interprofessional Collaboration

Actions/Interventions	Rationales
■ Note the frequency and tone of critical remarks directed toward the self regarding appearance or function.	The extent or severity of response is highly related to the value placed on a body part or function affected. Negative statements about the affected body part indicate a limited ability to integrate the change into the patient's self-concept. QSEN: Patient-centered care.
■ Assess the perceived impact of the actual change on ADLs, social behavior, personal relationships, and occupational activities.	This may give some perspective on any perceived misconceptions that could affect recovery. QSEN: Patient-centered care.

Therapeutic Interventions

Actions/Interventions	Rationales
■ Demonstrate positive caring in routine activities.	Professional caregivers are a "testing ground" for societal reaction to appearance; a supportive relationship facilitates coping with body image disturbance.
■ Acknowledge the normalcy of the patient's emotional response to the actual or perceived change in body structure or function.	Experiencing the stages of grief over change or loss of a body part or function is normal. The length of time varies between patients.
■ Encourage the verbalization of feelings about the changed body.	It is worthwhile to encourage the patient to separate feelings about changes in the body from feelings of self-worth. The expression of feelings can enhance the patient's coping strategies. QSEN: Patient-centered care.
■ Help the patient identify actual changes.	Patients may perceive changes that are not actually present. Scar maturation may take up to 2 years. Skin appearance may continue to improve during that time.
■ Assist the patient in identifying frightening or worrisome potential situations; role-play responses.	This technique gives the patient "practice" in responding to staring, questions, unwanted sympathy, and thoughtless behaviors that he or she may encounter.
■ Encourage attendance at a support group.	Participation in support groups may allow the patient to realize that others have the same problem and that he or she may use this as a means to find suggestions for specific care challenges.

Related Care Plans

Deficient fluid volume, Chapter 2
Ineffective coping, Chapter 2
Gastrointestinal bleeding, Chapter 8

Pressure Ulcers (Impaired Skin Integrity)

Pressure Sores; Decubitus Ulcers; Bedsores

Pressure ulcers are a major health problem. Nurses play a key role in prevention and successful treatment. The National Pressure Ulcer Advisory Panel defines pressure ulcer as "a localized injury to the skin and/or underlying tissue usually over a bony prominence, as a result of pressure or pressure in combination with shear and/or friction." Prolonged pressure occurs when tissue is between a bony prominence and a hard surface such as a mattress. The pressure compresses small blood vessels and leads to ineffective tissue perfusion. Loss of perfusion causes tissue hypoxia and eventually cellular death. In addition to prolonged pressure, friction and shearing force contribute to the development of pressure ulcers. These forces are present when a patient slides down in bed and is pulled

⊝volve For additional care plans, go to http://evolve.elsevier.com/Gulanick/.

up against the surface of the mattress. Pressure ulcers are usually staged to classify the degree of tissue damage observed.* Pressure ulcers stage I through III can heal with aggressive local wound treatment and proper nutritional support; stage IV pressure ulcers often require surgical intervention (e.g., flap closure, plastic surgery). Pressure ulcers affect persons, regardless of age, who are immobile, are malnourished, or have contributing conditions (e.g., incontinence, decreased level of consciousness). Wound care remains a challenge for nurses and the health care team. More research in wound healing is needed. This care plan is based on recommendations from the 2015 National Pressure Ulcer Advisory Panel, the National Guideline Clearinghouse, and the Agency for Healthcare Research and Quality Pressure Ulcer Prevention Guidelines. This care plan addresses care issues in hospital, long-term care, or home settings. The Joint Commission's National Patient Safety Goals require that all patients admitted to a health care facility or home care agency be assessed for pressure ulcer risk.

NANDA-I NDx Impaired Skin Integrity

Common Related Factors

Extremes of age
Inadequate nutrition
Mechanical factors (friction, shear, pressure)
Pressure over bony prominences
Impaired circulation
Alteration in sensation
Moisture
Radiation therapy
Chronic disease state
Immunodeficiency

Defining Characteristics

Destruction of skin layers
Disruption of skin surfaces
Invasion of body structures
Pressure ulcer stages
- Deep tissue injury (new stage):
  - Purple or maroon localized area of intact skin or blood-filled blister resulting from pressure damage of underlying soft tissue
- Stage I:
  - Nonblanchable redness of a localized area usually over a bony prominence; area may be painful, firm, soft, warmer or cooler than adjacent tissue
  - Epidermis intact
- Stage II:
  - Partial-thickness skin loss
  - Shallow, open ulcer with a red-pink wound but without slough; may have an intact or open or ruptured serum-filled blister
- Stage III:
  - Full-thickness tissue loss
  - Subcutaneous fat may be visible
  - Bone, tendon, or muscle is not exposed
  - Slough may be present; may include undermining and tunneling
- Stage IV:
  - Full-thickness tissue loss with exposed muscle, bone, joint, or body cavity
  - Usually has adherent necrotic material (slough)
  - Undermining and tunneling may develop
- Unstageable: Depth unknown
  - Full-thickness tissue loss in which actual depth of ulcer is completely obstructed by slough or eschar in the wound bed

*Panel for the Treatment of Pressure Ulcers. *Treatment of Pressure Ulcers: Clinical Practice Guideline, No. 15* (AHCPR Pub No. 95-0652). Rockville, MD, 1994, Agency for Health Care Policy and Research, Public Health Service, U.S. Department of Health and Human Services.

Integumentary Care Plans

■ = Independent   ▲ = Interprofessional Collaboration

Common Expected Outcomes

Patient receives stage-appropriate wound care, experiences pressure reduction, and has controlled risk factors for prevention of additional ulcers.

Patient experiences healing of pressure ulcers.

NOC Outcomes

Wound Healing: Secondary Intention; Tissue Integrity: Skin and Mucous Membranes

NIC Interventions

Pressure Ulcer Prevention; Pressure Ulcer Care; Positioning; Pressure Management

Ongoing Assessment

Actions/Interventions	Rationales
▪ Use an objective tool for pressure ulcer risk assessment: • Braden scale • Norton scale	These are validated tools for risk assessment. The Braden scale is the most widely used. It consists of six subscales: sensory perception, moisture, activity, mobility, nutrition, and friction and/or shear. *Acute care:* Assessment should be carried out on all patients on admission and every 24 to 48 hours or sooner if the patient's condition changes. *Long-term care:* Assess on admission, weekly for 4 weeks, then quarterly and whenever the resident's condition changes (www.NPUAP.org). QSEN: Evidence-based practice.
▪ Assess the specific risk factors for pressure ulcers:	Even patients who already have a pressure ulcer continue to be at risk for further injury. Centers for Medicare and Medicaid Services recommends that nurses consider all potential risk factors for pressure ulcers beyond those noted on standard tools. QSEN: Evidence-based practice; Safety.
• Determine the patient's age and general condition of the skin.	The skin of older patients is less elastic, has less padding and moisture, and has thinning of the epidermis, making for a higher risk for skin impairment.
• Specifically assess the skin over bony prominences (sacrum, trochanters, scapulae, elbows, heels, inner and outer malleolus, inner and outer knees, back of the head).	These areas are at highest risk for breakdown resulting from tissue ischemia from compression against a hard surface.
• Assess the patient's awareness of the sensation of pressure.	Normally individuals shift their weight off pressure areas every few minutes; this occurs more or less automatically, even during sleep. Patients with decreased sensation are unaware of unpleasant stimuli (pressure) and do not shift weight, thereby exposing the skin to excessive pressure.
• Assess the patient's ability to move (shift weight while sitting, turn over in bed, move from the bed to a chair).	Immobility is the major risk factor in skin breakdown.
• Assess the patient's nutritional status, including weight, weight loss, and serum albumin levels, if ordered.	An albumin level less than 2.5 g/dL is a grave sign, indicating severe protein depletion. Patients with pressure ulcers lose large amounts of protein in wound exudates and may require 4000 kcal/day or more to remain anabolic.
• Assess for a history of radiation therapy.	Irradiated skin becomes thin and friable, may have less blood supply, and is at a higher risk for breakdown.
• Assess for fecal and urinary incontinence.	The urea in urine turns into ammonia within minutes and is caustic to the skin. Stool may contain enzymes that cause skin breakdown. Diapers and incontinence pads with plastic liners trap moisture and hasten breakdown.

Integumentary Care Plans

Actions/Interventions

- Assess for environmental moisture (wound drainage, excessive perspiration, high humidity).
- Assess the surface that the patient spends a majority of time on (mattress for bedridden patients, cushion for patients in wheelchairs).
- Assess the amount of shear (pressure exerted laterally) and friction (rubbing) on the patient's skin.

- Assess the skin on admission and daily for an increasing number of risk factors.
- Assess for a history of preexisting chronic diseases (e.g., diabetes, malignancy, acquired immunodeficiency syndrome [AIDS], or peripheral and/or cardiovascular disease).

■ Assess and stage the pressure ulcers (see Defining Characteristics, earlier in care plan).

■ Measure the size of the ulcer, and note the presence of undermining.

■ Describe the condition of the wound or wound bed:
- Color

- Odor

- Presence of necrotic tissue

- Visibility of bone, muscle, or joints

■ Assess for wound exudate.

Rationales

Moisture may contribute to skin maceration.

Patients who spend the majority of time on one surface need a pressure reduction or pressure relief device to lessen the risk for breakdown.

Shearing forces are most commonly noted on the sacrum, scapulae, heels, and elbows from skin-sheet friction, from semi-Fowler's positioning and repositioning, and from lift sheets.

The incidence of skin breakdown is directly related to the number of risk factors present.

Patients with chronic diseases typically manifest multiple risk factors (see above) that predispose them to pressure ulceration. These include poor nutrition, poor hydration, incontinence, and immobility.

Staging is important because it determines the treatment plan. Staging should be assessed at each dressing stage. It reflects whether the epidermis, dermis, fat, muscle, bone, or joint is exposed. If the ulcer is covered with necrotic tissue (eschar), it cannot be accurately staged. Stage I ulcers are difficult to detect in darkly pigmented skin. The use of mirrors or a penlight may be helpful.

The ulcer dimensions include length, width, and depth. An ulcer begins in the deepest tissue layers before the skin breaks down. Therefore the opening of the skin's surface may not represent the true size of the ulcer.

The color of tissue is an indication of tissue viability and oxygenation. White, gray, or yellow eschar may be present in stage II and III ulcers. Eschar may be black in stage IV ulcers.

Odor may arise from infection present in the wound; it may also arise from necrotic tissue. Some local wound care products may create or intensify odors and should be distinguished from wound or exudate odors.

Necrotic tissue is tissue that is dead and eventually must be removed before healing can take place. Necrotic tissue exhibits a wide range of appearances: thin, white, shiny, brown, tough, leathery, black, hard.

In stage IV pressure ulcers, these may be apparent at the base of the ulcer. Wounds may demonstrate multiple stages or characteristics in a single wound (i.e., healthy tissue with granulation may be present along with necrotic tissue).

Exudate is a normal part of wound physiology and must be differentiated from pus, which is an indication of infection. Exudate may contain serum, blood, and white blood cells and may appear clear, cloudy, or blood-tinged. The amount may vary from a few cubic centimeters, which are easily managed with dressings, to copious amounts not easily managed. Drainage is considered "excessive" when dressing changes are needed more often than every 6 hours.

Integumentary Care Plans

■ = Independent   ▲ = Interprofessional Collaboration

Actions/Interventions	Rationales
■ Assess the condition of wound edges and surrounding tissue.	Surrounding tissue may be healthy or may have various degrees of impairment. Healthy tissue is necessary for the use of local wound care products requiring adhesion to the skin. The presence of healthy tissue demarcates the boundaries of the pressure ulcer.
■ Assess ulcer healing, using a pressure ulcer scale for healing (PUSH) tool. Consider also using picture-taking per institutional protocol.	This tool provides standardization in the measurement of wound healing. It quantifies surface area, exudate, and the type of wound tissue. It is located at the National Pressure Ulcer Advisory Panel website (www.NPUAP.org). Digital picture-taking of wound status facilitates ongoing comparisons of healing. QSEN: Evidence-based practice.
■ Assess the patient's pain level, especially related to dressing changes and procedures.	The Joint Commission mandates frequent and regular assessments of pain. Prophylactic medications may be indicated. QSEN: Patient-centered care.

Therapeutic Interventions

Actions/Interventions	Rationales
■ Change the patient's position frequently: bed-bound people every 2 hours and chair-bound people every hour.	Position changes relieve pressure, restore blood flow, and promote skin integrity.
■ Use pressure-redistributing beds, mattress overlays, and chair cushions.	These devices redistribute pressure when frequent position changes are not possible. Avoid using doughnut-type devices and sheepskin for accomplishing redistribution goals.
▲ Clean the ulcer with a nontoxic solution such as normal saline (0.9%).	Cleansing the ulcer removes debris and bacteria, which promotes healing.
▲ Provide local wound care as follows:	The type and level of wound treatment depend on the staging of the ulcer and the type of infection present. QSEN: Evidence-based practice.
Stage I:	The goal is to prevent further damage and shearing away of the epidermis.
• Apply a flexible hydrocolloid dressing (e.g., DuoDerm, Sween-A-Peel) or a vapor-permeable membrane dressing (e.g., OpSite, Tegaderm).	These dressings prevent friction and shear.
• Apply vitamin-enriched emollient to the skin every shift.	Emollient moisturizes the skin.
• Apply a topical vasodilator (e.g., Proderm, Granulex).	A topical vasodilator increases circulation to the skin.
Stage II:	The goal is to prevent further damage and shearing away of the epidermis. A moist environment can aid wound healing.
• Hydrogels (Aqua Skin, Carrasyn V)	Hydrogels are used for shallow ulcers without exudates and promote wound debridement and healing.
• Hydrocolloids or a vapor-permeable membrane dressing	Hydrocolloids promote wound debridement and healing. Do not use with heavy exudate–producing wounds.
• Alginates (Kalginate, Kaltostat, Sorbsan)	Alginates are used for ulcers with exudates or moderate drainage. Avoid in both dry and heavily bleeding ulcers. They can be used in stage II to IV ulcers.
• Gauze with sodium chloride solution	This maintains a moist environment but requires multiple dressing changes. Dressings must be removed *while still wet*. Dressings absorb small amounts of drainage.
Stage III and IV:	
• Consult a plastic surgeon to perform a sharp debridement (the surgical removal of eschar)	This surgical procedure removes any necrotic thick eschar to promote future healing.
• Gauze with sodium chloride solution	This maintains a moist environment but requires multiple dressing changes as described for stage II.

Integumentary Care Plans

ⓔvolve   For additional care plans, go to http://evolve.elsevier.com/Gulanick/.

Actions/Interventions	Rationales
• Foams	Foams reduce odor and repel bacteria and water. They can be used with moderate to heavy drainage. They may macerate surrounding skin.
• Wound fillers	Wound fillers are used in conjunction with other dressings. They absorb exudates, fill the wound, and cause autolytic debridement.
• Debridement	Debridement is an important step in the overall management of ulcers. See *Other therapies* in the following section.
• Negative pressure wound therapy	See *Other therapies* in the following section.
• Palliative wound care	See *Other therapies* in the following section.
Other therapies:	
• Sharp debridement	Sharp debridement uses a scalpel or laser to remove devitalized tissue. It is very effective, especially when cellulitis or sepsis is involved.
• Mechanical debridement	Mechanical debridement uses a physical method for removing necrotic tissue, such as wet-to-dry gauze, which adheres to tissue and is later removed. Unfortunately, healthy granulation tissue often is also removed.
• Autolytic debridement	Autolytic debridement uses enzymes already present in the wound to dissolve the necrotic tissue, usually with a hydrocolloid or hydrogel.
• Enzymatic debridement (collagenase, chlorophyll, papain)	Enzymatic debridement uses proteolytic enzymes to remove necrotic tissues. These agents work by selectively digesting the collagen portion of the necrotic tissue. Care should be taken to prevent damage to surrounding healthy tissues.
• Biosurgery	Biosurgery uses maggots for quick debridement.
• Negative pressure wound therapy	Negative pressure wound therapy involves a device for draining stage III and IV wounds that would require frequent dressing changes. It decompresses the interstitial fluid in the wound, thus improving blood flow, promoting granulation tissue, and increasing fibroblasts. Serious bleeding can occur with this device so close patient monitoring is required.
• Topical growth factors	Colony-stimulating factors, fibroblast growth factors, and nerve growth factors are currently under study for pressure ulcers, though they have been found to be effective in diabetic and venous ulcers.
• Electrical stimulation	The application of a low-voltage current to a wound area can increase blood vessel growth and promote granulation.
• Palliative wound care	Palliative wound care may be an option for a patient with a chronic, nonhealing wound. These wounds occur in patients with preexisting debilitating disease. This option requires a comprehensive history as well as evaluation of the patient's goals for comfort and independence. Goals include control of symptoms, control of caregiver strain, and reduction of stress in the patient and family. Education must be conveyed that while the wound is nonhealing and remains open indefinitely, it can remain stable. These cases may require referral to a wound specialist.

Integumentary Care Plans

■ = Independent   ▲ = Interprofessional Collaboration

NANDA-I
NDx Risk for Infection

Common Risk Factors

Open pressure ulcer
Poor nutritional status
Proximity of sacral wounds to perineum

Common Expected Outcomes

Patient remains free of local or systemic infection, as evidenced by absence of copious, foul-smelling wound exudate.
Patient maintains normal body temperature.

NOC Outcomes

Risk Detection; Nutritional Status: Food and Fluid Intake

NIC Interventions

Infection Protection; Wound Care; Nutrition Management

Ongoing Assessment

Actions/Interventions	**Rationales**
■ Assess pressure ulcers for drainage, color of tissue, and odor.	All wounds produce exudate; the presence of exudate that is clear to straw-colored is normal. Purulent green or yellow drainage in large amounts typically indicates an infection, as does foul-smelling drainage. Infected tissue usually has a gray-yellow appearance without evidence of pink granulation tissue. QSEN: Safety.
▲ Obtain wound cultures, if available.	All pressure ulcers are colonized (i.e., will culture out bacteria) because skin normally has flora that will be found in an open skin lesion; however, not all pressure ulcers are infected. Infection is present when there is copious, foul-smelling, purulent drainage and the patient has other symptoms of infection (fever, increased pain) and a bacteria count greater than 10^5. Swab cultures are not recommended. Rather, tissue biopsy should be used to quantify and qualify the aerobic and anaerobic organisms present.
■ Assess the patient for unexplained sepsis.	When septic workup is done, the pressure ulcer must be considered a possible cause. QSEN: Safety.
■ Assess the patient's nutritional status.	Patients who are seriously nutritionally depleted (e.g., serum albumin <2.5 mg/dL) are at risk for developing infection produced by a pressure ulcer. In addition, patients with pressure ulcers lose tremendous amounts of protein in wound exudate and may require 4000 kcal/day or more to remain anabolic.
■ Assess for urinary and fecal incontinence.	Sacral wounds, because of their proximity to the perineum, are at highest risk for infection caused by urine or fecal contamination. It is sometimes difficult to isolate the wound from the perineal area. QSEN: Safety.
■ Monitor temperature.	Fever may indicate infection, unless the patient is immunocompromised or diabetic. QSEN: Safety.
▲ Monitor the white blood cell (WBC) count.	Elevated WBC counts may indicate infection, although in very old individuals, the WBC count may rise only slightly during an infection, indicating a diminished marrow reserve. QSEN: Safety.

Integumentary Care Plans

Therapeutic Interventions

Actions/Interventions	Rationales
▲ Provide local wound care as prescribed (see Impaired Skin Integrity, earlier in this care plan).	The type and level of wound treatment depend on the staging of the ulcer and the type of infection present.
■ Provide thorough perineal hygiene after each episode of incontinence.	This measure minimizes pathogens in the area of sacral pressure ulcers. QSEN: Safety.
▲ Consult the dietitian for assistance with a high-calorie, high-protein diet.	These patients, because of their overall condition, often require enteral or parenteral nutrition to meet nutritional needs. QSEN: Teamwork and collaboration.
▲ Administer antibiotics as prescribed.	Complicated wounds may develop cellulitis or sepsis, requiring antibiotic therapy. Oral antibiotics or topical silver sulfadiazine can be effective.
▲ Provide hydrotherapy if available.	Hydrotherapy is needed to achieve wound cleansing and to promote circulation.

NANDA-I
NDx   **Risk for Ineffective Health Maintenance**

Common Risk Factors

Need for long-term pressure ulcer management
Lack of previous similar experience
Possible need for special equipment
Impaired functional status

Common Expected Outcome

Patient and caregiver verbalize understanding of the following aspects of home care: pressure relief, wound care, nutrition, and incontinence management.

NOC Outcomes
Knowledge: Treatment Regimen; Decision-Making; Coping; Family Functioning
NIC Interventions
Discharge Planning; Family Support; Decision-Making Support; Teaching: Prescribed Diet

Ongoing Assessment

Actions/Interventions	Rationales
■ Assess the patient's and caregiver's understanding of the long-term nature of wound healing of pressure ulcers and palliative wound care.	Pressure ulcers may take weeks to months to heal, even under ideal circumstances. Wounds heal from the base of the ulcer up, and from the edges of the ulcer toward the center. Palliative wound care may be appropriate for clean, chronic, nonhealing wounds.
■ Assess the patient's and caregiver's knowledge of and ability to provide local wound care.	Patients are no longer kept hospitalized until pressure ulcers have healed. The need for local wound care may continue for weeks to months. QSEN: Patient-centered care.
■ Assess for the availability of a pressure reduction or pressure-relief surface.	Patients may take thick, dense foam mattresses home from the hospital to place on their own beds. Rental provisions of low–air-loss beds (e.g., Flexicare, KinAir) and air-fluidized therapy beds (e.g., Clinitron, Skytron, FluidAir) may be arranged but often pose financial difficulty because few payer sources will cover the cost of these beds in the home. QSEN: Safety.

Integumentary Care Plans

■ = Independent   ▲ = Interprofessional Collaboration

Actions/Interventions

- Assess the patient's and caregiver's understanding of and ability to provide a high-calorie, high-protein diet throughout the course of wound healing.

- Assess the patient's and caregiver's understanding of the relationship between incontinence and further skin breakdown or complications of healing.

- Assess the patient's and caregiver's understanding of the prevention of further pressure ulcer development.

Rationales

Patients may require enteral feeding (through gastronomy tube, nasogastric feeding tubes, or the oral route), which requires knowledge of preparation and the use of special equipment (e.g., feeding pumps and administration sets).

Managing incontinence may be the most difficult aspect of home management and is often the reason decisions for nursing home placement are made.

Patients who are incapable of independent movement will need frequent repositioning to reduce the risk for breakdown in those areas that are intact. QSEN: Safety.

Therapeutic Interventions

Actions/Interventions

- Teach the patient and caregiver local wound care, and provide an opportunity for return demonstration.

- Teach the patient and caregiver to report the following signs indicating wound infection: purulent drainage, odor, fever, malaise.

- Provide written instructions with listed resources.

- ▲ Involve a social worker or case manager.

- Consider or discuss with the patient and caregiver the need for in-home nursing care or homemaker services.

- Consider or discuss with the patient and caregiver the possible need for respite care.

- Teach the patient and caregiver the importance of pressure reduction and relief:
  - Use of a specialty surface; if provision of specialty beds is a problem because of reimbursement issues, a water bed may be a reasonable alternative
  - Use of a pressure reduction and relief surface where the patient sits
  - A turning schedule that does not compromise other body areas

- ▲ Consult a wound specialist to evaluate care in the home.

Rationales

This allows the learner to use new information immediately, thus enhancing retention. Immediate feedback allows the learner to make corrections, rather than practice the skill incorrectly. QSEN: Patient-centered care.

Early assessment prompts early intervention. Providing information about signs of infection allows the patient to be a full partner in making decisions and reducing the risk of harm. QSEN: Safety.

Long-term management requires specific written plans to enhance adherence to treatment. Several Internet resources provide lay education.

Referral helps the patient and family determine whether placement in an extended care facility is needed. Because many patients with pressure ulcers are older, it is often an older spouse who is available to provide care; as a result of the intensive nursing care needs of these patients, discharge to home is often unrealistic. QSEN: Teamwork and collaboration.

These provide all or part of the patient's care and can be less costly to the patient. In addition, keeping the patient in his or her own environment (if possible) reduces the risk for nosocomial infection and keeps the patient in familiar surroundings. QSEN: Teamwork and collaboration.

Long-term responsibility for patient care in the home is taxing; those providing the care may need help to understand that their own needs for relaxation are essential to the maintenance of health and should not be viewed as "shirking responsibility."

Teaching content about the need for adherence to pressure prevention guidelines allows the patient to be a full partner in providing care and reduces the risk of harm to the patient. QSEN: Evidence-based practice; Safety.

Besides evaluating the ability to deliver care, the specialist may be useful in securing specialty equipment. QSEN: Teamwork and collaboration.

Integumentary Care Plans

Evolve **For additional care plans, go to http://evolve.elsevier.com/Gulanick/.**

Actions/Interventions

▲ Include a dietitian in teaching how to plan high-calorie, high-protein meals or how to supplement regular meals with dietary supplements.

■ Teach the patient and caregiver how to manage incontinence:
- Use of external catheters
- Care of indwelling catheters if no other option is feasible
- Use of underpads or linen protectors
- Use of moisture barrier ointments

Rationales

Specialty expertise may be required. Patients have high nutritional needs. QSEN: Teamwork and collaboration.

Teaching proper techniques can prevent leakage and skin problems. Reusable products such as underpads or linen protectors made of cloth with a waterproof lining are better for the patient's skin and are more economical but require laundering. Moisture barrier ointments protect intact skin from excoriation. QSEN: Safety.

Related Care Plans

Caregiver role strain, Chapter 2
Imbalanced nutrition: Less than body requirements, Chapter 2
Enteral nutrition, Chapter 4
Plastic surgery for wound closure, ⊖volve

Psoriasis

Psoriasis is a noninfectious common inflammatory skin disorder that results in an overproduction of epidermal cells that are evident as red, dry, itchy patches of thickened skin that may be associated with silvery scales. Symptoms vary from person to person. Patches are usually found on the arms, legs, trunk, or scalp but can occur anywhere, most commonly on the knees or elbows and usually in a symmetrical, bilateral pattern. Although the specific cause is not known, it seems to be related to an immunological process in which T cells malfunction, causing increased production of both normal skin cells and T cells that compete for space. The newly formed cells are shunted to the outer layer of skin while the older cells have yet to be removed. These combinations result in accumulation of thick patches on the skin's surface. Specific triggers have been identified, including infections, stress, injury to the skin, smoking, and cold weather.

Psoriasis is a chronic disease for which most people experience recurrent periods of flare-ups and remissions. There is no cure, but for most individuals the symptoms are more of an inconvenience; however, the more severe cases can be disabling when associated with psoriatic arthritis. Treatment is geared to disrupting the overproduction of cells and removing the dry scales to smoothen the skin. Therapy consists of combinations of topical medications, light therapy, and a variety of oral medications. This care plan focuses on nursing care in the outpatient setting.

NANDA-I NDx Knowledge Deficit

Common Related Factors

Insufficient information
Insufficient interest in learning
Misinformation presented by others
Insufficient knowledge of resources

Defining Characteristics

Insufficient knowledge
Inaccurate follow-through of instruction
Inappropriate behavior

Integumentary Care Plans

 = Independent ▲ = Interprofessional Collaboration

Common Expected Outcome

Patient verbalizes understanding of disease process, preventive care, and treatment plan.

NOC Outcomes
Knowledge: Chronic Disease Management; Knowledge: Disease Process; Knowledge: Treatment Regimen

NIC Interventions
Health Literacy Enhancement; Learning Facilitation; Teaching: Disease Process; Teaching: Prescribed Medication

Ongoing Assessment

Actions/Interventions	Rationales
■ Assess the patient's level of knowledge of psoriasis and its treatment.	Patients will be responsible for evaluating their condition on a daily basis to make determinations about preventive strategies and therapeutic intervention. QSEN: Patient-centered care
■ Assess how long psoriasis has been a problem and any patterns of remission and exacerbation, as well as any associated factors.	Information provides data as to how the patient may have handled flare-ups in the past or whether he or she has engaged in preventive measures that were successful. QSEN: Patient-centered care.

Therapeutic Interventions

Actions/Interventions	Rationales
■ Introduce or reinforce information about diagnosis, disease process, chronicity of skin disease, symptoms, remissions, and exacerbations: • Diagnosed by presentation of typical skin patches (plaque psoriasis) such as red, raised patches with silvery scales or peeling; can be itchy. Plaques tend to appear bilaterally on the same area of the body. • Chronic condition with periods of exacerbation then remission. For some this condition can be disabling. May develop psoriatic arthritis causing joint pain and/or stiffness.	Patients must have a comprehensive understanding of the disease to actively participate in their own care. QSEN: Patient-centered care.
■ Provide information about preventive home care strategies: • Maintain moisturized skin. • Soak in bathwater with oil or bath salts to moisturize skin, remove scales, and reduce inflammation. • Bathe with coal tar or similar agents to remove scales. • Avoid irritating cosmetics and soaps. • Consider light therapy such as daily exposure of the skin to natural sunlight (helps many but may exacerbate condition in others). • Avoid exposure to triggers such as stress, smoking, infections, local injury to the skin, intense sun exposure	Many home measures can help reduce flare-ups, treat symptoms, and improve the appearance of damaged skin. QSEN: Safety.

Integumentary Care Plans

Actions/Interventions

- Provide information about common medical treatments:

Topical agents:

- Corticosteroids—anti-inflammatory medications that slow cell turnover
- Coal tar—reduces itching and slows the production of excess skin cells; probably the oldest treatment
- Anthralin—tree bark extract found to be very effective; acts by normalizing DNA activity in skin cells
- Retinoids—normalize DNA activity, reduce the redness of skin and the size of patches
- Vitamin D_3 (calcipotriene)—slows the production of excess skin cells
- Salicylic acid—promotes sloughing of dead cells and reduces scaling
- Moisturizers—help reduce scaling and itching, although they do not heal psoriasis

Systemic medications:

- Methotrexate—suppresses the immune system and slows the production of skin cells
- Cyclosporine—suppresses the immune system and slows the production of skin cells
- Biologicals (immunomodulators) given by IV, intramuscular (IM), or subcutaneous (SQ) injections for psoriatic arthritis to reduce inflammation; examples include etanercept, infliximab, adalimumab, and ustekinumab.

Phototherapy:

- UVB ultraviolet light, which is usually combined with other medical therapies; newer narrow-band UVB may be more effective
- PUVA (photochemotherapy or psoralen plus UVA): Psoralen makes the skin more sensitive to light when combined with ultraviolet light therapy
- Excimer laser—treats only the involved skin area

- Stress the importance of long-term follow-up.

- Encourage the patient to discuss new or over-the-counter treatments with health care professionals.

- ▲ Suggest referral to an arthritis specialist for optimal treatment of psoriatic arthritis.

Rationales

The choice of which drug to use for one's condition depends on many factors. About 80% of patients with psoriasis have mild to moderate disease that generally can be managed with topical agents. Guidelines recommend starting with the mildest treatments such as topical creams and light therapy. There is not one drug that will work most effectively for all patients. Patients often rotate medications or combine them as needed. Oral or injected drugs may be used for short-term treatment because of severe side effects. Some medications such as the biologicals are expensive, costing several thousand dollars per year. Treatment should be tailored to meet an individual patient's need. QSEN: Evidence-based practice.

Psoriasis is a chronic condition currently with no cure. Ongoing research may find better treatments and possible cure in the future.

The patient may be vulnerable to fads or advertisements claiming the curative effects of high-dose vitamins, special health foods, or similar unproven therapies.

This practitioner may be in the best position to understand the nuances of a patient's disease and be aware of the latest treatment regimens. QSEN: Teamwork and collaboration.

NANDA-I
NDx Risk for Disturbed Body Image

Common Risk Factors

Visible skin plaques
Preoccupation with changed appearance
Psoriatic arthritis with joint deformity

Integumentary Care Plans

■ = Independent   ▲ = Interprofessional Collaboration

Common Expected Outcomes

Patient demonstrates positive body image, as evidenced by ability to look at, talk about, and care for skin lesions. Patient verbalizes ways to conceal skin plaques as required by personal preference.

NOC Outcome
Body Image

NIC Interventions
Body Image Enhancement; Coping Enhancement

Ongoing Assessment

Actions/Interventions	Rationales
■ Assess the patient's perception of his or her changed appearance.	Mild outbreaks of psoriasis may not affect one's appearance and resultant body image. However, more severe or chronic cases with flare-ups lasting weeks or months may significantly affect how patients view their appearance to others. The peeling and itching of the skin or the joint problems with related arthritis can be overwhelming for some, causing a preoccupation with their skin condition.
■ Assess the patient's behavior related to his or her appearance.	Patients with potential body image issues may reduce their socialization based on fear about reactions of others. QSEN: Patient-centered care.

Therapeutic Interventions

Actions/Interventions	Rationales
■ Allow patients to verbalize feelings regarding their skin condition.	Through talking, the patient can be guided to separate physical appearance from feelings of personal worth.
■ Assist the patient in identifying ways to enhance appearance.	Clothing, cosmetics, and accessories may direct attention away from the skin lesions. Careful use of concealing clothing may help the patient who is having problems adjusting to body image changes.
■ Assist the patient in articulating responses to questions from others regarding skin plaques and infectious risk.	Patients may need some guidance in determining what to say to people who comment about the appearance of their skin. The rehearsal of set responses to anticipated questions may provide some reassurance. QSEN: Patient-centered care.
■ Instruct the patient to avoid contact with harsh chemicals and triggers for psoriasis, as well as to use materials such as moisturizers that can reduce scaling and further inflammation (see Knowledge Deficit, earlier in this care plan).	The patient needs to be aware of therapies to reduce symptoms.
■ Suggest referral to a psoriasis support group.	Groups that come together for mutual goals can be supportive and often provide helpful information.

NANDA-I
NDx Impaired Skin Integrity

Common Related Factor	Defining Characteristics
Disease process	Inflammation Dry, scaly skin Erosions, fissures Pruritus, pain

Common Expected Outcome

Patient maintains optimal skin integrity within limits of the disease, as evidenced by intact skin.

NOC Outcomes
Knowledge: Treatment Regimen; Tissue Integrity: Skin and Mucous Membranes
NIC Interventions
Skin Care: Topical Treatments; Skin Surveillance

Ongoing Assessment

Actions/Interventions	Rationales
■ Assess the skin, noting areas affected by color changes, any raised areas with scaling and patches, along with any plaques.	Psoriasis has characteristic patterns of skin changes and lesions.
■ Assess the skin systematically.	Patches are usually found on the arms, legs, trunk, or scalp but can occur anywhere. Knees and elbows are most common. Psoriasis has a characteristic bilateral component.
■ Identify the signs of itching and scratching.	The patient who scratches the skin to relieve intense itching may cause open skin lesions with an increased risk for infection.

Therapeutic Interventions

Actions/Interventions	Rationales
▲ Encourage the patient to adopt skin care routines to decrease skin irritation:	One of the first steps in the management of psoriasis is to prevent further drying of the skin.
• Bathe or shower using lukewarm water and bath salts or oils.	Long bathing or showering in hot water causes drying of the skin and can aggravate itching through vasodilation. Bath oils and salts help moisturize the skin to reduce further cracking of plaque.
• After bathing, allow the skin to air dry or gently pat the skin dry. Avoid rubbing or brisk drying.	Rubbing the skin with a towel can irritate the skin and exacerbate the itch-scratch cycle.
• Apply topical lubricants immediately after bathing.	Lubrication with fragrance-free creams or ointments serves as a barrier to prevent further drying of the skin through evaporation. Moisturizing is the cornerstone of treatment.
▲ Apply topical steroid creams or ointments.	These drugs reduce inflammation and promote healing of the skin. These are discussed under Knowledge Deficit, earlier in this care plan.
■ Encourage the patient to avoid aggravating factors: long sun exposure, smoking, stress.	Some change in lifestyle may be indicated to reduce triggers.

Related Care Plans

Chronic pain, Chapter 2
Shingles, Chapter 14

Integumentary Care Plans

■ = Independent   ▲ = Interprofessional Collaboration

Shingles

Herpes Zoster

After chickenpox infection, the varicella-zoster virus (VZV) lies dormant in the ganglia of the spinal nerve tracts. Shingles is an infectious viral condition caused by a reactivation of this latent VZV. Reactivation usually occurs in individuals with impaired immunity; it is common among adults over age 50 years. VZV produces painful vesicular eruptions along the peripheral distribution of nerves from posterior ganglia and is usually unilateral and characteristically occurs in a linear distribution, abruptly stopping at the midline both posteriorly and anteriorly. Shingles is characterized by burning, pain, and neuralgia. Although VZV typically affects the trunk of the body, the virus may also be noted on the buttocks or face.

With facial involvement there is concern about involvement of the eye and cornea, potentially resulting in permanent loss of vision. Secondary infection resulting from scratching the lesions is common. One is considered contagious until the shingles blisters scab over. The course of the disease is usually 2 to 6 weeks. It is possible to get shingles more than once. Some individuals may experience painful postherpetic neuralgia long after the lesions heal. VZV infection can lead to central nervous system (CNS) involvement. This disease is routinely treated on an outpatient basis unless CNS involvement or pneumonia occurs. A herpes zoster vaccination is recommended for adults after age 50.

NANDA-I NDx Risk for Infection

Common Risk Factors

Skin lesions (papules, vesicles, pustules)
Crusted-over lesions
Itching and scratching

Common Expected Outcomes

Patient remains free of secondary infection, as evidenced by intact skin without redness or lesions.
Risk for disease transmission is minimized through use of universal precautions.

NOC Outcomes

Knowledge: Infection Management; Risk Control; Risk Detection; Tissue Integrity: Skin and Mucous Membranes

NIC Interventions

Infection Protection; Wound Care

Ongoing Assessment

Actions/Interventions

- Assess for the presence and location of skin lesions.

- Assess for lesions around the eye or ear.

Rationales

Lesions are fluid-filled, becoming yellow and finally crusting over, on one side of the trunk or buttock. Lesions follow the path of dermatomes and occur in bandlike strips. Lesions may occur also on the face, arms, and legs if nerves for these areas are involved. As lesions rupture and crust, they take on the appearance of the lesions associated with chickenpox.

Particular attention needs to be given to assessing lesions near the eyes and ears because the virus may cause serious damage to the eyes and ears. This can cause blindness or hearing difficulties. To detect lesions on the cornea, the physician or nurse practitioner will stain the cornea in the office with fluorescein stain and view the typical lesions under a Wood's lamp.

 volve For additional care plans, go to http://evolve.elsevier.com/Gulanick/.

Integumentary Care Plans

Actions/Interventions

- Assess for pruritus or irritation from the lesions, and the amount of scratching. Assess for the signs of localized infection: redness and drainage from the lesions.
- ▲ Obtain a culture and sensitivity test of the suspected infected lesions, as ordered.
- ▲ Obtain additional cultures and blood work, as ordered.

- Assess the patient's and family's immunization status and past history of chickenpox.

Rationales

Secondary infection can occur because scratching opens pustules introduces bacteria.

A culture and sensitivity test provides an indication for appropriate antibiotic therapy.
Viral cultures, Tzanck smear, or viral smear may be required for diagnosis. Serological diagnoses also may be obtained.
Patients with shingles are contagious to others who have not had chickenpox. Those who have had varicella vaccine are considered immune but should have varicella titers to confirm immunity.

Therapeutic Interventions

Actions/Interventions

- Discourage the scratching of lesions. Encourage the patient to trim fingernails.
- Suggest the use of gauze to separate the lesions in skin folds.
- Teach contact isolation.

- Instruct the patient in the use of antiviral agents, as ordered.

- Instruct the patient in the use of systemic steroids, if ordered, for anti-inflammatory effect.
- Use universal precautions in caring for the patient to prevent transmission of the disease to self or other patients.

- Instruct the patient to avoid contact with pregnant women and immunosuppressed individuals.

Rationales

These measures prevent the inadvertent opening of lesions, cross-contamination, and bacterial infection.
This reduces irritation, itching, and cross-contamination.

VZV is spread by contact with fluid from lesions containing viruses. A person with shingles can pass the virus to anyone who is not immune to chickenpox. QSEN: Safety.
Antiviral agents are most effective during the first 72 hours of an outbreak, when viruses are proliferating. Drugs of choice are acyclovir, famciclovir, or valacyclovir.
The use of steroids is controversial; they are most commonly used for severe cases.
VZV can be transmitted to others and cause chickenpox in the person who has not previously had the disease. QSEN: Safety.
Active lesions can be infectious, and immunosuppressed individuals are more susceptible. QSEN: Safety.

NANDA-I NDx   Acute/Chronic Pain

Common Related Factor

Nerve pain (most commonly thoracic, cervical, lumbar and sacral, or ophthalmic division of trigeminal nerve)

Defining Characteristics

Self-report of pain using a standardized pain scale
Facial expression of pain

Common Expected Outcomes

Patient is comfortable, as evidenced by ability to rest.
Patient reports satisfactory pain control at decreasing levels using a standardized pain scale.

NOC Outcomes
Pain Level; Pain Control
NIC Intervention
Pain Management

Integumentary Care Plans

■ = Independent   ▲ = Interprofessional Collaboration

Ongoing Assessment

Actions/Interventions	Rationales
■ Assess the patient's description of pain or discomfort: quality, severity, location, onset, duration, precipitating or relieving factors.	The patient may describe the pain as a tingling sensation, a burning pain, or extreme hyperesthesia in one area of the skin. These sensations usually precede the development of skin lesions by several days. Postherpetic neuralgia is a chronic pain syndrome that may continue after the skin lesions have healed. The patient may have constant pain or intermittent episodes of pain.
■ Assess for nonverbal signs of pain or discomfort.	Each individual has his or her own pain threshold and ways to express pain or discomfort. Some individuals may deny the experience of pain when it is present. Attention to associated signs may help the nurse evaluate pain. QSEN: Patient-centered care.

Therapeutic Interventions

Actions/Interventions	Rationales
■ Instruct the patient to do the following:	
• Apply cool, moist dressings to pruritic lesions with or without Burrow's solution several times a day. Discontinue once the lesions have dried.	This provides relief and reduces the risk for secondary infection.
• Use topical steroids (anti-inflammatory effect), antihistamines (anti-itching effect, particularly useful at bedtime), and analgesics.	A variety of medications may be required to provide relief.
• Avoid rubbing or scratching the skin or lesion.	Scratching stimulates the skin, which in turn increases itchiness. It also can increase the possibility of secondary infection.
• Avoid temperature extremes, in both the air and bathwater.	Tepid water causes the least itching and burning.
• Wear loose, nonrestrictive clothing made of cotton.	Constrictive, nonbreathing garments may rub lesions and aggravate skin irritation. Cotton clothing allows evaporation of moisture.
▲ Administer medications as prescribed.	Oral opioid analgesics (hydrocodone, codeine) are typically prescribed during the acute phase. Analgesics, antidepressants, and anticonvulsant medications may be used in the management of postherpetic neuralgia. Topical preparations for postherpetic neuralgia include capsaicin cream (Zostrix) and lidocaine-prilocaine cream (EMLA). QSEN: Evidence-based practice.

NANDA-I NDx Risk for Disturbed Body Image

Common Risk Factors
Visible skin lesions
Preoccupation with changed body part

Common Expected Outcomes
Patient demonstrates positive body image, as evidenced by ability to look at, talk about, and care for lesions.
Patient verbalizes feelings about lesions and continues daily activities.

NOC Outcome
Body Image
NIC Interventions
Body Image Enhancement; Coping Enhancement

Integumentary Care Plans

Ongoing Assessment

Actions/Interventions	Rationales
■ Assess the patient's perception of his or her changed appearance.	Because the course of an outbreak may span several weeks, patients typically need to work or carry out their usual routine; they may require assistance coping with changes in appearance. QSEN: Patient-centered care.
■ Note verbal references to skin lesions.	Scarring may occur with repeated outbreaks or if lesions are infected. This may cause a preoccupation with appearance.

Therapeutic Interventions

Actions/Interventions	Rationales
■ Assist the patient in articulating responses to questions from others regarding lesions and infectious risk.	Patients may need some guidance in determining what to say to people who comment about the appearance of their skin. The rehearsal of set responses to anticipated questions may provide some reassurance. QSEN: Patient-centered care.
■ Suggest the use of concealing clothing when lesions can be easily covered.	This approach may help the patient who is having problems adjusting to body image changes.

NANDA-I
NDx # Deficient Knowledge

Common Related Factors
Insufficient information
Insufficient interest in learning
Misinformation presented by others
Insufficient knowledge of resources

Defining Characteristics
Insufficient knowledge
Inaccurate follow-through of instruction
Inappropriate behavior

Common Expected Outcome
Patient or caregiver verbalizes needed information about disease, treatment, and possible complications of herpes zoster.

NOC Outcomes
Knowledge: Disease Process; Knowledge: Treatment Regimen

NIC Interventions
Health Literacy Enhancement; Learning Facilitation; Teaching: Disease Process; Teaching: Individual; Teaching: Prescribed Medication

---

Ongoing Assessment

Actions/Interventions	Rationales
■ Determine the patient's and caregiver's understanding of the disease process, complications, and treatment.	It is necessary for patients and caregivers to understand that an occult disease may have weakened the patient and allowed the expression of the herpes zoster.
■ Because of potential infectivity, determine whether the patient's caregiver or family has had chickenpox or varicella vaccine or is immunocompromised.	Even though varicella vaccine does not confer immunity to shingles, it is less common in varicella-vaccinated adults than those who have had chickenpox.

■ = Independent ▲ = Interprofessional Collaboration

Therapeutic Interventions

Actions/Interventions	Rationales
■ Provide necessary information to the patient and caregiver, including written information:	Patients may confuse terminology and confuse herpes zoster with genital herpes. Because the patient may be reluctant to ask, clarify this point for the patient. Patients must have a comprehensive understanding of their disease to actively participate in their own care. QSEN: Patient-centered care; Safety.
• Description of herpes zoster, including how the disease is spread	Fluid from lesions contains viruses, which are spread by direct contact.
• Explanation of the need for isolation	Patients should isolate their clothing and linen, including towels.
• Need to notify health professionals of the signs of central nervous system (CNS) inflammation (changes in the level of consciousness)	Early assessment facilitates prompt treatment of complications.
■ Encourage herpes zoster vaccination (Zostavax).	This vaccination is recommended for individuals 50 years or older. The vaccine does not guarantee you won't get shingles, but it will help reduce the course and severity of the disease and its complications. It is not recommended for pregnant women or those with primary or acquired immunodeficiencies or any allergy to its components. QSEN: Safety.

Skin Cancer

Basal Cell Carcinoma; Squamous Cell Carcinoma; Malignant Melanoma

Tumors of the skin may be benign, premalignant, or malignant. Malignant tumors are categorized as either nonmelanoma cancers (basal cell carcinoma and squamous cell carcinoma) or melanoma. Prolonged exposure to ultraviolet radiation is the primary cause of all forms of skin cancer. It has been estimated that more than 1 million cases of skin cancer are diagnosed each year. Basal cell carcinoma is the most common form of skin cancer and the least deadly. Squamous cell cancer more frequently occurs on sun-exposed skin and can be highly aggressive with the potential to metastasize. Both of these forms of skin cancer can be cured with early detection and intervention. Malignant melanoma is the most serious form of skin cancer and is ranked as the eighth most common cancer in the United States. Risk factors include personal or family history of skin cancer; having numerous moles, especially atypical ones; being fair skinned who freckles easily; having blond or red hair, and blue or green eyes; spending a lot of time outdoors; living or vacationing at high altitudes or in tropical climates; and having a gene mutation, such as the *BRAF* gene. Melanomas can metastasize to regional lymph nodes or to visceral organs if not diagnosed in the early stages. Premalignant skin conditions include actinic keratosis, solar keratosis, and actinic cheilitis. Most premalignant lesions later develop into squamous cell carcinoma. Actinic keratosis occurs most often in older adults. The skin lesions are usually rough, scaly raised growths that range in color from brown to red. The lesions of actinic cheilitis occur on the lower lip, causing dryness, and scaling. Less common forms of skin cancer can include Kaposi sarcoma, seen most often in people with human immunodeficiency virus (HIV) infection, and cutaneous lymphoma, commonly seen in people with weak immune systems such as those with acquired immunodeficiency syndrome (AIDS) or with HIV infection.

NANDA-I NDx Impaired Skin Integrity

Common Related Factor	Defining Characteristics
Tumors	Erosions of the skin with drainage or bleeding Destruction of the epidermis

Common Expected Outcome

Patient maintains optimal skin integrity within limits of the disease.

NOC Outcome
Tissue Integrity: Skin and Mucous Membranes

NIC Interventions
Skin Surveillance; Chemotherapy Management; Incision Site Care; Wound Care

Ongoing Assessment

Actions/Interventions	Rationales
■ Assess the skin lesions for changes in shape, size, color, bleeding, or exudates. *Basal cell carcinoma:* • An open sore that bleeds, oozes, or crusts and does not heal after 3 weeks • A persistent reddish patch on the chest, shoulders, arms, or legs that may crust or itch • A shiny nodule that is pearly or translucent and different in color than the surrounding skin • A pink growth with elevated borders and a crusted center; blood vessels may be prominent as the growth enlarges *Squamous cell carcinoma:* • A wartlike growth that crusts and bleeds • A persistent, scaly red patch with irregular borders that crusts or bleeds • An elevated growth with a central depression that may bleed and grows rapidly	Regular inspection of the skin over the entire body is important to identify skin cancers in their earliest stages. Melanoma can be found in places that do not have sun-exposed skin. Any change in the skin with development of a new growth or an open sore that fails to heal may be a precursor to skin cancer. Some skin cancers may resemble psoriasis or eczema in the early stages. These conditions need prompt referral to a physician for further evaluation and diagnosis.

Malignant melanoma:
• Evaluate for changes in existing moles or development of a new pigmented skin lesion, paying specific attention to the ABCDE guide:
  • *Asymmetry:* Most early melanomas are asymmetrical. A line through the middle does not create matched halves.
  • *Border irregularity:* Borders may be uneven.
  • *Color changes:* Normal moles are an even brown color. Melanomas may have many colors (brown, black, red, blue, pink).
  • *Diameter:* Moles greater than 6 mm should be evaluated for removal. This is larger than the eraser on a pencil.
  • *Evolving;* Melanomas change in color, shape, or size over a short period. Any changing moles need to be evaluated by a dermatologist.
	Risk for malignant melanoma is increased in people with a previous personal or family history of melanoma or in people with more than 50 larger or atypical (dysplastic) moles. Often these people have a genetic mutation.

▲ Assist with the tissue biopsy.	A biopsy of any skin growth is necessary to determine the type of cancer and guide treatment.

■ = Independent   ▲ = Interprofessional Collaboration

Therapeutic Interventions

Actions/Interventions	Rationales
▲ Anticipate and prepare the patient for surgical therapy:	Many of the surgical procedures used in the treatment of skin cancer can be done using local or regional anesthesia in an outpatient setting.
• Cryosurgery (cryotherapy)	With cryosurgery, liquid nitrogen is used to destroy the tumor by freezing. This is a bloodless procedure. Redness, swelling, blistering, and crusting may occur in the treatment area. This is primarily used for premalignant lesions.
• Mohs microscopic surgery used in nonmelanoma skin cancer	The surgeon removes a very thin layer of tissue. Each layer is examined under a microscope. Repeated layers are removed and examined until the area is free of tumor cells. This procedure is used in areas of recurring tumors or in areas on the face because it preserves the greatest amount of healthy tissue.
• Excisional surgery	The entire growth is removed with a surrounding border of normal tissue. The incision is closed with sutures. This procedure is used with any type of skin cancer.
• Reexcision and sentinel lymph node dissection (SLND)	Lymphoscintigraphy and SLND are recommended for patients with tumors greater than 1.1 mm. Complete lymph node dissection is indicated for patients with positive sentinel lymph nodes or palpable lymph nodes. Lymphoscintigraphy is used to map lymph system drainage and locate the sentinel nodes, which are the first one or two nodes that are closest to the tumor. These nodes can be removed and evaluated to detect early micrometastatic disease. Accurate staging and identification of early micrometastasis are important in identifying patients who would benefit from complete lymph node dissection and those eligible for adjuvant immunotherapy.
▲ Assist with the application of topical chemotherapeutic agents.	Topical application of 5-fluorouracil (5-FU) in a cream or lotion is effective in treating actinic keratosis and cancers that involve only the superficial layers of the skin. Intense inflammation may occur during treatment, but scarring afterward is rare.
▲ Administer immunotherapy, systemic chemotherapy, and/or targeted therapy in the adjuvant or metastatic melanoma patient.	For patients diagnosed with squamous cell cancer that has spread to the lymph nodes or other organs, and for stage III or IV melanoma, more aggressive treatments are indicated. Immunotherapy (α-interferon, PD-1 inhibitors, CTLA-4 inhibitors), systemic chemotherapy (cisplatin, doxorubicin, 5-FU, topotecan, and etoposide), and targeted therapy using such drugs as vemurafenib are often used in combination. Patients may be encouraged to participate in clinical drug trials. These treatments are rigorous, and patient teaching and nursing and medical support during treatment are critical. QSEN: Evidence-based practice.
▲ Anticipate and prepare the patient for radiation therapy.	Radiation therapy is indicated for patients who are not candidates for surgery because of preexisting health problems, or when the cancer cannot be removed during surgery. A series of treatments is usually given over several weeks. Permanent changes in skin color and texture may develop in the treatment area.
■ Instruct regarding skin grafting and reconstructive surgery as indicated.	These procedures may be required after removal of large basal or squamous cell cancers. Healthy skin is taken from another part of the body and grafted over the wound.

Integumentary Care Plans

NANDA-I NDx Disturbed Body Image

Common Related Factors
Alterations in structure:
- Visible tumor
- Surgical scars and grafts

Defining Characteristics
Alteration in view of one's body
Negative feelings about body
Nonverbal response to change in body appearance
Perceptions that reflect an altered view of one's body appearance
Preoccupation with change
Change in social involvement

Common Expected Outcome
Patient demonstrates positive body image as evidenced by ability to look at, touch, talk about, and care for altered body part.

NOC Outcomes
Body Image; Coping; Social Interaction Skills
NIC Intervention
Body Image Enhancement

Ongoing Assessment

Actions/Interventions

■ Assess the patient's perception of the changed appearance.

■ Assess the patient's behavior related to appearance.

Rationales

The nurse needs to understand the patient's attitudes about visible changes in the appearance of the skin that occur with skin cancer and its treatment. The extent of the response is more related to the value or importance the patient places on the appearance of the skin. QSEN: Patient-centered care.

There is a broad range of behavior associated with body image disturbance ranging from totally ignoring the alteration to preoccupation with it. Patients with body image issues may try to hide or camouflage their lesions. Their socialization may decrease based on their anxiety or fear about the reactions of others. QSEN: Patient-centered care.

Therapeutic Interventions

Actions/Interventions

■ Allow patients to verbalize feelings regarding their skin condition.
■ Assist the patient in identifying ways to enhance appearance.

■ Assist the patient in articulating responses to questions from others regarding the lesions.

▲ Assist the patient with a referral for plastic and reconstructive surgery.

Rationales

Through talking, the patient can be guided to separate physical appearance from feelings of personal worth.
Clothing, cosmetics, and accessories may direct attention away from skin lesions and scars. The patient should not aggravate skin lesions or healing surgical sites.
Patients may need guidance in determining what to say to people who comment about the appearance of their skin. The rehearsal of set responses to anticipated questions may provide some reassurance. QSEN: Patient-centered care.
The surgical excision of skin cancer of the head and neck may require the removal of extensive amounts of tissue. The patient may be a candidate for skin grafting and reconstructive surgery. QSEN: Teamwork and collaboration.

Integumentary Care Plans

■ = Independent ▲ = Interprofessional Collaboration

Deficient Knowledge

Common Related Factors

Insufficient information
Insufficient interest in learning
Misinformation presented by others
Insufficient knowledge of resources

Common Expected Outcome

The patient verbalizes knowledge about skin cancer prevention and treatment.

Defining Characteristics

Insufficient knowledge
Inaccurate follow-through of instruction
Inappropriate behavior

NOC Outcomes

Knowledge: Disease Process; Knowledge: Health Behavior; Tissue Integrity: Skin and Mucous Membranes

NIC Interventions

Health Literacy Enhancement; Learning Facilitation; Teaching: Disease Process; Teaching: Procedure/Treatment; Skin Surveillance; Skin Care: Topical Treatments

Ongoing Assessment

Actions/Interventions	Rationales
■ Assess the patient's knowledge of the diagnosis and its treatment options.	The patient needs information about skin cancer and treatment options to make informed decisions about care. QSEN: Patient-centered care.
■ Assess the patient's knowledge of skin cancer prevention and sun safety behaviors.	Skin cancers can recur, and the patient needs to know about methods to reduce exposure to ultraviolet light. QSEN: Safety.

Therapeutic Interventions

Actions/Interventions	Rationales
■ Provide information about methods to decrease skin exposure to ultraviolet light. • Avoid exposure to artificial sources of ultraviolet light such as sunlamps and tanning booths. • Limit sun exposure during midday hours (10 AM to 4 PM), when the sun's rays are most intense. • Apply sunscreen with a sun protection factor (SPF) of 15 or higher with UVA and UVB protection. Apply liberally to all sun-exposed areas, and reapply every 2 hours and after swimming or perspiring. • Wear sunglasses for eye protection. • Wear sun-protective clothing with tightly woven fabrics and wide-brimmed hats.	Ultraviolet light from natural and artificial sources is the contributing or primary cause of skin cancer. Reducing exposure can prevent the recurrence of tumors and the development of new lesions. QSEN: Safety.

Integumentary Care Plans

Actions/Interventions

- Teach the patient and a family member to do monthly skin self-examinations. Do the examination in a well-lighted room using a full-length mirror and a handheld mirror.
  - Become familiar with all birthmarks, moles, and skin blemishes. Look for changes in size, shape, or color using the ABCDE guide described earlier.
  - Monitor all skin sores that do not show signs of healing after 3 weeks.
  - Look at all body surfaces in the mirror, including the front and back of the body, both right and left sides, scalp, between fingers and toes, nail beds, and between skin folds including the buttocks.
  - Give special attention to all skin surfaces exposed to the sun.
  - Use a comb or blow dryer to move hair on the scalp for better visualization.
  - Ask a family member to examine the skin in hard-to-see areas.
  - Consider taking a picture of skin areas so changes are easier to detect

- Provide information regarding the importance of annual skin examination by a physician.

- Educate regarding websites with information for health care professionals and patients:
  - Skin Cancer Foundation: www.skincancer.org
  - American Cancer Society: www.cancer.org
  - American Academy of Dermatology: www.aad.org
  - National Institutes of Health: www.nih.gov
  - Melanoma Research Foundation: www.melanoma.org
  - Oncology Nursing Society: www.ons.org
  - National Comprehensive Cancer Network's Clinical Practice Guidelines: www.nccn.org

Rationales

Early diagnosis of skin cancer is associated with better chances for cure and less disfigurement from surgical interventions. The best time for skin self-examinations is after bathing or showering. Skin areas over the entire body need to be examined. QSEN: Safety.

Patients who have had a malignant melanoma are seen on a regular follow-up schedule with a physician at 3-, 6-, and 12-month intervals for a complete skin examination and lymph node examination and for additional diagnostic studies, if indicated. QSEN: Safety.

Several Internet resources provide useful lay education. Patients must have a comprehensive understanding of the disease to actively participate in their own care.

Integumentary Care Plans

■ = Independent ▲ = Interprofessional Collaboration

Page numbers followed by "*f*" indicate figures, "*t*" indicate tables, and "*e*" indicate online content.

Quick Care Plan Locator